Problem Solving in Musculoskeletal Imaging

Problem Solving in Musculoskeletal Imaging

William B. Morrison, MD

Associate Professor of Radiology, Director, Division of Musculoskeletal and General Diagnostic Radiology, Thomas Jefferson University Hospital, Philadelphia, PA

Timothy G. Sanders, MD

Director of Education and Research, National Musculoskeletal Imaging, Weston, FL, Professor, Department of Radiology, University of Kentucky, Lexington, KY

MOSBY

ELSEVIER

PROBLEM SOLVING

MOSBY
ELSEVIER

1600 John F. Kennedy Blvd.
Ste 1800
Philadelphia, PA 19103-2899

PROBLEM SOLVING IN MUSCULOSKELETAL IMAGING ISBN: 978-0-323-04034-1

Notice

Knowledge and best practice in this field are constantly changing. As new research and experience broaden our knowledge, changes in practice, treatment and drug therapy may become necessary or appropriate. Readers are advised to check the most current information provided (i) on procedures featured or (ii) by the manufacturer of each product to be administered, to verify the recommended dose or formula, the method and duration of administration, and contraindications. It is the responsibility of the practitioner, relying on their own experience and knowledge of the patient, to make diagnoses, to determine dosages and the best treatment for each individual patient, and to take all appropriate safety precautions. To the fullest extent of the law, neither the Publisher nor the Authors assume any liability for any injury and/or damage to persons or property arising out of or related to any use of the material contained in this book.

Library of Congress Cataloging-in-Publication Data
Morrison, William B.
Problem solving in musculoskeletal imaging / William B. Morrison, Timothy G. Sanders.—1st ed.
p. ; cm.
Includes bibliographical references and index.
ISBN 978-0-323-04034-1
1. Musculoskeletal system—Imaging. 2. Musculoskeletal System—Diseases—Diagnosis. 3. Problem solving. I. Sanders, Timothy G. II. Title.
[DNLM: 1. Musculoskeletal Diseases—diagnosis. 2. Magnetic Resonance Imaging—methods. 3. Musculoskeletal System. WE 141 M883p 2008]
RC925.7.M68 2008
616.7'075—dc22

2007042922

Acquisitions Editor: Rebecca Gaertner
Developmental Editor: Elizabeth Hart
Project Manager: Mary Stermel
Design Direction: Steven Stave
Marketing Manager: Catalina Nolte

Printed in China.

Last digit is the print number: 9 8 7 6 5 4 3 2 1

Contributors

Kenneth A. Buckwalter, MD
Professor
Department of Radiology
Indiana University School of Medicine
University Hospital
Indianapolis, IN

Angela Gopez, MD
Assistant Professor
Department of Radiology
Thomas Jefferson University Hospital
Philadelphia, PA

Eoin C Kavanagh, MRPCI, FFR, RCSI
Consultant Radiologist and Senior Lecturer
Mater Misericordiae Hospital
Dublin, Ireland

W. James Malone, DO
Academic Chief, Musculoskeletal Imaging
Department of Radiology
Geisinger Medical Center
Danville, PA

Levon N. Nazarian, MD, FACR
Professor and Vice Chairman for Education
Department of Radiology
Thomas Jefferson University Hospital
Philadelphia, PA

Imran M. Omar, MD
Assistant Professor
Department of Radiology
Northwestern Memorial Hospital
Chicago, IL

Paul Shieh, MD
Staff Radiologist
Community Medical Center
Saint Barnabas Health Care System
Toms River, NJ

Adam C. Zoga, MD
Associate Professor
Department of Radiology
Thomas Jefferson University Hospital
Philadelphia, PA

Preface

The "Problem Solving" series by Elsevier is a new type of teaching tool: a series of texts in different disciplines that strive to distill the authors' experience and approach to clinical challenges rather than merely index the imaging appearance of injury and disease.

This format is difficult to achieve in all areas, and therefore texts within this series will incorporate different variations of this concept. Our musculoskeletal edition, for example, is roughly divided into three areas: technical issues and optimization, approach to musculoskeletal diseases, and advanced joint imaging.

The first technical chapter teaches a practical methodology for improving image quality across modalities, as well as providing examples of how the radiologist can use the modality to answer specific clinical questions. The attached CD is an extension of this chapter; it includes material that aids the radiologist in day-to-day clinical operations—patient questionnaires, dictation templates, and MRI/CT protocols, including pictorial examples of positioning and plane selection. Additional chapters provide instruction on performance of arthrography and bone/soft tissue biopsy.

The approach chapters address general categories of disease, including arthritis, tumor and infection; these chapters attempt to provide the reader with tips and thought processes associated with diagnosis of these conditions.

The joint-oriented chapters strive to teach the reader how to interpret advanced imaging studies on a high level, similar to a dedicated musculoskeletal radiologist. Figures are formatted in an easy-to-read way analogous to a PowerPoint slide rather than traditional book figures with dozens of arrows and long legends.

Problem Solving in Musculoskeletal Imaging is intended to be read cover-to-cover. The entire work is an effort to enable readers to "get into the mind" of a bone radiologist, so that they may provide high-level service to their patients and referring clinicians. We hope that we have achieved this goal. We are eternally grateful to our teachers and contributors who helped make this book a reality.

William B. Morrison, MD
Timothy G. Sanders, MD

Acknowledgments

I am very grateful to David Karasick, MD, Diane Deely, MD, and Alex Dresner, PhD, for lending me their extensive expertise. I am also indebted forevermore to David and Diane, as well as Mark Schweitzer, MD, for providing teaching, mentoring, and continuing support throughout my career. All my other teachers, colleagues, and friends deserve credit for their guidance—you know who you are—your martini is waiting!

Thanks to dancers Phil Colucci and Emily Hayden of the Pennsylvania Ballet for modeling arthrographic technique. Special thanks to Anne Dugan for her assistance.

—WBM

I would like to acknowledge two very special mentors and friends, Robert Miller, MD, at the University of Florida for first sparking my interest in musculoskeletal radiology, and Phillip Tirman, MD, for helping to jumpstart my academic career. My time in radiology has been much richer as a result of these two individuals. I would like to acknowledge the entire Air Force community: for the fun, the education, and the varied opportunities during 25 great years.

Finally, I would like to thank my family; my parents for their steadfast support throughout the years, and of course my wife, DeAun, and daughters, Kelly and Courtney, for their continued understanding and support during the preparation of this book.

—TGS

Contents

SECTION I

ADVANCED MODALITIES: Protocols and Optimization

Chapter 1

OPTIMIZATION OF CLINICAL MUSCULOSKELETAL IMAGING

CHAPTER OUTLINE

MAGNETIC RESONANCE IMAGING

When protocols are created or altered for musculoskeletal magnetic resonance (MR) imaging examinations, consideration should be given to the type of MR scanner being used (e.g., high field or low field), available surface coils and their configurations, and technologist experience. Beyond that, thought should be given to what specific information is needed from the examination, taking into account the clinical history and what is the appropriate field of view to answer the question. Is high spatial resolution required to answer the question, or is high contrast between structures more important? Planes and sequences should be selected to optimize relevant anatomy and pathology, optimizing signal-to-noise ratio (SNR). Finally, consideration should be given as to whether intravenous or intra-articular contrast is necessary, and whether any specialized sequences, planes, or positions would be advantageous. This section deals with each of these issues in addition to artifacts and their minimization. Sample protocols with suggested plane selection are available on the accompanying CD.

High-Field versus Low-Field Scanners

Scanners come in a variety of field strengths, and options are available for various gradient strengths and slew rates intended to optimize scanning. Software options are often available at additional cost. These issues can cause confusion when selecting a scanner for purchase. In addition, different manufacturers have different terminology for sequences, magnet homogeneity, and other physical features that make it difficult to perform an "apples to apples" comparison. However, rarely does musculoskeletal imaging come into consideration when purchasing a scanner. Typically, neurologic and body imaging applications are those that guide scanner selection and purchase, and musculoskeletal imaging is a secondary consideration. A basic understanding of MR physics principles is generally all that is needed to optimize musculoskeletal imaging protocols, no matter what machine is used. The differences between high-field and low-field scanners are extremely important in musculoskeletal imaging; advantages and disadvantages are summarized in Table 1-1.

Low-field scanners, that is, lower than 0.7 tesla (T), have difficulty performing standard presaturation-type frequency selective fat suppression because the signal peaks for the protons in water and fat are closely approximated. This is very important because musculoskeletal radiologists generally prefer to apply fat suppression on T2-weighted images to highlight fluid and edema. In addition, because fat is ubiquitous in the musculoskeletal system, fat suppression is preferred when gadolinium is injected intravenously or into a joint. As such, this can be a significant limitation of low-field scanners. Instead of T2-weighted fast spin-echo fat-suppressed imaging, which is a standard in musculoskeletal radiology, short tau inversion recovery (STIR) imaging is used to achieve fluid conspicuity, but at the expense of lowered resolution or a larger field of view. Alternatively, fluid conspicuity can be achieved without fat suppression by increasing echo time (TE), about 100 to 120 msec. However, this is at the expense of the SNR, which decreases as TE is raised. This creates difficulty in visualizing small cartilage lesions. One should not expect to consistently see small cartilage defects on a low-field scanner.

Without fat suppression on T1-weighted images, visualization of intravenously or intra-articularly administered contrast can be difficult, limiting applications such as tumor/infection imaging and MR arthrography. Also, there is relatively lower signal overall. To compensate, this requires increasing the number of signal averages to increase signal at the expense of increased imaging time, which can increase motion artifact in the extremities. Length of examinations is generally much greater on low-field scanners and may not be as useful for uncooperative patients. Coil options are often limited on low-field scanners, with a small variety of multipurpose surface coils available for imaging various musculoskeletal struc-

Table 1-1 Low-Field MRI: Advantages and Disadvantages

Advantages
Lower magnetic susceptibility artifact
High T1 contrast
Ease of positioning
Obese patients (up to 500-pound weight limit)
Eccentric body parts easier to center
Disadvantages
Difficulty performing "standard" fat suppression
Lower overall signal—longer scan times needed (motion artifact can be an issue)
Low resolution (imaging of cartilage, small structures such as labrum limited)

tures. This can result in an inappropriately large field of view and low resolution.

Nevertheless, there are some advantages to musculoskeletal imaging on low-field scanners. T1 contrast is actually superior to that of high-field scanners, although this is a relatively minor advantage in practice; in fact, improved T1 contrast can be disadvantageous. Consider evaluation of the knee on a low-field system; on a T1-weighted sequence fluid may appear black, blending with signal of the menisci (Fig. 1-1). Because of lower field strength, artifact from metal may be decreased compared with high-field scanners, and imaging patients who have prostheses, screws, or other orthopedic hardware can actually be improved by directing these patients to a low-field scanner. Keep in mind that advances in gradient technology at high fields have offset many of these advantages for high-field scanners. Chemical shift artifact is also decreased at low field.

Moreover—and what is possibly the most important consideration—is the gantry size and table weight limit of low-field scanners, which generally offer an open environment and a weight limit of up to 500 pounds. For obese patients, no other imaging options may be available. This is mainly an issue in the United States. Regarding fat suppression, many low-field scanners offer a software option based on the Dixon technique, which acquires an in-phase and out-of-phase image, and through subtraction post-processing, obtains a fat-suppressed image (Fig. 1-2). If the subtraction is performed from images acquired in the same series no subtraction errors occur, and the images and degree of fat suppression are generally excellent. In fact, if the radiologist's intention is to perform MR arthrography on a low-field scanner, strong consideration should be given to acquiring this post-processing software. Newer generations of low-field scanners can actually separate the fat and water peaks, performing true fat saturation, but this has been suboptimal compared with the Dixon technique.

Extremity scanners are also available, which are generally low field at about 0.2 T; although they are low cost and provide a high degree of patient comfort, low image quality corresponds to the low strength. Also, the narrow bore of the magnet limits scanning

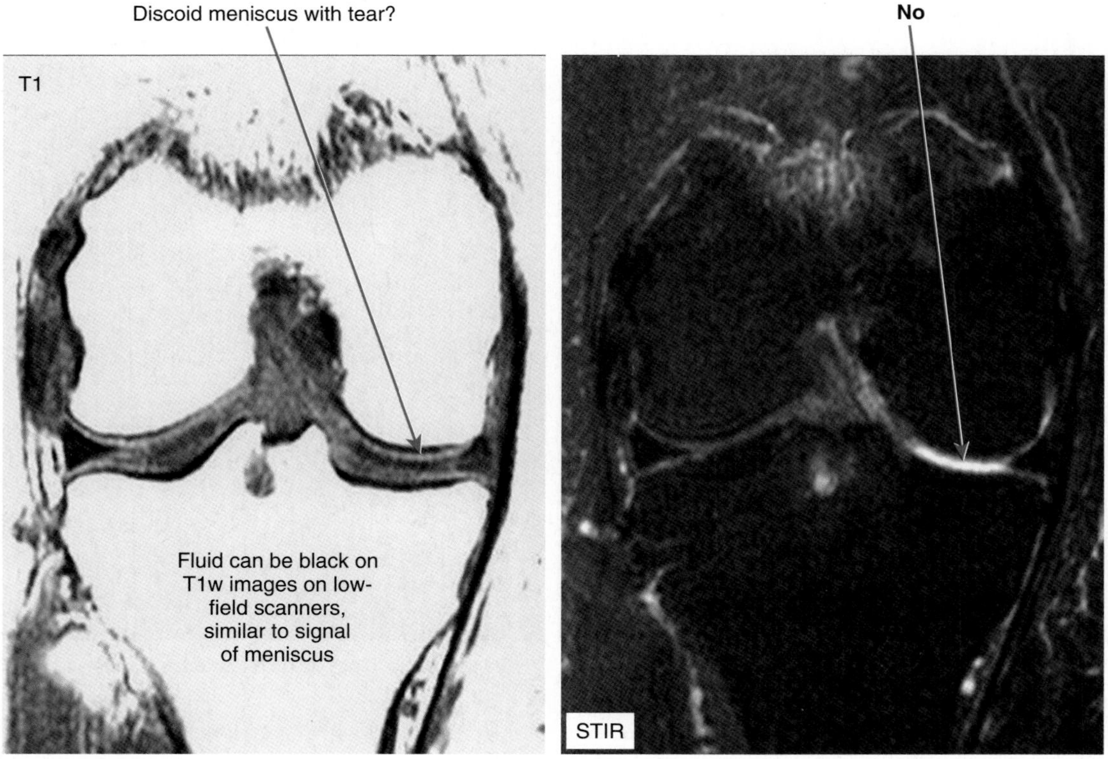
Discoid meniscus with tear?
No
T1
Fluid can be black on T1w images on low-field scanners, similar to signal of meniscus
STIR

Figure 1-1 0.3 T MRI of the knee. Low-field scanners have better T1 contrast than high-field units. However, this can have a detrimental effect on joint imaging.

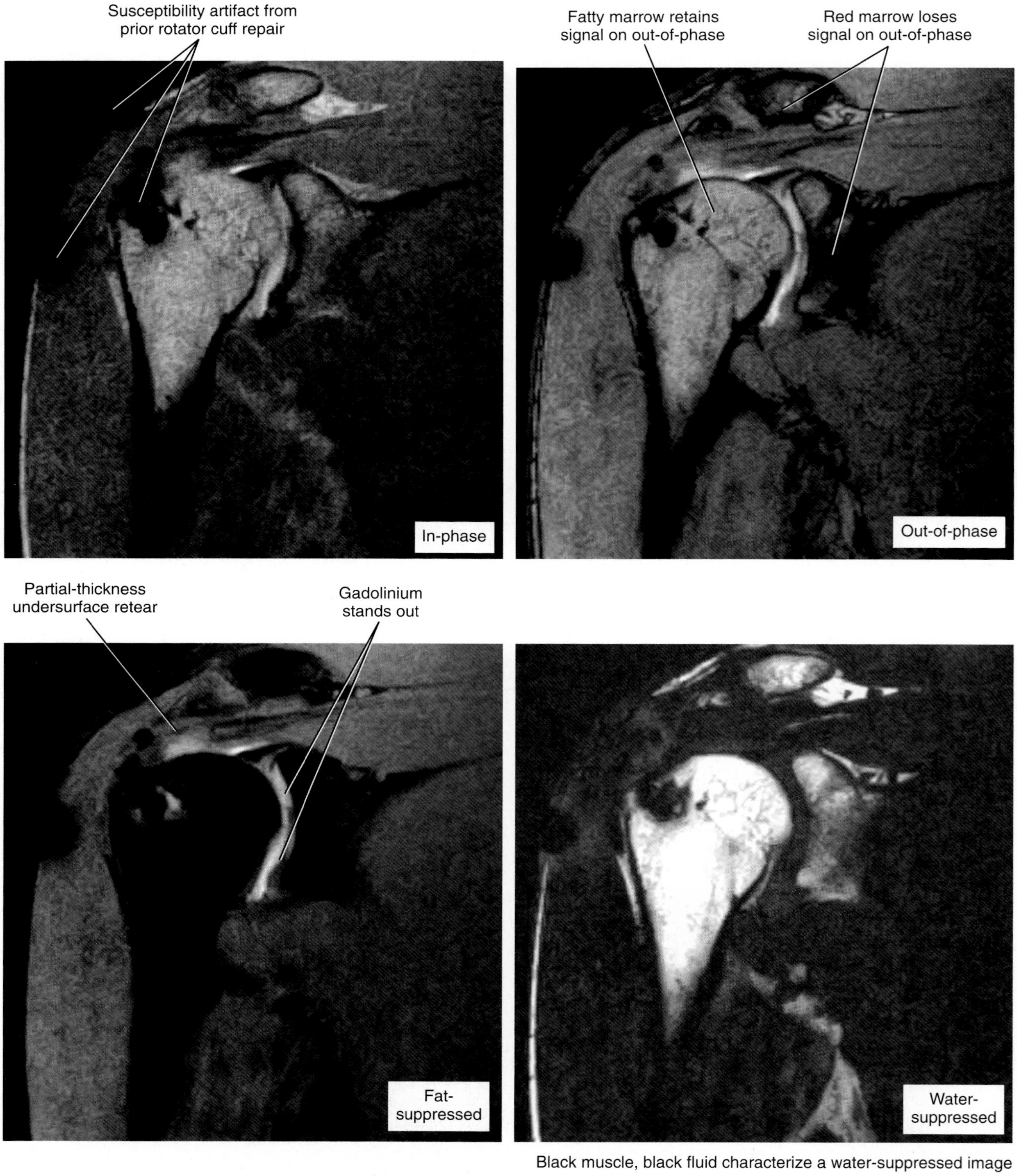
Susceptibility artifact from prior rotator cuff repair
Fatty marrow retains signal on out-of-phase
Red marrow loses signal on out-of-phase
In-phase
Out-of-phase
Partial-thickness undersurface retear
Gadolinium stands out
Fat-suppressed
Water-suppressed
Black muscle, black fluid characterize a water-suppressed image

Figure 1-2 ***MR arthrogram on a 0.3 T system.*** *Dixon technique for fat-water separation. An in-phase and out-of-phase image is acquired (useful for marrow evaluation) as well as a fat-suppressed and a water-suppressed image. The fat-suppressed image is ideal for use in MR arthrography on low-field scanners. However, as a gradient-echo sequence, it is prone to susceptibility artifact from metal, air, blood products, and calcium.*

to wrists/hands, elbows, ankles/feet and knees. However, a 1.0 T extremity scanner is available that provides good image quality comparable to that achieved with closed 1.5 T scanners (Fig. 1-3). Other open configuration 1.0 T scanners are also available.

Advantages and Disadvantages of 3 T Scanners for Musculoskeletal Imaging

There are some distinct advantages of 3 T MRI for musculoskeletal imaging. The high field strength provides high SNR over all imaging sequences, allowing an increase in the matrix, a decrease in slice thickness, and a decrease in field of view, providing increased resolution; ultimately, high resolution is a major key to success in musculoskeletal radiology (Fig. 1-4). Alternatively, one can use the signal surplus to decrease number of excitations (NEX), thereby shortening examination time and increasing patient throughput. However, protocols must be altered somewhat to account for the different physical properties of the 3 T environment. For example, the high field strength at 3 T accentuates susceptibility artifact from metal, limiting evaluation of orthopedic hardware. In addition, chemical shift artifacts may be increased, resulting in black-white effect at fat–water

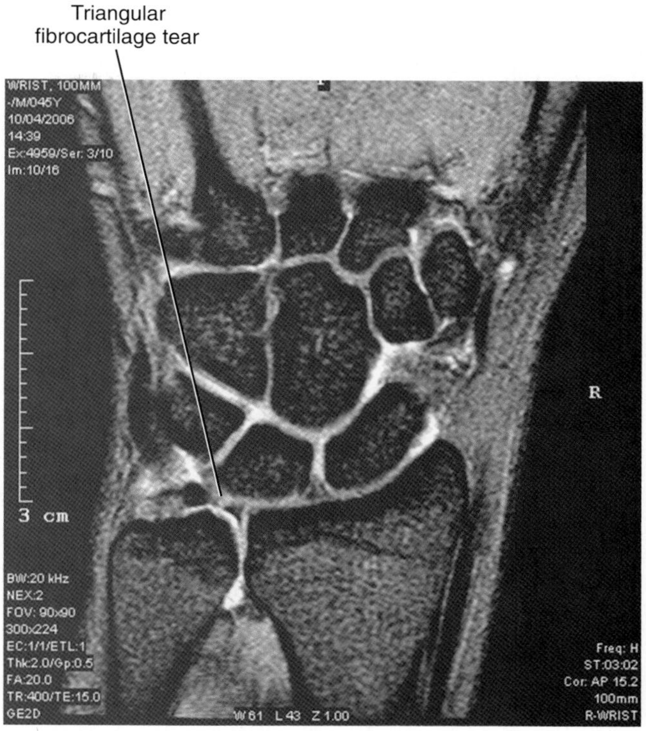
Triangular fibrocartilage tear
3 cm
R

Figure 1-3 Coronal gradient-recalled echo image of the wrist acquired with a 1.0-T dedicated extremity scanner. (Courtesy of ONI and Joel Newman, Boston, MA.)

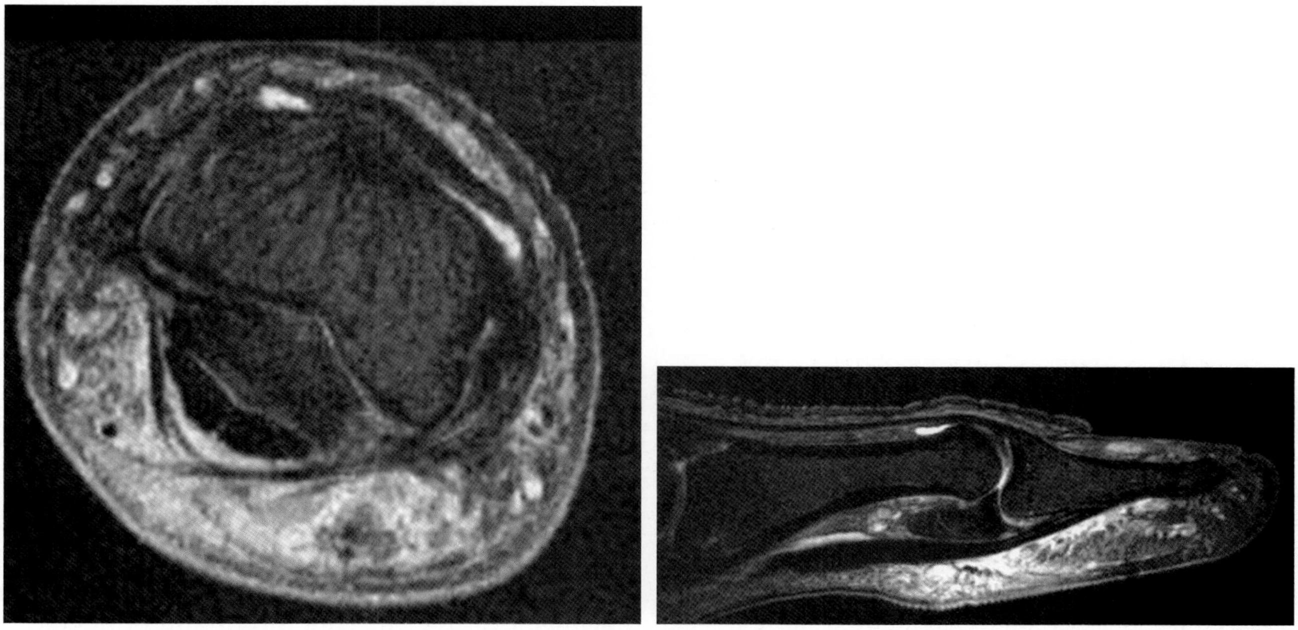

Figure 1-4 High-resolution 3 T imaging of the thumb using a small solonoid coil. Improved knowledge of anatomic detail and microstructural pathology will be required once this degree of resolution is routinely achieved. (Courtesy of Ivan Dimitrov, Best, the Netherlands, Philips.)

interfaces. This can be eliminated if fat suppression is used; alternatively, one can make the pixels smaller to reduce this artifact by increasing matrix or decreasing the field of view. Manipulation of the receiver bandwidth is a third strategy that can be used to address the problem.

Coils

Although an understanding of MR imaging physics and basic sequence optimization is essential, purchasing a wide range of coils is the easiest way to optimize musculoskeletal imaging (Fig. 1-5), regardless of scanner type. Unlike coils designed for the abdomen, head, and spine, there is a tremendous degree of variation in configuration and quality of various surface coils used for extremities. A rule of thumb is that the smallest coil possible should be used for imaging an extremity to achieve the desired field of view (Box 1-1). Basically, the coil is analogous to an ear trying to hear a faint noise coming from the body part being imaged. The farther the ear is from the body part, the softer the noise (i.e., weaker the signal) will be. Therefore, the more closely the coil fits against the body part, the better the images will be. It follows that an extremity coil used for the knee will not be as optimal for imaging the ankle, which is smaller and not cylindrically shaped.

One common mistake is to attempt to image both ankles at the same time within a head coil, which provides inadequate imaging for both ankles. A similar error is to attempt to image the foot and ankle at the same time without moving the coil (although newer coil designs have a chimney for the forefoot and provide satisfactory images). A send-receive coil is preferred to a receive-only coil; a receive-only coil requires the body coil to send the radiofrequency signal, so a larger area is exposed to the energy, which can create issues of specific absorption rate (SAR) (body energy deposition) and also aliasing artifact. Quadrature or phased-array coils are also preferred, as are multichannel coils. When a particular coil does not fit a body part, a combiner box can be used to link two coils positioned around the anatomy, but this partitions signal from each coil such that signal returning from each coil is reduced. This can be a limitation if the body part being imaged is thick, leading to signal drop-off in the center of the image.

Occasionally, patient limitations require an alternate coil configuration. For example, it is optimal to image the elbow above the head in an extremity coil, but this position may be difficult for patients to achieve, particularly those who have shoulder problems. A reasonable alternative would be imaging the arm at the side wrapped in a flex coil; at least the patient will be able to tolerate the examination with less motion. Similarly, some newer shoulder coil configurations are fitted to shoulder shape, but this can also create drawbacks. A shoulder coil design that is cuplike may not fit all patients, resulting in field cutoff (Fig. 1-6). This may also not allow positional imaging, such as the abduction–external rotation (ABER) position.

BOX 1-1 COIL BASICS

- Try to use smallest coil possible, closest to area of concern (maximize signal)
- Prefer phased array coil
- Prefer send/receive coil
- Small parts: Try taping 3-inch temporomandibular joint coils or 5-inch surface coil to the area
- Coil must be positioned correctly! (Look at scout to check)
- If patient cannot tolerate position, it may be best to go with second option to avoid motion

IMAGING SEQUENCE SELECTION

In selecting a sequence to be used for musculoskeletal imaging, decisions should be made concerning the speed necessary for imaging and whether contrast resolution or spatial resolution is more important to detect the pathology in question. Also, some scanners offer greater advantages using some sequences. For example, in a very homogeneous magnet, standard "presaturation-type" fat suppression may provide very homogeneous fat saturation, compared with a scanner with a relatively nonhomogeneous magnetic field, in which STIR may be a better option.

Spatial Resolution versus Contrast—Which to Choose?

Sequences that offer high spatial resolution are useful for evaluating small structures, such as interosseous ligaments of the wrist and the labrum of the hip, or for evaluation of the articular cartilage. These sequences require high SNR, allowing the radiologist to decrease field of view and increase matrix size. Gradient-echo imaging (see Fig. 1-3) can provide

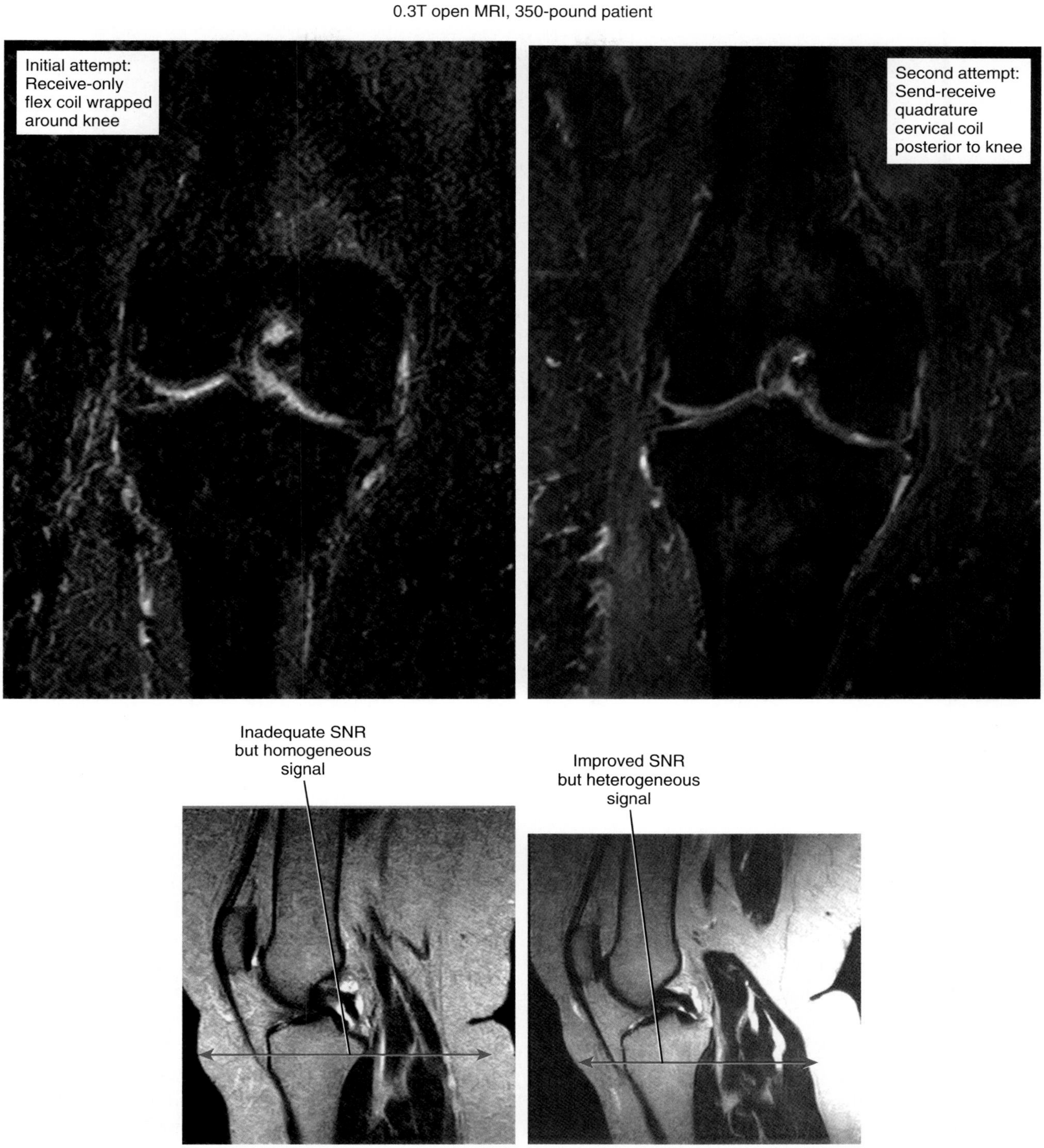
0.3T open MRI, 350-pound patient
Initial attempt: Receive-only flex coil wrapped around knee
Second attempt: Send-receive quadrature cervical coil posterior to knee
Inadequate SNR but homogeneous signal
Improved SNR but heterogeneous signal

Figure 1-5 Optimizing coil selection and placement is a major factor in optimizing image quality. This knee of an obese patient was imaged on a 0.3 T scanner; the knee did not fit in the extremity coil. The flex coil (*left*) yielded unacceptable signal-to-noise ratio (SNR). Use of a quadrature cervical coil (*right*) improved overall signal. However, note asymmetric distribution of signal on the sagittal image.

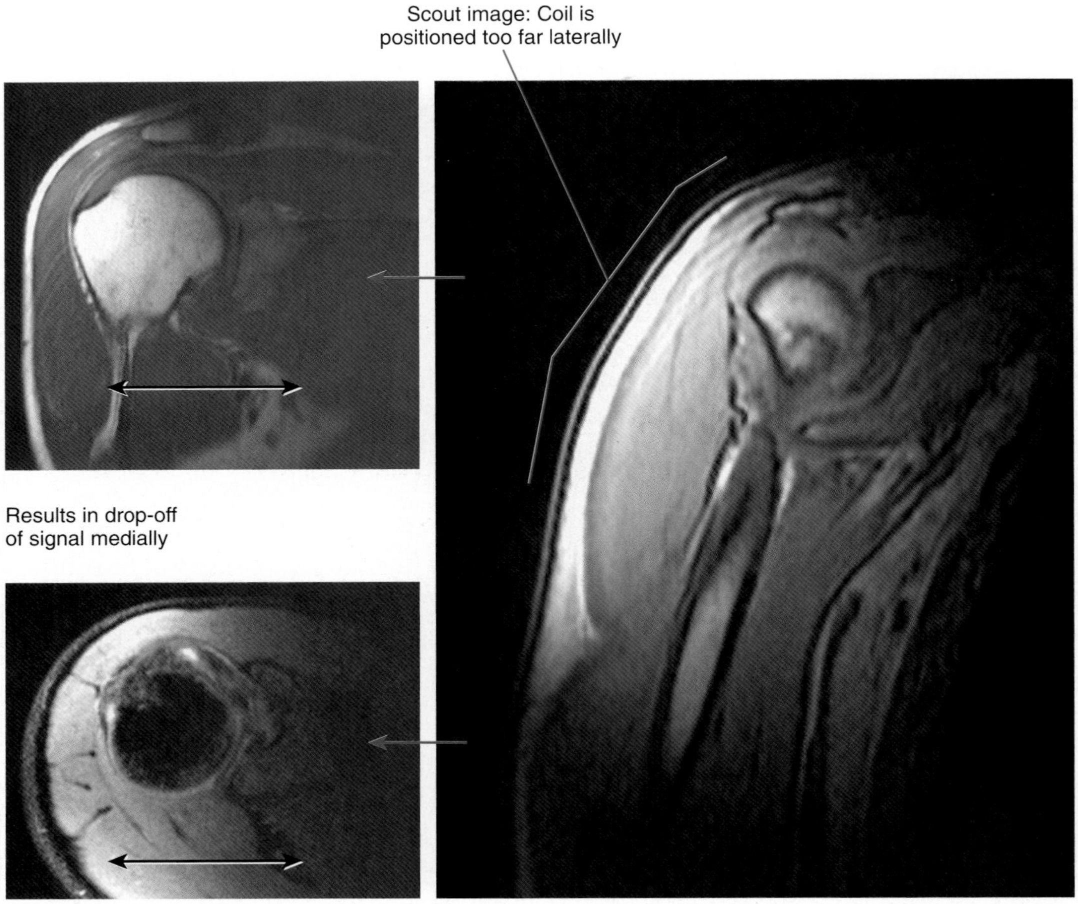
Scout image: Coil is positioned too far laterally
Results in drop-off of signal medially

Figure 1-6 Optimizing coil placement is also essential. Here, the shoulder coil is malpositioned, leading to dropoff of signal medially; the labrum is barely visible. Coil position is easily gleaned from the scout image (*right*). If the image is inadequate, the technologist should reposition the coil or use a better-fitting coil.

high in-plane and out-of-plane resolution; in-plane resolution is related to SNR, field of view, and matrix (i.e., discrimination of adjacent structures in the X/Y plane), and out-of-plane resolution is related to slice thickness and interslice gap. Three-dimensional gradient sequences can be acquired at very narrow slice thickness, without a gap. Proton density imaging provides high SNR, since fat and fluid both have high signal (Fig. 1-7). This added signal can be used to decrease field of view and increase image matrix size, thus increasing spatial resolution (Fig. 1-8).

Sequences with high contrast resolution provide a large difference in signal between the anatomic structures being imaged and the surrounding tissues. For example, a fat-suppressed T2-weighted image of the wrist has high contrast resolution, with fluid being very bright and the triangular fibrocartilage being very dark. STIR imaging has high contrast, but may be limited by lower spatial resolution. One way to increase contrast resolution is to perform MR arthrography using fat-suppressed T1-weighted images (Fig. 1-9), which, when performed with spin-echo or gradient-echo imaging, also can be optimized for spatial resolution. This is one advantage for performing MR arthrography for internal derangement. Although it may be desirable to combine high contrast and spatial resolution, often these cannot be achieved in the same sequence, and protocols should be set up with some sequences optimized for spatial resolution (high matrix, small field-of-view proton density for gradient-echo imaging) and others designed for high contrast (fat-suppressed T2-weighted imaging or STIR). Newer scanners provide an estimate of SNR when changing sequence parameters from the stan-

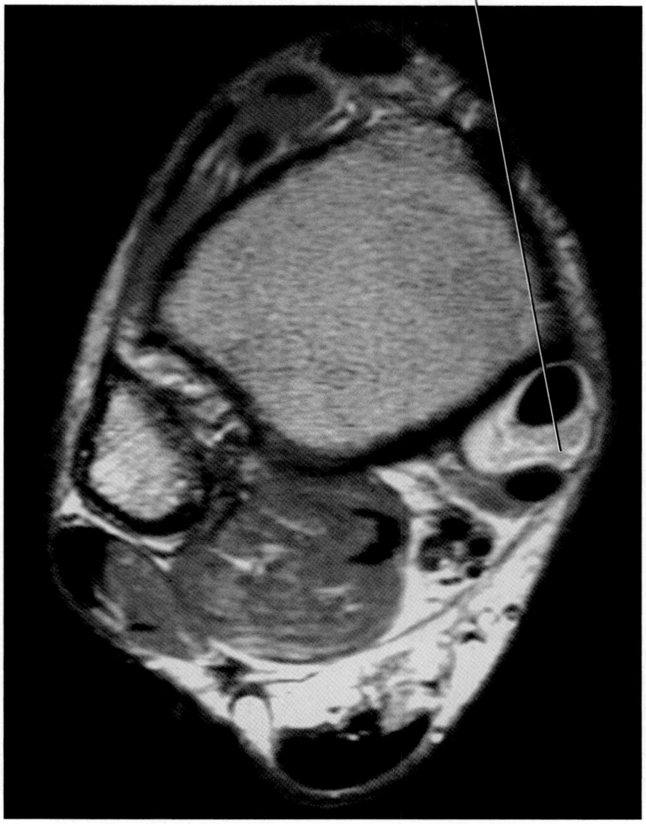
Synovial proliferation within posterior tibialis tendon sheath

Figure 1-7 Sequence emphasizing spatial resolution. Proton density (intermediate-weighted) sequences are very useful in musculoskeletal imaging; high signal allows alteration of other parameters such as acquisition of thinner slices or higher matrix in order to achieve high resolution. Gradient-echo sequences can also be used to provide high resolution.

dard settings, allowing the technologist to alter those parameters to adjust SNR to a satisfactory level. This can take some of the guesswork out of protocol management.

SPIN-ECHO IMAGING

Spin-echo imaging provides high SNR T1-weighted images and also is very useful when combined with fat suppression for MR arthrography or post-contrast imaging. In addition, T1-weighted images can be acquired using fast gradient sequences, and, if susceptibility artifact is not a consideration, gradient-echo T1-weighted imaging such as a radiofrequency spoiled sequence (SPGR from GE, T1-FFE from Philips; FLASH from Siemens) can be useful as a faster substitute. T1-weighted images are necessary in musculoskeletal imaging to evaluate the subcutaneous tissues and bone marrow. Evaluation of muscle atrophy, detection of fascial abnormalities, and evaluation of subsynovial fat also is facilitated by T1-weighted imaging. In addition, detection of ossified intra-articular bodies is improved when using T1-weighted imaging. Therefore, most institutions incorporate at least one non–fat-suppressed T1-weighted sequence into all musculoskeletal imaging protocols.

FAST SPIN-ECHO IMAGING

For many years, the fast spin-echo pulse sequence has dominated musculoskeletal imaging. The majority of centers use fast spin-echo imaging for acquisition of T2-weighted images because of its increased efficiency relative to spin-echo imaging. Acquisition of multiple echoes per time to repetition (TR; typically 8) speeds the acquisition process, enabling higher image matrix sizes to enhance resolution. Alternatively, fast spin-echo can be used to shorten scan time. The echoes are acquired at a variety of TEs, which are used to fill K space and form the image; echoes decrease in strength as the TE increases. Image contrast is determined by echoes acquired around the desired TE, whereas resolution is determined by the other echoes.

The presence of lower TEs cause fat to be relatively bright on T2-weighted fast spin-echo images compared with spin-echo images. For this reason, T2-weighted fast spin-echo images should be acquired with fat suppression or with long TR and TE times (nominally 4000 and 100 msec, respectively). Otherwise, fluid may not be conspicuous in contrast to surrounding fat signal. An alternative strategy is the use of driven equilibrium pulse sequences, which allow for shorter TR and TE settings while maintaining image contrast (FRFSE on GE, RST on Siemens, DE on Philips equipment).

When using fast spin-echo imaging, care should also be taken to avoid blur artifact. This is less of a consideration in newer scanners, but can still be seen with a combination of a high echo train length and low TE. In this situation, the low selected TE is used to plot the center of K space (resulting in contrast at

SECTION I

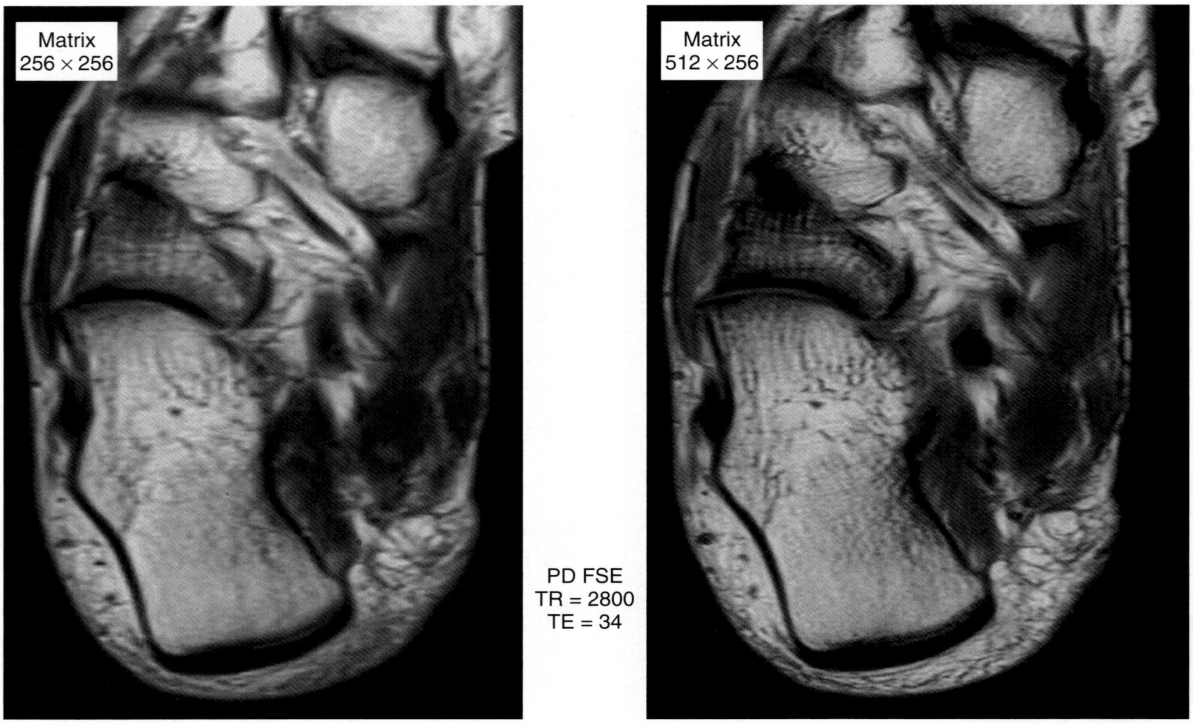
Matrix
256 × 256
Matrix
512 × 256
PD FSE
TR = 2800
TE = 34

Figure 1-8 If the image has adequate signal, increasing the matrix and/or decreasing the field of view improves resolution. Note improved detail of trabeculae as well as soft tissue structures as the matrix is increased. However, as the voxel size decreases, signal-to-noise ratio decreases, so this must be titrated. FSE, fast spin-echo; PD, protein density; TE, echo time; TR, time to repetition.

the desired TE), whereas the higher TEs, which are low in amplitude, are used for the periphery of K space (which determines image sharpness). The low amplitude of the TEs used for resolution results in lack of sharpness of the image, or blur artifact. For this reason, some authors have suggested that fast spin-echo imaging should not be used for proton density imaging, such as for evaluation of the knee menisci. However, if the echo train length is limited to 4 and TE is not below 20 msec, this artifact is generally not noticeable. In addition, the use of a higher receiver bandwidth setting to reduce the interecho spacing will reduce blurring artifacts: 20- to 24-kHz bandwidth settings on gradient echo and 150- to 200-Hz/pixel settings on Siemens; and 1 to 1.5-pixel shift on Philips equipment work well. Fast spin-echo imaging can even be used to acquire T1-weighted images. At such a low TE, the echo train length must be decreased further, generally to 2 echoes.

Another common mistake is using similar parameters that were historically used for T2-weighted spin-echo imaging for fast spin-echo imaging, which results in unsatisfactory images. When spin-echo technique is used to acquire T2-weighted images, a TE of 100 to 120 msec is used to achieve high fluid conspicuity. Fast spin-echo imaging with fat suppression at the same TE results in a very black-and-white image with low SNR and a grainy appearance. The recommended TE for T2-weighted fast spin-echo fat-suppressed images is about 40 to 60 msec (Figs. 1-10 and 1-11). Although this borders on proton density imaging parameters, lowering the TE recaptures signal and provides a high-quality anatomic image while retaining fluid conspicuity. As long as all these factors are taken into consideration, fast spin-echo imaging can be used to acquire both high spatial resolution proton density images, in addition to high-contrast fat-suppressed T2-weighted images for evaluation of the musculoskeletal system (Table 1-2).

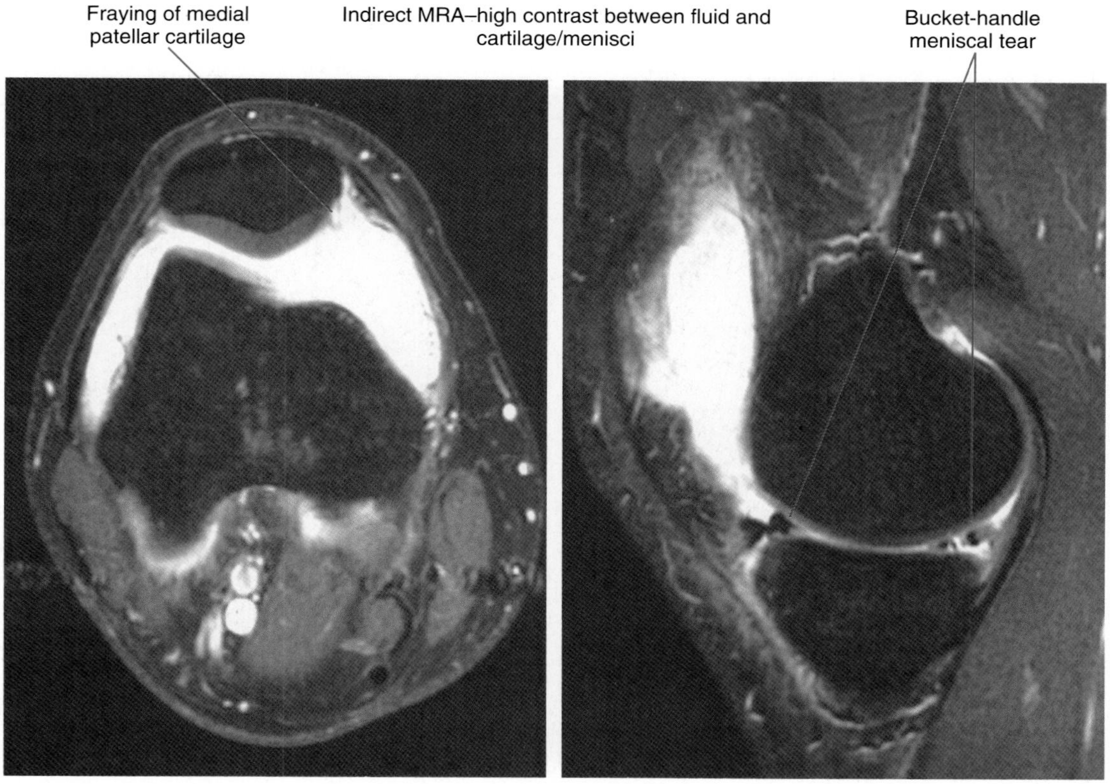
Fraying of medial patellar cartilage
Indirect MRA–high contrast between fluid and cartilage/menisci
Bucket-handle meniscal tear

Figure 1-9 High-contrast sequence. Intravenous contrast dye was administered with T1-weighted fat-suppressed spin-echo imaging performed after a 30-minute delay (indirect MR arthrogram [MRA]). High-signal joint fluid provides high contrast from the adjacent intermediate-signal hyaline cartilage and low-signal fibrocartilage.

Table 1-2 Altering Echo Time

Increase	Decrease
Advantages	
Increased fluid brightness	Recapture signal-to-noise ratio (SNR)
Reduce blur artifact	Reduce metal artifact
Disadvantage	
Lose SNR	Decreased fluid brightness

SHORT TAU INVERSION RECOVERY

STIR imaging is like the bone scan of MRI—very sensitive but with relatively low resolution. The STIR sequence incorporates a 180-degree inversion pulse followed after a certain time interval (the inversion time, TI) by a spin-echo or fast spin-echo sequence. After the 180-degree pulse, protons in different tissues relax through the transverse plane at different rates. The tissue crossing the transverse plane gets dephased by the 90-degree pulse that initiates the rest of the sequence, and the result is no signal from that tissue. Selection of the inversion time is generally based on relaxation of fat through the transverse plane to achieve a fat-suppressed image. Because T1 relaxation rates are different at different field strengths, the inversion time also must be adjusted at different field strengths. Table 1-3 lists optimal inversion times at various field strengths. STIR imaging can be acquired at any field strength and is particularly advantageous at low field strengths, where other forms of fat suppression are limited. STIR also is useful at higher field strengths when using a large field of view (Fig. 1-12) in which the anatomy does not fit the coil (Fig. 1-13), or in situations with a heterogeneous magnetic field, either inherent in the scanner or created by metal in the adjacent tissues.

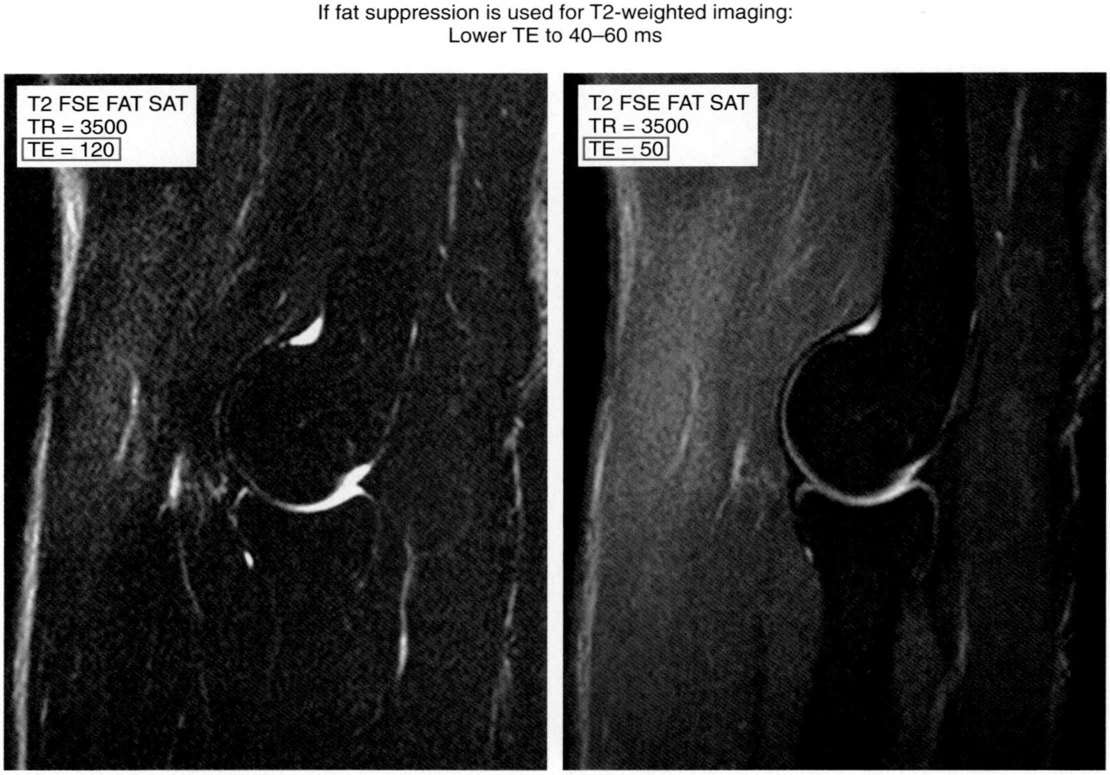
If fat suppression is used for T2-weighted imaging:
Lower TE to 40–60 ms
T2 FSE FAT SAT
TR = 3500
TE = 120
T2 FSE FAT SAT
TR = 3500
TE = 50

Figure 1-10 If fat suppression is used in conjunction with T2-weighted fast spin-echo imaging, the echo time (TE) must be lowered to achieve adequate signal. Note that fluid remains conspicuous, even at proton density–type TE. FSE, fast spin-echo.

Table 1-3 Optimizing Inversion Time (TI) Different Field Strengths

Field Strength (Tesla)	TI (msec)
0.3	80
0.5	110
1.0	130
1.5	150
3.0	180

To summarize, examples of the use of the STIR sequence include imaging of the thorax, pelvis, thighs, and calves (large field of view); imaging of the hands and feet (coils not configured to match anatomy); imaging on an open scanner; imaging around metal prostheses or other orthopedic hardware: and imaging as an alternate technique when fat suppression is not functioning properly. STIR imaging is also commonly useful as an adjunct to other fluid-sensitive sequences, since very high contrast can be useful even without high spatial resolution in certain situations. For example, in wrist imaging it may be useful to detect fluid passing through the ligaments, diagnostic for tear despite low resolution. An important limitation for musculoskeletal imaging is that gadolinium contrast at concentrations used for MR arthrography results in dark signal on STIR images (Fig. 1-14). Similarly, STIR should not be used after intravenous contrast administration.

GRADIENT-ECHO IMAGING

Gradient-recalled echo imaging can be performed as a two-dimensional or three-dimensional sequence. With no refocusing pulse like spin-echo and fast spin-echo imaging, gradient-echo sequences are prone to magnetic susceptibility artifact. This artifact can be created by air, calcium, or iron in the form of hemosiderin, but is particularly problematic when dealing

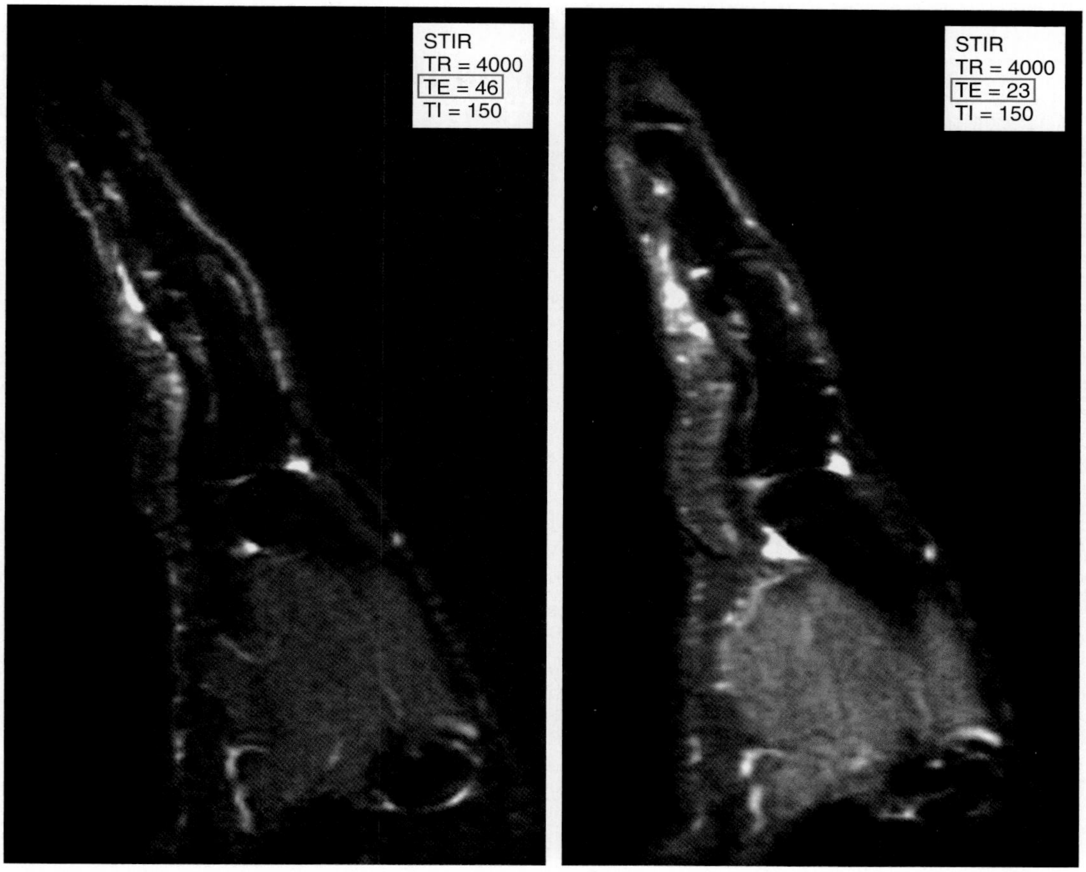
STIR
TR = 4000
TE = 46
TI = 150
STIR
TR = 4000
TE = 23
TI = 150

Figure 1-11 Lowering echo time (TE) can also improve signal-to-noise ratio on STIR sequences. Like fat-suppressed T2 fast spin-echo imaging, because of inherent fat suppression on STIR images, there is little signal left apart from fluid. Lowering the TE can improve overall signal without diminishing conspicuity of fluid. Alternatively, the inversion time (TI) can be changed slightly off what is considered optimal for the scanner field strength (i.e., at 1.5 T optimal fat nulling is achieved at a TI of 150 msec; changing to 140 or 160 msec may provide a more pleasing image). TR, time to repetition.

with metal implants or even with microscopic metal fragments left behind by surgical instruments. This creates a misregistration artifact with low signal drop-off adjacent to intense increased signal in a region surrounding the metal. Severity of artifact depends on a number of factors, including type of metal (titanium: minimum artifact; stainless-steel/cobalt chrome: severe artifact), complexity of the surface (pin/rod: minimal artifact; screw: moderate artifact; shrapnel: maximal artifact) and to a lesser degree, orientation in the magnet (aligned with B0: less artifact).

Gradient-echo sequences can be performed as T1 or fluid-sensitive (T2*-weighted) sequences, as well as intermediate-weighted sequences. Although contrast is determined partly by TR and TE, the flip angle has an impact as well. Higher flip angles (40–90 degrees) have more T1 weighting, whereas lower flip angles (e.g., 20 degrees) have less T1 weighting. For most sequences, longer TE times are associated with more T2* weighting. Thus, T1-weighted gradient-echo imaging is optimal using the shortest possible TE in conjunction with a high flip angle. Conversely, T2* weighting is achieved with longer TE times (20–40 msec at 1.5 T) and lower flip angles (less than 20 degrees).

Gradient-echo sequences are versatile. They can be used in situations in which high resolution is necessary, particularly where thin slices are needed. Very thin slices without skip can be achieved with three-dimensional gradient-echo sequences. For small structures such as the wrist interosseous ligaments,

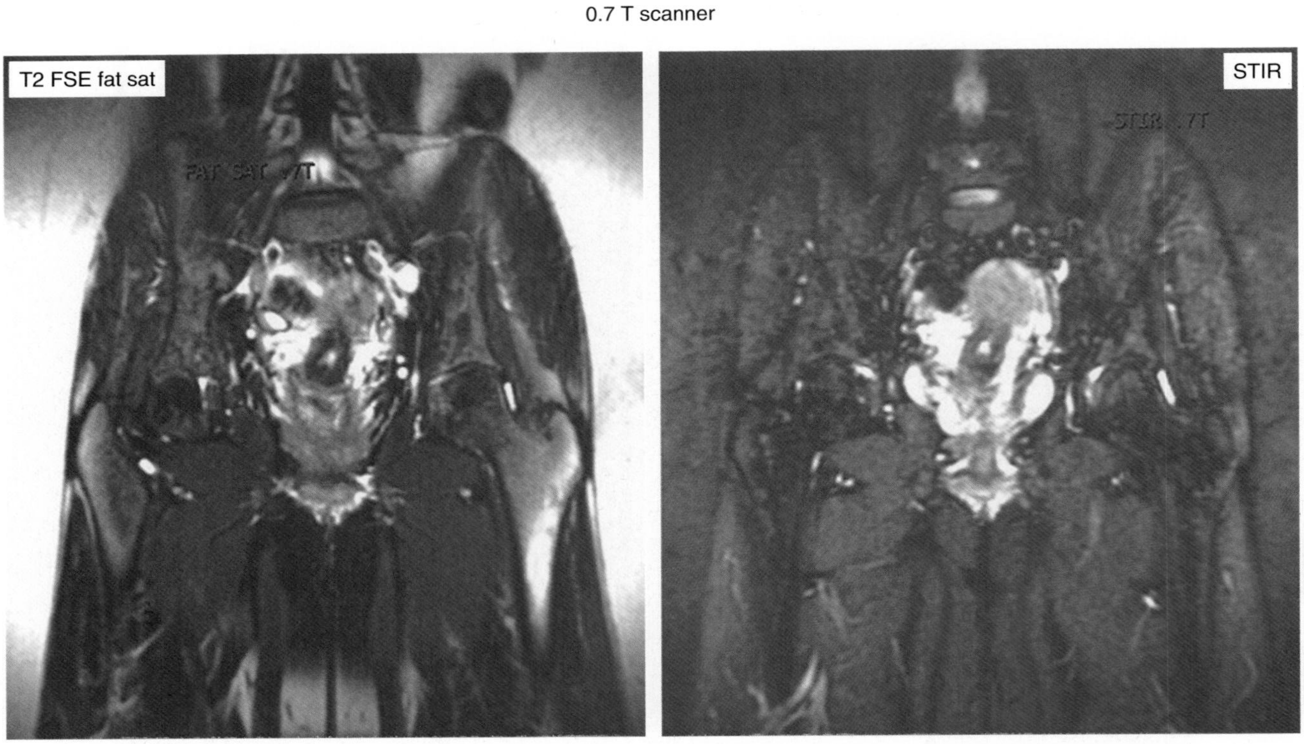
0.7 T scanner
T2 FSE fat sat
STIR

Figure 1-12 Use of STIR to achieve more homogeneous fat suppression over a large field of view.

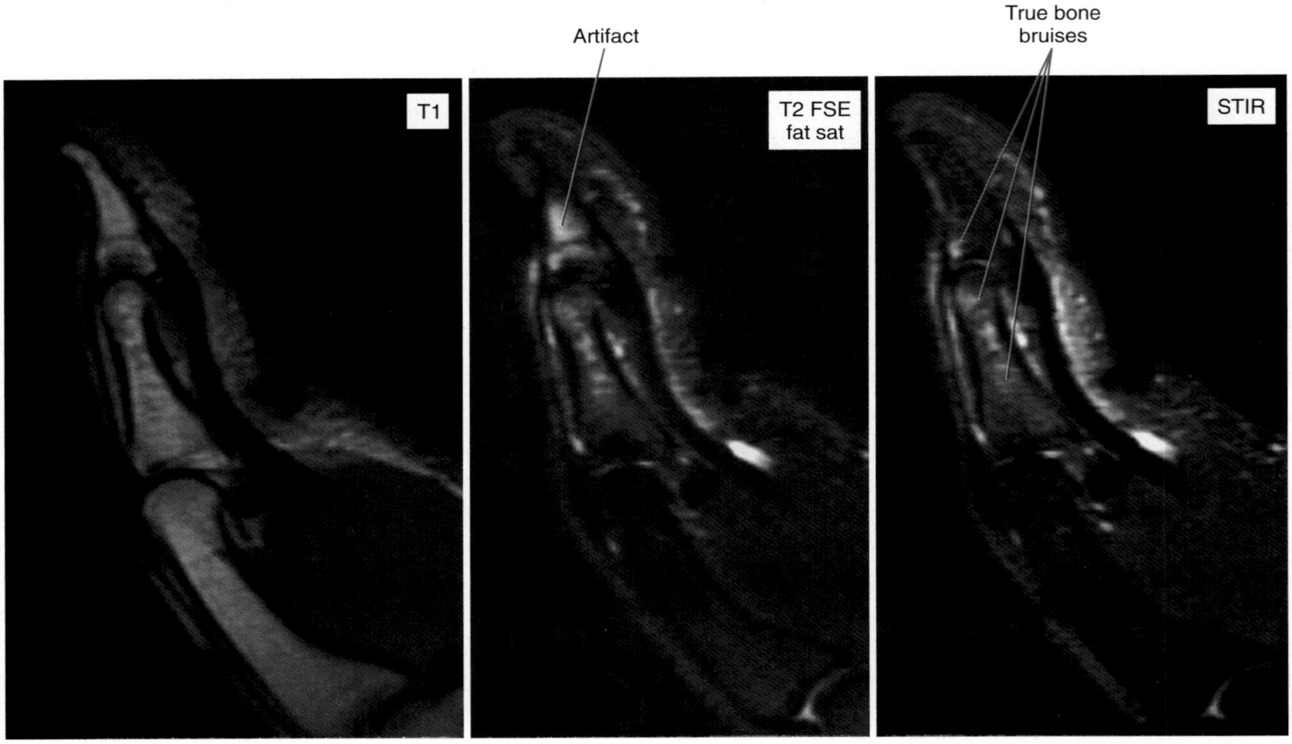
Artifact
True bone bruises
T1
T2 FSE fat sat
STIR

Figure 1-13 Professional baseball player with subacute injury. STIR provides improved homogeneity of fat suppression compared with T2 FSE fat sat in situations in which large field of view is required (i.e., the pelvis) or in which the anatomy does not closely match the coil configuration (i.e., hands and feet).

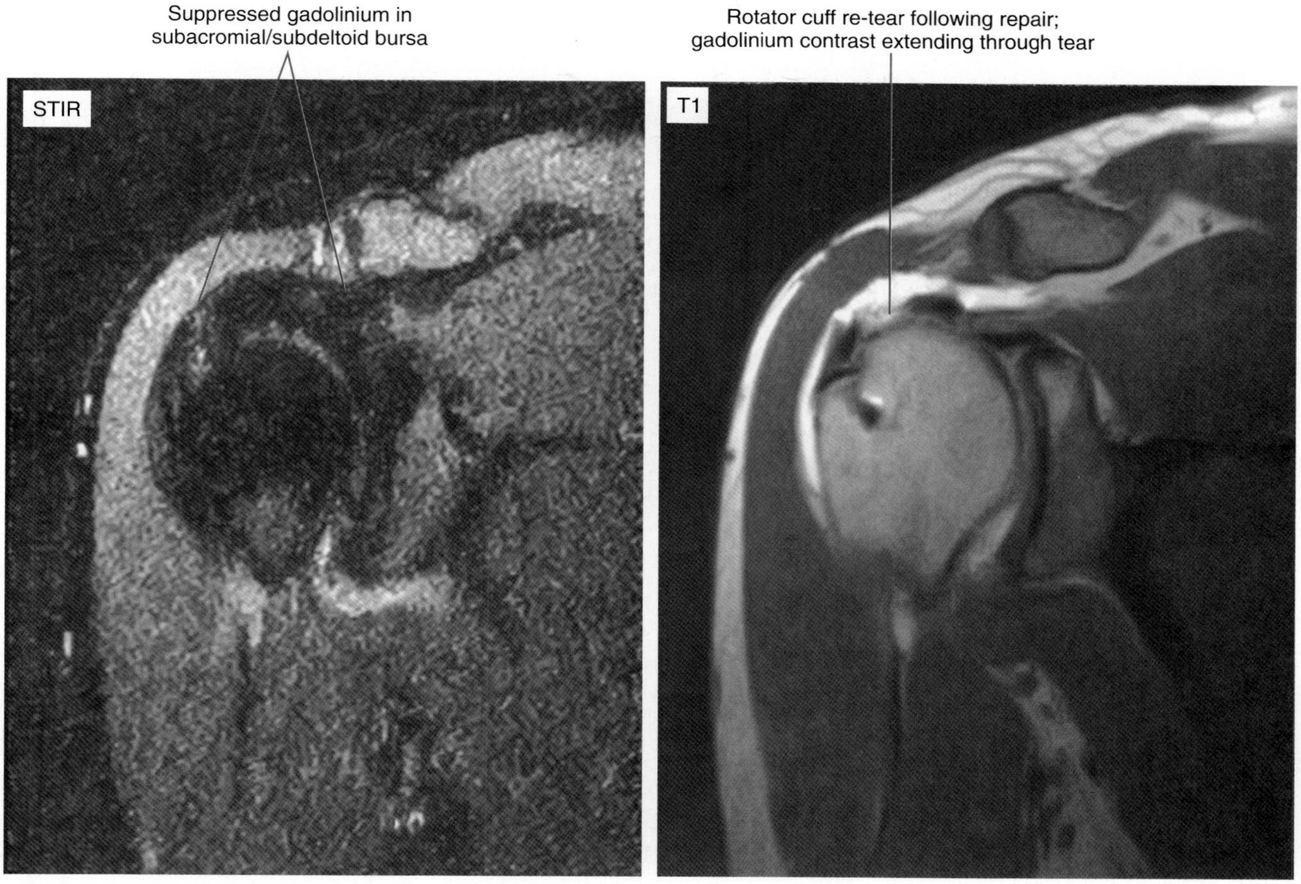
Suppressed gadolinium in subacromial/subdeltoid bursa
Rotator cuff re-tear following repair; gadolinium contrast extending through tear
STIR
T1

Figure 1-14 **Gadolinium contrast can result in low signal on STIR images.** MR arthrogram on 0.3 T MRI.

numerous slices can be acquired compared with a spin-echo sequence the thickness of which yields only three or four slices through the anatomy. Fast gradient-echo sequences also can be used in situations in which speed is important, such as with fat suppression and radiofrequency spoiling to acquire T1-weighted dynamic contrast-enhanced images (i.e., for tumor vascularity or soft tissue or bone necrosis; Fig. 1-15) or for acquiring contrast-enhanced images in three planes in a very short time period. Because of the rapid capability of these sequences, they also can be used to acquire images at very short TEs, facilitating in-phase and out-of-phase imaging.

Although metal creates the most problematic artifact, on gradient-recalled echo images images artifact is also created by calcium, so marrow signal on a gradient-echo image is partially related to local trabecular density; in general, unless comparing pre- and post-contrast or in-phase and out-of-phase images, marrow findings on gradient-recalled echo images should be interpreted with care. Similarly, owing to the low TE generally used in gradient-echo imaging, magic angle phenomenon is often observed in tendons and ligaments on these sequences. These latter factors can limit the overall usefulness of gradient-echo imaging for global joint evaluation.

The disadvantages also come with some advantages (Figs. 1-16 through 1-22). Knowing how to use gradient-echo artifact to your advantage is important for problem solving in musculoskeletal imaging (Box 1-2).

MR ARTHROGRAPHY

Direct and indirect MR arthrography and optimization of these techniques are discussed in Chapter 2.

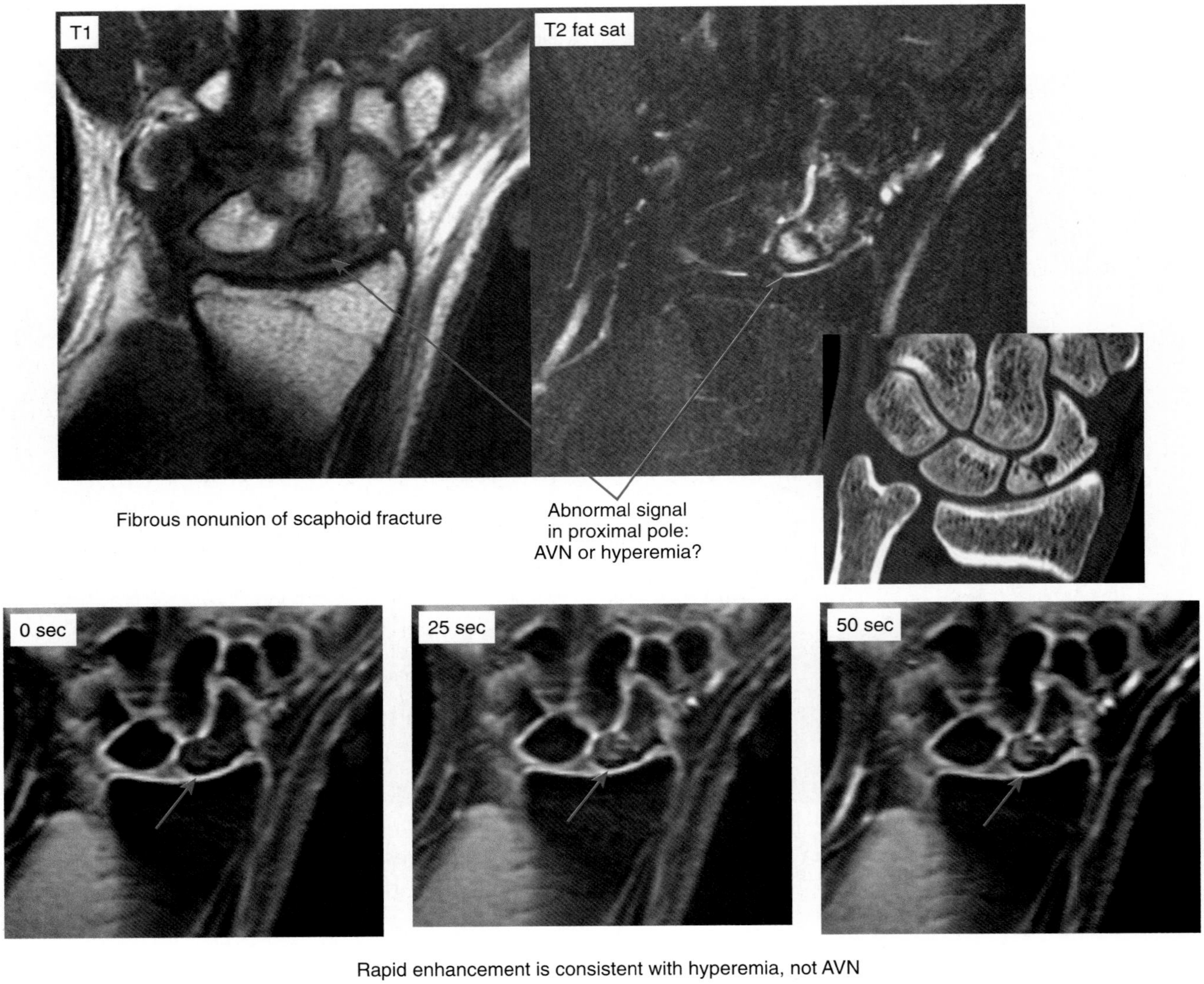
T1
T2 fat sat
Fibrous nonunion of scaphoid fracture
Abnormal signal
in proximal pole:
AVN or hyperemia?
0 sec
25 sec
50 sec
Rapid enhancement is consistent with hyperemia, not AVN

Figure 1-15 Fast gradient-recalled echo sequences are excellent for acquiring dynamic contrast-enhanced images, rapidly imaging and re-imaging the same region before and immediately after an intravenous bolus of contrast. This technique is useful in musculoskeletal imaging for determining the vascularity of tumors and whether edematous tissue is hyperemic or necrotic. In the case above, the surgeons can be informed preoperatively that fusion across the nonunion has a better chance of success given presence of blood flow to the proximal pole. AVN, avascular necrosis.

OPTIMIZING SIGNAL-TO-NOISE RATIO

Once the sequence has been selected, parameters should be optimized to maximize the SNR while achieving desired resolution and field of view. If a particular set of images appears grainy, even in the adjacent air, most likely the problem is low signal, high noise, or both (Box 1-3). Common problems are that the TE is too high or the voxel size is too small; both decrease signal, and since noise is constant, SNR decreases. SNR is especially a problem on signal-starved sequences, such as fat-suppressed, fluid-sensitive sequences. Suppressing the fat signal lowers the overall signal in the image, and unless there is marked edema, there will be little signal relative to background noise. The most common protocol problem on fat-suppressed T2-weighted fast spin-echo and STIR images is to use a TE that is too high, which further decreases overall signal and results in unacceptably low SNR.

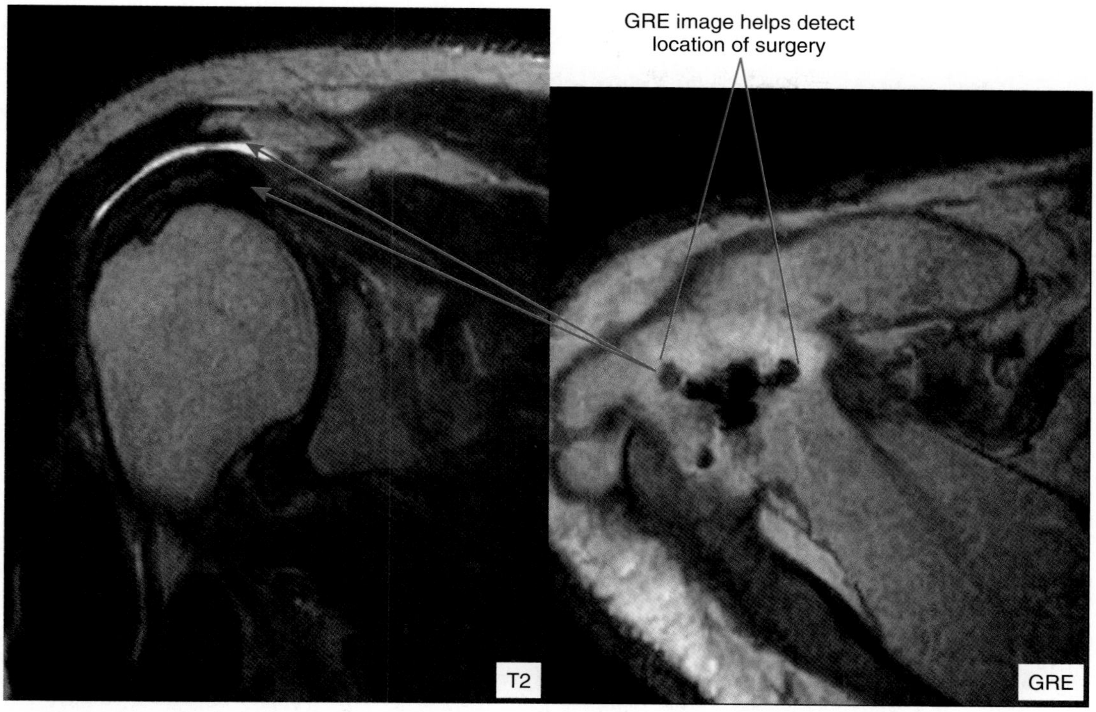
GRE image helps detect location of surgery
T2
GRE
Acromioplasty and tendon-to-tendon cuff repair

Figure 1-16 Gradient-recalled echo (GRE) sequences can help find the site of surgery in cases where provided history is limited. Microscopic metal fragments from surgical instruments exhibit blooming artifact and become more obvious.

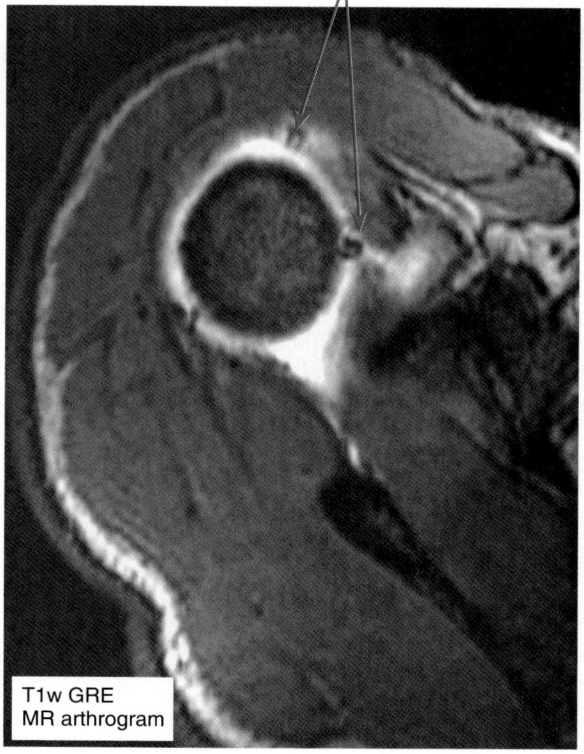
After rotator cuff repair displaced, suture anchors are seen in the joint
T1w GRE
MR arthrogram

Figure 1-17 Gradient-recalled echo (GRE) images are excellent for detection of slight susceptibility artifact created by bioabsorbable sutures and implants.

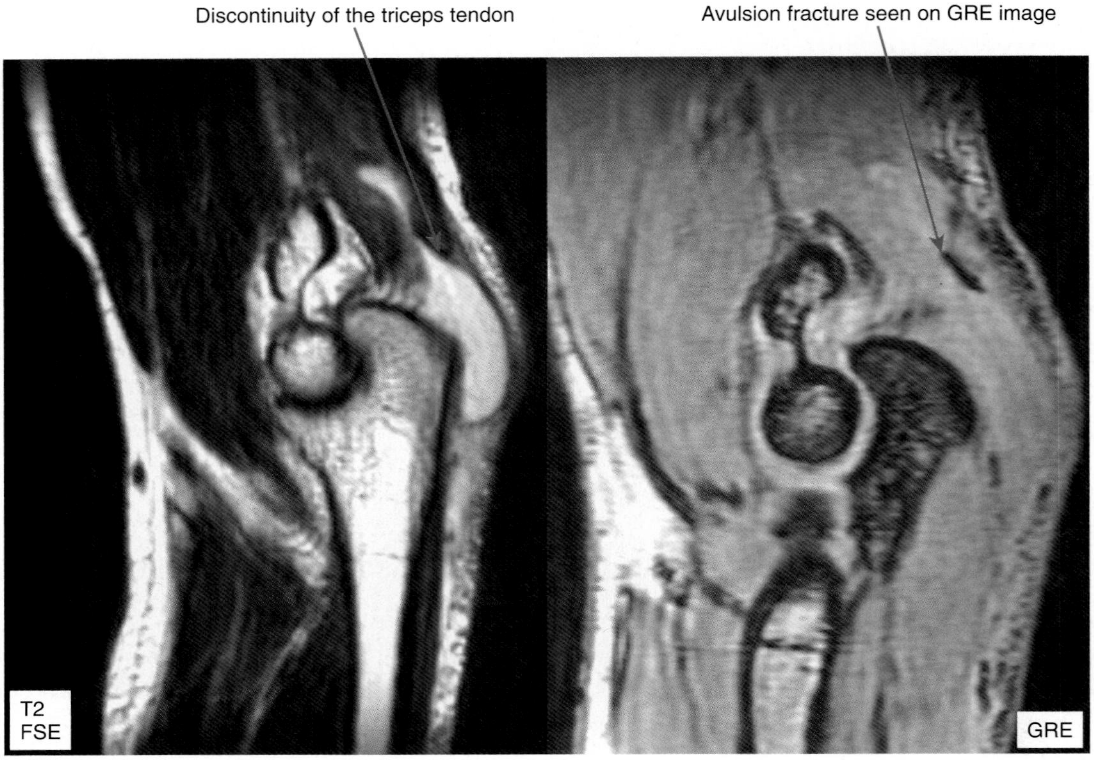
Discontinuity of the triceps tendon
Avulsion fracture seen on GRE image
T2
FSE
GRE

Figure 1-18 Gradient-recalled echo (GRE) images are useful for detecting foci of calcification in the soft tissues, such as avulsion fractures. FSE, fast spin-echo.

BOX 1-2 USE OF GRADIENT-RECALLED ECHO (GRE) SEQUENCES TO TAKE ADVANTAGE OF SUSCEPTIBILITY ARTIFACT*

- Detection of hemosiderin
  - Pigmented villonodular synovitis, hemophilia, hematoma, hemorrhagic tumor
- Detection of calcification
  - Myositis ossificans/heterotopic bone, calcified mass, intra-articular bodies/synovial osteochondromatosis, calcific tendinosis, avulsion/chip fracture
- Detection of metal
  - Finding location of surgical bed
- Detection of foreign body
- Detection of air/gas (e.g., necrotizing fasciitis)

*When using GRE images for detection of susceptibility artifact, in general avoid fat suppression because dark fat may obscure the finding.

BOX 1-3 WAYS TO INCREASE SIGNAL-TO-NOISE RATIO (SNR)

- Grainy image and uniformly low SNR
  - Lower echo time
  - Remove fat sat
  - Lower bandwidth
  - Thicken slices
  - Widen field of view/decrease matrix
  - Use different coil
  - Increase number of excitations (inefficient and may increase motion artifact)
- Grainy image on one side
  - Reposition coil
  - Use different coil (e.g., with larger field of view)

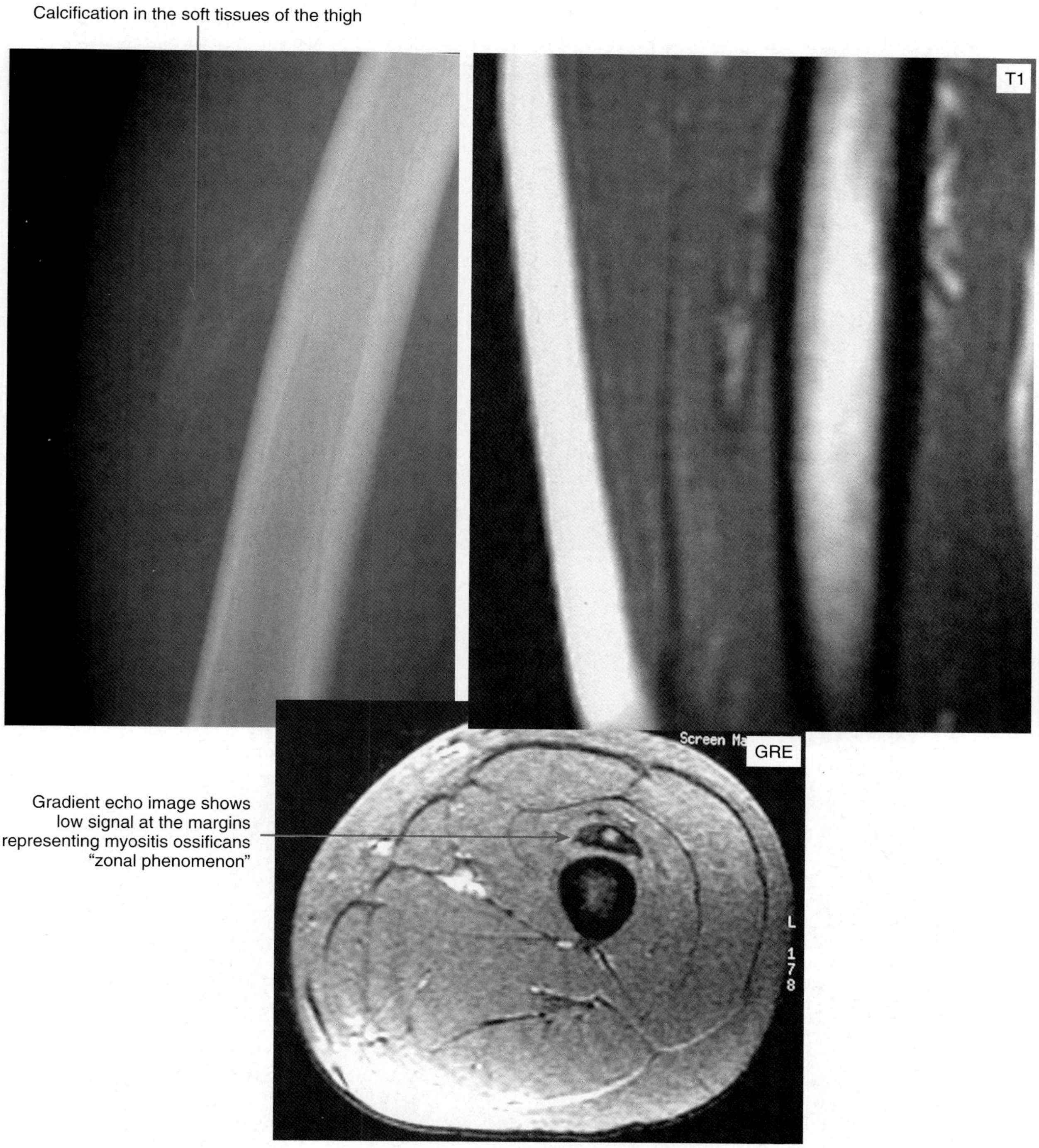
Calcification in the soft tissues of the thigh
T1
GRE
Gradient echo image shows low signal at the margins representing myositis ossificans "zonal phenomenon"
L
178

Figure 1-19 *Gradient-echo (GRE) imaging can be useful for evaluating distribution of calcification in a suspected mass.*

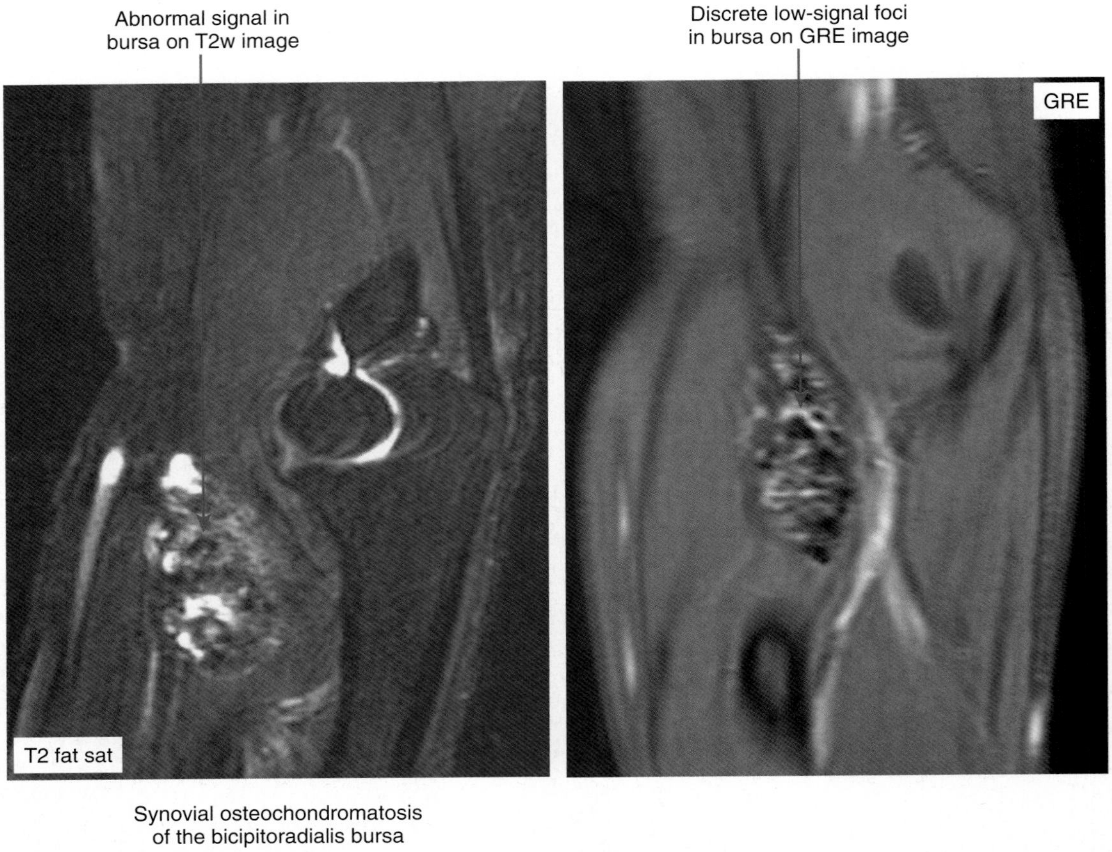
Abnormal signal in
bursa on T2w image
Discrete low-signal foci
in bursa on GRE image
GRE
T2 fat sat
Synovial osteochondromatosis
of the bicipitoradialis bursa

Figure 1-20 Foci of calcification are more apparent on gradient-echo images.

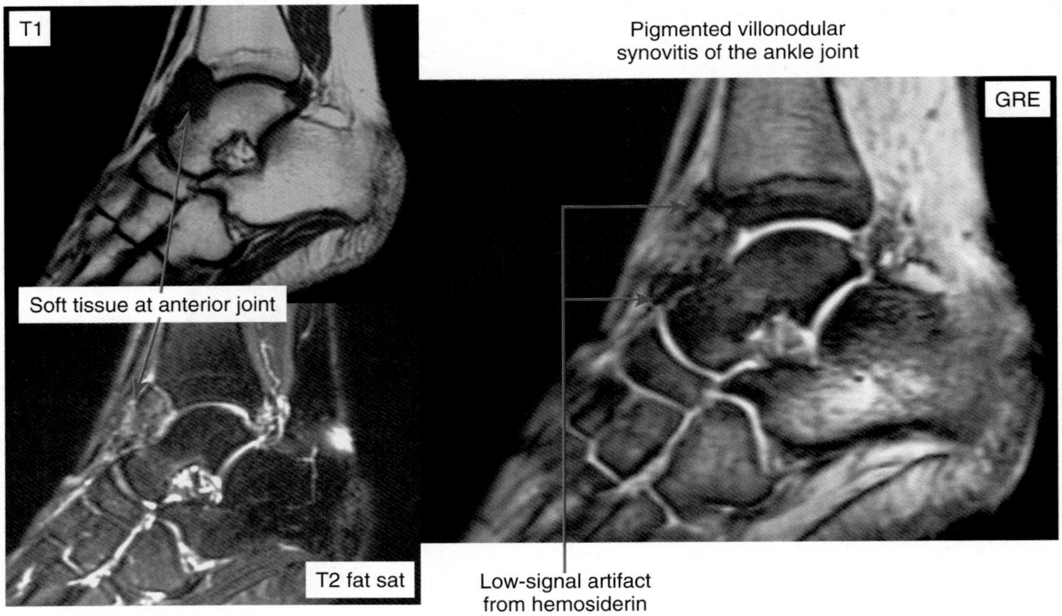
T1
Pigmented villonodular
synovitis of the ankle joint
GRE
Soft tissue at anterior joint
T2 fat sat
Low-signal artifact
from hemosiderin

Figure 1-21 Gradient-echo (GRE) sequences are useful for detection of hemosiderin in hematomas and conditions such as hemophilia and pigmented villonodular synovitis.

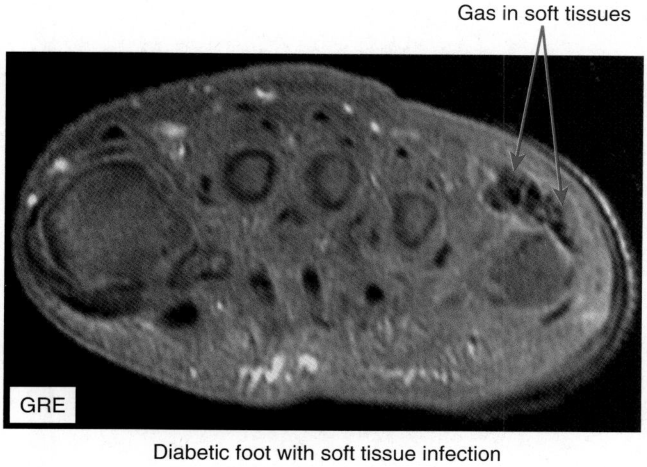
Gas in soft tissues
GRE
Diabetic foot with soft tissue infection

Figure 1-22 Gradient-echo (GRE) imaging is also useful for detection of gas in the soft tissues, as seen in necrotic tissue and sinus tracts/fistulas.

The first steps that the radiologist should take to improve SNR should be those that do not result in a loss of time or resolution. The most obvious change is to use a better or smaller coil, or one that better accommodates the anatomy. As previously discussed, if the sequence is fat-suppressed, T2-weighted fast spin-echo or STIR, first try lowering the TE to 40 to 60 for fast spin-echo or 20 to 40 for STIR. Although these times border on proton density, because of fat suppression, fluid will still be conspicuous. If the slices are too close together, cross-talk from adjacent slices can decrease contrast due to residual dephasing; increasing the interslice gap to 20% to 25% of slice thickness removes the problem. On newer scanners, cross-talk is less of a problem, and 10% interslice gap (e.g., 3 mm with a 0.3-mm gap) is often acceptable. Interleaving slices removes cross-talk and removes the need for a gap but doubles scan time and

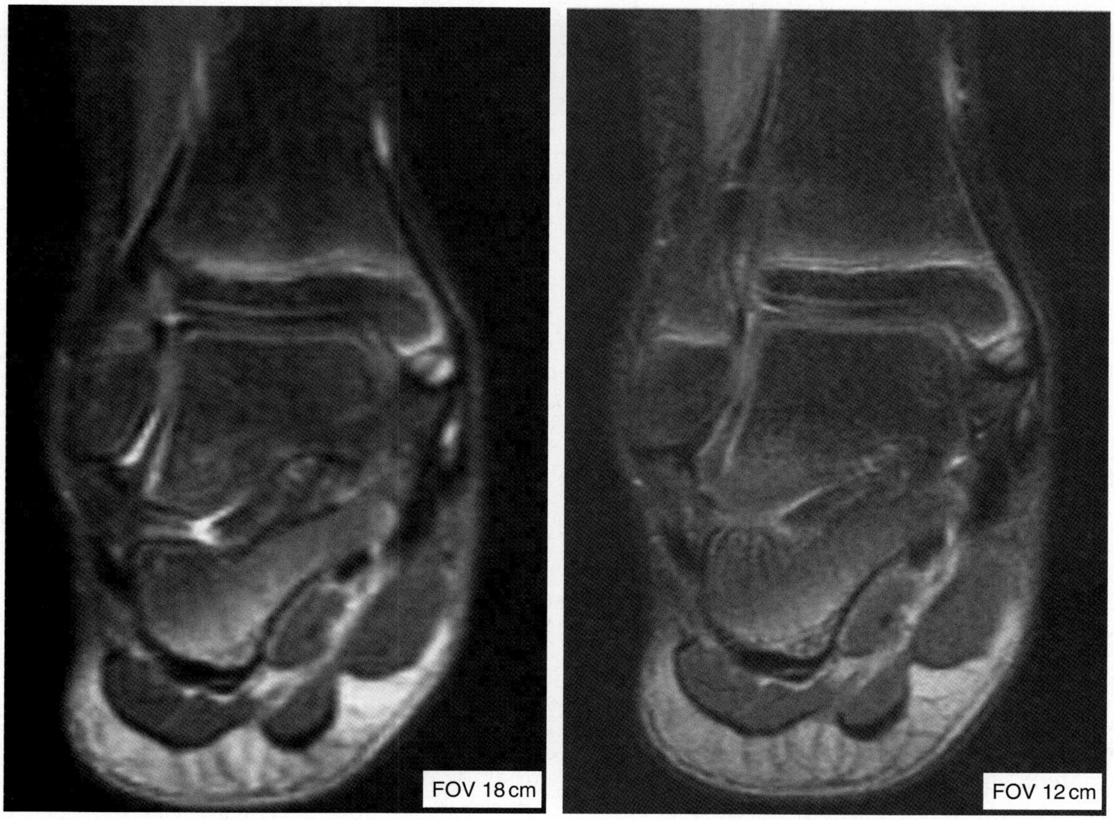
FOV 18 cm
FOV 12 cm

Figure 1-23 **Change in field of view (FOV).** T2-weighted fast spin-echo images with identical parameters and coil; only alteration was from 18 to 12 cm FOV. Note improved detail with small FOV. However, it is important to ensure that there is high enough signal-to-noise ratio to accommodate the smaller voxel dimension. Conversely, to improve a signal-poor image, it may be necessary to increase FOV or slice thickness, or to decrease the matrix.

SECTION I

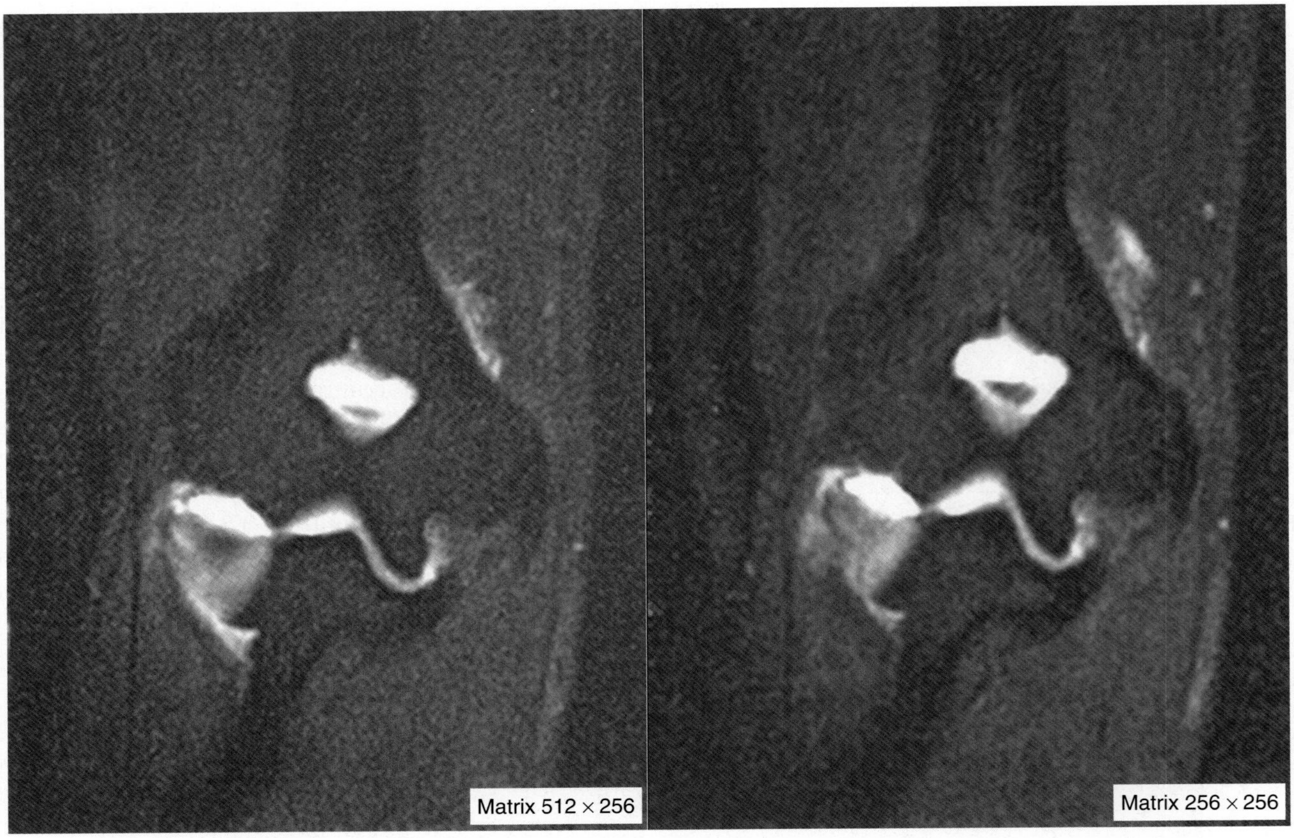
Matrix 512 × 256
Matrix 256 × 256

Figure 1-24 Effect of changing matrix. Similar to lowering field of view, increasing matrix makes voxel dimensions smaller. This can improve resolution, but if there is inadequate signal the image will become too noisy.

is generally not used except in situations in which imaging of small structures (e.g., the wrist ligaments) makes a gap undesirable.

Second, one can try altering voxel dimension (Figs. 1-23 and 1-24). Unlike signal, noise is uniform across the image, so increasing voxel dimension solves the problem but at the expense of resolution. Try incrementally increasing slice thickness, decreasing the matrix, or increasing field of view until acceptable SNR is achieved. Increasing number of excitations increases SNR but is an inefficient method relative to the increase in imaging time, and motion artifact will be accentuated. Similarly, lowering the radiofrequency receiver bandwidth improves SNR (Fig. 1-25) but has disadvantages, including a potential increase in scan time and accentuation of chemical shift artifacts. Finally, if the changes just mentioned are not working, removing fat suppression or trying a different sequence may be necessary.

HOW TO REDUCE ARTIFACTS SEEN ON MUSCULOSKELETAL MR IMAGING

Artifacts Related to Fat Suppression

Heterogeneous Fat Suppression

Occasionally, images with standard fat saturation (presaturation of lipid-resonant frequency) result in a heterogeneous effect with parts of the images showing little to no fat suppression (Fig. 1-26). This may be due to heterogeneity of the magnetic field of the scanner and is typically seen when performing this type of fat suppression on a large field of view. This effect can create a "harlequin" pattern, with poor fat suppression at opposite edges of the field (see Fig. 1-12). It may also occur if the patient has metal implants or artifact-producing material in retained

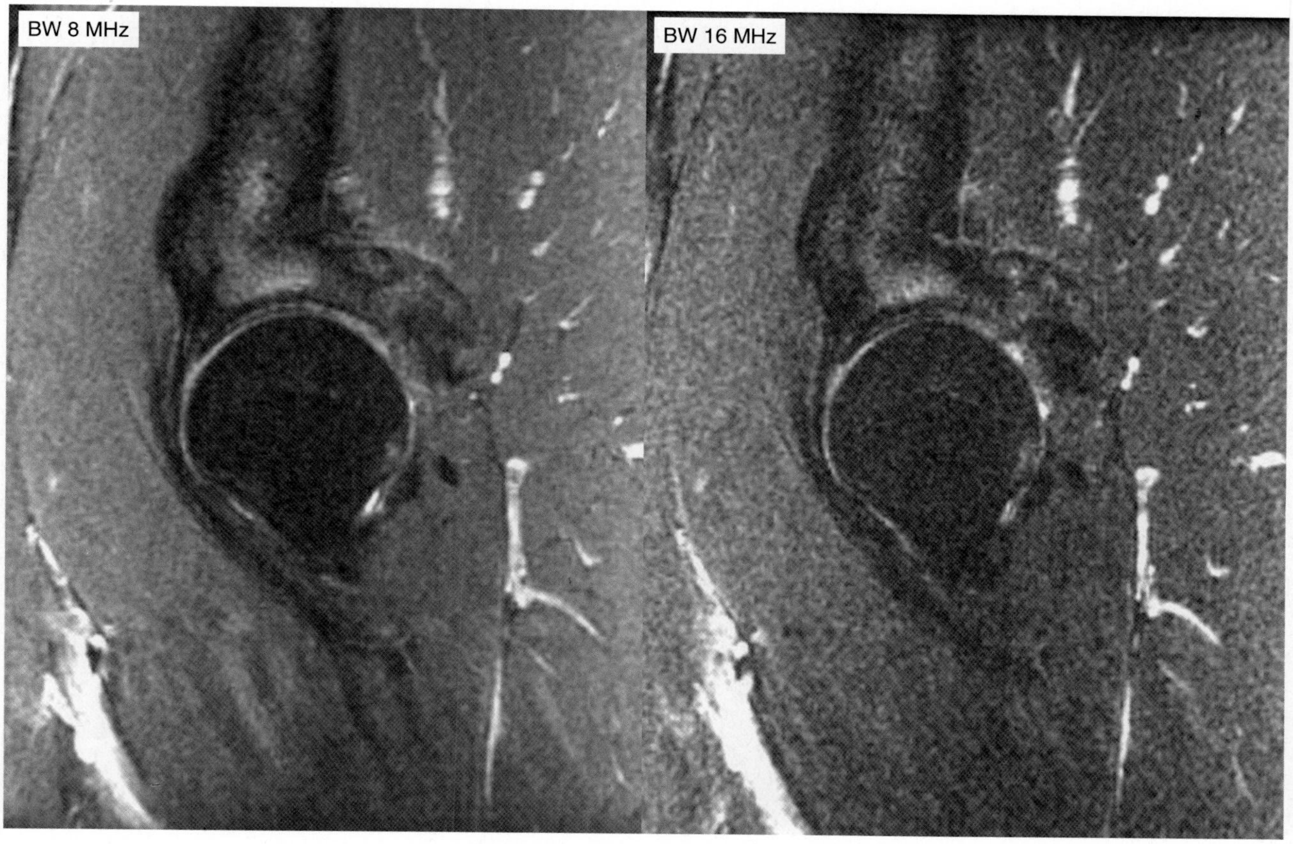
BW 8 MHz
BW 16 MHz

Figure 1-25 Effect of altering bandwidth (BW). Lowering bandwidth improves signal; note better definition of articular surfaces in the 8-MHz image compared with the 16-MHz image. The 16-MHz image appears grainier, reflecting lower signal-to-noise ratio.

BOX 1-4 HETEROGENEOUS FAT SUPPRESSION

Coil not positioned well—reposition
Remove fat saturation
Use STIR instead: STIR is more reliable than fat sat for large field of view

clothing. In addition, this heterogeneous effect can be created by poorly fitting coils on particular body parts and is commonly seen when the foot and ankle are imaged in a cylindrical coil.

One of the simplest ways to correct the problem of heterogeneous fat suppression is to use STIR imaging rather than standard fat-suppressed T2-weighted imaging (Box 1-4). Alternatively, the technologist can change the field of view, reposition the coil, or reposition the body part within the coil (e.g., plantar flexion of the foot in the extremity coil). Standoff pads may also help to prevent near-field brightening, which can accentuate the heterogeneity of fat suppression. Surrounding the body part with bags of water has been reported to be effective. The problem also may be due to poor selection of the fat peak for suppression, in which case the peak can be selected manually by the technologist (on some scanners) and the sequence repeated.

Water Suppression

Water suppression can mimic heterogeneous fat suppression because it often only partially affects the image. However, in water suppression, the water peak rather than the fat peak is suppressed, leading to a region of artifactually abnormal signal in which fluid is black. Muscle, containing large amounts of water, is also typically dark, which helps identify water suppression as being the problem. Again, this is often due to heterogeneity of the magnetic field, and coil repositioning or manual selection of the fat peak may

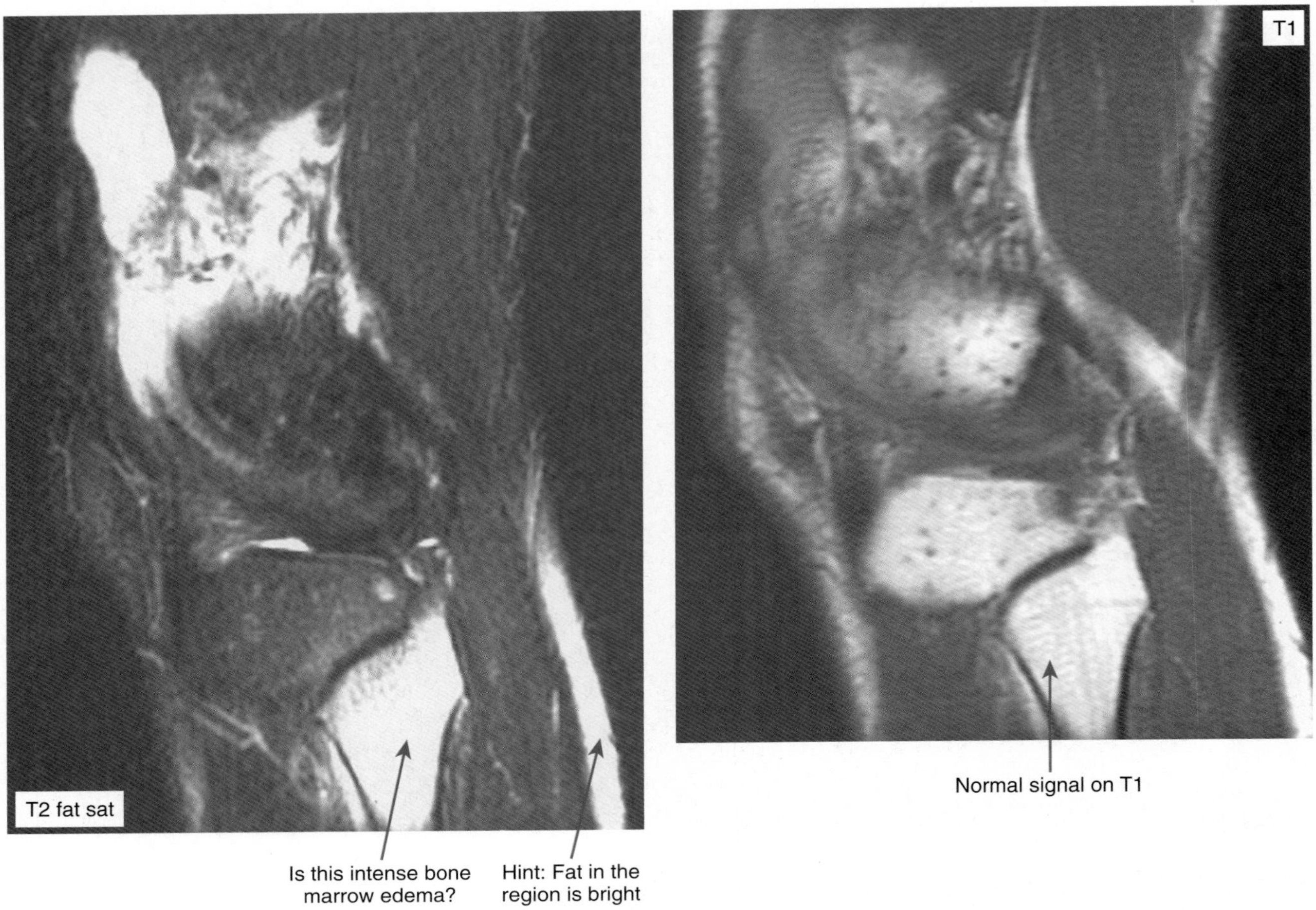
T2 fat sat
Is this intense bone marrow edema?
Hint: Fat in the region is bright
T1
Normal signal on T1

Figure 1-26 Heterogeneous fat suppression. Look at the adjacent fat as a clue to this artifact.

resolve the problem. On the other hand, the artifact may be due to a hardware malfunction. The best way to correct this problem is to remove fat suppression (Fig. 1-27) or to use an alternate method for fat suppression such as STIR imaging (Box 1-5).

Occasionally, STIR images appear even more visually displeasing than normal, either with very low signal and very bright fluid (a "black and white" image), or the fluid in cerebrospinal fluid, bladder, or joint does not appear bright (Box 1-6). The latter is a good internal control, indicating that pathology in the marrow or soft tissues may not be bright either. This may be due to poor selection of the inversion time leading to inadequate fat suppression, or signal loss due to a variety of other factors. Rescanning with slightly different inversion time (such as 140 or 160 msec rather than 150 msec at 1.5 T) may solve the problem. Alternatively, a variety of parameters can be altered that are aimed at increasing signal, such as acquiring thicker slices or altering TR or TE to recapture signal. This may be required if the problem is persistent over multiple patients.

Artifacts Related to Motion

Periodic versus Nonperiodic

Motion artifact can be divided into periodic and nonperiodic motion (Box 1-7). Periodic motion includes internal motion such as vascular flow, respiration, and cardiac motion. Cardiac motion can be a problem when imaging the ribs, in which case swapping phase and frequency encoded directions may help. However, cardiac gating can be performed. Respiratory compensation can be enabled for some scan sequences (spin-echo and gradient echo), although it may be more effective and simpler to place the area of abnormality dependently against the

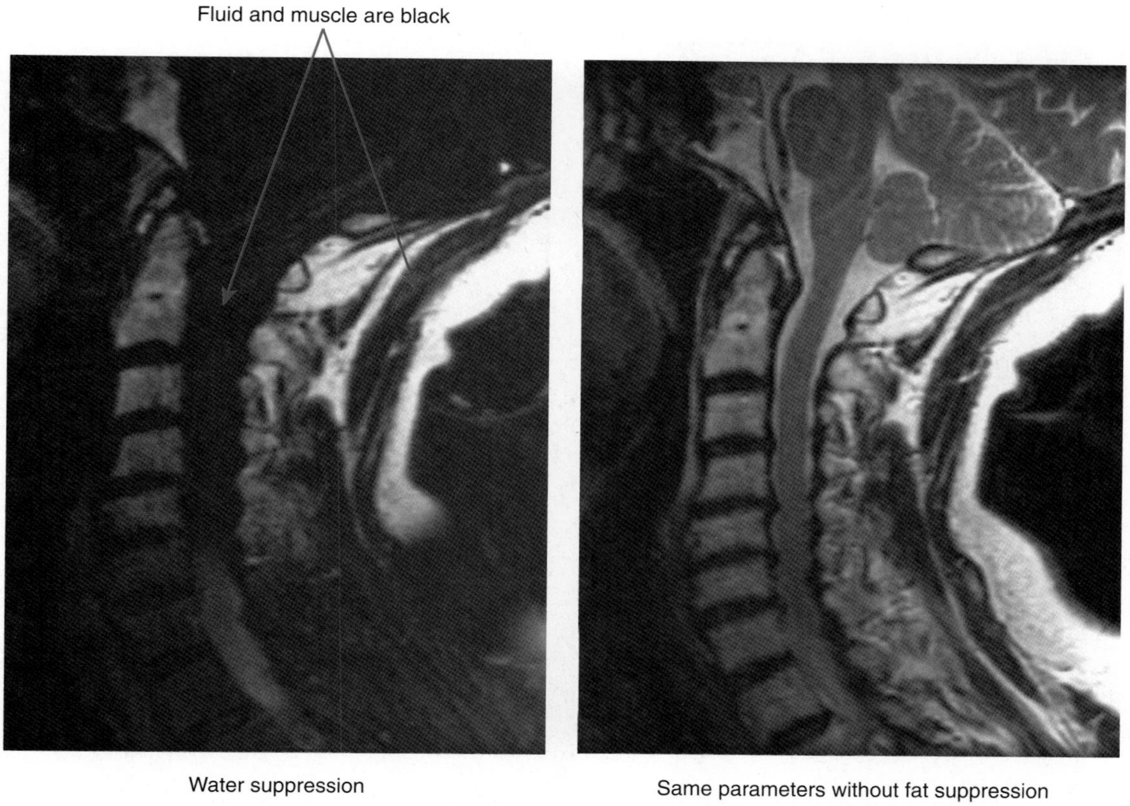
Fluid and muscle are black
Water suppression
Same parameters without fat suppression

Figure 1-27 **Water suppression.** Note that fat is bright but unlike with heterogeneous fat suppression, fluid and muscle are black. The fat peak can be manually selected, or the sequence can be repeated without fat suppression.

BOX 1-5 WATER SUPPRESSION

Problem: Heterogeneous signal; fluid and muscle dark
Solution
- Remove metal
- Manually select fat peak
- Re-do without fat saturation

BOX 1-6 STIR IMAGE TOO DARK, BLACK AND WHITE

Alter TI by about 10 msec to recapture anatomic signal
Decrease echo time
Reposition coil
Thicken slices
Decrease bandwidth

Use bladder, joint fluid, cerebrospinal fluid, and so on, as internal control for fluid conspicuity. If not bright, the pathology may not be bright either; this may require an increase in echo time.

coil to limit motion artifact, swapping phase, and frequency to place the respiratory motion in the transverse plane. Respiratory-triggered scans can be used with fast spin-echo sequences and are useful when the patient is unable to lie prone.

Vascular motion can be a problem in extremity imaging, with phase ghosting extending through areas of anatomic interest (such as the cruciate ligaments of the knee on sagittal images and the patellar cartilage on axial images). This is typically controlled with saturation bands above and below the field of view, to presaturate arterial and venous blood signal traversing the slice, swapping phase, and frequency as needed to place residual ghosting artifact away from the area of interest (Fig. 1-28). Flow compensation also can be enabled to refocus spins from moving blood into the vascular structure. Some of these strategies increase scan time or cause an alteration in TEs,

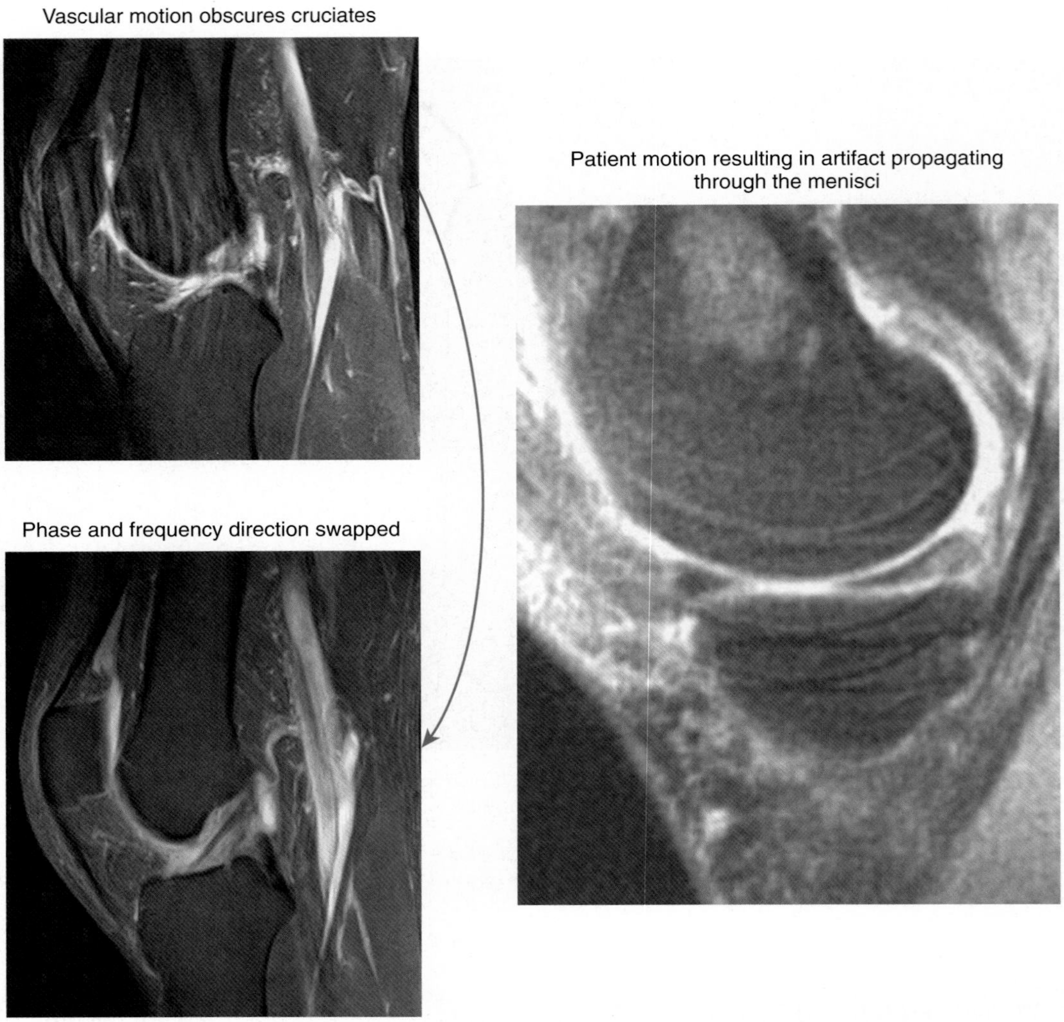
Vascular motion obscures cruciates
Patient motion resulting in artifact propagating through the menisci
Phase and frequency direction swapped

Figure 1-28 Dealing with motion artifact. Swapping phase and frequency can help move artifact away from the area of interest. Vascular motion artifact can be minimized by presaturating tissue above and below the field of view. Patient motion is best dealt with by packing the extremity tighter, lightly sedating the patient or using a faster sequence.

so be aware that each of these techniques has a downside.

Nonperiodic motion includes motion of the bowel (this is not usually a problem in musculoskeletal imaging) as well as patient motion. This motion is often easily controlled by immobilizing the limb within the coil using Styrofoam or towels. If this does not work, sedation can be used. In addition, faster sequences can be used such as fast spin-echo in place of standard spin-echo, or individual sequences can be shortened by altering parameters such as shortening the TR (although this yields fewer slices). However, the most important parameter to alter in this situation is reduction of number of excitations, since increasing the number of acquisitions accentuates motion artifact. Reduction of motion artifact may improve the image quality, even at the expense of signal.

Blur Artifact

Blur artifact is created when a low TE is performed along with a high echo train length during fast spin-echo imaging. Basically, you got greedy and tried to crank up signal and speed, and all you got was a blurry image. Blur artifact is seen as indistinctness of the image, appearing as low resolution, rather than

BOX 1-7 REDUCING MOTION ARTIFACT

- Patient external motion (nonperiodic)
  - Use tight-fitting coil; immobilize limb
  - Use faster sequence (fast spin-echo, gradient-recalled echo; avoid spin-echo, STIR)
  - Sedation
  - Shorten sequence, even at the expense of signal (decrease number of excitations)
- "Internal" motion (vascular flow, cerebrospinal fluid flow, respiration, cardiac motion)—periodic
  - Faster sequences
  - Swap-phase/frequency
  - Saturation bands (inside versus outside field of view)
  - Respiratory/cardiac gating
  - Introduce randomness in signal acquisition, K-space filling

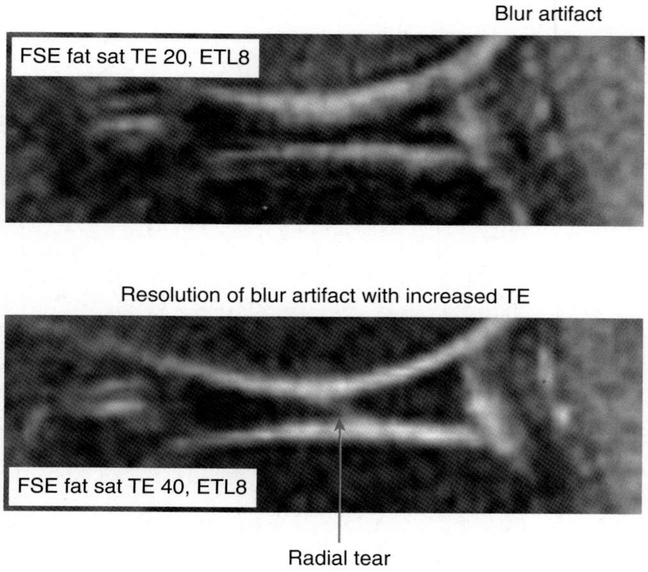
Blur artifact
FSE fat sat TE 20, ETL8
Resolution of blur artifact with increased TE
FSE fat sat TE 40, ETL8
Radial tear

Figure 1-29 Blur artifact is a consequence of using a short echo time (TE) and high echo train length (ETL). This can be an issue on proton density fast spin-echo (FSE) sequences, which are popular in musculoskeletal MR imaging. To eliminate this artifact, increase the TE and/or decrease the echo train length.

low SNR, which appears as a grainy image. This is mainly a problem when proton density fast spin-echo images are acquired, such as for meniscal imaging. The best ways to address this problem is to raise the TE, lower the echo train length, or increase the receiver bandwidth setting (Fig. 1-29). For proton density imaging, a TE of 25 to 30 msec and an echo train length of 3 to 5 should virtually remove blur artifact.

Artifacts Related to Signal Loss: Field Cutoff/Coil Malposition

If the image looks bright nearer to the coil, this is an effect known as "near-field brightening"; it is usually inconsequential, especially on picture archiving and communication systems (PACS), where dynamic windowing is available. However, if the coil is malpositioned or if a coil that is too small for the anatomy is used, this effect can become pronounced and problematic, with loss of signal in important anatomic areas farther from the coil. Coil malpositioning can be suspected if, on review of the scout localizer image, intense signal is seen a distance from relevant anatomy, such as over the lateral aspect of the deltoid with rapid drop-off in signal over the glenohumeral joint (see Fig. 1-6). The image may be windowed so that the signal appears high, but the image will appear progressively more grainy farther from the coil indicating lower and lower SNR. If this effect is observed, it should be recognized that important pathology is likely to be missed in the area of low SNR. The coil should be repositioned. If the problem persists, elements or channels of the coil may be malfunctioning.

Cross-talk is another potential reason for diminished signal and image contrasts. This is due to radiofrequency "leakage" from one slice to another, leading to partial dephasing of the slice being imaged. This can be seen globally across the image if the spacing between slices is too low; to solve this problem, increase the spacing or interleave slices (acquire every other slice, and then scan remaining slices). The effect also can be seen focally within an image if adjacent slices intersect one another; for example, when slices are angled through the disks of the lumbar spine, lines of low signal are seen at the areas of slice overlap due to dephasing.

Magic Angle Phenomenon

Magic angle phenomenon is a common artifact in musculoskeletal imaging and should be recognized as a normal finding. When monotonous, coherently aligned structures with few mobile protons (e.g., ligaments and tendons, which are composed of tightly arranged and anisotropically aligned collagen fibers) are positioned at 55 (54.7) degrees to the main

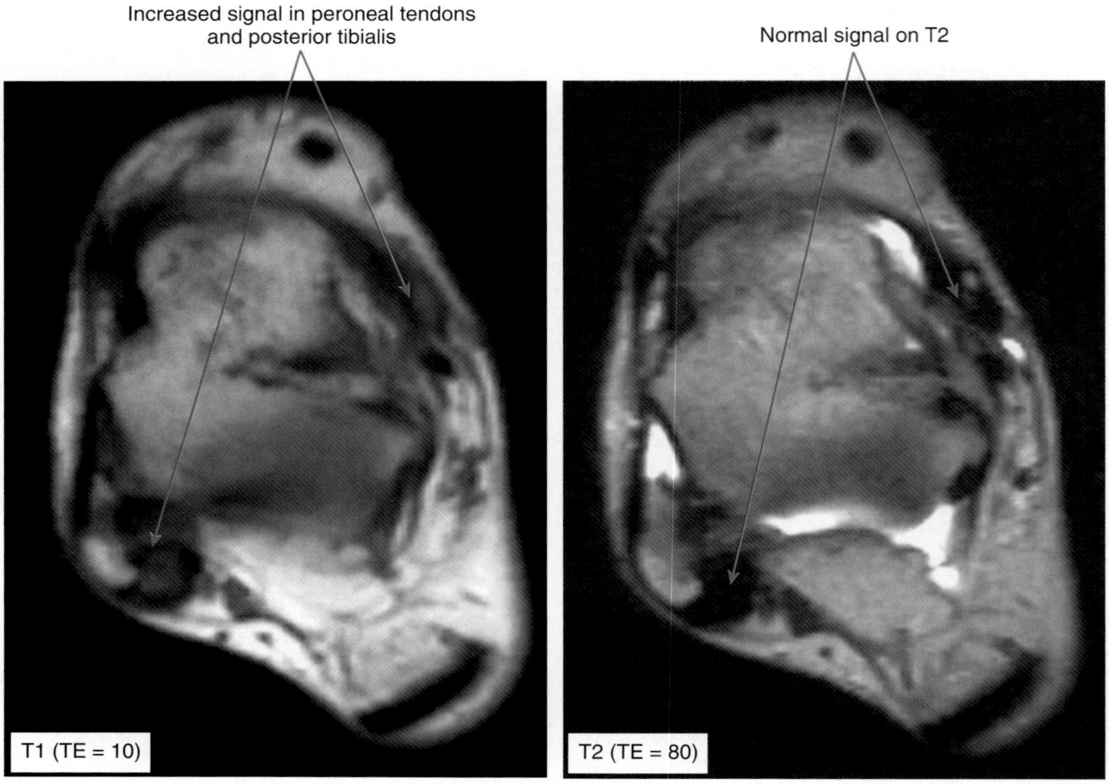
Increased signal in peroneal tendons and posterior tibialis
Normal signal on T2
T1 (TE = 10)
T2 (TE = 80)

Figure 1-30 Magic angle phenomenon. When tendons (or ligaments) are angled at 55 degrees relative to the main magnetic field, artifactual signal is observed at low echo time (TE). This can be avoided by raising the TE, although degeneration is also intermediate in signal on T1-weighted images, so when observed, other objective findings of tendinosis such as thickening, intermediate T2 signal, or synovial fluid should be sought.

magnetic field, signal artifactually increases at low TE (Fig. 1-30). This effect is commonly observed in tendons that curve or angle through the plane, such as the distal rotator cuff tendons, the ankle tendons, and the patellar tendon. On T1-weighted and proton density images, therefore, one should be careful not to overcall tendinopathy, but verify the abnormality on high TE images or note coexisting tendon thickening.

Magnetic Susceptibility Artifact

Some paramagnetic and ferromagnetic substances found in the body, most notably air, calcium, iron and metal, create field heterogeneity resulting in misregistration of signal and a black void known as magnetic susceptibility artifact. A refocusing pulse, such as that used in spin-echo imaging, corrects for some of the field heterogeneity and reduces the effect. Therefore, gradient-echo images are most prone to this effect. On longer TE sequences, this effect also is more pronounced than at shorter TE. Conventional fat saturation, which relies on a homogeneous magnetic field to presaturate the fat peak, accentuates the artifact. Therefore, to reduce the artifact, one can remove fat suppression (using STIR instead, for example), lower TE, and avoid using gradient-echo imaging. However, one of the most important parameters to change is bandwidth; high bandwidth reduces metal artifact (Box 1-8). Artifact from metal implants has been shown to be related to the type of metal (e.g., titanium is better than steel) and complexity of the metal surface (e.g., rods are better than screws) as well as the orientation of the metal (Box 1-9). Artifact can be reduced if the long aspect of the implant is oriented along the main magnetic field (however, even in extremities this is not very practical). In addition, the shape of the artifact can be altered somewhat by swapping phase and frequency, which can be attempted to recapture signal adjacent to the implant (Fig. 1-31). It should be recognized that automatic

BOX 1-8 IMAGING METAL: METHODS FOR OPTIMIZATION

Remove fat saturation
Avoid gradient-recalled echo
STIR instead of fat saturation T2
Increase bandwidth
Use fast spin-echo rather than spin-echo
Increase matrix (especially in frequency-encoding direction)
Swap phase and frequency
Turn body part in gantry if possible (align length of component with B0)
Add IV contrast, image pre- and postcontrast with same parameters

BOX 1-9 HARDWARE ARTIFACT—SEVERITY

Type/complexity of metal can be used to predict quality of MRI
No/little artifact
- Bioabsorbable components
- Silastic implants
- Coral/bone graft substitutes
- Cement

Low artifact
- Material: Titanium
- Low surface complexity: Rods/pins

High artifact
- Material: Steel/cobalt chrome/iron (e.g., shrapnel)
- High surface complexity: Screws/burr/shrapnel

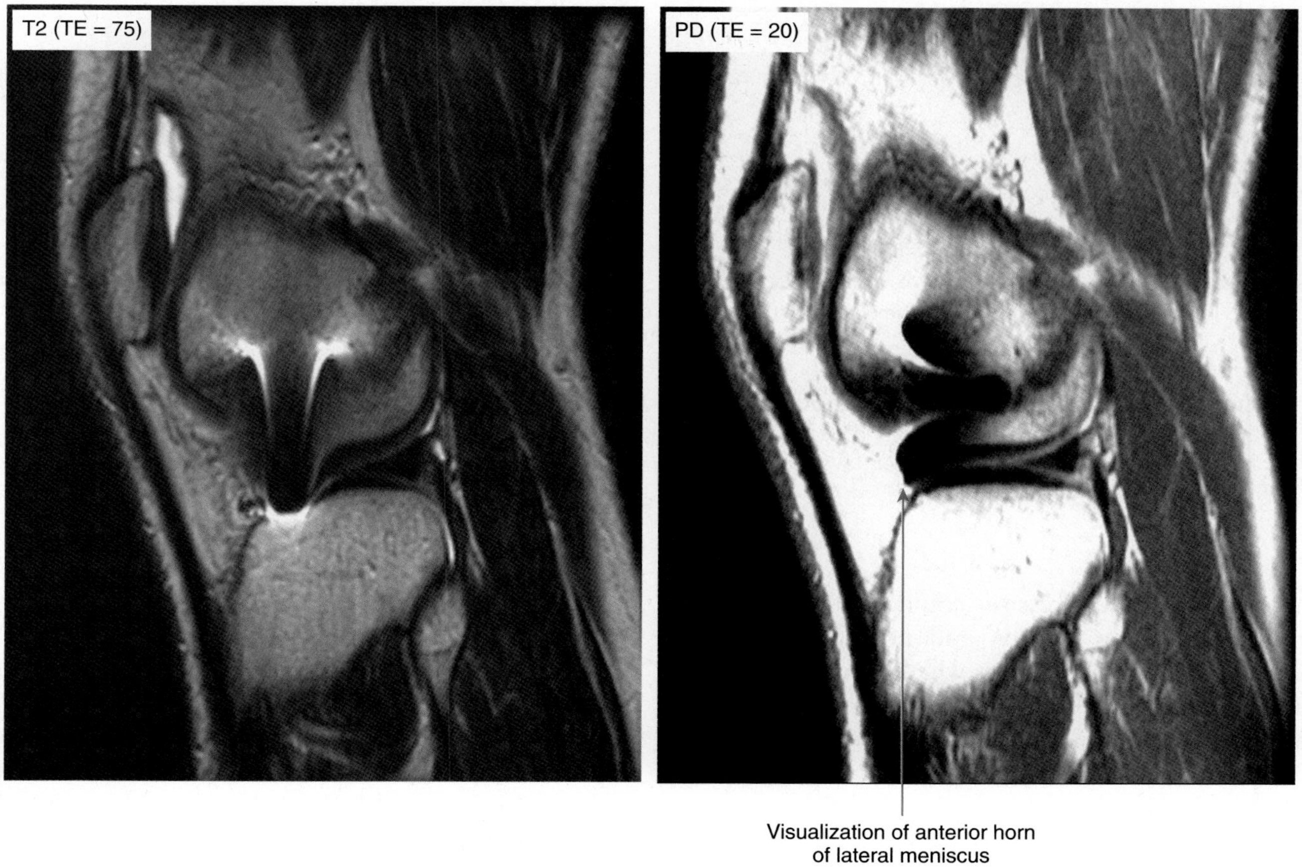
T2 (TE = 75)
PD (TE = 20)
Visualization of anterior horn of lateral meniscus

Figure 1-31 Metal artifact often has a morphology that can be turned 90 degrees by swapping phase and frequency. In this case, from the T2-weighted image to the proton density image phase and frequency directions were switched, allowing visualization of the anterior horn of the lateral meniscus. Lowering echo time (TE) also decreases metal artifact.

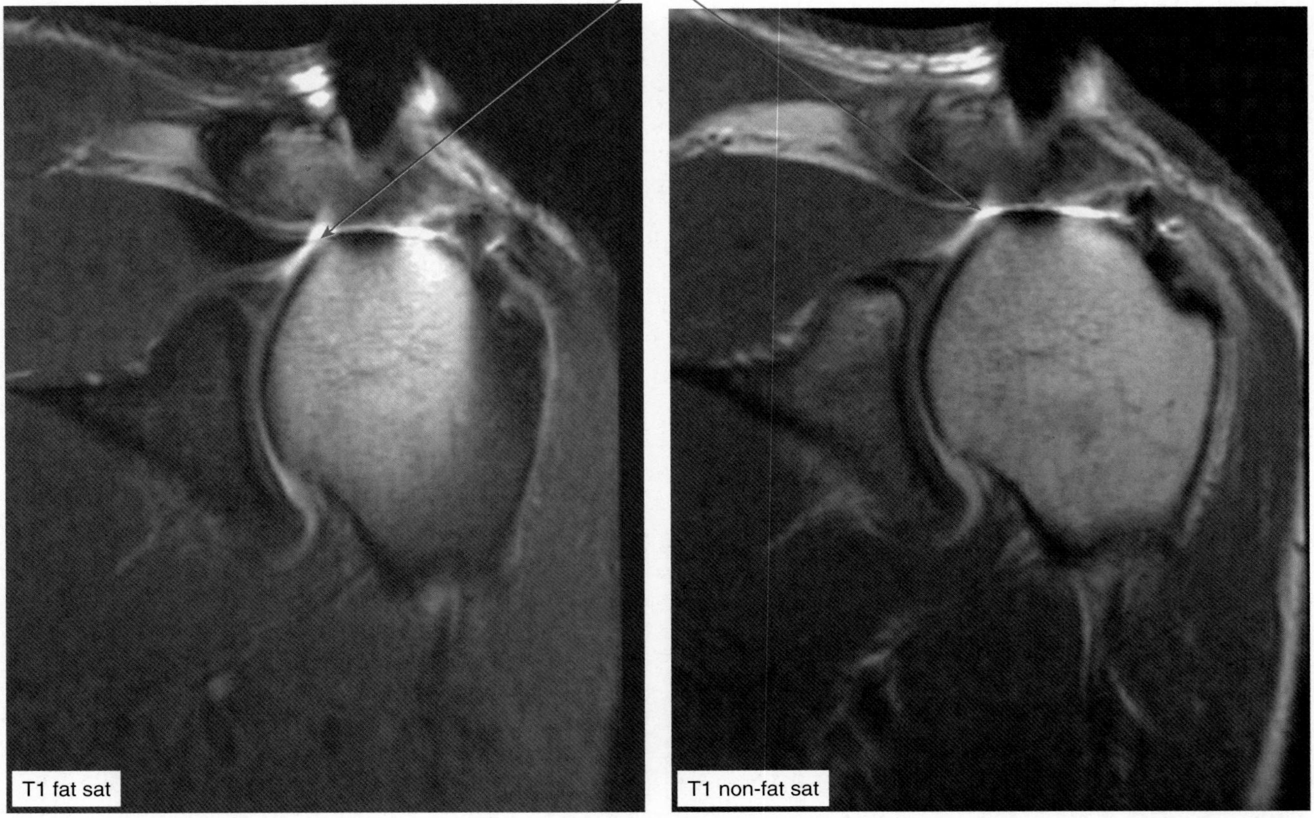
Cuff re-tear with retraction
T1 fat sat
T1 non-fat sat
Removal of fat suppression results in more homogeneous signal, but no change in diagnosis in this case

Figure 1-32 MR arthrogram of the shoulder. Evaluation of rotator cuff repair. Acromioplasty results in susceptibility artifact. Image on left is fat-suppressed, image on right is without fat suppression using same parameters. It is better to monitor cases to check whether removal of routine fat suppression could result in better visualization of relevant anatomy. Often there is no difference in diagnostic accuracy or there is even a detrimental effect.

removal of fat suppression could actually be detrimental to image quality, and postoperative cases should be monitored to see whether protocol alteration is necessary (Fig. 1-32). Increasing bandwidth has a significant impact on reduction of metal artifact (Fig. 1-33) with a slight, usually imperceptible, decrease in signal.

Chemical Shift Misregistration Artifact

Chemical shift artifact is created by slight differences in precession frequencies of protons in fat and water. Because the computer expects all protons to have the same precession frequencies, signals from fat and water are slightly malpositioned ("misregistered") relative to each other, with one shifted a small amount to one side (in the frequency-encoding direction), creating a bright line on one side and a dark line on the other side. This is seen, for example, when fat is adjacent to muscle, which contains a large amount of water. The artifact is minimized by decreasing pixel size by increasing the matrix; it is also reduced by raising the bandwidth. It is eliminated by using fat suppression (Box 1-10). The effect is accentuated at

BOX 1-10 CHEMICAL SHIFT ARTIFACT

- Signal from fat; water gets misregistered
- Makes bright/dark line at interfaces
- More pronounced at higher field strength
- Minimize by increasing matrix/increasing bandwidth
- Eliminate by using fat suppression

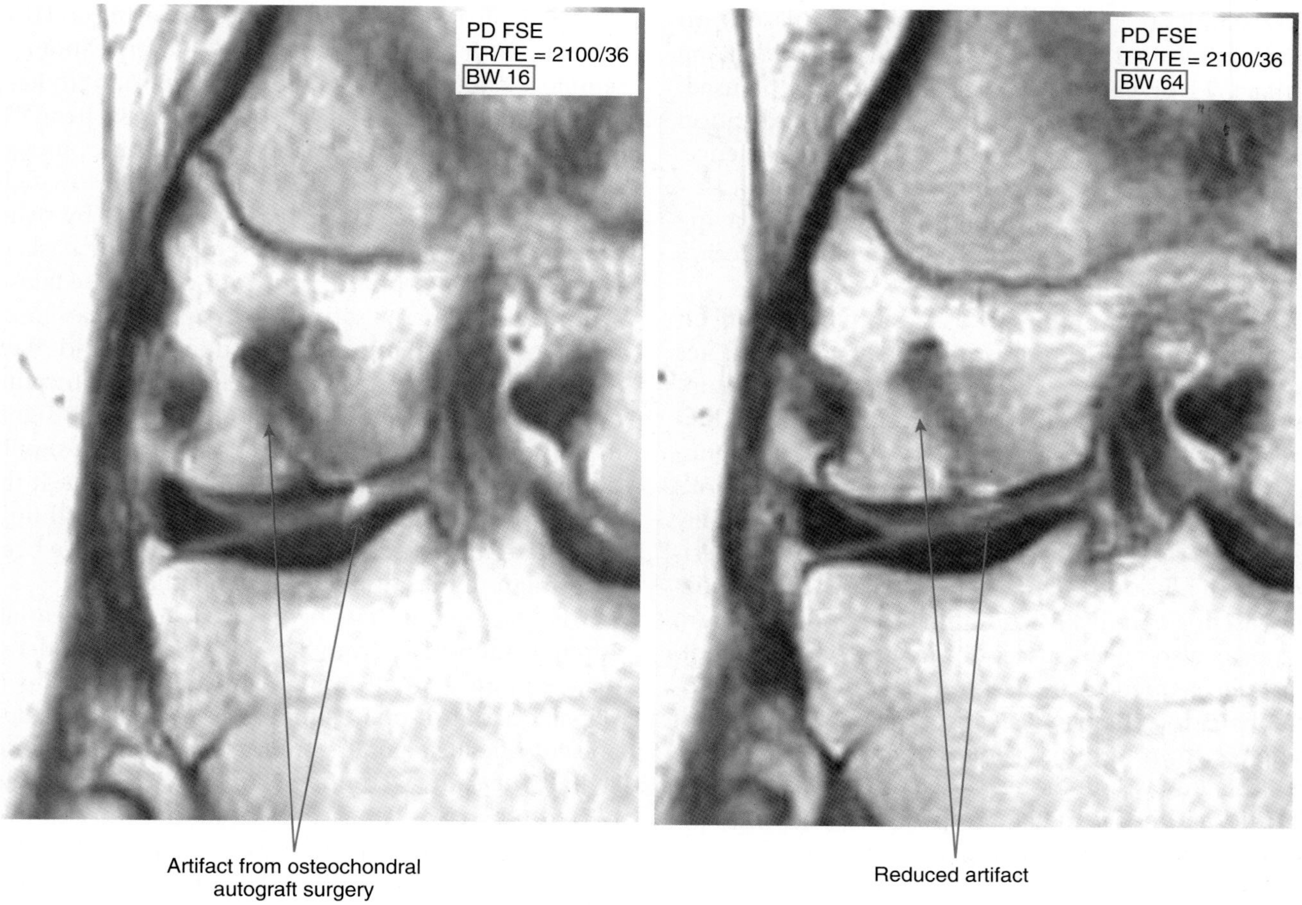
PD FSE
TR/TE = 2100/36
BW 16
PD FSE
TR/TE = 2100/36
BW 64
Artifact from osteochondral autograft surgery
Reduced artifact

Figure 1-33 Effect of alteration of bandwidth (BW). Increasing bandwidth reduces metal artifact. FSE, fast spin-echo; PD, proton density; TE, echo time; TR, time to repetition.

higher field strengths, in which the precession frequency differences between fat and water are more pronounced.

USING ARTIFACTS TO YOUR ADVANTAGE

How to Take Advantage of Magnetic Susceptibility Artifact

Artifacts generally should be avoided, but there are occasions where the radiologist can use them to an advantage, gleaning additional useful pieces of information (see Figs. 1-16 through 1-22). Magnetic susceptibility artifact is especially useful to the bone radiologist! Since gradient-echo imaging sequences are fast and provide the most susceptibility artifact, these are the best sequences to use for this purpose. For postoperative cases of virtually any kind, it is useful to include a gradient-recalled echo sequence to "find the surgery." If time is an issue, the localizer sequence often serves this purpose. Often it is not evident what kind of surgery the patient had. In fact, the patient may not know, and frequently neither does the referring doctor. You will save a lot of time at the workstation and look like Sherlock Holmes to the referring clinician if you can easily see where the surgical fingerprints are.

Similarly, gradient-echo images can be useful to find displaced anchors and sutures within the joint; even if nonmetallic, they usually stand out. It may be useful to include a non–fat-saturated gradient-echo sequence if the history includes acute trauma and if radiographs are not available. Small avulsion fractures can be difficult to see on most sequences, but they stand out against surrounding soft tissues on gradient-recalled echo images because of blooming artifact. T1 or T2*-weighted sequences may be used. Detecting intra-articular bodies is another indication for the addition of a gradient-recalled echo sequence. In this case, T2*-weighted images better depict calcified bodies next to the surrounding joint fluid. Leaving fat suppression off is helpful to differentiate bodies from subsynovial fat.

Foreign bodies in the soft tissues often are difficult to find, but most contain some material that creates susceptibility artifact. In this situation, add fat suppression to remove potentially confusing signal heterogeneity from fat, and use a T1-weighted sequence to avoid fluid signal. The remaining image looks bland, with the artifact standing out against a gray background. The same sequence is useful for detecting small amounts of air, such as in cases of necrotizing fasciitis and disk vacuum phenomenon. Calcium deposits also create susceptibility artifact, and gradient-echo sequences are useful in the absence of radiographs to document any calcification within structures, ranging from tumors (bone, e.g., enchondromas, osteosarcomas; soft tissue, e.g., synovial sarcomas) to calcific tendinosis, to heterotopic bone/myositis ossificans. Hemosderin deposits (e.g., pigmented villonodular synovitis, giant cell tumor of tendon sheath) also bloom on gradient-echo images, but it is best to avoid using fat suppression so that the blood products can be distinguished from surrounding fat (see Box 1-2).

How to Take Advantage of Chemical Shift Artifact

In-phase/out-of-phase imaging uses the slight differences in precession frequencies between fat and water to advantage (Fig. 1-34). Because fat and water protons are spinning at different rates, their vectors become aligned periodically. If imaging data are collected when the protons in fat and water in the same voxel are aligned (in-phase), signal will be additive; if data are collected when protons in fat and water are completely opposite in direction (out-of-phase), their signals will cancel. This effect is seen at multiples of a certain base TE, which varies by field strength. At 1.5 T, the first out-of-phase event occurs at 2.2 msec, followed by in-phase at 4.4 msec, followed by out-of-phase at 6.6 msec, and so on. A fast gradient-echo sequence is used. The effect is strongest at lower TEs, but since the effect continues to repeat, it can also be achieved on 0.3 T scanners, by comparing a TE of 20 msec with a TE of 40 msec. Whatever scanner or sequence parameters are used, it is important to keep all other parameters that are identical apart from TE; optimally, the in-phase and out-of-phase images should be acquired in the same series. On low-field scanners, this effect can be easily achieved by using the Dixon fat-water separation sequence, the basis of which is an in-phase and out-of-phase dataset acquired in the same series. Always perform an internal control—the out-of-phase image should have dark lines at fat/muscle interfaces owing to canceling of signal. This tells you it's working! Also, the signal in monotonous fat or fluid should not change significantly because there is nothing to cancel it out. If the region of interest (ROI) values of cerebrospinal fluid are different on the two phases, there may have been a problem undermining the intended effect.

This technique has been used to differentiate adrenal adenomas from adenocarcinomas. Adenomas contain a small amount of fat, and a drop in signal on out-of-phase images is a clue that fat is present and its signal is subtracting from the water signal. The same technique is used by musculoskeletal radiologists to image the bone marrow. Conveniently, hematopoietic marrow contains about equal parts of fat and water. If a focus of marrow signal is considered suspicious on T2-weighted or STIR images, a drop in signal on out-of-phase images compared with the in-phase images is a sign that some fat is present. Tumors generally exclude or metabolize fat and do not drop significantly in signal. It is rare for tumors to drop in signal more than 20%, with the exception being infiltrative processes such as myeloma, which can preserve small amounts of marrow fat. Therefore, although the technique is useful to provide an additional piece of information, like most things it is not 100% reliable. It should also be recognized that lesions containing all or mostly fat (e.g., lipomas, fatty marrow, some degenerative endplate changes, some hemangiomas) do not drop much or at all in signal.

Special Planes/Positions

In musculoskeletal imaging, it may be advantageous to image the anatomy using "nonstandard" planes, placing the body part in different positions, or exposing the anatomy to stress. For example, to visualize the ulnar collateral ligament of the thumb requires an imaging plane coronal to the thumb; imaging the

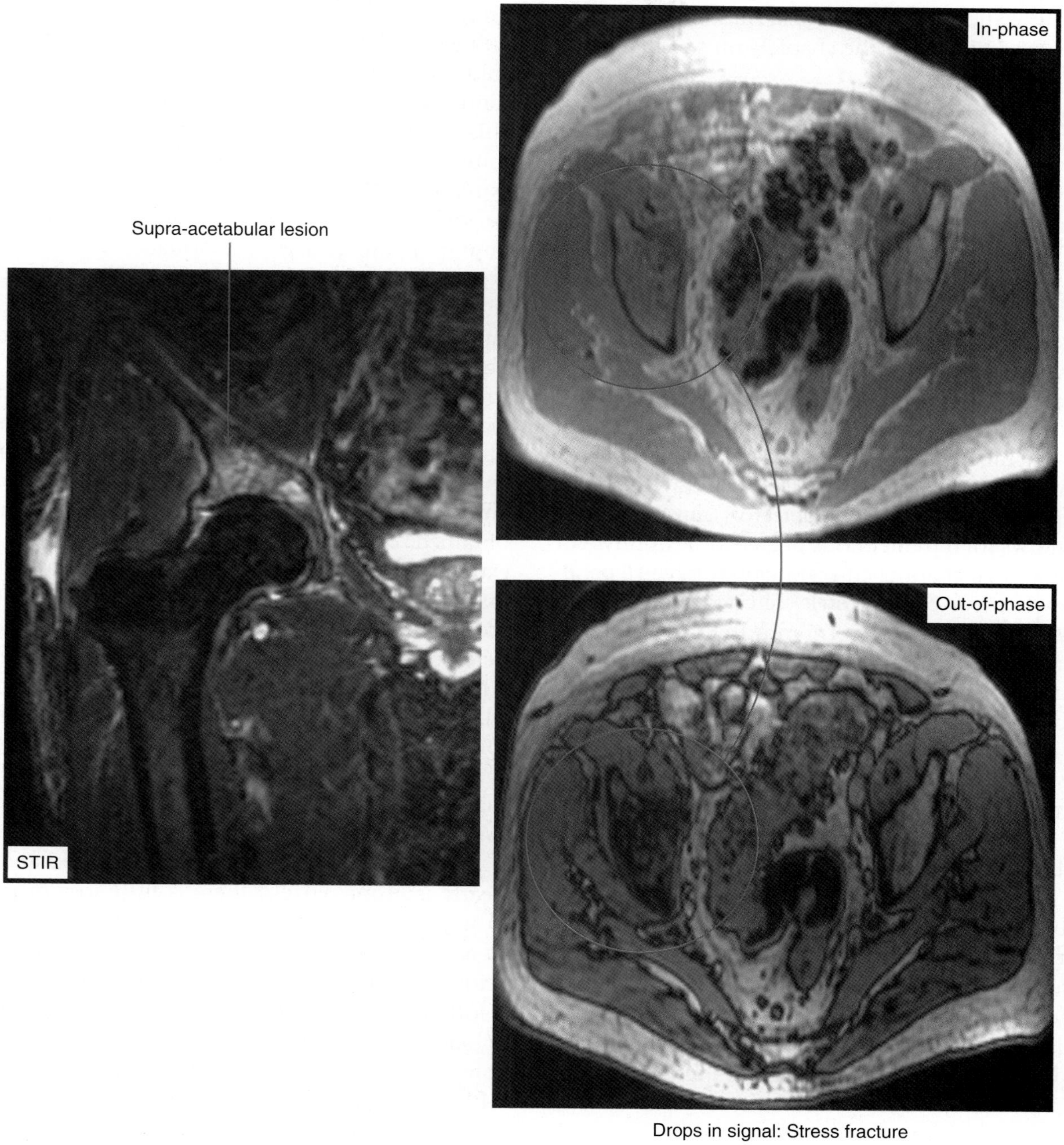
Supra-acetabular lesion
STIR
In-phase
Out-of-phase
Drops in signal: Stress fracture

Figure 1-34 Chemical shift imaging is very useful for evaluation of bone marrow. Acquiring a pair of fast gradient-echo sequences with short TEs catches water and fat protons in-phase (signal adds) and out-of-phase (signal subtracts). Suspected tumor on routine sequences would be expected to replace marrow fat and should not drop in signal significantly, whereas hematopoietic marrow (approximately half fat and half water) drops a great deal as do benign lesions with marrow edema such as fracture.

shoulder in abduction and external rotation (ABER position) can help diagnose labral tears; imaging digits with flexion stress can assist in detection and characterization of pulley lesions. These "special situations" are discussed in the chapters on specific joints.

COMPUTED TOMOGRAPHY

Sample protocols for general indications are available on the accompanying CD.

Basics of Multidetector CT

Unlike conventional single-slice CT scanners, which have a single detector row, multidetector CT (MDCT) uses a stacked array of detector rows. Therefore, multiple slices can be acquired during each rotation of the x-ray tube. In addition, multiple channels transmit information from the detector array, and the alignment of channels and detectors can be altered; this allows for a tremendous degree of flexibility. For example, a 16-channel CT scanner may have 16 parallel rows of 0.75-mm thick detectors sandwiched between 4 and 4 rows of 1.5-mm thick detectors for a total detector complement of 24 rows. However, this machine configuration allows for only 16 simultaneous channels, resulting in two scan modes: 16 × 0.75 mm and 16 × 1.5 mm. The end result enables a wide variety of slice thickness choices. Different machines have different arrangements of detectors and channels, and scanner configurations change rapidly as technical advancements are made. Discussion of such configurations is beyond the scope of this book. However, as in MRI, a working knowledge of basic physical principles of MDCT is all that is needed to achieve high-quality musculoskeletal CT images and reformats.

With the development of multi-channel technology, CT is enjoying a renaissance in musculoskeletal imaging. MDCT scanners are able to achieve slices thin enough to approach isotropic voxels, in which the slice thickness is equal to the pixel dimensions in the transverse plane. Why is this important? Basically, on old scanners the pixel resolution in the axial plane was excellent, but slices were too thick to provide high-quality reformatted images, with resultant stair-step pattern or appearance of low resolution on reconstructed sagittal and coronal images. Voxels looked like columns, not cubes. If slices are acquired thin enough, voxels become cubes, and the data contain the same resolution from whatever perspective it is viewed; the result is a near three-dimensional dataset, with reformatted images in any plane with similar resolution as the axial images.

Speed is another advantage to MDCT. Because a volume of information can be acquired in a single gantry rotation, large areas can be scanned quickly. This is useful, for example, for scanning an entire spine in the setting of trauma, or an entire lower extremity for surgical planning. Motion artifact can be virtually eliminated by rapid scanning, further improving the quality of reformats.

Another benefit of advances in CT is reduction in streak artifact. Previously, this was a significant limitation in interpretation of studies in which metal was present (especially prostheses), or even when full-strength iodinated contrast was present. Artifact would virtually obscure tissue surrounding plates and prostheses. CT arthrography had to be performed with dilute contrast, or a combination of contrast and air. Currently, very high-quality images can be obtained of metal implants, and now MDCT is extremely useful for evaluation of complications associated with prostheses, as well as healing of bone around fixation. This advance essentially has rendered conventional tomography obsolete. Moreover, CT arthrography has made a comeback (see Chapter 2). Full-strength contrast can be used without concern for streak artifact. Similarly, imaging of large patients is improved using MDCT; in large patients or for large joints, the kilovolt peak (kVp) can be increased to improve photon penetration.

Reformats can be performed in any plane, and with nearly isotropic voxels, there is little loss in resolution. One advantage to newer systems is the ability to acquire curved reformats. For example, a coronal reformat of the spine can be plotted off the sagittal reformatted image, curved along the course of the spinal column so that the coronal "straightens" the spine. The reverse can be done in cases of scoliosis, with artificial straightening of the spine in the sagittal plane, simplifying interpretation of abnormalities such as fusion or segmentation anomalies. This also can be used to advantage in evaluation of acutely injured joints. Often joints (e.g., elbow) are scanned in a cast, or the patient simply cannot comfortably straighten the extremity long enough to scan. With MDCT, the axial images are reformatted into the plane of the joint best showing the curvature or deformity, and a curved reformat in that plane can be acquired (Fig. 1-35).

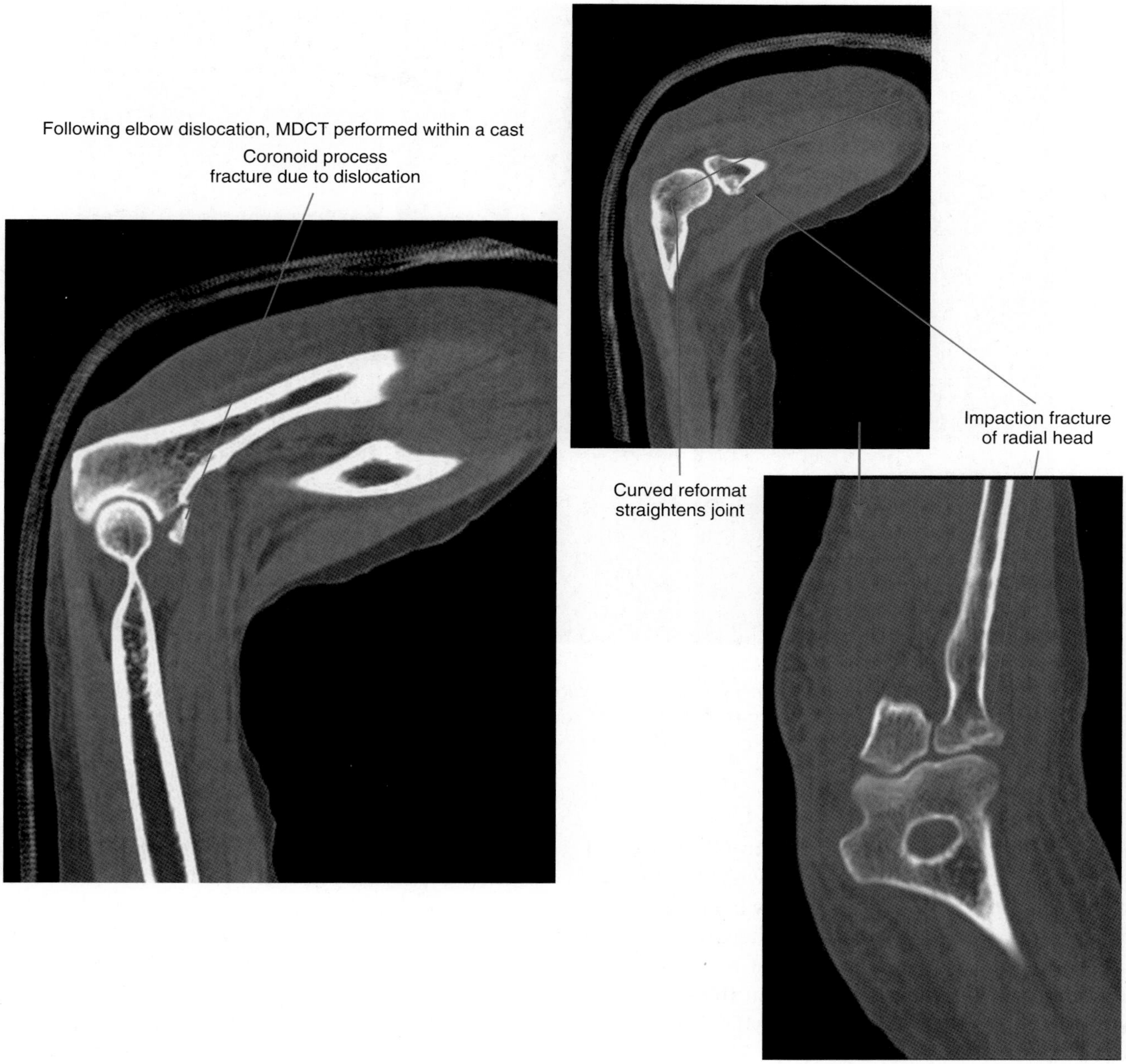
Following elbow dislocation, MDCT performed within a cast
Coronoid process fracture due to dislocation
Impaction fracture of radial head
Curved reformat straightens joint

Figure 1-35 *Capability of acquiring high-quality curved reformats is important in situations, such as imaging of joints in flexion, as well as curved structures, such as in spinal trauma.*

Reconstruction of high quality three-dimensional shaded surface displays may be of benefit in preoperative surgical planning (Fig. 1-36).

Historically, CT has been very useful for answering specific musculoskeletal questions, such as preoperative evaluation of alignment and anatomy, evaluation of intra-articular bodies, bone tumors (for matrix, margins, and cortical breakthrough), and rim calcification for diagnosis of myositis ossificans. MDCT has led to increased use of CT for a variety of indications.

To perform high-quality MDCT of the musculoskeletal system, like MRI, certain physical principles are helpful to know. The basis for high-quality MDCT images (and CT in general) is proper technique. Up to a point, the more photons that pass through the

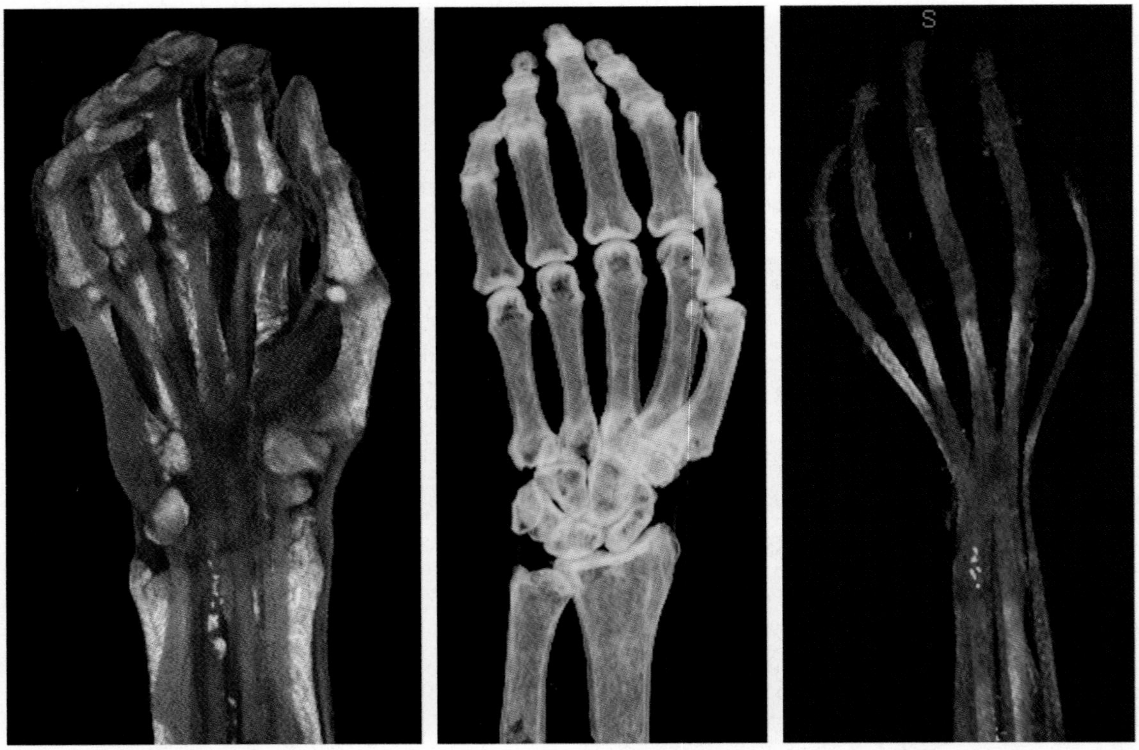
S

Figure 1-36 Application of three-dimensional reconstruction programs and subtraction methods to multidetector CT can provide highly detailed anatomic information useful for surgical planning. (Courtesy of Angela Gopez, MD, Philadelphia, PA.)

patient (photon flux), the better the CT image. Of course, this means a higher dose, which should be taken into consideration, particularly in pediatric and young adult patients. However, when imaging the extremities, radiation exposure is of somewhat less concern. In addition, radiation from the penumbra of the x-ray beam is diminished on MDCT; the radiation is used more efficiently.

Focal Spot

A small focal spot is desired to optimize spatial resolution, but a small focal spot can limit current and lead to excessive tube heating on low-slice MDCT scanners (less than 16-slice). For large patients or body parts or where a wide anatomic coverage is necessary, it may be necessary to use a larger focal spot.

Pitch

Pitch is defined as table motion (per gantry rotation) divided by width scanned (in the Z-axis). Therefore, a pitch of 1 or greater means that there is no overlap of slices; a pitch less than 1 means that there is overlap. Overlap is good for musculoskeletal imaging for a variety of reasons. With MDCT, manufacturers have different definitions of pitch, so don't get confused. Some define pitch based on the width of the beam (roughly equivalent to the width of the active detectors as a group, called "beam pitch"), whereas others define it based on width of a single detector ("detector pitch"). Basically, the definition doesn't matter as much as the concept that the goal is to acquire images with overlap of information.

mAs

mAs is the amount of current used to generate x-rays during scanning. The more mAs, the more photons are sent into the patient. Higher photon flux can result in a better image, so higher scan techniques may be helpful in musculoskeletal imaging. Dose is proportional to mAs, so higher settings increase patient exposure in a linear fashion.

kVp

kVp is the peak energy of the photons being sent into the patient. Higher energy photons pass through more tissue or denser tissue before being absorbed. Therefore, just as in conventional radiography, when imaging obese patients or dense body regions like the pelvis or shoulders, it is helpful to increase the kVp. Keep in mind that patient dose increases 30% to 40% when increasing the exposure from 120 to 140 kVp.

Filter (Reconstruction Algorithm)

To create an image from the data acquired, the computer applies reconstruction algorithms intended to enhance certain features. The detail or bone algorithm sharpens edges, which makes cortices and trabeculae prominent but also accentuates artifact and noise. For peripheral musculoskeletal imaging, the detail algorithm makes the image more pleasing, but it can reduce the quality of the image if there is high soft tissue density, metal, or high-density contrast. In these situations, a "standard" or "soft tissue" algorithm is recommended.

Optimizing image quality in musculoskeletal MDCT is found in Figures 1-37 through 1-48.

For musculoskeletal CT imaging, high resolution is key, and acquisition of isotropic voxels is essential to reformat high-quality images in any plane. Therefore, use of the thinnest slices possible is typically recommended for joint imaging. However, body thickness and dose are considerations. For large body parts such as the hip and shoulder, the photon flux generally needs to be increased (by increasing kV and mAs) to penetrate the tissues, and slice thickness generally needs to be increased. Decreasing pitch so that there is overlap of slices (e.g., pitch less than 1) also increases photon flux. These are also the basic principles in imaging metal: A higher photon flux provides better image quality around the plate or prosthesis, with decreased streak artifact. This is less of a consideration with MDCT, but a slight incremental benefit can still be achieved by optimizing parameters. This is particularly true when imaging stainless-steel or cobalt-chrome components, which create significantly more streak artifact than titanium. Dose is especially a consideration for imaging the more central joints, and thought should be given to decreasing photon flux (and thereby dose) in situations in which additional diagnostic benefit of higher resolution is marginal.

Angulation

Imaging joints at an angle can also improve the quality of reformatted images. Even when using thin axial sections, only a few slices may pass through small joints, like those in the hands, limiting quality of reformats. By angling joints in the scanner whenever possible, more slices pass through the articular

Text continued on page 47

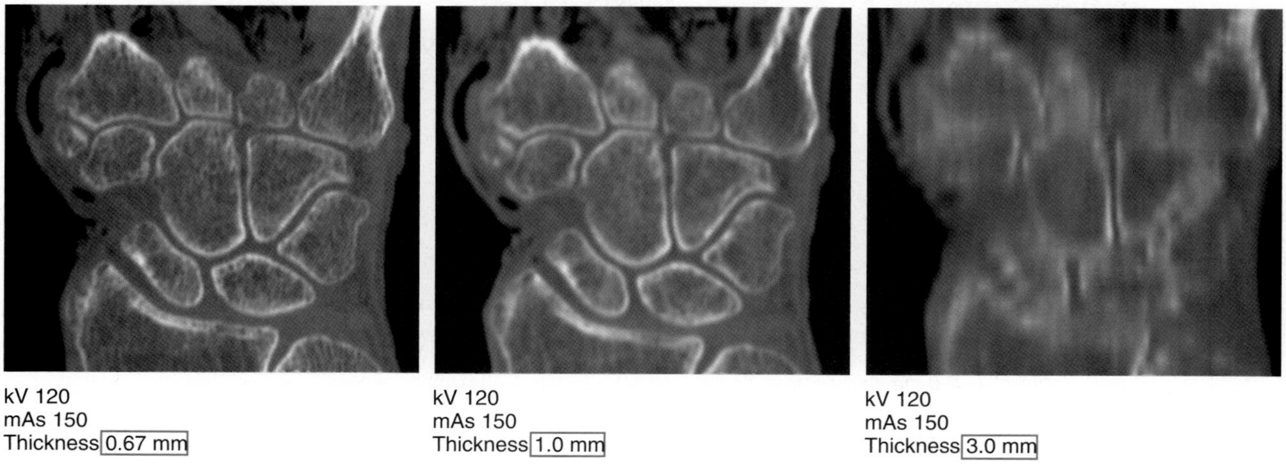
kV 120
mAs 150
Thickness 0.67 mm
kV 120
mAs 150
Thickness 1.0 mm
kV 120
mAs 150
Thickness 3.0 mm

Figure 1-37 Small parts: effect of changing slice thickness. Thinner slice acquisition results in improved detail. With large body parts such as the hip, thin slices can result in increased noise unless other parameters such as kV are increased.

SECTION I

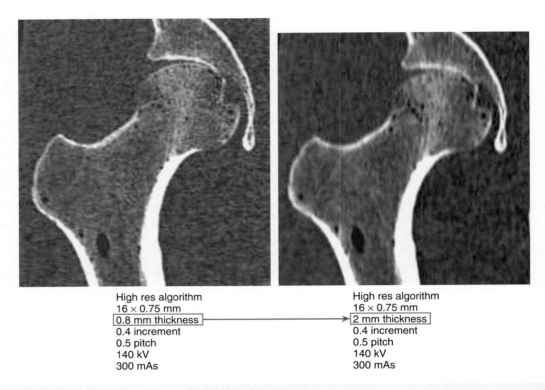

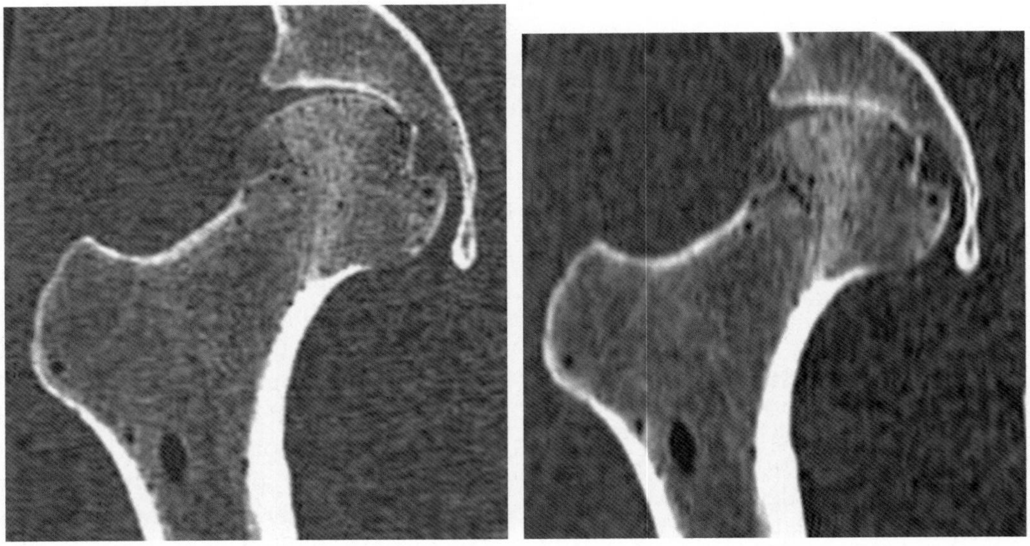
High res algorithm
16 × 0.75 mm
0.8 mm thickness
0.4 increment
0.5 pitch
140 kV
300 mAs
High res algorithm
16 × 0.75 mm
2 mm thickness
0.4 increment
0.5 pitch
140 kV
300 mAs

Figure 1-38 **Effect of increasing slice thickness.** Note sharper image with thinner slices. However, if the body part is large, noise may degrade the image when using thinner slices unless other parameters (kV, mAs) are altered to increase photon flux.

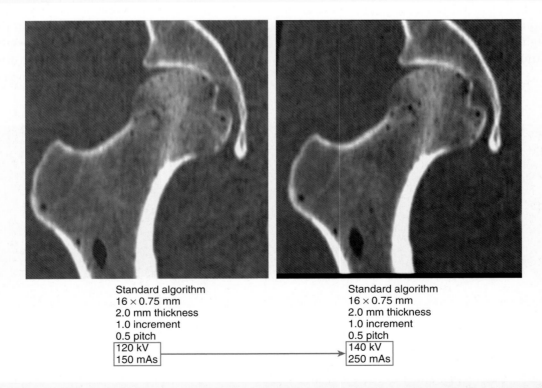

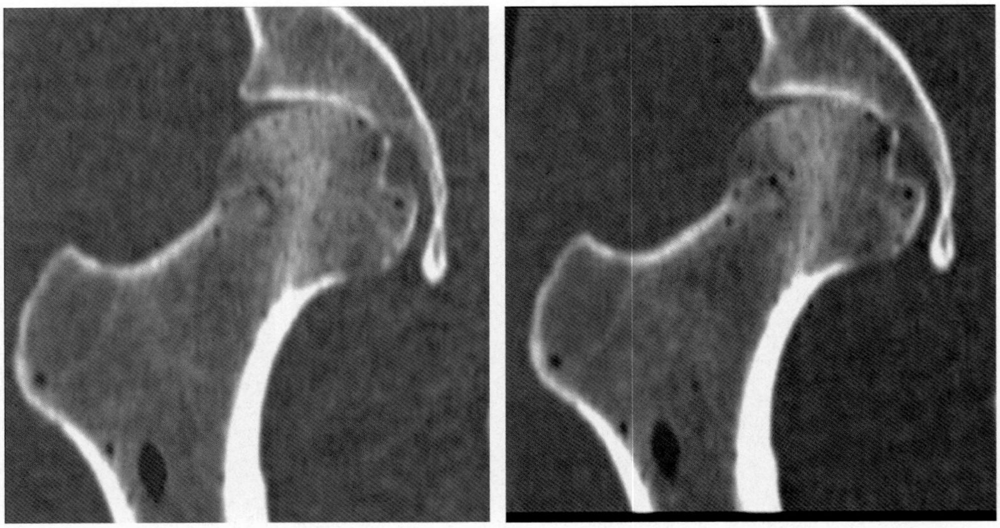
Standard algorithm
16 × 0.75 mm
2.0 mm thickness
1.0 increment
0.5 pitch
120 kV
150 mAs
Standard algorithm
16 × 0.75 mm
2.0 mm thickness
1.0 increment
0.5 pitch
140 kV
250 mAs

Figure 1-39 Increasing mAs and kV increases photon flux through the patient and improves image quality (Note lower noise around the hip). Dose is increased, however.

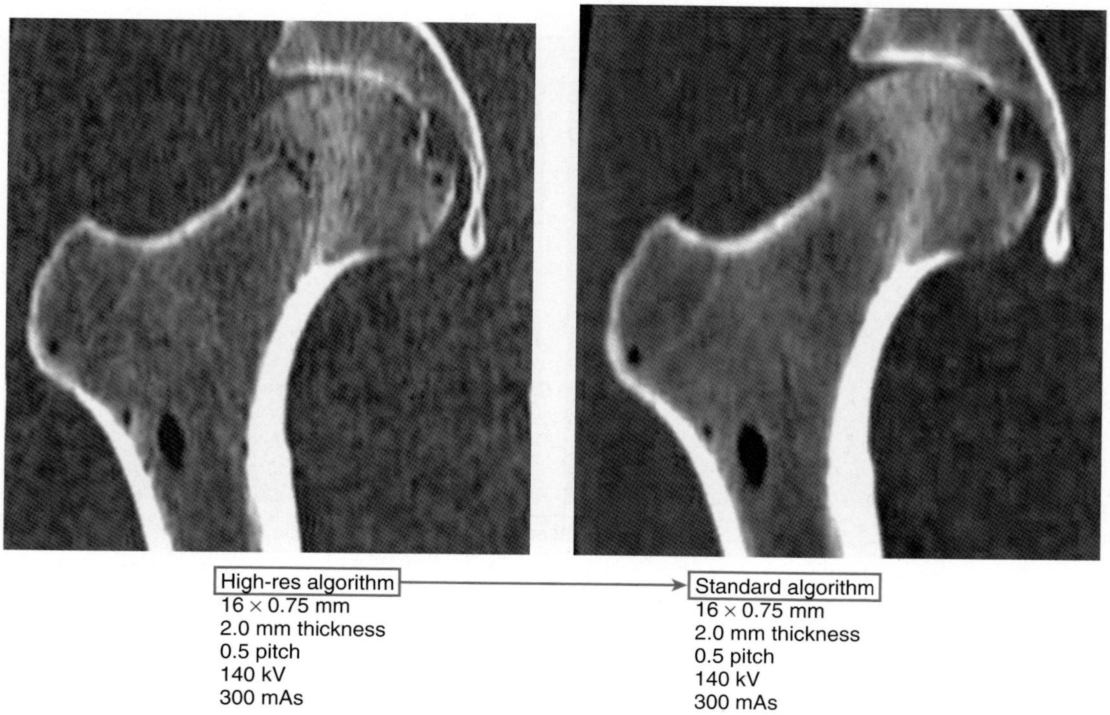
High-res algorithm
16 × 0.75 mm
2.0 mm thickness
0.5 pitch
140 kV
300 mAs
Standard algorithm
16 × 0.75 mm
2.0 mm thickness
0.5 pitch
140 kV
300 mAs

Figure 1-40 Effect of change in reconstruction algorithm. The detail ("high res") filter sharpens the image but can accentuate artifact. Therefore, in the presence of metal use of the detail filter can lower image quality.

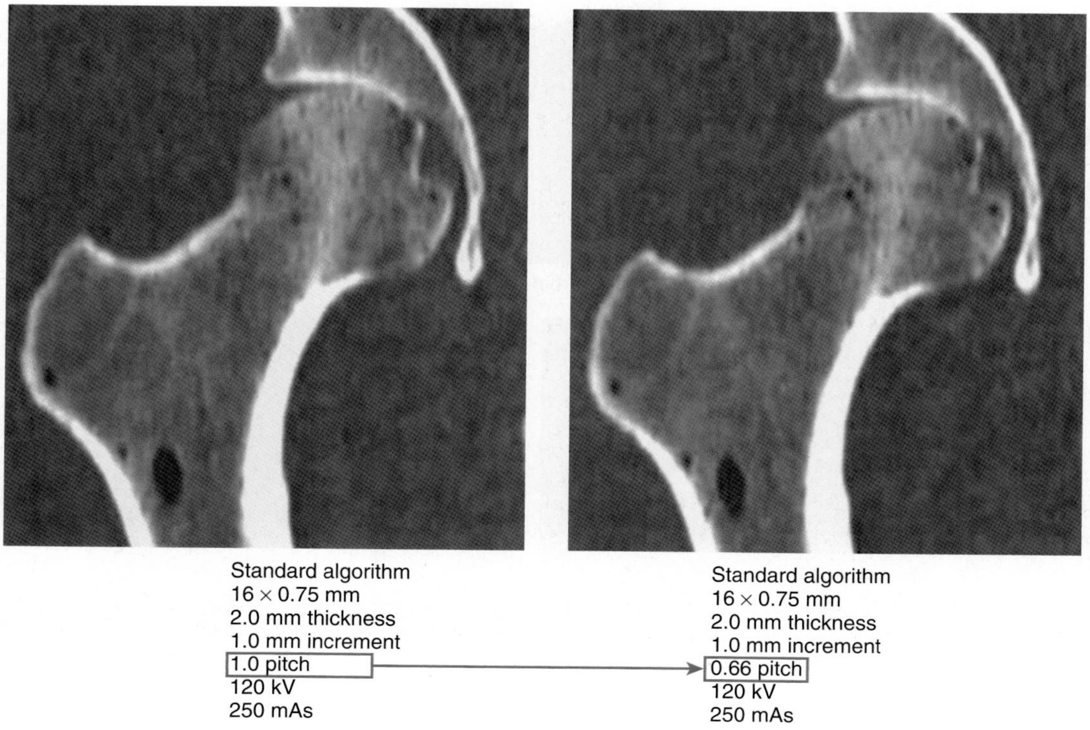
Standard algorithm
16 × 0.75 mm
2.0 mm thickness
1.0 mm increment
1.0 pitch
120 kV
250 mAs
Standard algorithm
16 × 0.75 mm
2.0 mm thickness
1.0 mm increment
0.66 pitch
120 kV
250 mAs

Figure 1-41 Effect of decreased pitch. A pitch less than 1 typically means that there is overlap of slices, resulting in higher image quality.

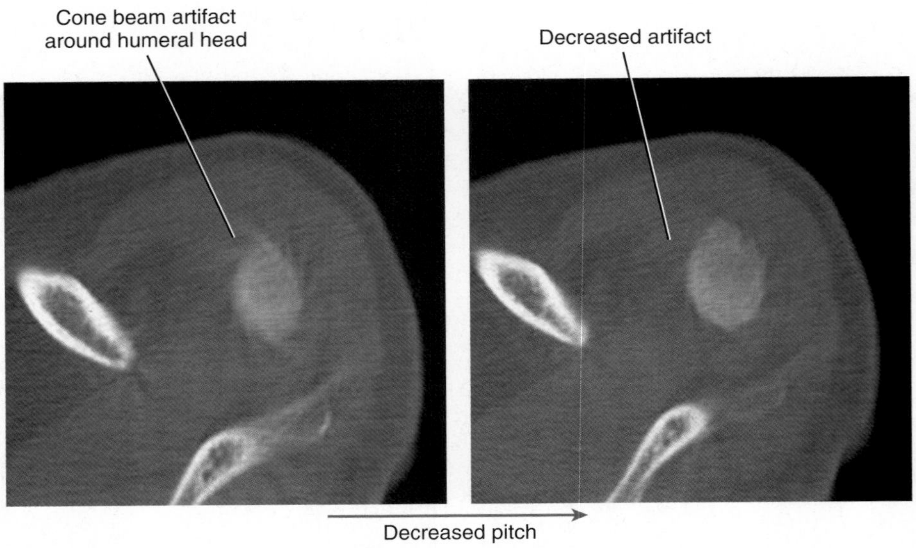
Cone beam artifact
around humeral head
Decreased artifact
Decreased pitch

Figure 1-42 Cone beam artifact can be seen on multidetector CT images, especially when high pitch is used.

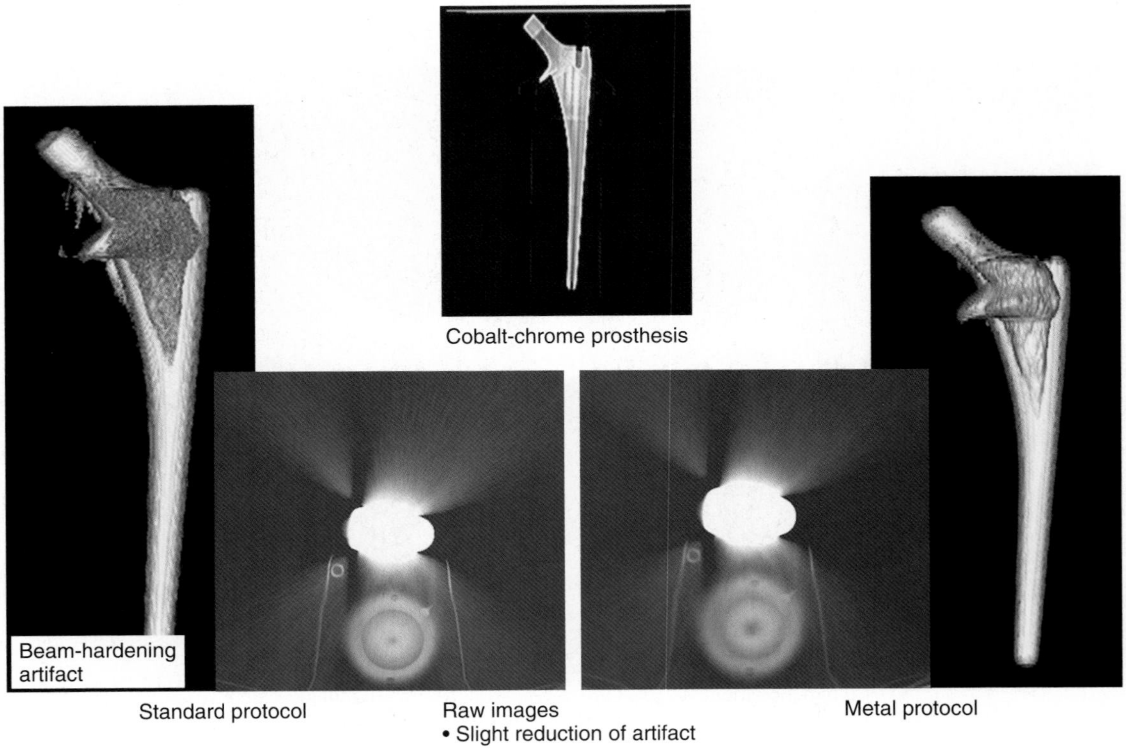
Cobalt-chrome prosthesis
Beam-hardening
artifact
Standard protocol
Raw images
• Slight reduction of artifact
Metal protocol

Figure 1-43 **Cobalt-chrome prosthesis.** This material creates significant streak ("beam-hardening") artifact. Use of multidetector CT (MDCT), even with a standard protocol, has markedly reduced this effect, which previously rendered CT ineffective for imaging prostheses. Even with MDCT, an incremental benefit can be seen using a metal protocol.

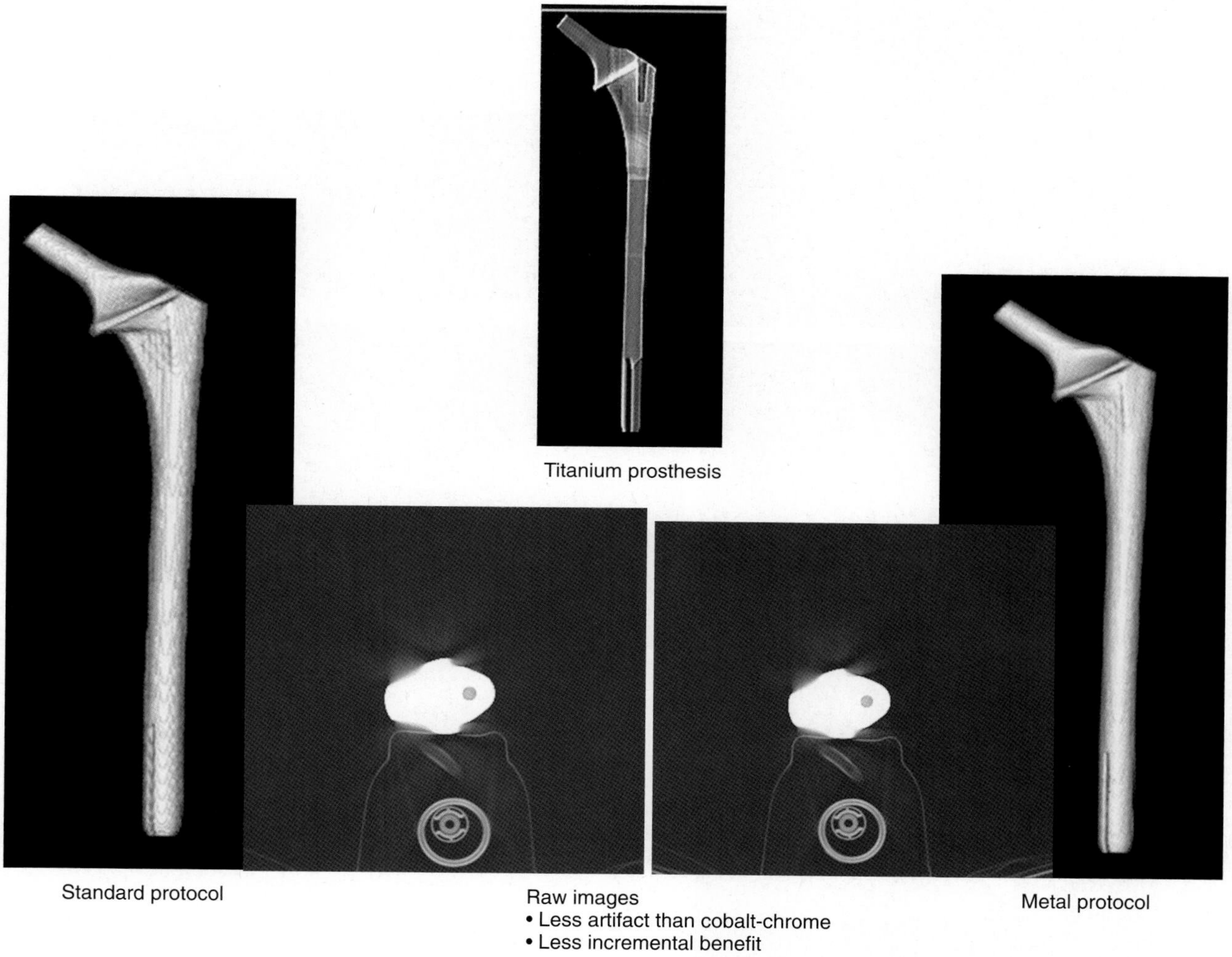
Titanium prosthesis
Standard protocol
Raw images
• Less artifact than cobalt-chrome
• Less incremental benefit
Metal protocol

Figure 1-44 Titanium prosthesis. This material creates less artifact than cobalt-chrome. The incremental benefit of using a metal protocol therefore is smaller and may not be needed if reduction of radiation dose is a consideration.

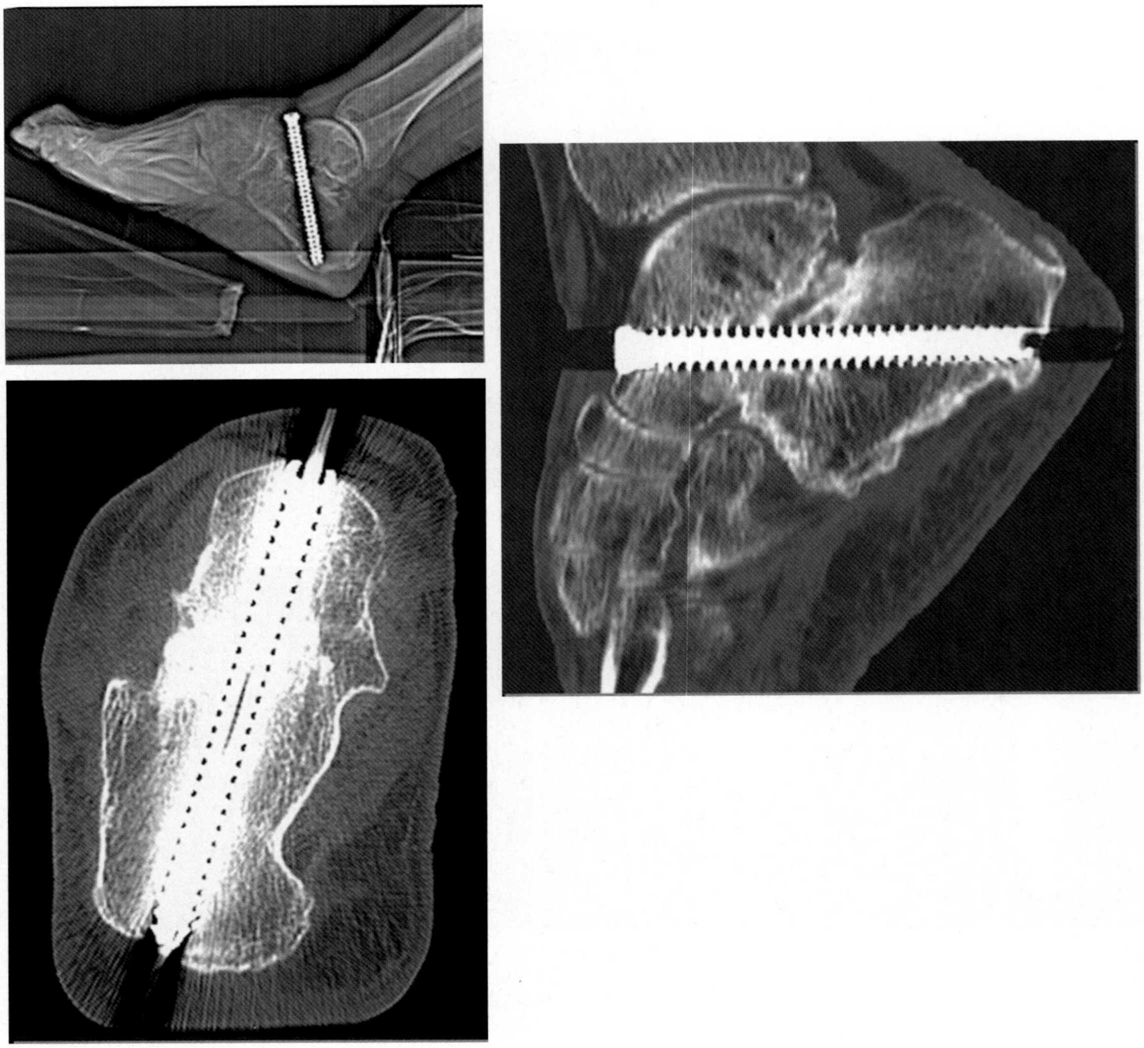

Figure 1-45 If possible, orienting metal implants along the x-ray beam results in an improvement in beam-hardening artifact. (Courtesy of Catherine Roberts MD, Mayo, Scottsdale, AZ.)

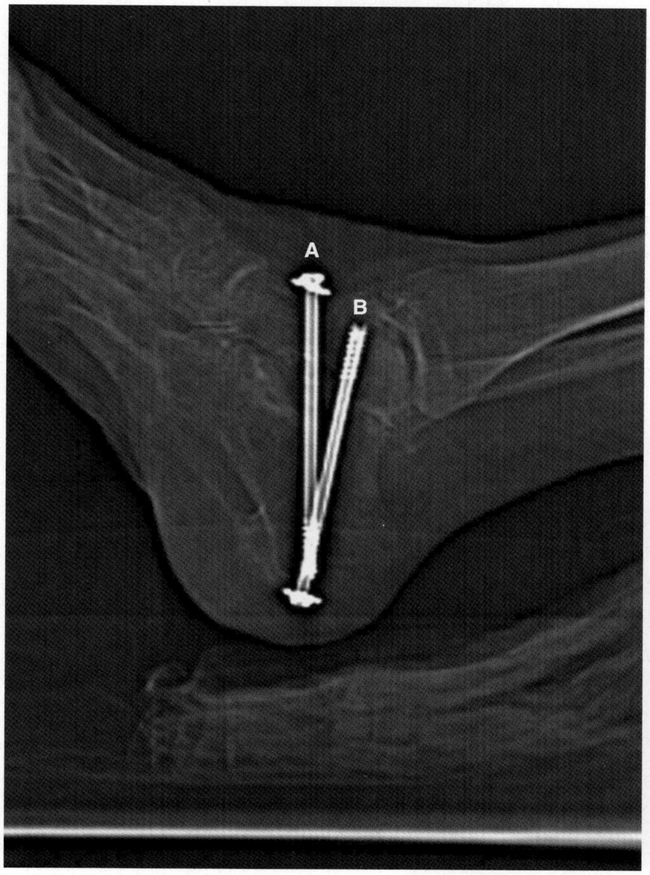
A
B

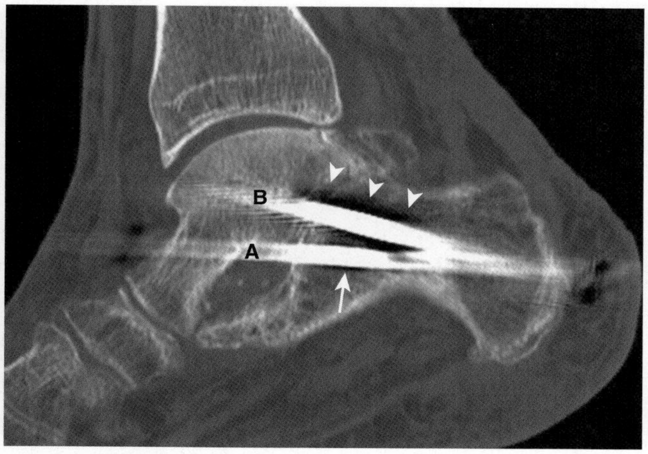
B
A

Figure 1-46 Orienting metal implants oblique to the x-ray beam results in accentuation of beam-hardening artifact (screw A: in line with beam; screw B: off-line). (Courtesy of Catherine Roberts, MD, Mayo, Scottsdale, AZ.)

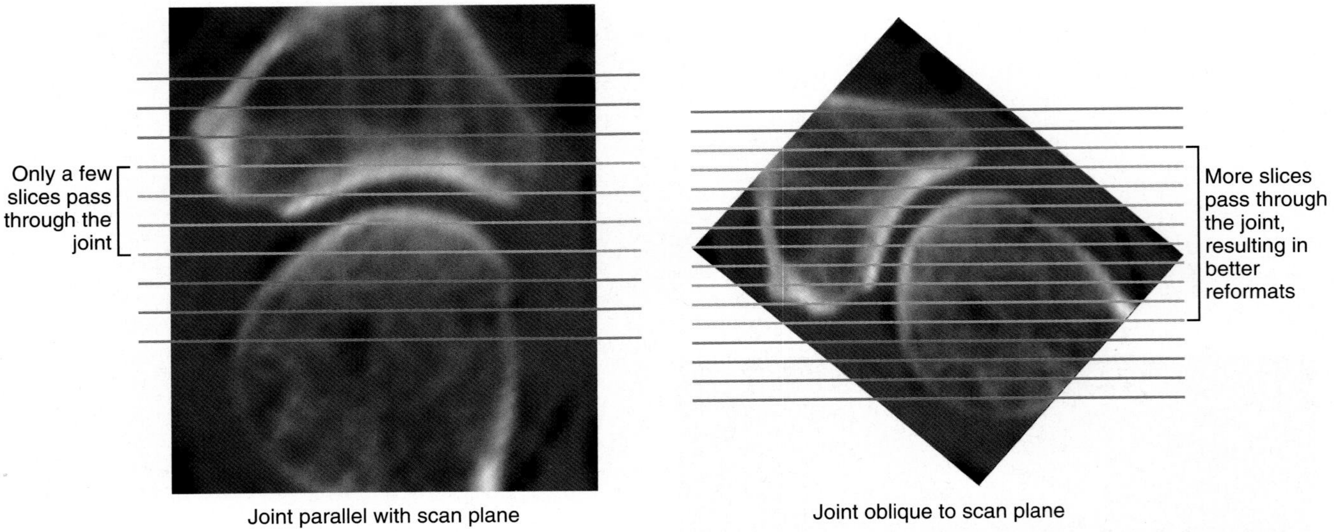
Only a few slices pass through the joint
More slices pass through the joint, resulting in better reformats
Joint parallel with scan plane
Joint oblique to scan plane

Figure 1-47 Principle of obliquity. If source images are acquired oblique to a joint, more slices cut through the joint, resulting in improvement in reformatted images. This effect is greater when thicker cuts are used or when the joint is smaller. With modern multidetector CT scanners, very thin slices are routinely acquired, minimizing the need for such pre-exam planning and creative positioning.

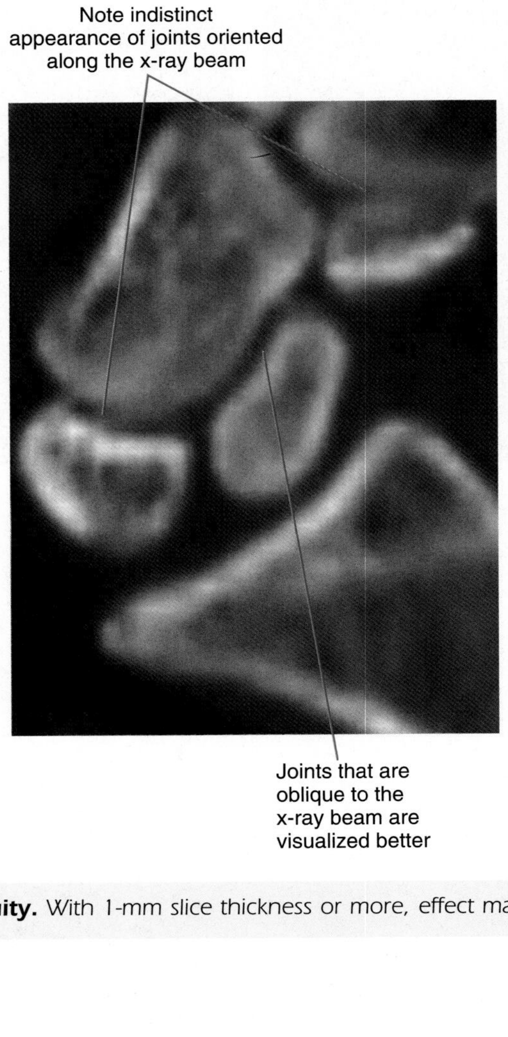
Note indistinct appearance of joints oriented along the x-ray beam
Joints that are oblique to the x-ray beam are visualized better

Figure 1-48 Principle of obliquity. With 1-mm slice thickness or more, effect may be observed in smaller joints.

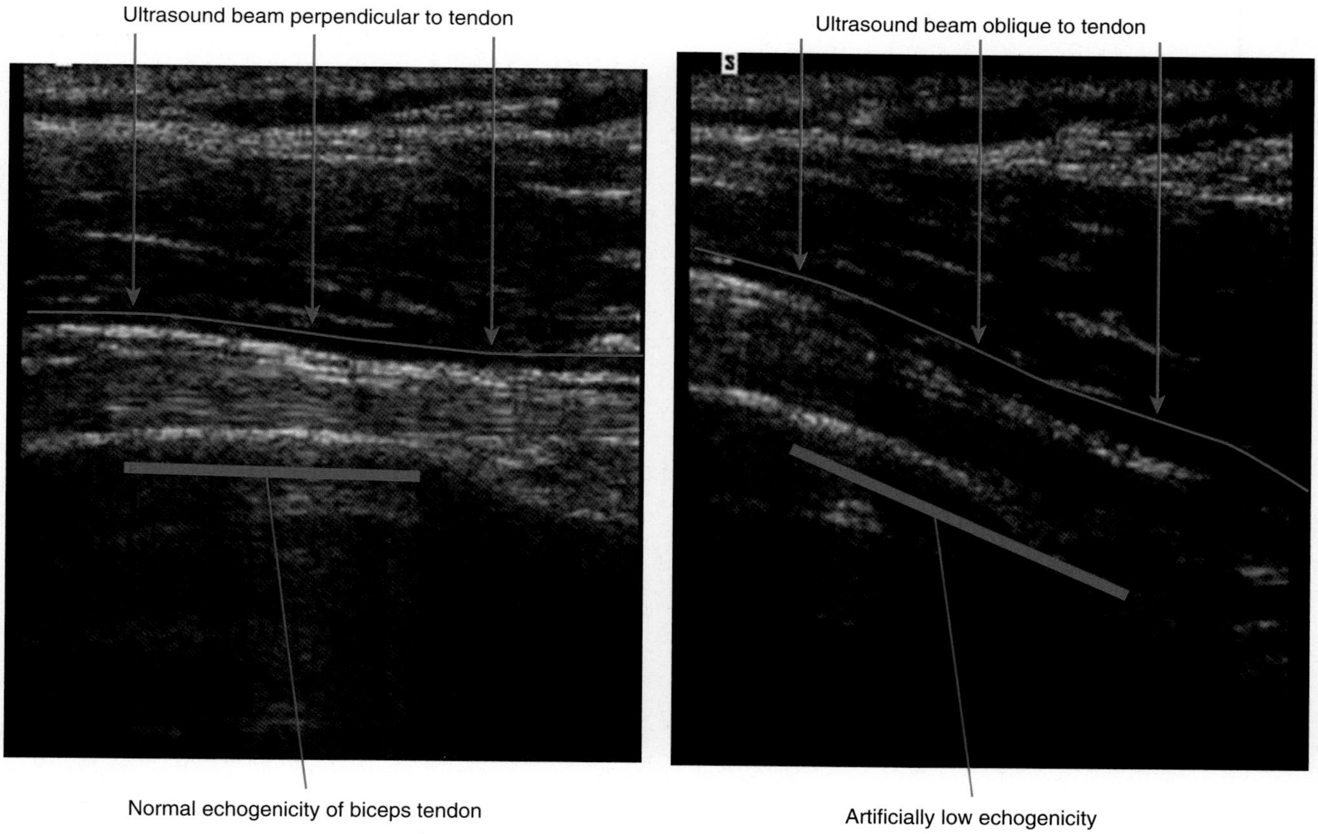
Ultrasound beam perpendicular to tendon
Ultrasound beam oblique to tendon
S
Normal echogenicity of biceps tendon
Artificially low echogenicity

Figure 1-49 Anisotropy depicted on an ultrasound study of the biceps long head tendon at the shoulder. When the ultrasound beam is obliqued, one can see artifactual low echogenicity within the tendon, simulating pathology.

surfaces, providing more data for reformatting. In cases in which metal is present, if the component (i.e., screw) can be aligned with the x-ray beam, streak artifact in the adjacent tissues is reduced.

MUSCULOSKELETAL ULTRASOUND

The musculoskeletal ultrasound examination depends on the experience and skill of the examiner as well as the quality of the equipment. There are also several key technical considerations. The higher the frequency of the ultrasound probe, the better the resolution. Generally, for musculoskeletal ultrasound, the frequency should be at least 7.5 MHz to yield diagnostic quality images. A linear array should be used to minimize anisotropy. Anisotropy occurs when imaging specular reflectors such as tendon fibers (Fig. 1-49); if the ultrasound beam is not perpendicular to a specular reflector, then no echo is produced. The solution to anisotropy is to manipulate the ultrasound probe to keep the probe face parallel with the structure of interest. Other important considerations include minimizing the depth of the image to include only the region of interest, placing the focal zone(s) at the correct location, and, when available, using technical advances such as harmonic imaging, compound imaging, and extended field of view.

SECTION II

PROCEDURES

Chapter 2

ARTHROGRAPHY AND JOINT INJECTION AND ASPIRATION: Principles and Techniques

CHAPTER OUTLINE

Joint injection/aspiration is a commonly performed procedure in many radiology practices, but in some practices it is uncommon and radiologists have variable experience. This chapter outlines simplified techniques for performing these procedures as well as different approaches to joints that have been described.

GENERAL TECHNIQUES

Conventional Arthrography

Conventional arthrography involves the percutaneous injection of contrast material into a joint, followed by a series of radiographs with specific views, depending on the joint being imaged. As a diagnostic technique, conventional arthrography has been replaced by other imaging modalities in nearly all cases. Conventional athrography is rarely performed today; however, it is essential for the practicing radiologist to be familiar with the techniques used because the injection methods can be applied to any advanced form of arthrographic imaging. In patients with severe claustrophobia and in centers without CT or MRI technology, it may be necessary to use conventional arthrography. Many textbooks have addressed the nuances of the art of arthrography, and these provide a useful reference guide if one of these procedures needs to be performed.

The techniques used in conventional arthrography can also be applied to joint aspiration. For joint aspiration, fluoroscopy, ultrasound, or CT guidance can be used. However, fluoroscopy is used most commonly because of its versatility, relatively low cost, and ease of use.

For aspiration of suspected septic arthritis, an 18-gauge needle or larger is recommended for joint access, since infected joint fluid usually has a higher viscosity compared with that of regular joint fluid. When performing a joint aspiration, it is essential to inject a small volume of iodinated contrast material to verify the intra-articular location of the needle tip and to assess any potential abnormal communications of the joint space. If aspiration of a suspected septic joint yields no fluid, it may be useful to instill sterile saline into the joint, followed by aspiration, thereafter sending any aspirated material for culture. When infection is suspected, it is best to avoid the initial intra-articular administration of iodinated contrast material, which has bacteriostatic properties.

CT Arthrography

CT arthrography (CTA) is useful for demonstration of cartilaginous and osseous intra-articular bodies, cartilage defects, fracture fragments, synovial abnormalities, and ligamentous disruption (Figs. 2-1 through 2-7). CTA is usually reserved for patients with contraindications to MRI, but is being performed more commonly recently owing to improved scanner technology that provides isotropic volumetric data.

The most common contraindications to MRI are patients with claustrophobia, patients with implanted pacemaker/defibrillator devices, and patients with any other internal metallic objects that specifically exclude the possibility of MRI because of their composition or location.

CTA involves the intra-articular injection of iodinated contrast material typically followed by axial CT scanning. With multidetector CT technology, very thin sections allow for acquisition of volumetric data, thereby allowing reconstructions to be performed in any plane without loss of resolution. The newer-generation multidetector CT scanners generate a higher photon flux, thus decreasing the streak artifact that often limited CTA on older scanners. Therefore, 300 mg/mL nonionic iodinated contrast can be used without the need for intra-articular air injection when a multidetector scanner is used and excellent quality images can be acquired. With older-generation CT scanners, it is prudent to dilute contrast (typically 50:50) with sterile saline or to use a less concen-

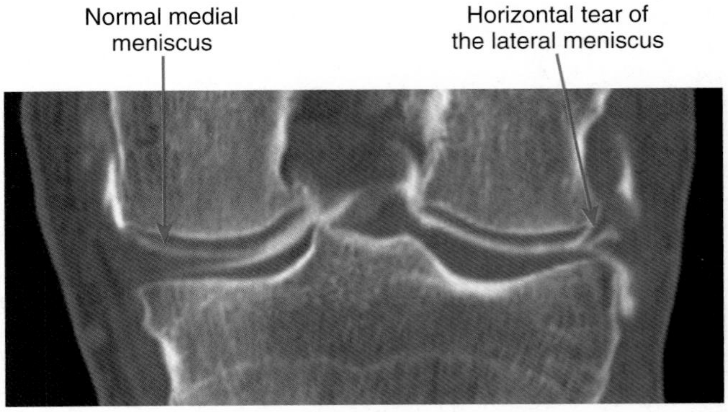
Normal medial meniscus
Horizontal tear of the lateral meniscus

Figure 2-1 CT arthrogram of the knee showing a meniscal tear.

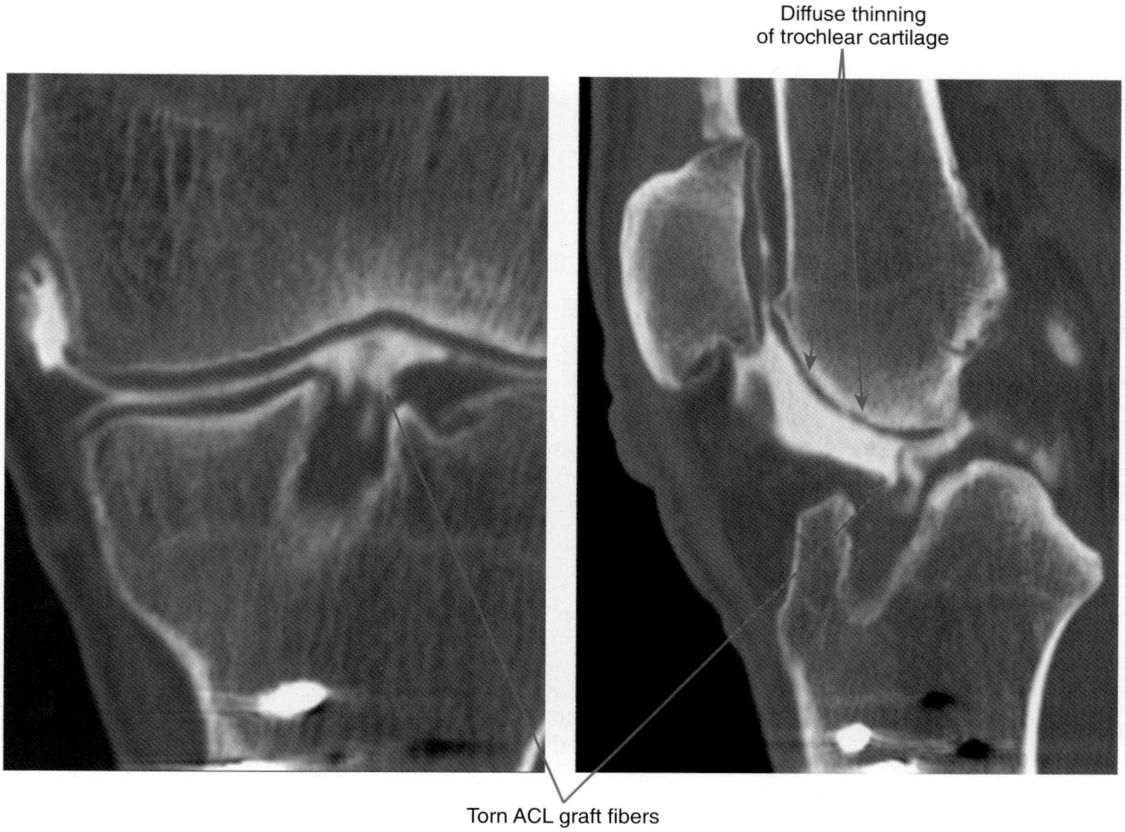
Diffuse thinning
of trochlear cartilage
Torn ACL graft fibers

Figure 2-2 *CT arthrogram of the knee showing tear of the anterior cruciate ligament (ACL) graft and trochlear cartilage erosion.*

trated iodinated contrast preparation to avoid streak artifact. Many authors in the past have advocated injection of variable amounts of air as a negative contrast agent. This is useful to distend the joint without creating significant artifact, and the air can be moved about the joint by putting the patient in different positions. Some authors "coat" the synovium with only a few milliliters of contrast, filling the rest of the joint with air. These techniques have fallen by the wayside with the advent of multidetector CT technology.

The techniques used for accessing the joint are the same as those used for conventional arthrography and MR arthrography (MRA). Contraindications to CTA include patients with a history of severe contrast allergy and pregnant women. Because the spatial resolution that can be achieved with CTA is high, some authors feel that CTA is excellent for the detection of subtle cartilage surface lesions. CTA has been studied in the evaluation of the postoperative knee, with visualization of meniscal re-tears indicated by contrast entering the meniscal substance. CTA is also very useful in patients who have metallic orthopedic hardware in the region of interest. Using high mAs techniques, beam-hardening artifact from implanted metal hardware can be almost completely eliminated. Such patients would typically not be candidates for MRA owing to the distortion of MR images secondary to metallic susceptibility artifact. In the near future, multidetector CTA is likely to be increasingly used for imaging postoperative joints.

MR Arthrography

Direct MR Arthrography

Conventional MRI has enjoyed great success in imaging the musculoskeletal system and has deservedly become the "gold-standard" imaging technique for suspected internal derangement of joints. There

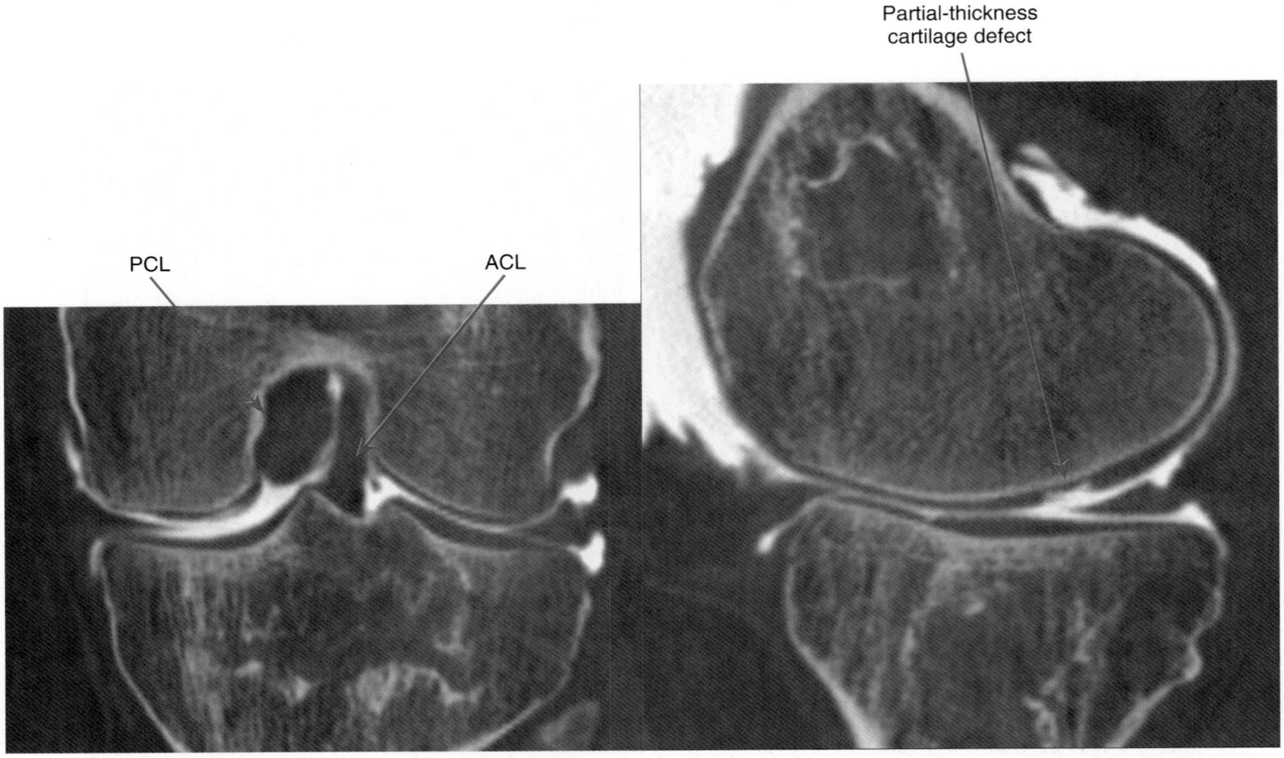
Partial-thickness
cartilage defect
PCL
ACL

Figure 2-3 CT arthrography using multidetector CT yields high resolution and can visualize small cartilage defects; however, unlike MRI it is difficult to see the cartilage unless contrast is directly adjacent. Therefore, the joint must be adequately filled with contrast. Note sharp calcification within the medullary cavity representing chronic bone infarctions. ACL, anterior cruciate ligament; PCL, posterior cruciate ligament.

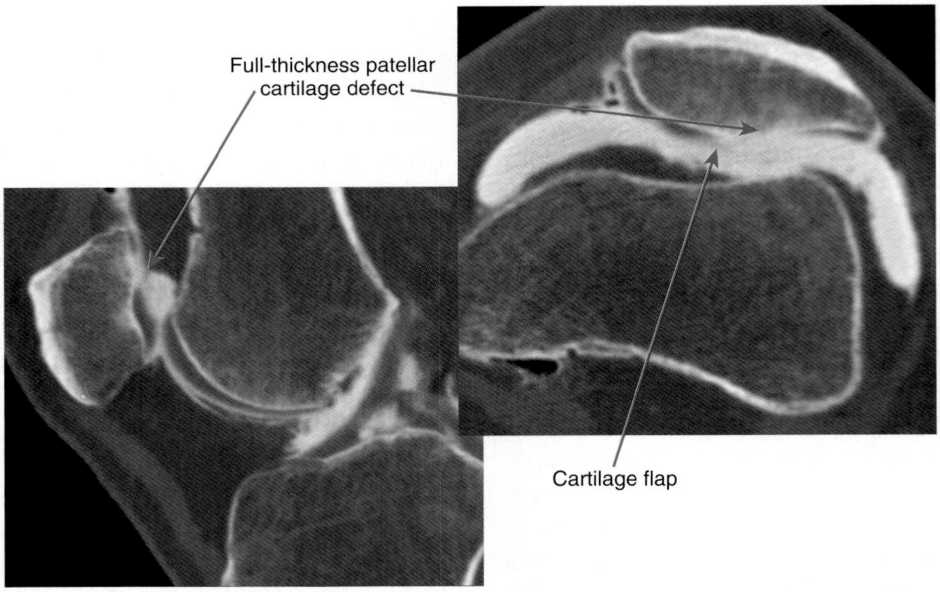
Full-thickness patellar
cartilage defect
Cartilage flap

Figure 2-4 In CT arthrography, a full-thickness cartilage defect results in blending of cortical and intra-articular contrast density.

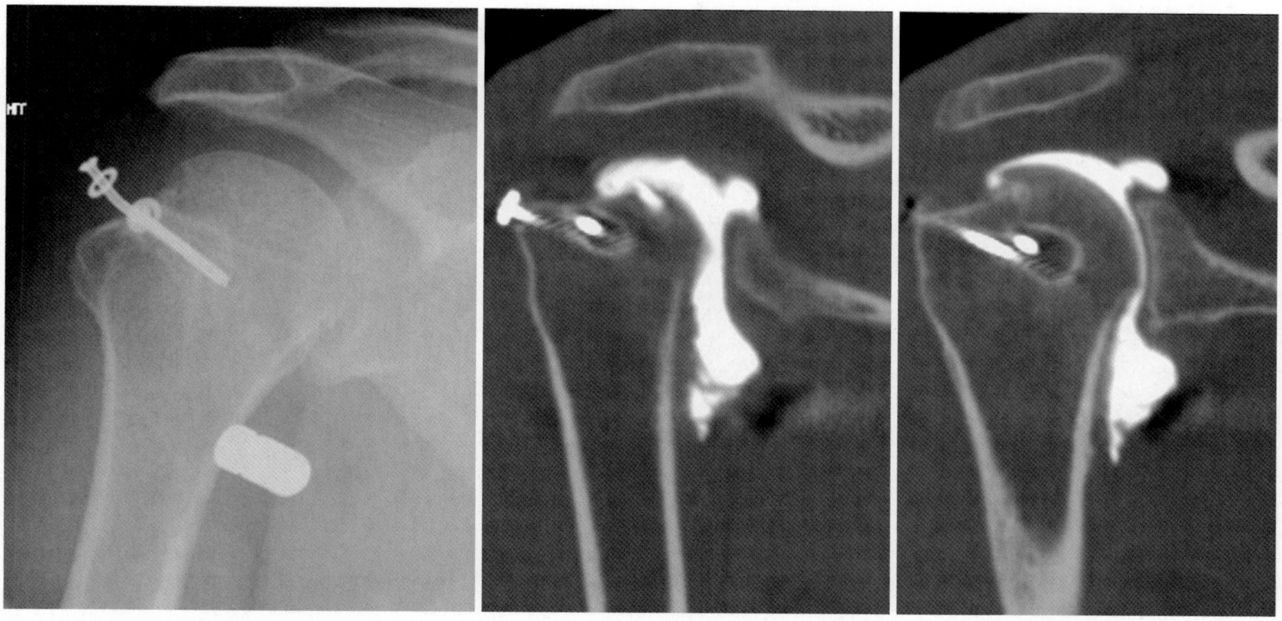

RT

Figure 2-5 CT arthrography shows excellent detail despite the presence of metal. In this case, the screws appeared loose radiographically, but CT arthrography shows that the rotator cuff repair remains water-tight.

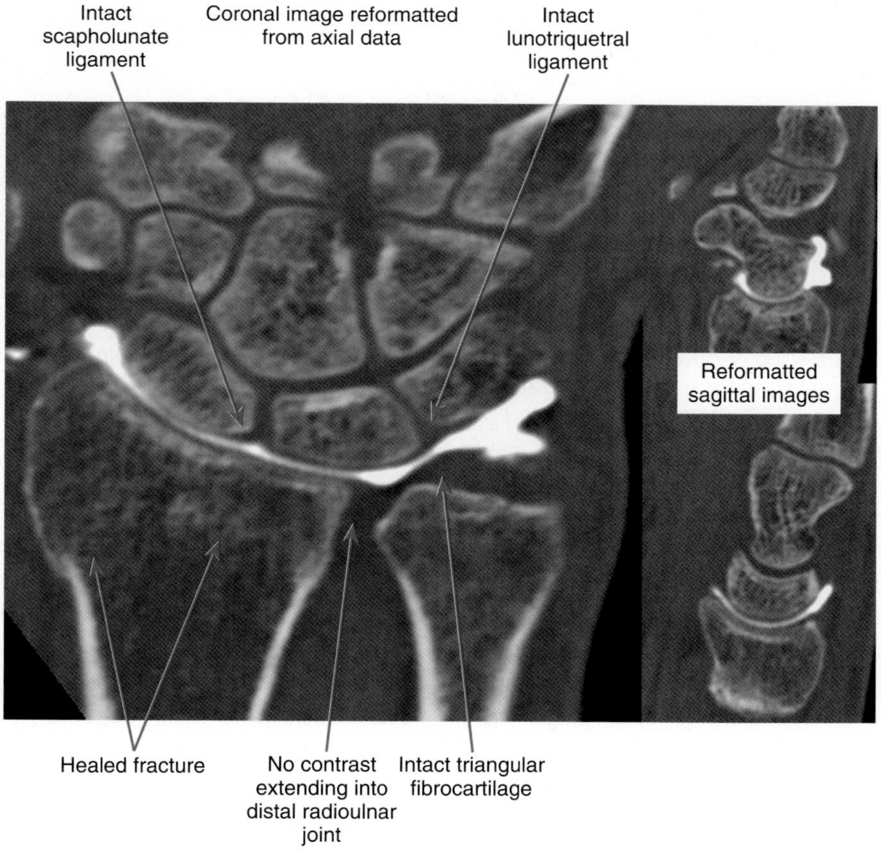

Intact scapholunate ligament
Coronal image reformatted from axial data
Intact lunotriquetral ligament
Reformatted sagittal images
Healed fracture
No contrast extending into distal radioulnar joint
Intact triangular fibrocartilage

Figure 2-6 With the advent of multidetector CT, CT arthrography has become more popular. Acquisition of thin slices yields isotropic voxels, which can be reformatted in any plane without loss of resolution.

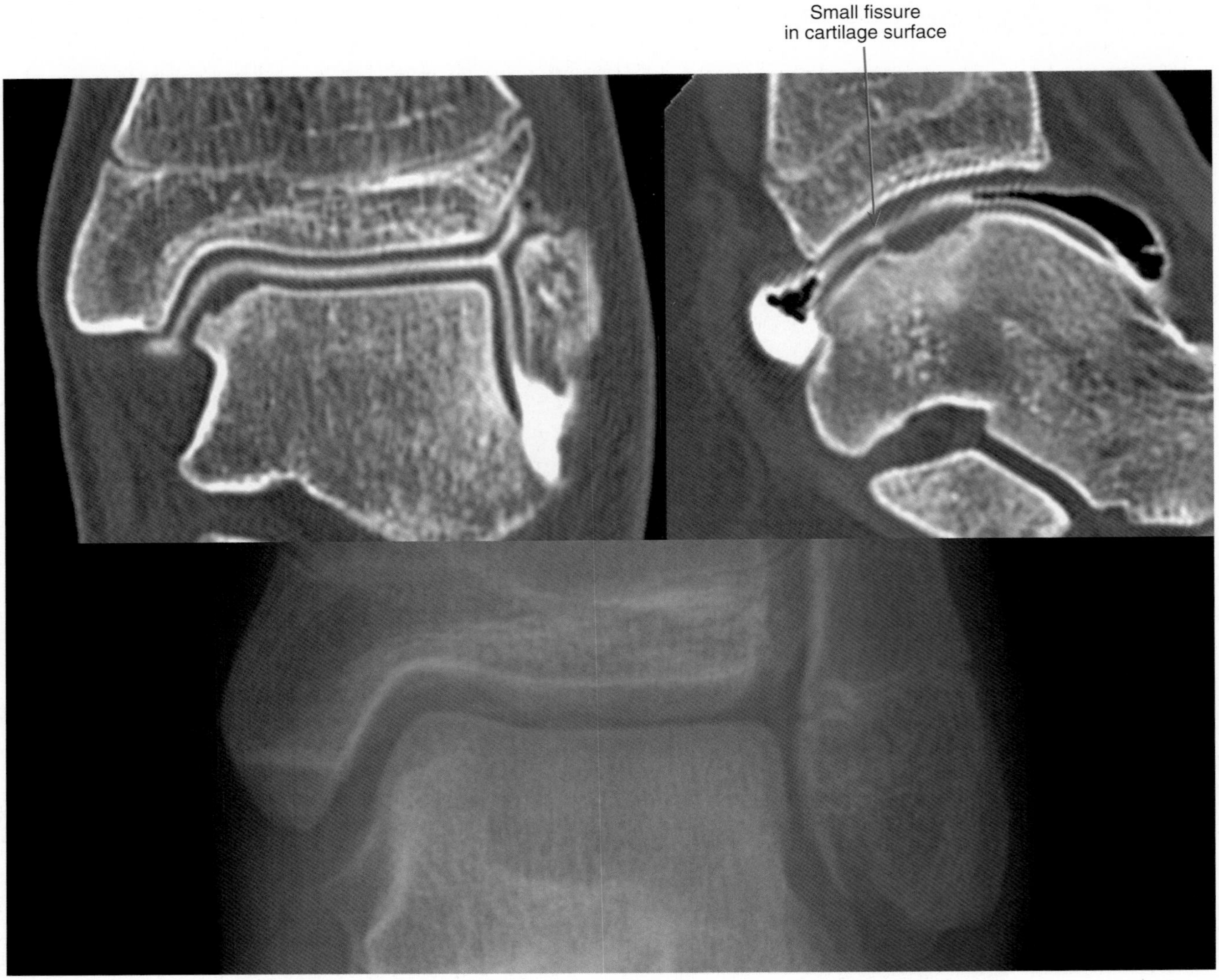
Small fissure
in cartilage surface

Figure 2-7 Multidetector CT arthrography is good for imaging surface detail of cartilage. In this example, a CT arthrogram of the ankle joint shows an osteochondral lesion of the medial talar dome with only slight fissuring of overlying cartilage.

are, however, several limitations of conventional MRI examinations, including the inability to visualize small intra-articular structures and the fact that many pathologic processes have similar signal intensity to normal anatomic structures. Postoperative findings may also be similar in signal intensity to pathologic changes. Unless there is an effusion, conventional MRI may be somewhat limited owing to nondistention of the joint.

Direct MRA involves the direct injection of dilute gadolinium, followed by MR imaging. This type of MRA leads to improved intra-articular contrast owing to the T1 shortening effect of gadolinium and also provides distention of the joint, which allows smaller intra-articular structures to be visualized (Figs. 2-8 through 2-12). The distention effect alone of saline injection has proved to be better than conventional MRI in some studies. The distention effect also forces intra-articular contrast through and around pathologic entities. With adequate distention, intra-articular gadolinium enters any pathologic entity in communication with the joint space. MRA provides excellent soft tissue contrast and demonstrates many abnormalities beyond the resolution of conventional

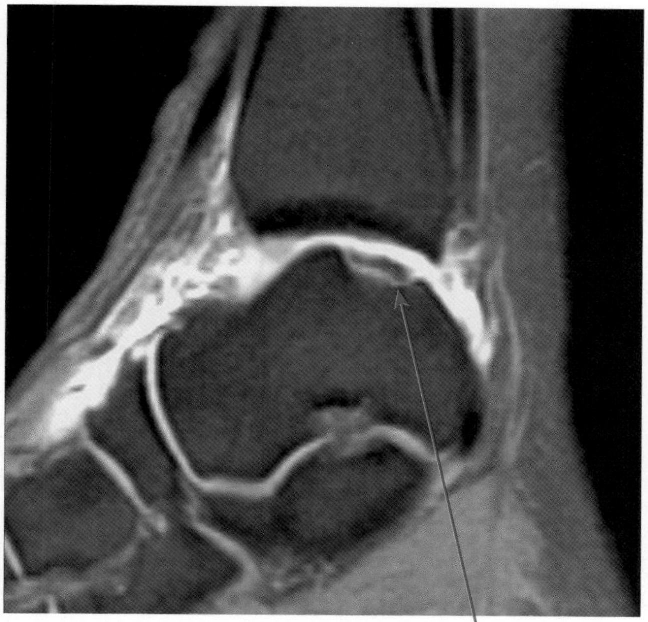
Contast extends
under OCD

Figure 2-8 Direct MR arthrography of the ankle documenting instability of an osteochondral lesion of the talus.

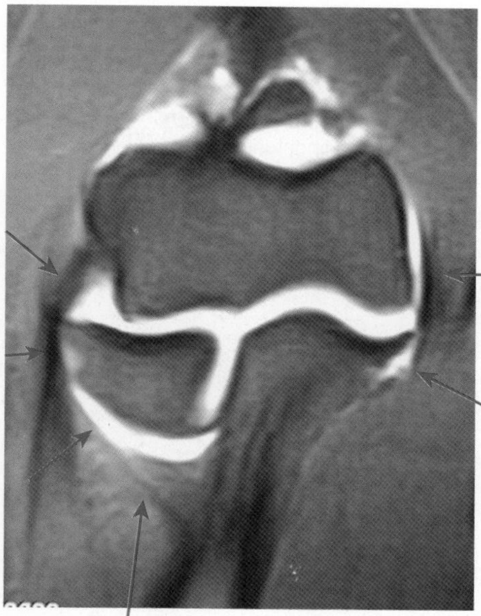
Medial
collateral
ligament
Undersurface
partial-
thickness
tear
Normal lateral ulnar
collateral ligament

Figure 2-9 Direct MR arthrography showing an undersurface partial-thickness tear of the distal aspect of the medial collateral ligament (the T sign).

MRI. One of the main disadvantages of MRA is the presence of artifacts seen in patients with implanted prostheses and metallic hardware.

To perform direct MRA, the gadolinium injected should be diluted to 2.5 mM. To achieve this concentration we add 0.1 mL of gadopentetate dimeglumine to 20 mL of normal saline. The final gadolinium dilution ratio should be 1:200 to achieve maximal signal (Fig. 2-13). It has been demonstrated that iodinated contrast reduces the T1 shortening effect of gadolinium. This effect is seen on both high and low field-strength systems. It is therefore advisable to use as little iodinated contrast as needed when performing direct MRA examinations. The quality of the examination on direct MRA does not appear to be affected by patient exercise. We therefore encourage patients to ambulate normally to the MRI suite after injection, but we do not routinely prescribe nor avoid exercise after injection for direct MRA.

Current indications for direct MRA include assessment of the glenoid labrum in the shoulder and acetabular labral tears in the hip. Direct MRA is also useful for the imaging of cartilage lesions. MRA can also be used for accurate determination of the congruity of the rotator cuff and for distinguishing between rotator cuff tendinosis and a full-thickness tear (when gadolinium pathologically enters the subacromial-subdeltoid bursa). Direct MRA is useful in imaging the postoperative joint (especially the shoulder and knee). It is also useful for assessment of intraosseous ligament tears in the wrist and for assessment of ligament tears about the elbow joint. Direct MRA in the ankle can determine the patency of the anterior talofibular ligament in patients with ankle sprain. Direct MRA is a safe procedure with minimal to no adverse effects reported over almost two decades.

Indirect MR Arthrography

Indirect MRA involves the injection of a standard dose of 0.1 mmol/kg of intravenous gadolinium followed by delayed imaging to create an "arthrographic effect" as the contrast diffuses into the joint (Fig. 2-14). As the gadolinium diffuses from the bloodstream into the synovial compartment of the joint being imaged, the degree of arthrographic effect depends on the volume of synovial fluid within the joint and on the degree of synovial vascularity.

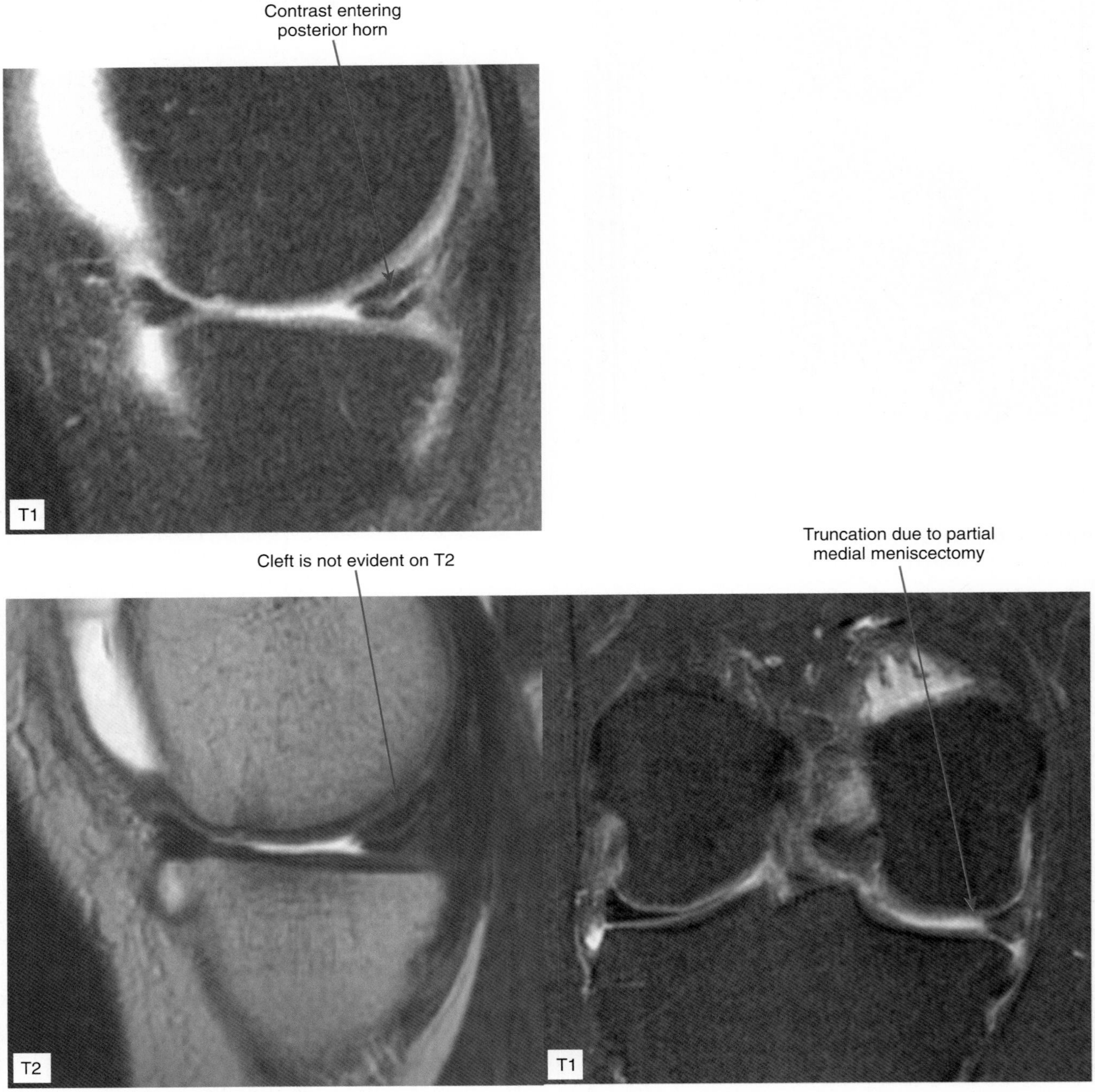
Contrast entering
posterior horn
T1
Cleft is not evident on T2
Truncation due to partial
medial meniscectomy
T2
T1

Figure 2-10 MR arthrography showing contrast entering the posterior horn. MR arthrography visualizes communications better than noncontrast MRI owing to a distention effect as well as use of higher SNR (signal-to-noise ratio) T1-weighted technique. However, keep in mind that a horizontal cleft *(top image)* may not represent a re-tear; some surgeons leave these if they are stable, debriding only the unstable flaps rather than performing a more extensive resection that might accelerate joint degeneration.

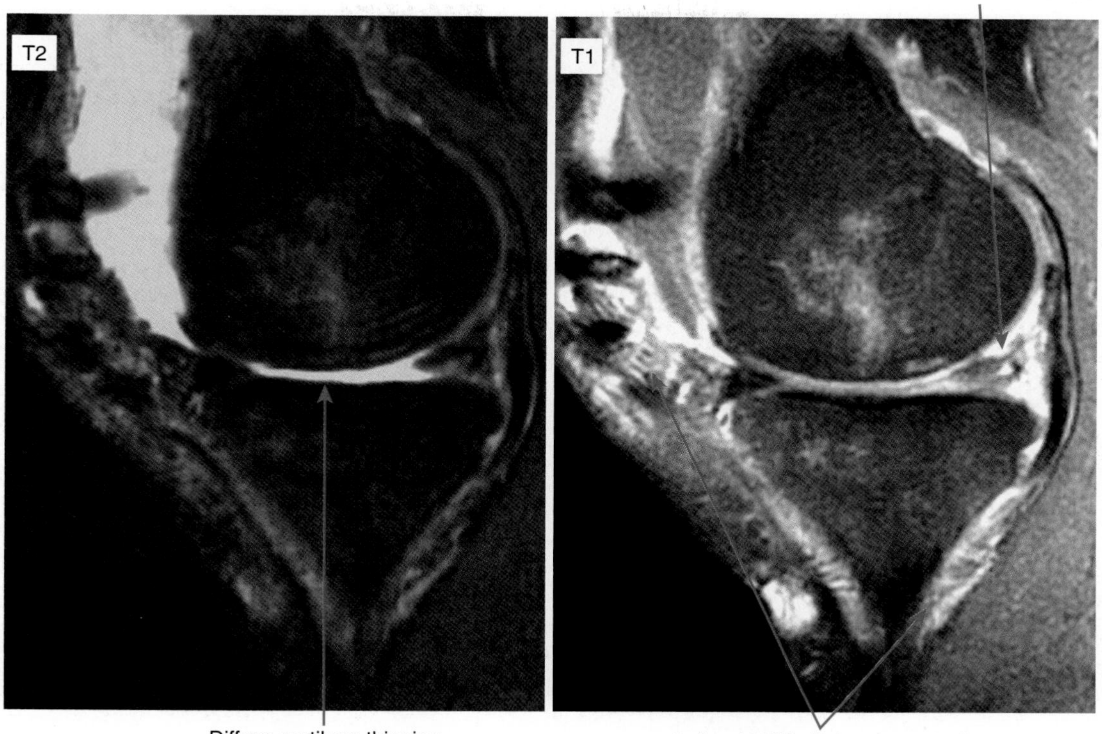
Irregular enhancement
meniscal tear or re-tear
T2
T1
Diffuse cartilage thinning
with subchondral edema
Indirect MRA: Enhancement of
synovium and operative site

Figure 2-18 Indirect MR arthrography of the postoperative knee. Note that on an indirect MR arthrogram, vascular structures within and outside the joint enhance; therefore, there is a separate learning curve associated with their interpretation. In this case there is enhancement of the posterior horn of the medial meniscus. Although enhancing granulation tissue can be seen after surgery, the irregular morphology of the meniscus and irregular enhancement make it more likely to be a tear or re-tear. However, the patient is more likely to be symptomatic because of the associated cartilage loss, seen better on the T2-weighted image.

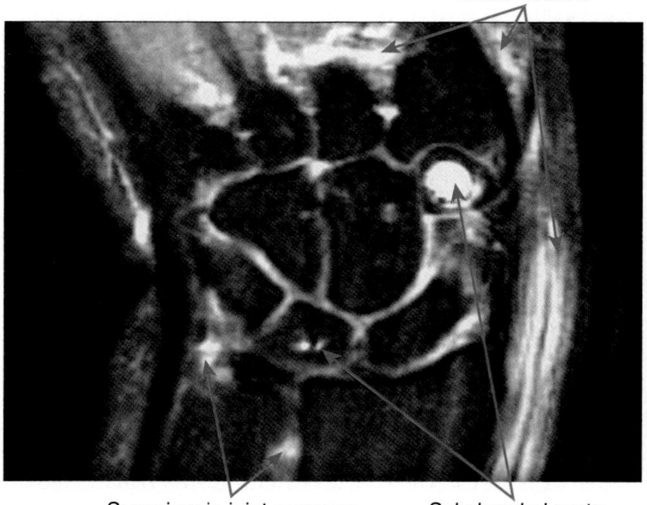
Indirect MR arthrography:
Other vascular structures enhanced
Blood vessels
Synovium in joint recesses
Subchondral cysts

Figure 2-19 Pitfalls of indirect MR arthrography. Other vascular structures, such as blood vessels, synovium, and subchondral cysts, enhance, both within and outside the joint.

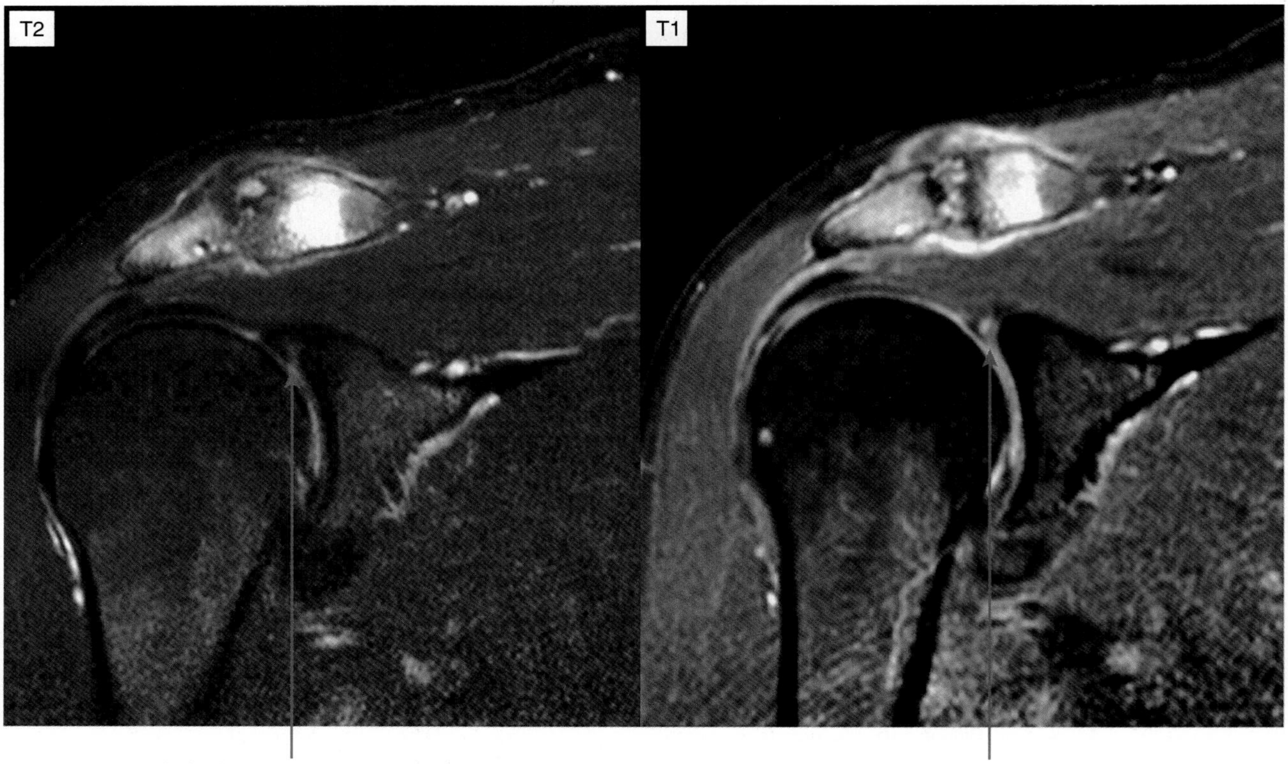
Enhancement of other pathology:
AC joint chronic injury
T2
T1
Labral tear: Not seen on T2
Enhancement of chronic SLAP lesion

Figure 2-20 On indirect MR arthrography, scar enhances; therefore, this technique may prove to be very useful for detection of chronic injuries containing granulation tissue. Such injuries, when intra-articular such as the labral tear in Figure 2-15, may not allow contrast injected directly into the joint to enter if scar has formed. AC, acromioclavicular.

contrast, it is advisable to prescribe pretreatment with 32 mg of oral methylprednisolone at 12 and 2 hours before the procedure. Pregnancy is also a relative contraindication to arthrography because of the potentially teratogenic effects of radiation. In pregnant patients who require arthrography, consideration should be given to ultrasound-guided joint injection.

There are very few absolute contraindications to arthrography, but they include an unwillingness or inability of the patient/caretaker to consent to the procedure and active infection at the site of skin puncture.

Equipment Needed for Fluoroscopic Guidance (Fig. 2-22)

- Flouroscopy table or C-arm with facility for spot radiographs
- Various sizes and shapes of cushions, bolsters, and weights for patient positioning
- Metallic marker/pen
- Skin cleanser
- 2 × 5- to 10-mL syringes (for lidocaine and iodinated contrast)
- 1 × 20-mL syringe (for the injectate—depending on the arthrography technique)
- Insulin syringe (for drawing gadolinium)
- Soft connector tubing
- Sterile gloves
- Sterile gauze
- Sterile drapes, one fenestrated
- Adhesive bandage
- Various 1.5-inch needles, 25- to 26-g mosquito, 23 g, 20 g, and 18 g
- 3-inch 18- to 22-g needle for arthrogram (length/gauge depends on the joint and indication)
- 20 mL sterile saline
- 10-mL 1% lidocaine
- 10-mL iodinated contrast 300 mg/mL

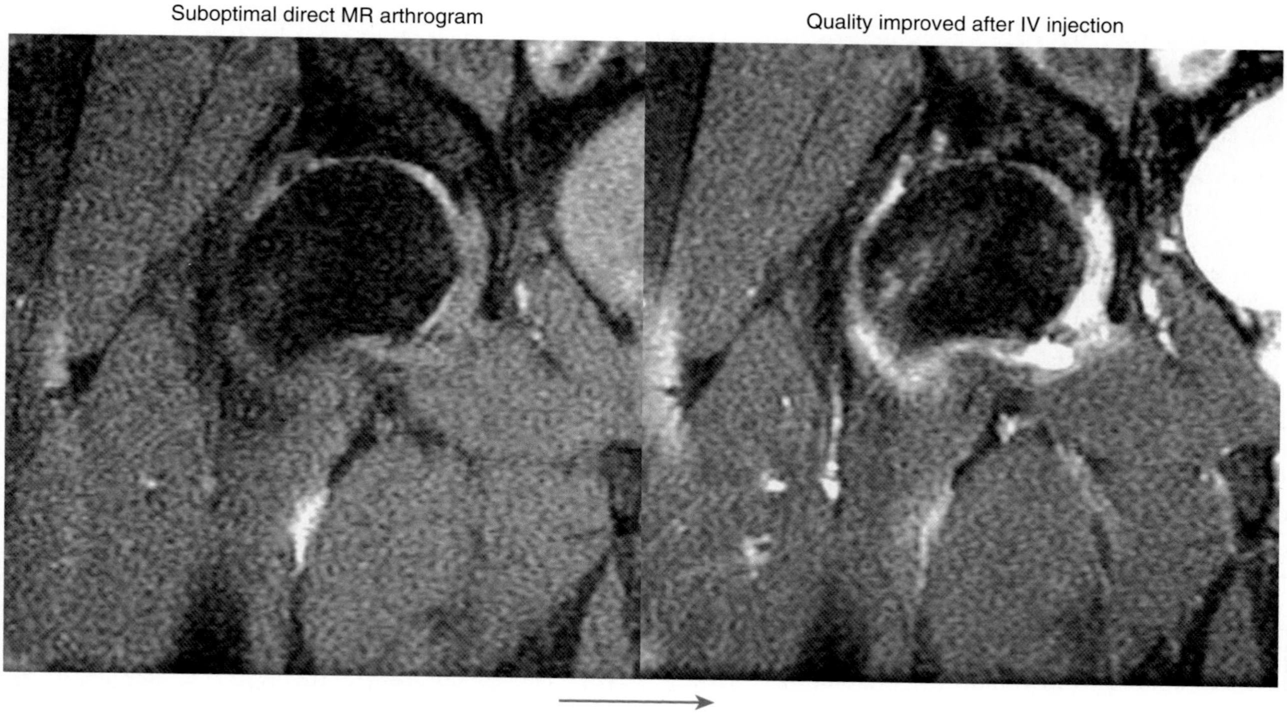
Suboptimal direct MR arthrogram
Quality improved after IV injection

Figure 2-21 Indirect MR arthrography can also be used to salvage a suboptimal direct MR arthrogram. This image follows an attempted intra-articular injection, in which most contrast appeared in the iliopsoas bursa after initial MR imaging. Improved image quality resulted when the patient was given an intravenous injection using a standard dose and imaged after 30 minutes.

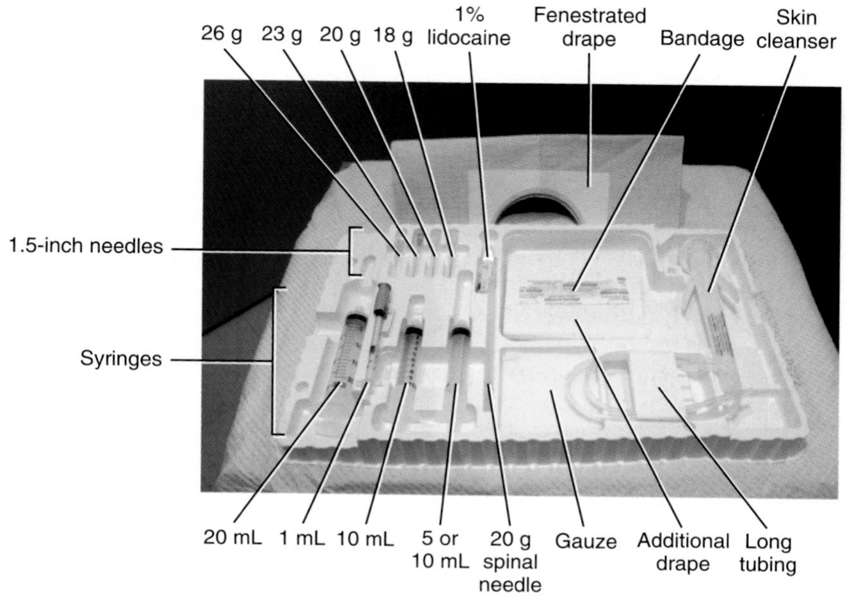
26 g
23 g
20 g
18 g
1% lidocaine
Fenestrated drape
Bandage
Skin cleanser
1.5-inch needles
Syringes
20 mL
1 mL
10 mL
5 or 10 mL
20 g spinal needle
Gauze
Additional drape
Long tubing

Figure 2-22 Standard arthrogram tray.

BOX 2-1 ADVANTAGES AND DISADVANTAGES OF INDIRECT MR ARTHROGRAPHY (MRA) COMPARED WITH DIRECT MRA

Advantages

Better patient acceptance
Logistical considerations
- No need for fluoroscopic-guided arthrography
- Easier to schedule
- Better for "satellite" centers
- Potential "off hours" and weekend examinations
- Can be used to accommodate the "unscheduled arthrogram"

Intra-articular and extra-articular enhancement
- Can be indicator of hyperemia, soft tissue processes

Granulation tissue enhances (an advantage in the nonoperative joint)
Higher reimbursement in some markets

Disadvantages

Intra-articular and extra-articular enhancement
- Most pathology will enhance; may result in overcalls (e.g., tendinosis versus tear)
- Enhancement of normally vascular structures occurs (e.g., peripheral TFCC and peripheral meniscus)
- Fluid in all compartments enhances (e.g., subacromial contrast is not necessarily indicative of a rotator cuff tear)

Granulation tissue enhances (a potential disadvantage in the postoperative joint)
Reliance upon preexisting joint effusion
Tense effusion or synovial scarring can result in slower uptake of contrast into the joint.
Imaging too soon after injection results in a suboptimal examination.
- Particularly problematic in large joints

Decreased overall contrast compared with direct MRA
- Often limited on low-field MRI without fat suppression
- Limited in situations with low SNR (e.g., deep structures such as the hip)

No IV access = no indirect MRA

SNR, signal-to-noise ratio; TFCC, triangular fibrocartilage complex.

General Fluoroscopic Technique

The procedure, its risks, alternatives, and potential complications are explained to the patient. A consent form is signed. The patient is positioned on the fluoroscopy table; when the desired patient position is achieved, preliminary radiographs are obtained. It is essential to review the preliminary radiographs before commencing the arthrographic procedure. A metallic marker is placed over the expected needle entry site. Using real-time or intermittent fluoroscopy, the desired position is marked with a pen or a skin impression is made using, for example, the circular end of a needle cover. The skin over the needle entry site is prepped and draped in the usual fashion. Lidocaine is administered to the skin and subcutaneous tissues. The arthrography needle is then advanced into the joint using real-time or intermittent fluoroscopy. When the needle has achieved entry into the joint, a small volume of iodinated contrast material can be injected via soft tubing to confirm intra-articular placement of the needle tip. If an effusion is present, it should be drained to completion. Some authors advocate the intra-articular injection of a small (1–3 mL) volume of lidocaine or bupivacaine (Marcaine) to provide additional diagnostic information as to whether pain relief is achieved post-arthrography. Thereafter, the injectate of choice is administered to the joint, depending on the desired arthrographic technique.

Some centers advocate the addition of a small volume of epinephrine to the injectate if imaging is to be performed after a delay (e.g., at an off-site MRI facility). The administration of intra-articular epinephrine results in synovial vasoconstriction and delays resorption of the injectate. To add epinephrine, draw 0.1 mL of 1:1000 epinephrine using an insulin syringe and add it to the injectate, or simply draw epinephrine into the syringe and squirt it out before drawing up the gadolinium mixture (analogous to use of vermouth in a dry martini).

In general, low resistance is a useful sign of intra-articular position (which is why a 20-gauge needle is recommended for most joint injections), but this sign is limited in obese patients who have a large amount of loose connective tissue. If fluoroscopy shows the needle tip to lie within the joint but high resistance is encountered, then the operator should try turning the needle tip while injecting. If this is not successful, the needle should be pulled back 1 to 2 mm because the needle tip may be embedded in cartilage. However, more often the joint has not yet been reached; the capsule in many cases feels firm and can simulate bone. With proper technique, injury to the articular structures is extremely rare; such concern should not dissuade the radiologist from advancing the needle farther. The capsule is often sensitive, and an additional 1 to 2 mL of lidocaine injected at the site can be useful. As above, if this injection of lidocaine is met with little resistance, one should suspect intra-articular positioning and commence with iodinated contrast injection for confirmation, followed by gadolinium in the case of MRA. Injection should be stopped if any significant pain is encountered or when the capsule is fully distended (the operator will note a rapid increase in resistance). Injection should also be terminated when the target intra-articular injection volume has been achieved.

Ultrasound Guidance Technique

Many practicing radiologists use ultrasound-guided techniques for joint aspiration or for arthrographic joint injection (prior to CT or MRA). The advantages of ultrasound are that it is readily available, it does not use ionizing radiation, and it is a relatively quick and simple technique.

The procedure, its risks, alternatives, and potential complications are explained to the patient. A consent form is then signed. Next, the patient is placed in a comfortable position on the examination couch to allow for easy access to the joint for injection. Typically, a 5- to 12-MHz linear array transducer is used for ultrasound-guided joint access techniques. The appropriate location and window are then chosen based on known joint recesses or by targeting a specific pocket of joint fluid. Doppler evaluation is recommended to assess for vascular structures surrounding the joint for injection or along the projected potential needle approach path. Some operators find it useful to mark the chosen transducer position with indelible ink on the skin surface. The skin is then prepped and draped in the usual fashion. A sterile cover is placed over the ultrasound probe. With strict aseptic technique, 1% lidocaine is administered to the skin and subcutaneous tissues; then a 20- to 22-gauge needle is inserted oblique to the skin and along the long axis of the probe to achieve optimal needle visualization under direct ultrasonic guidance. The needle tip itself should be identified as a moving reflector (Figs. 2-23 through 2-25). The needle can be "jiggled" slightly and if not immediately observed, movement of the surrounding tissues can be easily detected. The path of the needle is then adjusted under real-time ultrasonic guidance. Passage of the needle tip into a joint is generally associated with a feeling of transient capsular resistance followed by a sensation of a resistance-free space. Joint injection can then be performed under real-time sonographic observation.

SPECIFIC FLUOROSCOPIC JOINT ACCESS TECHNIQUES

Shoulder

Approximately 12 to 14 mL injectate is instilled into the shoulder joint when assessing the glenoid labrum (depending on the volume of the capsule). Volumes of 16 mL or more (until increased capsular resistance is felt) can be used when assessing the integrity of the rotator cuff.

The most common technique used is the straight anterior approach (Fig. 2-26) with insertion of a needle at the junction of the middle and lower thirds of the glenohumeral joint. A 20-gauge, 3.5-inch spinal needle is used. The patient is positioned in the supine position with the arm in external rotation. A sandbag is placed in the patient's upturned palm to maintain this position. The preferred access point is marked with a metallic marker at the lower third of the glenohumeral joint, slightly on the humeral side of the joint. After administration of local anesthetic to the skin and subcutaneous tissues, the needle is placed straight down to the joint erring to the side of the humeral head to avoid transgressing the glenoid labrum. With this technique, the needle must traverse the subscapularis myotendinous junction and the inferior glenohumeral ligament. Therefore, there are associated potential risks of distorting or damaging anatomic structures, although this has not proved to be a significant issue.

Some authors advocate a modified anterior approach via the rotator interval (Fig. 2-27). With this technique, the needle is directed from a position on the skin just anterior to the acromion toward the medial upper quadrant of the humeral head, entering the joint capsule via rotator interval. We have found this technique to be useful in obese patients in whom breast tissue overlies the shoulder in the supine position. A smaller 22- to 25-gauge needle is used for joint access. The potential difficulty with this technique of injection is that the subacromial-subdeltoid bursa overlies the superior aspect of the rotator interval, and this may result in inadvertent puncture of the bursa leading to difficulties with diagnostic interpretation.

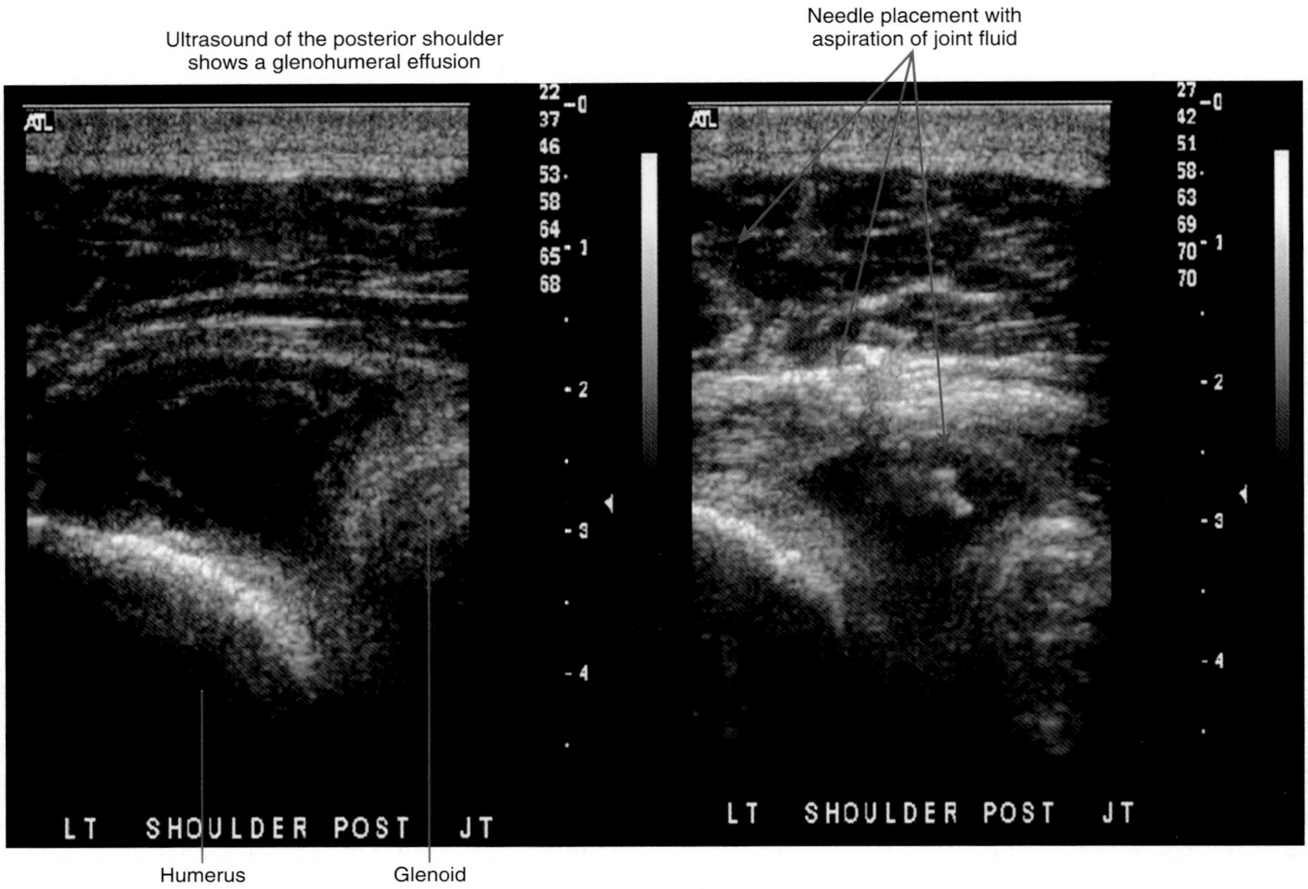
Ultrasound of the posterior shoulder shows a glenohumeral effusion
Needle placement with aspiration of joint fluid
LT SHOULDER POST JT
LT SHOULDER POST JT
Humerus
Glenoid

Figure 2-23 Ultrasound guidance for glenohumeral joint aspiration and injection. Glenohumeral effusion in posterior shoulder. *Arrows* show needle placement with aspiration of joint fluid.

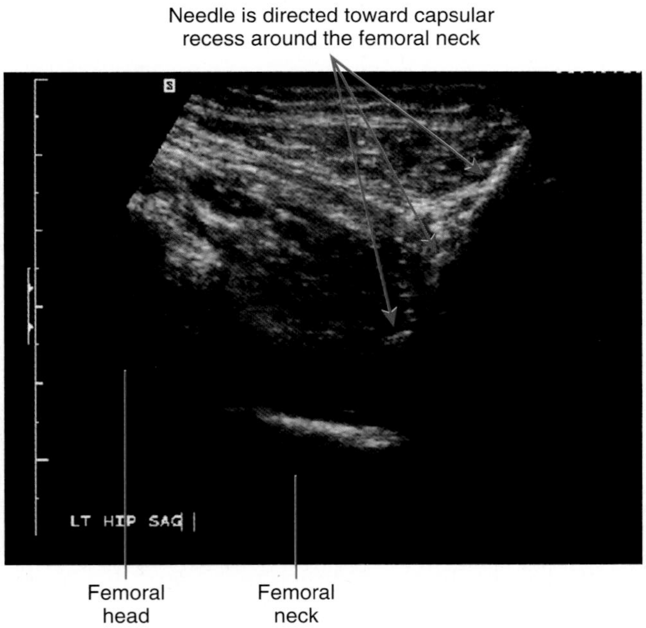
Needle is directed toward capsular recess around the femoral neck
LT HIP SAG
Femoral head
Femoral neck

Figure 2-24 Ultrasound guidance for hip aspiration and injection.

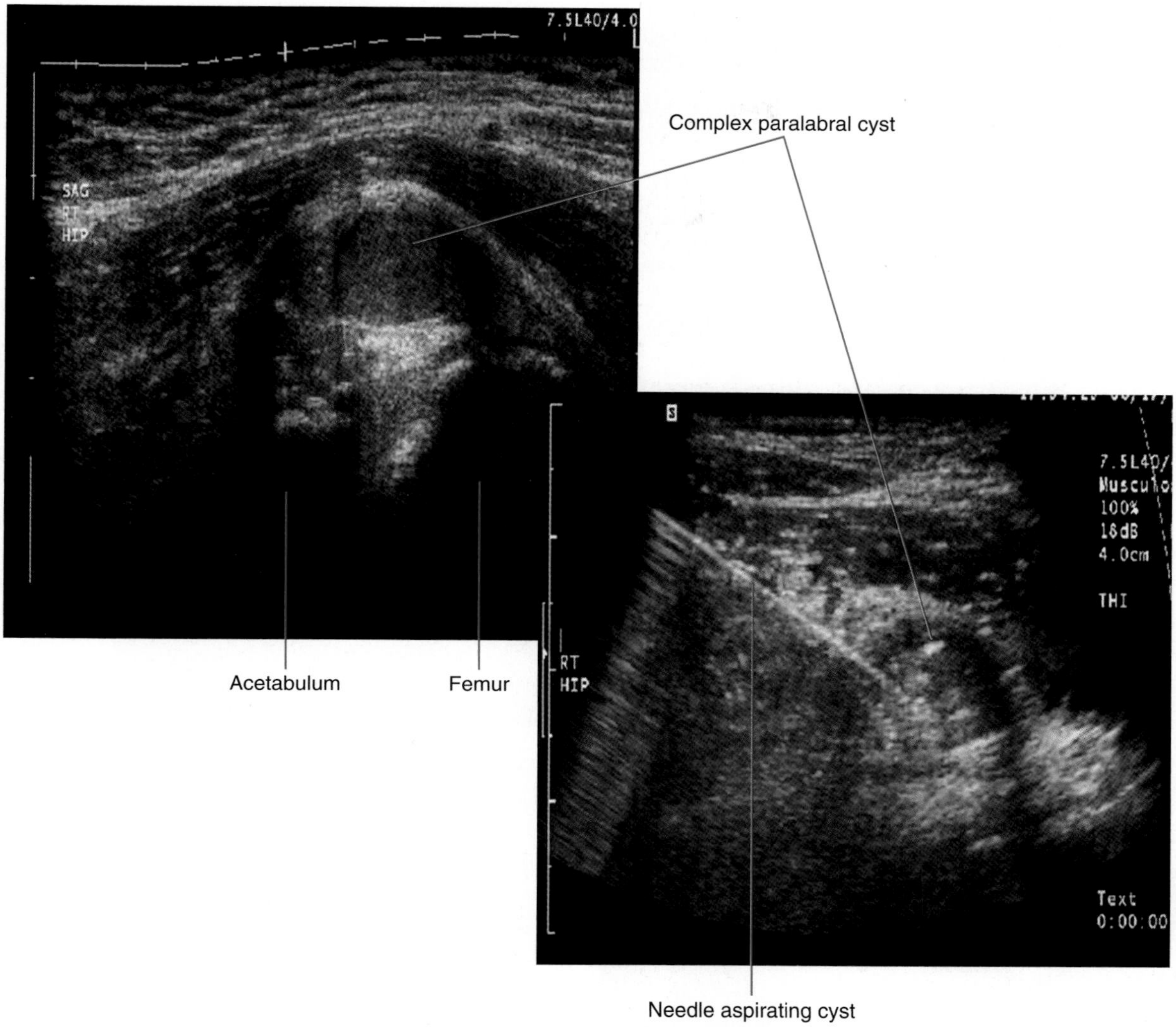
Complex paralabral cyst
Acetabulum
Femur
Needle aspirating cyst
SAG
RT
HIP
RT
HIP
7.5L40/4.0
100%
18dB
4.0cm
THI
Text
0:00:00

Figure 2-25 **Aspiration of a paralabral cyst of the hip.**

A posterior approach to the joint capsule is most commonly used by non-radiologists without image guidance; this often leads to inadvertent injection of the overlying muscle or subacromial-subdeltoid bursa. However, a modified fluoroscopic approach has been advocated by some authors, especially for patients with suspected anterior instability and for muscular patients (Fig. 2-28). The needle tip is aimed at the upper third of the posterior glenohumeral joint. Positioning for fluoroscopic guidance is more challenging than for anterior approaches because an oblique view along the glenohumeral joint must be acquired with the patient in the prone position. This position can be achieved with bolsters under the shoulder and by use of a C-arm.

Conventional shoulder arthrography is still used for the detection of full-thickness rotator cuff tears. For this technique, 8 mL of intra-articular contrast is administered followed by 8 mL of intra-articular air. Both the contrast and the air can be drawn into a 20-mL syringe and injected without disconnecting the tubing. Once the air is injected and the intra-articular position is verified, the needle is withdrawn without disconnecting the syringe and tubing (otherwise air will leak through the needle). The patient is then exercised by swinging the arm. Anteroposterior views of the shoulder are obtained in internal and external rotation with and without the use of counterweights. If a full-thickness rotator cuff tear is present, then contrast and air will be seen to extend

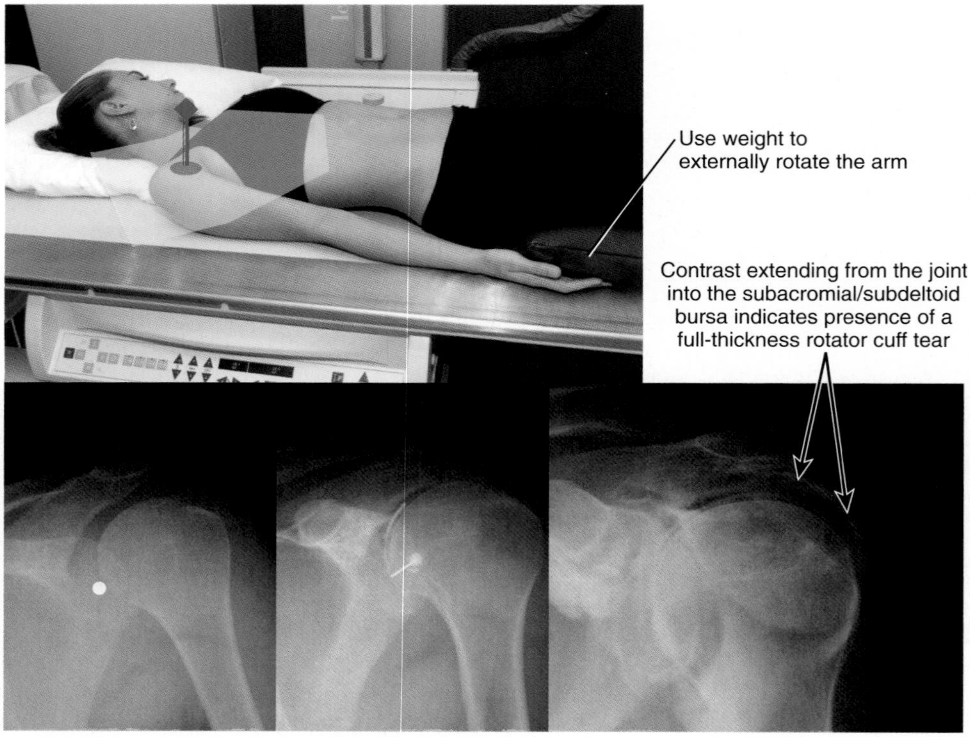
Use weight to
externally rotate the arm
Contrast extending from the joint
into the subacromial/subdeltoid
bursa indicates presence of a
full-thickness rotator cuff tear

Figure 2-26 **Shoulder arthrogram, anterior approach.**

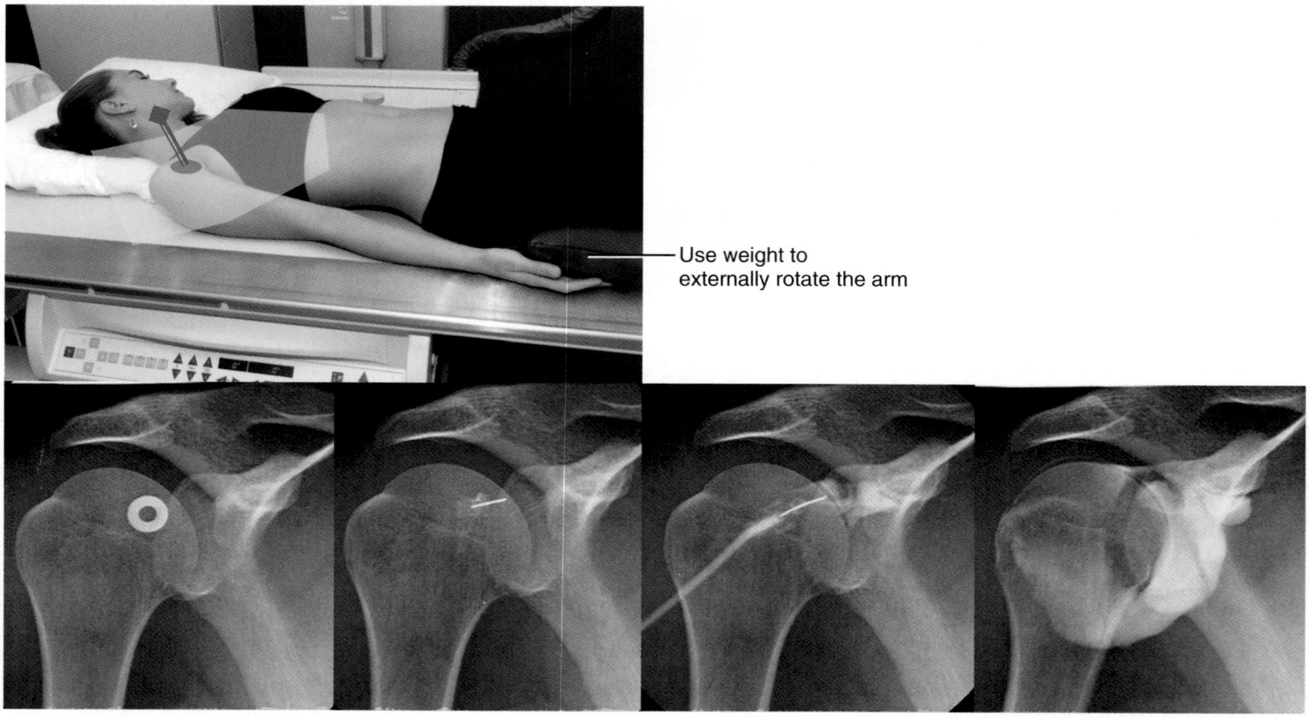
Use weight to
externally rotate the arm

Figure 2-27 **Shoulder arthrogram, rotator cuff interval approach.** (Images courtesy Arthur Newberg, MD, and Joel Newman, MD, Boston, MA.)

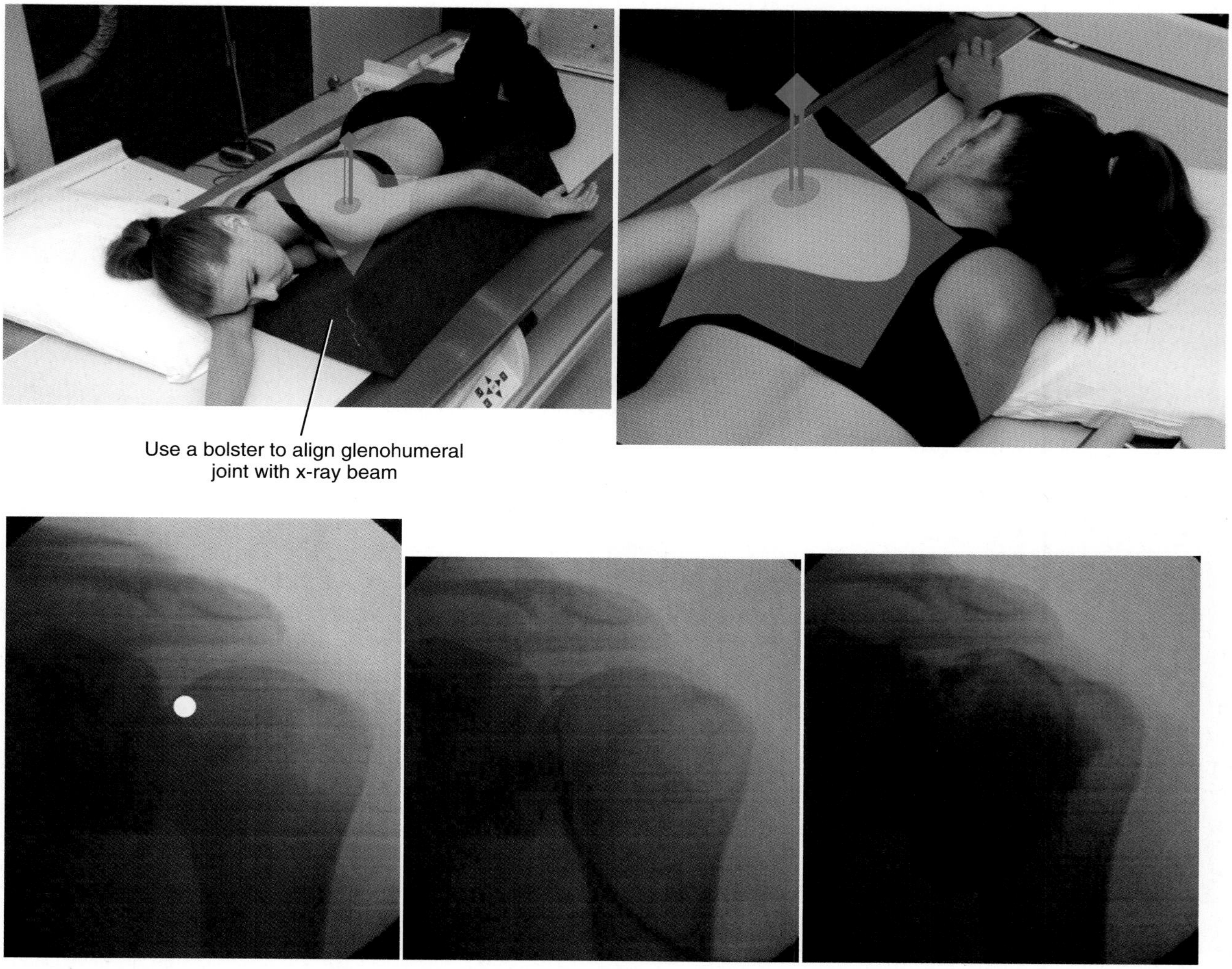
Use a bolster to align glenohumeral joint with x-ray beam

Figure 2-28 **Shoulder arthrogram, posterior approach.** (Images courtesy Douglas Beall, MD, Oklahoma City, OK.)

from the glenohumeral joint into the subacromial-subdeltoid bursa.

Sonography and MR guidance have also been used for needle positioning in shoulder arthrography.

Elbow

For arthrographic access to the elbow joint, the patient should be lying prone with the arm over the head or sitting in a chair with the arm placed on a table and the elbow flexed to 90 degrees (Fig. 2-29). The prone position is preferred to reduce the risk of vasovagal response and to avoid temptation for the patient to view the procedure. The joint is entered laterally over the radiocapitellar joint using fluoroscopic guidance or posterolaterally between the olecranon and the humerus. The latter can be performed when a question of radial collateral ligament injury is present. A 1.5-inch, 20- or 22-gauge needle is used to access the radiocapitellar joint and 7 to 10 mL of injectate is then instilled.

Wrist

Wrist arthrography is typically performed for assessment of a suspected triangular fibrocartilage complex tear or an interosseous ligament tear of either the scapholunate or lunatotriquetral ligament. Tears of these small ligaments are diagnosed by direct visualization of the tear or by extension of contrast into an adjacent compartment. There are three joint components that can be potentially evaluated in a complete

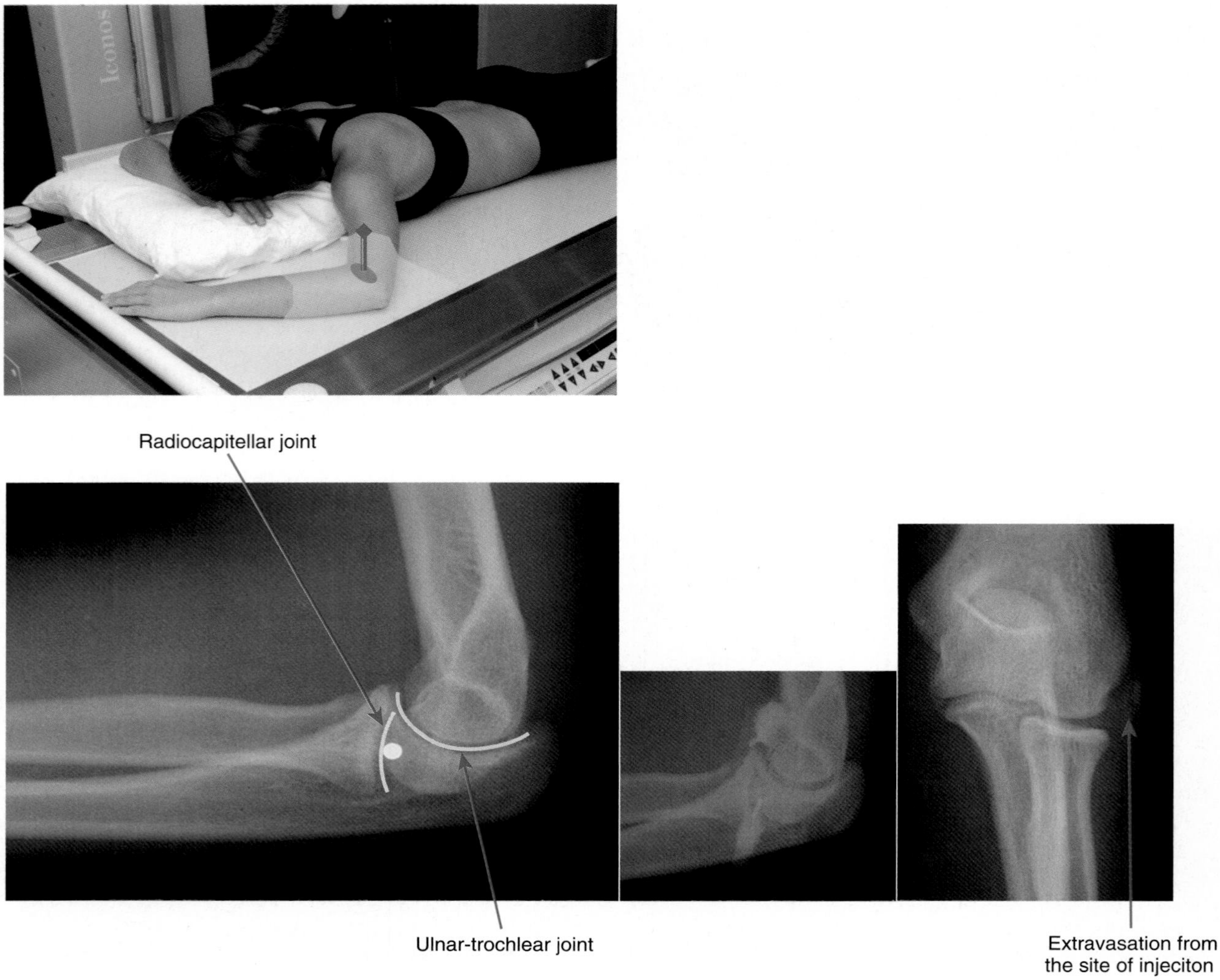
Radiocapitellar joint
Ulnar-trochlear joint
Extravasation from the site of injeciton

Figure 2-29 Elbow arthrogram.

wrist arthrogram: the radiocarpal joint, the midcarpal joint and the distal radioulnar joint. Since there are multiple sites of potential communication, it is beneficial to radiographically evaluate the early flow of iodinated contrast (whether performing conventional, MR, or CT athrography). Small perforations and abnormal communications can be detected on early spot radiographs. Compartmental communication will also be evident on later films but the exact location of a perforation may have become obscured. Although some authors have recommended three-compartment arthrography to detect one-way communication, this practice has become uncommon because of the rare nature of such communication as well as the advent of MR imaging. Most practitioners now inject only the radiocarpal joint for conventional arthrography as well as for CT and MRA. Exercise after injection forces fluid through ligament tears and can potentially reduce the risk of missing a one-way communication.

The administration of subcutaneous lidocaine is optional when accessing the radiocarpal joint because the needle used is typically a short 25-gauge needle. The patient's hand is placed with the palm facing downward (Fig. 2-30). For injecting the radiocarpal joint, a roll can be used to place the wrist in a small degree of flexion. The needle is then advanced into the radiocarpal joint via a dorsal approach, aiming between the distal radius and the mid-scaphoid. Pitfalls of radiocarpal injection include injection into

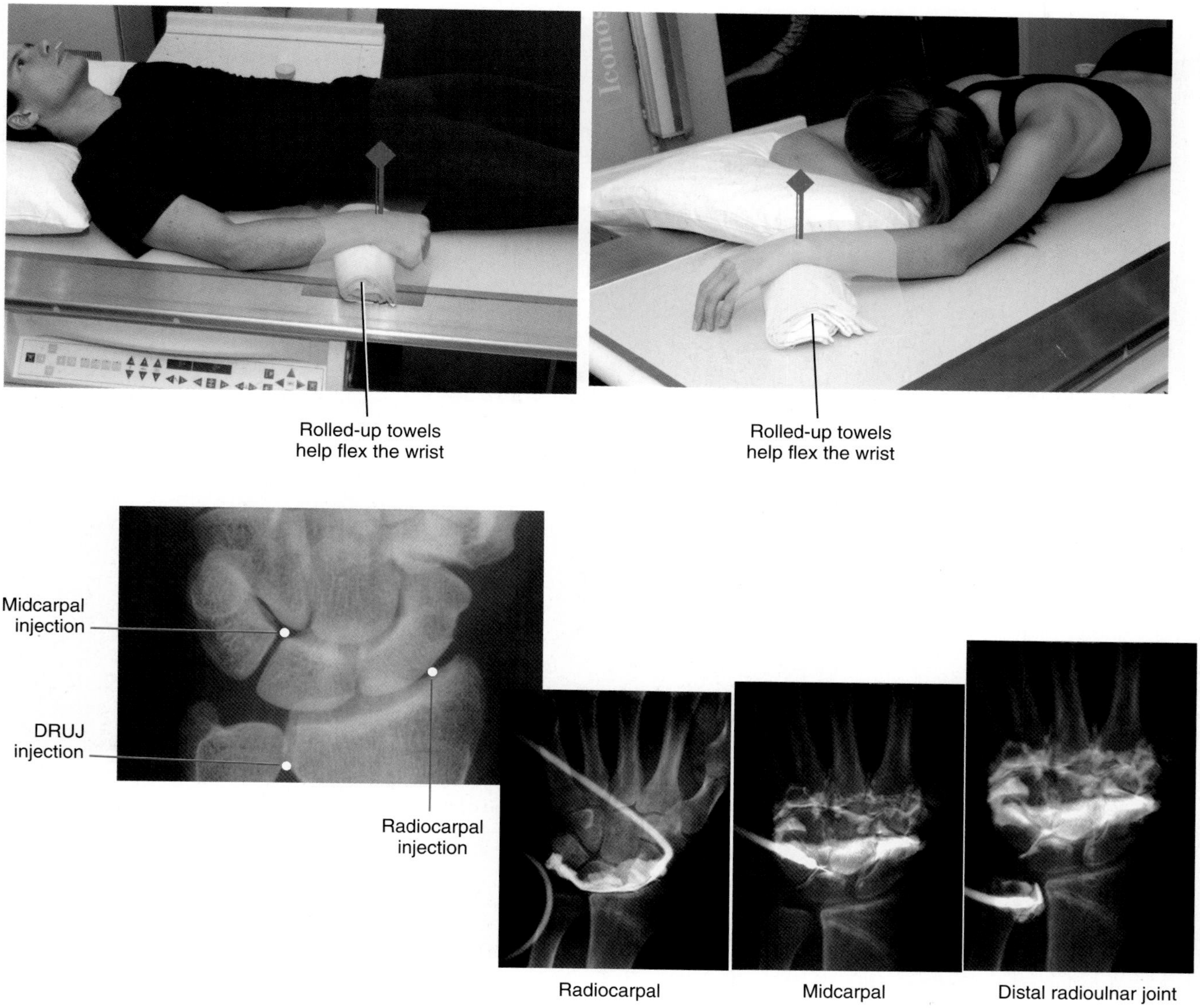
Rolled-up towels help flex the wrist
Rolled-up towels help flex the wrist
Midcarpal injection
DRUJ injection
Radiocarpal injection
Radiocarpal
Midcarpal
Distal radioulnar joint

Figure 2-30 ***Wrist arthrogram.*** *Supine versus prone positioning. DRUJ, distal radioulnar joint.*

the superficial extensor tendons and targeting the osseous surface of the radial rim. A three-compartment wrist arthrogram involves initial injection of the radiocarpal joint followed by exercise. The patient is then brought back 3 to 4 hours later, and injection of the midcarpal joint, followed by injection of the distal radioulnar joint, is carried out. Each injection is followed by exercise. The target location for injection of the midcarpal joint is at the joint space at the junction of the triquetral, capitate, hamate, and lunate bones (this is usually a relatively capacious region, except where a type 2 lunate exists, resulting in lunate/hamate articulation). The location for injection of the distal radioulnar joint is at the proximal aspect, where a recess is present. If the distal radioulnar joint requires injection, it should be performed last because it can be a painful procedure owing to the sensitivity of the adjacent periosteum.

Typical injection volume is 3 mL for the radiocarpal joint, 2 to 3 mL for the midcarpal joint, and 1 mL for the distal radioulnar joint (the latter two joints are typically injected until resistance is felt).

Another recently described method for accessing the radiocarpal joint is via the pisotriquetral recess. The same positioning is performed as in Figure 2-15, but the needle is directed toward the proximal

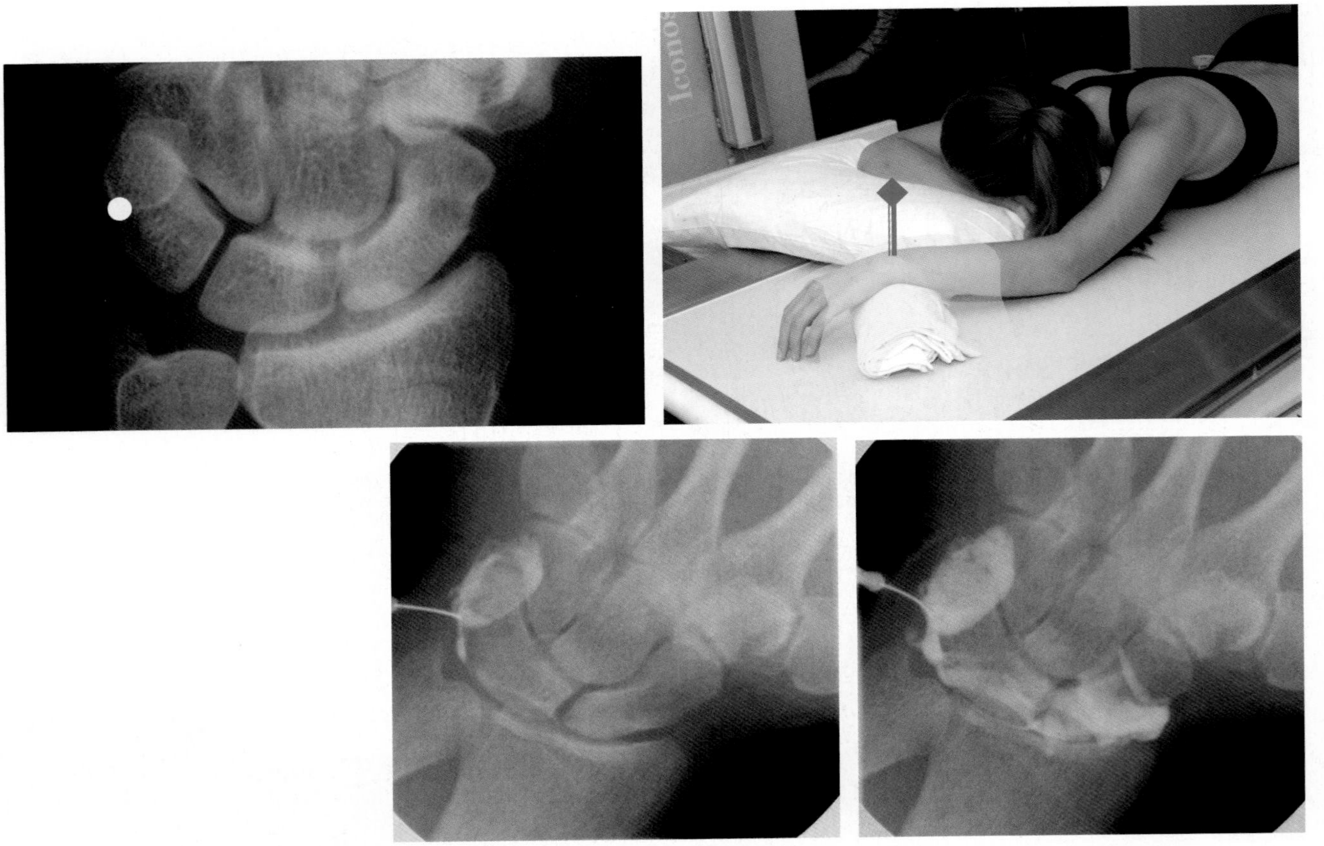

Figure 2-31 **Alternate access to the radiocarpal joint via the pisotriquetral recess.** (Images courtesy Kira Chow, MD, Los Angeles, CA.)

pisotriquetral joint distal to the expected location of the triangular fibrocartilage (Fig. 2-31).

Sacroiliac Joint

Arthrography of the sacroiliac (SI) joint is rarely performed. Therapeutic injection and/or aspiration of the SI joint are much more commonly requested. The techniques used for access to the joint for arthrography can be applied to therapeutic injection or aspiration of the SI joint. Image guidance is essential to achieve accurate intra-articular needle placement.

The anterior/inferior half to two thirds of the SI joint is a synovium-lined cartilaginous joint, and the posterior/superior portion of the joint consists of a fibrous articulation. Therefore, the inferior aspect of the joint should be targeted for aspiration or injection.

Arthrography of the SI joint is typically performed under fluoroscopic guidance (Fig. 2-32). Experience is essential for successful injection under fluoroscopy, since the joint has a complex shape and different areas of the joint appear at different degrees of obliquity. The patient is placed prone on the fluoroscopy table, and access to the SI joint is obtained using a posteroinferior to anterosuperior approach. The C-arm is rotated to best visualize the inferior aspect of the joint. A 22-gauge spinal needle is directed straight down along the beam to the inferior aspect of the SI joint. Intra-articular placement of the needle tip can be confirmed with an injection of a small volume of iodinated contrast material.

CT guidance can facilitate injection if fluoroscopic guidance is unsuccessful. This is often required when there is underlying osteoarthritis and joint space narrowing. The patient is also placed prone on the CT table. Using CT guidance, a 22-gauge spinal needle is advanced into the inferior aspect of the SI joint. Arthrography, aspiration, or therapeutic injection of the SI joint can then be performed.

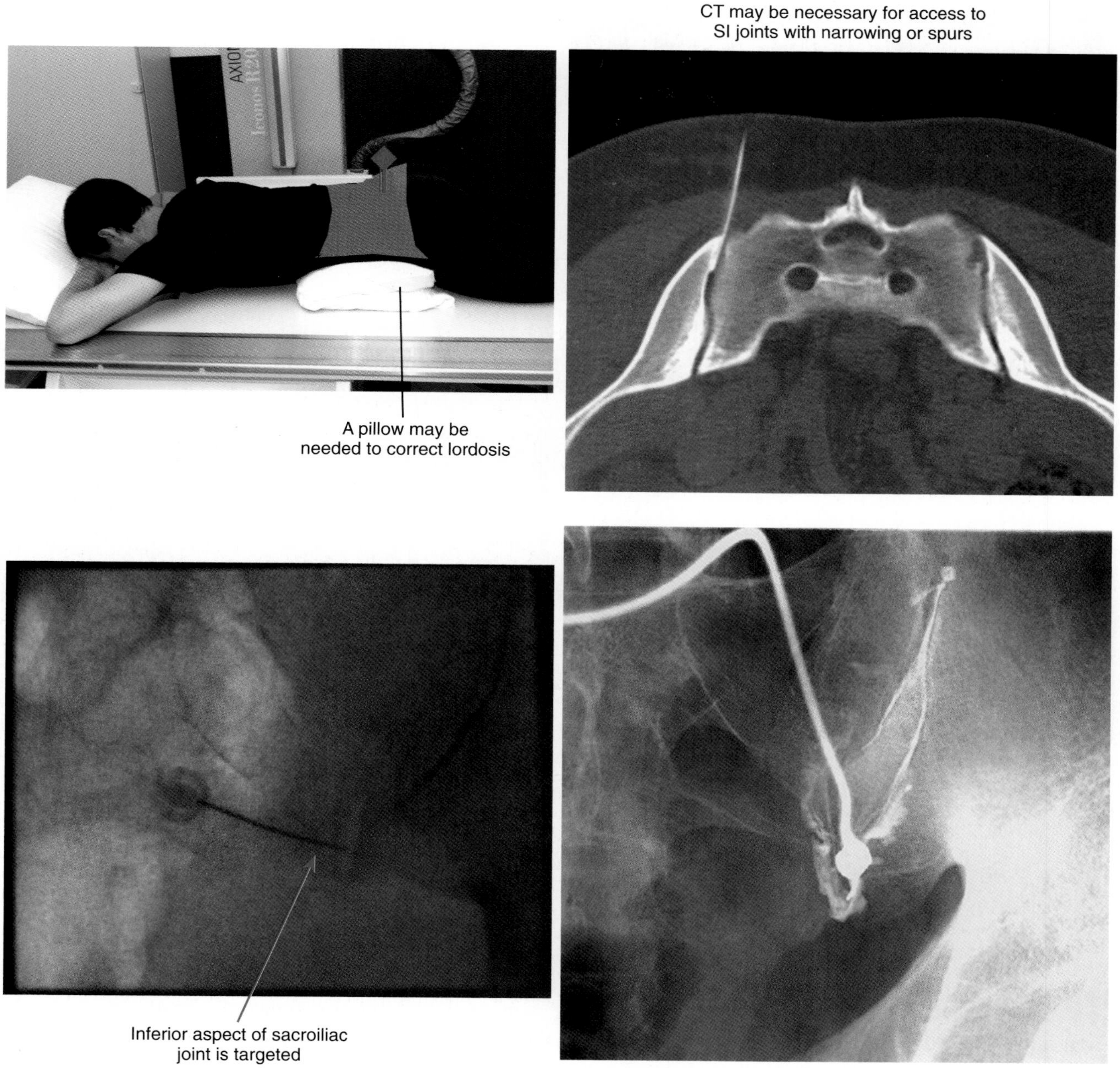
CT may be necessary for access to SI joints with narrowing or spurs
A pillow may be needed to correct lordosis
Inferior aspect of sacroiliac joint is targeted

Figure 2-32 ***Positioning for sacroiliac injection and aspiration.***

Pubic Symphysis

Arthrography of the pubic symphysis is best performed under sonographic or fluoroscopic guidance (Fig. 2-33). After subcutaneous injection of local anesthesia, a 22-gauge needle is targeted toward the symphyseal cleft at the upper margin of the joint, using a cranial to caudal approach. When the needle reaches the outer margin of the joint, signified by increased resistance with a firm consistency, the needle is advanced 1 cm farther into the cleft of the fibrocartilaginous disk. After positioning the needle, 1 mL of nonionic contrast material is injected into the symphyseal cleft to confirm the needle's position. For treatment of osteitis pubis or for diagnosis of the source of pain, an aqueous suspension composed of steroid and long-acting local analgesic can be injected into the cleft.

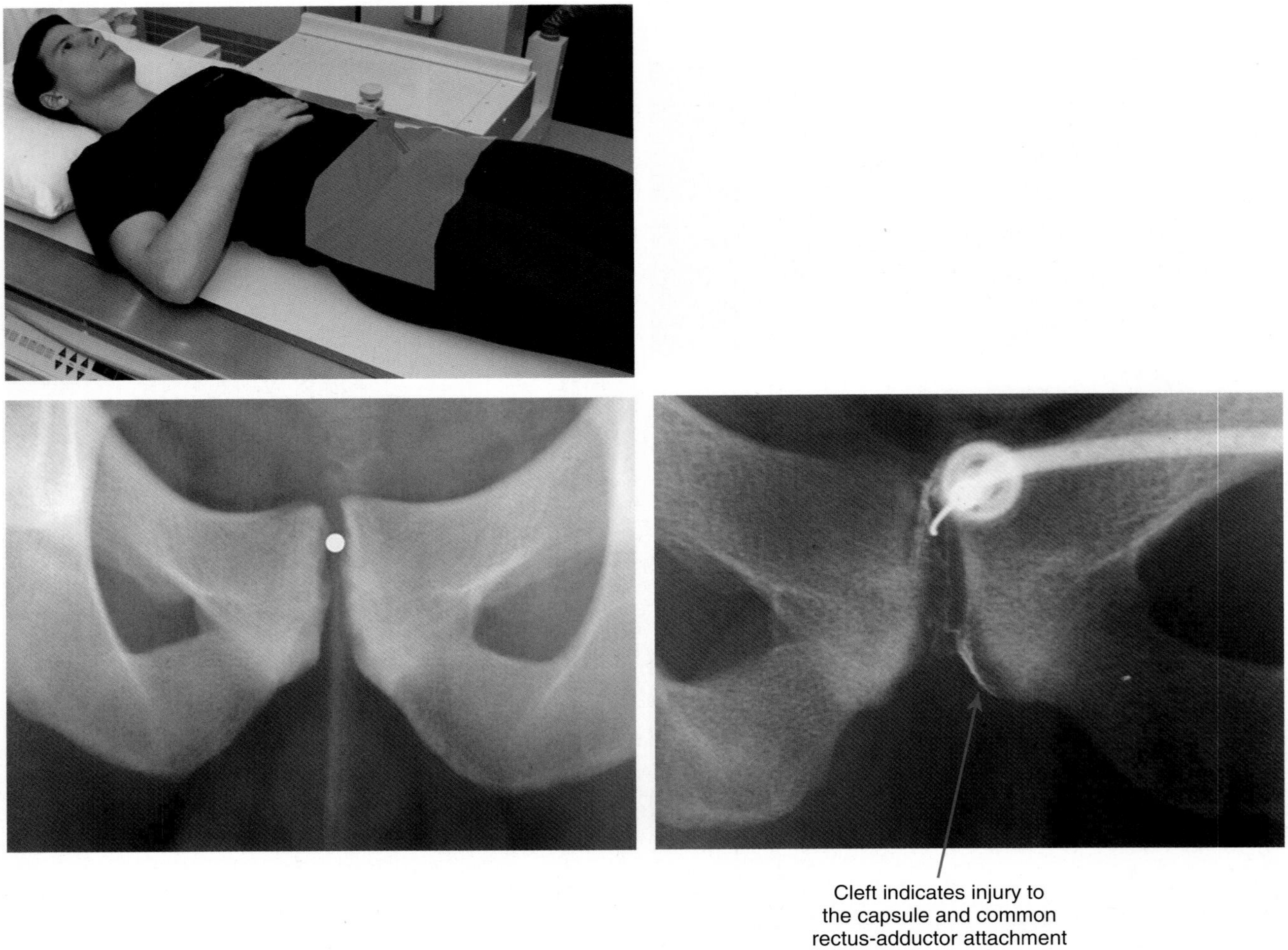
Cleft indicates injury to
the capsule and common
rectus-adductor attachment

Figure 2-33 **Pubic symphysis injection.**

Hip

When addressing the topic of hip arthrography, it is essential to review the anatomy of the femoral canal (Fig. 2-34). The femoral canal overlies the medial hip joint and is the passageway by which femoral neurovascular structures exit from the abdomen into the upper thigh. The boundaries of the femoral canal are anteriorly the inguinal ligament, medially the pubic bone and the lacunar ligament, laterally the iliopsoas muscle, and posteriorly the pubic ramus and pectineus muscle. The femoral canal is divided into two compartments by the medial border of the femoral vein. The medial compartment is termed the *femoral ring*. The lateral compartment contains the following structures from medial to lateral; lymphatic channels, the femoral vein, the femoral artery, and most laterally the femoral nerve. The femoral artery and vein are enclosed by the femoral sheath, an extension of the transversalis fascia. It is useful to palpate and mark the course of the femoral artery in each patient undergoing hip arthrography to ensure that inadvertent puncture of these vessels does not occur. Reliance on anatomic landmarks is not safe practice because variations in this region can occur and differences in the patient's body habitus can lead to misjudgment of where the femoral vessels lie.

Hip arthrography is commonly used to assess the articular cartilage, intra-articular bodies, and labral tears that may be associated with femoral-acetabular impingement. Therapeutic hip injection and diagnostic aspiration are also major indications for this technique.

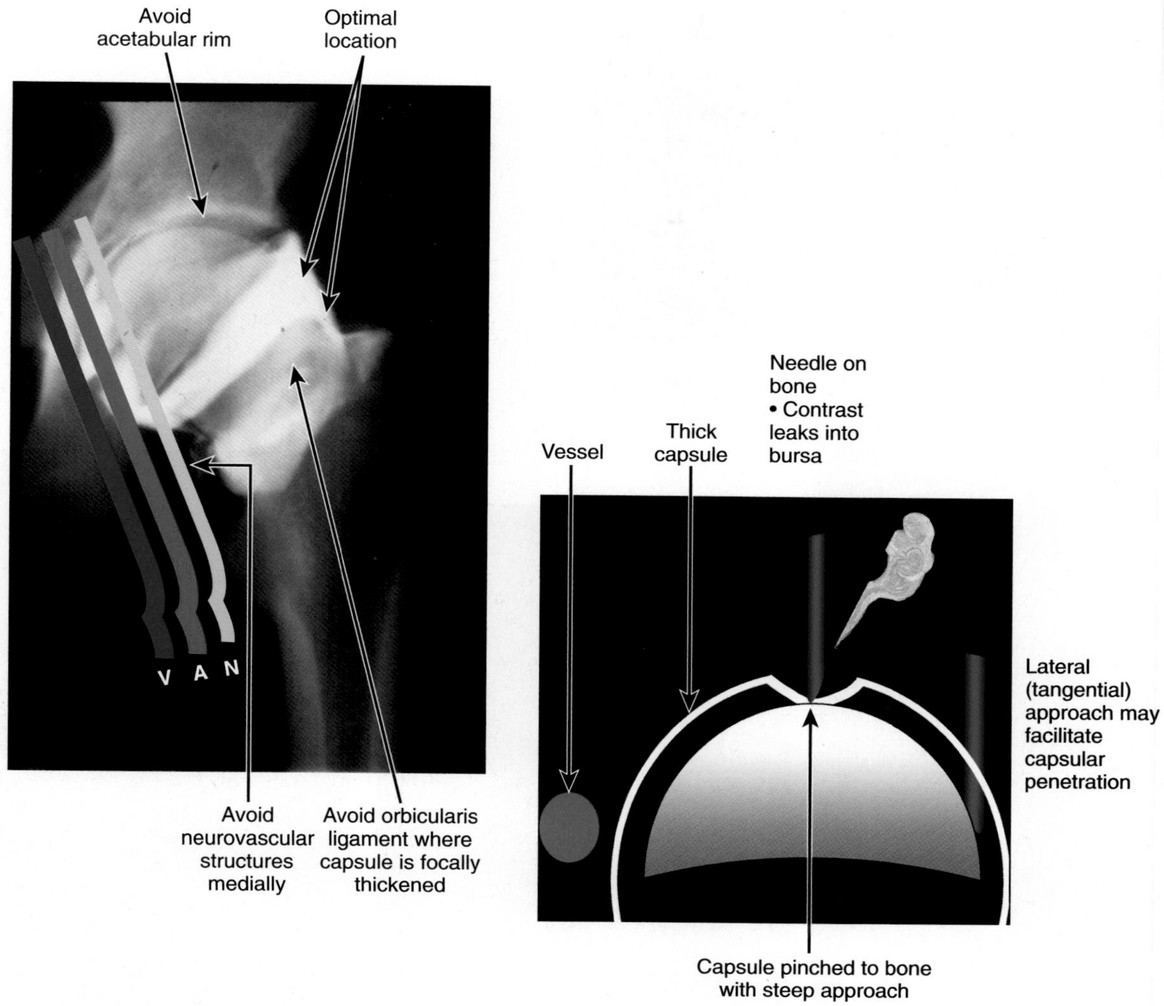
Avoid
acetabular rim
Optimal
location
V A N
Avoid
neurovascular
structures
medially
Avoid orbicularis
ligament where
capsule is focally
thickened
Vessel
Thick
capsule
Needle on
bone
• Contrast
leaks into
bursa
Lateral
(tangential)
approach may
facilitate
capsular
penetration
Capsule pinched to bone
with steep approach

Figure 2-34 Location of neurovascular structures around the hip joint and optimal location for injection. V, femoral vein; A, femoral artery. N, femoral nerve.

Hip arthrography is most commonly performed using a direct anterior approach, with the needle inserted toward the lateral aspect of the junction of the femoral head and neck (Fig. 2-35). The reason for this approach is that the joint capsule is a thick structure that is best approached at an angle (see Fig. 2-34). The medial joint should be avoided, since the femoral nerve and vessels overlie this region. Many different techniques for hip arthrography have been reported in the radiology literature. Some authors have recommended a lateral or steep oblique supratrochanteric approach, which may be useful in obese patients with abdominal pannus. Targeting the center of the femoral neck is a commonly used technique; however, a direct approach onto the femoral neck can pinch the capsule onto the bone, resulting in high resistance or injection into the bursa. Some authors recommend caudal or cranial angulation of the needle tip during its approach. For hip arthrography 10 to 12 mL of injectate is instilled into the hip joint, depending on the tolerated volume of the joint.

Total Hip Arthroplasty Aspiration

Aspiration of a total hip arthroplasty (THA) is a frequently requested radiologic exam. Postoperative patients with sepsis or pain may be referred for this technique. The technique of total hip aspiration is relatively straightforward, with fluoroscopic guidance (Fig. 2-36).

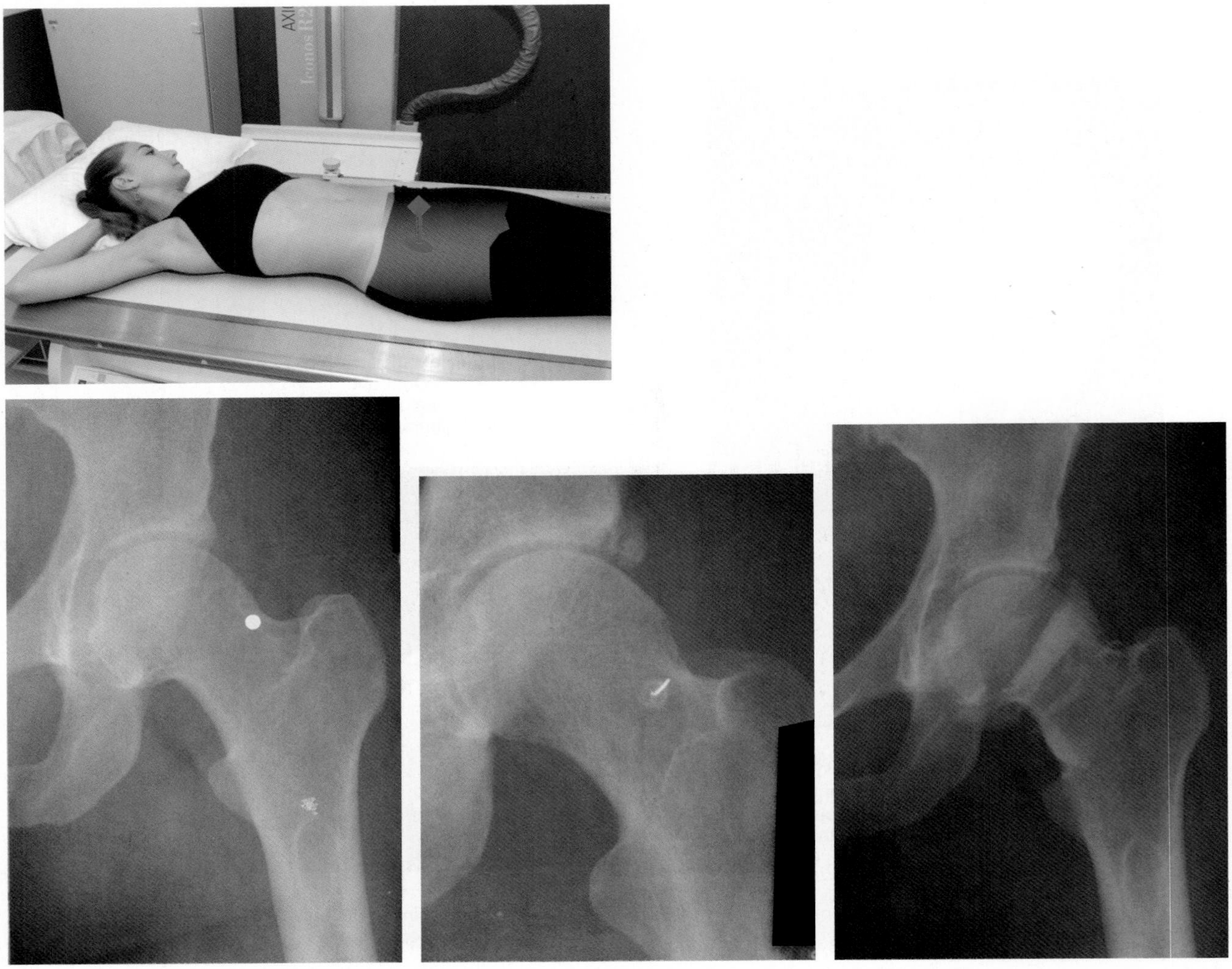

Figure 2-35 **Hip joint injection technique.**

The course and position of the femoral artery are marked on the patient's skin. This is important since anatomic markers may have changed in a postoperative patient as a result of scarring of the superficial tissues. After the skin is marked, an 18-gauge needle is advanced toward the metallic femoral head or neck component of the hip prosthesis. It may be difficult to visualize the needle on the fluoroscopic images because of the metallic nature of the total hip prosthesis. Angulation of the tube may aid visualization of the needle tip.

Once the needle is felt to impress on a metallic surface, an aspiration sample is obtained. If no fluid can be obtained, the needle should be "walked" around the medial and lateral aspects of the femoral neck. An alternative access method has been described which involves advancing the aspiration needle past the lateral aspect of the shaft of the prosthesis and into the dependent portion of the joint.

If still no fluid is obtained, 10 mL of sterile saline should be injected and an immediate aspiration taken. Fluid obtained is then sent for culture. Once the aspiration is completed, iodinated contrast is injected (7–15 mL) to verify intra-articular position and to evaluate for abnormal communication into any pathologic entities such as sinus tracts and abscesses, as well as around the prosthesis, indicating loosening. Postaspiration radiographs are then

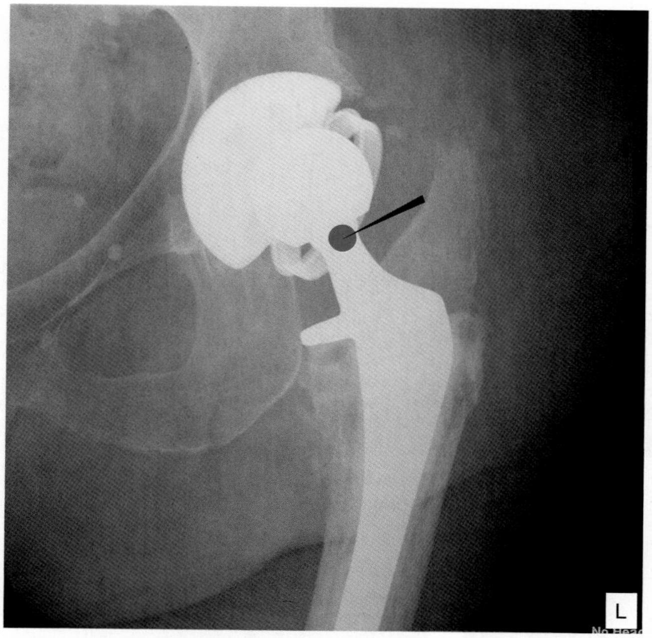
L

Figure 2-36 Total hip arthroplasty aspiration and injection. The prosthetic femoral head-neck junction is targeted. A characteristic metal-on-metal clink is felt as the needle hits the prosthesis.

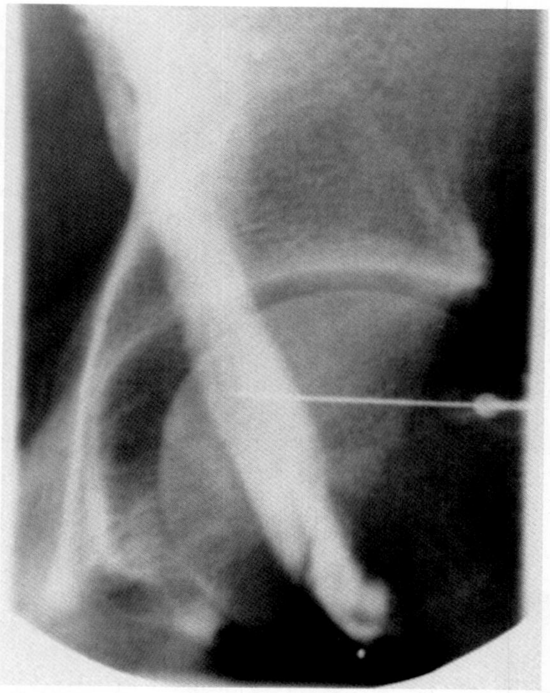

Figure 2-37 Iliopsoas bursagram.

obtained, including the whole prosthesis. Contrast extending around the prosthesis or bone-cement interface of the femoral component distally or the central aspect of the acetabular component is diagnostic of loosening.

Iliopsoas Bursagram

Occasionally it can serve a purpose to perform an iliopsoas bursagram. This can be performed for symptomatic iliopsoas bursitis and for differential diagnosis of snapping hip symptoms. The procedure is similar to a hip arthrogram as described previously, with two differences. First, the needle should be directed more medially (Fig. 2-37), corresponding to the course of the iliopsoas tendon. Second, the joint should be "missed": that is, the needle is passed to the bone but pulled back as contrast is injected. When decreased capsular resistance is noted and contrast is seen extending in an oblique vertical fashion above the hip joint, the correct location is documented. Anesthetic and steroid can be injected to test for symptom relief; also, the patient can perform the maneuver that causes the snapping sensation and the iliopsoas tendon (the lucent stripe within the contrast) is observed fluoroscopically for sudden snapping across the anterior acetabulum.

Knee

Conventional arthrography of the knee is now rarely performed because of the superiority of conventional MRI for the detection of internal derangement; however, injection of the knee remains common as a part of MR or CT arthrography. There are a few methods for access to the knee joint. The most popular method is via the patellofemoral joint, either medial or lateral. Many radiologists prefer the lateral approach, but the medial approach can be easier, especially when lateral patellar subluxation or spurs are present. However, if a lateral approach is used, the patella can be manually deflected medially during needle placement. A 1.5-inch, 20-gauge needle is used, and, whether medial or lateral, it is directed posterior to the mid-patella. One method of patellofemoral access involves placing the patient in the

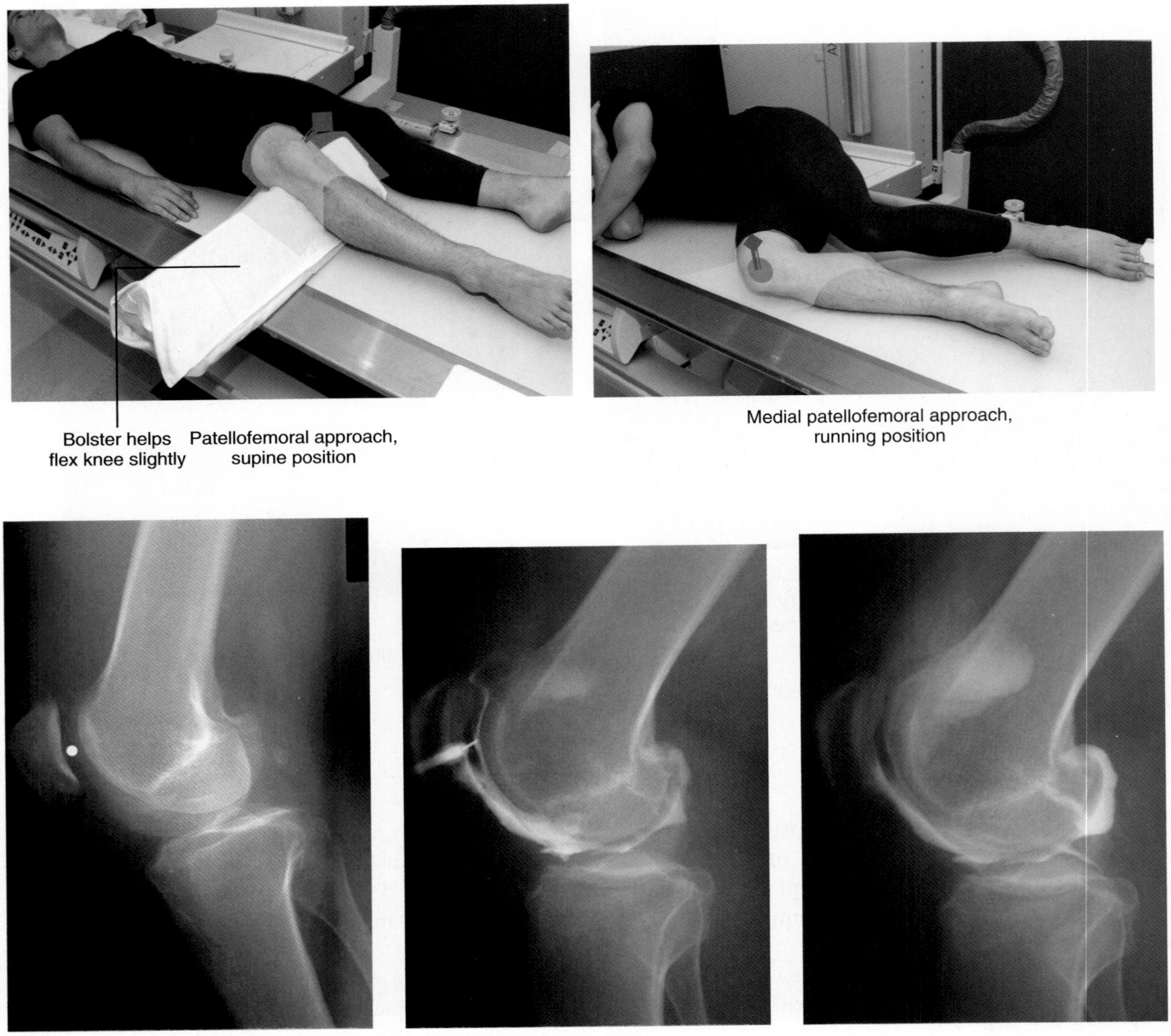
Bolster helps
flex knee slightly
Patellofemoral approach,
supine position
Medial patellofemoral approach,
running position

Figure 2-38 Knee arthrogram. Patellofemoral approach, supine position. Medial patellofemoral approach, running position.

supine position in which the knee is placed in slight flexion with a roll positioned under the popliteal fossa (Fig. 2-38). Some operators find that placing the patient on the side in the "running man" position is useful for this approach.

An anterior approach for knee arthrography, which mimics the route used for arthroscopy, has also been used with success (Fig. 2-39). With this technique, the knee is imaged in the lateral plane (in the running-man position), and following palpation of the patellar tendon the needle is advanced medial to the tendon in the direction of the trochlear sulcus. To perform knee arthrography via an anterior approach, a 3.5-inch, 20-gauge needle is recommended.

The total amount of injectate for knee arthrography is 20 to 30 mL, although generally the more the

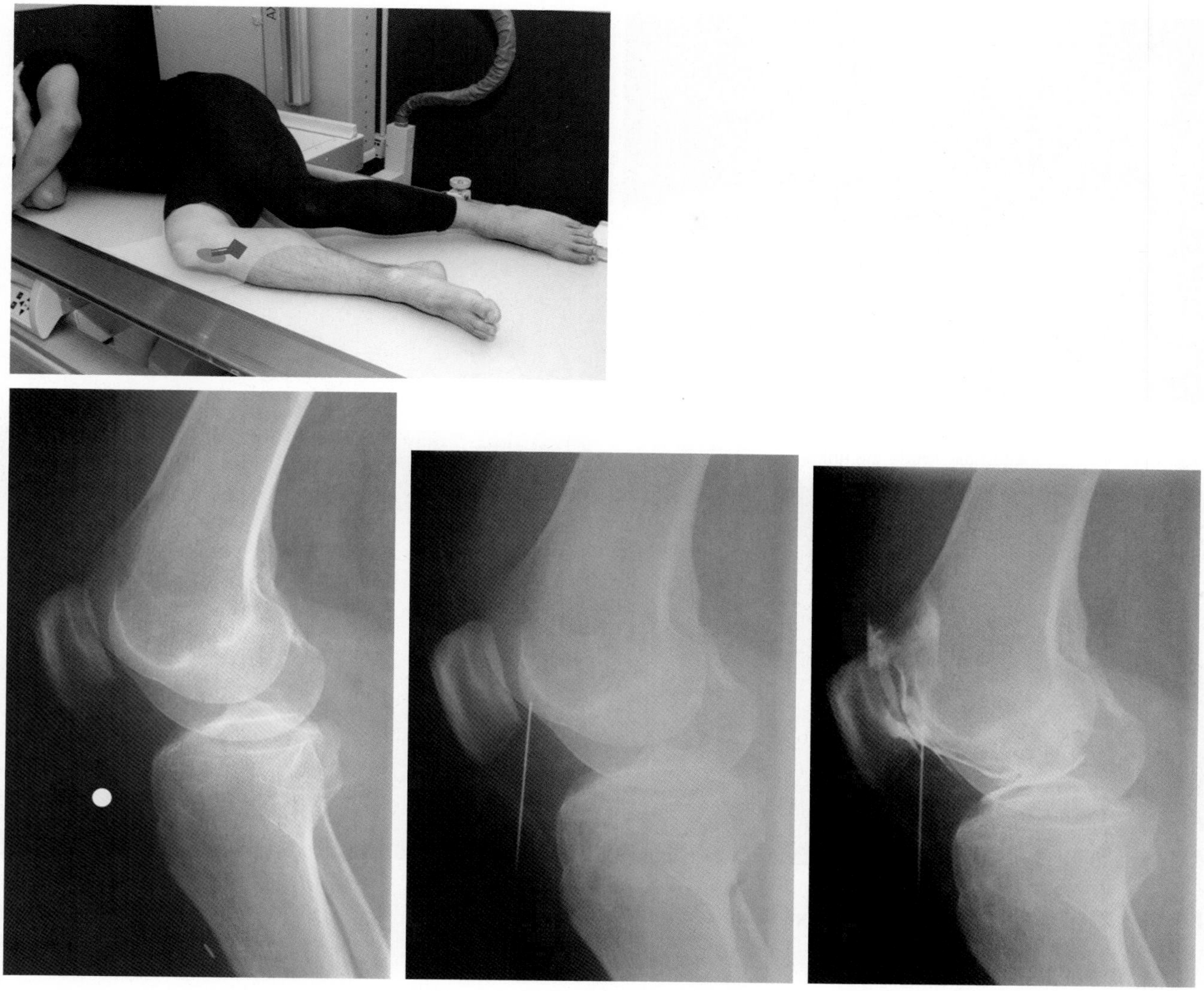

Figure 2-39 Knee arthrogram. Arthroscopic approach, running position.

better in terms of image quality. After injection, an elastic bandage can be wrapped around the knee above the patella to prevent contrast from pooling in the suprapatellar recess.

One of the main indications for direct MRA of the knee is in assessment of the postoperative knee. Meniscal re-tears are manifested as areas in which gadolinium penetrates the substance of the meniscus. Joint distention is therefore critical when performing direct MRA of the knee, to allow for passage of gadolinium into meniscal re-tears. It is also useful for evaluation of osteochondral lesions and intra-articular bodies.

Ankle—Tibiotalar Joint

For ankle arthrography, the course of the dorsalis pedis artery first should be marked. The artery is positioned lateral to the anterior tibialis tendon (ATT). If the patient dorsiflexes the foot against resistance, the ATT will become easy to palpate as a cord anteromedially. The optimal site for needle placement is just medial to the ATT. A running-man position is also useful to gain access while acquiring a lateral position for fluoroscopic monitoring (Fig. 2-40). After injection of a small volume of subcutaneous lidocaine and under fluoroscopic guidance, a 1.5-inch,

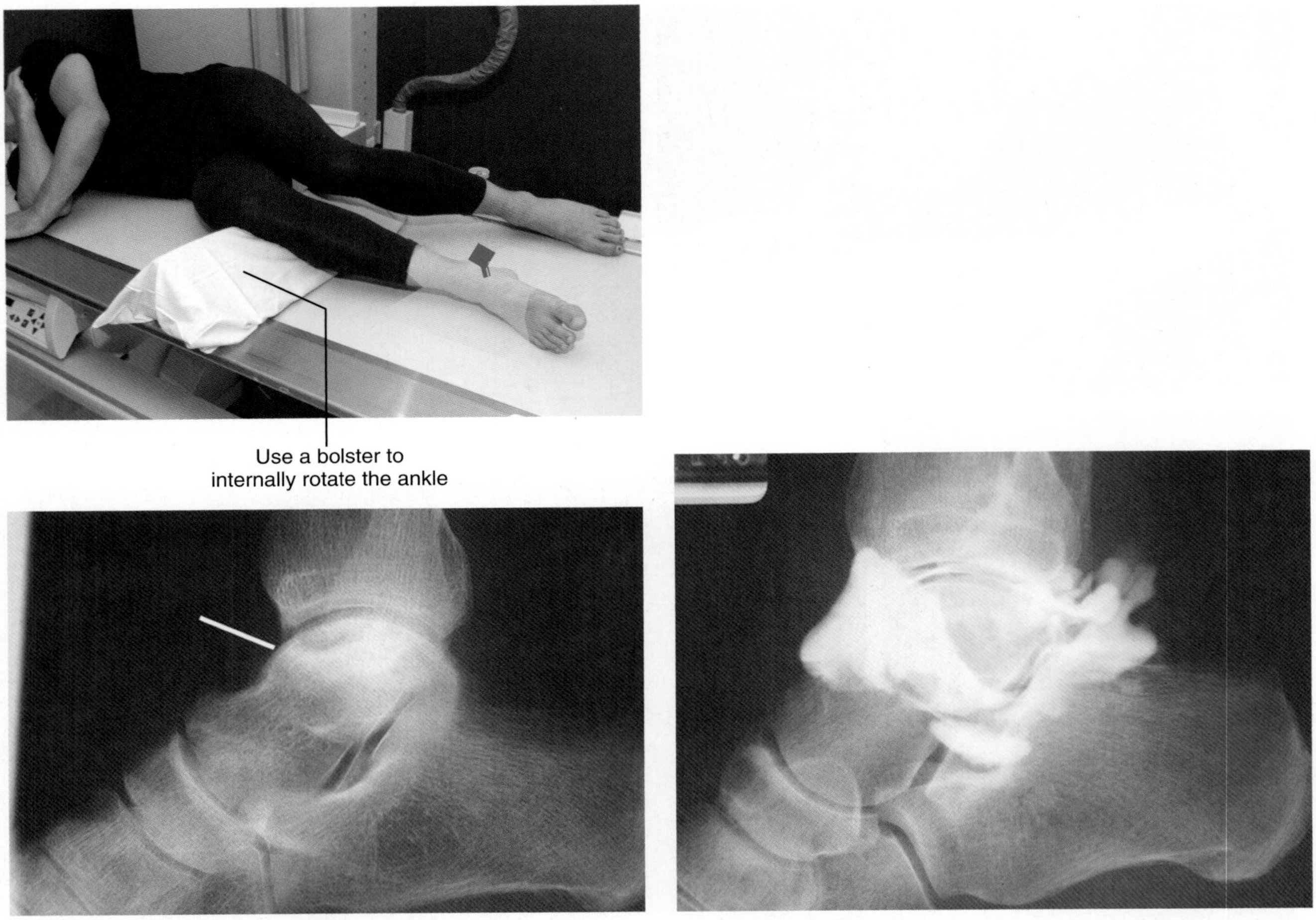
Use a bolster to
internally rotate the ankle

Figure 2-40 Ankle (tibiotalar) arthrogram technique.

20-gauge needle is introduced medial to the ATT, aiming laterally for the talar dome. Approximately 7 to 12 mL of injectate are injected into the joint. Contrast material may extend into the flexor hallucis longus tendon sheath and may also extend into the subtalar joint (6–25% of individuals). If this occurs then a greater volume of contrast may be required to distend the joint adequately.

Metatarsophalangeal Joint

Diagnostic arthography of the metatarsophalangeal joints is rarely performed but can be very useful for accurate evaluation of plantar plate tears and other pathologic conditions affecting these joints. With fluoroscopic guidance, a 1.5-inch, 22-gauge needle is advanced into the joint using a dorsal approach (Fig. 2-41). Similar technique is used for other small distal extremity joints, with positioning as needed to gain access.

Acromioclavicular Joint

Arthrography of the acromioclavicular joint is typically performed under fluoroscopic guidance with a 1.5-inch, 22-gauge needle introduced anterosuperiorly using cranial to caudal angulation. The patient is placed in the supine position. A tiny volume of contrast is injected into the joint to confirm intra-articular placement of the needle tip. This procedure is usually performed for administration of local anesthesia to the joint for documentation of symptom relief.

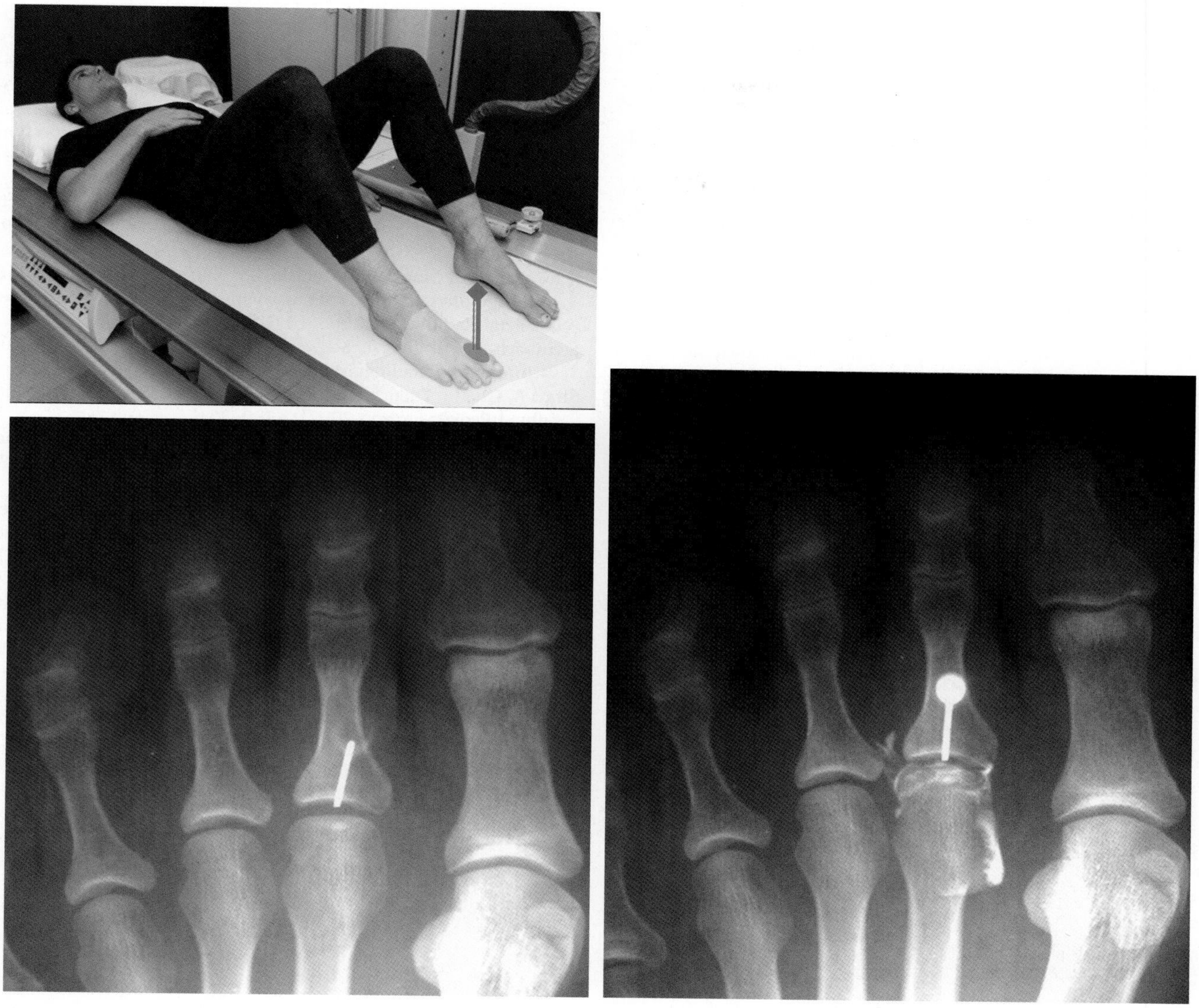

Figure 2-41 **Metatarsophalangeal arthrogram.**

Suggested Readings

Aliabadi P, Baker ND, Jaramillo D. Hip arthrography, aspiration, block, and bursography. Radiol Clin North Am 1998;36: 673–690.

Bergin D, Schweitzer ME. Indirect magnetic resonance arthrography. Skeletal Radiol 2003.32(10):551–558.

Brandser EA, El-Khoury GY, FitzRandolf RL. Modified technique for fluid aspiration from the hip in patients with prosthetic hips. Radiology 1997;204:580–582.

Brenner ML, Morrison WB, Carrino JA, et al. Direct MR arthrography of the shoulder: is exercise prior to imaging beneficial or detrimental? Radiology 2000;215(2):491–496.

Brown RR, Clarke DW, Daffner RH. Is a mixture of gadolinium and iodinated contrast material safe during MR arthrography? Am J Roentgenol2000;175:1087–1090.

Chung CB, Dwek JR, Feng S, Resnick D. MR arthrography of the glenohumeral joint: a tailored approach. AJR Am J Roentgenol 2001;177(1):217–219.

Cicak N, Matasovic T, Barraktarvic T. Ultrasonographic guidance of needle placement for shoulder arthrography. J Ultrasound Med 1992;11:135–137.

Depelteau H, Bureau NJ, Cardinal E, et al. Arthrography of the shoulder: a simple fluoroscopically guided approach for targeting the rotator cuff interval. AJR Am J Roentgenol 2004;182:329–332.

Dussault RG, Kaplan PA, Anderson MW. Flouroscopy-guided sacroiliac joint injection. Radiology 2000;214:273–277.

Farber JM. CT arthrography and postoperative musculoskeletal imaging with multichannel computed tomography. Semin Musculoskelet Radiol 2004;8(2):157–166.

Farmer KD, Hughes PM. MR arthrography of the shoulder: fluoroscopically guided technique using a posterior approach. AJR 2002;178:433–434.
Freiberger RH. Arthrography. Upper Saddle River, NJ: Prentice Hall, 1979.
Haims A, Katz LD, Busconi B. MR arthrography of the hip. Radiol Clin North Am 1998;36:691–702.
Hendrix RW, Anderson TM. Arthrographic and radiologic evaluation of prosthetic joints. Radiol Clin North Am 1981;19: 349–364.
Kenin A, Levine J. A technique for arthrography of the hip. Am J Roentgenol Radium Ther Nucl Med 1952;68:107–111.
Kilcoyne RF, Kaplan P. The lateral approach for hip arthrography. Skeletal Radiol 1992;21:239–240.
Kim KS, Lachman R. In vitro effects of iodinated contrast media on the growth of staphylococci. Invest Radiol 1982;17(3): 305–309.
Kramer J, Recht MP. MR arthrography of the lower extremity. Radiol Clin North Am 2002;40(5):1121–1132.
Masi JN, Newitt D, Sell CA, et al. Optimization of gadodiamide concentration for MR arthrography at 3 T. Am J Roentgenol 2005;184:1754–1761.
Miller TT. MR arthrography of the shoulder and hip after fluoroscopic landmarking. Skeletal Radiol 2000;29:81–84.
Montgomery DD, Morrison WB, Schweitzer ME, et al. Effects of iodinated contrast and field strength on gadolinium enhancement: implications for direct MR arthrography. J Magn Reson Imaging 2002;15(3):334–343.
O'Connell MJ, Powell T, McCaffrey NM, et al. Symphyseal cleft injection in the diagnosis and treatment of osteitis pubis in athletes. AJR Am J Roentgenol 2002;179(4):955–959.
Ozonoff MB. Controlled arthrography of the hip: a technique of fluoroscopic monitoring and recording. Clin Orthop 1973;93:260–264.
Resnick D. Shoulder arthrogrpahy. Radiol Clin North Am 1981;19: 243–253.
Salvati EA, Freiberger RH, Wilson PD Jr. Arthrography for complications of total hip replacement. A review of thirty-one arthrograms. J Bone Joint Surg Am 1971;53:701–709.
Schneider R, Ghelman B, Kaye JJ. A simplified injection technique for shoulder arthrography. Radiology 1975;114: 738–739.
Schwartz AM, Goldberg MJ. The medial adductor approach to arthrography of the hip in children. Radiology 1979; 132:483.
Schweitzer ME, Natale P, Winalski CS, Culp R. Indirect wrist MR arthrography: the effects of passive motion versus active exercise. Skeletal Radiol 2000;29(1):10–14.
Steinbach LS, Palmer WE, Schweitzer ME. Special focus session. MR arthrography. Radiographics 2002;22(5):1223–1246.
Straw R, Chell J, Dhar S. Adduction sign in pediatric hip arthrography. J Pediatr Orthop 2002;22:350–351.
Strife JL, Towbin R, Crawford A. Hip arthrography in infants and children: the inferomedial approach. Radiology 1984;152: 536.
Strobel K, Pfirrmann CW, Zanetti M, Nagy L, Hodler J. MRI features of the acromioclavicular joint that predict pain relief from intraarticular injection. AJR Am J Roentgenol 2003;181(3): 755–760.
Trattnig S, Breitenseher M, Rand T, et al. MR imaging-guided MR arthrography of the shoulder: clinical experience on a conventional closed high-field system. AJR Am J Roentgenol 1999; 172(6):157.
Valls R, Melloni P. Sonographic guidance of needle position for MR arthrography of the shoulder. AJR Am J Roentgenol 1997; 169(3):845–847.
Zurlo JV, Towers JD, Golla S. Anterior approach for knee arthrography. Skeletal Radiol. 2001;30(6):354–356.

Chapter 3

MUSCULOSKELETAL PERCUTANEOUS BIOPSY: Techniques and Tips

CHAPTER OUTLINE

Image-guided percutaneous biopsy of bone and soft tissue lesions has become integral to modern medical care and is an essential part of the practice of musculoskeletal radiology. This technique has a number of advantages. For example, imaging guidance increases the likelihood of the biopsy being acquired from the lesion if it is small or from viable regions of the lesion if it is large. Imaging also facilitates avoidance of vessels, nerves, organs, and other sensitive structures. Conscious sedation (or in some cases just local anesthetic) may be used rather than the general anesthesia that is associated with surgery. Therefore, percutaneous biopsy can also reduce risk of complications. Percutaneous biopsy has been shown in numerous studies to be safe and effective. However, biopsy must be performed by a radiologist with knowledge of equipment, use of the imaging modalities and relevant anatomy, approaches and potential complications, and limitations of the procedure. This chapter outlines these issues but cannot substitute for practical experience.

EVALUATION OF THE PRE-BIOPSY IMAGING STUDIES

A number of issues should be raised when a percutaneous biopsy is requested. The next step is strongly influenced by findings on recent imaging examinations on which the lesion was diagnosed. These exams should always be reviewed, without exception. The clinical service requesting a biopsy should provide all relevant imaging exams that were performed, and the institutional radiology information system should be searched for prior studies. The following questions should be considered:

1. Should the lesion be biopsied at all? Since there is a risk of morbidity and even mortality with biopsy and sedation, the onus is on the radiologist to make sure that the biopsy is indicated. The fact that the clinician demands it or wants peace of mind should not enter into the decision-making process. If the lesion is clearly benign, a biopsy may cause more harm, and the radiologist is the one who will be held accountable if a complication results.

   Conversely, the radiologist interpreting an exam should keep in mind that a report suggesting the presence of infection or tumor may obligate the surgeon to request biopsy, either surgical or percutaneous. If the lesion is clearly benign or noninfectious on imaging, an ambiguous report may be detrimental to the patient and could leave the radiologist at risk for litigation if a complication arises from the resultant invasive procedure. The two main situations in which this occurs are a bone lesion clearly demonstrating nonaggressive features and degenerative disk disease, which is often related to segmental instability. Ways to be more specific about these diagnoses are reviewed in Chapters 5 and 6.
2. Is the lesion too dangerous to biopsy (Box 3-1)? Of course, danger is in the eye of the beholder. Some radiologists are comfortable acquiring biopsies from lesions that others wouldn't touch (the body of C2 can be accessed through the oral cavity—would you try it?). For each lesion, the radiologist must weigh the benefits and risks based on the level of suspicion and experience in performing the particular approach required. This should be discussed with the referring clinician and the patient. In some cases, although the percutaneous biopsy approach is technically challenging, open surgery may carry even greater risk. This brings up the next principle.
3. Is there a better lesion to biopsy? The clinician often requests biopsy of the lesion that was found on prior exams, but this is not necessarily the best or safest lesion to sample. In suspected metastases, for example, there may indeed be a lesion at C5, but if a pelvic lesion or a lesion at L4 exists, the risk of complication from biopsy of one of these other lesions is clearly reduced. The clinician is often adamant that a particular lesion be biopsied. This may stem from the inexperience of the clinician, and some education is in order. However, sometimes there is good reason to sample the more challenging lesion. For example, for a spine lesion that is to be irradiated or surgically stabilized, one may need to document beforehand the histology of that particular lesion. Reports of patients receiving radiation therapy

BOX 3-1 HIGHER-RISK BIOPSIES

- Upper cervical spine
- Position adjacent to major vessels
- Highly vascular lesions in noncompressible tissues
- Spinal lesion with posterior wall compromise
- Uncooperative patient

for spine infection, or for lesions subsequently proven to be benign, support this. If an alternate site is chosen, care must be taken to document that the "safe" lesion being targeted is the same as the other lesion(s) that generated the clinical concern.

4. Does the patient have a bleeding problem? Is the platelet count adequate to initiate clot formation? Are the prothrombin time (PT) and activated partial thromboplastin time (PTT) adequate? The PT and PTT values are usually expressed as a combined value—the international normalized ratio (INR). It is difficult to provide definite cutoff values for biopsy since tolerance of abnormal values depends on a variety of factors, including whether the lesion appears highly vascular on imaging, whether there are adjacent blood vessels, and whether the lesion is deep or in a noncompressible location. If there is a concern, fresh frozen plasma (FFP) can be infused 1 to 2 hours before the procedure to temporarily normalize the values.
5. Is it infection or tumor? Could it be amyloid? These questions rarely influence the decision to biopsy once the lesion has been identified by the radiologist as being of concern. However, after the sample is acquired, decisions must be made regarding whether to send the sample to microbiology, pathology, or both. In general, it is prudent to also consider infection when tumor is the working diagnosis and to consider tumor when the lesion is suspected to be infection. Of course, if there is articular or disk involvement, tumor is much less likely; this rule of thumb applies mostly to atypical infections such as fungal and mycobacterial infections, which can appear masslike and simulate tumor. If the patient has renal failure and amyloid is suspected, the pathologist needs to be alerted to this because Congo red stain may be needed to test for amyloid.
6. In the case of tumor, could the course of the biopsy needle result in contamination of a potential myocutaneous flap? This is especially important when biopsy of a primary bone or soft tissue tumor is performed. Metastasis and myeloma are mainly treated systemically. In a primary lesion, the approach must always be discussed with the physician who will perform the definitive surgery because he or she will be the one deciding (assuming the worst-case scenario such as sarcoma) what flap to use during resection. Often this necessitates a more complicated and technically difficult biopsy approach. The surgeon may request that the tract be marked with methylene blue as the needle is removed. Also, based on the suspected tumor type, the pathologist may need a larger quantity of tissue (e.g., a larger core) to study the lesion architecture.
7. In the case of infection, could the needle course spread infection to bone, joint, or tendon sheath? In a common clinical scenario, a patient may have cellulitis, and a bone biopsy or joint aspiration is requested. If the needle passes through the infected tissue into uninvolved bone or synovium, these tissues can become infected as well. Therefore, the approach should always avoid overlying infected tissue. Again, this may complicate the procedure and requires more planning. The exception to this is when the bone or joint is clearly infected on imaging and when biopsy/aspiration is being performed to document the infecting organism.
8. Can the patient tolerate the biopsy? The patient should be asked beforehand whether he or she can tolerate the position required for biopsy. Occasionally, a biopsy is planned only to find out that the patient cannot lie on the stomach for more than a few minutes (e.g., because of recent surgery). A moving target makes for a dangerous biopsy, and whether voluntary or involuntary, motion should be minimized. Altering patient position to accommodate comfort can complicate the procedure (e.g., taking a biopsy of the spine with the patient on his/her side). Respiratory problems can not only cause problems with positioning but may also prevent use of conscious sedation. Patients who are uncooperative may need to be sedated more deeply to avoid excess movement.

EQUIPMENT

Guidance Modalities

An essential aspect to keep in mind when planning a biopsy is that the lesion should be visible on the guidance modality. Alternatively, if the lesion is extensive or infiltrative, the lesion itself need not be visible, just the region involved. Fluoroscopy has definite advantages over other modalities. For example, imaging is easily performed in real time. The limitation of projectional radiographic imaging is not a major one considering how easy it is to alter the angle craniocaudally or transversely to acquire a different

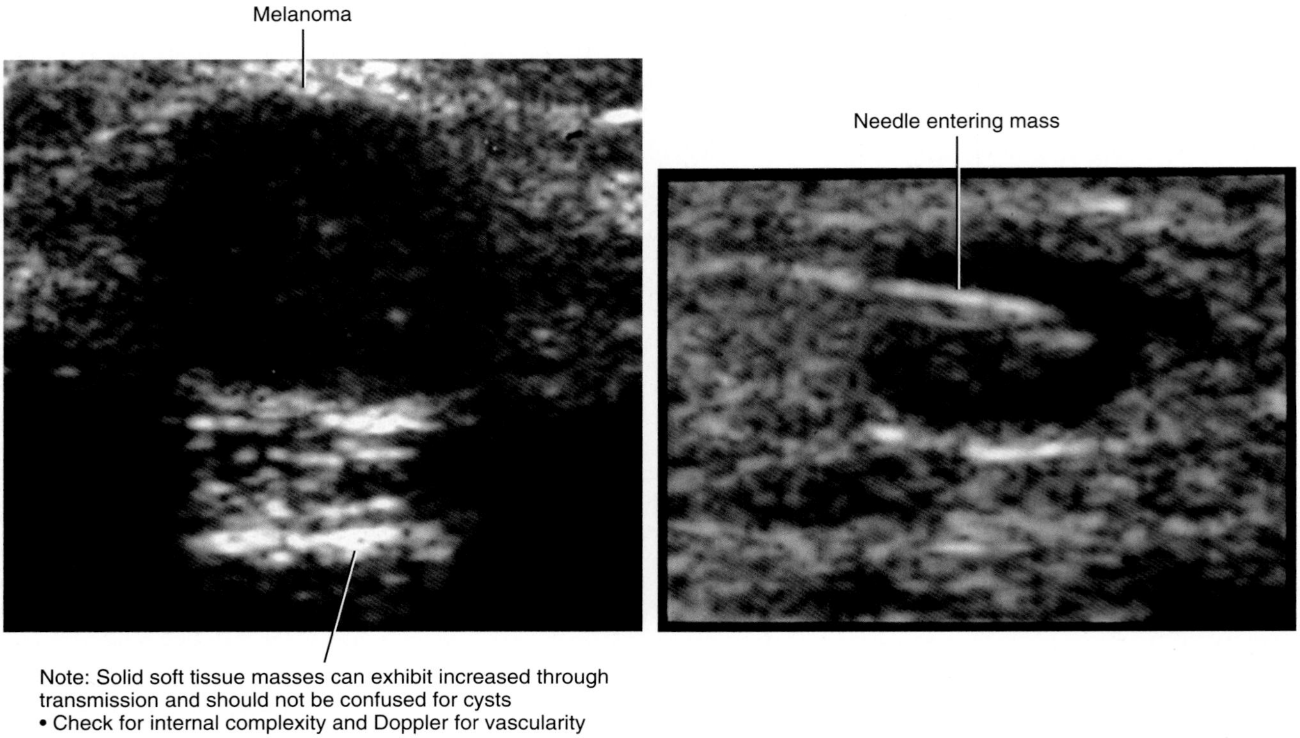
Melanoma
Needle entering mass
Note: Solid soft tissue masses can exhibit increased through transmission and should not be confused for cysts
• Check for internal complexity and Doppler for vascularity

Figure 3-1 **Ultrasound-guided biopsy.**

viewpoint. Biopsies using fluoroscopy are often easier to schedule as well. However, the room and configuration of the fluoroscopy equipment (C-arm, fixed-image intensifier, angiography room) can create problems with access to the biopsy area and must be considered in advance. Many angiography units have a narrow work area, which can cause problems when a long biopsy needle is used. Also, some C-arms and angiography units cannot achieve the angulations needed for the desired approach.

For most lesions, CT is the preferred guidance method. Simultaneous visualization of the lesion and soft tissue structures such as blood vessels is extremely helpful for planning the approach, especially for small or deep lesions. The angle of approach can be planned to avoid vital structures, and assessment of the depth to the lesion assists in needle selection. Repeat scans can be acquired in the plane of the needle when changes in needle position are made. CT fluoroscopy assists in speeding this process: Instead of leaving the suite for each scan, the operator remains in protective lead and steps on a foot pedal to almost instantly acquire a small series of images through the needle. Disadvantages of CT include relatively high radiation dose and limitation regarding craniocaudal angulation.

Ultrasonography is very versatile and can also be used for localization of soft tissue lesions (Fig. 3-1). Obviously, because ultrasound does not visualize within bone, it generally cannot be used for bone biopsy localization except for superficial lesions or those with cortical breakthrough. Ultrasound with Doppler easily visualizes blood vessels and can improve the safety of the desired approach. Solid and vascular regions of soft tissue masses can also be accurately targeted. The needle passage can be directly visualized in real time rather than periodically after repositioning.

MRI is used in some centers for localization but requires special preparation (Fig. 3-2). If equipment is needed (e.g., to provide sedation and monitoring) it must be MRI-compatible (e.g., all components must be nonferromagnetic). In addition, needles must be MRI-compatible and made of a material that creates relatively little artifact so that the needle tract is well visualized with reference to surrounding anatomy. MRI can be useful for ablation because the destroyed tissue can be visualized (e.g., ice ball formation in cryoablation).

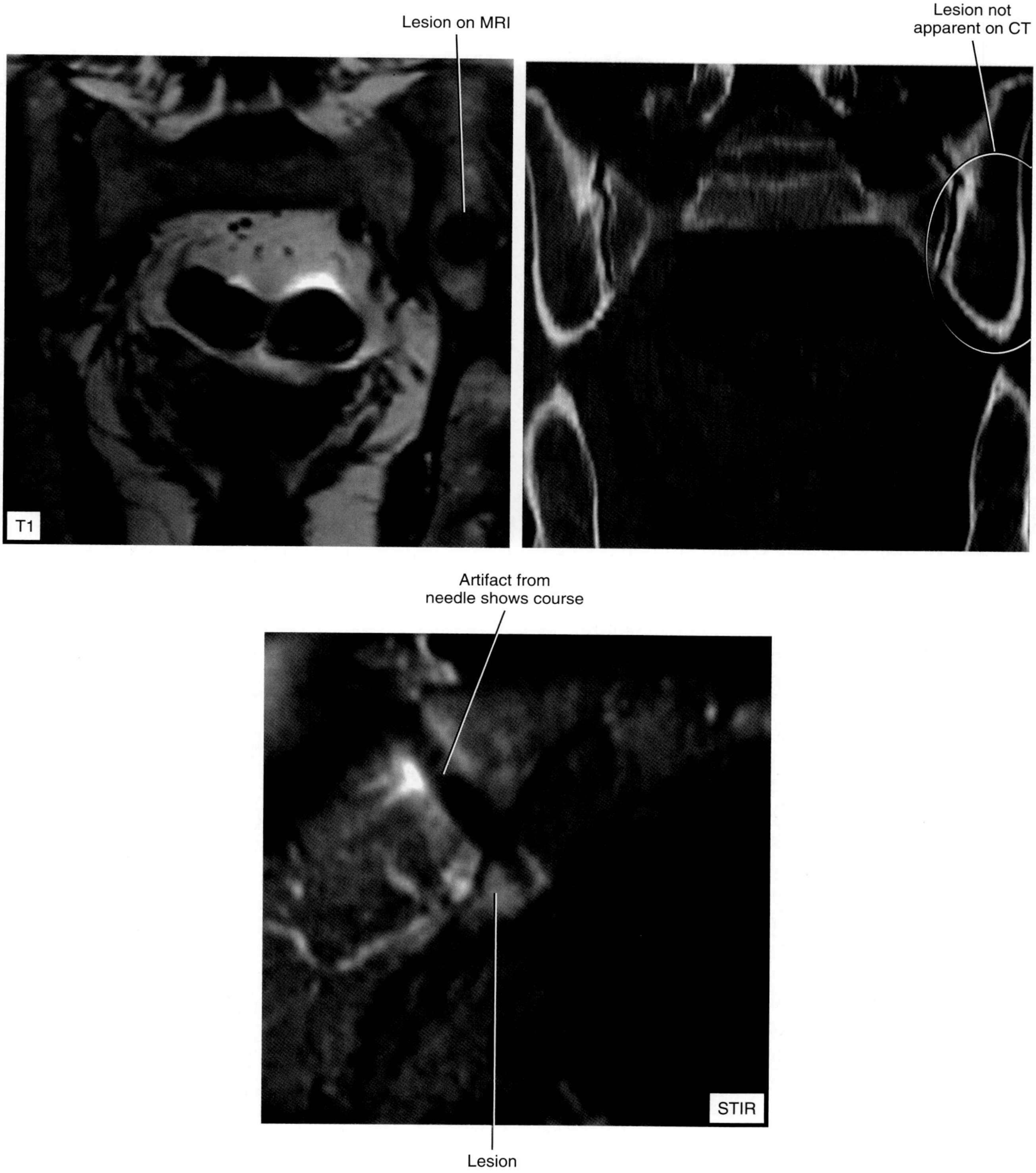
Lesion on MRI
Lesion not apparent on CT
T1
Artifact from needle shows course
STIR
Lesion

Figure 3-2 MRI-guided biopsy. MRI-compatible needles are available. Using T1 spin echo or STIR, lesions are visible and artifact is kept to a minimum, facilitating biopsy. This technique is useful for cryoablation as well as biopsy, the latter especially when the lesion is only visualized on MRI. (Courtesy of John Carrino, MD, MPH, Baltimore. (Carrino JA, Blanco R: Magnetic resonance-guided musculoskeletal interventional radiology. Semin Musculoskelet Radiol 2006;10[2]:159–174.)

Needles

Fine-Needle Aspiration Fine-needle aspiration needles are used for collection of cytology samples; needles are small gauge and collect groups of cells rather than core samples. The needle is placed within the lesion with stylet in place. The stylet is removed while using an "in-and-out" motion within the lesion; changing direction with each pass while pulling the stylet out collects the sample. Alternatively, a syringe can be attached to the needle hub and aspiration performed while the needle is manipulated. The sample is placed into cytology fluid; in the lab the sample is spun down into a block and evaluated.

Fine-needle aspiration is especially useful because low-profile needles may reduce the risk of damage to adjacent tissues. However, unless real-time imaging is performed during needle manipulation (i.e., ultrasound) the in-and-out motion is performed blindly and may not be advised for lesions near vital structures. Another disadvantage is that the architecture of the lesion is altered and the sample volume is small, making it more difficult to make the diagnosis, especially for primary lesions. Nevertheless, some authors have recommended that a cytology sample be acquired in addition to the core biopsy sent to the histology department for increased diagnostic yield overall.

Diagnostic yield is highly dependent on the experience of the interpreting cytologist or pathologist. Close communication between the radiologist and the pathologist is important to give feedback in both directions. The radiologist should discuss radiologic findings with the pathologist, especially for atypical cases, and the pathologist should provide feedback to the radiologist regarding the quality of the samples acquired that may require a change in needle type or methodology.

Needles have a variety of configurations and tips designed to offer different advantages. Since there are many needles and vendors are continually modifying them, it is difficult to discuss the specific features of each. However, some general features can be outlined with reference to their intended purpose.

Coaxial Systems Coaxial systems are needles that have an outer sheath and an inner cutting needle and are intended for either soft tissue or bone (Figs. 3-3 and 3-4). The cutting needle extends a certain distance beyond the sheath. This is almost universally used in musculoskeletal biopsies because it requires only one localization/placement procedure to position the sheath/stylet at the margin of the lesion, after which multiple passes can be obtained. The only situation in which a non–coaxial system may be used is a very superficial lesion that is easy to localize and that is not near any vital structures (Figs. 3-5 and 3-6).

Soft Tissue Guns Soft tissue guns collect a core of tissue unlike with fine aspiration needles (Fig. 3-7). They are larger gauge—typically 14 to 18 G. Rather than having a hollow cutting needle design, they incorporate a solid inner core with a recess near the tip. This portion of the needle is advanced into the lesion, after which an inner sheath "shoots" over it, cutting the tissue filling the recess. The system is then withdrawn from the outer sheath and the sample is collected. Therefore, two components are advanced in succession: the solid inner needle and the inner sheath. In some needles this is automated, triggered by a button that is pressed when the needle is in position. However, it is not always desirable to shoot the inner needle without feel or control. For example, if the lesion is near a vital structure or not as large as the "throw" of the needle, it is better to retain control of the first step. Some needles have a setting or alternate triggering mechanism that allows the radiologist to slowly advance the inner needle as far as desired; when in position, the sheath is triggered to advance.

Bone Biopsy Needles Various techniques are used to cut and hold the sample in the needle. The Elson and Ackermann needles (Cook; see Fig. 3-3) have a serrated tip that is useful for cutting through cortex. Trephine needles such as the Jamshidi have a simple, beveled tip that facilitates purchase on bone. These needles have a straight inner bore without tapering. However, most needles have a tapered tip, in which the end of the needle is curved slightly inward. After the needle is advanced into the lesion, the end is "wobbled" or rotated to cut the tip of the core. The disadvantage of this is that the actual inner gauge of the needle is smaller than advertised on the package. If the needle is used as a sheath for another needle, this must be taken into account; there may be a 2- to 3-gauge difference in what can actually fit through the needle. The Ostycut needle (Bard, Tempe, Ariz; see Fig. 3-6) has a threaded tip that is screwed into the lesion; altering the course and advancing farther are supposed to result in cutting the sample. A syringe

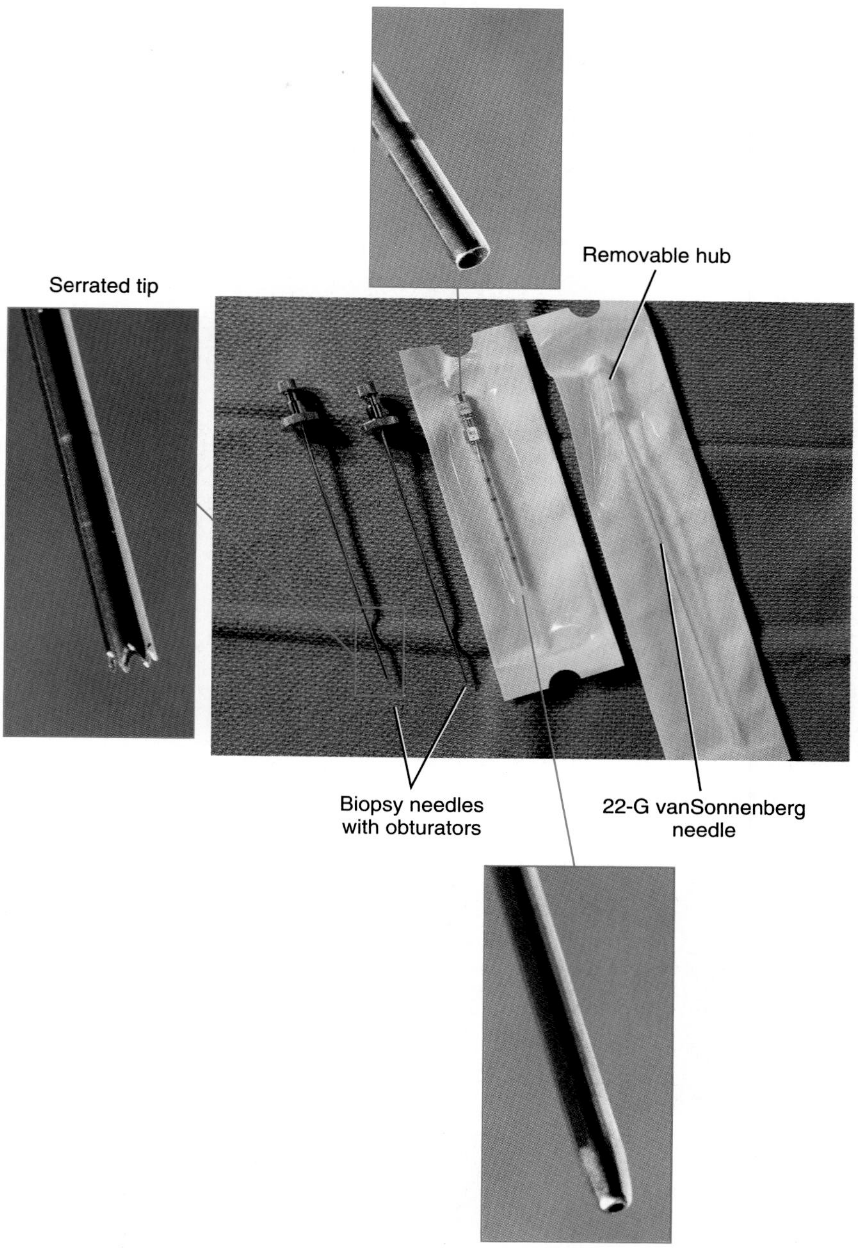
Sheath
Serrated tip
Removable hub
Biopsy needles
with obturators
22-G vanSonnenberg
needle
Hollow stylet

Figure 3-3 Coaxial bone biopsy needles. Cook Elson/Ackermann 14 G pictured. Available with solid or hollow stylet. Hollow version is especially useful for accessing difficult lesions; after a 22-G vanSonnenberg needle is passed safely to the site, the entire hub can be removed and the Ackermann needle passed over the needle down to the lesion. Multiple biopsies can be acquired coaxially through the sheath. (Courtesy of Catherine Roberts, MD, Scottsdale, AZ.)

can be used to provide negative pressure in the needle to assist in retention of the core. The TrapLok system (MD Tech, Gainesville, FL; see Fig. 3-5) has a thin, curved implement that hugs the inner margin of the needle and is advanced around the core, "trapping" it in as the needle is withdrawn.

The Bonopty needle system (Radi, Uppsala, Sweden; see Fig. 3-4) is a coaxial system in which the radiologist can substitute the stylet for a small drill. The drill is slightly eccentric and wobbles, thereby cutting a hole large enough to accommodate the sheath. The drill is excellent for accessing lesions within sclerotic bone or through thick cortex. Also, lesions that are deep within bone (e.g., anterior vertebral body lesion approached through the pedicle) can be difficult to access coaxially with other systems. With Bonopty, the sheath/stylet is placed at the outer margin of bone, lined up with the lesion; the stylet is replaced

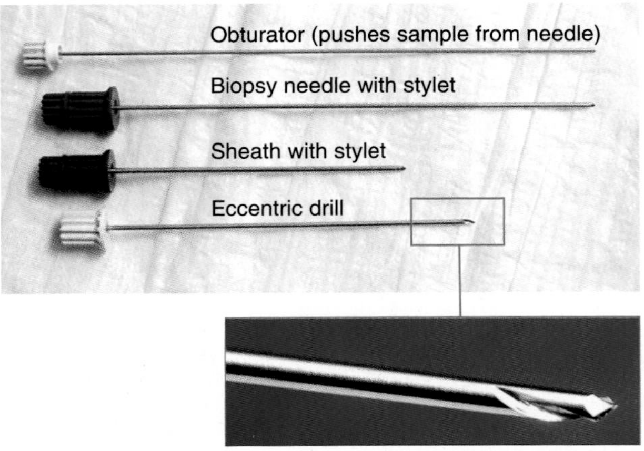
Obturator (pushes sample from needle)
Biopsy needle with stylet
Sheath with stylet
Eccentric drill

Figure 3-4 Bone biopsy needles. RADI Bonopty 15 G with eccentric drill. This is a coaxial system that is very advantageous for penetrating thick cortex. (Courtesy of Catherine Roberts, MD, Scottsdale, AZ.)

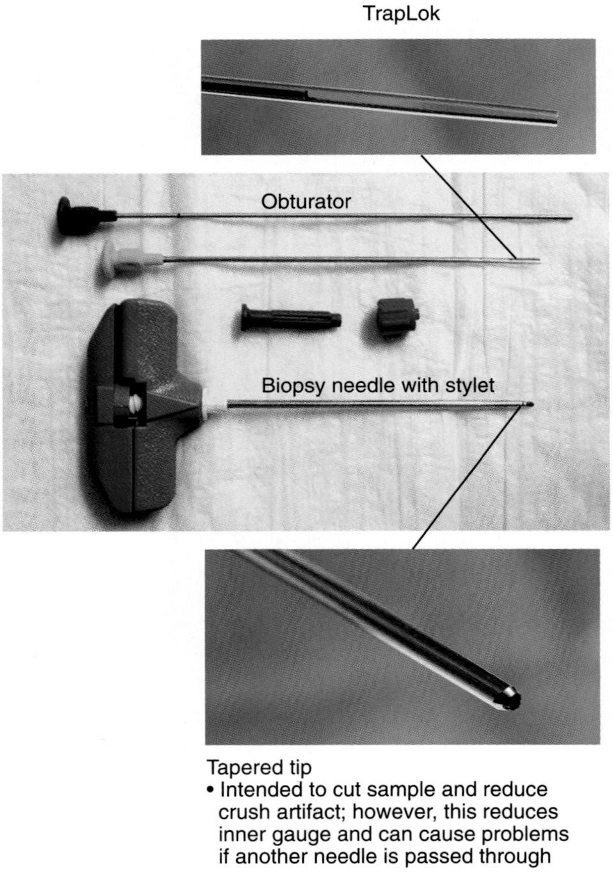
TrapLok
Obturator
Biopsy needle with stylet
Tapered tip
• Intended to cut sample and reduce crush artifact; however, this reduces inner gauge and can cause problems if another needle is passed through

Figure 3-5 Noncoaxial bone biopsy needles. MD Tech 11 G with TrapLok pictured. This is not a coaxial system, therefore it is disadvantageous for most image-guided biopsies. After advancing the biopsy needle into bone, inserting the TrapLok device is intended to hold the sample in place. (Courtesy of Catherine Roberts, MD, Scottsdale, AZ.)

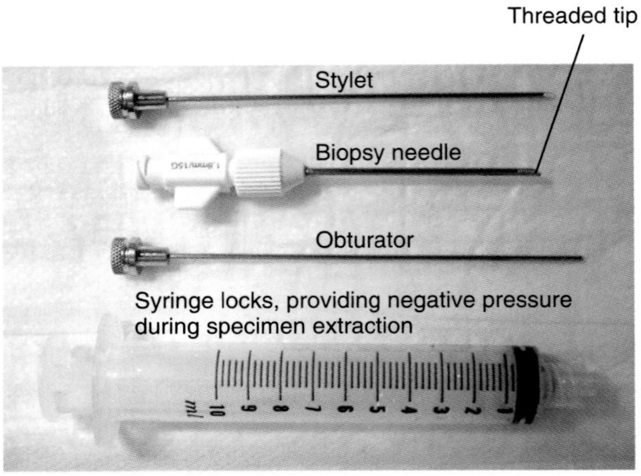
Threaded tip
Stylet
Biopsy needle
Obturator
Syringe locks, providing negative pressure during specimen extraction

Figure 3-6 Noncoaxial bone biopsy needles. Bard Ostycut 15 G pictured. This system has been limited by lack of a coaxial design. However, the short version is useful for biopsy of superficial bones.(Courtesy of Catherine Roberts, MD, Scottsdale, AZ.)

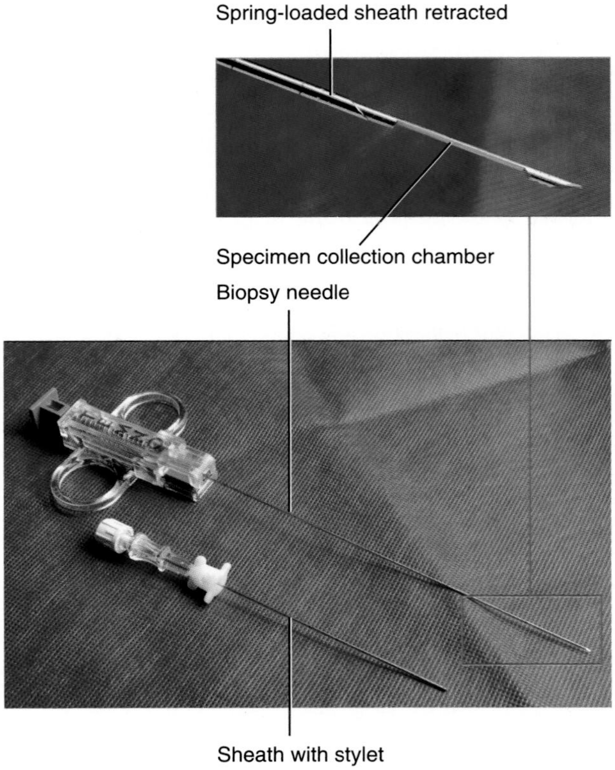
Spring-loaded sheath retracted
Specimen collection chamber
Biopsy needle
Sheath with stylet

Figure 3-7 Soft tissue guns. There are many types available (Temno, Cardinal Health, Inc., Dublin, OH, pictured). A spring-operated sheath shoots over the stylet containing a cutout portion for collecting the sample. Soft tissue guns may also be used coaxially through a trocar bone biopsy sheath, which can punch through cortex to sample lytic lesions within bone.

with the drill, which creates a pathway. The sheath is advanced over the drill, and this process is continued until the lesion is reached. Next, the drill is replaced with the cutting needle, and multiple samples are acquired through the sheath.

With all bone biopsy needles, the core can occlude the needle, making it difficult to advance. This is especially true when a thick cortex is penetrated. If it is difficult to advance the needle at any point, the bore may be occluded and the needle should be withdrawn and cleared. If this is not done, the biopsy is made more difficult and the sample can be damaged with crush artifact seen at histology.

Stylets Stylets are kept in the needle and function to occlude the barrel (avoiding extraneous tissue damage and sampling), help guide the needle in place (for beveled stylets), and achieve "purchase," or initiation of entry into bone (Fig. 3-8). Although different vendors sell a number of configurations, the point can be either in the center (diamond tip) or at the edge with a flat, tilted surface (bevel).

Diamond point tips make the needle more difficult to steer. However, this type of tip has the advantage of being deflected less than a beveled tip by fascia and muscle. The diamond tip may also be easier to achieve purchase in bone.

A beveled tip can be very useful to guide the needle in place by directing the open aspect of the bevel away from the desired direction. This can be useful for deflection within bone as well, especially for vertebroplasty. When the desired angle of approach is achieved, some needles allow for trading with a diamond tip stylet, facilitating straight advancement toward the lesion.

When guiding a needle into place through soft tissue, it should be recognized that the fascia serves as a fulcrum. If proper guidance cannot be achieved

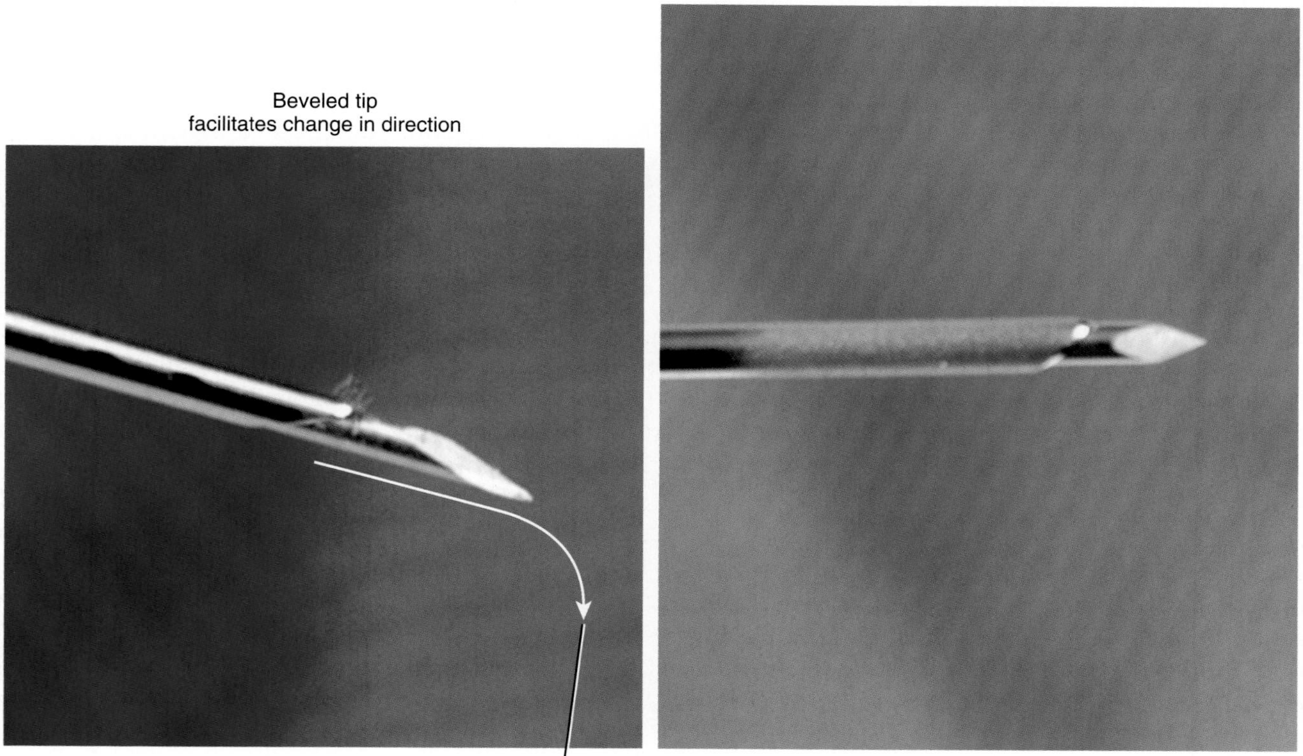
Diamond tip
optimally achieves purchase in bone
Beveled tip
facilitates change in direction
Direction needle
will tend to go

Figure 3-8 **Stylet types and function.**

and the needle continues along the same course, it may need to be pulled back beyond the primary fascia, or a deeper skin/fascial cut should be made (rather than just a skin nick).

Selection of Appropriate Needle The optimal needle should always be selected before the procedure, with an alternate choice kept to the side. The pre-biopsy imaging is very useful for planning needle selection. Axial CT or MR images are especially useful; the angle and distance from the skin can be evaluated. The depth of the lesion within bone and thickness of the cortex should be noted (a drill-type needle may be needed). If the lesion is lytic and near the cortex, a combination of bone and soft tissue biopsy needles can be used. For example, a large-bore bone biopsy needle can be used to punch a hole in the intact cortex positioned at the superficial margin of the lesion; the stylet is removed and a soft tissue gun is passed coaxially into the lesion and samples are acquired. If this method is used, care should be taken *not* to use the automatic needle throw. Some soft tissue guns function by cocking the needle back and pressing a button, causing the needle to shoot out 2 to 4 cm followed immediately by the sheath, cutting the sample. If this is done within or onto bone, the end of the needle can bend or break.

It can be difficult to acquire a solid sample from very aggressive, lytic lesions using a bone biopsy needle alone. One technique is to pass the needle completely through the lesion (assuming the opposite cortex is intact), impacting bone into the tip of the needle, holding the sample in the needle. If the lesion is lytic and the cortex is permeated or thinned, a soft tissue gun inserted through a sheath may be the best option. The sheath of a soft tissue gun with stylet in place can be used to punch through the weakened cortex and the sample acquired as previously described.

Length On the preliminary imaging studies, an estimation should be made regarding the depth of the lesion through soft tissue and regarding how much bone should be traversed to reach the lesion at the planned angle of approach. Obviously, the needle selected should be long enough to reach the bone. Some needles can more easily traverse bone than others. For lesions deep within bone, an eccentric drill system (Bonopty) is very useful, for example, for a lesion in the anterior vertebral body for which a transpedicle approach is planned. However, the needle is short, which may be a limiting factor in obese patients.

Needle Gauge and Number of Passes In general, for all lesions, the larger the cores and the more cores are acquired, the better. The core sent to histology shrinks 25% to 50% during decalcification, so the actual sample size is smaller than the needle width would suggest. However, thought should always be given to the safety of the patient, and if the lesion is near vessels, nerves, or other important structures, a smaller-gauge needle may be a better choice. Similarly, more passes with the needle may increase the potential for complications if the lesion is near a vital area. Typically, three to five passes are taken.

The smaller the sample size, the less architecture is available for evaluation. Often, an associated soft tissue or periosteal reaction is intermingled with the biopsy material. If the biopsy is small, the neoplastic component may not be adequately represented and an erroneous diagnosis may result. On the other hand, some aggressive tumors such as Ewing sarcoma and osteosarcomas often have a soft tissue extension that can be easily sampled, is less calcified than the intramedullary component, and is amenable for frozen section analysis. Histologic grading can also be affected owing to variations in tumor sampling from field to field (cartilaginous tumors, dedifferentiation within a neoplasm). In addition, some biphasic lesions (i.e., fibrous dysplasia, secondary ABC change) may contain a predominance of one component in one area while another component may predominate elsewhere. Sampled tissue must be adequate to perform ancillary studies (immunohistochemical, culture, molecular diagnostics, flow cytometry) if needed.

Whenever possible, it is beneficial to have a cytologist present to verify that an adequate sample has been acquired. Although this increases the time of the procedure, it helps to prevent the need for re-biopsy. The experience of the pathologist is important as well. If there is no bone pathologist at the institution, "yield" or success of biopsy may be artificially low because of hedging with a high ratio of "inadequate samples." On the other hand, the radiologist can help to prevent this by providing as much relevant clinical information as possible on the request. A good pathologist reviews imaging studies of cases that are not clear-cut. Similarly, for cases of infection, yield may be increased if the sample is sent for both histologic and microbiologic evaluation. Even if no bacteria are cultured from the sample, histologic evaluation can confirm the presence of osteomyelitis. Lidocaine, once thought to be inhibitory toward the growth of bacteria, has been found to have no significant effect on growth.

Always check the needles before penetrating the skin. Check for the following:

- *Soft tissue guns:* Measure how far through the sheath the cutting needle goes. When the sheath is in place within the lesion and is 2 cm from the aorta, this is not the time to be guessing.
- *Combinations of needles* (i.e., using one biopsy needle as a sheath for a smaller cutting needle, creating a coaxial system from separate vendors): Make sure the needles fit together and that the cutting needle can pass far enough through the bone to reach the lesion. Usually, a 2-gauge difference between the outer and inner needle is enough to ensure a proper fit. However, if the outer needle selected has a tapered tip (see Fig. 3-5), the effective caliber of the inner channel is constricted at the tip and the needle may not fit all the way through. In this case, a thinner inner needle can be selected or a nontapered outer needle used. Some needles indicate on the package an accurate inner core diameter, which facilitates selection of the biopsy needle; however, this is variable and should always be tested before patient use.

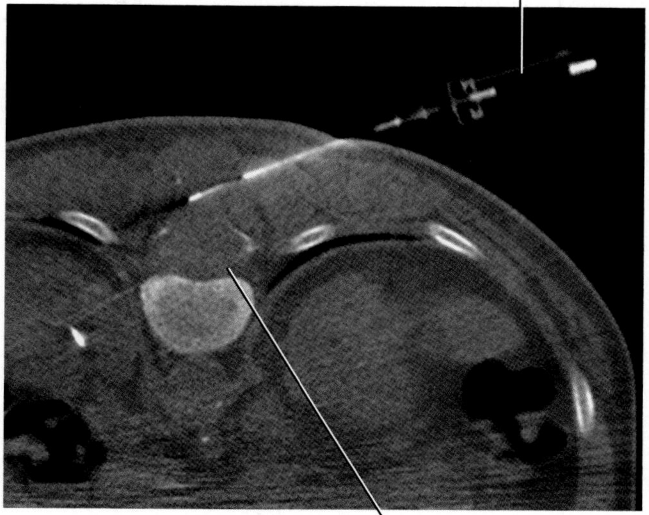
Superficial lesion
• Tangential approach can help anchor the needle
Soft tissue gun
This approach also helps avoid the spinal canal
Metastastic lesion of the spinous process

Figure 3-9 Superficial lesion. This can be difficult if the needle has to be held in place while scanning in between passes. Solutions are (1) to use a shorter, smaller needle; (2) to use a tangential approach (see figure); (3) to achieve a longer course through the soft tissues, which can anchor the needle better, and (4) to use an external holder.

LESION TYPES AND APPROACHES

Many techniques and approaches have been described for various lesion types and locations. The needle or needle combination used depends on the location and type of lesion as well as on practitioner comfort and experience. One general concept is that the adjacent vital structures, such as the spinal canal, pleura, or aorta, must be directly visualized or location easily surmised using the modality selected. For all lesions under CT guidance, one must always measure from the skin straight to the closest "danger point" (e.g., pleura, aorta, and so on). The needle must not be inserted beyond this point before checking position and angle.

Superficial Lesions (Figs. 3-9 through 3-11)

The problem with superficial lesions is that the needle flops against the skin and doesn't stay in line after positioning. If imaging is truly needed for localization, this can be a challenging situation. Ultrasound guidance may be the best option in this circumstance. If CT or fluoroscopy is used, it is helpful to use the shortest needle available (e.g., 5 cm) and park the sheath at the lesion, acquiring samples via coaxial technique. If the small sheath will not stay in place, a small needle (e.g., 22 G, 1.5 inch) can be localized at the margin of the lesion by imaging and the orientation of this needle can be used as a guide for the biopsy needle orientation. If the lesion is large enough, a coaxial technique may not be needed at all, and a simple biopsy needle can be passed repeatedly into the lesion and samples collected through the same skin site.

Rib Lesions

Rib lesions can be challenging to biopsy (see Fig. 3-11). The bone is small and rounded, and needles can slip off with pleura and lung underneath. In addition, the ribs pass obliquely through the axial plane,

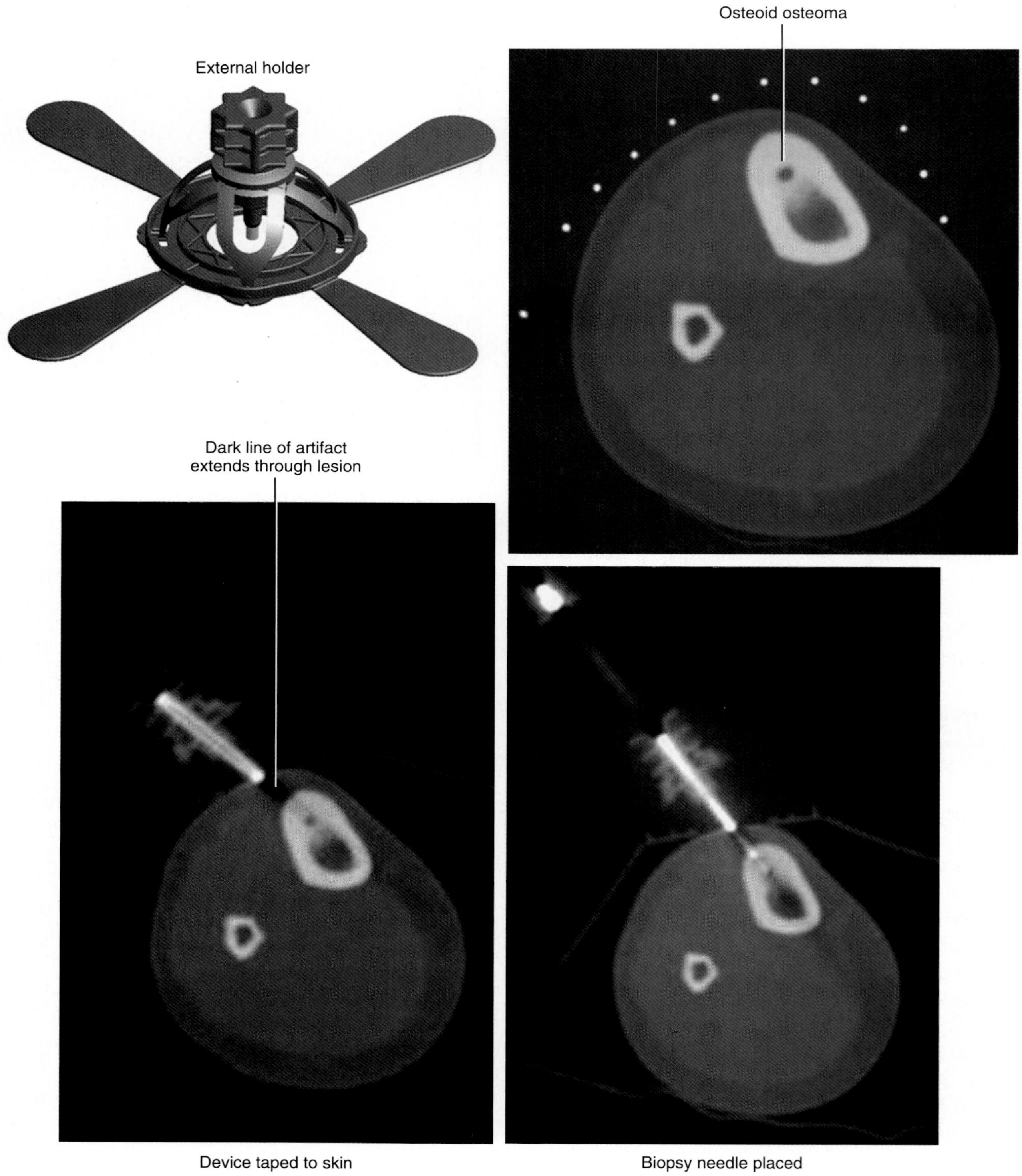
External holder
Osteoid osteoma
Dark line of artifact extends through lesion
Device taped to skin
Biopsy needle placed

Figure 3-10 External holder (SeeStar; Radi, Uppsala, Sweden) taped to the skin facilitates some biopsies and other percutaneous procedures (in this case, radiofrequency ablation of an osteoid osteoma of superficial lesions). The metal holder creates a dark line of artifact on CT, which facilitates needle alignment before placement.

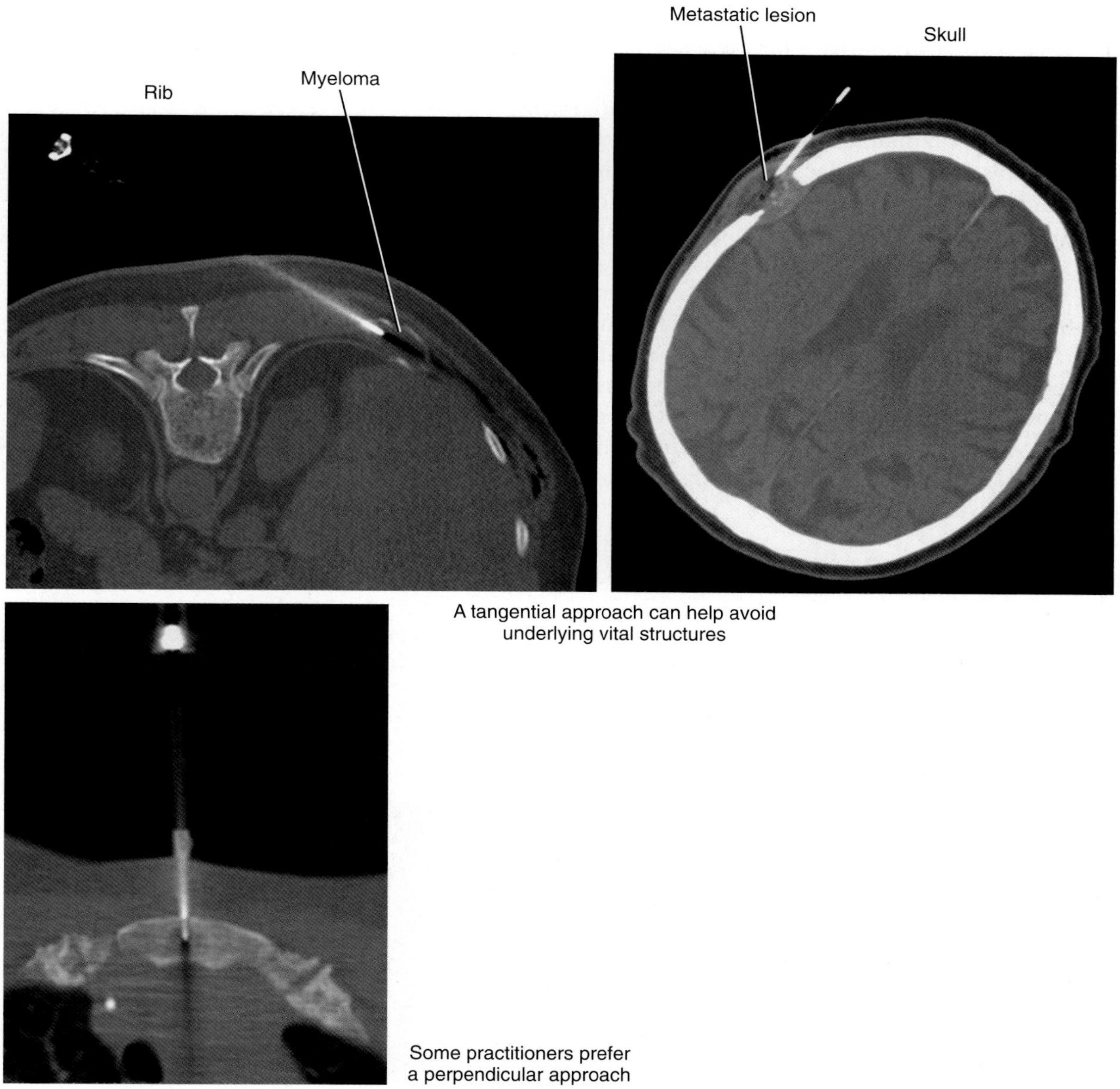
Metastatic lesion
Skull
Myeloma
Rib
A tangential approach can help avoid underlying vital structures
Some practitioners prefer a perpendicular approach

Figure 3-11 Lesion in the rib/sternum/skull. These bones are challenging compared with other superficial bones due to the proximity to vital structures beneath. A tangential approach is often used to minimize the risk of deep needle transgression. However, some practitioners favor a perpendicular approach, especially for rib lesions; the rationale is that ribs are rounded and a tangential approach can result in "slipping off" the lesion. A perpendicular approach can be used to achieve better purchase in bone. Care must be taken not to transgress the inner cortex or slip off!

making them hard to localize on CT, especially with breathing motion. Fluoroscopy can be difficult as well; a C-arm can be used to triangulate the needle tip relative to the lesion, but this technique requires some experience. If the lesion can be seen by ultrasound, this may be useful. CT is commonly used by musculoskeletal radiologists because the pleural margin is most easily seen. Two popular approaches are directly perpendicular to the rib, and tangential. The tangential approach is useful to avoid the pleura, but it may be more difficult to acquire a core sample. Depending on the location, there may be limited choice. Rib lesions under the scapula to a certain extent can be uncovered by changing arm position.

Rib lesions present different problems in thin people (superficial location) compared with obese people (deep location). In thin people, it can be tough to keep the sheath in place between sampling or scanning. As previously mentioned, it may be helpful to place a small needle at the lesion for orientation, which will remain in place better. In obese people, it can be difficult to place the needle on the rib with confidence that the pleural margin has not been transgressed. Measuring the depth of the pleura from the skin using the desired approach is essential, with the needle marker or block placed to prevent entry to this depth. CT fluoroscopy can be very useful for rapid checks of needle tip position. For CT, breath holding during scanning can be detrimental because the degree of inspiration varies, especially with conscious sedation, and this can move the rib out of the scanned field. It is often better to have the patient just breathe shallowly and naturally.

Lesions Near a Vital Structure

For lesions near vital structures, careful planning of the approach is essential. Use of a smaller-gauge needle is prudent (Figs. 3-12 and 3-13). Frequent checks using the guidance modality are recommended.

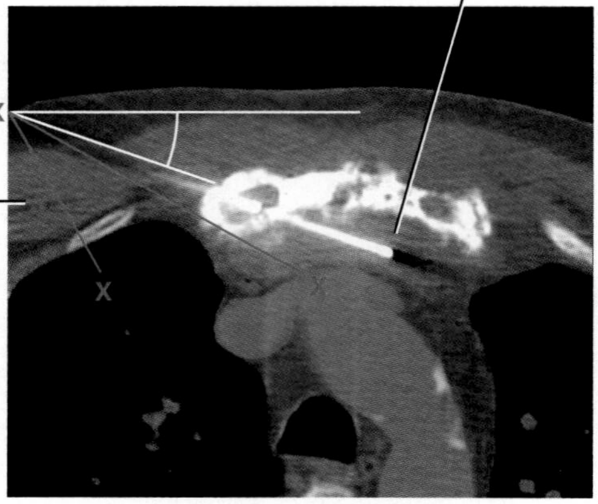
Needle entry site and angle are planned to avoid major vessels
Soft tissue mass
X
Always know the distance to vital structures; check needle position frequently
X
Metastatic prostate cancer

Figure 3-12 Lesion near vital structures. The tangential approach can be used in any part of the body, planning the course of the needle to avoid vascular and other important structures, even if the needle goes farther than expected. Distance that the needle extends from the sheath should always be measured before the procedure and planned accordingly based on measurements from CT.

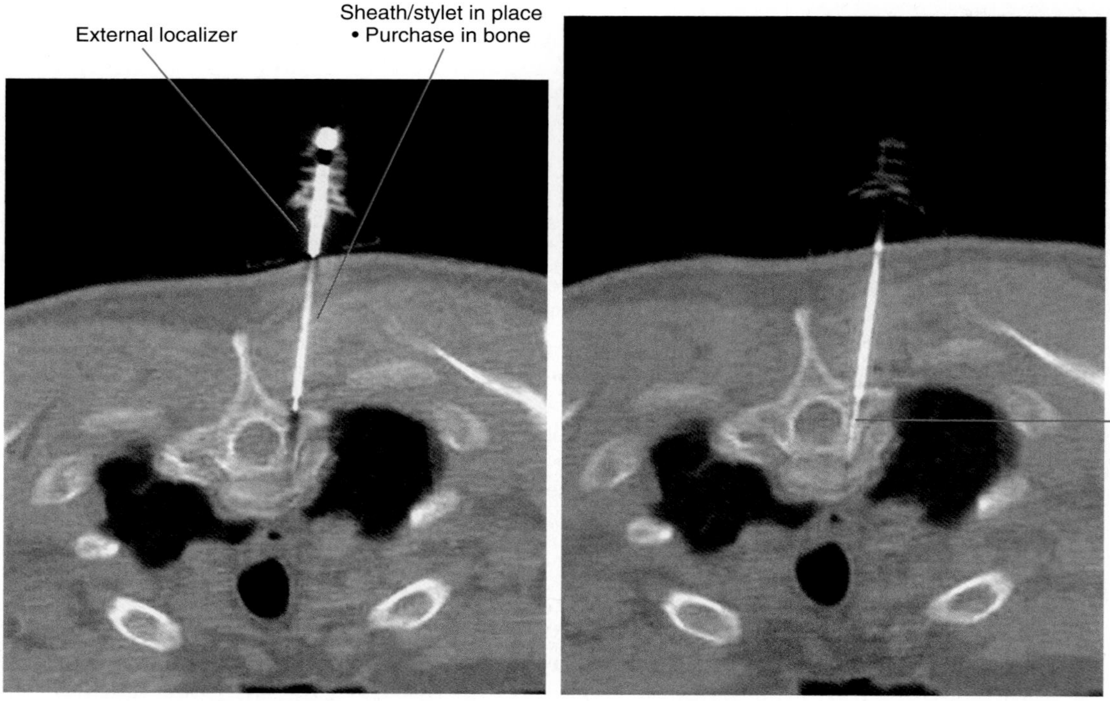
External localizer
Sheath/stylet in place
• Purchase in bone
Passage of biopsy needle
T1 transpedicle biopsy

Figure 3-13 An external localizer (see Fig. 3-10) can be used to guide the needle to the optimal position prior to passage of the biopsy needle.

If a soft tissue gun is used, the "manual throw" setting is best; instead of the needle shooting out of the sheath, the manual throw setting allows the user the slowly push the needle out manually as far as desired. The sheath is triggered, which shoots over the needle cutting the sample. The needle tip advances no farther than manually placed.

Deep Soft Tissue Lesions

For deep soft tissue lesions (Fig. 3-14), a soft tissue gun is generally used and a coaxial system is essential. The outer sheath is placed at the margin of the lesion and multiple samples can be acquired.

Deep, Small Lesions in Bone

A lesion deep within bone presents a special challenge (Fig. 3-15). A coaxial system is essential, again,

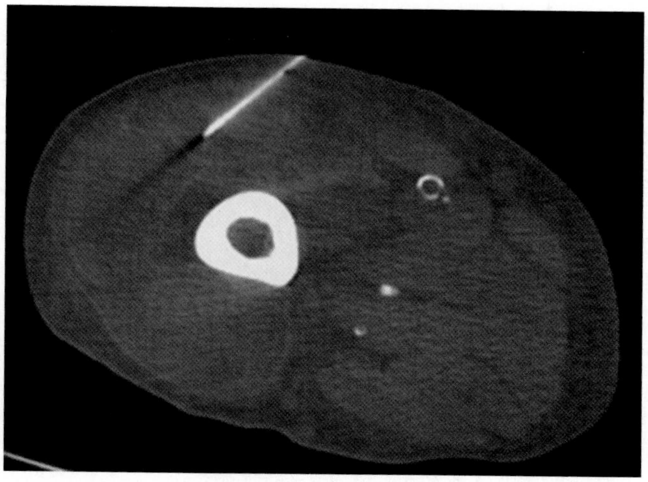
Diabetic myonecrosis

Figure 3-14 **Deep soft tissue biopsy.** A soft tissue gun is used.

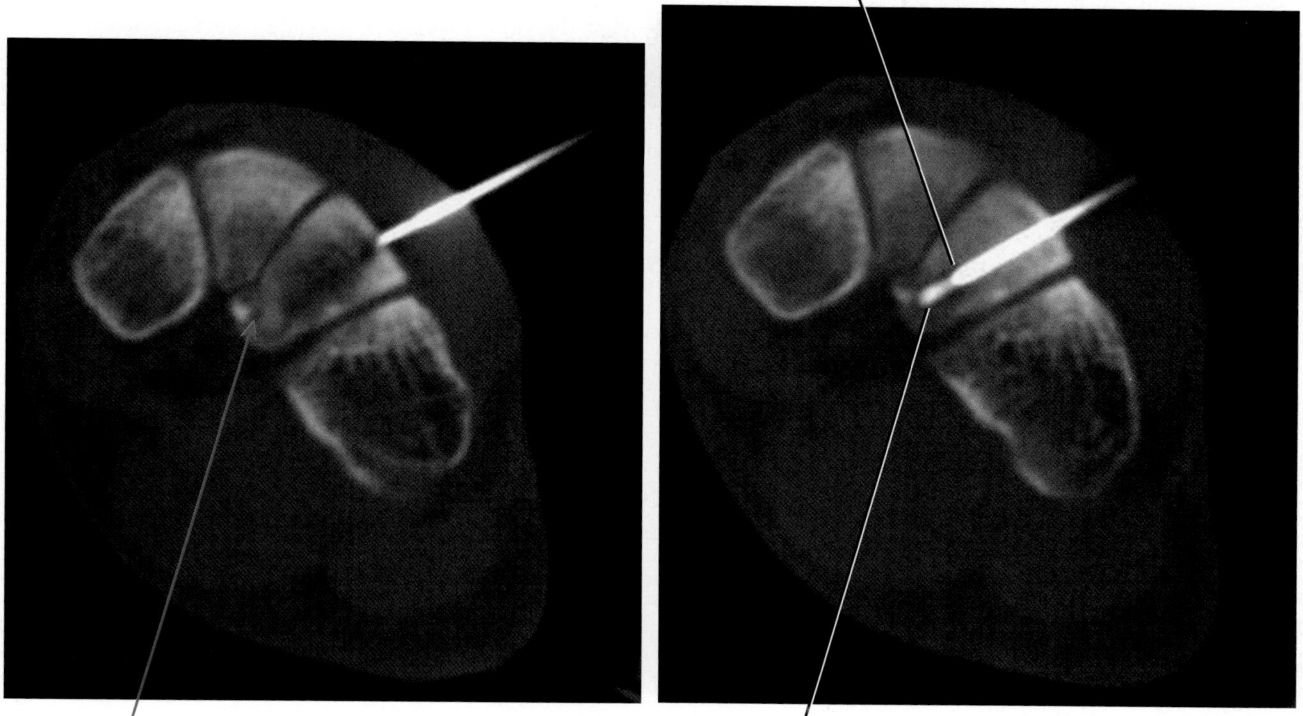
End of sheath
Osteoid osteoma
Drill

Figure 3-15 Small lesion, deep in a bone. This can be challenging because with most biopsy systems the outer sheath is difficult to advance into bone, limiting sampling to the length of needle that extends from the end of the sheath. The Bonopty system has an eccentric drill and the sheath can be passed into the bone facilitating sampling. However, the system has no beveled stylet and therefore it may be difficult to guide the needle once it is within bone.

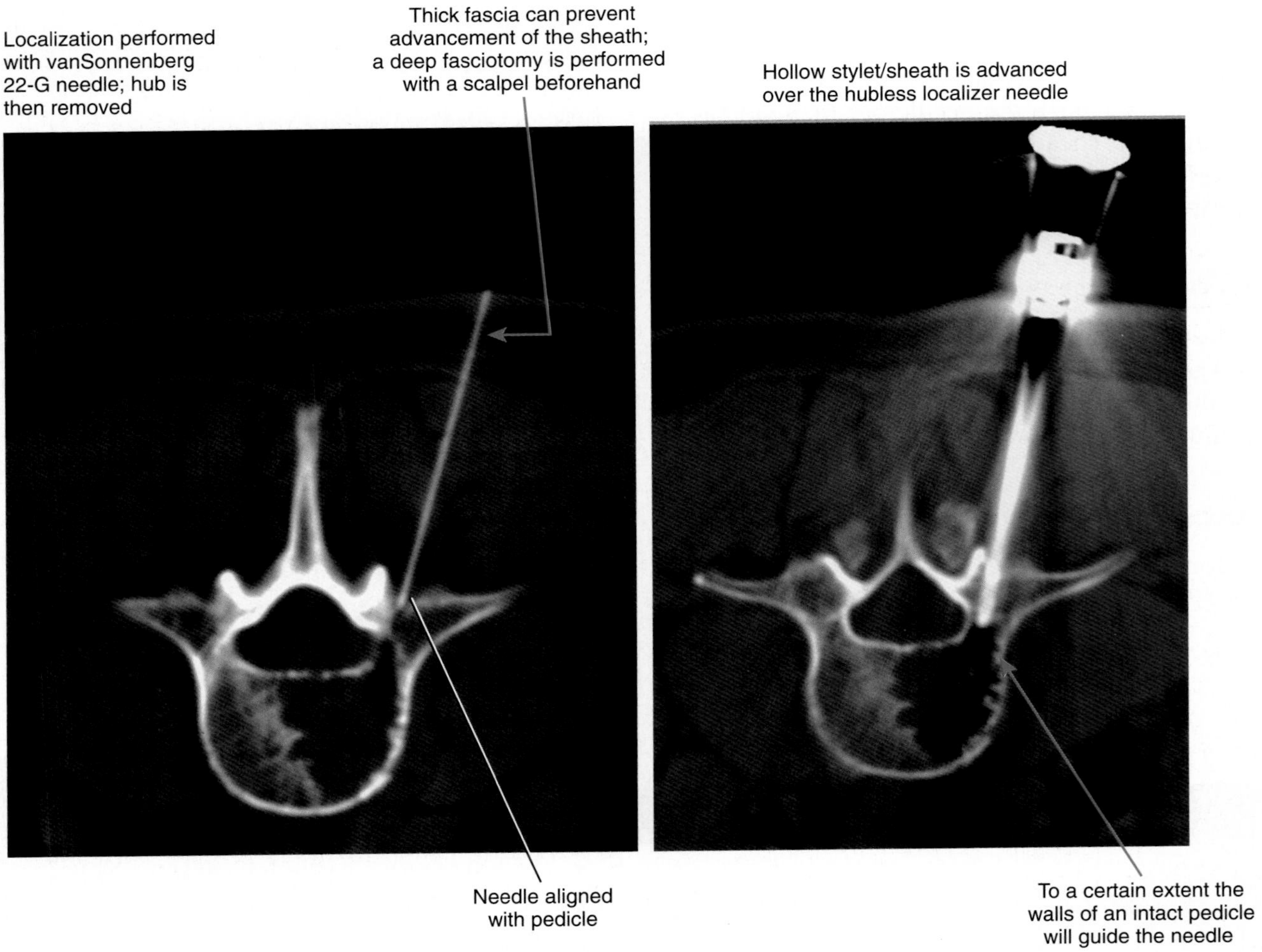
Localization performed with vanSonnenberg 22-G needle; hub is then removed
Thick fascia can prevent advancement of the sheath; a deep fasciotomy is performed with a scalpel beforehand
Hollow stylet/sheath is advanced over the hubless localizer needle
Needle aligned with pedicle
To a certain extent the walls of an intact pedicle will guide the needle

Figure 3-16 Spine–transpedicular approach. Hollow Ackermann-type needle is used.

to allow acquisition of multiple samples through the same sheath. However, most sheaths cannot be advanced into bone, but rather are "parked" at the outer margin of the bone with the cutting needle placed into the lesion. With many coaxial systems, the cutting needle cannot pass a long way through the sheath, making it difficult to reach the lesion through the sheath. The radiologist must make sure that the cutting needle is long enough to access the lesion with the system used. An alternative to this is the Bonopty drill system, in which an eccentric drill makes a channel larger than the sheath, allowing advancement of the sheath into bone and thus facilitating access of deep lesions.

Spine Lesions: Approaches

Transpedicular Approach

The transpedicular approach (Figs. 3-16 and 3-17) is very useful for lesions in the anterior vertebral body. With use of this route, the radicular nerves, major blood vessels, and spinal canal are avoided. In addition, the walls of the pedicle, tangential to the needle course, tend to keep the needle/stylet on track, with the medullary cavity being the path of least resistance to needle advancement. The disadvantage is that the needle can be difficult to guide toward the lesion once in the pedicle, and unless the lesion is

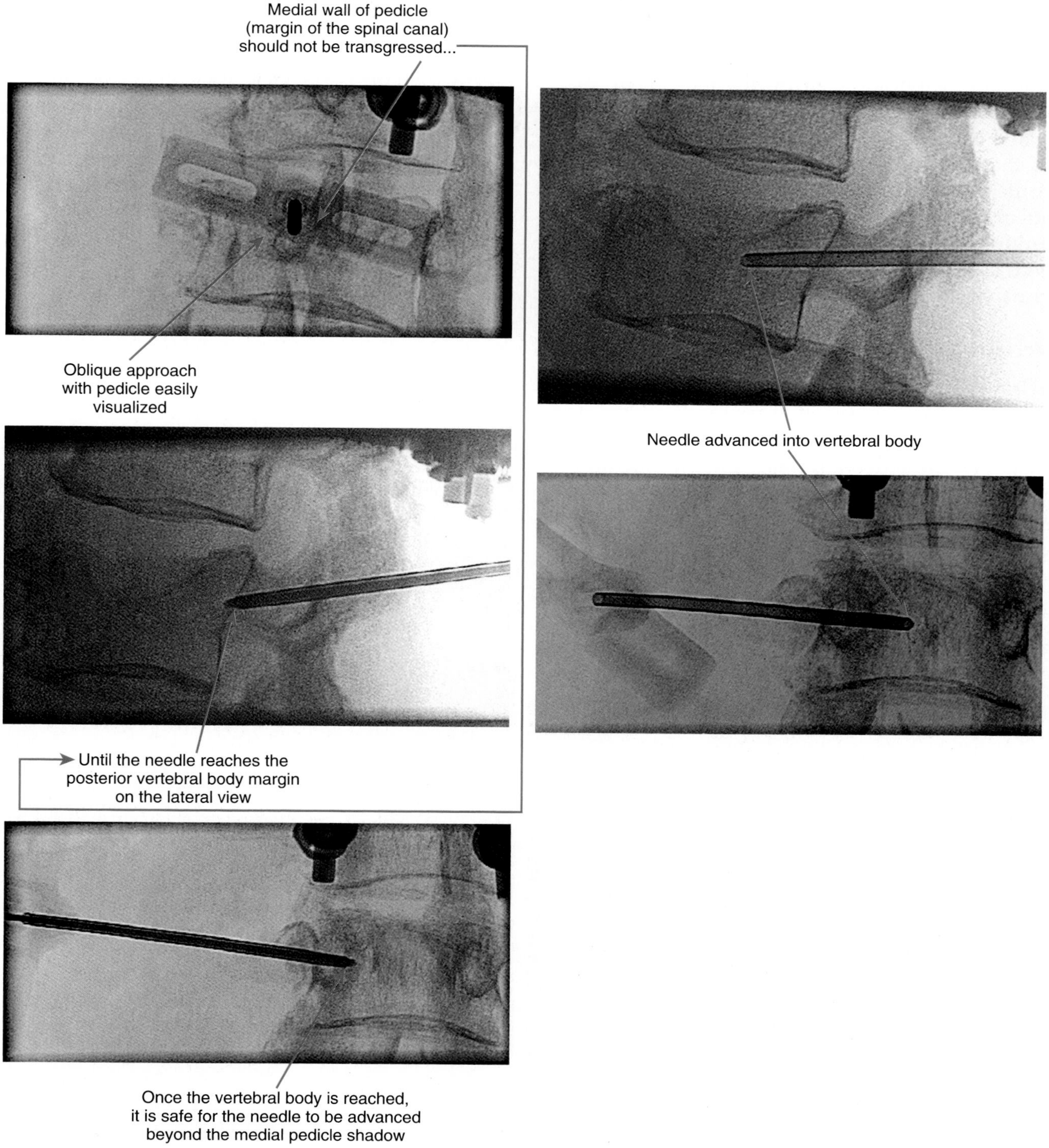
Medial wall of pedicle (margin of the spinal canal) should not be transgressed...
Oblique approach with pedicle easily visualized
Until the needle reaches the posterior vertebral body margin on the lateral view
Once the vertebral body is reached, it is safe for the needle to be advanced beyond the medial pedicle shadow
Needle advanced into vertebral body

Figure 3-17 Transpedicle approach using fluoroscopy. Biopsy is acquired during vertebroplasty procedure.

lined up with the pedicle, a different approach may be needed. A beveled stylet can be useful for guiding the needle once it is in bone. Another disadvantage is that the needle passes close to the walls of the pedicle, and if the wall is transgressed there is a high risk of complication involving the spinal canal (medial wall) or neural foramen (superior or inferior wall). Whether CT or fluoroscopy is used, the walls of the pedicle must not be transgressed. This gets harder to accomplish the higher in the spine it is attempted because pedicle size diminishes significantly above the mid-thoracic region. Also, in patients with kyphosis and osteoporosis, it can be difficult to visualize the upper thoracic pedicles.

Vertebroplasty Fluoroscopic Approach

Using fluoroscopy, the vertebral body can be accessed using a transpedicle approach using a steep or shallow trajectory (see Fig. 3-17). For the steep trajectory, the vertebra is imaged in the anteroposterior (AP) plane, angled craniocaudally so the pedicles come sharply into view. A slight degree of rotation can help visualize the pedicle on the side being accessed. The needle is advanced to the lateral margin of the pedicle, midway from top to bottom. The needle is advanced into the bone, and the correct orientation of the needle in craniocaudal direction is assessed on the lateral view. Back on the AP view, the needle is advanced farther toward the center of the pedicle more medially. When the medial wall of the pedicle is approached, the lateral projection is again checked to make sure that the needle tip is at or beyond the posterior vertebral body margin. If so, the needle can be advanced into the vertebral body without fear of traversing the spinal canal. However, if on the AP view the tip of the needle is near the medial wall of the pedicle and on the lateral view it is not yet at the posterior vertebral body wall, the needle must be repositioned more laterally to avoid the canal.

Paravertebral Approach

The paravertebral approach is very straightforward (Figs. 3-18 through 3-21). The needle can be started

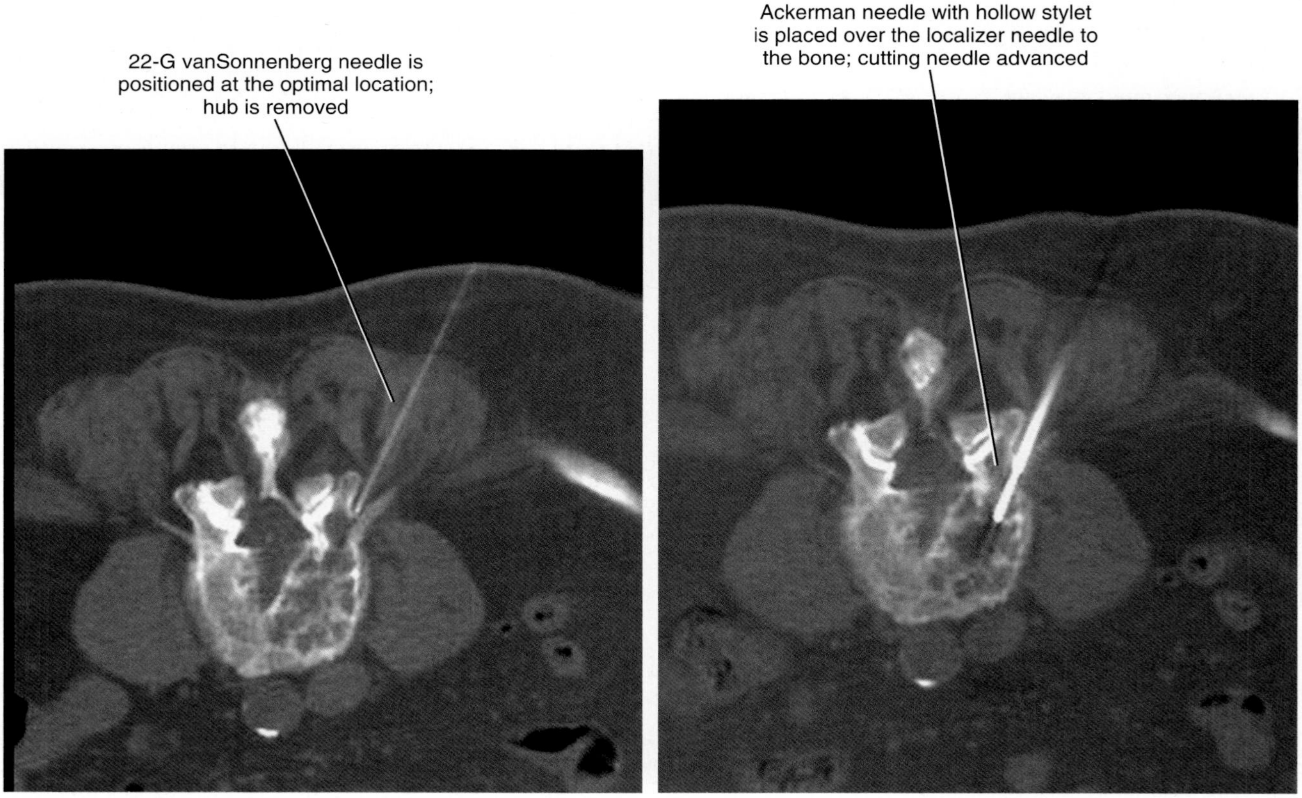
22-G vanSonnenberg needle is positioned at the optimal location; hub is removed
Ackerman needle with hollow stylet is placed over the localizer needle to the bone; cutting needle advanced

Figure 3-18 Paravertebral approach via the crux between the facet joint and the transverse process.

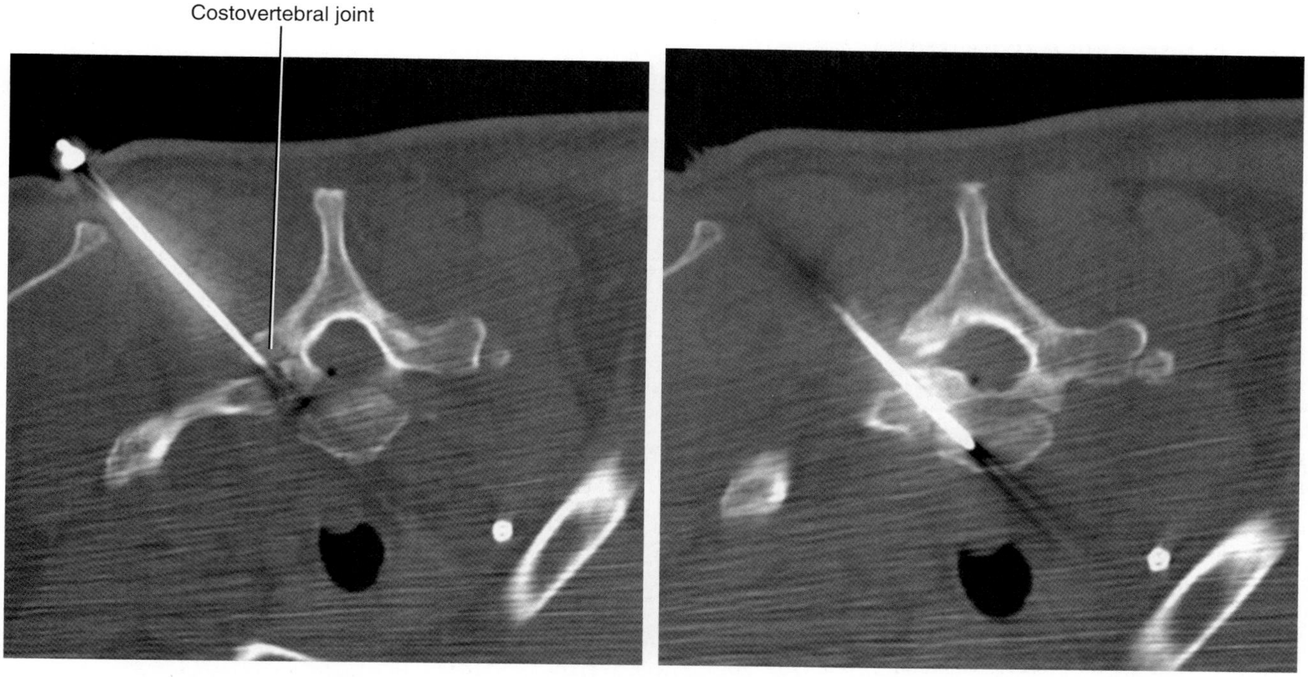
Costovertebral joint

Figure 3-19 Paravertebral approach. Use of the costovertebral junction at the upper thoracic spine.

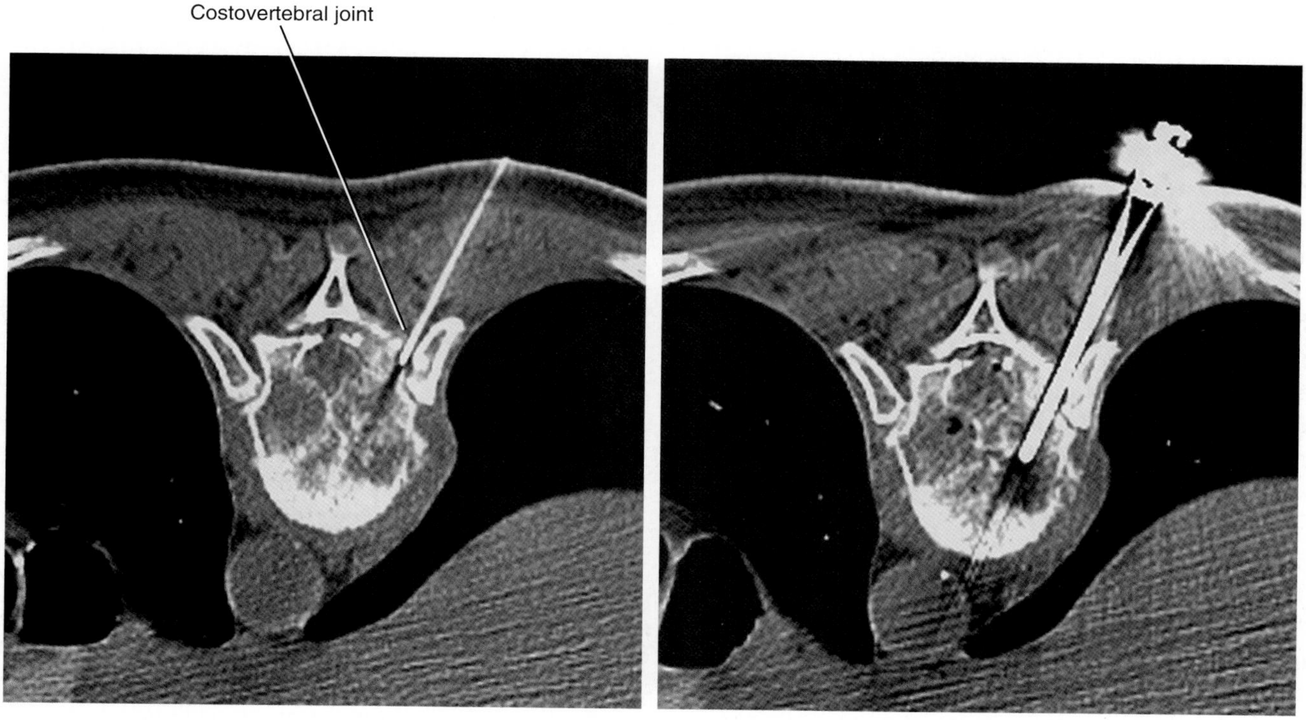
Costovertebral joint

Figure 3-20 Paravertebral approach. Use of the costovertebral junction at the lower thoracic spine.

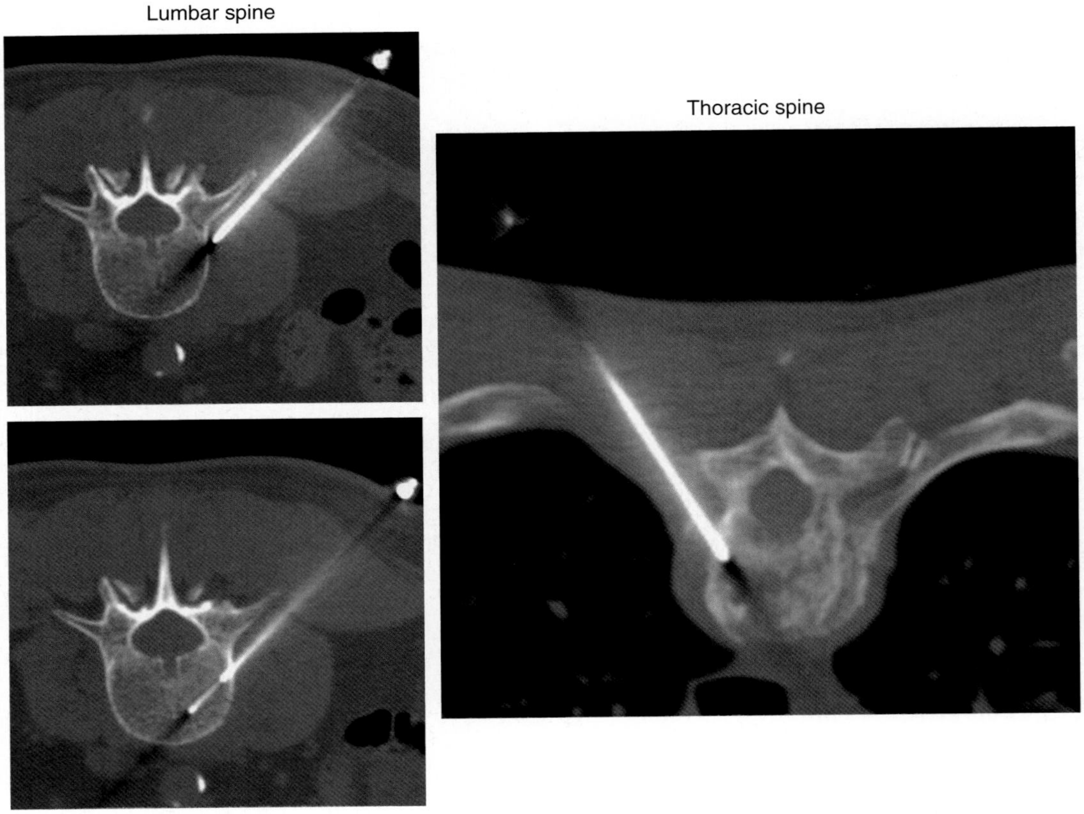
Lumbar spine
Thoracic spine

Figure 3-21 Far lateral paravertebral approach. The spinal canal is maximally avoided but it may be difficult to achieve purchase in the bone using a relatively tangential approach. In the thoracic spine where the pedicles are small, this approach can be very useful. Also, if the desired biopsy site is near the midline this approach can facilitate central positioning compared to a transpedicle approach.

just lateral to the facet joint at the crux, between the facet joint and the transverse process, or through the costovertebral joint. These locations are excellent for achieving needle purchase into bone. From these locations, the needle enters the lateral pedicle and then into the vertebral body. The needle can alternatively be started lateral to the transverse process, avoiding bone altogether until the posterolateral margin of the vertebral body is reached. This approach makes it easier to guide the needle toward a focal lesion in the vertebral body, since less bone must be passed to get to the lesion. However, this approach is feasible only when there is enough paraspinal soft tissue to accommodate the needle track. In the thoracic spine, the pleural margin may prevent this approach. Some authors have reported injecting saline or air into the paraspinal soft tissues to push the pleural surface away from the needle tip (Fig. 3-22). In addition, in some cases it may be necessary to perform a nerve block before continuing passage of the needle; however, this should be reserved for situations in which the nerve cannot be avoided (Fig. 3-23).

Diskographic Approach

When using fluoroscopy, the diskographic approach is an excellent way to access intervertebral disks for aspiration (Fig. 3-24). With the patient in the prone position, the image intensifier is obliqued so that the superior articular process is near the junction of the middle and posterior thirds of the vertebral body at the level to be aspirated. Next, the image intensifier is angled craniocaudally to make the disk tangential to the beam. The needle is passed straight down the beam just anterior to the superior articular process into the center of the disk. This approach is straightforward in the lumbar spine, except that it may be difficult at L5-S1. Some individuals have a low L5-S1 junction, and during rotation and angulation of the image intensifier to the appropriate position, the iliac

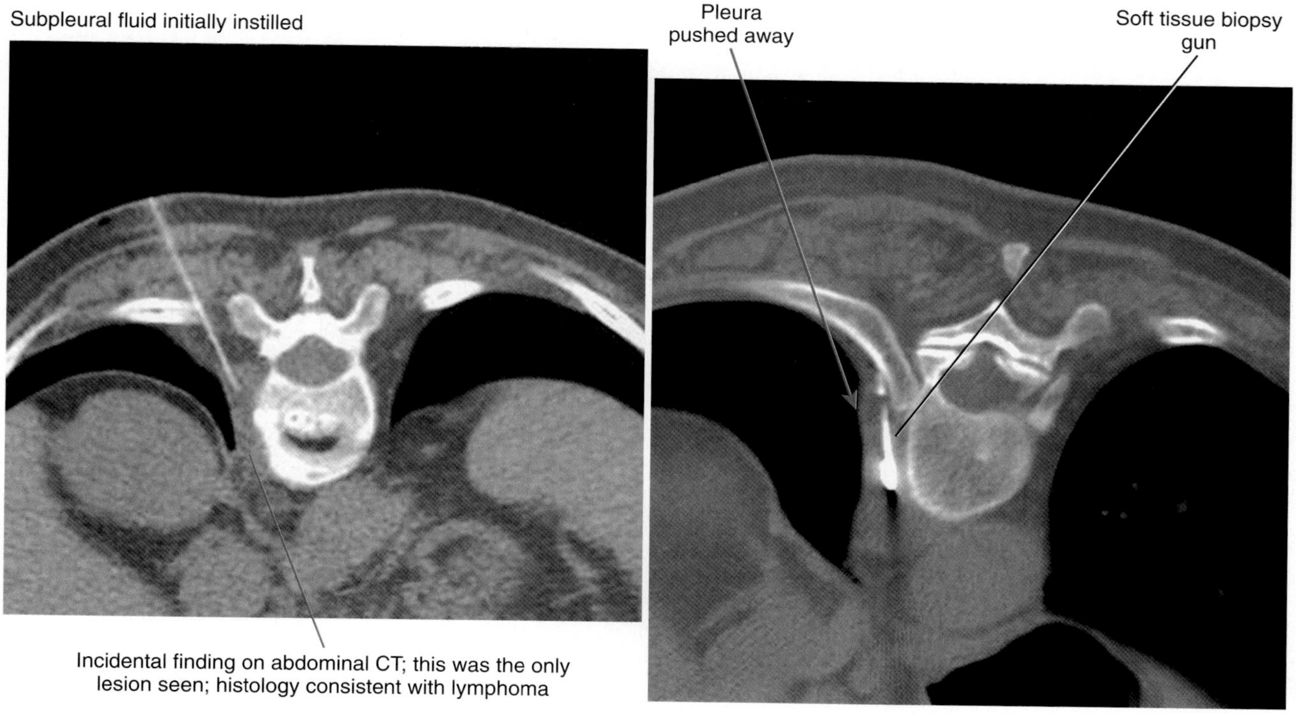
Subpleural fluid initially instilled
Pleura pushed away
Soft tissue biopsy gun
Incidental finding on abdominal CT; this was the only lesion seen; histology consistent with lymphoma

Figure 3-22 Subpleural fluid installation. For situations in which the pleural surface is near the path of the needle, saline can be instilled initially to push the pleura away. However, the effect may be minimal and fluid could even obscure fat planes surrounding the lesion.

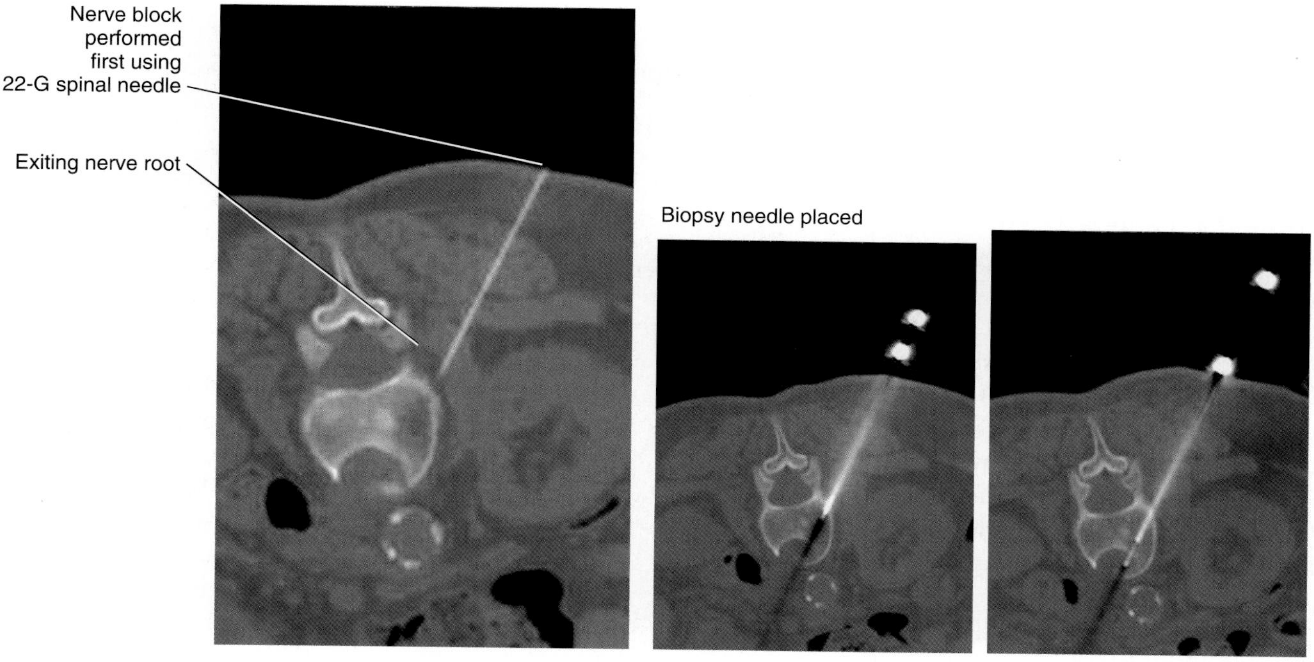
Nerve block performed first using 22-G spinal needle
Exiting nerve root
Biopsy needle placed

Figure 3-23 Initial nerve block facilitating paravertebral approach.

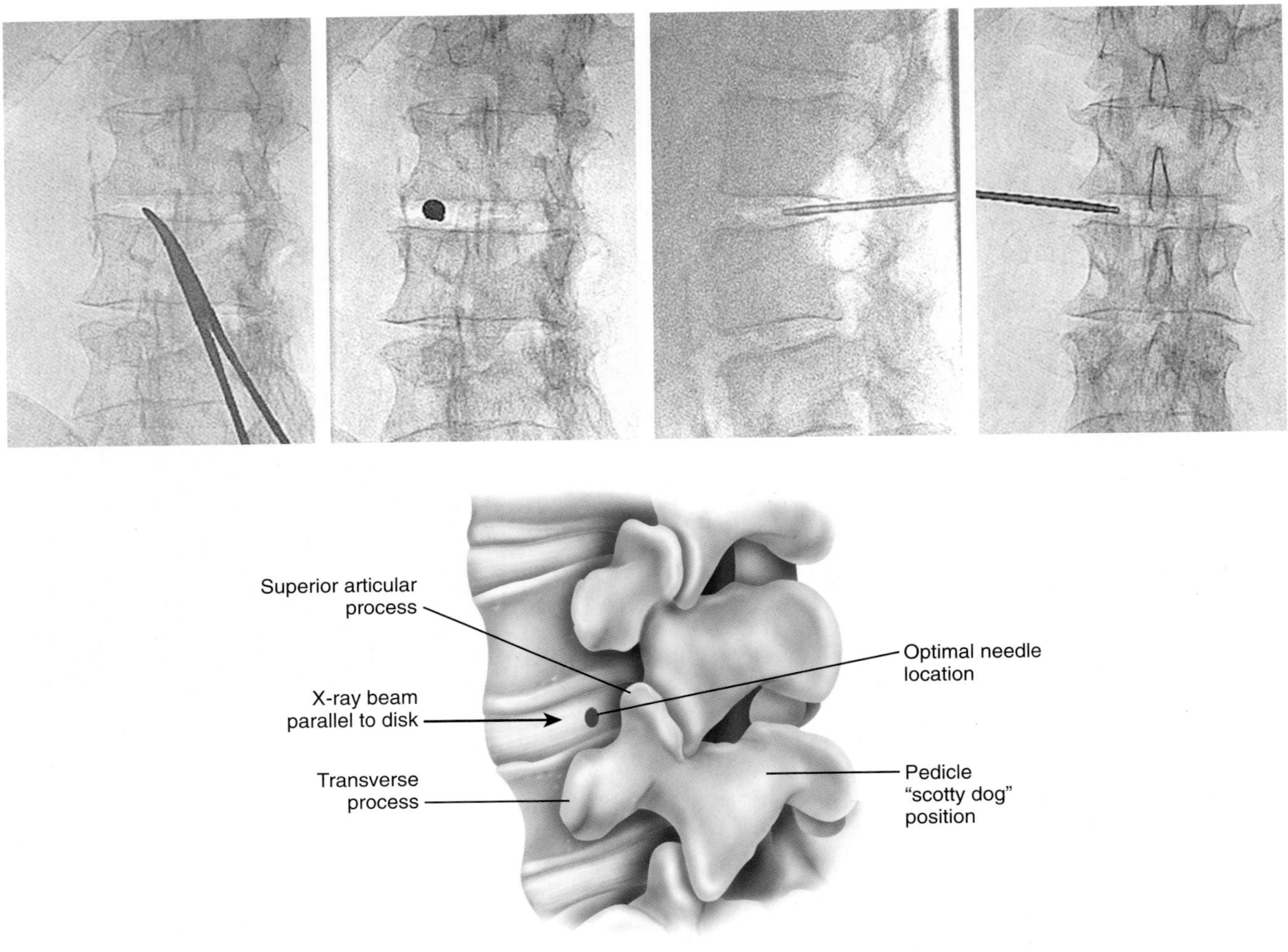
Superior articular process
X-ray beam parallel to disk
Transverse process
Optimal needle location
Pedicle "scotty dog" position

Figure 3-24 Disk aspiration/endplate biopsies: diskography approach. The patient is placed prone and the x-ray beam is obliqued craniocaudally such that the target disk is best visualized, and mediolaterally such that the superior articular process is halfway from front to back of the vertebral body. The biopsy needle is advanced toward the disk just anterior to the superior articular process, checking position periodically on the anteroposterior view. At the margin of the disk, the biopsy needle stylet is removed, and a long 18-G needle is advanced coaxially into the disk for aspiration. The stylet is replaced, and the biopsy needle deflected toward the endplate, where a bone biopsy is taken. A nerve block may need to be performed by injecting 1 mL preservative-free lidocaine just outside the disk margin. Biopsy of infected disks can be painful, so conscious sedation and intravenous pain medication are essential.

crest overlies the disk. In this case, the beam is progressively rotated to a steeper approach until a small triangle appears, bounded by the iliac bone, the superior articular process, and the inferior L5 endplate. In the thoracic spine, a similar approach can be used, but the ribs and pleural margin must also be avoided.

Cervical Spine Approach

In the cervical spine, the posterior elements can be accessed using an oblique posterior approach under CT (Figs. 3-25 and 3-26). The vertebral bodies can be difficult to access with a posterior or lateral approach because there is little space in the soft tissues without important blood vessels or nerves. Pedicles are usually too small to use as a needle guide. The anterior approach is limited by the trachea as well as vessels and nerves. CT is very useful for these biopsies, since the major structures can be seen. An intravenous contrast bolus can be used to delineate the major vessels before biopsy, but this is usually not needed. The route is determined by the location of the lesion

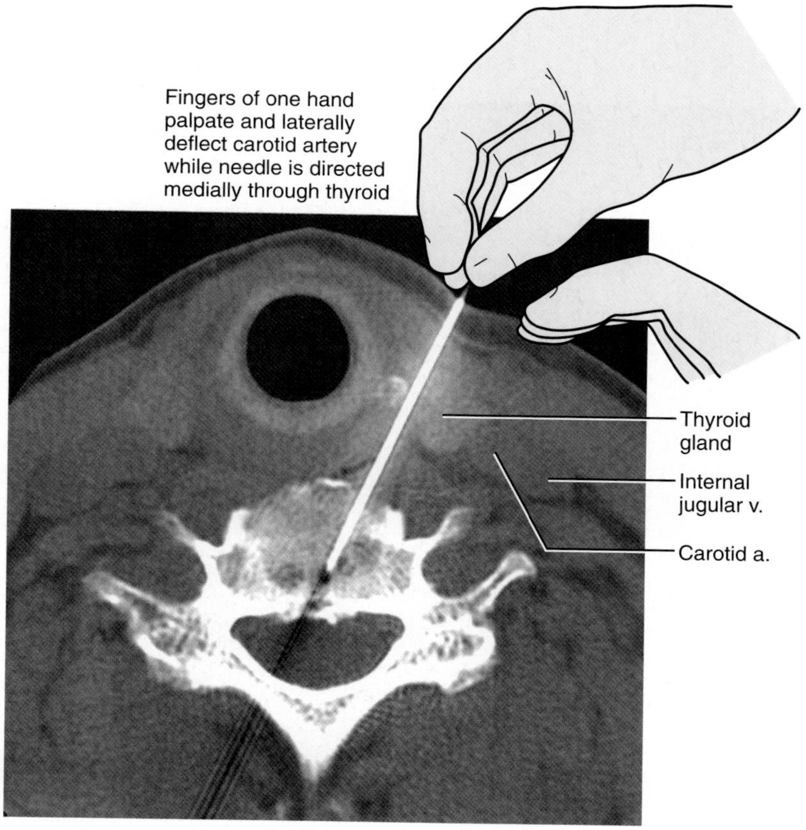
Fingers of one hand palpate and laterally deflect carotid artery while needle is directed medially through thyroid
Thyroid gland
Internal jugular v.
Carotid a.

Figure 3-25 **Anterior approach to the cervical spine.**

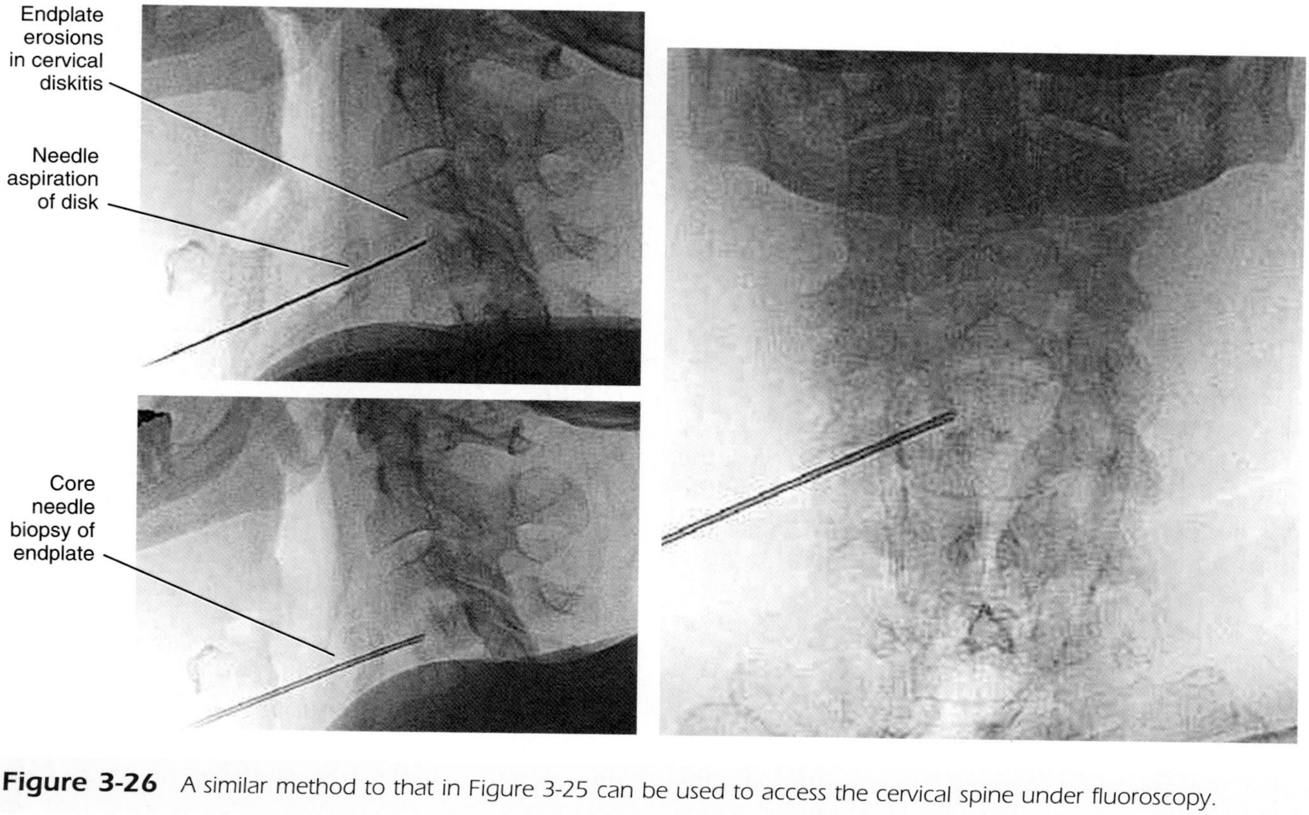
Endplate erosions in cervical diskitis
Needle aspiration of disk
Core needle biopsy of endplate

Figure 3-26 A similar method to that in Figure 3-25 can be used to access the cervical spine under fluoroscopy.

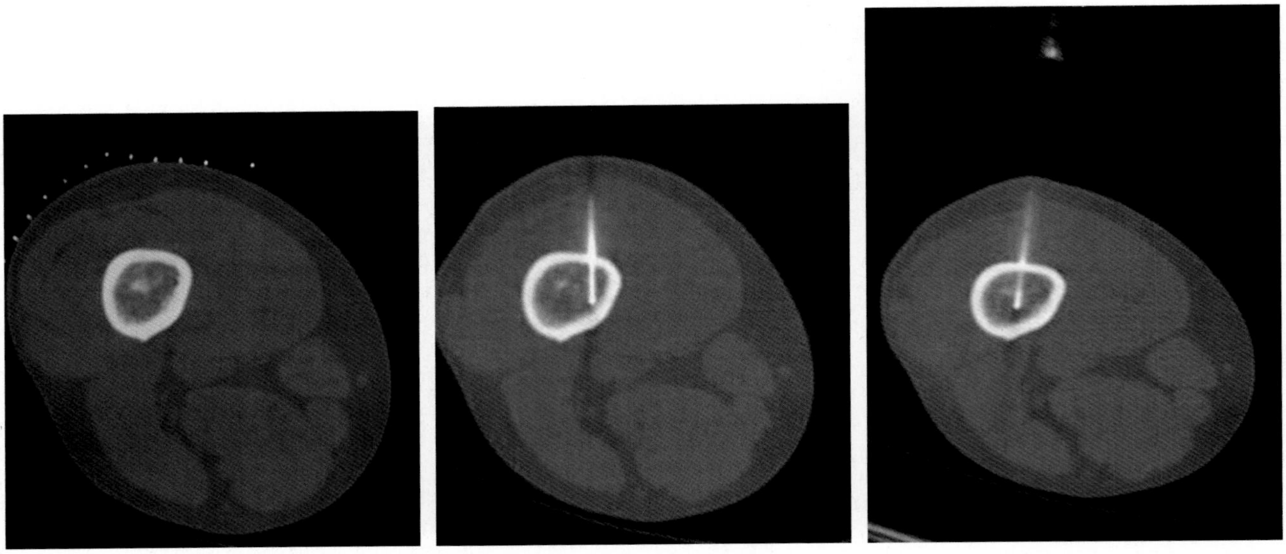

Figure 3-27 Biopsy through a thick cortex. A coaxial drill system is optimal. In this case, because the differential diagnosis included a chondroid lesion, multiple sites were sampled by angling the needle using the cortex as a fulcrum.

relative to overlying structures. An anterior approach has been described and is similar to the technique used for placing needles into the disks for cervical diskography. The carotid is palpated with the tips of the fingers of one hand while the needle is held in the other. The carotid is deflected laterally with gentle pressure, and the needle is placed just medial to it, lateral to the trachea. The thyroid may be transgressed, but this is not usually problematic and often cannot be avoided. Obviously, a coaxial needle is necessary and a small-gauge needle is recommended.

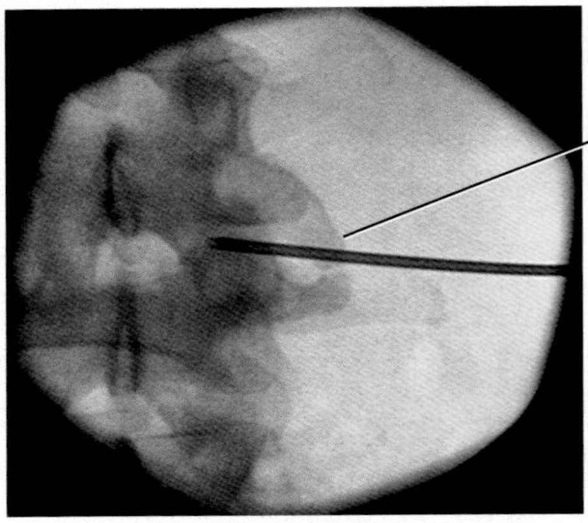
Spurs drilled through using bonopty needle
Chronic diskitis/osteomyelitis; a thick shell of spurs initially blocked entry to the disk

Figure 3-28 Occasionally the best location to biopsy appears inaccessible because of overlying normal bone or spurs. In this case, it may be necessary to drill through normal bone to get to the site. However, care must be taken in the setting of primary tumors or infection not to seed uninvolved bone.

Thick Bone

Biopsy of a thick bone (e.g., femur) requires a coaxial system because it often takes multiple passes at the same point to traverse the cortex into the medullary cavity (Fig. 3-27). A needle with serrated tip (e.g., the Cook Ackermann or Elson) can be helpful, as can the Radi Bonopty drill system. This can also be useful to drill through endplate spurs to reach a disk (Fig. 3-28).

Small Bone

Biopsy of a small bone (e.g., toe) that is superficially located may not require a coaxial system. Often the approach is fairly obvious through the same skin entry site, and initial fluoroscopic verification of needle position may be all that is needed, followed by multiple passes along the same approach. A short needle is usually desirable in this situation because it is easier to control and position.

Disk Aspiration and Biopsy

Disk aspiration is performed for infection. However, for aspiration alone, yield of Gram stain/culture is low, about 20% to 50%. If the patient is already on antibiotics, this figure is even lower. A trial period of 48 hours off antibiotics may be used if the patient is stable enough, to increase yield. As with joint aspiration, if no fluid can be aspirated, a few milliliters of sterile saline can be injected and re-aspirated immediately. This is common practice, but it is unclear whether it is effective; also similar to septic arthritis, a dry tap of a disk may imply lack of infection. To ensure that the fluid present will be aspirated, a larger-gauge needle (at least 18 G) must be used. Infected fluid is often very viscous and may not be able to be drawn through smaller needles. Because of the low yield of aspiration alone, most authors advocate acquiring samples of the area of signal abnormality in the endplate as well. To accomplish this, it is useful to use a bone biopsy needle and a paravertebral approach (by CT, as previously described) or a diskography approach (by fluoroscopy). Advantages of fluoroscopy are (1) imaging to check needle position is performed more quickly; (2) the plane can be more easily tilted parallel with the disk, especially useful at L5-S1; and (3) the needle can be observed in real time while it is deflected toward the endplate for bone biopsy. The pleural margin is seen easily using both techniques.

Biopsy of a Primary Tumor

Primary tumors of bone or soft tissue may require definitive surgery by a specialized bone tumor surgeon. If amputation or limb-salvage surgery is required, the surgeon may need adjacent tissue for a myocutaneous flap, covering the resected area or stump. If the passage of the biopsy needle traverses this adjacent tissue, it may be considered contaminated and necessitate a more extensive surgical procedure. Therefore, it is essential for the radiologist to discuss the intended approach to a presumed primary lesion with the surgeon who will perform the definitive surgery. Often the agreed-upon approach is more technically difficult than the direct approach through the myocutaneous flap tissue.

Biopsy Assist Devices

Some institutions have developed tracking software linked to pre-procedure imaging that establishes fiducial markers and allows dynamic localization without frequent re-scanning. These systems are predominantly used for placement of screws, but in the future may be available commercially for biopsy procedures. The SeeStar (Radi, Uppsala, Sweden; see Fig. 3-10) is an external guide that holds the needle in position outside the patient (preventing deflection of the needle when let go during scanning), making it very useful for biopsy of superficial lesions or for biopsy of lesions using a horizontal approach. In addition, the metallic needle guide creates a dark, linear artifact on CT images, which can be aligned to the lesion, facilitating the approach before needle placement.

Percutaneous Needle Localization

Occasionally a lesion is in a dangerous location, or a lesion is in the soft tissues and is hard or calcified; thus, a core biopsy is difficult or inadvisable. Other situations occur in which the patient is scheduled for an open surgical biopsy, but the anatomy is distorted by scar tissue, or the lesion is small enough that it may be difficult to localize at surgery and preoperative localization may be preferred. This is accomplished by using a hookwire-type breast localization needle (Fig. 3-29). The needle is placed (within the sheath) into or adjacent to the lesion using the guidance modality. Needle tip position is verified and the sheath is withdrawn. The hook deploys as it is unsheathed, holding the needle in position. The wire extending from the skin is coiled and steri-stripped against the sterilized skin and is covered with a sterile gauze cover. A final scan is acquired and printed for the surgeon to use for planning in the operating room.

BIOPSY SAMPLE PREPARATION

Once you acquire the sample, it is important to prepare it correctly. Some lesions are best sent on a saline-soaked Telfa pad. These include any lesion suspected of being hematopoietic or lymphoproliferative in nature (i.e., T-cell lymphoma). This allows for touch preparation/smear preparation to be performed for cytologic evaluation. In addition, material can be sent for flow cytometry or molecular analysis prior to frozen section or routine processing. Cultures can be taken within the pathology laboratory if indications are properly conveyed to the lab before reception of the material. Sterility has to be maintained for

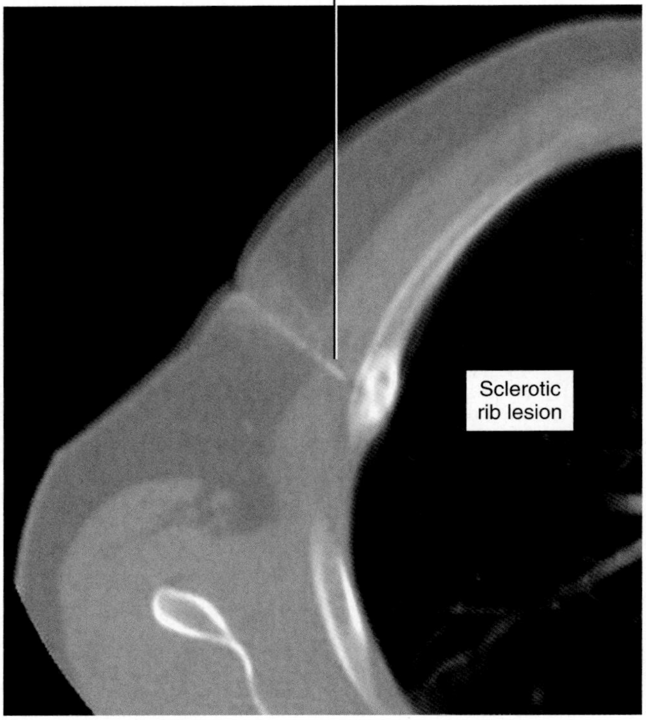
Hookwire needle
• When the needle tip is positioned properly, the hook is deployed
Sclerotic rib lesion

Figure 3-29 Needle localization. A hookwire needle typically used for breast lesions can also be used for preoperative musculoskeletal lesion localization.

microbiologic cultures as well as tissue culture and cytogenetics. Most other lesions can be sent in formalin for routine processing and microscopic evaluation after decalcification. If there is a possibility of a delay in delivery of the specimen to the pathology lab, then the material should be placed in formalin. Frozen section may be performed to evaluate adequacy of material and also to address primary diagnostic questions. Most intramedullary tumors can be frozen despite the presence of trabecular bone. Touch preparations can also be performed to enhance diagnostic yield.

SEDATION AND MONITORING

Choice of local anesthetic only versus conscious sedation versus monitored anesthesia care depends on a number of factors, including location of the biopsy, inherent level of sensation (e.g., diabetic neuropathy or paraplegia), cardiopulmonary status, ability to cooperate, and patient pain tolerance, among other things. For most musculoskeletal biopsies, conscious sedation is used, with a combination of midazolam (Versed) and fentanyl. In the event of oversedation, midazolam can be reversed, and fentanyl is short-acting. Monitoring patients is important to assess for oxygenation and heart rate and rhythm.

Suggested Readings

Ahrar K, Himmerich JU, Herzog CE, et al. Percutaneous ultrasound-guided biopsy in the definitive diagnosis of osteosarcoma. J Vasc Interv Radiol 2004;15(11):1329–1333.

Blanco Sequeiros R, Carrino JA. Musculoskeletal interventional MR imaging. Magn Reson Imaging Clin N Am 2005;13(3): 519–532.

Gangi A, Guth S, Imbert JP, et al. Percutaneous vertebroplasty: indications, technique, and results. Radiographics 2003;23(2):10.

Geremia G, Joglekar S. Percutaneous needle biopsy of the spine. Neuroimaging Clin N Am 2000;10(3):503–533.

Gil-Sanchez S, Marco-Domenech SF, Irurzun-Lopez J, et al. Ultrasound-guided skeletal biopsies. Skeletal Radiol 2001; 30(11):615–619.

Hadjipavlou AG, Kontakis GM, Gaitanis JN, et al. Effectiveness and pitfalls of percutaneous transpedicle biopsy of the spine. Clin Orthop Relat Res 2003;411:54–60.

Jelinek JS, Murphey MD, Welker JA, et al. Diagnosis of primary bone tumors with image-guided percutaneous biopsy: experience with 110 tumors. Radiology 2002;223:731–737.

Kelekis AD, Somon T, Yilmaz H, et al. Interventional spine procedures. Eur J Radiol 2005;55(3):362–383.

Liu JC, Chiou HJ, Chen WM, et al. Sonographically guided core needle biopsy of soft tissue neoplasms. J Clin Ultrasound 2004;32(6):294–298.

Mathis JM, Wong W. Percutaneous vertebroplasty: technical considerations. J Vasc Interv Radiol 2003;14(8):953–960.

Moller S, Kothe R, Wiesner L, et al. Fluoroscopy-guided transpedicular trocar biopsy of the spine—results, review, and technical notes. Acta Orthop Belg 2001;67(5):488–499.

Morrison WB, Sanders TG, Parsons TW, Penrod BJ. Preoperative CT-guided hookwire needle localization of musculoskeletal lesions. AJR Am J Roentgenol 2001;176(6):1531–1533.

Roberts CC, Morrison WB, Leslie KO, et al. Assessment of bone biopsy needles for sample size, specimen quality and ease of use. Skeletal Radiol 2005;34(6):329–335.

Saifuddin A, Mitchell R, Burnett SJ, et al. Ultrasound-guided needle biopsy of primary bone tumours. J Bone Joint Surg Br 2000;82(1):50–54.

Schweitzer ME, Deely DM. Percutaneous biopsy of osteolytic lesions: use of a biopsy gun. Radiology 1993;189(2):615–616.

Schweitzer ME, Deely DM, Beavis K, Gannon F. Does the use of lidocaine affect the culture of percutaneous bone biopsy specimens obtained to diagnose osteomyelitis? An in vitro and in vivo study. AJR Am J Roentgenol 1995;164(5):1201–1203.

Schweitzer ME, Gannon FH, Deely DM, et al. Percutaneous skeletal aspiration and core biopsy: complementary techniques. AJR Am J Roentgenol 1996;166(2):415–418.

Sequeiros RB, Ojala R, Kariniemi J, et al. MR-guided interventional procedures: a review. Acta Radiol 2005;46(6):576–586.

Vieillard MH, Boutry N, Chastanet P, et al. Contribution of percutaneous biopsy to the definite diagnosis in patients with suspected bone tumor. Joint Bone Spine 2005;72(1): 53–60.

White LM, Schweitzer ME, Deely DM. Coaxial percutaneous needle biopsy of osteolytic lesions with intact cortical bone. AJR Am J Roentgenol 1996;166(1):143–144.

White LM, Schweitzer ME, Deely DM, Gannon F. Study of osteomyelitis: utility of combined histologic and microbiologic evaluation of percutaneous biopsy samples. Radiology 1995;197(3): 840–842.

SECTION III

PROBLEM SOLVING: Disease Categories

Chapter 4

ARTHRITIS

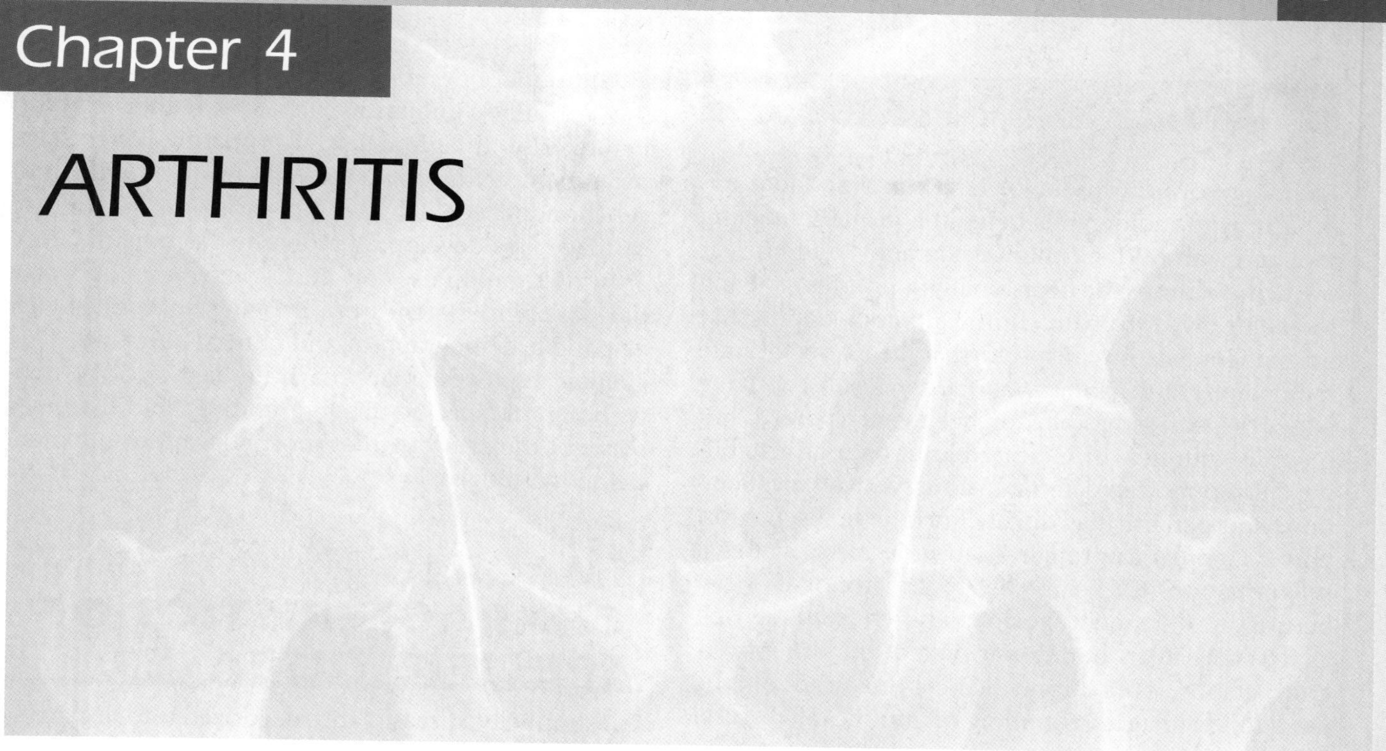

CHAPTER OUTLINE

MODALITIES

Radiology of arthritis involves a multimodality approach, with radiographs being the primary imaging tool and with MRI, CT, ultrasonography, and nuclear medicine being useful occasionally as problem-solving tools. Ideally, two main clinical situations occur: (1) the patient has an unspecified arthropathy despite radiography and clinical/laboratory results; (2) the patient's arthritis has already been characterized, but presents with new or increased joint pain or instability. Ultrasound can detect effusion, synovial proliferation, and periarticular disease such as tenosynovitis; power Doppler can roughly gauge degree of synovial inflammation. CT (especially multidetector CT) can be used to document erosions and effusion, as well as intra-articular bodies facilitated by use of CT arthrography. Nuclear medicine bone scan can be used to evaluate distribution of multifocal disease. MRI is useful to evaluate effusion, erosion, cartilage loss, bodies, ligament and fibrocartilage tear, and periarticular disease. Contrast-enhanced MRI is especially useful for evaluation of extent of synovitis, and MR arthrography is most useful for detection of intra-articular bodies. MRI has also been used to track response to arthritis drugs, documenting changes objectively.

In many clinical settings, MR imaging is commonly ordered as the initial exam, or advanced imaging is ordered because radiographic findings were subtle or merely overlooked. Radiographs are often not available, so the musculoskeletal radiologist must be familiar with the appearance of basic arthropathies on MRI. The findings may not be specific, but in many cases the differential diagnosis can be narrowed based on the MR imaging appearance.

Regardless of the modality used, the first decision is whether the imaging findings in question actually represent arthritis or some other pathology. If the process involves both sides of the joint, an arthropathy should be suspected. However, injury can cause kissing bone bruises on MRI, so obviously the clinical context is important. Joint effusion is a hallmark of arthritis but is nonspecific as well. Even synovial proliferation can be seen after injury or surgery and is not necessarily indicative of arthritis. However, if one can identify that the origin of a process is from within a joint, malignancy can virtually be excluded, since tumors rarely arise within joints. In fact, joints (and disks) act as a barrier to tumor spread.

Additional questions to consider concern whether the arthritis is monarticular and whether it is inflammatory. Inflammatory arthropathies often have prominent effusion, synovial proliferation, and subchondral edema; later on, erosions and diffuse cartilage loss develop. A monarticular inflammatory arthritis should raise concern for infection. Differential possibilities stem from imaging findings as well as patient demographics and clinical situation. This chapter discusses an approach to diagnosis of arthritis based on specific imaging findings and discusses some of the arthropathies most relevant to the practicing radiologist.

IMAGING CHARACTERISTICS OF SPECIFIC DISEASES

For simplicity, diseases are categorized into degenerative processes, inflammatory arthropathies, connective tissues diseases, crystalline disorders, metabolic conditions and noninflammatory monarticular diseases.

DEGENERATIVE DISEASE

Osteoarthritis

Osteoarthritis is defined by the hallmarks of osteophytes, joint narrowing, subchondral cysts and subchondral sclerosis (Fig. 4-1). However, these hallmarks are not specific for osteoarthritis.

In primary osteoarthritis, joint degeneration occurs as a result of a primary abnormality of the articular cartilage, usually due to overuse or old age. In weight-bearing joints, distribution of joint narrowing typically reflects the line of force (e.g., superomedial in the hip). Joints that undergo chronic stress or overuse such as the joints of the hand also commonly exhibit primary osteoarthritis. Patients with acromegaly experience premature primary osteoarthritis related to lack of nutrition of abnormally thickened cartilage. Similarly, paralyzed patients may acquire degenerated joints, which result from chondrolysis or decreased pumping action of nutrient-filled synovial fluid into the avascular hyaline cartilage. Patients with developmental joint conditions (e.g., epiphyseal dysplasias) are also more susceptible to hyaline cartilage wear.

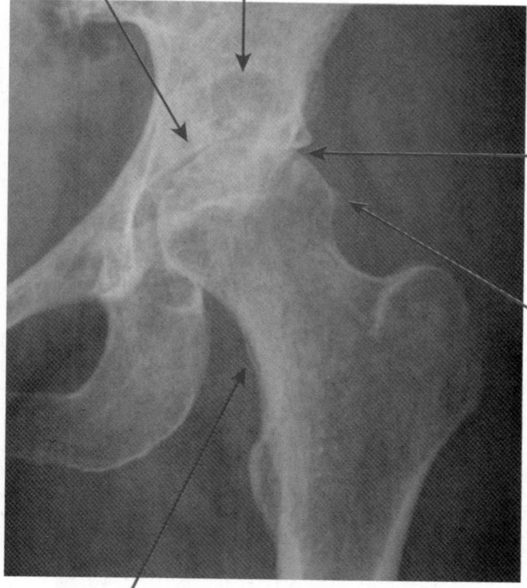
Large supra-acetabular subchondral cyst
Sclerosis
Superior-lateral joint narrowing
Osteophytes
"Buttressing" or bone formation in response to altered stresses

Figure 4-1 Hallmarks of osteoarthritis. The cortex thickens because of slow periosteal apposition, called "buttressing." Similarly, osteophyte formation and subchondral sclerosis are responses to internal derangement and instability or altered stress, an adaptive phenomenon that secondarily may help support the joint.

Secondary osteoarthritis is seen as a delayed consequence of some joint insult (Box 4-1). This includes diverse mechanisms such as (1) fibrocartilage or ligament injury (e.g., medial meniscal tear with medial compartment osteoarthritis; anterior cruciate ligament tear with osteoarthritis; glenoid labral tear with instability and subsequent osteoarthritis; acetabular labral tear with superolateral hip osteoarthritis); (2) articular incongruity (e.g., intra-articular fracture with malunion and articular stepoff; avascular necrosis with articular surface collapse; developmental deformity such as hip dysplasia; progressive deformity of bone as with Paget disease; malalignment such as scapholunate advanced collapse of the wrist); or (3) cartilage destruction (e.g., septic arthritis, rheumatoid arthritis or hemophilia with primary chondrolysis and subsequent osteoarthritis) (Fig. 4-2). Secondary osteoarthritis due to cartilage destruction may cause confusion because there are signs of the primary process as well as the hallmarks of osteoarthritis. A common example is chronic rheumatoid arthritis with marginal erosions and diffuse joint narrowing due to hyaline cartilage destruction and with superimposed osteophytes.

BOX 4-1 CAUSES OF SECONDARY OSTEOARTHRITIS

Joint Incongruity/Instability

Internal derangement/instability (e.g., meniscal tear, anterior cruciate ligament tear)
Intra-articular fracture
Paget disease
Developmental deformity
Avascular necrosis with collapse

Cartilage Destruction

Septic arthritis
Noninfectious inflammatory arthropathies (e.g., rheumatoid arthritis)
Hemophilia
Crystalline arthropathies (gout, crystalline calcium pyrophosphate dehydrate [CPPD] arthopathy)
Pigmented villonodular synovitis
Synovial osteochondromatosis

Cartilage Descriptors and MR Imaging Protocol

Detecting hyaline cartilage defects can be a challenge in certain joints even with high-field MRI. Low-field scanners are at a great disadvantage owing to low resolution, signal, and limited fat suppression. Cartilage is bright on most imaging sequences in which fat suppression is used (without fat suppression, hyaline cartilage appears intermediate to dark); the key is using a sequence with high resolution and signal-to-noise ratio (SNR) with sufficient contrast between joint fluid and cartilage. On high-field scanners the most common sequences used are protein density (PD) or T2-weighted sequences with fat suppression and two- or three-dimensional fat-suppressed T1-weighted spoiled gradient-recalled echo (GRE) sequences. The T2-weighted sequence should optimally have a PD-like echo time (TE) of around 40 to 60 msec to increase SNR while retaining high fluid conspicuity. The GRE sequence can be acquired with a flip angle of 40 to 60 degrees, using the same value for time to repetition (TR) (40–60 msec) and minimum TE, combined with fat suppression. This yields a T1-weighted sequence in which cartilage is bright and fluid is dark. Both are sensitive for cartilage loss,

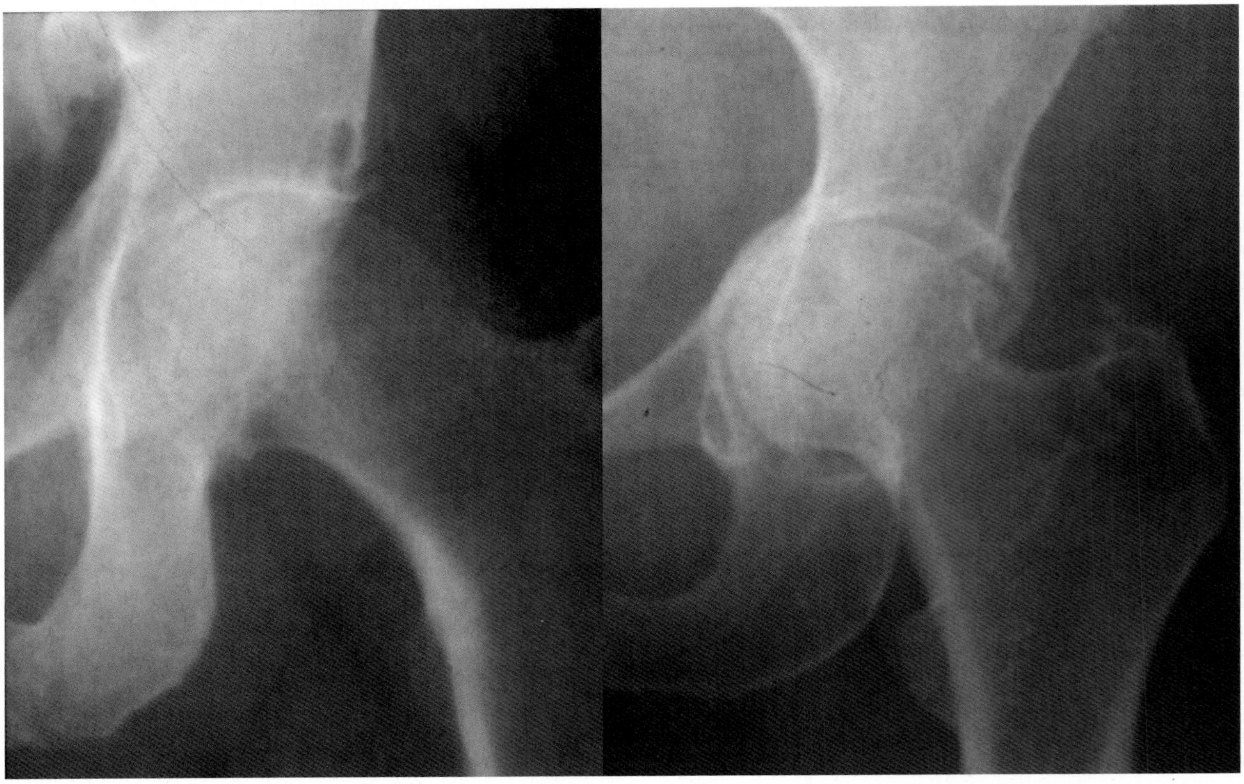
Secondary OA (mechanical)
Secondary OA (post-inflammatory)
Superolateral narrowing
• Related to impingement and labral tear
Concentric narrowing axial migration
• Related to prior rheumatoid arthritis

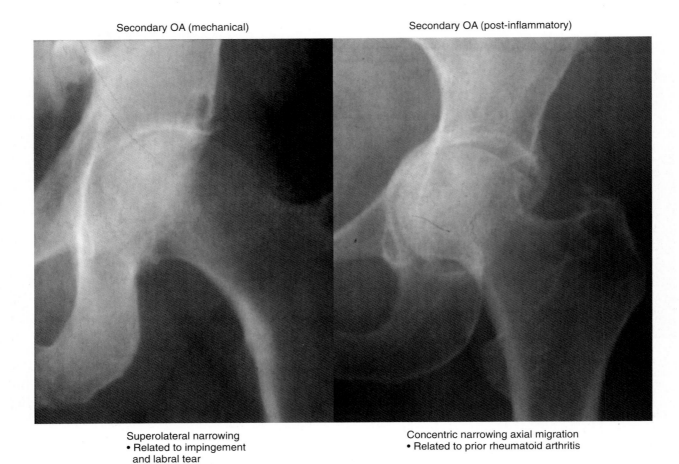

Figure 4-2 Osteoarthritis (OA) can be separated into primary and secondary forms. Secondary osteoarthritis can be from mechanical causes such as joint incongruity or instability or other acute or chronic joint insult. Sequelae of inflammatory conditions (e.g., septic arthritis, rheumatoid arthritis) result in diffuse loss of cartilage. These chondrolytic processes as well as other processes resulting in diffuse cartilage loss (e.g., chemical, recurrent joint hemorrhage) are distinguished by diffuse (concentric) joint narrowing; mechanical causes of osteoarthritis often result in joint narrowing distributed asymmetrically in the joint.

but the PD T2-weighted sequence is more versatile and is also useful for ligaments, tendons, and marrow. The GRE sequence is very useful in situations in which cartilage is thin or the joint is small, as in the wrist and elbow. Intra-articular contrast can be useful to demonstrate cartilage defects, but there is often insufficient difference in signal between cartilage and joint fluid containing gadolinium. Newer sequences improve detection of cartilage defects; these generally involve steady-state GRE techniques and their nomenclature is vendor-specific. Physiologic imaging techniques including T2-mapping, T1-rho imaging, spectroscopy, and delayed gadolinium-enhanced MR imaging of cartilage (dGEMRIC) can be used to map areas of dehydration and proteoglycan depletion indicative of early cartilage degeneration. These techniques are used mainly for research studies but may be incorporated into routine MR protocols in the future as treatments for early cartilage damage evolve.

Radiologists interpreting MRI should use a common language with referring doctors and strive to be accurate and precise in describing cartilage damage. A commonly used grading system in the orthopedic nomenclature is the Outerbridge system (Box 4-2), which dates back to the late 1950s and was subsequently modified in 1975. The system was based on probing of the cartilage surface at surgery: grade 1 is cartilage softening; grade 2 is a cartilage defect smaller than half-inch wide (the width of the probe end; later

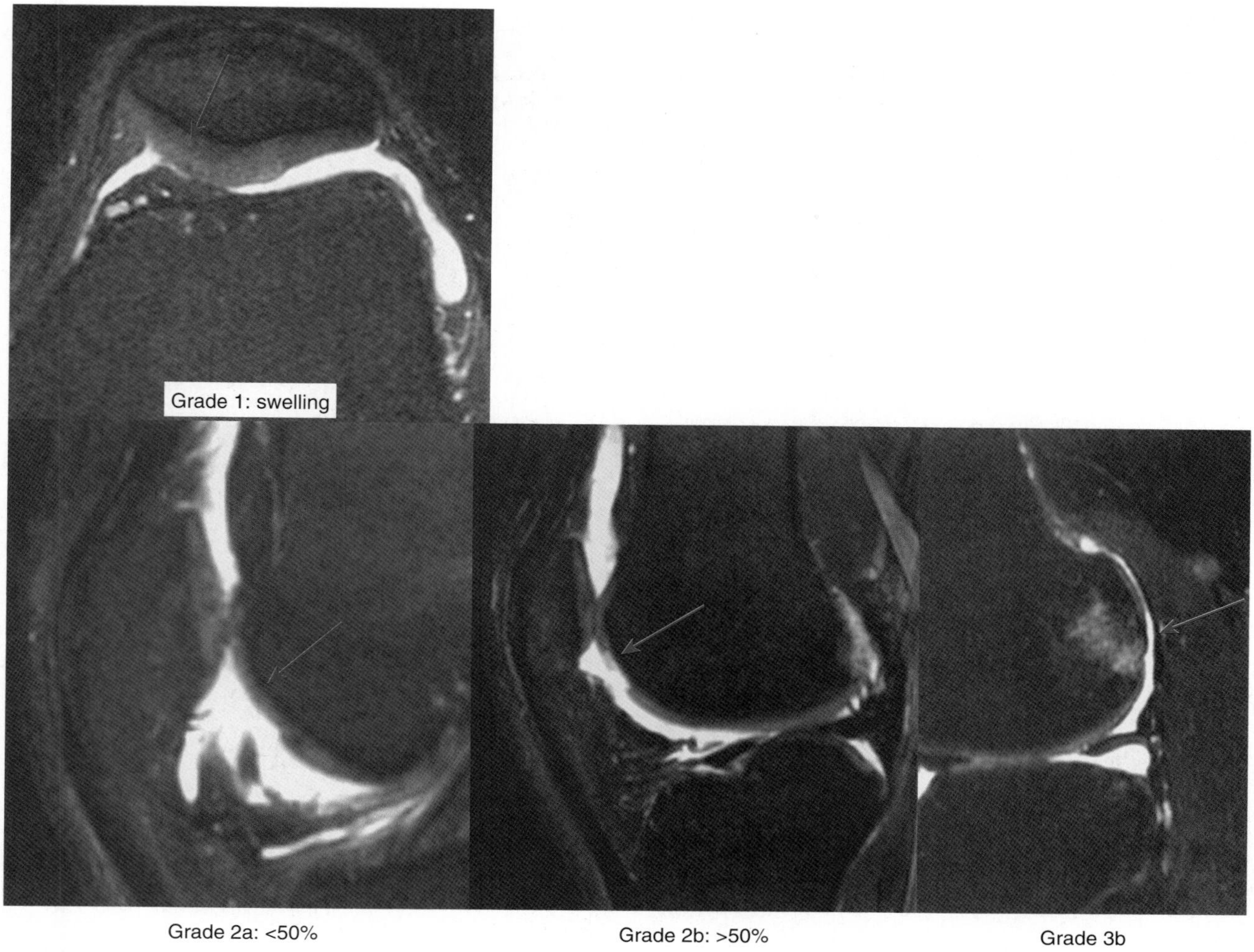
Grade 1: swelling
Grade 2a: <50%
Grade 2b: >50%
Grade 3b

Figure 4-3 Examples of different Noyes grades of chondromalacia (see Box 4-2).

changed to 1.5 cm); grade 3 is a defect greater than or equal to half-inch wide; and grade 4 is a full-thickness defect with exposed bone (Fig. 4-3). This system is awkward to apply to MRI because a combination of grades is usually present, and the surgical grading is based on surface analysis.

Other classification systems have subsequently been developed (see Box 4-2). The commonly used term chondromalacia is particularly useless and nondescriptive. The most useful method of characterizing cartilage loss is to be descriptive in location, size, and depth of cartilage defects seen. Cartilage loss can be divided into diffuse and focal lesions (Figs. 4-4 and 4-5). Some useful descriptors are listed in Box 4-3.

Cartilage flaps and delamination deserve special consideration. These represent unstable cartilage lesions and should be described separately. A cartilage flap is an oblique linear defect (see Fig. 4-4), causing the fragment to be potentially mobile; this can result in pain and locking, and the fragment can break off to form a body. Delamination is separation of the hyaline cartilage from underlying bone (Figs. 4-6 and 4-7). Fluid undermines the cartilage, and although the lesion may not be observed on arthroscopy, the "bubble" of fluid can propogate and form a flap.

Cartilage lesions of all types can exhibit subchondral edema on MRI; this may occur only on one side of the joint in the early stages, later progressing to cyst formation (Fig. 4-8). Cartilage lesions almost always progress but occasionally spontaneously fill in with dark fibrocartilage or bone (Fig. 4-9). In the knee, a typical progression of cartilage loss is observed. A common presentation is tearing of the medial meniscus with extrusion; the altered forces cause

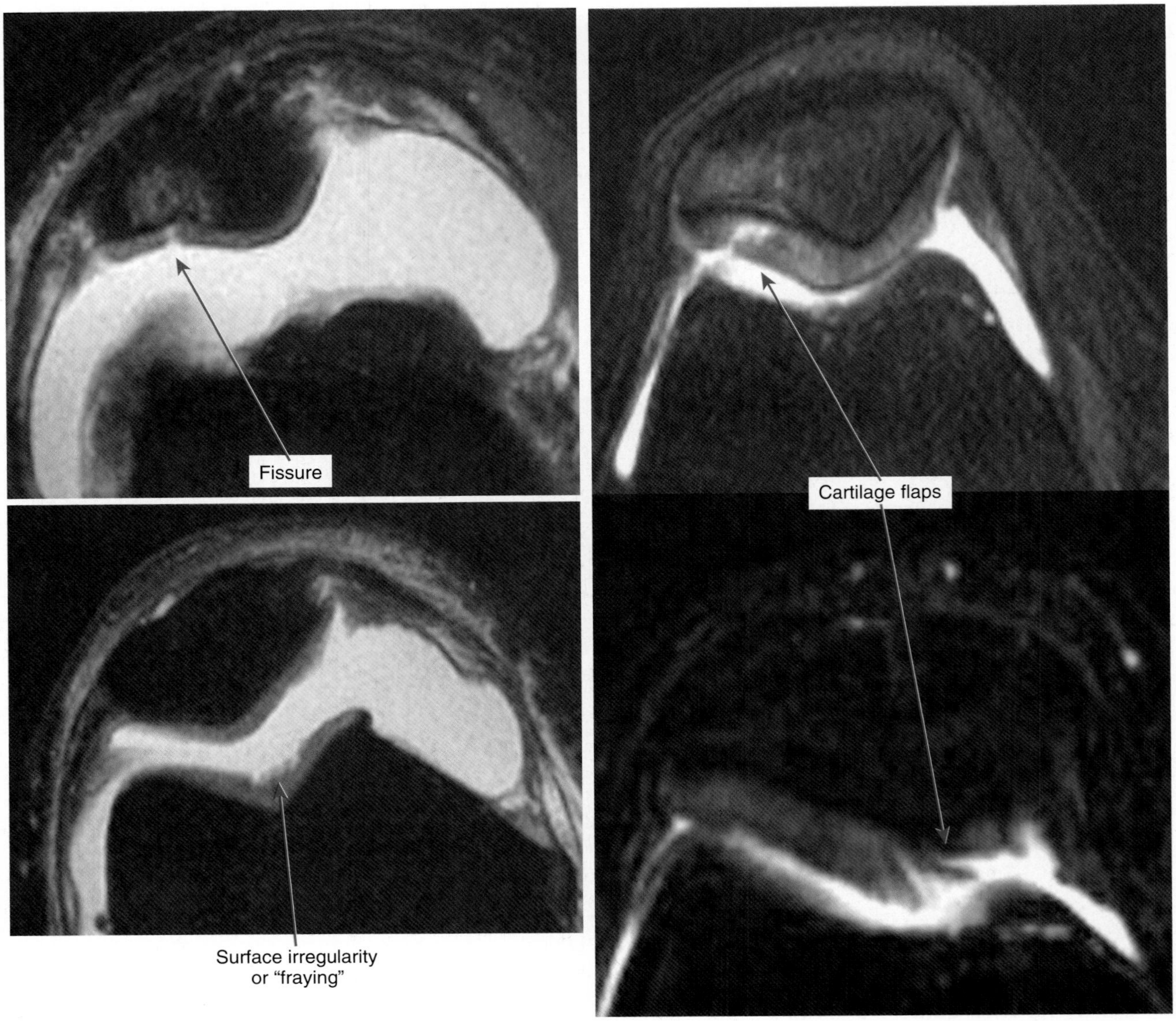
Fissure
Cartilage flaps
Surface irregularity
or "fraying"

Figure 4-4 Cartilage descriptors (see Box 4-3).

diffuse cartilage loss in the medial compartment and osteophyte formation. Lateral compartment spurs form, with cartilage loss beginning near the tibial spines and eventually distributed throughout the compartment with a degenerative tear of the lateral meniscus following thereafter (Fig. 4-10). Meniscal extrusion and unstable meniscal tears (especially complex tears and radial tears) can result in rapid compartmental cartilage loss (Figs. 4-11 and 4-12) and should be described in the radiology report. Impingement and instability in other joints are also associated with osteoarthritis. Early osteoarthritis can also occur at the hip related to impingement and labral tear, for example.

Erosive Osteoarthritis

Erosive osteoarthritis, also called EOA or inflammatory osteoarthritis, is seen in patients with underlying osteoarthritis of the hands. Patients are typically elderly and often female. Arthritic interphalangeal joints (especially the distal interphalangeal joints)

BOX 4-2 POPULAR GRADING SYSTEMS FOR DEGENERATIVE ARTHRITIS

Kellgren-Lawrence Radiographic Grading Scale of Osteoarthritis of the Tibiofemoral Joint

Grade 0: No radiographic findings of osteoarthritis
1: Minute osteophytes of doubtful clinical significance
2: Definite osteophytes with unimpaired joint space
3: Definite osteophytes with moderate joint space narrowing
4: Definite osteophytes with severe joint space narrowing and subchondral sclerosis

Outerbridge Arthroscopic Classification of Chondrosis (Modified)

Grade 0: Normal cartilage
1: Cartilage with softening and swelling
2: A partial-thickness defect with fissures on the surface that do not reach subchondral bone or exceed 1.5 cm in diameter
3: Fissuring to the level of subchondral bone in an area with a diameter more than 1.5 cm
4: Exposed subchondral bone

Noyes Arthroscopic Classification of Chondrosis

Grade 0: Normal articular cartilage
1a: Mild softening or discoloration of articular cartilage
1b: Severe softening or discoloration of articular cartilage
2a: Partial-thickness defect of <50% of the total thickness of articular cartilage
2b: Partial-thickness defect of >50% of the total thickness of articular cartilage
3a: Full-thickness articular cartilage defect with normal subchondral bone
3b: Full-thickness articular cartilage defect with erosion of subchondral bone

become tender, painful, and swollen. Central erosions occur and lead to the classic "seagull" pattern of the joint surface (Fig. 4-13). The joint may eventually undergo ankylosis.

Neuropathic Osteoarthropathy

Neuropathic osteoarthropathy, also known as Charcot arthropathy, can be considered a severe, aggressive form of osteoarthritis with a component of instability. Some features of osteoarthritis are often present,

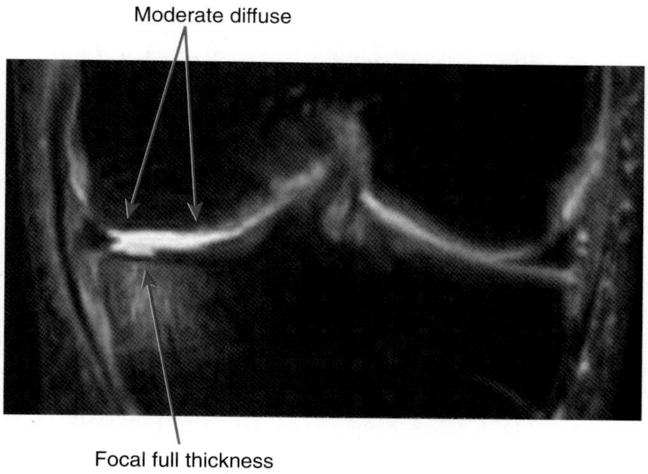
Moderate diffuse
Focal full thickness

Figure 4-5 Cartilage descriptors (see Box 4-3).

BOX 4-3 USEFUL CARTILAGE DESCRIPTORS FOR MRI

Diffuse

Diffuse surface irregularity
Diffuse partial-thickness cartilage loss
Diffuse severe cartilage loss

Focal

Fissuring/fraying (vertical linear defect)
Flap (oblique linear defect)
Delamination (fluid underneath otherwise intact cartilage)
Partial-thickness defect (some cartilage signal left); measure size
Full-thickness defect (no more cartilage signal); measure size

including sclerosis, osteophytes, and bodies. However, often subluxation, erosion, and joint destruction are seen, which may be extreme and deforming. The arthropathy begins as a sensory neuropathy, which may be from diabetes, syringomyelia, tabes dorsalis, leprosy, or other conditions (Box 4-4). Joints in the insensate region undergo unrecognized injury with ligament damage, osteochondral and capsular disruption and even fracture. The joint injury persists and progresses as a result of continued stress, and the arthropathy ensues. Loss of sympathetic control with neuropathy, or hypovascularity in the case of diabetic vasculopathy, may also play a role in disease progression.

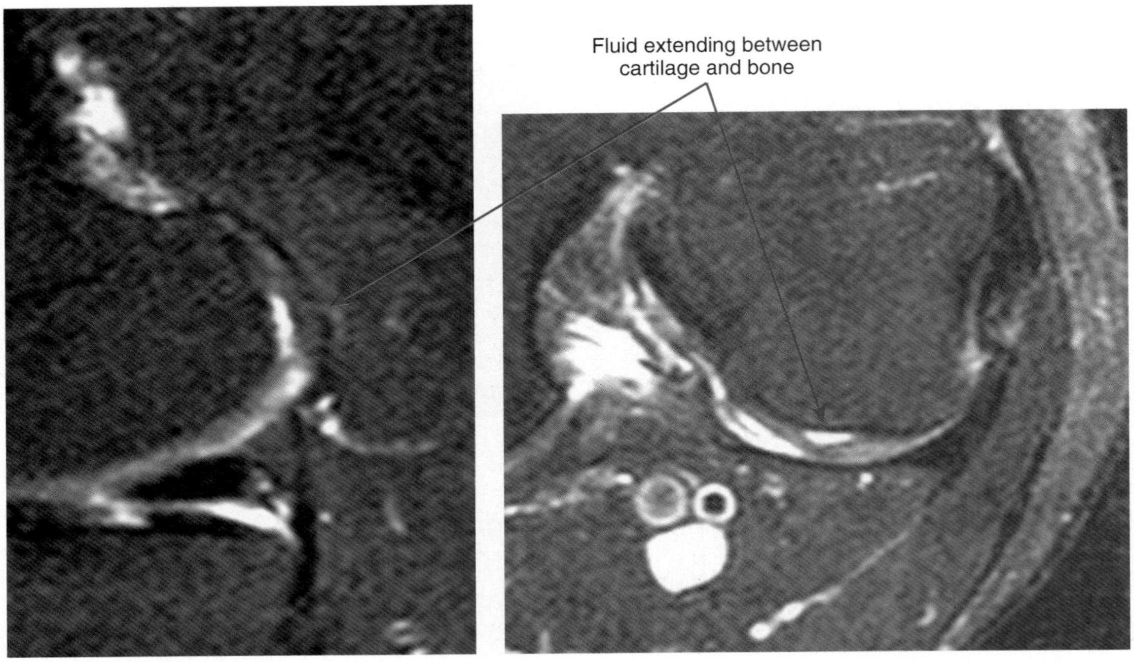
Fluid extending between
cartilage and bone

Figure 4-6 Delamination is separation of the hyaline cartilage from underlying bone. Fluid undermines the cartilage, and although the lesion may not be observed on arthroscopy, the "bubble" of fluid can propogate and form a flap.

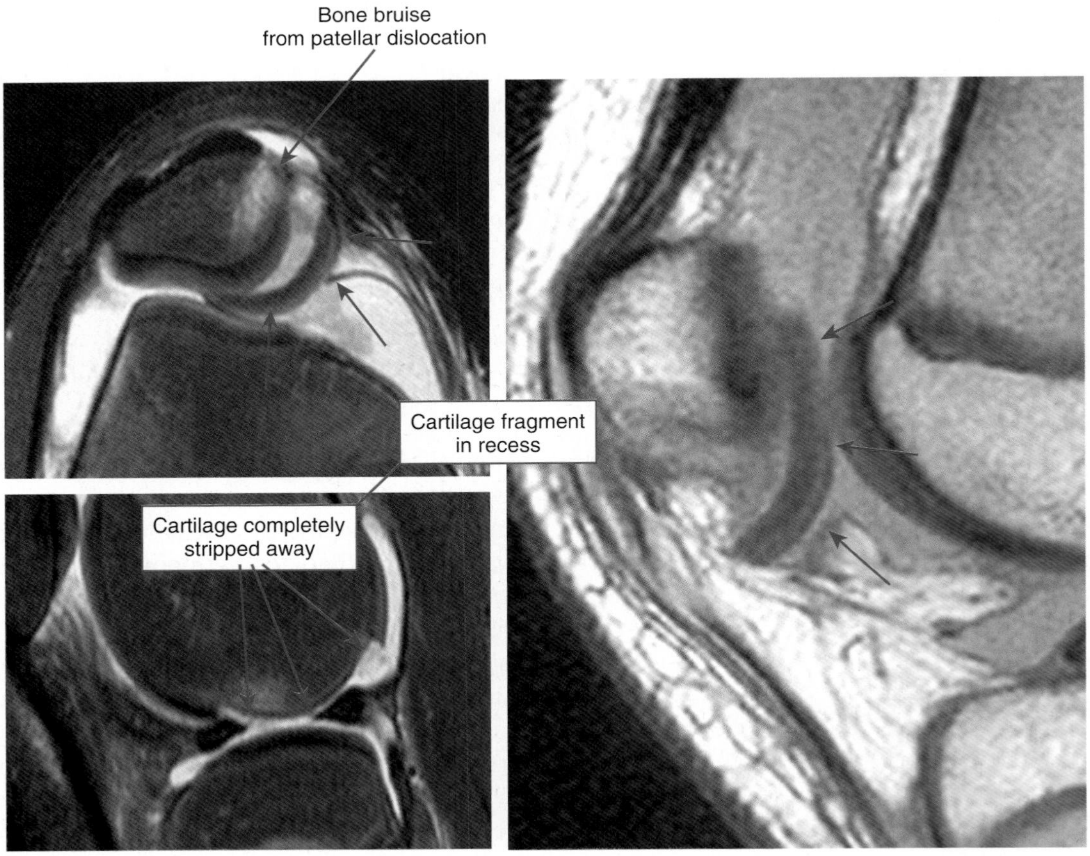
Bone bruise
from patellar dislocation
Cartilage fragment
in recess
Cartilage completely
stripped away

Figure 4-7 *Acute cartilage delamination in a 13-year-old boy following patellar dislocation.*

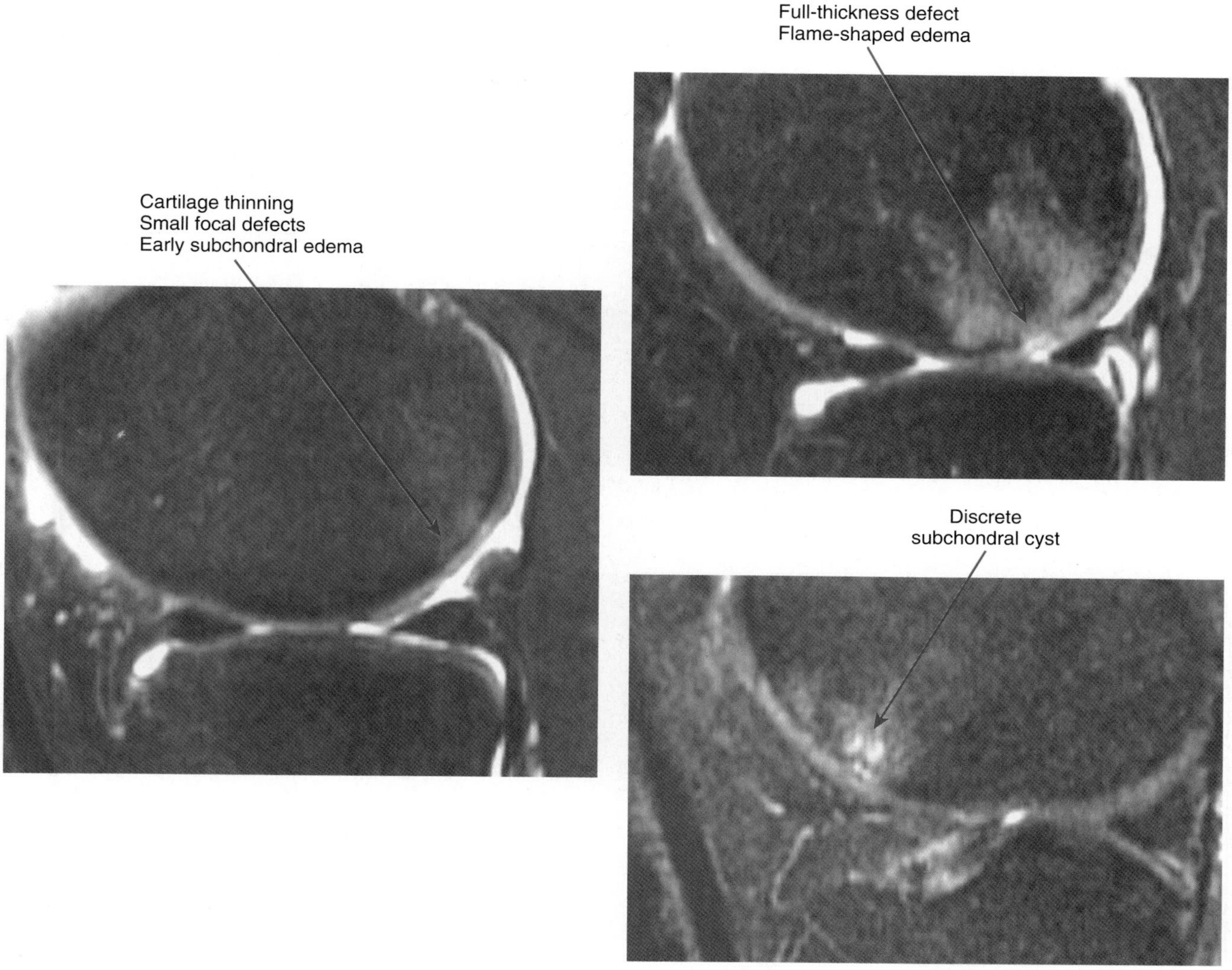
Full-thickness defect
Flame-shaped edema
Cartilage thinning
Small focal defects
Early subchondral edema
Discrete
subchondral cyst

Figure 4-8 *Subchondral changes associated with cartilage lesions of different stages.*

Neuropathic osteoarthropathy can be described in three forms: atrophic, hypertrophic, and mixed (Figs. 4-14 and 4-15). The atrophic form appears as well-defined osteolysis with a "surgical–like" appearance. Proliferative response is absent, but the remaining bones are normally mineralized and the margins may be sclerotic. This pattern is classically seen in the shoulders associated with a spinal cord syrinx. The hypertrophic form appears as a severe osteoarthritis with new bone production, sclerosis, fragmentation, and often subluxation. The mixed form has features of bone destruction and production.

BOX 4-4 NEUROPATHIC DISEASE: ETIOLOGY AND TYPICAL LOCATION

Leprosy: Distal extremities (hands and feet)

Diabetes: Feet (Lisfranc, hindfoot, metatarsophalangeal joints)

Syrinx: Upper extremities (esp. shoulder, bilateral symmetric)

Paralysis: Spinal segment (esp. at junction with fixation)

Tabes dorsalis (uncommon): Spine, hips, knees, ankles

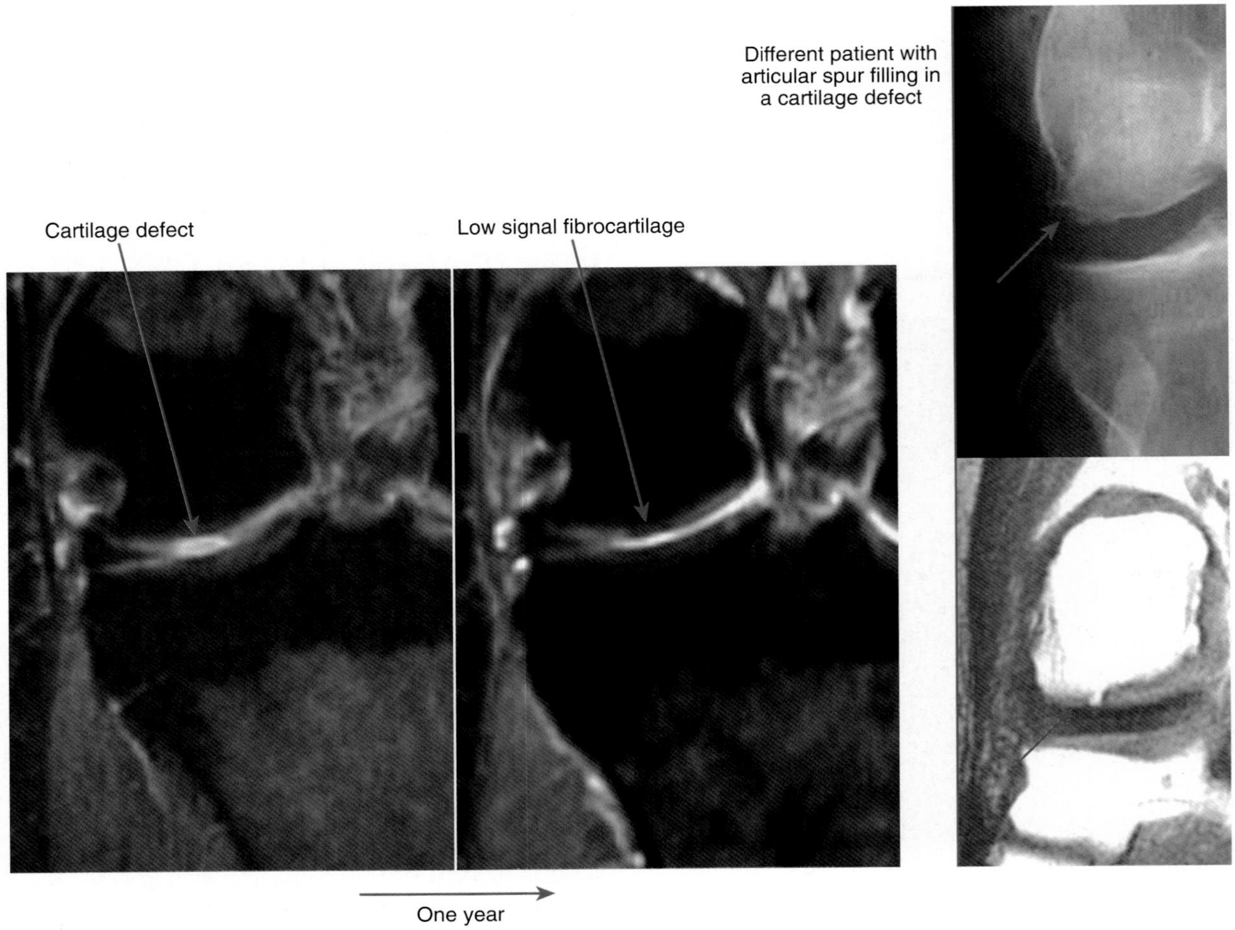
Different patient with articular spur filling in a cartilage defect
Cartilage defect
Low signal fibrocartilage
One year

Figure 4-9 Cartilage is avascular and has an intricate internal collagen architecture; therefore, it does not heal with the same structural makeup. However, cartilage defects can "fill in" naturally, with disorganized dark signal fibrocartilage or with bone. A similar outcome is seen after surgical microfracture technique.

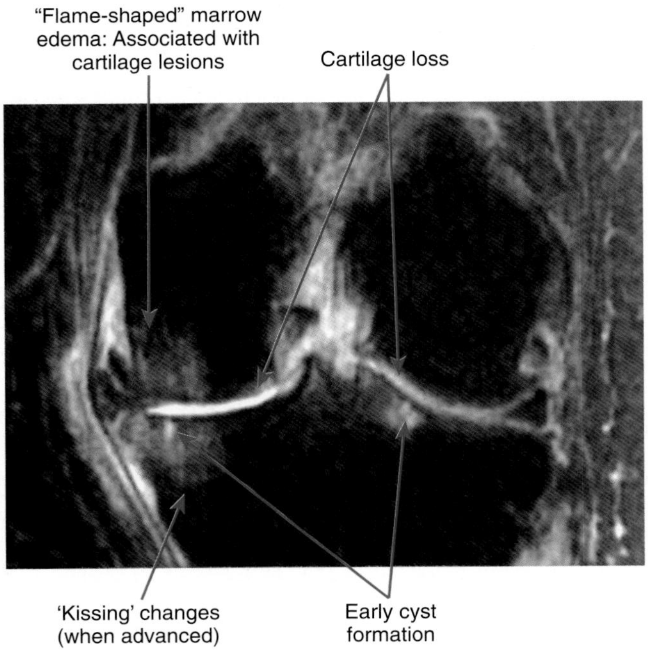
"Flame-shaped" marrow edema: Associated with cartilage lesions
Cartilage loss
'Kissing' changes (when advanced)
Early cyst formation

Figure 4-10 Subchondral cyst formation and progression are important to recognize on MRI, so as not to confuse findings with bone bruise, avascular necrosis, or other process.

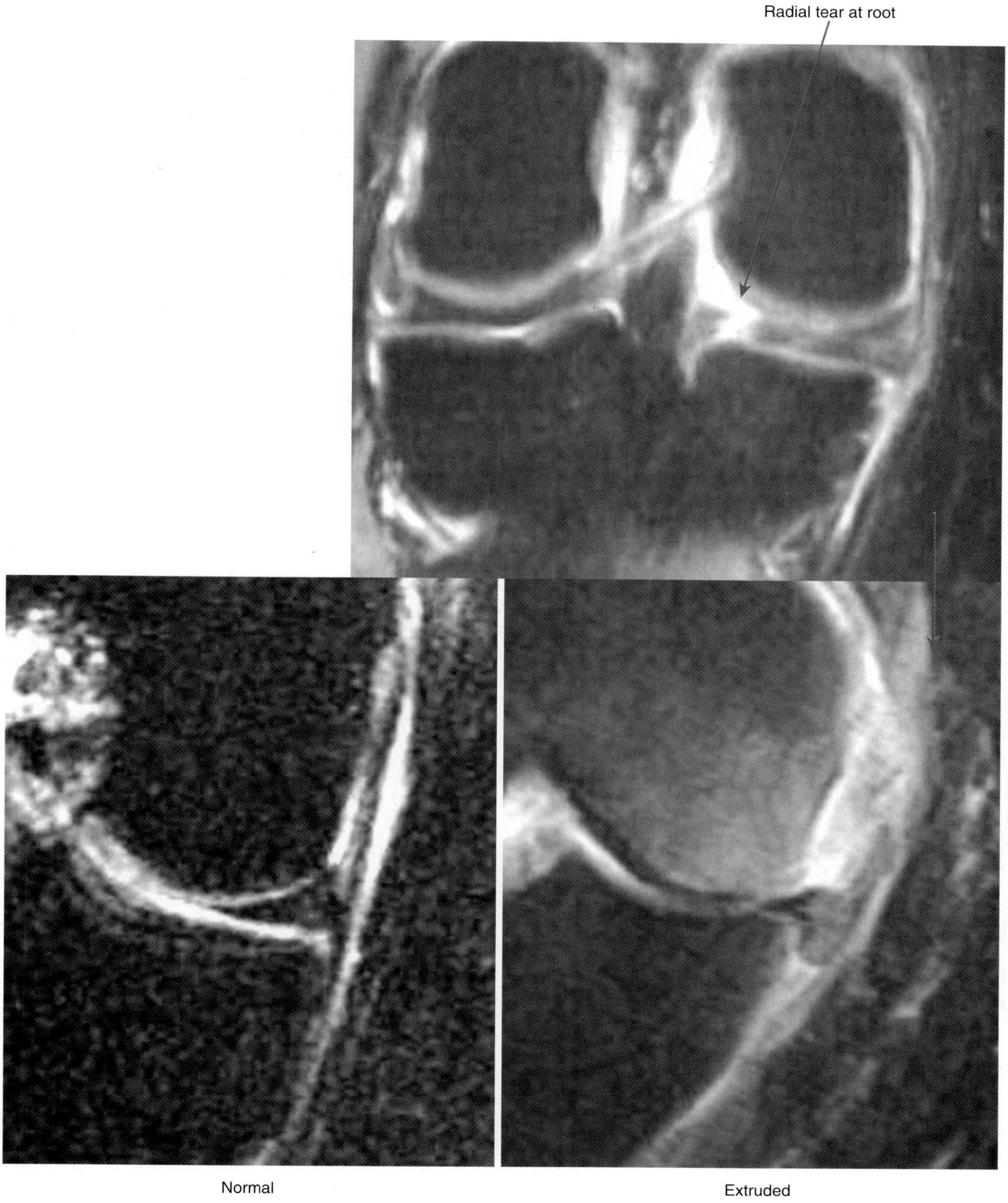
Radial tear at root
Normal
Extruded

Figure 4-11 Meniscal extrusion. Disruption of circular central meniscal fibers destabilizes the meniscus and leads to extrusion. Complex tears, large radial tears, and tears at the root attachments are associated with major (>3 mm) meniscal extrusion. Extrusion leads to compartmental osteoarthritis.

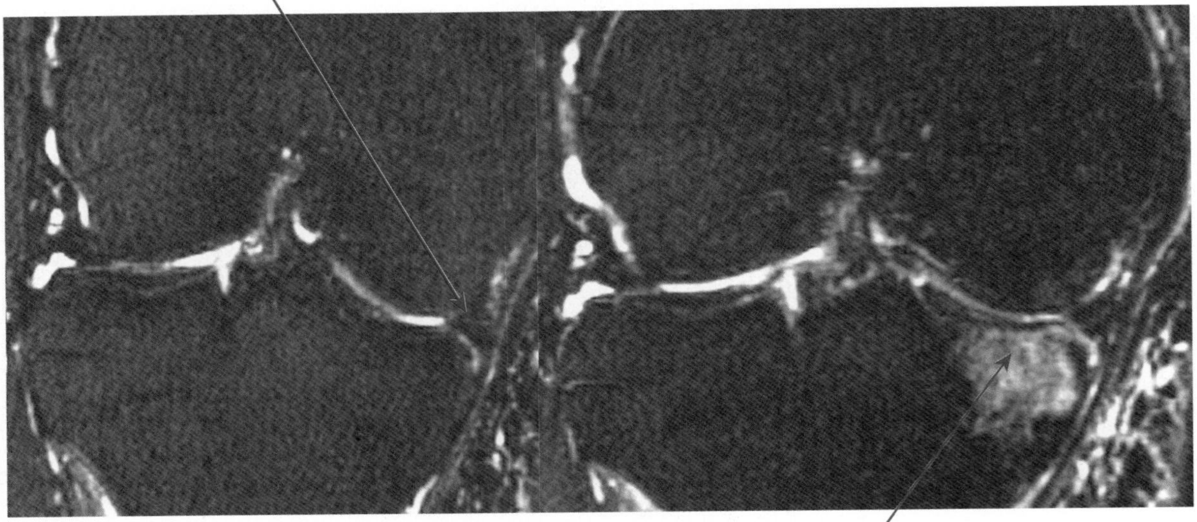
Meniscal extrusion
following tear
— 6 months →
Osteoarthritis

Figure 4-12 Rapid development of arthritis due to meniscal tear and extrusion.

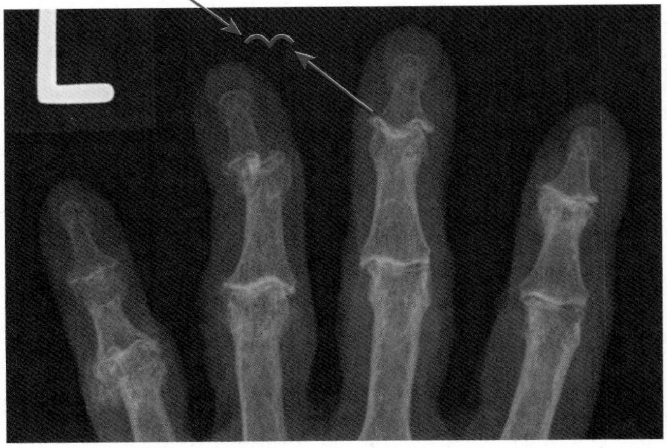
Central erosions
with underlying OA
"seagull" pattern

Figure 4-13 **Erosive osteoarthritis (OA).**

Neuropathic disease can also be described in terms of acute, chronic, or acute-on-chronic (Fig. 4-16). In acute neuropathic osteoarthropathy, the patient presents with diffuse swelling and erythema; clinically this can simulate infection. The involved joints in this early stage of disease often show little deformity or malalignment, and radiographs may show just soft tissue swelling. On MRI, joint effusions are common, with prominent subchondral edema that may extend far into the medullary cavity. Signal intensity changes in the bone marrow consisting of low signal intensity on T1-weighted images and high signal on T2-weighted images may be identical to those observed in septic arthritis and osteomyelitis. Erosions may be seen at the margins of the joint. On gadolinium-enhanced images, marrow enhancement is typically present, with predominantly subchondral distribution. Periarticular soft tissue enhancement may also be seen. Recent fractures related to neuropathic osteoarthropathy may create intense bone marrow edema, which lead to potential diagnostic pitfalls. In chronic neuropathic osteoarthropathy, radiographic features have been summarized by words beginning with "D": **d**estruction, **d**ebris, preserved bone **d**ensity, **d**isorganization, and **d**islocation (or subluxation) (Box 4-5).

The most commonly involved articulation is the Lisfranc joint. Involvement here causes the metatarsal

BOX 4-5 NEUROPATHIC DISEASE: THE "D"S

Deformity
Destruction
Dislocation/subluxation
Debris
Density (preservation of)

Follow-up
Atrophic neuropathic disease: Surgical-type margins

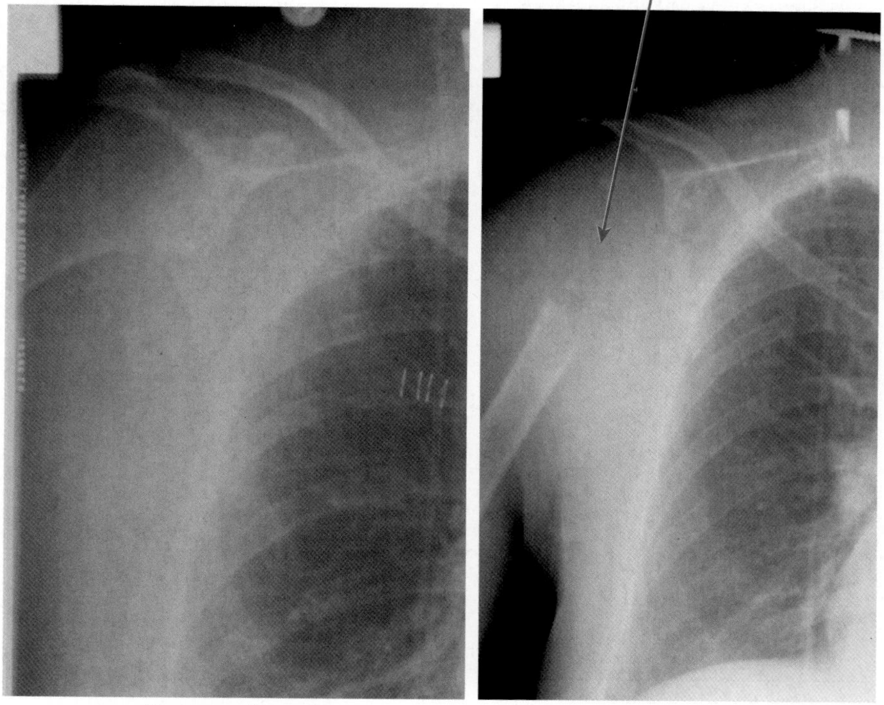

Post-op radiograph following shunt placement

Figure 4-14 *Atrophic neuropathic disease of the shoulder in a patient with a syrinx that was lost to follow-up for a period after ventriculoperitoneal shunting and subsequent shunt malfunction.*

Mixed atrophic/hypertrophic disease of THR ankle and hindfoot

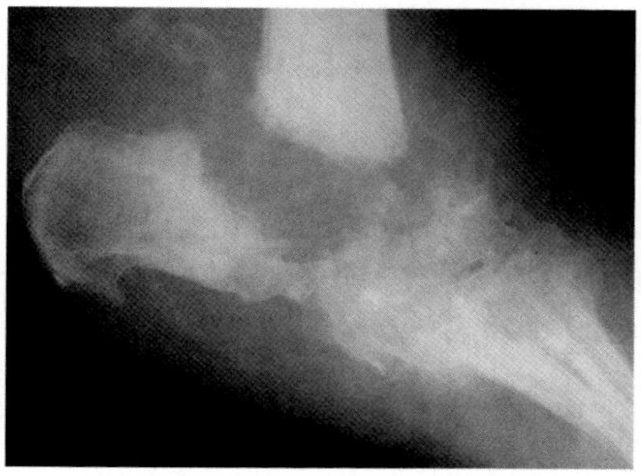

Hypertrophic pattern in the midfoot

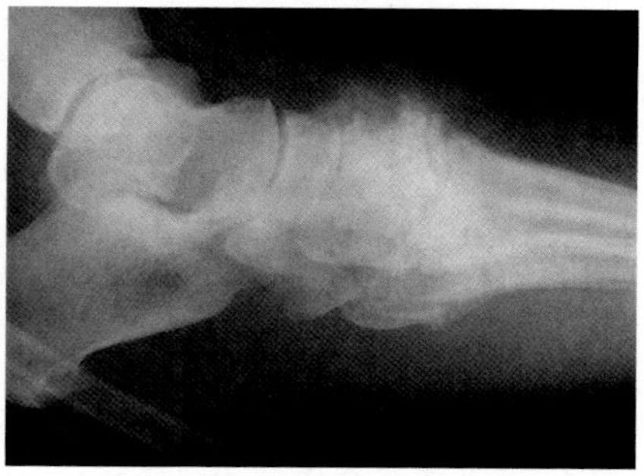

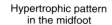

Hallmarks of neuropathic disease:
<u>The "D"s</u>

- Dislocation (or subluxation)
- Destruction
- Density (preservation of)
- Debris
- Disorganization

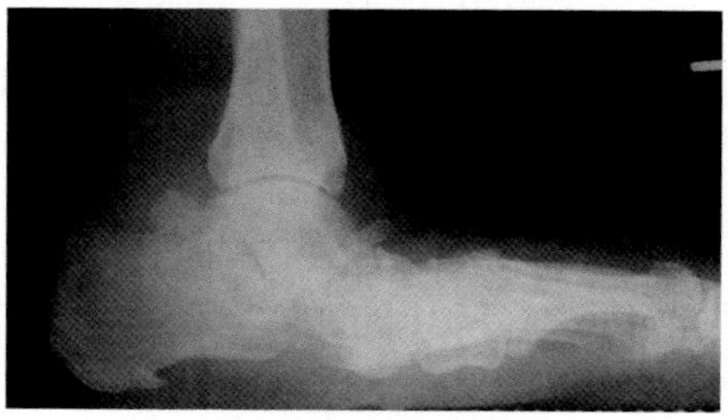

Hypertrophic pattern in the midfoot and hindfoot

Figure 4-15 Hypertrophic and mixed forms of neuropathic disease, common in feet of diabetic patients.

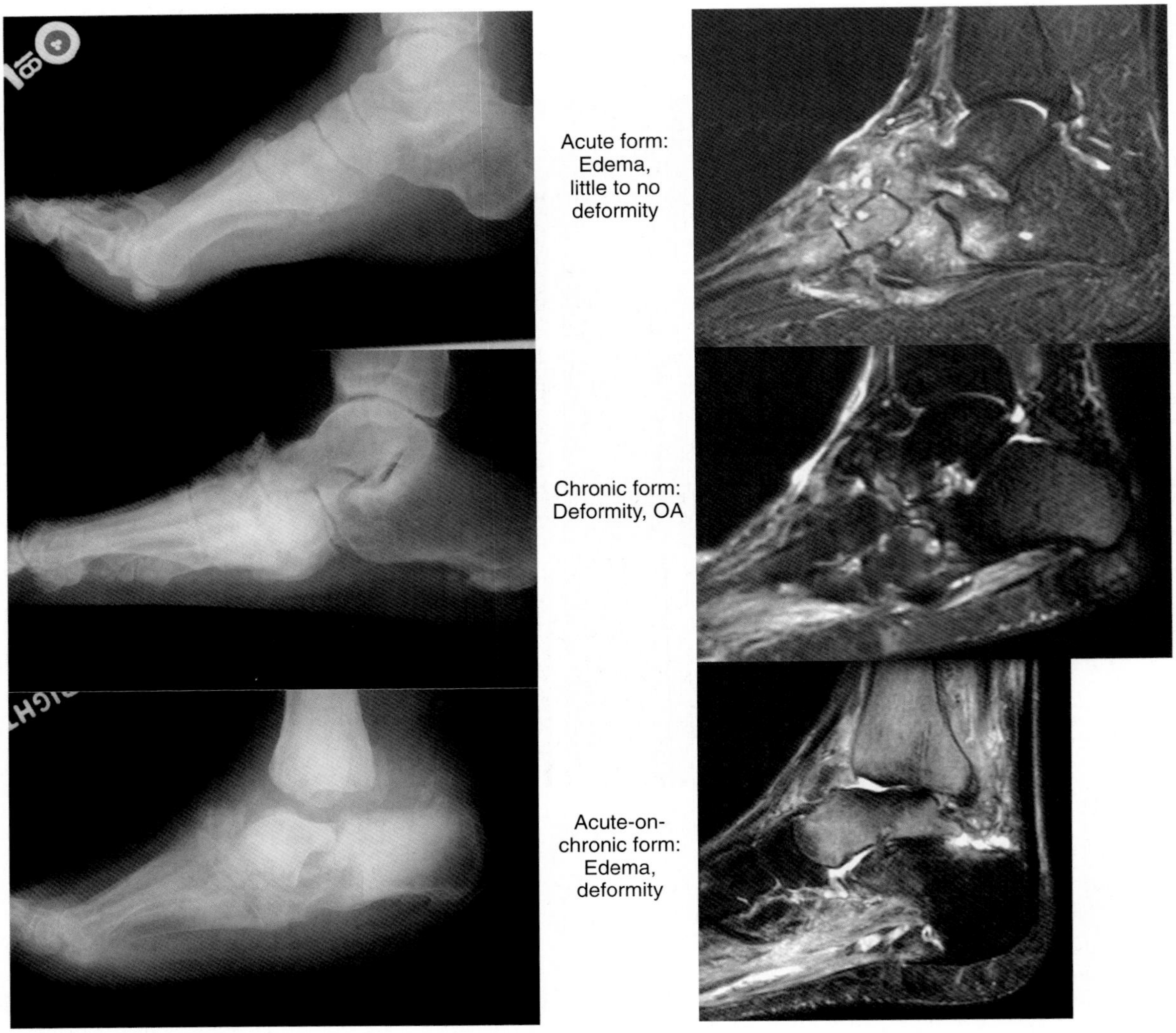
Acute form:
Edema,
little to no
deformity
Chronic form:
Deformity, OA
Acute-on-
chronic form:
Edema,
deformity

Figure 4-16 Neuropathic disease can also be described in terms of acute, chronic, or acute-on-chronic forms. OA, osteoarthritis.

bases to migrate dorsally, and the longitudinal arch collapses, resulting in a rocker-bottom deformity. MR imaging features are more typical of osteoarthritis, with bone production and subchondral cystic change. Acute clinical presentation may be superimposed on chronic neuropathic disease, resulting in features of both on radiographs and MRI. In any phase of neuropathic disease, in the setting of diabetes there is often underlying diffuse soft tissue edema or diffuse muscle atrophy, which in the absence of contrast can appear similar to diffuse cellulitis. Marrow changes can simulate infection.

In addition, osteomyelitis is frequently associated with neuropathic disease of the foot. Chronic neuropathic deformity causes osseous protuberances that can produce increased friction with ill-fitting footwear and results in adjacent skin callus formation, breakdown, and ulceration; osteomyelitis ensues from contiguous spread. Typical locations for this to occur are the metatarsal heads, midfoot, and calcaneus. Differential features between neuropathic disease and infection are discussed in detail in Chapter 5.

INFLAMMATORY DISORDERS

Septic Arthritis

Infection should always be considered when a monarticular arthropathy is seen. Imaging can appear identical to other inflammatory arthropathies such as rheumatoid arthritis or gout. Specific findings are discussed in more detail in Chapter 5.

Rheumatoid Arthritis

Rheumatoid arthritis (Figs. 4-17 through 4-22) affects females more often than males at a ratio of 2–3 to 1. Typically, adult-onset rheumatoid arthritis occurs in the 20s to 40s. Symptoms at presentation classically include joint stiffness, especially in the morning, with pain and swelling—most commonly polyarticular and symmetric. Systemic manifestations include fatigue and weight loss. Clinical criteria for diagnosis include at least four of the following (criteria 1 through 4 must have been present for at least 6 weeks): (1) morning joint stiffness lasting at least 1 hour; (2) soft tissue swelling of at least three joints; (3) swelling of the proximal interphalangeal, metacarpophalangeal, or wrist joints; (4) symmetric involvement; (5) subcutaneous nodules; (6) positive rheumatoid factor; (7) radiographic evidence of erosions of the joints of the hand or wrist. Most patients (approximately 85%) have positive serum rheumatoid factor.

The basic pathology of rheumatoid arthritis is inflammation and proliferation of synovium (pannus), which leads to the various radiographic appearances. Periarticular swelling is due to a combination of pannus and joint effusion. Fusiform soft tissue swelling is characteristic at the proximal interphalangeal joints of the hands, with focal soft tissue swelling at the metacarpophalangeal joints, at the dorsum of the wrist, and over the ulnar styloid. In the feet, soft tissue swelling is common at the metatarsophalangeal joints, especially the fifth. Rheumatoid arthritis can affect any synovial structure, including bursae and tendon sheaths. Bursitis can cause areas of ill-defined soft tissue planes or focal soft tissue prominence; this is most evident radiographically in the retrocalcaneal bursa and olecranon bursa. Tenosynovitis is evident radiographically as diffuse or longitudinally oriented soft tissue swelling, commonly involving the tendons of the wrist. Inflammatory nodular soft tissue lesions may occur, called "rheumatoid nodules." Rheumatoid nodules can occur in patients with rheumatoid arthritis and appear as focal soft tissue masses, usually at sites of chronic friction, such as the extensor surfaces of the forearm, as well as the hands and feet.

Periarticular osteopenia is a classic radiographic feature, especially in early stages of rheumatoid arthritis of the hands and feet, although a generalized pattern of osteopenia can also occur. Involved joints

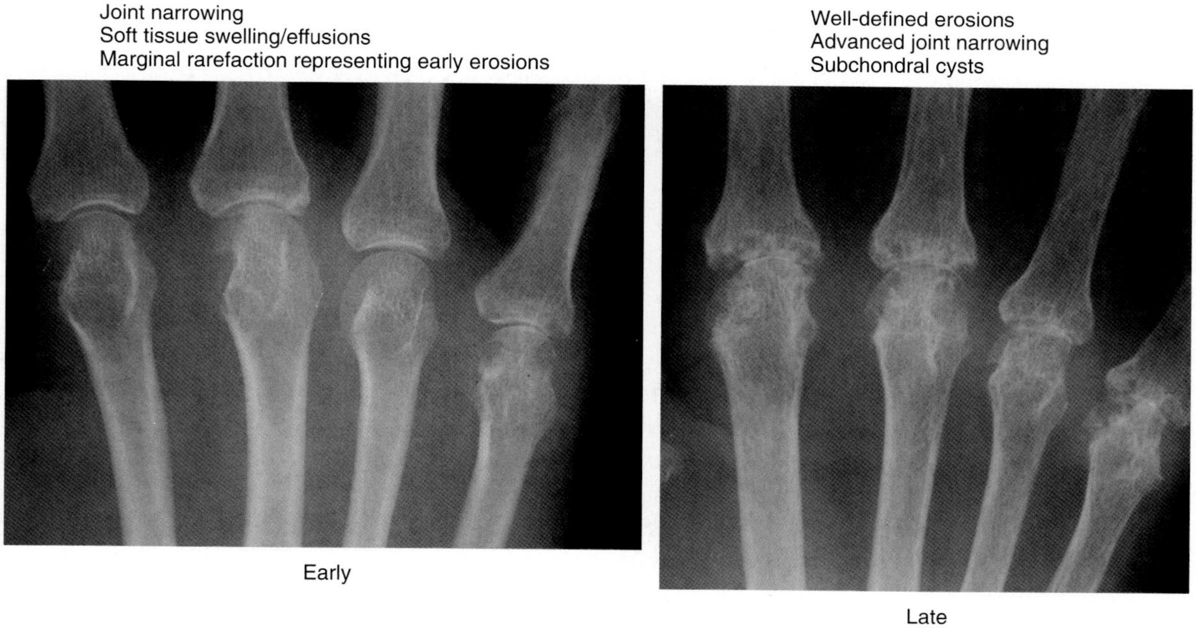
Joint narrowing
Soft tissue swelling/effusions
Marginal rarefaction representing early erosions
Early
Well-defined erosions
Advanced joint narrowing
Subchondral cysts
Late

Figure 4-17 Rheumatoid arthritis—progression of disease. Involved joints generally demonstrate concentric or uniform joint narrowing related to diffuse cartilage loss.

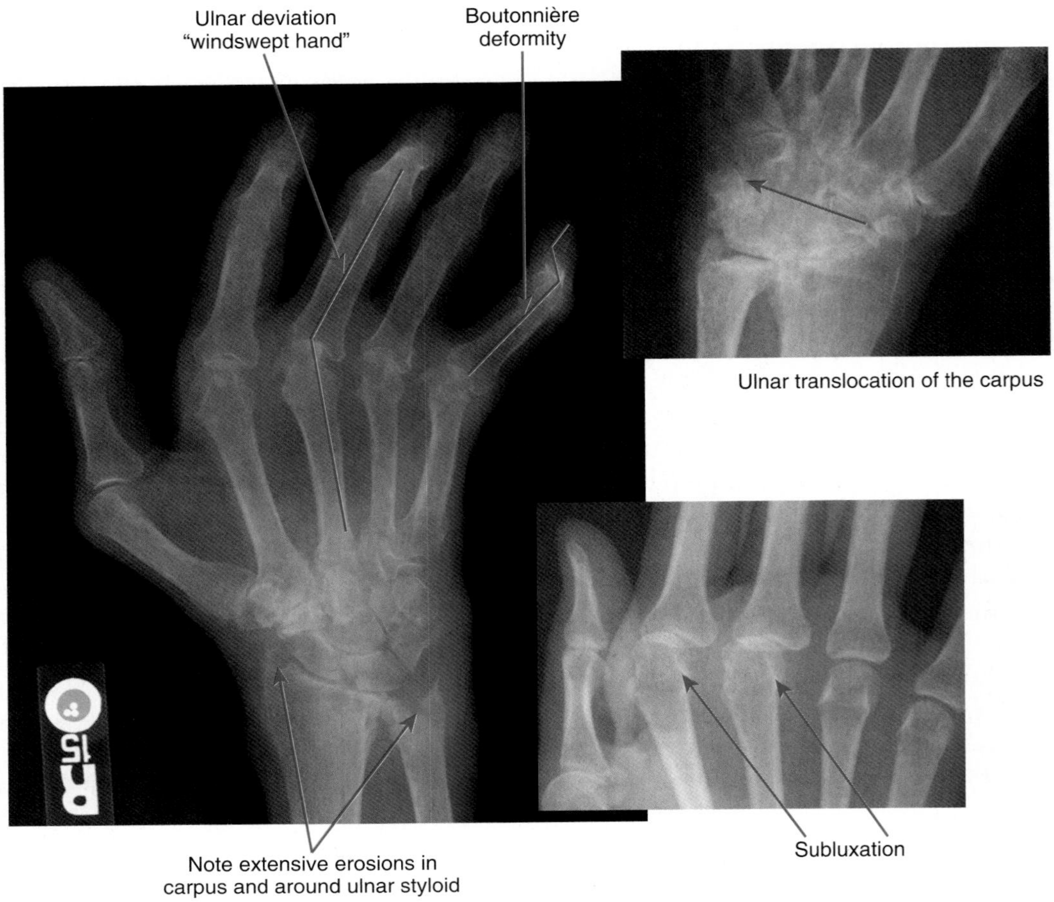

Ulnar deviation
"windswept hand"
Boutonnière
deformity
Ulnar translocation of the carpus
Subluxation
Note extensive erosions in
carpus and around ulnar styloid

Figure 4-18 Hand deformities in rheumatoid arthritis. Boutonnière deformity is flexion at the proximal interphalangeal (PIP) joint and extension at the distal interphalangeal (DIP) joint; swan-neck deformity is extension at the PIP and flexion at the DIP. Deformities are due to stretching or erosion of joint cartilage and capsular structures and supporting ligaments with imbalance of forces across the regions. Also not pictured are dorsal intercalated segmental instability and volar intercalated segmental instability deformity and other carpal malalignments that occur with intercarpal and capsular ligament insufficiency (see Chapter 9). Ulnar translocation occurs when the extrinsic ligaments erode, allowing the carpus to shift over the ulna.

generally demonstrate concentric or uniform joint narrowing related to diffuse cartilage loss. However, in weight-bearing joints there may be more severe narrowing at the weight-bearing surface. Axial migration can occur at the hips because of bone remodeling at the central portion of the acetabulum, with inward bowing of the iliopectineal line, called *protrusio acetabuli*. Characteristic marginal erosions result from thickened, inflammatory synovial tissue (pannus) eroding the bone at the bare area adjacent to the margin of the articular cartilage. Osseous proliferation is not a feature of rheumatoid arthritis; however, osteophyte formation can occur in longstanding rheumatoid arthritis as a result of superimposed secondary osteoarthritis.

Deformities of the hands and feet are common in rheumatoid arthritis for a variety of reasons: laxity and distention of the joint capsule, ligamentous laxity or disruption, tendinopathy or tendon tears, and altered muscle tone. The "swan neck" deformity is hyperextension at the proximal interphalangeal joint and flexion at the distal interphalangeal joint. The "boutonière" deformity is flexion at the proximal interphalangeal joint and hyperextension at the distal interphalangeal joint. These deformities result from imbalance of the flexor and extensor tendons. Subluxations at the metacarpophalangeal and metatarsophalangeal joints are also common: The digits of the hands deviate in an ulnar direction ("windswept hand" appearance); in the foot, hallux valgus is very

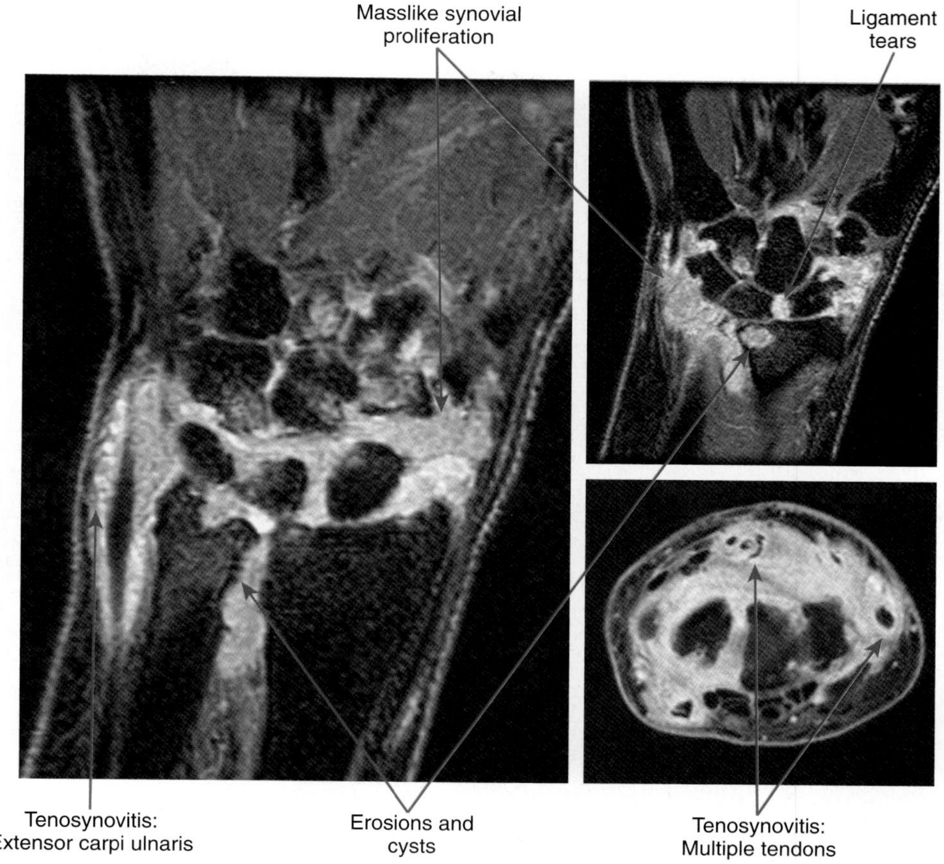
Masslike synovial proliferation
Ligament tears
Tenosynovitis: Extensor carpi ulnaris
Erosions and cysts
Tenosynovitis: Multiple tendons

Figure 4-19 MRI is useful for evaluation of rheumatoid arthritis, to detect early erosions and track extent of synovial proliferation; MRI findings have been used to document response to treatment objectively. Intravenous contrast is helpful in that synovial pannus enhances brightly and is easily evaluated. Dynamic contrast can be used to document degree of synovial hyperemia by plotting the time-uptake curve. MRI is also helpful in diagnosing various complications of the disease and its treatment, including ligament tears and avascular necrosis.

common and may be severe, leading to overlap of the first and second toes. In the hands, the carpal bones commonly erode (carpal-dominant involvement), with ligamentous disruption and laxity causing carpal instability patterns. In more severe cases, the process of erosion and instability may reach a point at which there is "carpal collapse," with the metacarpal bases nearly apposed to the radius. The entire carpus and hand may slip in an ulnar direction, referred to as "ulnar translocation." Carpal collapse and dissociation, in addition to mass effect from pannus, can cause impingement on the median nerve as it passes through the carpal tunnel, resulting in carpal tunnel syndrome.

Rheumatoid arthritis is most commonly recognized in the hands and feet; in fact, if there is a finding on a foot exam that is of questionable significance, it is often useful to evaluate radiographs of the hands, and vice versa. Distribution in the hands is characteristically more proximal than distal, commonly involving the carpus, as well as the metacarpophalangeal and proximal interphalangeal joints. In the feet/ankles, the distribution mimics that of the hands/wrists, with the metatarsophalangeal joints most commonly involved. Distribution is bilateral and symmetric; however, extent of involvement may not be the same from side to side.

Spine Involvement

A major site of serious musculoskeletal complications from rheumatoid arthritis is the cervical spine. The dens is surrounded by synovial tissue, anteriorly at the junction of the dens with the anterior arch of C1, and posteriorly at the transverse ligament. Pannus at these synovial locations and at the facet joints can cause laxity of the transverse ligament and erosion of the dens itself, leading to excessive motion and instability at C1-C2. The instability may not be apparent on a neutral lateral view; lateral views in flexion and extension are generally indicated to gauge the degree of instability, although the flexion/extension motion must be performed with great caution, always allowing patients to flex and extend the neck voluntarily, determining their own limitation. This instability is very important to identify in individuals at risk,

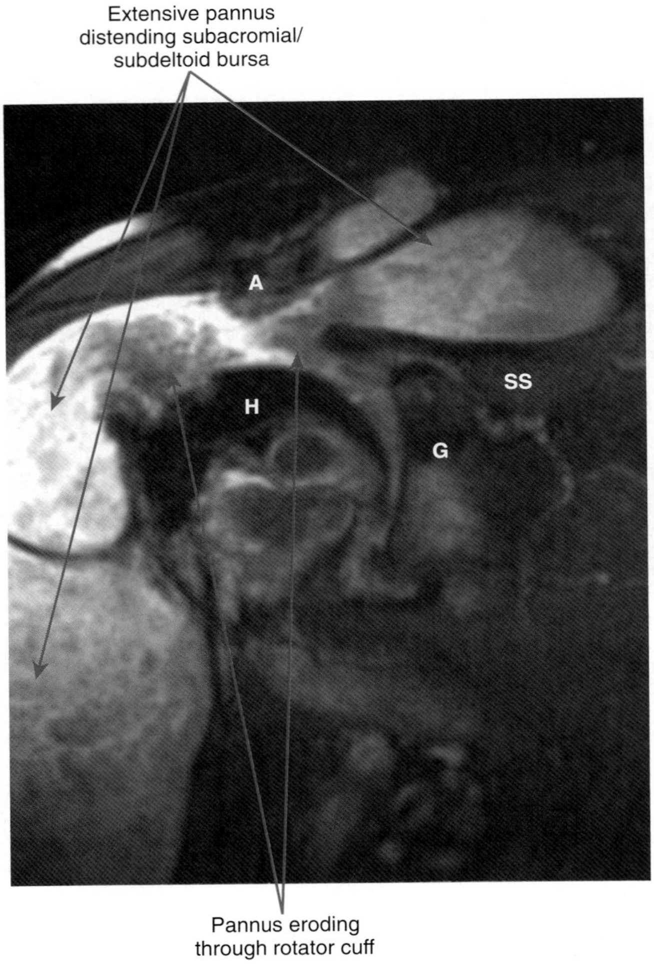
Extensive pannus distending subacromial/ subdeltoid bursa
A
SS
H
G
Pannus eroding through rotator cuff

Figure 4-20 Rheumatoid arthritis of the shoulder depicting how inflammatory synovial pannus can erode through intra-articular and capsular ligaments as well as periarticular structures. A, acromion; G, glenoid; H, humeral head; SS, supraspinatus.

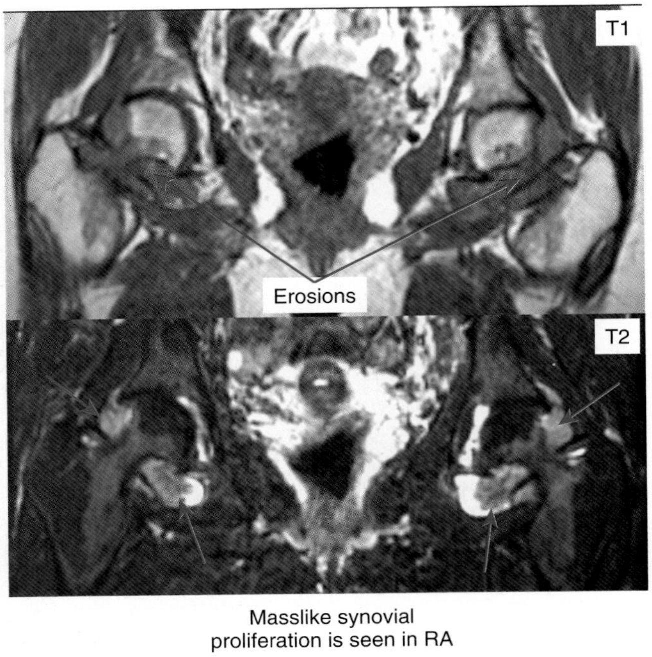
T1
Erosions
T2
Masslike synovial proliferation is seen in RA

Figure 4-21 Rheumatoid arthritis (RA) of the hips with masslike pannus and symmetric involvement.

because relatively minor trauma in this setting can cause a high cervical cord injury. This is especially a concern in the preoperative patient, since before and during surgery the neck is extended and flexed during intubation and anesthesia.

On MRI, effusions are commonly seen in joints affected by rheumatoid arthritis, and synovial pannus is a characteristic finding. Pannus is seen on MR images as intermediate signal on T1- and T2-weighted images with a masslike quality in the joint, distending the recesses. Intravenous contrast typically results in intense enhancement of proliferative, hyperemic synovium. Synovial pannus may erode through intra-articular or periarticular ligaments (e.g., causing wrist interosseous ligament tears) and tendons (e.g., causing rotator cuff tear). Ganglion cysts may arise from the joint or tendon sheaths and are often multiple and of large size.

Tenosynovitis and bursitis are common in persons with rheumatoid arthritis. Often multiple tendon sheaths are involved around the joint. If synovitis of a joint and of multiple adjacent tendon sheaths is observed, a diagnosis of rheumatoid arthritis should be entertained. In rheumatoid arthritis, synovial pannus can be observed within the tendon sheaths, with complex fluid seen on T2-weighted images, with marked distention of the sheath. Similarly, distention of periarticular bursae, such as the olecranon bursa and retrocalcaneal bursa may occur, seen on MRI as complex fluid signal representing pannus within the bursal capsule. In chronic rheumatoid arthritis, intra-articular bodies are occasionally observed and may be seen as multiple fibrous ovoid structures within the joint or tendon sheath known as "rice bodies" because of their shape, quantity, and whitish appearance at surgery. Rheumatoid nodules may be observed. On MRI rheumatoid nodules are well-defined, located in the subcutaneous fat, with low signal on T1-weighted images and variable T2 signal. Diffuse enhancement may also be seen. In the spine, MRI is

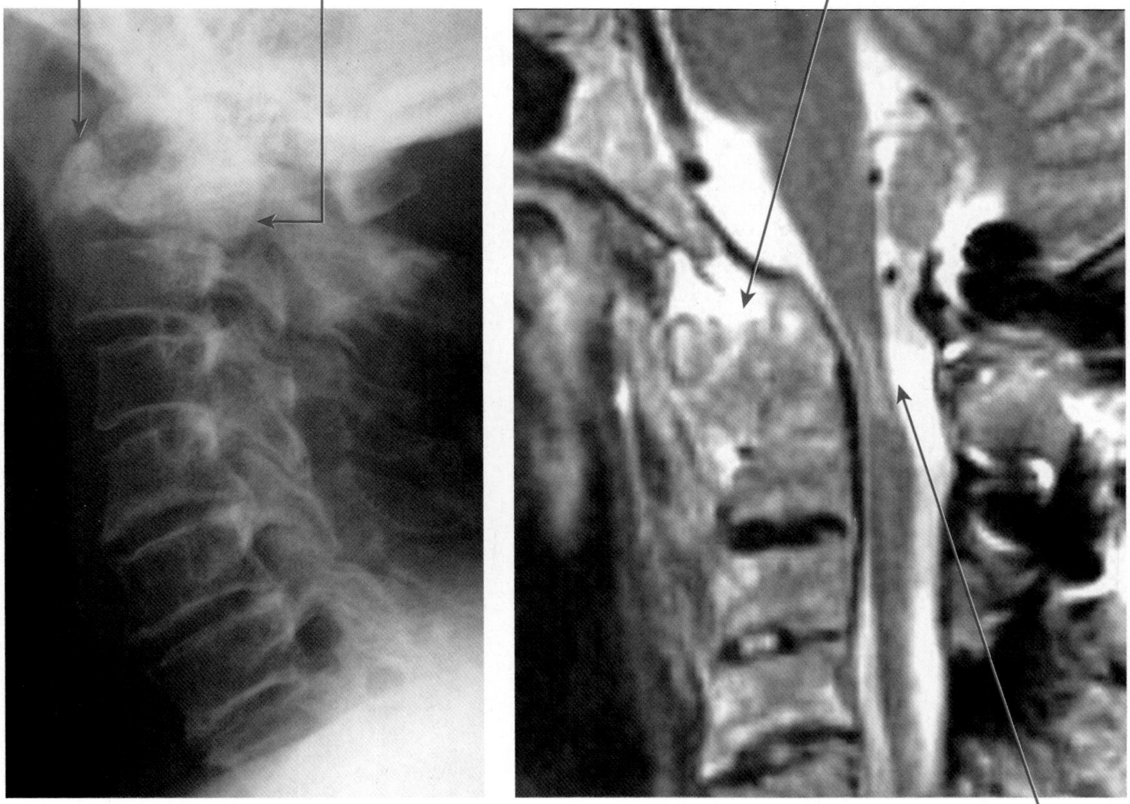
C1 anterior
neural arch
C2 body
Synovial proliferation
"pannus" at the C1-2 interval
with widening representing instability
Axial migration of dens into
the foramen magnum
Associated
myelomalacia

Figure 4-22 Rheumatoid arthritis involving the cervical spine. There are five separate synovial compartments at C1-C2, any of which can be involved by the inflammatory pannus. Resulting erosion of the dens and ligamentous insufficiency causes atlantoaxial instability and even axial migration.

useful for determining the extent of pannus formation at C1-C2, as well as the degree of compromise of the spinal canal.

Juvenile Chronic Arthritis (Fig. 4-23)

Juvenile chronic arthritis (JCA), more often called JRA, or juvenile rheumatoid arthritis, actually includes a number of subsets of articular disease with the common characteristic that they present before adulthood. These subcategories include juvenile-onset adult-type (seropositive) rheumatoid arthritis, seronegative chronic arthritis (Still disease), juvenile-onset ankylosing spondylitis, psoriatic arthritis, arthritis associated with inflammatory bowel disease, and miscellaneous categories. All tend to occur in an adolescent population and mimic the manifestations of the adult-onset disease except for Still disease, which typically occurs in younger children and is the most common form of JCA (approximately 70%). People affected with JCA at a young age have certain manifestations on radiographic examinations related to the chronic inflammation and hyperemia that occurs in growing joints; these manifestations are particularly associated with Still disease, likely in part related to the earlier age of onset of this disease.

Patients with Still disease can present with a variety of forms: systemic (10%), polyarticular (40%), and pauci- or monarticular (50%). Onset of the systemic

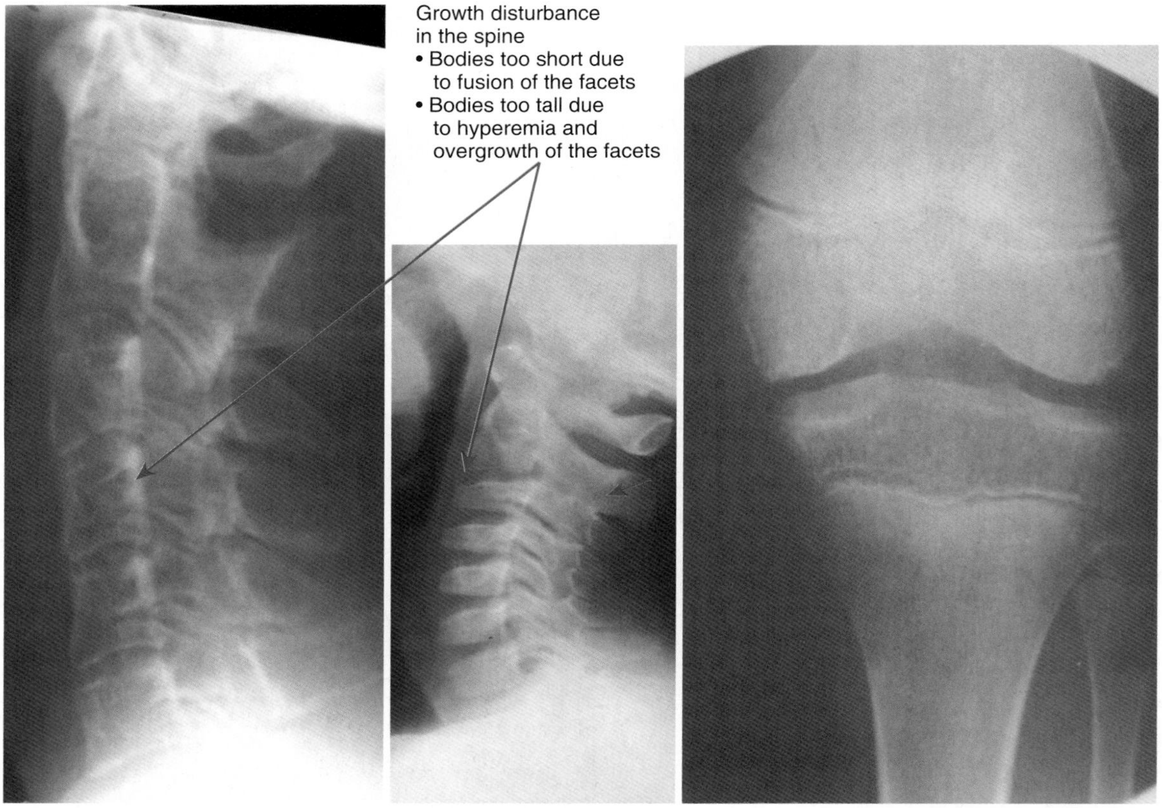
Growth disturbance
in the spine
• Bodies too short due
to fusion of the facets
• Bodies too tall due
to hyperemia and
overgrowth of the facets
Tall bodies
"caninization"
Short bodies
Epiphyseal overgrowth due
to hyperemia during development

Figure 4-23 **Juvenile chronic arthritis.** Chronic hyperemia during development can lead to overgrowth of the epiphyses in the appendicular skeleton as well as spinal deformity. Fusion is often seen, unlike in adult rheumatoid arthritis.

form is acute and often occurs in children younger than 5 years old. Systemic manifestations of the disease include fever, anorexia, rash, lymphadenopathy, hepatosplenomegaly, pericarditis/myocarditis, arthralgias and myalgias, and anemia/leukocytosis with increased sedimentation rate. Symmetric articular involvement is typical in the polyarticular form, with wrist joints, metacarpophalangeal and proximal interphalangeal joints of the hands, knee and ankle joints, intertarsal, metatarsophalangeal and interphalangeal joints of the feet, and the cervical spine articulations commonly involved. A monarticular or pauciarticular (four or fewer joints) pattern is often seen initially, which may progress to the polyarticular form. There are early-onset and late-onset subtypes; early-onset may occur in a child as young as 1 to 5 years of age. Joints commonly involved include the knee, ankle, elbow, wrist, and cervical spine. Systemic involvement is infrequent.

Some radiographic findings mimic the adult form of rheumatoid arthritis and include fusiform periarticular soft tissue swelling, periarticular osteoporosis, and concentric or uniform joint narrowing (although joint narrowing is typically seen only late in the disease course). However, unlike adult-onset rheumatoid arthritis, erosions are not a prominent feature. Also, in Still disease there is often periostitis adjacent to affected joints, whereas proliferation is uncommon in adult rheumatoid arthritis. Because the disease affects growing joints, other radiographic characteristics become prominent.

Hyperemia leads to overgrowth and an enlarged appearance of the epiphyses compared with the metaphyses and diaphyses (hemophilia can result in the same pattern). The hyperemic effect can also result in early fusion of the growth plate, causing an abrupt transition between the epiphysis and diaphysis. Early physeal fusion can cause growth disturbance, with bone shortening if the plate fuses uniformly or with deformity if the fusion affects only part of the growth plate. The diaphyses of affected extremities may be gracile, and the combination of thin diaphyses and epiphyseal overgrowth with abrupt transition results in an overtubulated pattern.

Juvenile chronic arthritis causes joint ankylosis much more frequently than does adult-onset rheumatoid arthritis. Any affected joints can fuse; in the cervical spine fusion of the facet joints may lead to a growth disturbance of the vertebral bodies. Because of the lack of space for the vertebral bodies to grow, they may become broad and flat or small and miniaturized. Fusion of the carpal or tarsal bones is also common. The deformity and effects of cartilage damage often result in development of secondary osteoarthritis in early adulthood.

As in adults, MR imaging of a joint affected with JCA shows a joint effusion that may be large, as well as synovial proliferation, which is best seen after contrast administration. Even without demonstration of synovial proliferation, a Baker cyst of the knee or ganglion cyst in other joints in a child should raise concern for JCA, since this finding is associated with chronic or recurrent effusion. Although synovial proliferation in a child should automatically prompt consideration of JCA, a careful history should be obtained because infection can look similar. For instance, Lyme disease can cause a chronic synovitis and is common in the spring in the northeastern United States. Of course, internal derangement can also result in synovial proliferation and is being seen increasingly as athletic activities are emphasized.

The rheumatoid factor–positive polyarticular form of JCA tends to occur later in life and behaves like adult rheumatoid arthritis. Other manifestations of JCA include a pattern resembling psoriatic arthritis and a chronic arthropathy associated with inflammatory bowel disease. Imaging characteristics of these forms of JCA are similar to the corresponding adult forms.

THE SERONEGATIVE SPONDYLOARTHROPATHIES

Seronegative spondyloarthropathy refers to a group of inflammatory conditions of the joints of the extremities and spine that are rheumatoid factor–negative. This group includes psoriatic arthritis, Reiter disease, ankylosing spondylitis, and arthropathy associated with inflammatory bowel disease.

Rheumatoid arthritis and seronegative spondyloarthropathies can be thought of as existing along a spectrum. Rheumatoid arthritis is primarily a synovial process, rarely involving entheses; so it "likes" joints, tendon sheaths, and bursae. Ankylosing spondylitis is primarily an enthesial disease; so it likes to involve the spine and sacroiliac joints, where ligamentous attachments are plentiful. Psoriatic and Reiter disease are in the middle, involving both synovial tissues and enthesial attachments.

Psoriatic Arthritis (Figs. 4-24 and 4-25)

Approximately 2% to 6% of patients with skin involvement from psoriasis have arthralgias; conversely, most patients with articular disease have skin involvement. Peak age range of presentation with psoriatic arthritis is 20 to 40 years, similar to that in rheumatoid arthritis. Patients may present initially with psoriatic involvement of one, a few, or many joints. Distribution consists of the distal joints of the hands and feet, but large joints of the extremities as well as the sacroiliac joints and spine can also be involved. In the distal extremities, some rays may be involved severely with sparing of other adjacent rays. Males and females are equally affected, but females predominate in cases of polyarticular disease and males predominate in cases with spinal disease.

Radiographically, psoriatic arthritis is characterized by erosions with bone proliferation, similar to Reiter disease. In fact, these two diseases are almost indistinguishable on radiographs alone. One useful differentiating feature is that psoriatic arthritis commonly involves the hand, whereas Reiter disease rarely involves the upper extremity. Correlation with clinical history is essential.

Diffuse joint narrowing is similar to that in the inflammatory arthropathies and is related to uniform cartilage loss. Erosions occur at the bare areas of the joint margins. These erosions classically have a proliferative appearance, with a fluffy or whiskered quality. If the disease progresses, the erosions can become severe, with a "sharpened pencil" appearance of the end of the bone. The articular surface at the opposite side of the joint can become cupped, and shortening of the digit from telescoping of one bone into the other may exist. With severe involvement, the articular surfaces can undergo complete destruction, referred to as "arthritis mutilans."

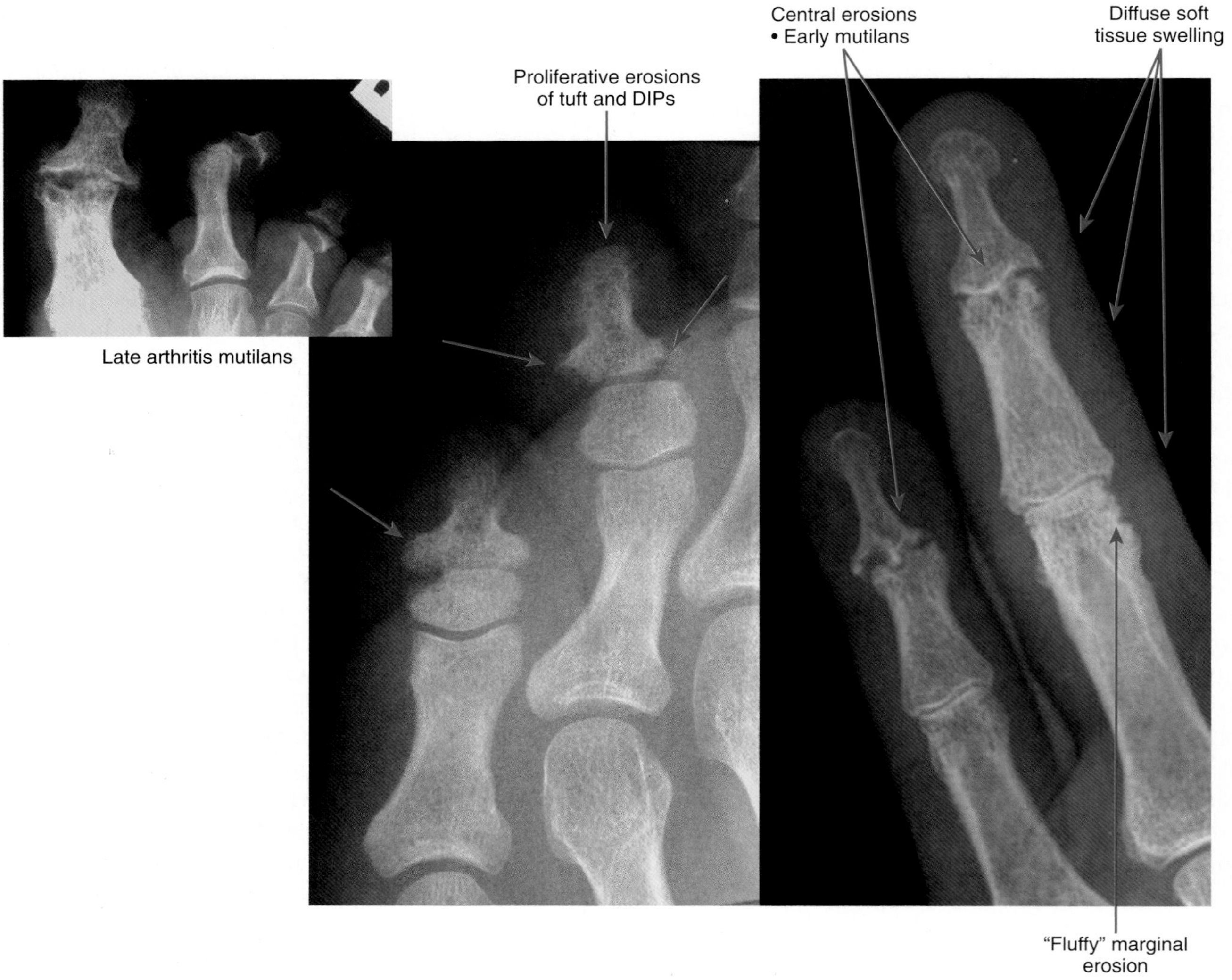
Central erosions
• Early mutilans
Diffuse soft
tissue swelling
Proliferative erosions
of tuft and DIPs
Late arthritis mutilans
"Fluffy" marginal
erosion

Figure 4-24 Psoriatic arthritis. Erosions classically have a proliferative appearance, with a fluffy or whiskered quality. Central erosions can lead to joint destruction with a "pencil-in-cup" pattern. DIP, distal interphalangeal joints.

Ankylosis can occur at any involved joint, but most commonly the interphalangeal joints, sacroiliac joints, and facet joints of the spine. At the sacroiliac joints, there is early loss of the thin subchondral white line and marrow edema, which progresses to form discrete erosions and surrounding reactive bone on both sides of the joint representing sacroiliitis. Sacroiliac involvement may be unilateral or bilateral but asymmetric. In addition to proliferative-type erosions, there is often periostitis adjacent to an involved joint. In the spine, lateral and asymmetric osseous bridging between vertebral bodies can occur. Erosions can also occur at the entheses. Affected entheses commonly have a fluffy appearance on radiographs, and on MRI they demonstrate soft tissue and marrow edema, an appearance mimicking injury (e.g., plantar fasciitis).

Distribution is characteristically distal extremities, especially the interphalangeal, metacarpophanalgeal and metatarsophanalgeal joints of the hands and feet, the spine, and sacroiliac joints. However, other joints including the wrist, ankle, elbow, knee, and shoulder can also be involved. Hip involvement is relatively uncommon. Unlike rheumatoid arthritis,

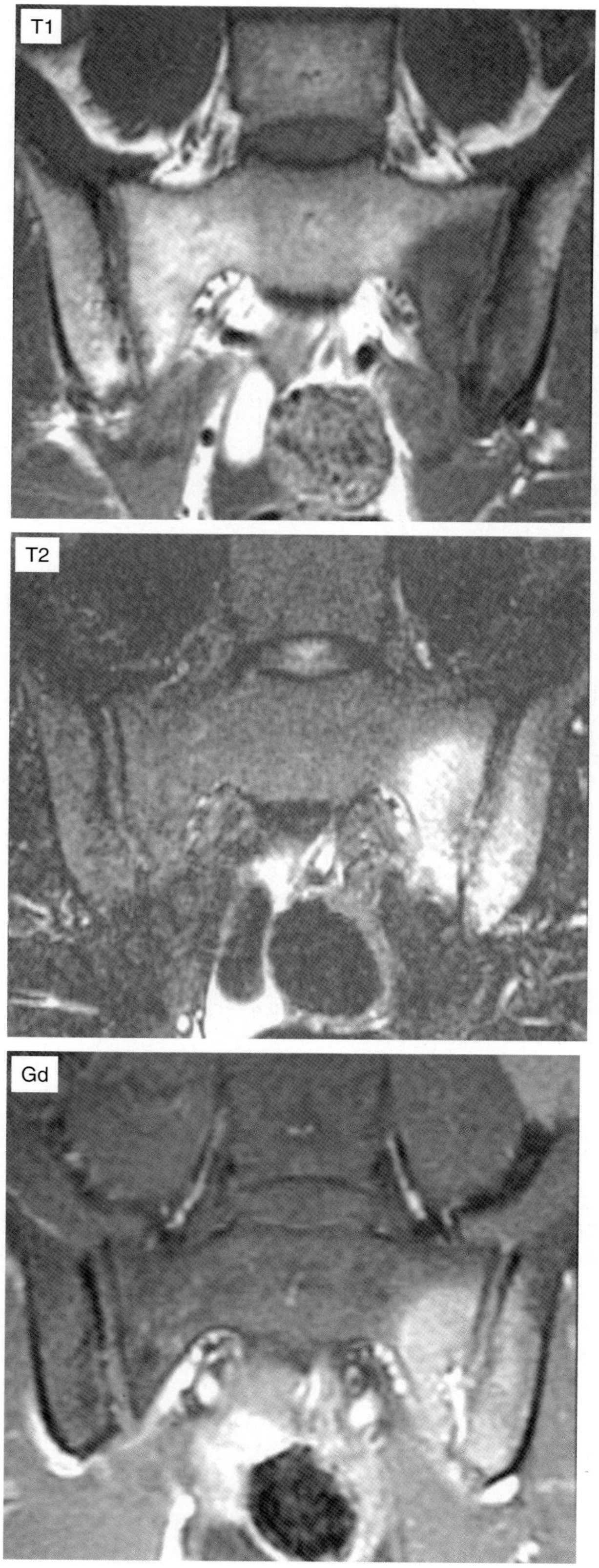
T1
T2
Gd

Figure 4-25 Psoriatic arthritis involving the sacroiliac joint unilaterally.

involvement of the hand/wrist is more distal than proximal, and there can be dramatic difference in involvement of adjacent rays in psoriatic arthritis, unlike in rheumatoid arthritis, in which involvement tends to be more uniformly distributed. Asymmetry of involved joints also differentiates distribution of psoriatic arthritis from the classic bilateral symmetric distribution of rheumatoid arthritis.

Deformity in psoriatic arthritis is generally limited to the digits related to underlying bone destruction. Fusiform soft tissue swelling occurs around the joints. With more severe involvement, the whole digit can become swollen, an appearance referred to as a "sausage digit." Focal soft tissue swelling can also be seen at entheses owing to inflammatory involvement, and in periarticular tissues due to bursitis. Pitting of the nails may occasionally be seen on radiographs in more severe cases. Bone mineralization is generally preserved, although early in the disease there may be some periarticular demineralization.

Reiter Disease (Reactive Arthritis) (Figs. 4-26 and 4-27)

Reiter disease, now referred to as reactive arthritis, is an oligoarticular arthritis and enthesopathy that follows an infectious condition, usually of the genitourinary or gastrointestinal tract). Age of onset varies from adolescence to middle age, but peaks in the third decade. The clinical syndrome classically includes urethritis, conjunctivitis, and arthritis; however, frequently one of the first two conditions is absent. The clinical symptoms usually begin within 1 month of the infection, which is typically *Chlamydia trachomatis* (if genitourinary) and can be a number of organisms including shigella, campylobacter, or salmonella (if gastrointestinal). The arthritis related to genitourinary disease affects men approximately nine times more frequently than women, whereas the syndrome that follows gastrointestinal disease is seen in men and women equally. Caucasians make up approximately 80% of patients, and the HLA-B27 antigen is seen in over 50% of people with the disease.

Lower extremity joints are most commonly affected in Reiter disease; the upper extremities are rarely involved. Distribution is usually distal, primarily involving the metatarsophalangeal and interphalangeal joints and is characterized by proliferative, or fluffy marginal erosions and joint narrowing. As in psoriatic arthritis, severe involvement may occur, with central erosions, joint destruction, or ankylosis.

SECTION III

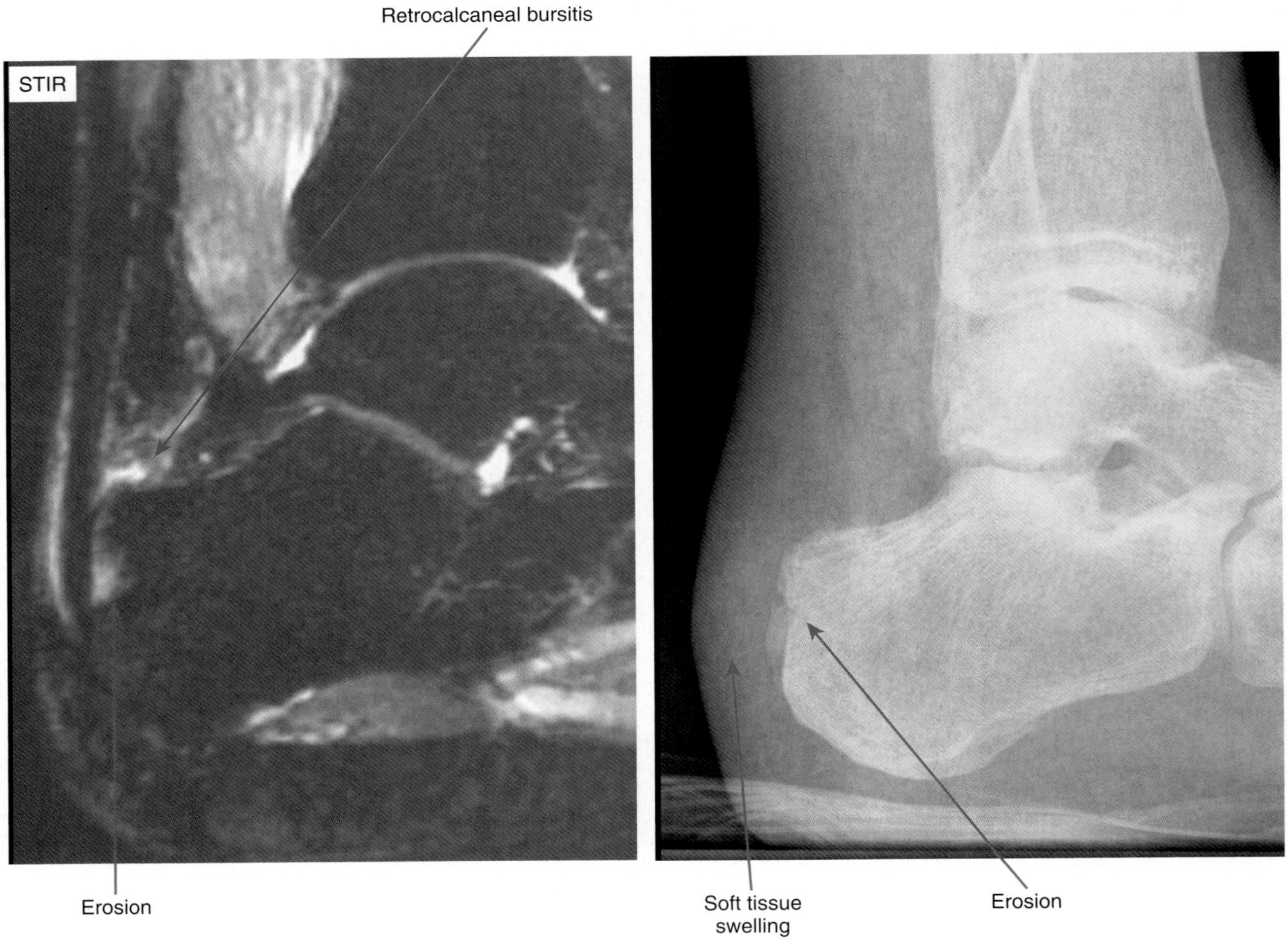
Retrocalcaneal bursitis
STIR
Erosion
Soft tissue swelling
Erosion

Figure 4-26 Reiter disease with reactive changes at the Achilles insertion. Like psoriatic arthritis, Reiter disease often involves tendons sheaths, attachment sites of tendons/ligaments/fascia (entheses), and adjacent bursae.

The sacroiliac joints may also be involved, similar to psoriasis. Diffuse soft tissue swelling can occur in one or a number of the digits, causing a "sausage digit." This appearance can be indistiguishable from psoriatic arthritis; however, most patients with psoriatic arthritis have the characteristic skin rash of psoriasis. Also, psoriatic arthritis commonly involves the hand, whereas in Reiter disease hand involvement is rare. Involved entheses becomes thickened, with poor definition of the adjacent fat planes. Bursae may be involved and appear distended with fluid and inflammatory synovium. With more chronic disease, bursitis and enthesitis can cause erosions and bone proliferation, resulting in a classic fluffy appearance.

Ankylosing Spondylitis (Figs. 4-28 through 4-31)

Ankylosing spondylitis is an inflammatory arthropathy and enthesopathy predominantly affecting the spine and pelvis; peak age is 20 to 40 years. Men are affected three to seven times more frequently than women. There is a strong association (90%) with the HLA-B27 antigen. Ankylosing spondylitis typically presents as back pain and stiffness, worse in the morning, improving with exercise. Patients may attempt to alleviate symptoms by avoiding bending and twisting of the spine. The disease can follow an intermittent course with recurrent flares. As ankylosis progresses the pain subsides, but stiffness obviously

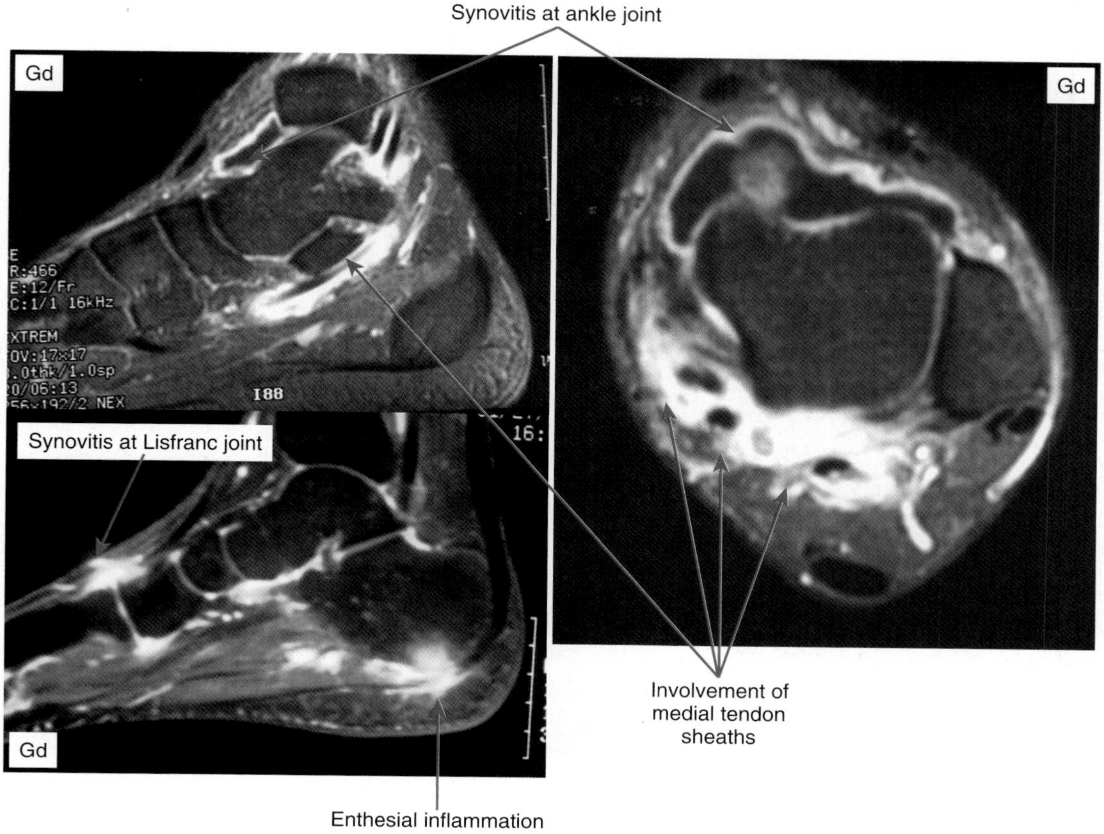
Synovitis at ankle joint
Gd
Gd
Synovitis at Lisfranc joint
Gd
Involvement of medial tendon sheaths
Enthesial inflammation

Figure 4-27 Reiter's disease involving synovium of joints and tendon sheaths as well as enthesis of plantar fascia.

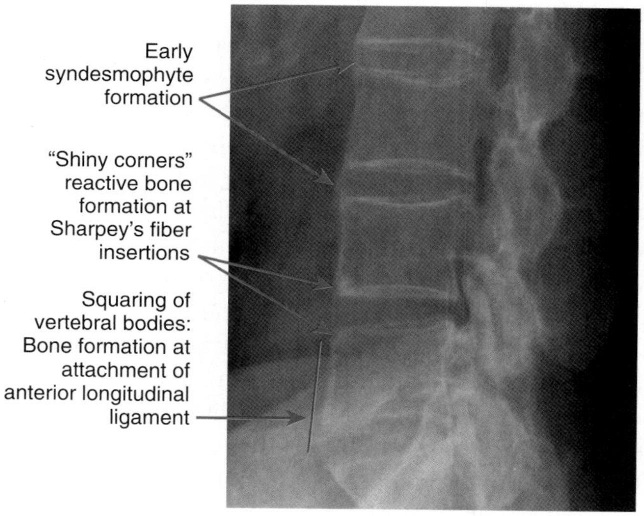
Early syndesmophyte formation
"Shiny corners" reactive bone formation at Sharpey's fiber insertions
Squaring of vertebral bodies: Bone formation at attachment of anterior longitudinal ligament

Figure 4-28 Ankylosing spondylitis. Early radiographic manifestations should be sought in any young patient with typical symptoms. In the spine, these include squaring of the anterior vertebral bodies, usually beginning at L5 due to enthesitis and proliferation at the anterior longitudinal ligament insertion; and sclerosis at the anterosuperior endplates related to reactive bone formation at Sharpey's fiber insertions ("shiny corners").

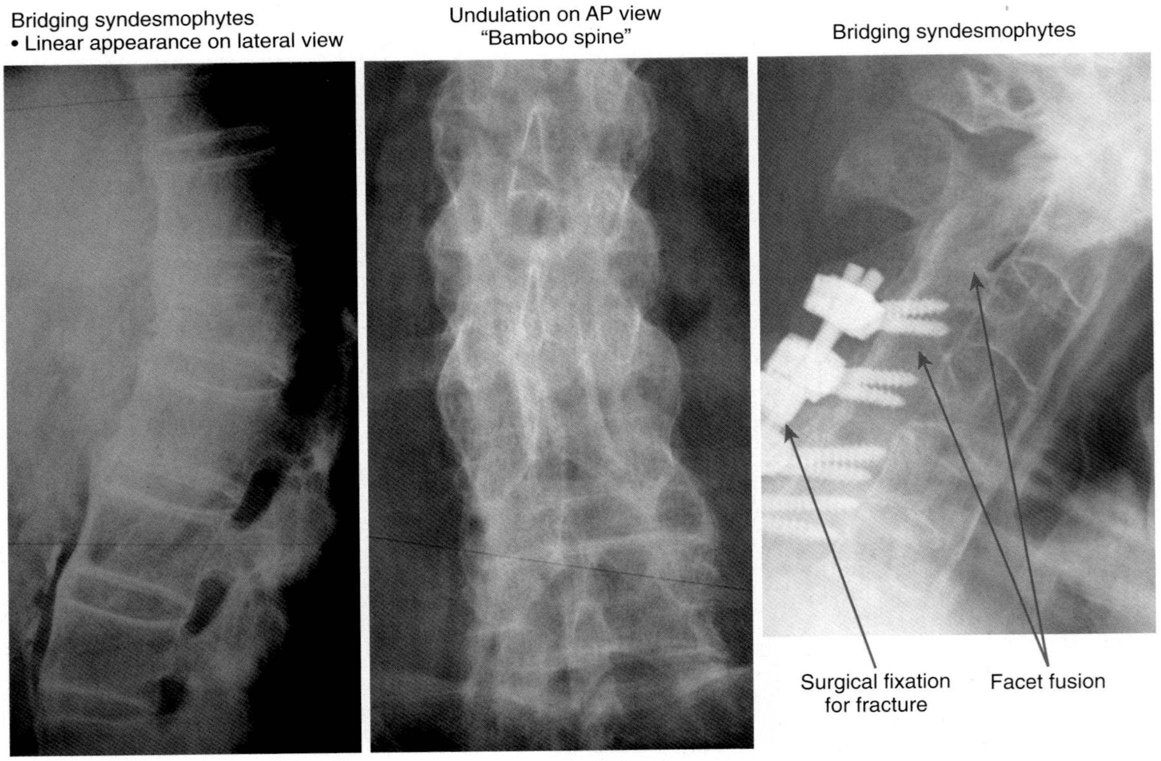
Bridging syndesmophytes
• Linear appearance on lateral view
Undulation on AP view
"Bamboo spine"
Bridging syndesmophytes
Surgical fixation for fracture
Facet fusion

Figure 4-29 Late changes. Fusion with syndesmophytes; linear, close to vertebral bodies on lateral view. "Bamboo" appearance on anteroposterior (AP) view. Fusion of facet and costovertebral joints may also occur.

does not. Fractures can occur obliquely through the fused segments, and patients can suffer from a restrictive respiratory disorder caused by fusion of costovertebral joints.

Early radiographic manifestations should be sought in any young patient with typical symptoms. In the spine, these include squaring of the anterior vertebral bodies, usually beginning at L5 resulting from enthesitis and proliferation at the anterior longitudinal ligament insertion; and sclerosis at the anterosuperior endplates related to reactive bone formation at Sharpey's fiber insertions ("shiny corners"). On MR imaging, edema may be seen at the anterior endplates at the sites of inflammation. Contrast enhancement can help detect subtle inflammation. Eventually, syndesmophytes form, bridging the disk; ossification is straight and closely opposed to the vertebrae on the lateral view and can be subtle. On the anteroposterior view, the ossification undulates ("bamboo spine").

Fusion in kyphosis often occurs in ankylosing spondylitis. Cervical spine fusion can lead to laxity at C1-C2 and instability. Facet joints and costovertebral joints often fuse as well. Fractures typically involve the disk space and run obliquely through the fused segments. Often the first imaging manifestations of ankylosing spondylitis occur at the sacroiliac joints; initially there is poor definition of the subchondral white line and subsequently discrete erosions, which make the joint look widened. Erosions occur initially at the iliac side of the anteroinferior aspect of the joint, which is the synovial portion. CT is excellent for detecting early erosions, and MR imaging with contrast is excellent for detecting sacroiliac synovitis. Later, reactive bone at the margins of the joint causes ill-defined sclerosis. Eventually the joint fuses and the reactive sclerosis may eventually subside. Both synovial and ligamentous portions of the joint fuse in time.

Sacroiliitis in ankylosing spondylitis (and inflammatory bowel disease) is characteristically bilateral and symmetric; sacroiliitis associated with psoriatic arthritis and Reiter disease can be unilateral or bilateral, but asymmetric. Septic arthritis is unilateral.

In the appendicular skeleton, the hips are the most common site of involvement, typically bilateral and

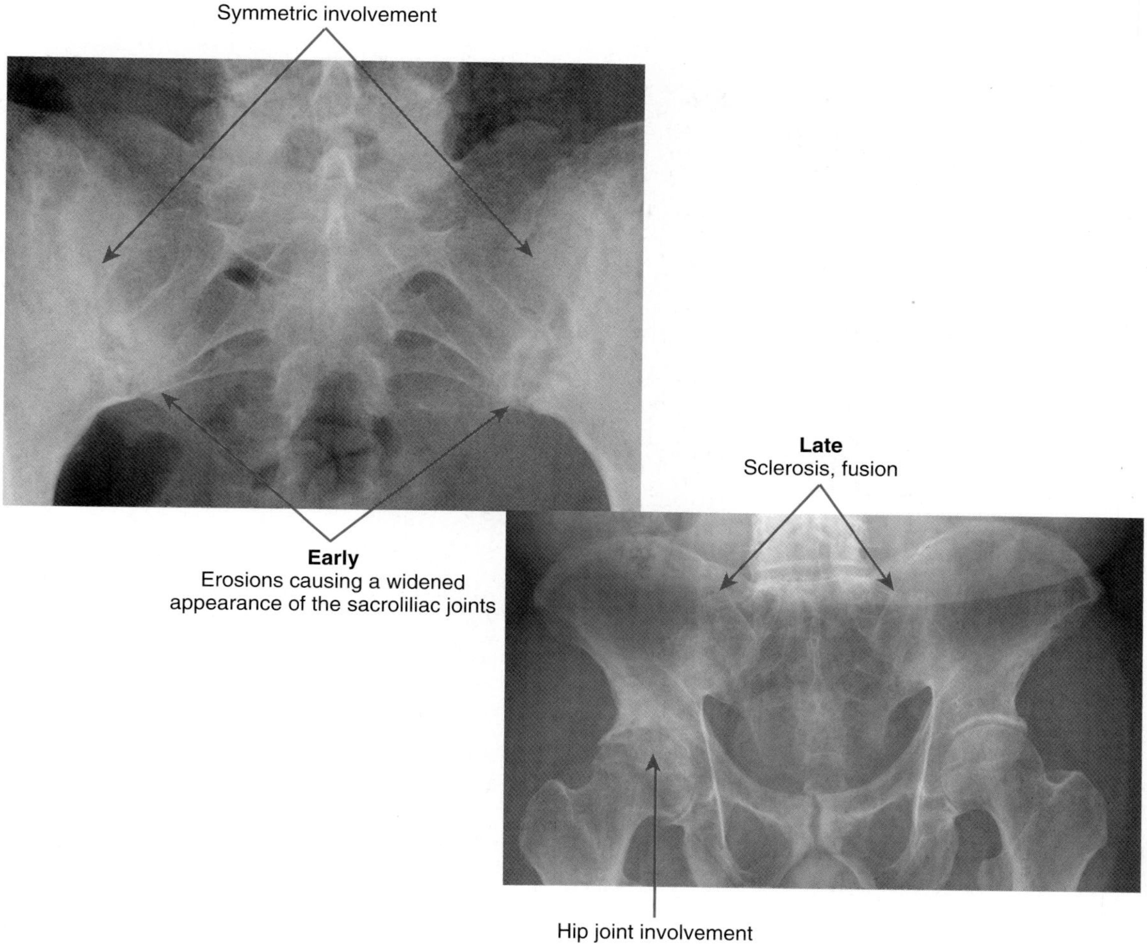
Symmetric involvement
Early
Erosions causing a widened appearance of the sacroiliac joints
Late
Sclerosis, fusion
Hip joint involvement

Figure 4-30 Often the first manifestations of ankylosing spondylitis occur at the sacroiliac joints. Initially, there is poor definition of the subchondral white line and subsequently discrete erosions, which make the joint look widened. Later in the course of disease, reactive sclerosis occurs around the sacroiliac joints, which ultimately may undergo fusion. Hip joint involvement may also occur.

symmetric. Concentric bilateral joint narrowing with axial migration with minimal to no erosion is common. The peripheral large joint pattern resembles rheumatoid arthritis.

Differential Diagnosis: DISH and OPLL

Radiographic findings can occasionally resemble those of diffuse idiopathic skeletal hyperostosis (DISH) (Figs. 4-32 and 4-33). However, DISH is seen in an older population and is distributed mainly in the thoracic spine, generally sparing the lumbar spine and sacroiliac joints. Also, whereas syndesmophytes in ankylosing spondylitis are closely applied to the spine on the lateral view, anterior ossification in DISH is undulating, arising from the anterior longitudinal ligament rather than Sharpey's fibers. Ossification of the posterior longitudinal ligament (OPLL) is another condition resulting in bone formation; this has special significance because it causes central spinal stenosis and cord impingement. DISH and OPLL may coexist, and patients with either condition also commonly exhibit prominent enthesophyte formation as well as excess heterotopic bone formation after arthroplasty. An overlap syndrome may also exist with ankylosing spondylitis, since a small proportion of patients exhibit common imaging characteristics.

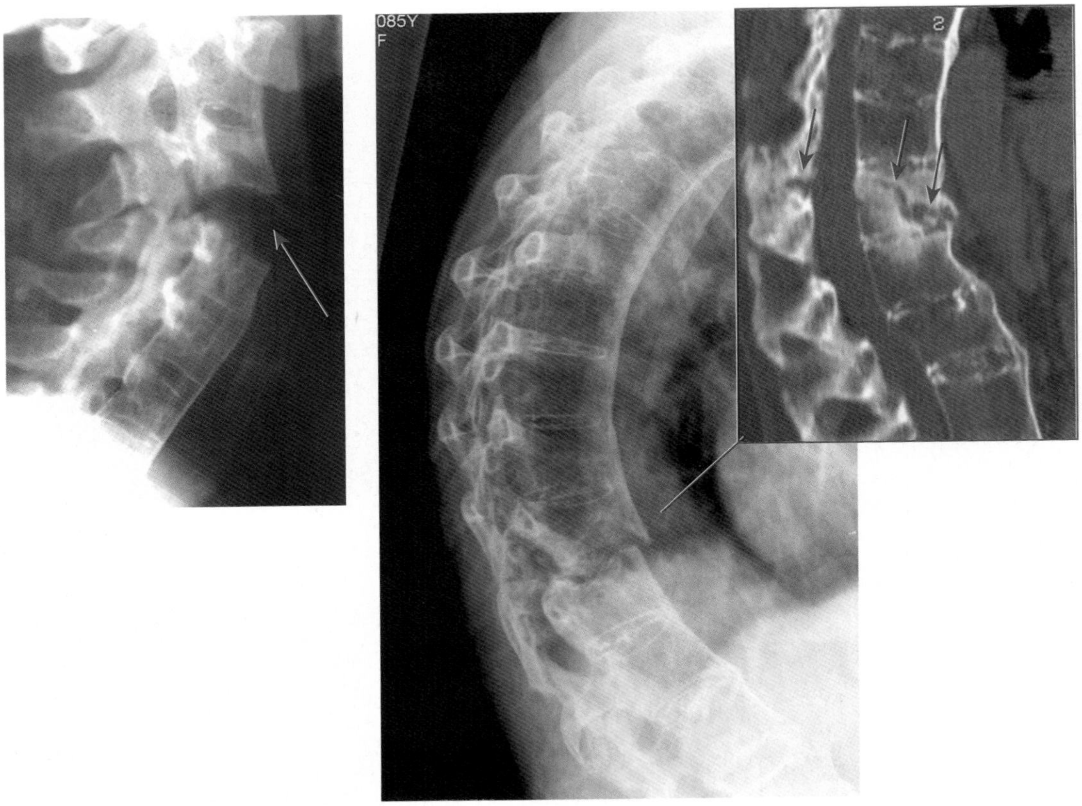
085Y
F
2

Figure 4-31 Fractures associated with ankylosing spondylitis typically involve the disk space and run obliquely through the fused segments.

Arthropathy Associated with Inflammatory Bowel Disease

Patients with either Crohn disease or ulcerative colitis may present with appendicular arthritic symptoms, which often mirror activity of the bowel disease. Changes in the spine and sacroiliac joints progress independently and appear identical to those in ankylosing spondylitis. The HLA-B27 antigen is found in approximately 50% of patients with spinal involvement. Spinal involvement is about three times more common in males.

Small Particle Disease (Figs. 4-34 and 4-35)

After joint replacement, materials can fragment or shed, and the small particles that are released may induce an inflammatory reaction, osteoclast migration, and osteolysis. In metallic joint prostheses, this is referred to as particle disease, aggressive granulomatous response, or histiocytic reaction. In the case of silicone plastic (Silastic) implants such as those used in the small joints, this process is termed "Silastic synovitis." Osteolysis and loosening are features of both large and small joint implants. Silastic is only partially radiopaque, but often fragmentation is observed radiographically. For large joint prostheses, there may be shedding of metal or cement components or wear of the radiolucent spacer. Other signs of loosening can also indicate particle disease, including protrusio (in the hip), lucency at the bone/cement interface, fractured cement or metal, or subsidence of the prosthesis into the underlying bone. On MR images, metallic implants obviously create significant artifact; multidetector CT is an excellent way to verify osteolysis and loosening. Silastic implants, on the other hand, are void of signal on all MR imaging sequences and the periprosthetic bone and soft tissue are easily evaluated. Areas of osteolysis are seen to be

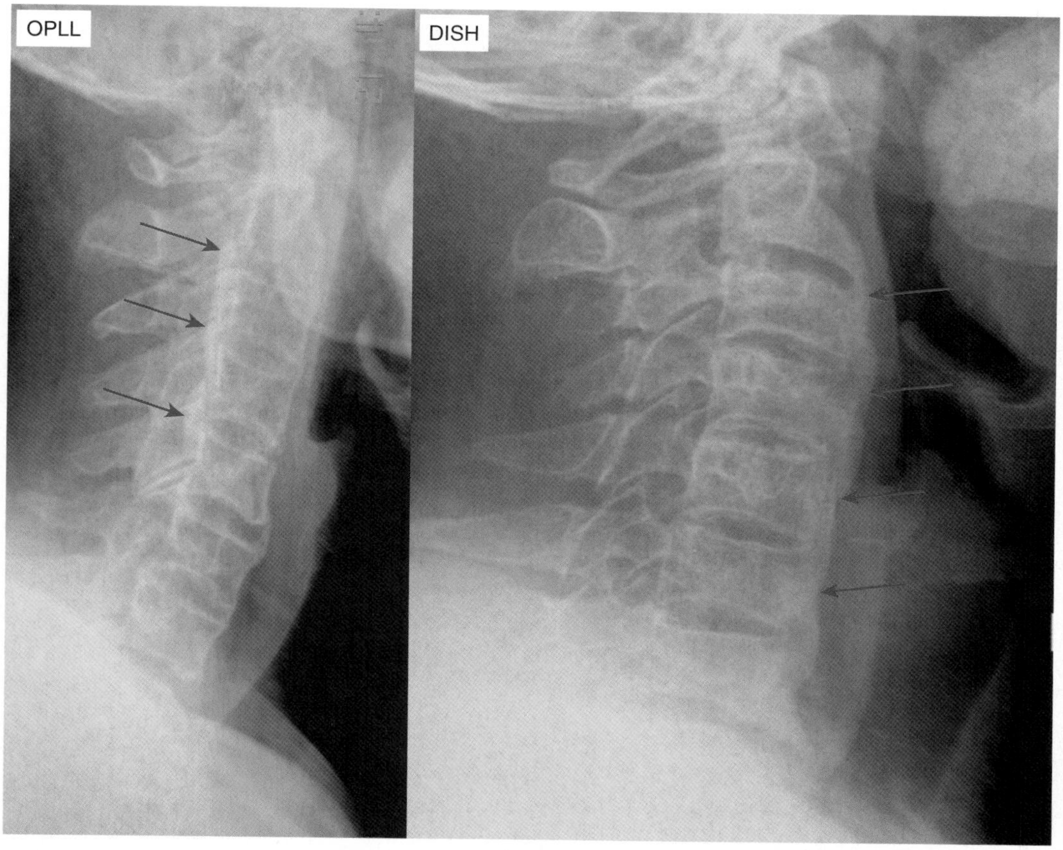
OPLL
DISH

Figure 4-32 Contrast findings of anklyosing spondylitis with ossification of the posterior longitudinal ligament (ossification of the posterior longitudinal ligament [OPPL]; note linear ossification along the posterior vertebral bodies) and diffuse idiopathic skeletal hyperostosis (diffuse idiopathic skeletal hyperostosis [DISH]; note undulating anterior ossification). Occasionally, there is overlap of these disorders.

filled with tissue having inflammatory or fibrous signal characteristics, rather than fluid, with significant gadolinium enhancement. Surrounding fluid collections are also common.

Connective Tissue Diseases

Scleroderma

Systemic sclerosis (scleroderma) is a rare, idiopathic disorder that consists of vasculopathy and fibrosis occurring in various parts of the body, most noticeably the skin and smooth muscle (Fig. 4-36). Musculoskeletal symptoms typically manifest as arthralgias, myalgias, and limited range of motion due to fibrosis. Radiography may show dense, linear soft tissue calcifications as well as acroosteolysis and tuft atrophy. A true arthritis occurs in 50% of people with scleroderma, which is similar in appearance to rheumatoid arthritis and may be related to development of an overlap disorder or mixed connective tissue disease. CREST syndrome is a limited form of scleroderma. The acronym stands for calcinosis (soft tissue calcification), Raynaud phenomenon, esophageal dysmotility, sclerodactyly, and skin telangectasias.

Systemic Lupus Erythematosus (Fig. 4-37)

Systemic lupus erythematosus (SLE) is an autoimmune disease occurring in a younger population (15–40 years old) with a predisposition for females (5:1 over males). Antibody screen shows positive antinuclear antibody (ANA). Arthralgias are common. The arthritis is a nonerosive but deforming disease characterized on radiography by subluxations without

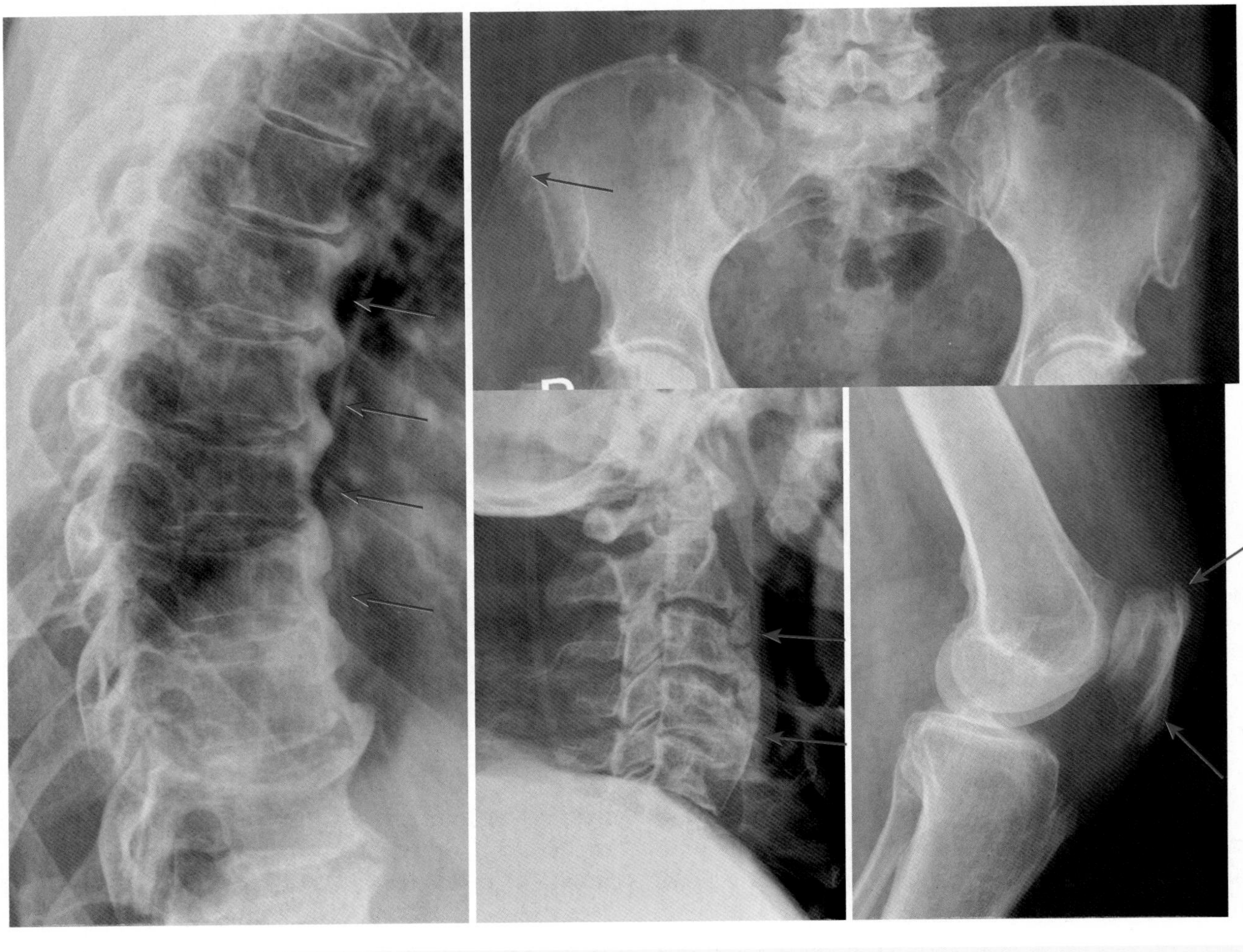

Figure 4-33 Diffuse idiopathic skeletal hyperostosis (DISH). DISH is seen in older individuals, predominantly involving the thoracic spine with flowing anterior ossification (at least four levels); associated with enthesophytes elsewhere (especially pelvis). Patients are at increased risk for heterotopic bone formation after joint replacement. Differentiated from anklyosing spondylitis by age (older), location (C, T spine > L spine, no sacroiliac involvement) and morphology (loosely flowing ossification on lateral view).

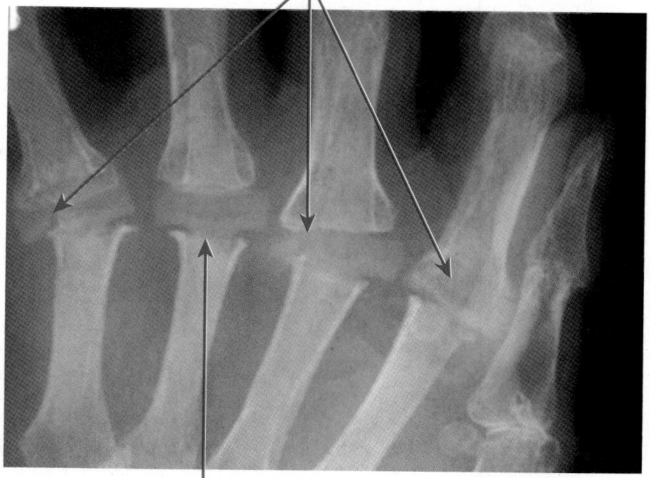
Fractured implants
Intact implant

Figure 4-34 Silastic implants at the metacarpophalangeal joints in a patient with rheumatoid arthritis.

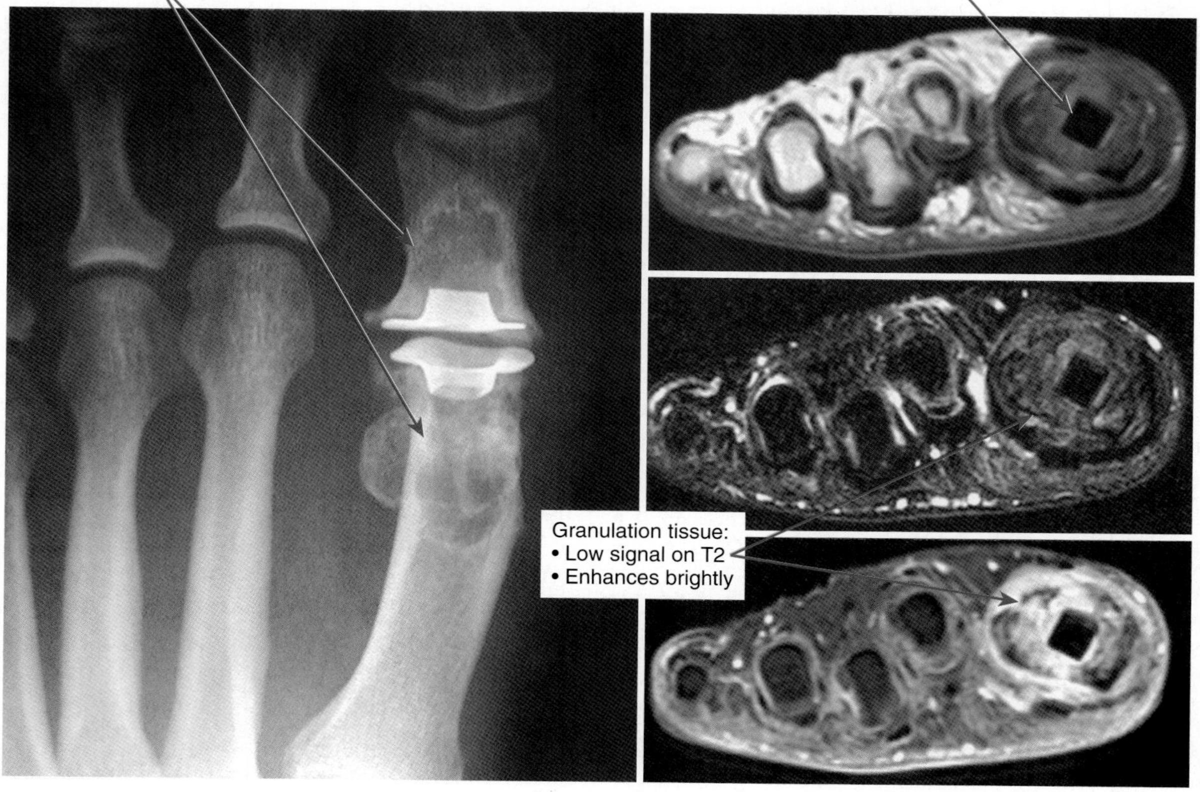
Osteolysis
Different patient: Silastic implant
Granulation tissue:
• Low signal on T2
• Enhances brightly

Figure 4-35 **Small particle disease.** Areas of osteolysis are seen to be filled with tissue having inflammatory or fibrous signal characteristics rather than fluid, with significant gadolinium enhancement.

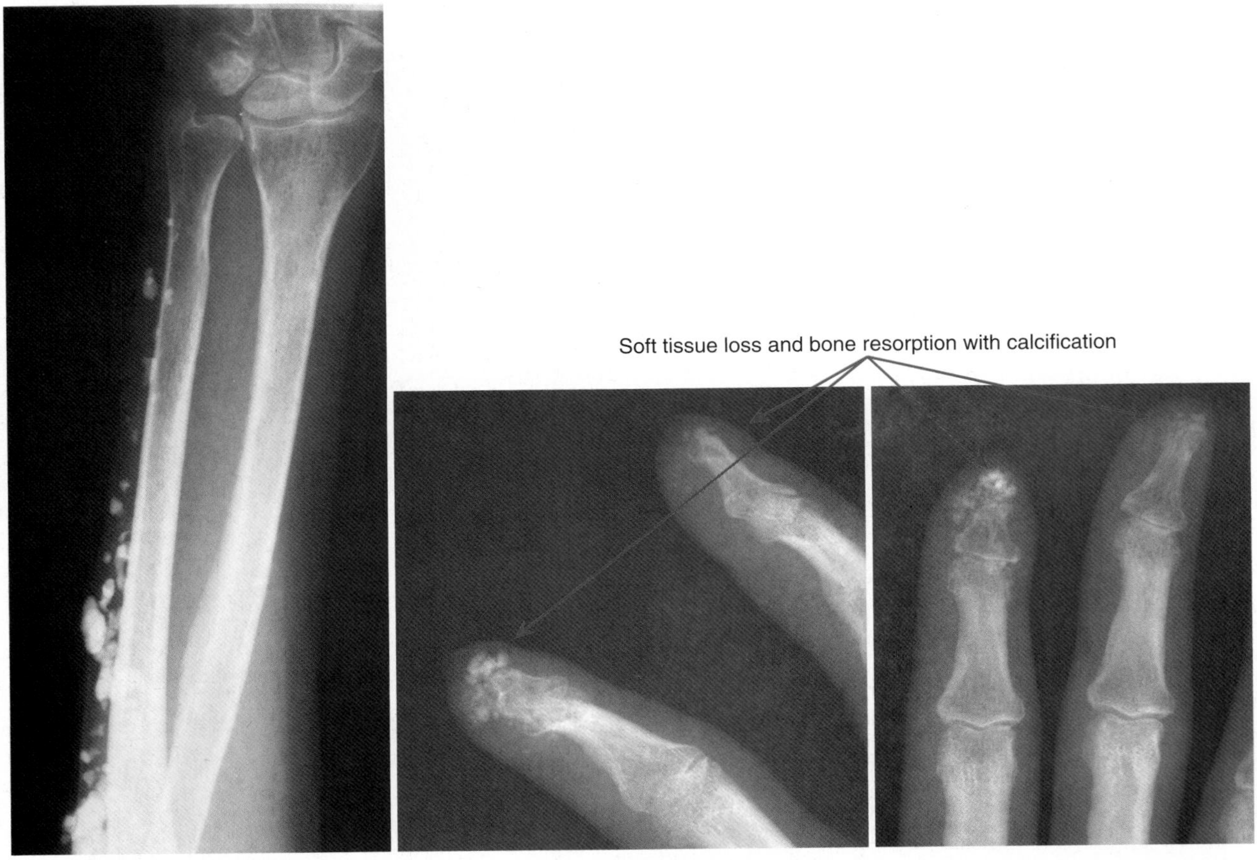
Soft tissue loss and bone resorption with calcification

Figure 4-36 Scleroderma. Dense, linear soft tissue calcifications are observed as well as acroosteolysis and tuft atrophy.

erosions. The subluxations reduce as the joints are flattened against the radiography plate and may be seen only on lateral and oblique views.

Mixed Connective Tissue Disease and Overlap Syndromes (Fig. 4-38)

Occasionally, a connective tissue disorder does not fall into a particular disease category, or includes features of multiple disorders. Terms used include mixed connective tissue disease (a combination of scleroderma, SLE, and polymyositis); overlap syndromes (satisfying criteria of more than one disease, such as SLE and rheumatoid arthritis, scleroderma and rheumatoid arthritis, scleroderma and SLE, scleroderma and polymyositis); and undifferentiated connective tissue syndromes (those that do not satisfy criteria for any specific diagnosis). Laboratory evaluation often helps to establish the diagnosis. Ninety-five percent of patients with mixed connective tissue disease are ANA-positive and 50% are rheumatoid factor–positive, for example.

Imaging features reflect the disease subsets represented by the combined disease process. Soft tissue swelling and coarse calcification are common. The distal digits may be "whittled" as in scleroderma, and acroosteolysis may be present. Joint narrowing occurs as part of the inflammatory arthropathy. Synovial marginal erosions develop as in rheumatoid arthritis. Flexion deformities and subluxations occur. Ankylosis is a late finding typically occurring at the metacarpophalangeal and interphalangeal joints. Mixed connective tissue disease favors small joints such as those in the hand and wrist. The radiologist should be aware of these overlap findings when the imaging findings do not fit neatly into a particular

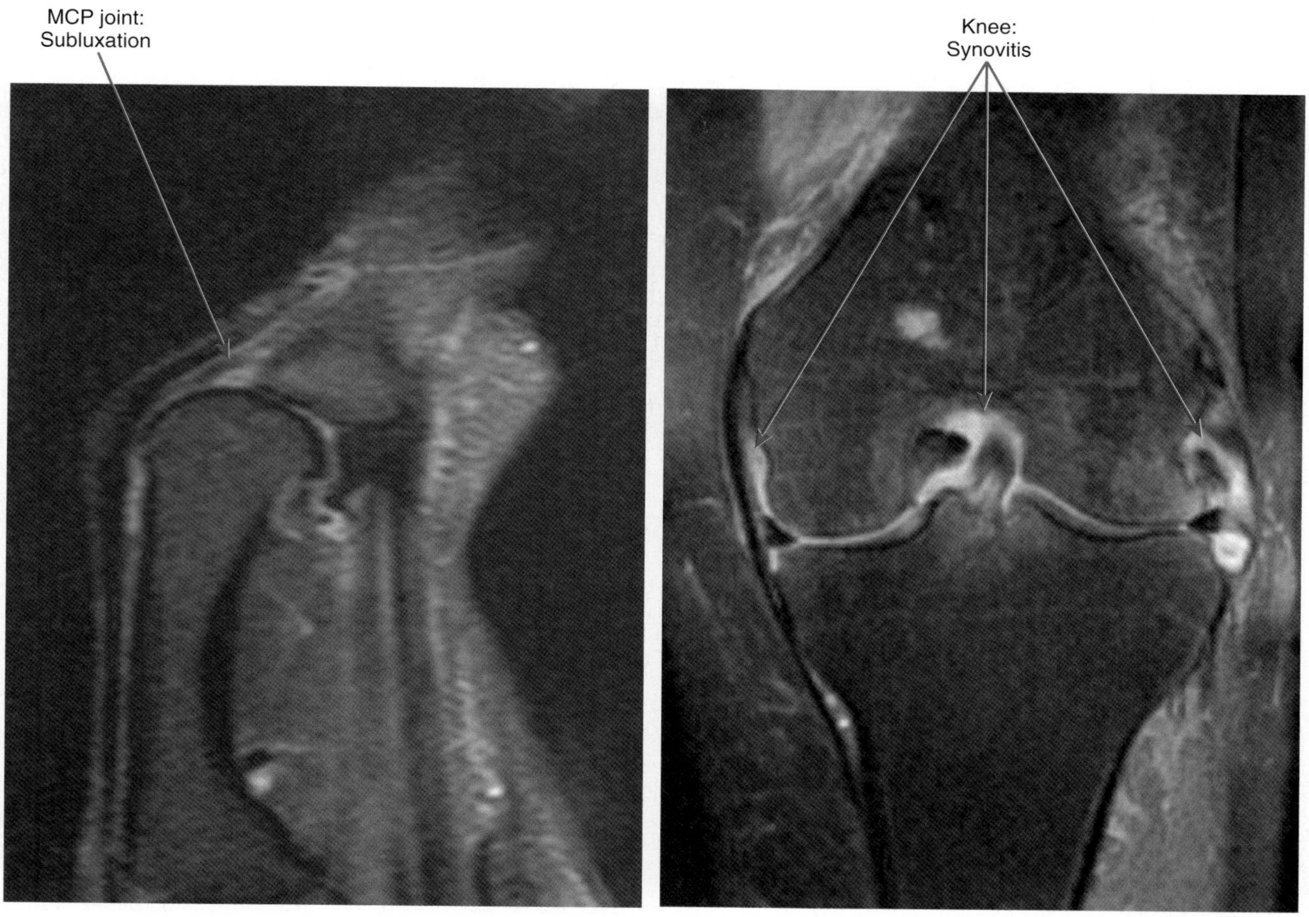
MCP joint:
Subluxation
Knee:
Synovitis

Figure 4-37 **Systemic lupus erythematosus. MCP, metacarpophalangeal joint.** The arthritis is a nonerosive but deforming disease characterized on radiography by subluxations without erosions. Effusions and synovitis may be seen.

disease, as when rheumatoid-like changes are seen at the wrist while calcifications are observed in the digits.

CRYSTALLINE AND DEPOSITION DISEASES

Gout (Figs. 4-39 through 4-45)

Uric acid is a normal degradation product of the metabolism of exogenous and endogenous purines and is not further degraded because of the lack of a uricase enzyme in humans. Renal excretion is the main route of elimination of uric acid. Hyperuricemia may be due to overproduction, underexcretion, or, more commonly, a combination of the two. Most patients with gout have a relatively deficient renal excretion mechanism. Factors that affect renal excretion include heredity, drugs (diuretics, cyclosporine, salicylates), and underlying chronic renal disease (most commonly hypertensive and/or diabetic nephropathy). Excessive alcohol use results in both uric acid overproduction and underexcretion. Gout typically occurs in middle-aged or elderly men, although it may also affect women after menopause. There is an elevated incidence in countries with a high standard of living, probably owing to a diet high in purines. The pathology consists of a foreign body granulomatous reaction surrounding the urate crystals. Tophi represent a focal accumulation of crystals, proteinaceous matrix, and inflammatory cells.

Patients present clinically with recurrent attacks of articular and periarticular inflammation and later with tophaceous deposits in soft tissues and joints. Peripheral joints (hands and feet) are most

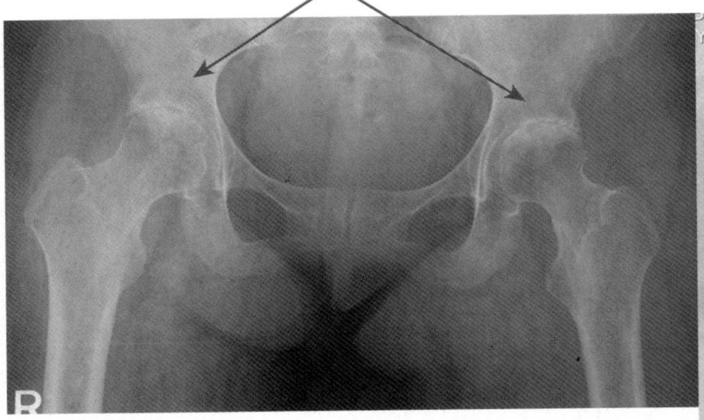
Symmetric diffuse cartilage loss
suggesting rheumatoid arthritis

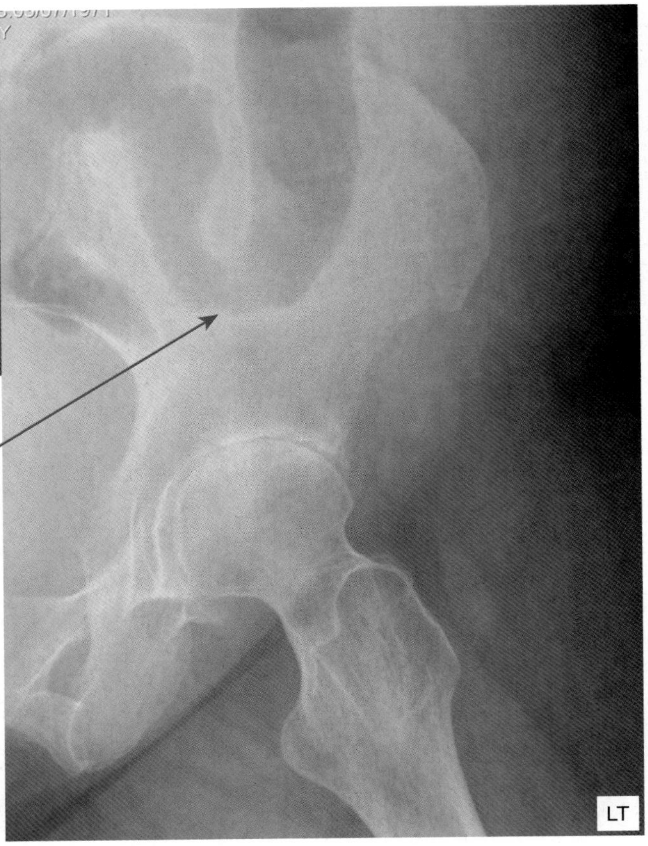
Bowel pattern
compatible
with scleroderma

Figure 4-38 Overlap syndrome. Patient exhibiting clinical, serologic, and imaging features of rheumatoid arthritis and scleroderma.

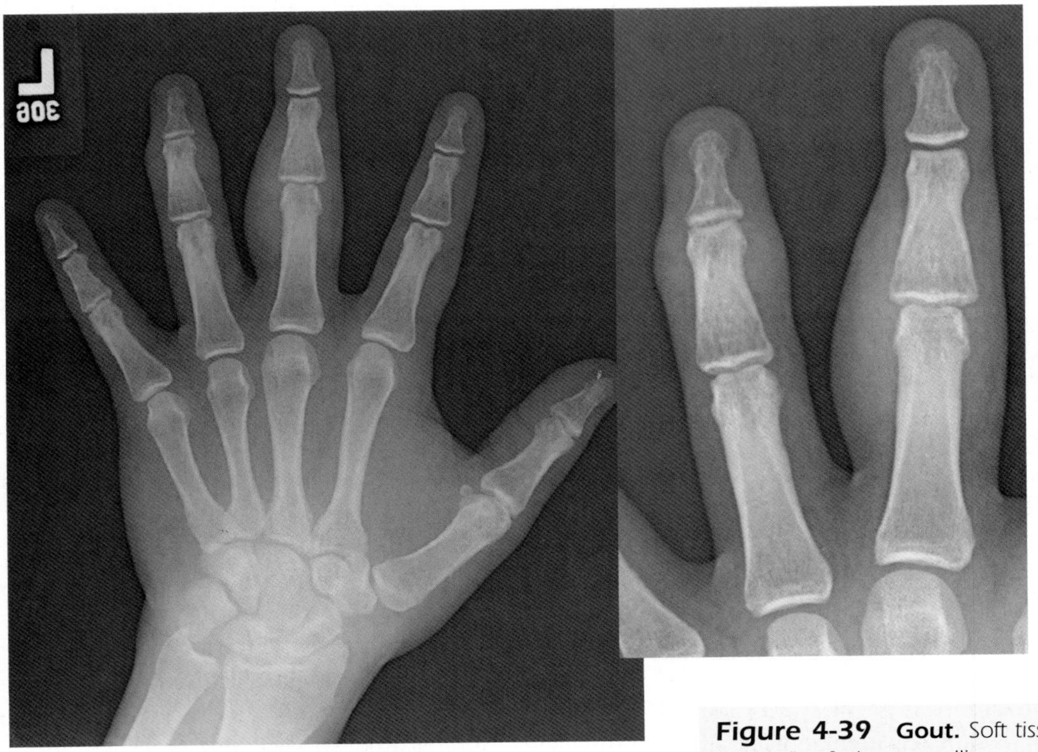
Asymmetric "lumpy bumpy"
soft tissue swelling

Figure 4-39 Gout. Soft tissue tophi result in "lumpy-bumpy" soft tissue swelling.

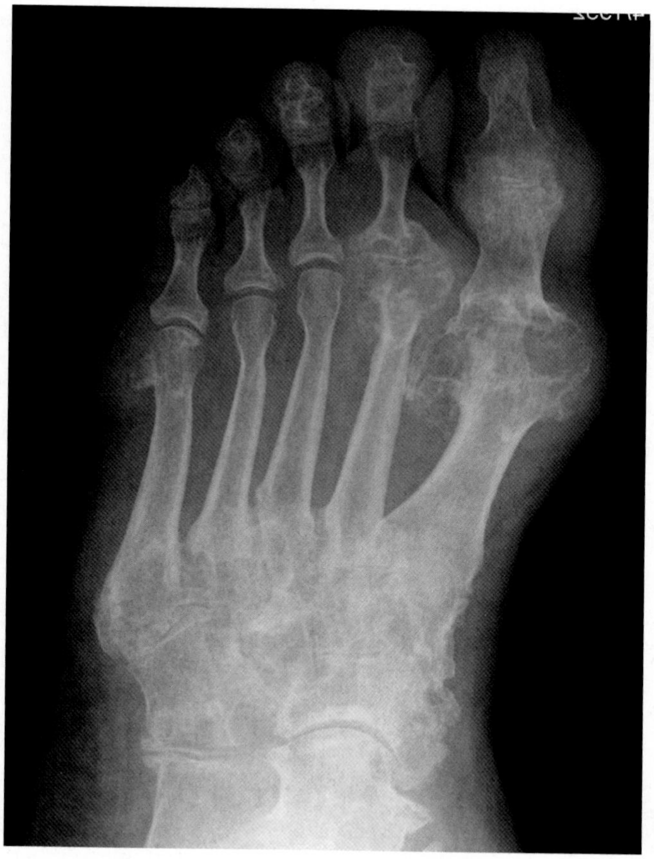

Figure 4-40 Tophi cause characteristic periarticular erosions with overhanging edges. Classic distribution in the foot includes the first ray (first interphalangeal and metatarsophalangeal joints) as well as the Lisfranc joint. Tophi are denser than surrounding tissue but are not commonly calcified. However, chondrocalcinosis may be seen within joints, and calcific bursitis (hydroxyapatite deposition disease [HADD]) is also occasionally seen.

commonly involved, where lower temperatures cause uric acid to crystallize out of solution.

Initially, acute attacks show nonspecific radiographic findings of soft tissue swelling without articular abnormalities. Occasionally, periostitis occurs. Chronic recurrent intra-articular deposition and resultant inflammation can cause marginal or central erosions and joint narrowing, eventually causing osteoarthritis in the involved joints. Severe involvement may cause a destructive arthropathy. Imaging can appear similar to septic arthritis. Classic periarticular rat-bite erosions with overhanging edges are seen in chronic tophaceous gout resulting from extra-articular deposits. These soft tissue tophi result in "lumpy-bumpy" soft tissue swelling. The tophi are dense but are generally not calcified on radiographs.

Classic joints involved in the feet are the first metatarsophalangeal and interphalangeal joints and the Lisfranc joint. The hands may show scattered involvement. The ankle, knee, and elbow are less commonly affected. Bursae may be involved (especially the olecranon), and unlike tophi, involvement often results in calcification of the bursa. Tendon infiltration may occur and results in tendon thickening and a predisposition to tendon tear.

On MR images, the gouty deposits are generally low to intermediate signal on T1- and T2-weighted images and do not enhance. The surrounding inflammatory synovium and soft tissue show edema and fluid collections with enhancement, the degree of which is dependent on the extent of hyperemia. This appearance, together with the common occurrence of joint effusion and subchondral edema, can simulate infection on MR images. However, history and low-signal periarticular or intra-articular gouty aggregates suggest the correct diagnosis.

Chondrocalcinosis and CPPD Arthropathy (Pseudogout)
(Figs. 4-46 and 4-47)

Chondrocalcinosis refers to deposition of crystalline calcium pyrophosphate dihydrate (CPPD) within hyaline cartilage or fibrocartilage. An important concept is that chondrocalcinosis is *not* synonymous with CPPD arthropathy. Chondrocalcinosis is usually asymptomatic and can be associated with a variety of degenerative and metabolic processes, including old age (most common), gout, renal failure, diabetes, hemochromatosis, and Wilson disease. In a subset of patients, chondrocalcinosis is associated with recurrent arthralgias appearing clinically similar to gouty attacks. This syndrome is referred to as CPPD arthropathy or pseudogout. Aspirate analysis is important in making the diagnosis, but some features can be used to suggest the cause.

CPPD arthropathy is most common at the knee and wrist, whereas gout is more common in the feet; however, there is considerable overlap in distribution. Both conditions are common in older individuals. In patients with clinical symptoms in which pseudogout is being considered, a chondrocalcinosis survey can be useful. This consists of anteroposterior radiographs of the knees, pubic symphysis/hips, and hands/wrists to look for typical calcification. In

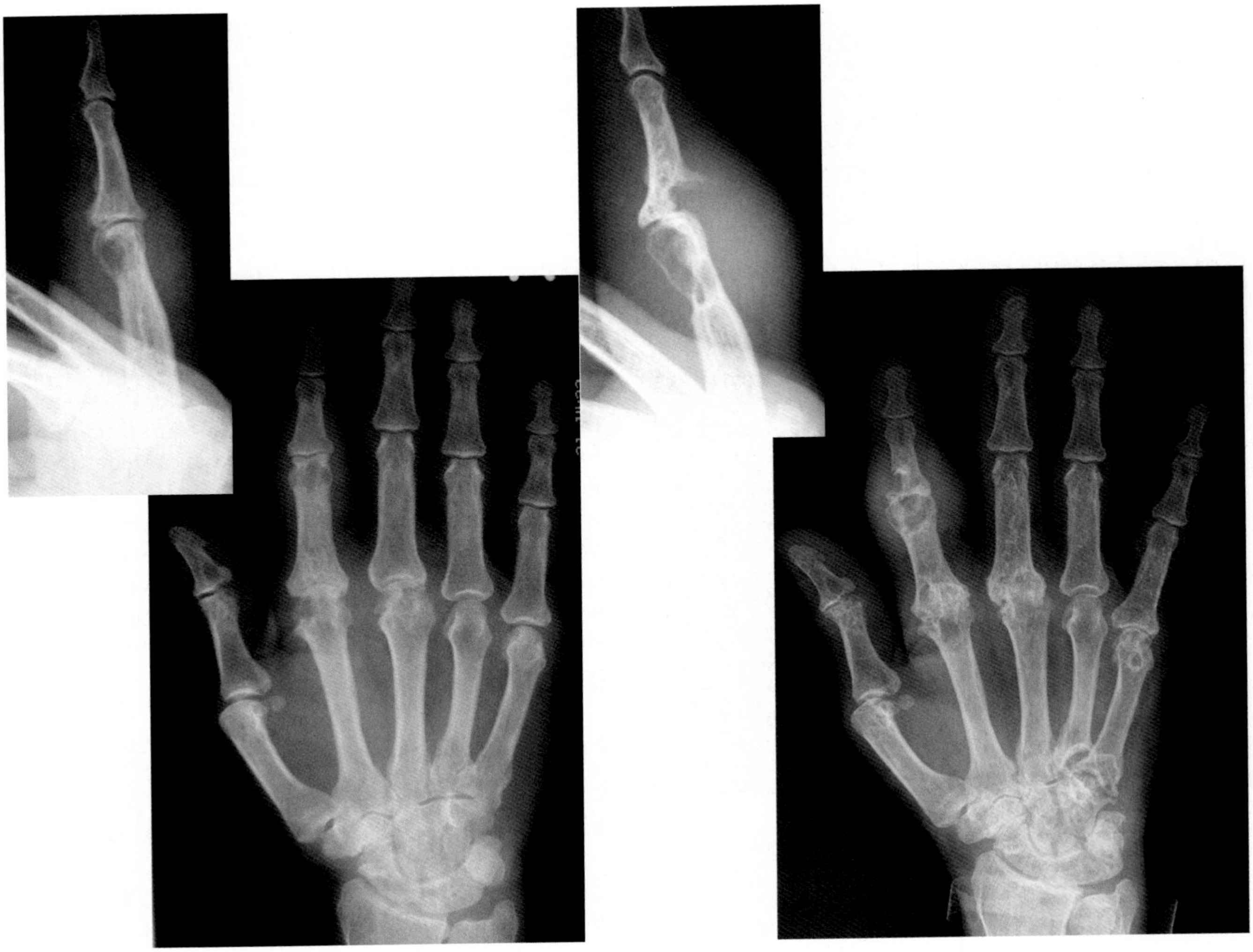

Figure 4-41 Progression of gouty erosions over time.

patients with radiographic signs of an effusion or periarticular soft tissue swelling in which chondrocalcinosis is present, pseudogout should be considered. Chronic CPPD arthropathy can result in secondary osteoarthritis. However, the classic feature used to diagnose CPPD arthropathy, namely, osteoarthritis in an atypical location such as the patellofemoral joint or radioscaphoid joint, is not helpful. Osteoarthritis at the patellofemoral joint, for example, is very common and is multifactorial, being by far more commonly related to a tracking disorder or repetitive injury and subsequent degeneration.

On MRI, chondrocalcinosis can be confusing; although calcium mineral is low signal on all sequences, the CPPD crystal has been reported to have intermediate or even high signal. Therefore, the calcium can cause areas of heterogeneity of hyaline cartilage signal, and, more important, hyperintensity against a background of dark fibrocartilage, potentially simulating a tear. Arthroscopically, the crystals are seen jutting from the meniscal surface and can appear on MRI as signal extending to the superior or inferior margin. Radiographic correlation or even multidetector CT can be useful to document the location of CPPD compared with the MR findings. Subchondral cysts are common in CPPD arthropathy, but this is a nonspecific finding.

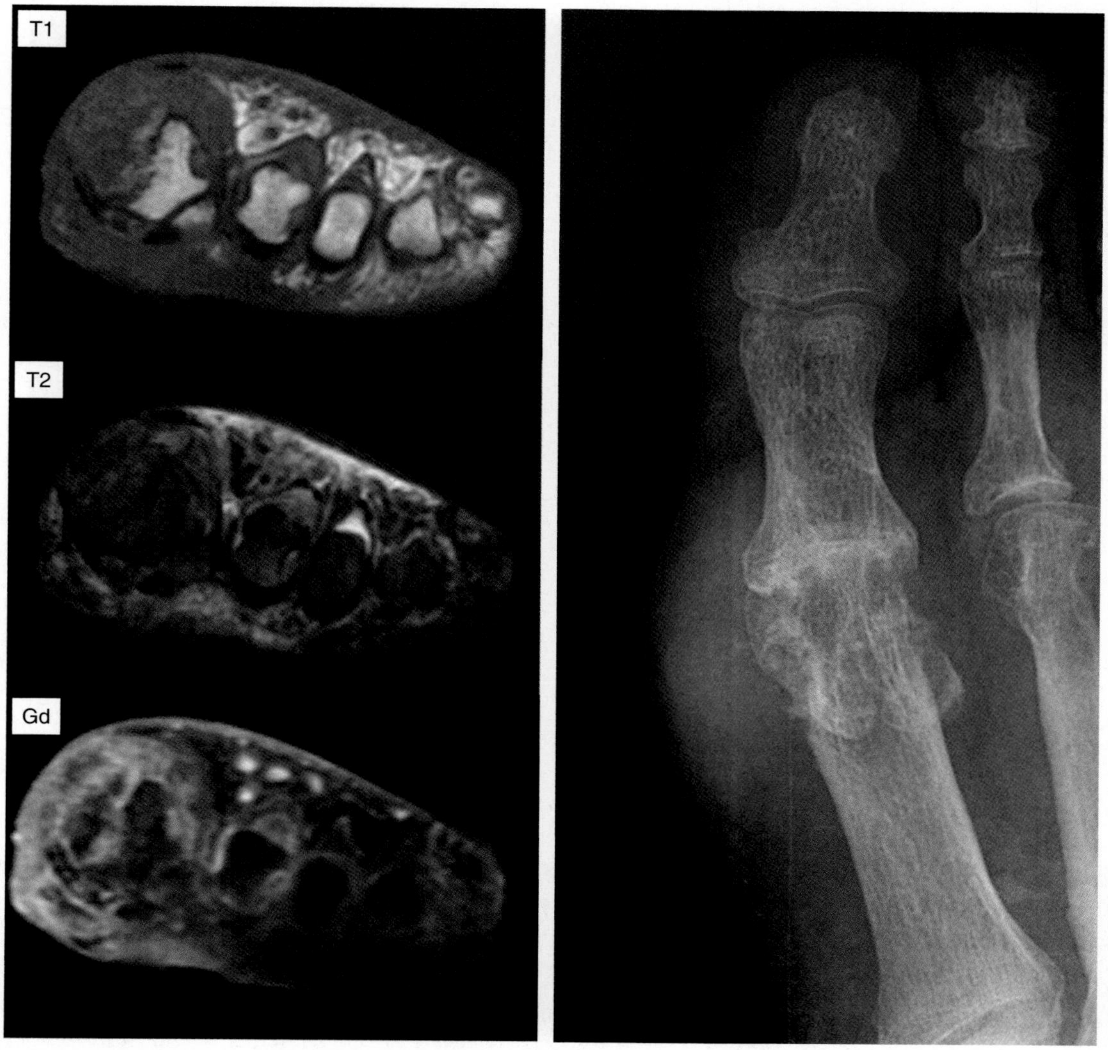
T1
T2
Gd

Figure 4-42 On MR images, the gouty deposits are generally low to intermediate signal on T1- and T2-weighted images and do not enhance.

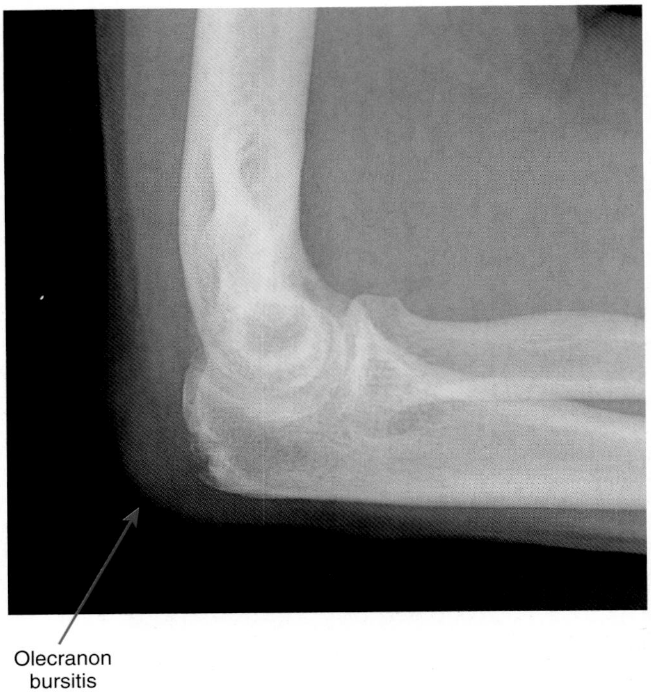
Olecranon
bursitis

Figure 4-43 Gout. Associated bursitis is common.

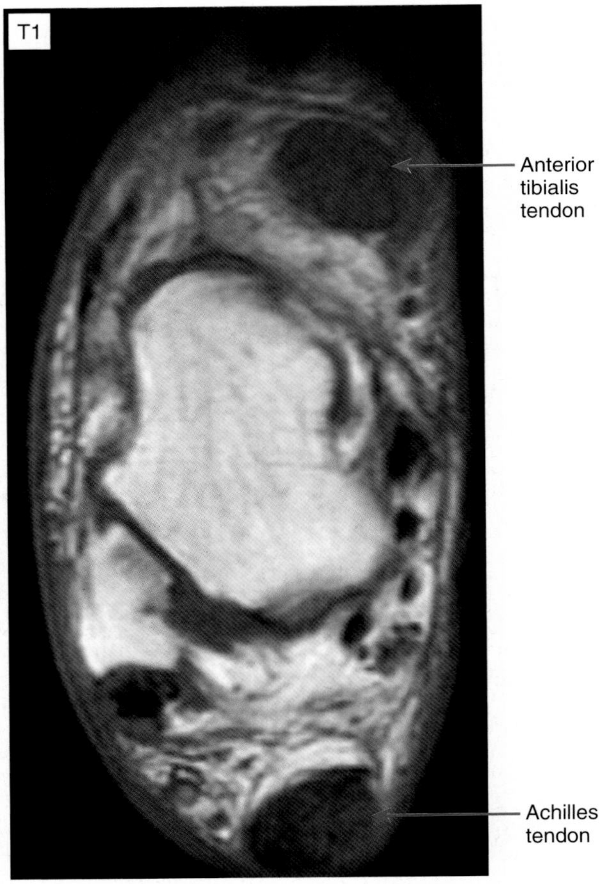
T1
Anterior
tibialis
tendon
Achilles
tendon

Figure 4-45 Gout with tendon infiltration. Tendon infiltration may also be seen in amyloidosis. Tendinosis and tears are more common in these conditions as well as with steroid and fluoroquinolone use, diabetes, and overuse.

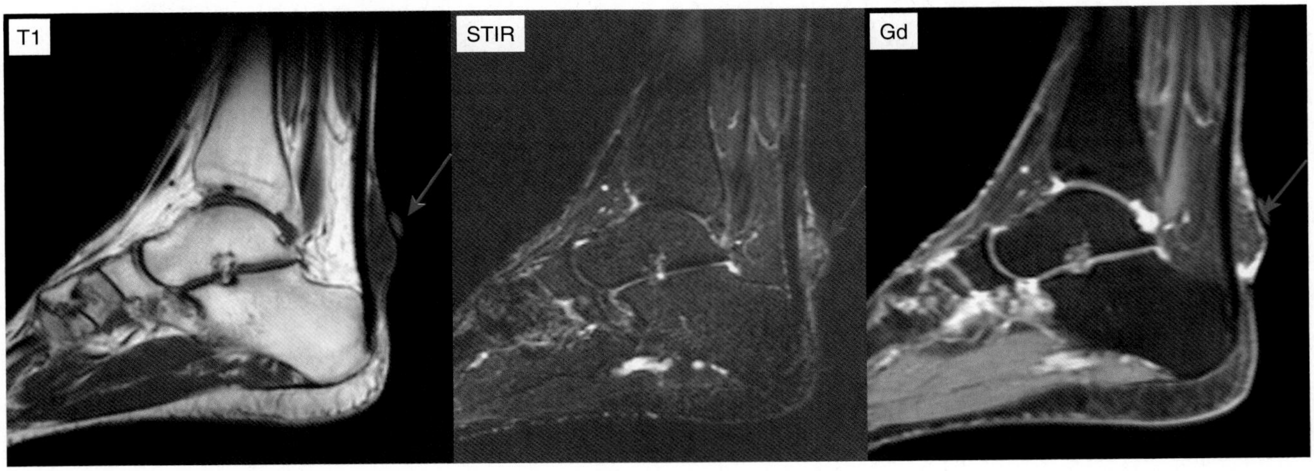
T1
STIR
Gd

Figure 4-44 Gouty deposit along the Achilles tendon. Tophi are characteristically low signal on T1- and T2-weighted sequences. However, they may be associated with fluid collections and bursitis.

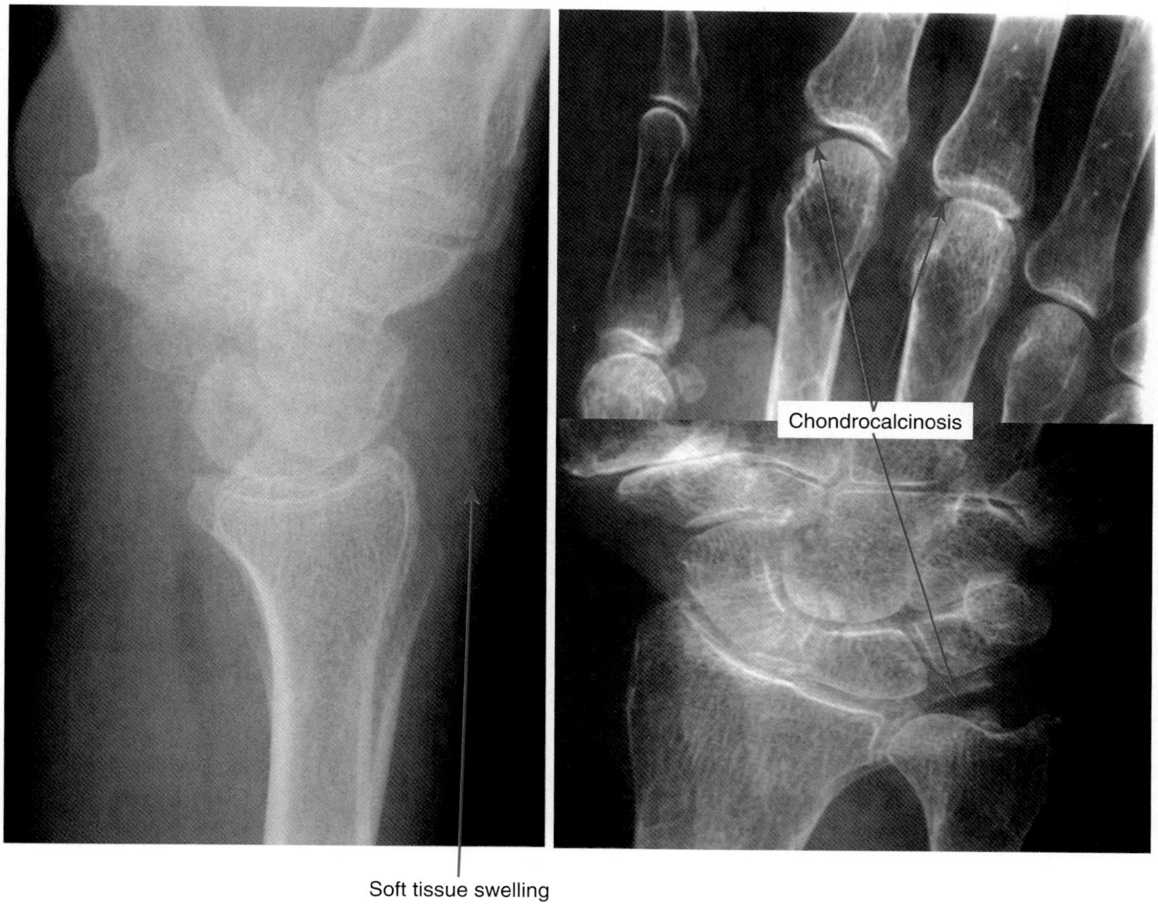
Chondrocalcinosis
Soft tissue swelling

Figure 4-46 In patients with arthralgia and radiographic signs of an effusion or periarticular soft tissue swelling and chondrocalcinosis, pseudogout should be considered.

Hydroxyapatite Deposition Disease (Figs. 4-48 through 4-51)

Hydroxyapatite deposition causes calcific tendinosis, calcific bursitis, and calcific periarthritis. Radiographically, the calcification tends to be small, focal, dense, and somewhat cloudlike. It is most common at the rotator cuff but may be observed in virtually any tendon. The more unusual the location, the more commonly it is unrecognized. For instance, calcific tendinosis of the longus colli tendon at the inferior margin of C1 can simulate retropharyngeal abscess and is often overlooked. Hydroxyapatite contained within a tendon is often asymptomatic until it bursts into the surrounding tissues; then it incites an inflammatory reaction and acute symptoms that range from pain, crepitus, erythema, swelling, and even a low-grade fever. Hydroxyapatite at the rotator cuff ruptures into the subacromial/subdeltoid bursa and then may be observed to be diffusely distributed within the space. After the rupture, hyperemia induced by the crystals results in rapid resorption of the calcification, often within 1 or 2 weeks. Rupture of hydroxyapatite or basic apatite crystals into the joint has been reported to cause a destructive arthropathy ("Milwaukee shoulder"). When hydroxyapatite causes symptoms in an atypical location such as around the hip or in the hand, it may be mistaken clinically as an infection. Calcific tendinosis may also cause erosion of bone at the insertion, simulating a tumor. Regardless of location and clinical presentation, typical calcification in the region of a tendon or bursa or in periarticular soft tissues should prompt the radiologist to suggest hydroxyapatite deposition disease (HADD). Treatment involves nonsteroidal anti-inflammatory drugs and is augmented by aspiration

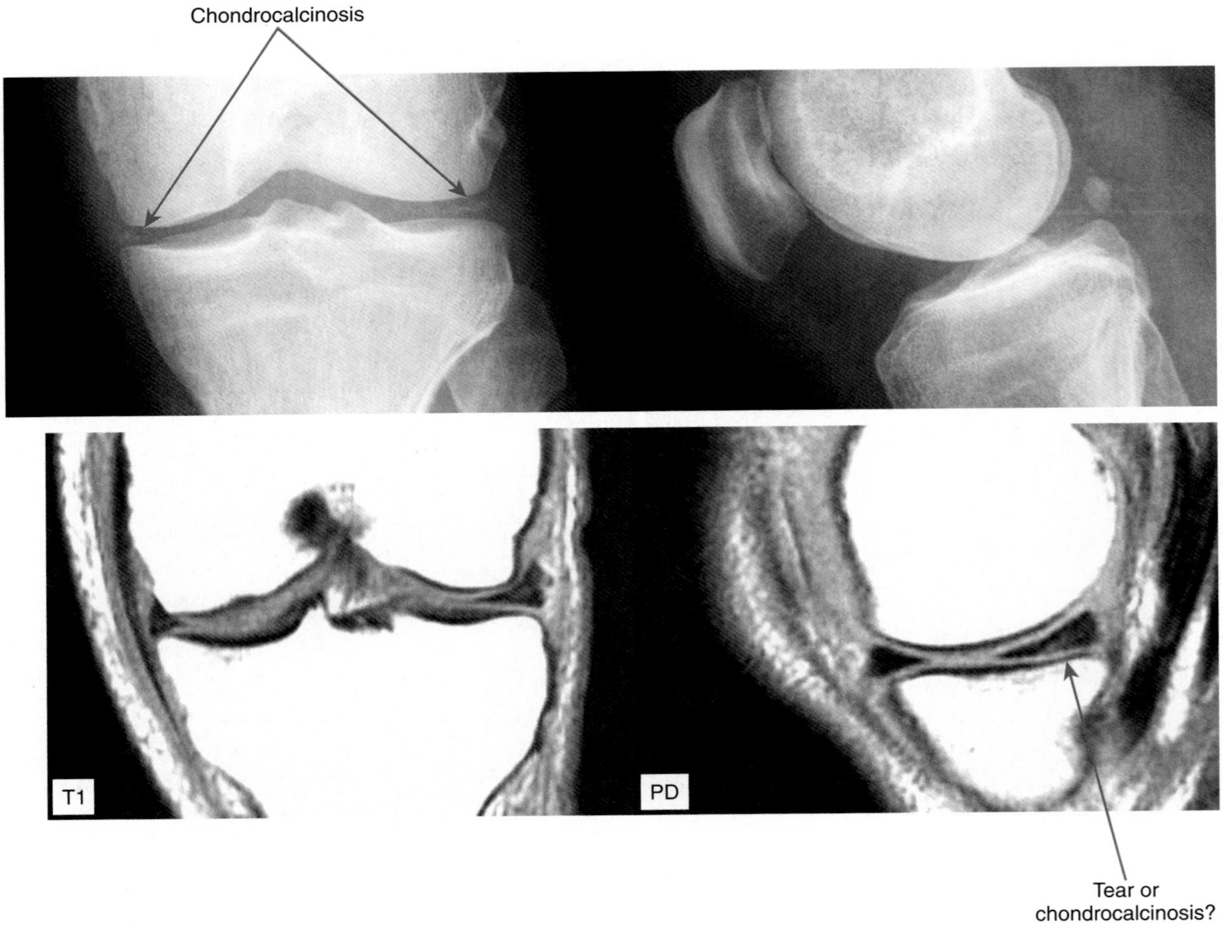
Chondrocalcinosis
T1
PD
Tear or
chondrocalcinosis?

Figure 4-47 Chondrocalcinosis can be hyperintense compared with normal meniscus on T1-weighted and proton density images and can potentially be misinterpreted as a meniscal tear if it appears near the superior or inferior surface.

of the pastelike material through a large-gauge needle. After appropriate treatment, symptoms improve rapidly and the patient may be saved from unnecessary antibiotics or surgery.

Calcification associated with hydroxyapatite deposition disease suspected on radiographs can be confirmed on CT, but this is not usually necessary. MRI is often ordered by referring clinicians who are not aware of this entity, after typical findings are missed on radiographs or if the clinical picture simulates infection. Hydroxyapatite contained within a tendon is often found incidentally, but is frequently overlooked on MRI because the calcification is dark and the tendon is dark, too. More commonly there is underlying tendinosis with intermediate signal, and the hydroxyapatite stands out as a focal "lump" of low signal. The calcification can be confirmed on gradient-echo sequences; the calcium stands out because of "blooming" artifact. When the MRI is acquired in the setting of an acute inflammatory reaction to hydroxyapatite, there is often bursitis (which may contain lumpy foci of low signal, a tip-off of the correct diagnosis) and surrounding edema. If contrast is given, the surrounding soft tissues enhance avidly, again simulating infection. Generally, if one looks closely, a small focus of low signal is observed within the area of intense enhancement. If the hydroxyapatite has ruptured from a tendon, on MRI it appears that there is a partial-thickness tear of the tendon, and again, the underlying cause may be overlooked. Bone marrow edema is occasionally observed at the insertion of the involved tendon, and discrete erosion is seen as a large focus of fluid signal; in this rare case, CT is very helpful for confirmation of the typical calcification, which may obviate the need for biopsy. Ultrasound may also be useful, demonstrating an

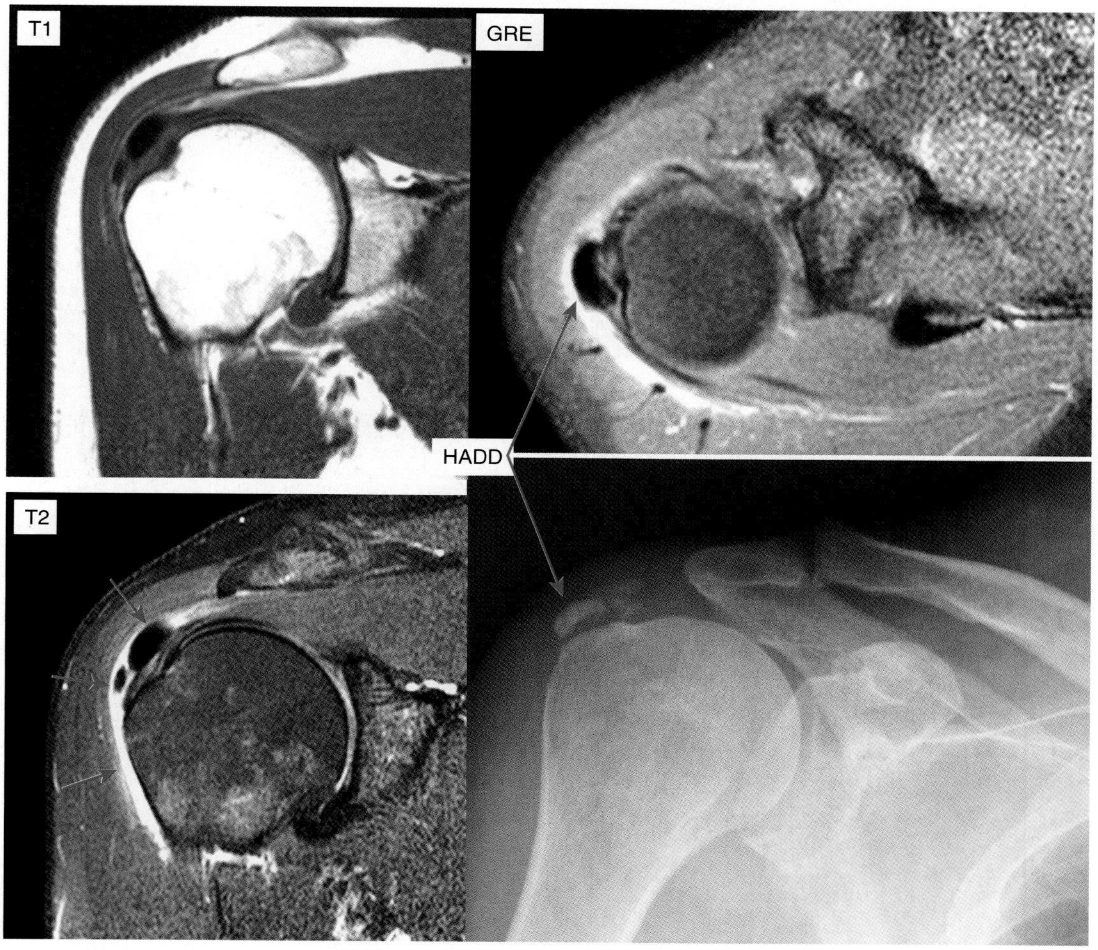
T1
GRE
HADD
T2
Calcification is within the bursa
with surrounding inflammation:
Likely recent rupture from tendon

Figure 4-48 Hydroxyapatite deposition disease (HADD). Hydroxyapatite deposition causes calcific tendinosis, calcific bursitis, and calcific periarthritis. Radiographically, the calcification tends to be small, focal, dense, and somewhat cloudlike.

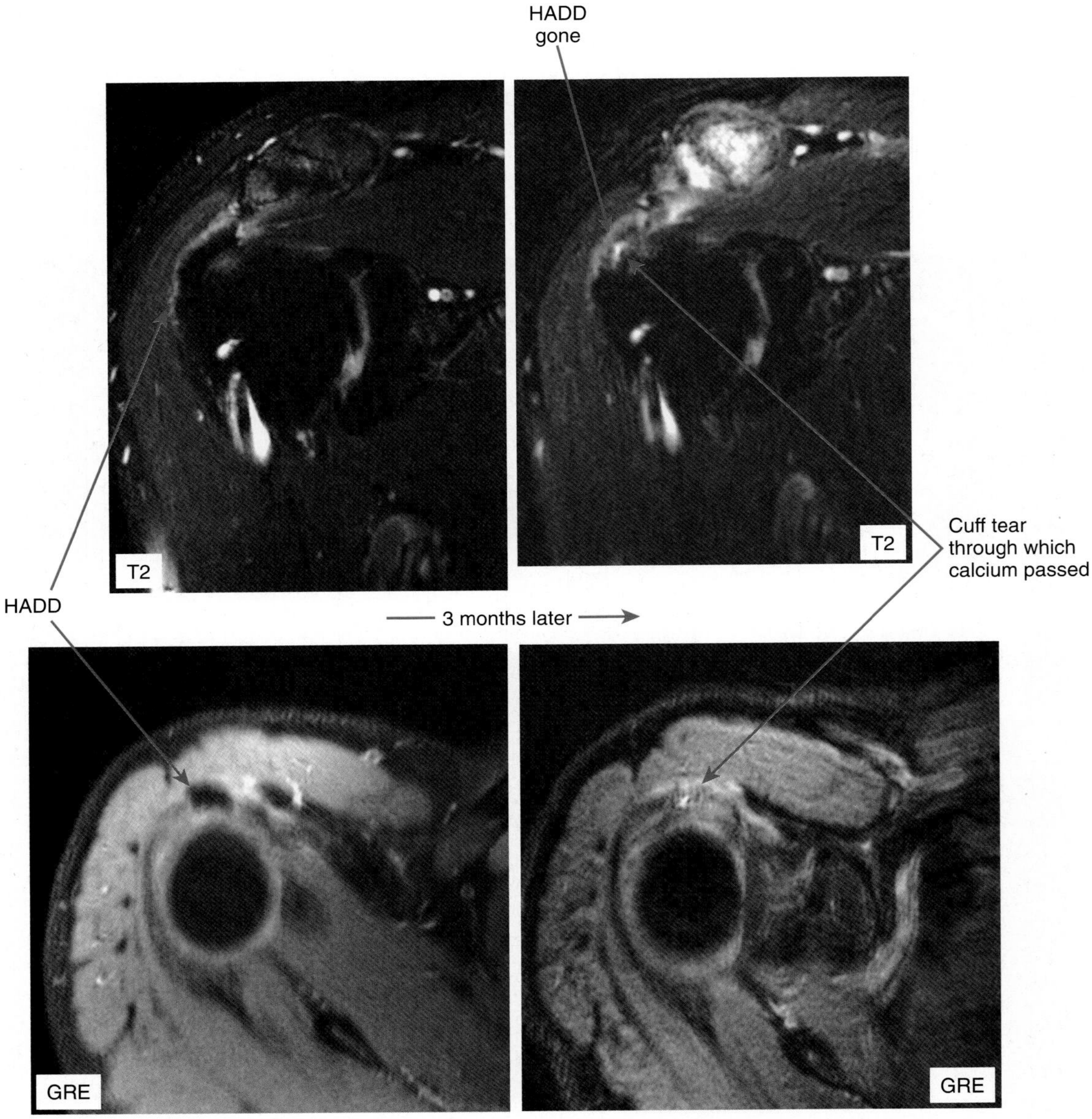
HADD
gone
T2
T2
Cuff tear
through which
calcium passed
HADD
3 months later
GRE
GRE

Figure 4-49 **Natural history of hydroxyapatite deposition disease (HADD).**

amorphous focus of increased echogenicity with variable degrees of acoustic shadowing.

METABOLIC CONDITIONS

Hemophilic Arthropathy
(Figs. 4-52 through 4-55)

Hemophilia is a group of inherited genetic disorders characterized by abnormal bleeding secondary to deficient or nonfunctional coagulation factors. The two most common forms are hemophilia A ("classic" hemophilia, factor VIII) and hemophilia B (Christmas disease, factor IX). The gene responsible is on the X chromosome, so the disease is fully manifested in males and carried by females. The musculoskeletal manifestations of hemophilia result from repetitive bleeding episodes.

Acute hemorrhagic effusions are seen as dense on radiographs and CT and as hyperintense on T1-weighted MR images. Subacute hemarthrosis may

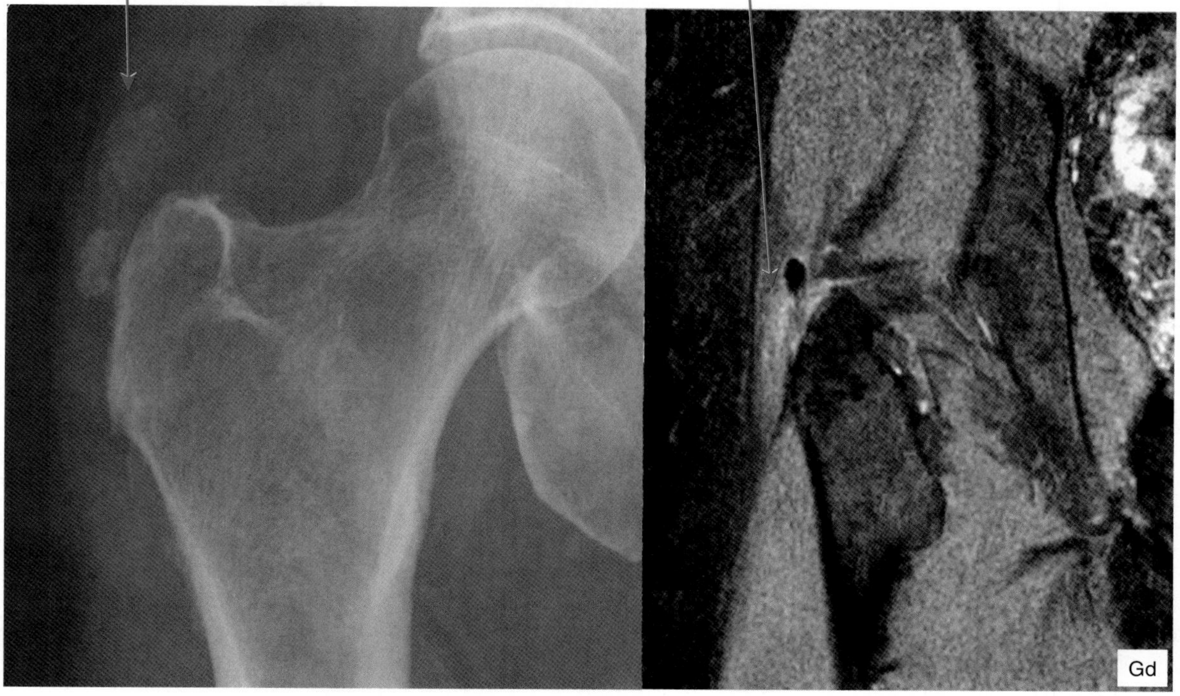
HADD at gluteus medius
Surrounding inflammation
Gd

Figure 4-50 When hydroxyapatite deposition disease (HADD) causes symptoms in an atypical location such as around the hip or in the hand, it may be mistaken clinically as an infection.

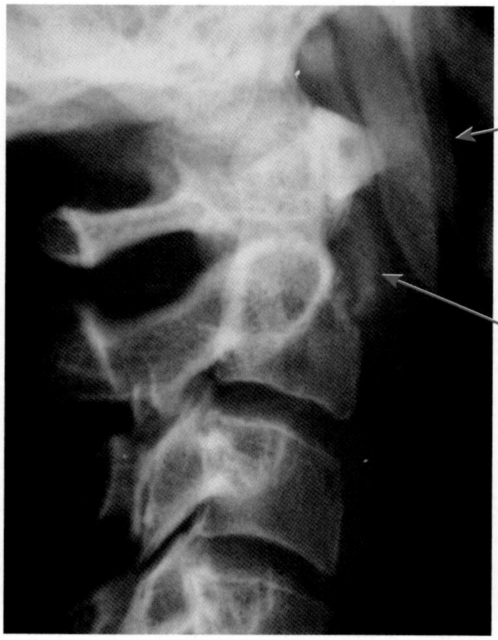
Prevertebral soft tissue swelling
HADD

Figure 4-51 Hydroxyapatite deposition disease (HADD) of the longus colli tendon inferior to the C1 anterior arch. Inflammation in this location can be misinterpreted clinically and on MRI as retropharyngeal abscess. Radiographs or CT can document the correct diagnosis, facilitating prompt, appropriate treatment with nonsteroidal anti-inflammatory drugs rather than aggressive therapy.

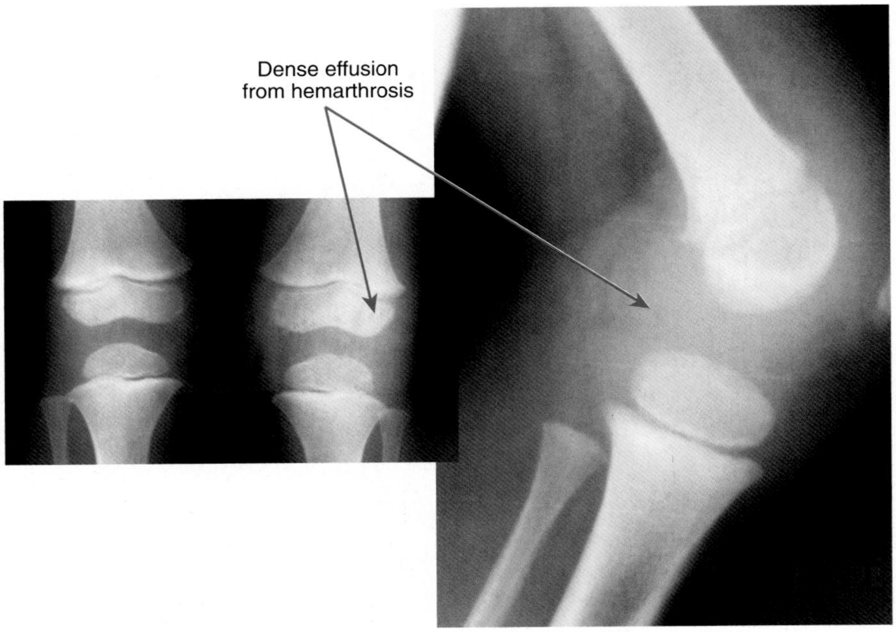
Dense effusion
from hemarthrosis

Figure 4-52 Hemophilia. Hemarthrosis is dense on radiographs. Hemarthrosis induces synovial hypertrophy, seen in the early phase of the disease.

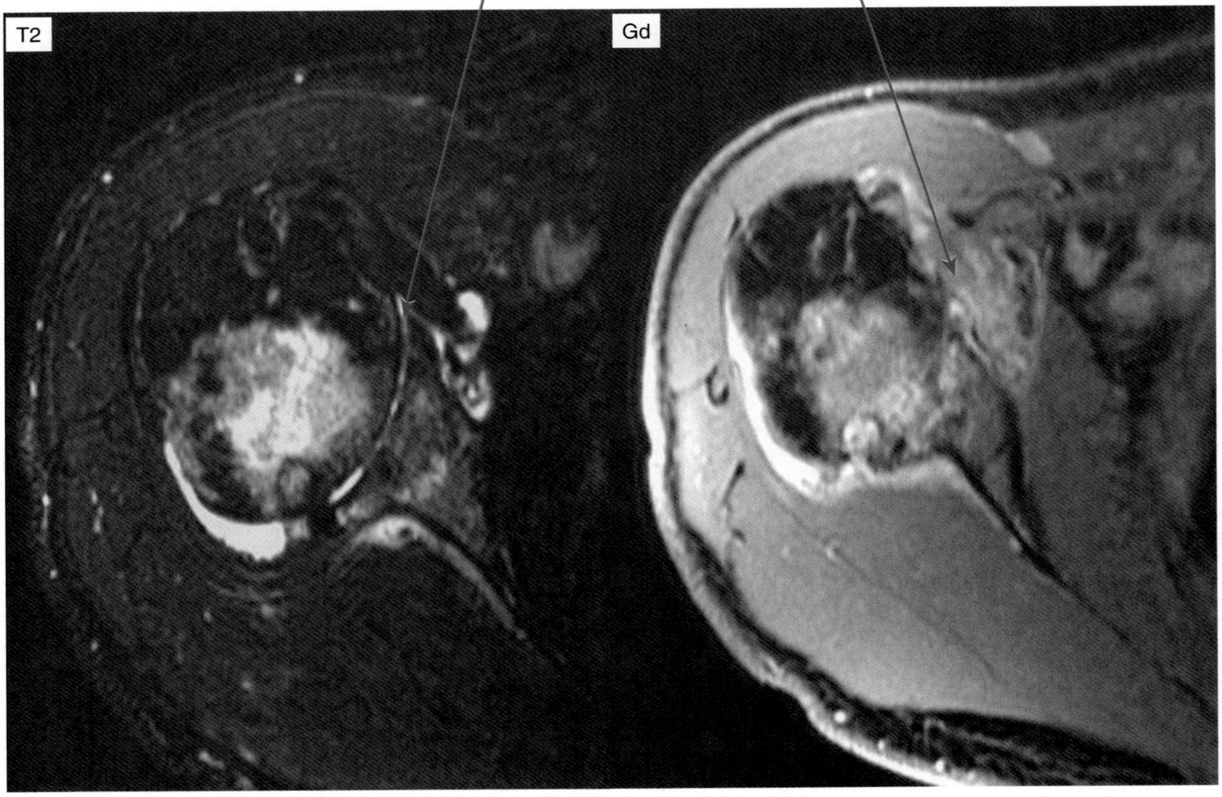
Diffuse cartilage loss
Enhancing synovitis
T2
Gd

Figure 4-53 Hemophilia. On MRI, synovium can appear thick and enhancing similar to inflammatory arthropathies. In later stages, synovial fibrosis ensues.

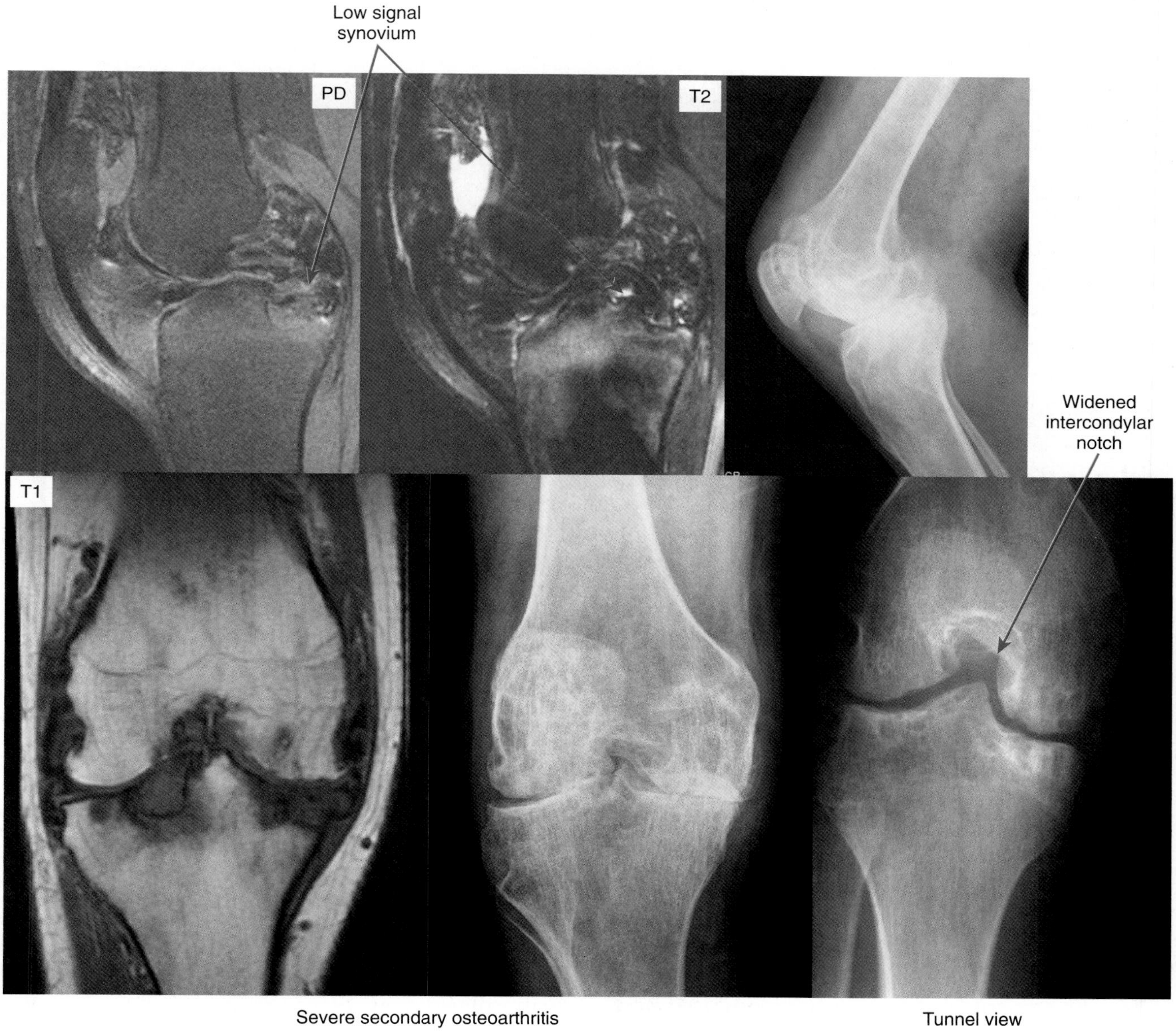
Low signal
synovium
PD
T2
Widened
intercondylar
notch
T1
Severe secondary osteoarthritis
Tunnel view

Figure 4-54 Hemophilic arthropathy, late findings. Radiographs and MRI show diffuse cartilage loss, secondary osteoarthritis, and widened intercondylar notch, with low-signal synovium on MRI.

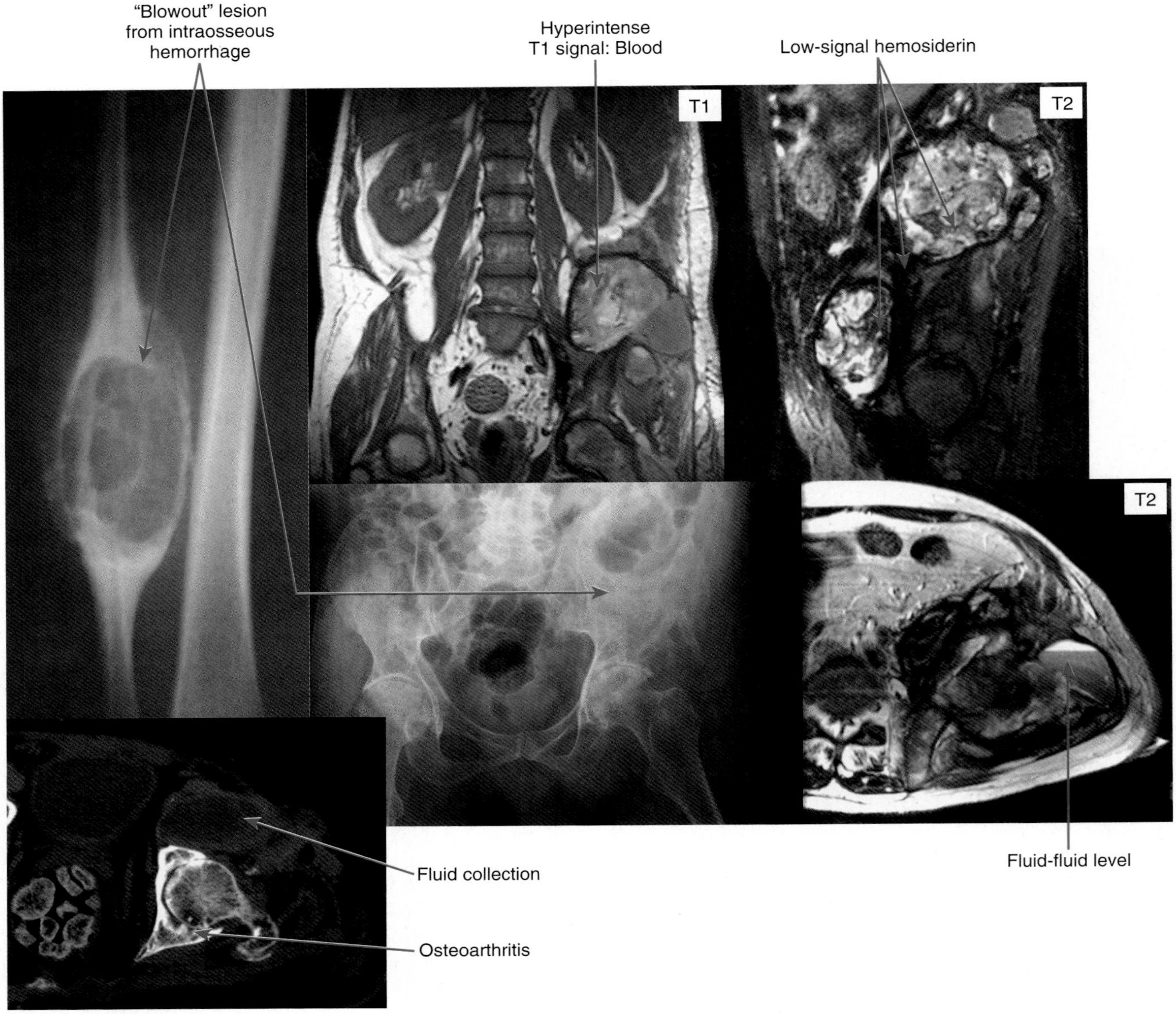
"Blowout" lesion from intraosseous hemorrhage
Hyperintense T1 signal: Blood
Low-signal hemosiderin
T1
T2
T2
Fluid collection
Osteoarthritis
Fluid-fluid level

Figure 4-55 Intraosseous hemophilic pseudotumors may mimic the radiographic appearance of a neoplasm.

show a hematocrit level. Hemarthrosis induces synovial hypertrophy, seen in the early phase of the disease. At this stage, synovium can appear thick and enhancing, similar to inflammatory arthropathies. The synovium is vascular and predisposes the joint to recurrent bleeds. Hemosiderin (low signal on MRI) deposits in the synovium, which eventually fibroses, thus limiting range of motion. In the late stage, the synovium may not enhance much. In between, recurrent episodes of hemorrhage result in diffuse articular cartilage loss and secondary osteoarthritis. Because hemorrhages may occur during childhood, hyperemia often results in hypertrophy of the epiphyses (a similar process occurs in juvenile chronic arthritis). The result is a ballooned appearance of the epiphyses, with overtubulation. Frequently traumatized joints are the most commonly involved; joints of the lower extremities are often involved bilaterally, though not necessarily symmetrically.

Other musculoskeletal involvement includes hemophilic pseudotumors due to osseous, subperiosteal or soft tissue (typically intramuscular) hemorrhage and contractures, which may result from the fibrotic response to intramuscular bleeding. Intraosseous hemophilic pseudotumors may mimic the radiographic appearance of a neoplasm. Radiographically, pseudotumor appears as a well-defined bone lesion. These lesions may progress rapidly with expansion. Subsequently, they develop a sclerotic border, and healing with re-ossification typically ensues. On MR imaging, the signal characteristics depend on the stage of the blood breakdown products: early stage, high T1 signal; late stage, low T2 signal. Maturation of the hematoma often progresses to ossification.

Amyloid Arthropathy (Figs. 4-56 through 4-59)

Amyloidosis refers to deposition of protein fibrils in organs and tissues, leading to organ enlargement and loss of function. It may be related to proteins elaborated from abnormalities of several different organ systems including the liver, spleen, and basement membranes of various structures. Amyloid fibrils are amorphous under light microscopy, but when stained with Congo red, a pathognomonic apple-green birefringence is observed under polarized light microscopy. Amyloidosis can be classified as primary or secondary and may be considered as either a localized or global phenomenon. A classification system based on the predisposing condition and the type of amyloid chains present has become the accepted convention. Immunostaining may allow classification into the different subtypes. Amyloid of the musculoskeletal system most often occurs in the setting of end-stage renal disease or plasma cell dyscrasias. Imaging demonstrates similar findings regardless of the origin or type.

The imaging findings in amyloidosis consist of erosions and soft tissue masses with preservation of the articular cartilage until late in the disease process. Subchondral lucent lesions are common, resembling cysts but often representing solid amyloid deposits.

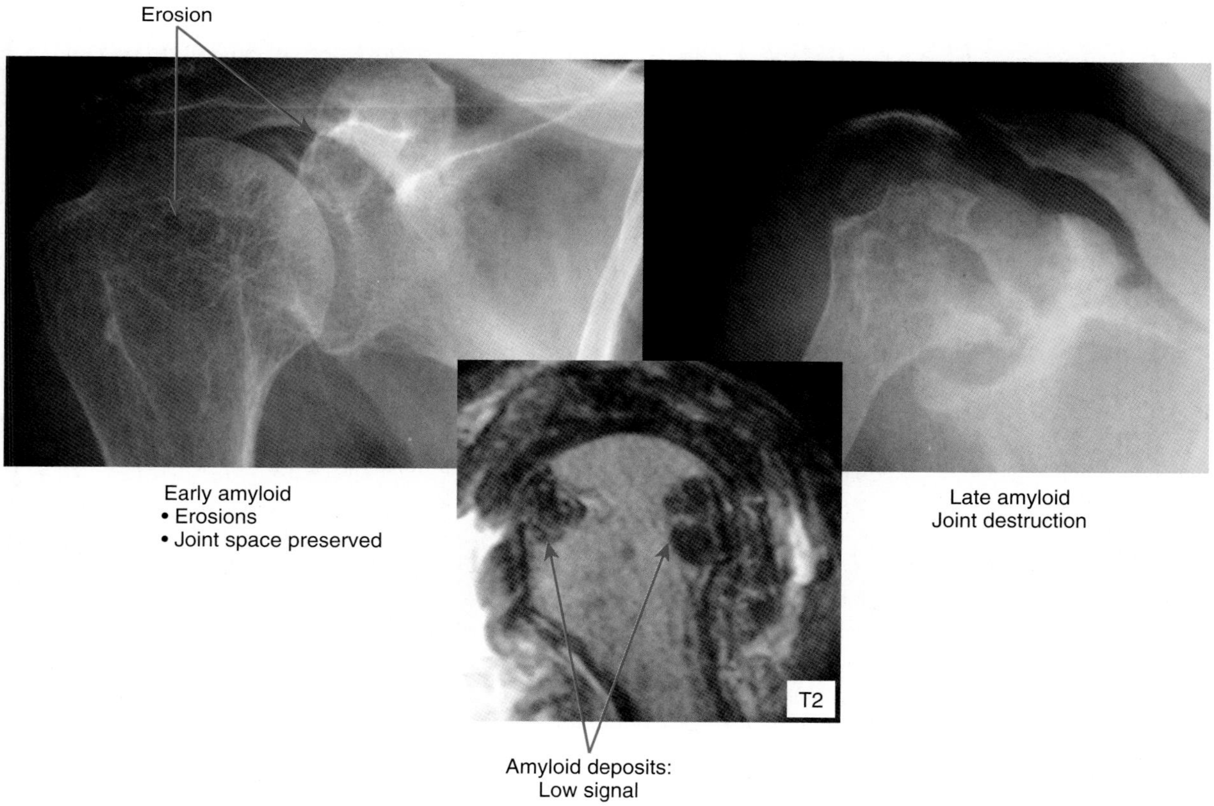
Erosion
Early amyloid
• Erosions
• Joint space preserved
T2
Late amyloid
Joint destruction
Amyloid deposits:
Low signal

Figure 4-56 Amyloid arthropathy. The imaging findings consist of erosions and soft tissue swelling or masses, with preservation of the articular cartilage until late in the disease process. Amyloid itself is low signal on T1- and T2-weighted images but may be associated with fluid collections.

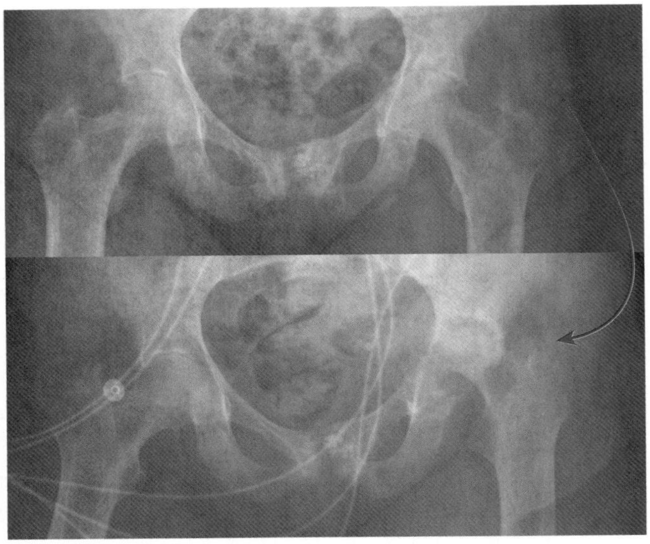
3 months

Figure 4-57 Progressive joint destruction in amyloid.

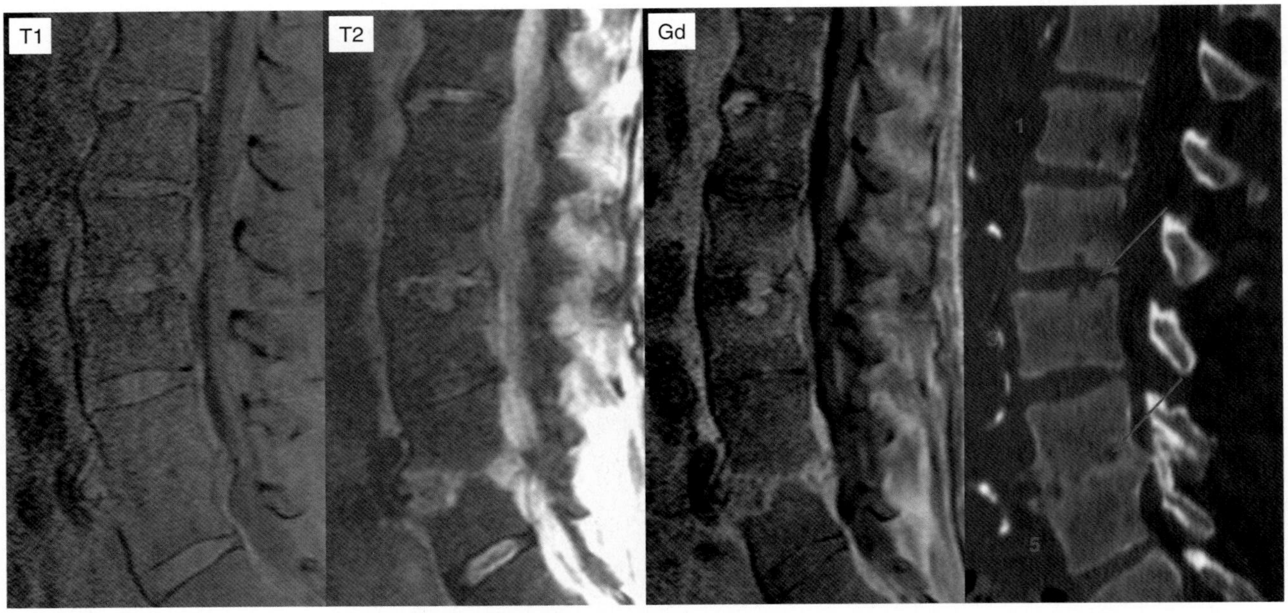
Amyloid exhibits low T1
and T2 signal; however,
fluid signal and adjacent
enhancement are also common
• Biopsy may be required
Endplate erosions can
simulate infection
T1
T2
Gd
Spondyloarthropathy of renal failure with amyloid deposition

Figure 4-58 Amyloid. Involvement of the spine may cause destructive changes at the disk (erosive azotemic osteodystrophy), which may mimic infection or neuropathic disease on all modalities. Disk narrowing is seen with endplate erosions and sclerosis, which can rapidly progress to endplate destruction resulting in spondylolisthesis.

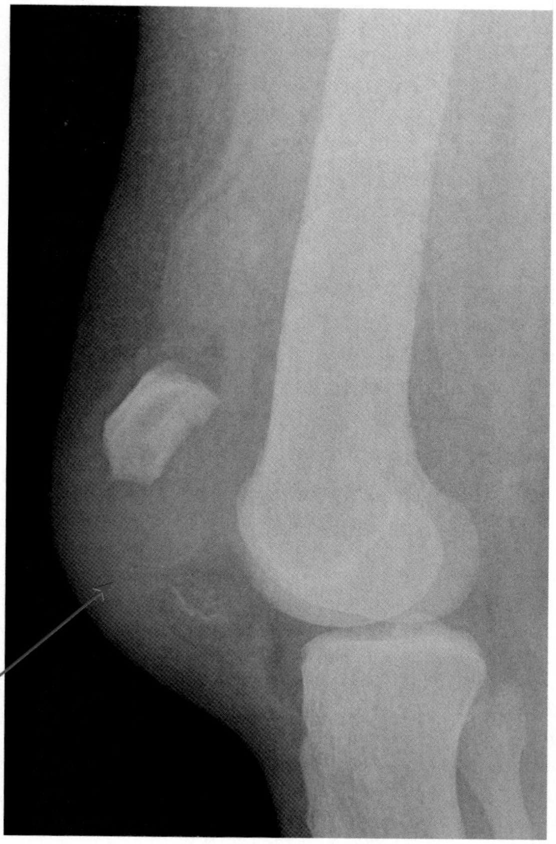
Avulsion of the
inferior patella
in a patient with
chronic renal failure

Figure 4-59 Amyloid. Involvement of tendons, ligaments, and, rarely, muscles may also occur. Also, chronic renal failure and osteomalacia predisposes to avulsions.

The shoulder, hip, knee, spine, and wrist are most commonly involved. When an erosive arthropathy is present, this disorder should be considered if there is a history of renal failure or suggestive radiographic signs, including vascular calcification, tuft resorption, radial side phalangeal resorption, distal clavicular or sacroiliac resorption, or "rugger jersey" spine. On MR imaging, amyloid is low-to-intermediate signal intensity on all pulse sequences, which helps differentiate this disease from inflammatory arthropathies and infection. However, there are often joint effusions or soft tissue fluid collections also associated with amyloidosis. The MR imaging picture may be confusing if interpreted without history or radiographs. Always consider that amyloidosis is a systemic disorder with multifocal involvement. Therefore, the other exams in the patient's file should be reviewed when the diagnosis of amyloid is entertained to search for signs of chronic renal failure and osteodystrophy.

Involvement of the spine in amyloidosis may cause destructive changes at the disk (erosive azotemic osteodystrophy), which may mimic infection or neuropathic disease on all modalities. Disk narrowing is seen with endplate erosions and sclerosis, which can rapidly progress to endplate destruction resulting in spondylolisthesis. Vertebral collapse and paraspinal soft tissue masses also occur. Multilevel involvement, which may or may not be contiguous, is typical of amyloidosis and reflects the underlying systemic process. Again, multifocal involvement and areas of low-signal amyloid should suggest the proper diagnosis. If biopsy is considered necessary, the pathologist should be alerted to the possibility of amyloid, so that a Congo red stain is used.

Soft tissue involvement is typified by masslike deposits of amyloid in subcutaneous and periarticular tissues. Calcification is rare. Involvement of tendons, ligaments, and rarely muscles may also occur. Carpal tunnel syndrome is a complication of wrist involvement. Tendon involvement can predispose to tendon tear; in addition, patients with renal failure are susceptible to avulsion fractures due to weakening of the underlying bone.

NONINFLAMMATORY MONARTICULAR ARTHROPATHIES

Synovial Osteochondromatosis (Figs. 4-60 through 4-62)

Synovial osteochondromatosis involves synovial metaplasia of unknown etiology resulting in formation of cartilaginous bodies that often ossify. It is seen in females twice as frequently as males and is a monarticular disorder usually affecting large joints, knee being most common. Extra-articular locations, particularly a bursa or tendon sheath, are occasionally involved. The disease most commonly presents in young adults. Symptoms include swelling, pain, locking, and decreased range of motion. In long-standing disease, secondary osteoarthritis often occurs, which may cause confusion in distinguishing this process from conventional osteoarthritis with multiple bodies.

If the bodies are calcified or ossified, radiographs show numerous bodies of similar small size, disproportionate to the degree of osteoarthritis. Osteoarthritis can form multiple bodies as well, but these typically vary in size and are few in number. CT is usually not necessary to make the diagnosis of synovial osteochondromatosis, but occasionally the bodies are so small and faintly calcified that they may

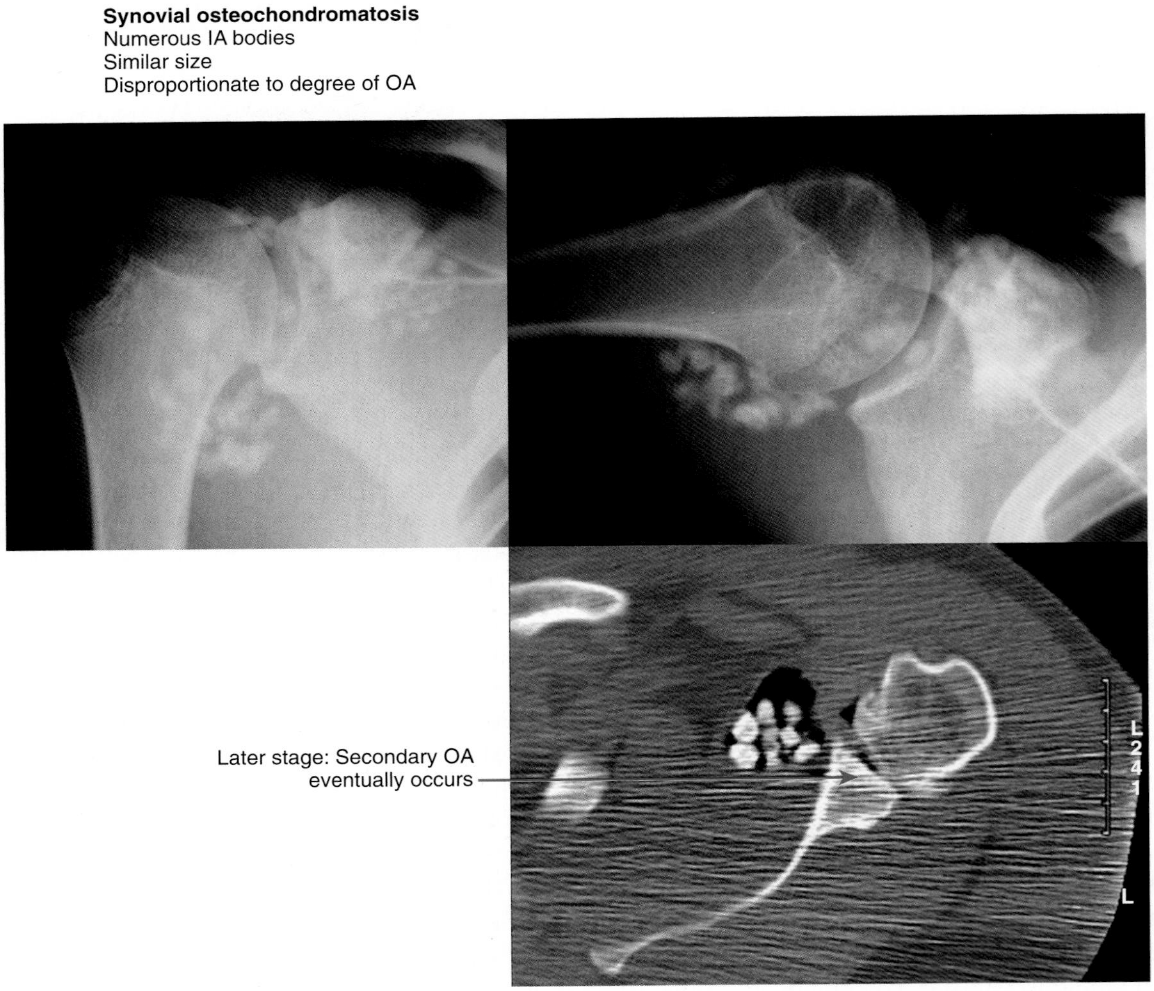
Synovial osteochondromatosis
Numerous IA bodies
Similar size
Disproportionate to degree of OA
Later stage: Secondary OA
eventually occurs
L
2
4
1
L

Figure 4-60 Synovial osteochondromatosis. If the bodies are calcified or ossified, radiographs show numerous bodies of similar small size, disproportionate to the degree of osteoarthritis (OA). IA, intra-articular.

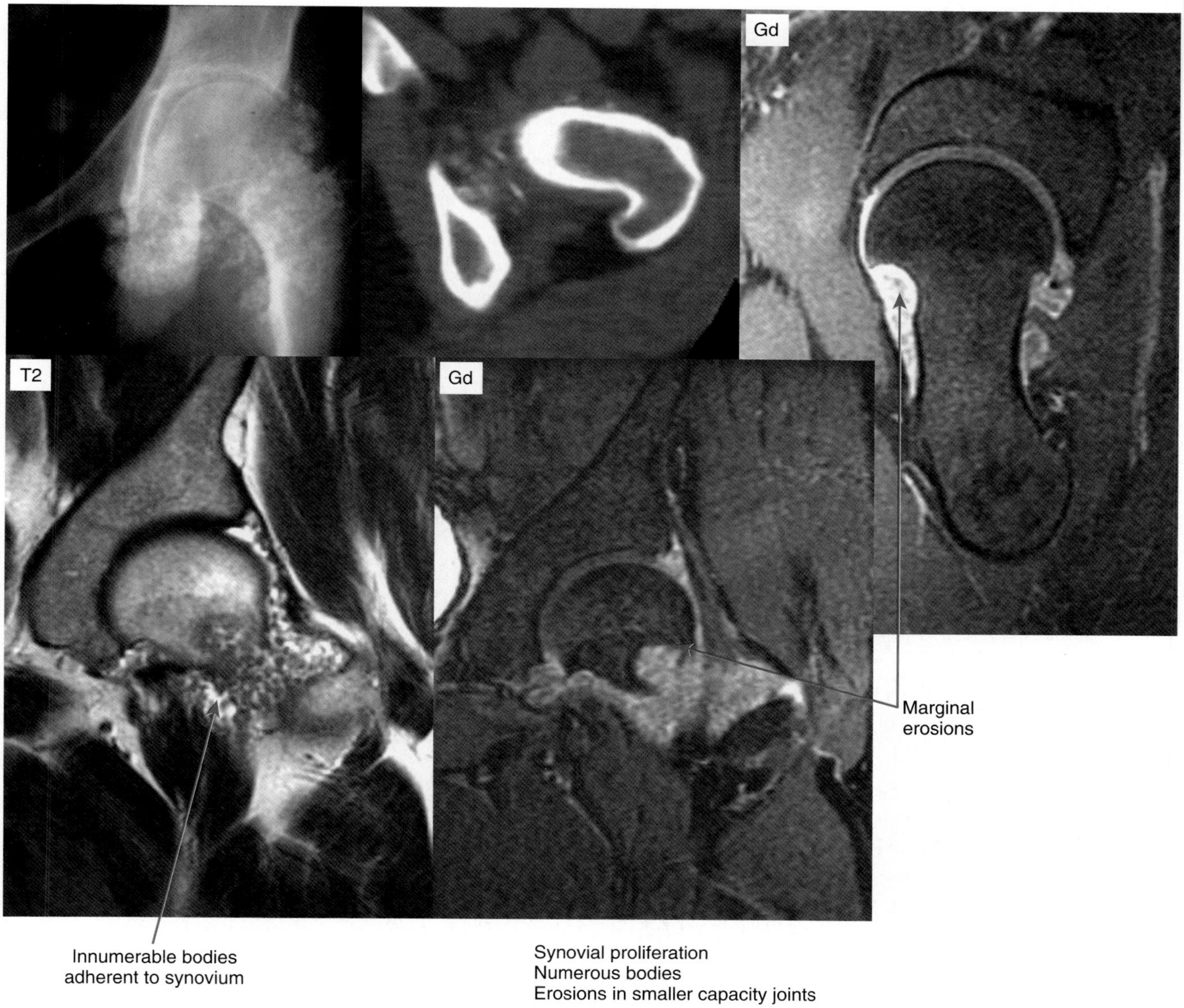
Gd
T2
Gd
Marginal erosions
Innumerable bodies adherent to synovium
Synovial proliferation
Numerous bodies
Erosions in smaller capacity joints

Figure 4-61 Synovial osteochondromatosis. Erosions can occur in joints with smaller capacity such as the hip; occasionally, the bodies are so small and faintly calcified that they may be missed on radiographs.

be missed on radiographs in large joints such as the hip. On MR imaging, the bodies are easily seen against a background of joint fluid, the calcification being low signal on all sequences. The articular cartilage is preserved until late in the course of the disease, and therefore the joint space is typically normal at initial presentation. Erosions may occur in articulations with tight capsules (e.g., the hip). No periosteal reaction is associated with uncomplicated synovial osteochondromatosis. The disorder may involve only a portion of the synovium (localized form) or may be diffuse. Bodies that form are usually adherent to the synovium but may break loose and collect in recesses. Cross-sectional imaging is particularly useful when there are no apparent calcified or ossified bodies (synovial chondromatosis). In this case there may be an effusion and well-defined erosions simulating inflammatory arthropathies.

CT is excellent for demonstrating erosions and detecting small amounts of calcification. However, small bodies can be obscured by intra-articular

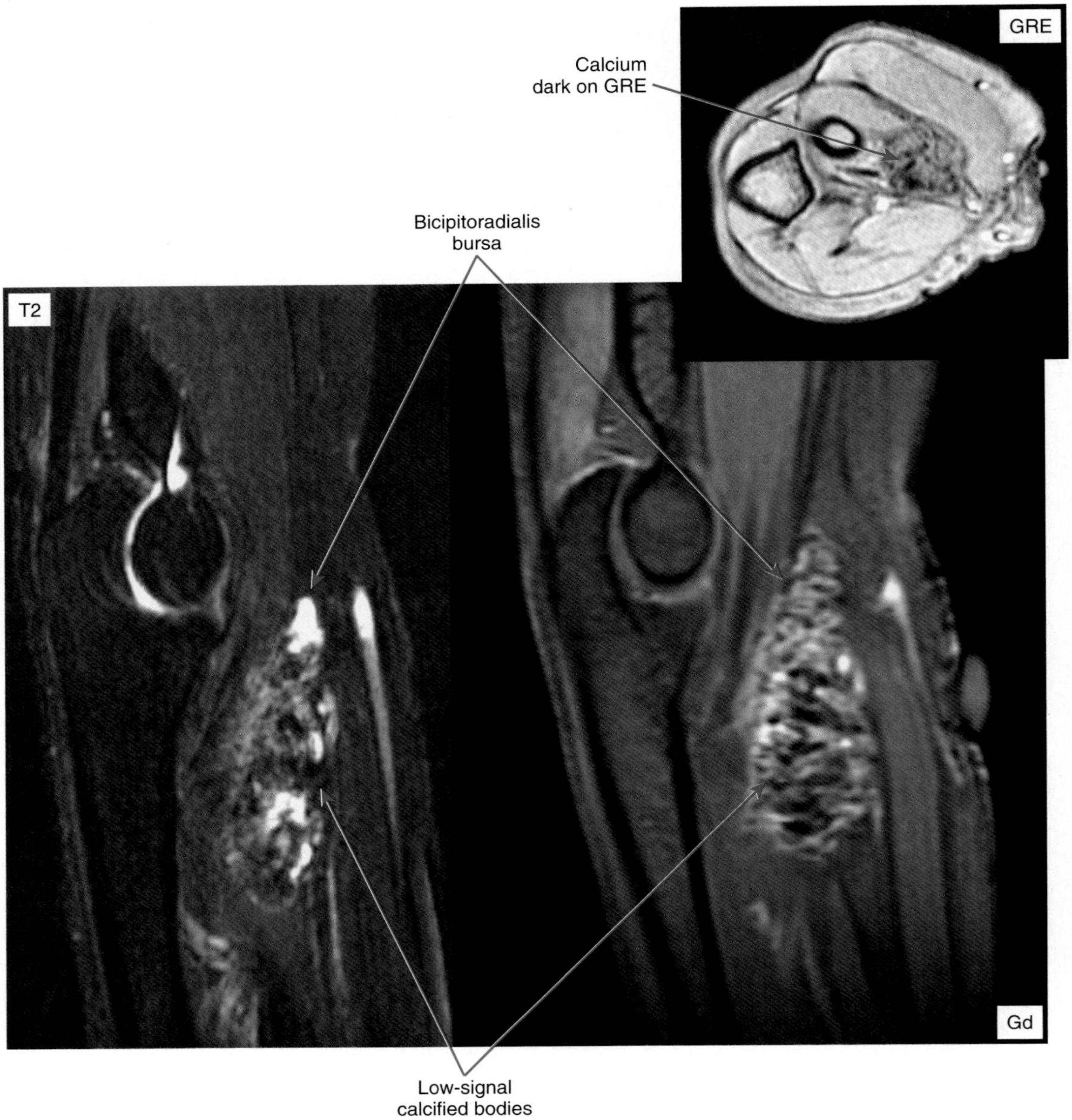
GRE
Calcium
dark on GRE
Bicipitoradialis
bursa
T2
Gd
Low-signal
calcified bodies

Figure 4-62 Rarely, synovial osteochondromatosis can involve a bursa or tendon sheath. Gradient–recalled echo (GRE) imaging is useful to detect calcium, or correlation with radiographs can be performed.

contrast. MR imaging can also detect small amounts of calcium in the synovium if gradient-echo images are used; fat suppression should not be used, however, because suppressed fat blends with the low signal of the calcium. Chondroid tissue is bright on T2-weighted sequences and can blend with joint fluid; gadolinium contrast can be useful to visualize areas of synovial proliferation associated with the disease process. After synovectomy, the disease may recur in recesses or periarticular locations, with characteristic small, numerous calcifications.

Pigmented Villonodular Synovitis (Figs. 4-63 through 4-66)

Like synovial osteochondromatosis, pigmented villonodular synovitis (PVNS) is a benign proliferative synovial disease of unknown etiology, occurring as a

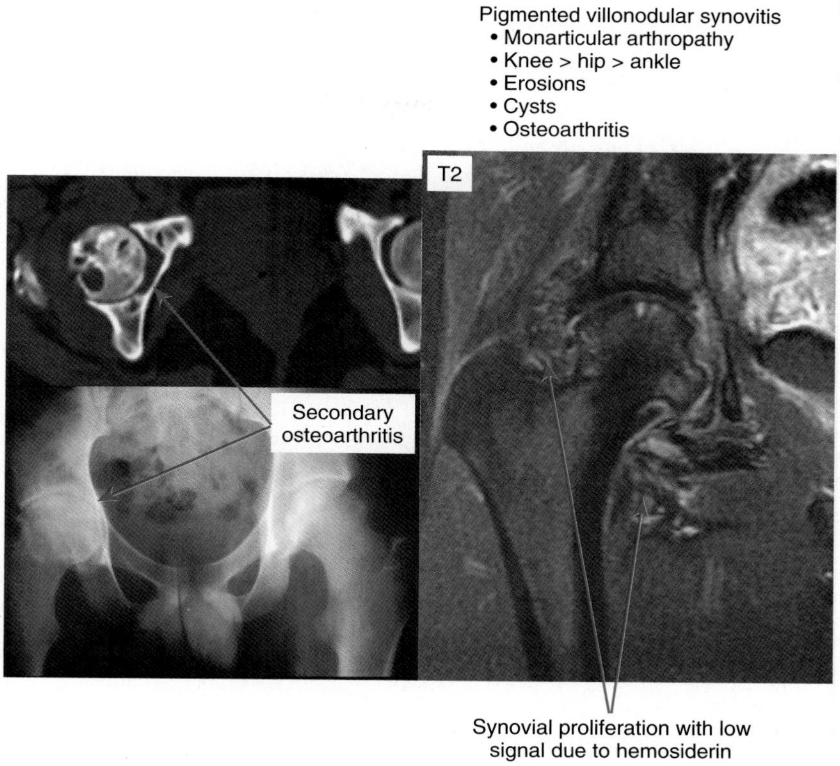
Pigmented villonodular synovitis
• Monarticular arthropathy
• Knee > hip > ankle
• Erosions
• Cysts
• Osteoarthritis
T2
Secondary osteoarthritis
Synovial proliferation with low signal due to hemosiderin

Figure 4-63 Pigmented villonodular synovitis (PVNS). Like synovial osteochondromatosis, PVNS should be considered whenever a young adult presents with a monarticular noninflammatory arthropathy. Similarly, the degree of erosion is inversely proportional to the joint capacity and is also related to extent/distribution of synovial proliferation. Unlike synovial osteochondromatosis, calcification is not a characteristic of PVNS.

diffuse or localized form. Extra-articular involvement may occur in a tendon sheath (common) or a bursa (uncommon). PVNS of a tendon sheath is more commonly referred to as giant cell tumor of the tendon sheath (GCTTS), which has no relation to giant cell tumor of bone. At gross inspection, the synovium has a reddish appearance due to hemosiderin deposition. Microscopically, synovial cell hyperplasia and surface proliferation are present. There is also subsynovial accumulation of hemosiderin-laden macrophages, multinucleated giant cells, and fibroblasts. The extra-articular localized form has the same histology but typically contains less hemosiderin than the articular counterpart.

Patients with PVNS present with a monarticular arthropathy or chronic joint effusion with insidious onset, most frequently in one of the large joints of the lower extremity: knee > hip > ankle. The age of presentation is typically in the 20- to 40-year age range with no gender predilection. Arthrocentesis may demonstrate serosanguineous fluid. The presence of a bloody effusion without trauma suggests PVNS. Treatment consists of synovectomy, which may be supplemented with intra-articular radioisotope treatment using a beta emitter.

Patients with GCTTS most commonly present with an extra-articular soft tissue mass or focal swelling, typically in the hand or foot and usually related to a flexor tendon. The age at presentation is older than with intra-articular PVNS, occurring in the fifth to sixth decades of life with a female predilection. It is the second most common soft tissue lesion of the hand after a ganglion.

On radiographs, PVNS typically shows a joint effusion. PVNS rarely calcifies, which helps to separate it from synovial osteochondromatosis. Scalloped erosions with thin, sclerotic margins may be observed; degree of erosion is inversely proportional to the joint capacity and is also related to extent/distribution of synovial proliferation. In a small-capacity joint such as the hip, erosions are often prominent. In the knee, erosions may be subtle, even with extensive joint involvement. As in synovial osteochondromatosis, gradual cartilage loss occurs, progressing to secondary osteoarthritis. CT may not be very useful except to exclude calcifications associated with synovial osteochondromatosis. MRI is fairly characteristic, showing synovial proliferation with dark signal on T2-weighted images from hemosiderin deposition. Gradient-echo imaging is especially useful to

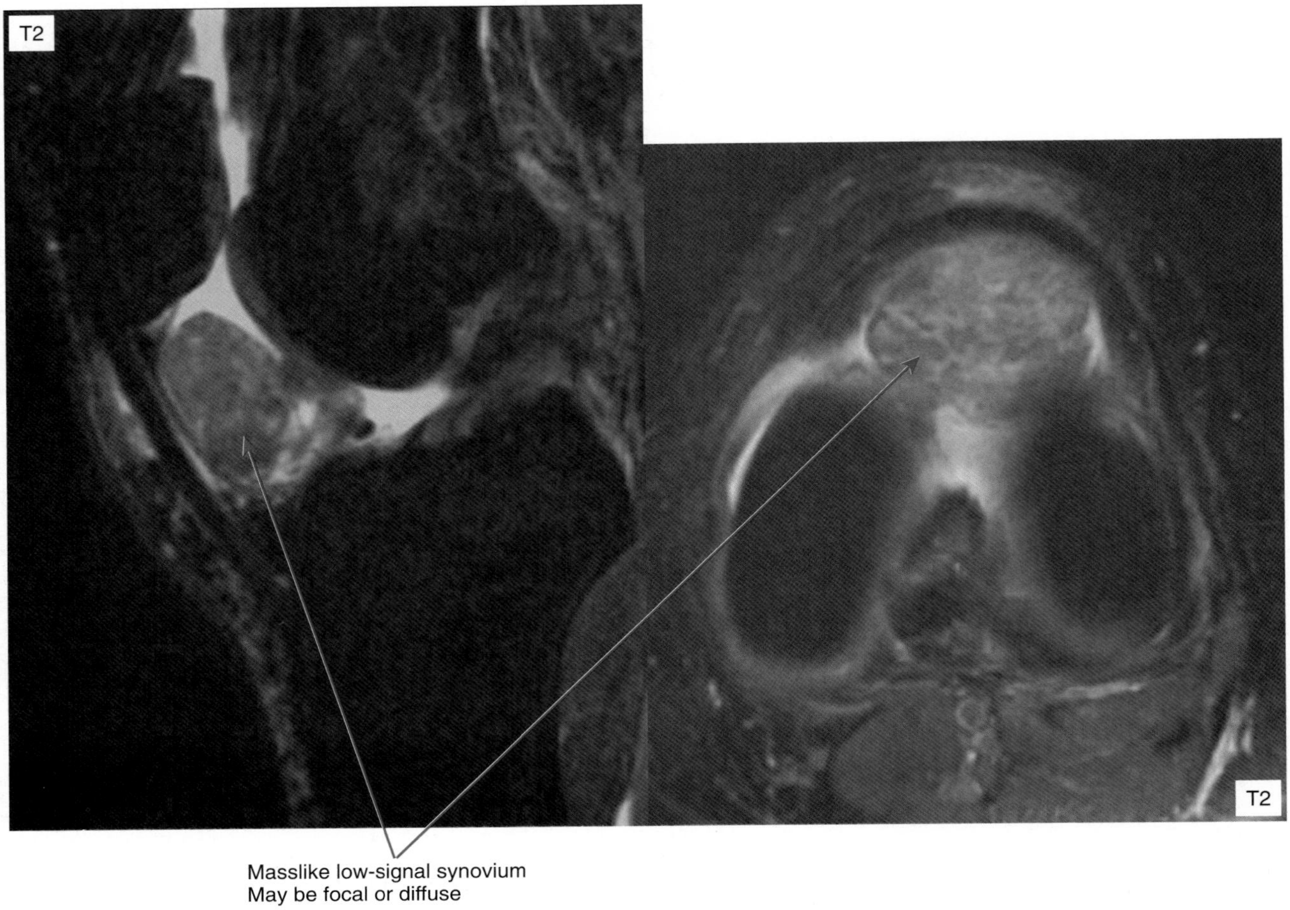
T2
T2
Masslike low-signal synovium
May be focal or diffuse

Figure 4-64 Pigmented villonodular synovitis (PVNS) can be focal or diffuse; also, the amount of hemosiderin and therefore signal intensity on T2-weighted images varies. The differential for dark synovium includes PVNS, synovial osteochondromatosis, gout, hemophilia, amyloid, post-op, and chronic arthropathy with scarring.

document blooming artifact from the hemosiderin, to help separate it from other causes of dark synovium (Box 4-6).

Lipoma Arborescans

Lipoma arborescans refers to proliferation of lipomatous tissue within the synovium (Fig. 4-67). It may result from a chronic inflammatory synovitis with resultant hyperplasia of the fatty subsynovial tissue, but often there is no recognized history of arthropathy. It presents as chronic masslike enlargement of the joint and most commonly affects the knee. MR imaging shows masslike synovial proliferation with signal corresponding to fat, with numerous frondlike excrescences.

BOX 4-6 DARK SYNOVIUM ON T2-WEIGHTED MR IMAGES

Post-operative fibrosis (usually non-masslike)
Hemosiderin (blooms on gradient-recalled echo [GRE] images):
- Pigmented villonodular synovitis (masslike)
- Hemophilia

Gout (masslike)
Rheumatoid arthritis (masslike)
Calcification (blooms on GRE images)
- Synovial osteochondromatosis (masslike with bodies)

Amyloid (masslike)

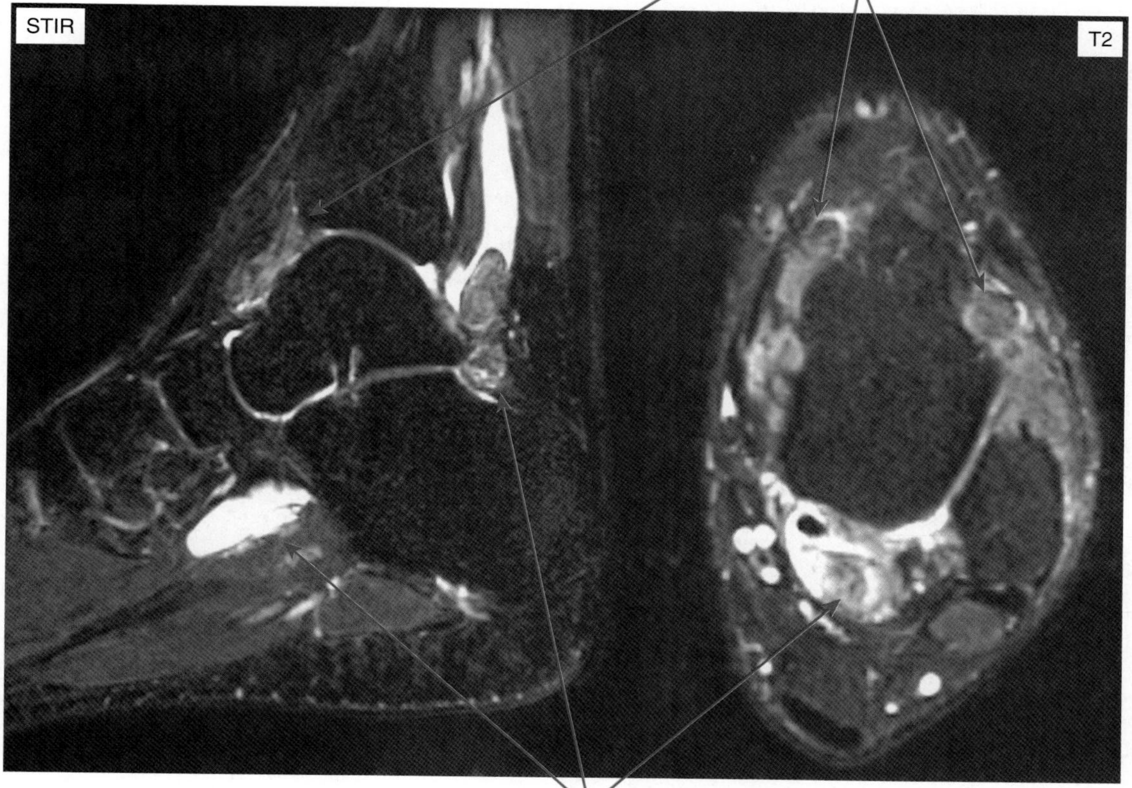
PVNS involving ankle joint
STIR
T2
Involvement of flexor hallucis longus sheath

Figure 4-65 *As with other arthropathies, pigmented villonodular synovitis (PVNS) can extend into contiguous compartments.*

DIFFERENTIAL DIAGNOSIS: APPROACH TO AN ARTHRITIS

It is useful to go through a checklist (Box 4-7) whenever an arthritis is suspected, so that all findings are considered. A standard approach involves evaluation of (1) the soft tissues, (2) bone mineralization, (3) the joint and subchondral bone, (4) erosion, (5) proliferation, (6) deformity, and (7) distribution of disease. This finding-based approach is extremely useful in generating a differential diagnosis, particularly when combined with the problem-solving capabilities of advanced modalities. On MRI, additions to the checklist include (1) effusion, (2) synovial

BOX 4-7 CHECKLIST FOR RADIOGRAPHIC EVALUATION OF ARTHRITIS

Soft tissues
Bone mineralization
The joint and subchondral bone
Erosion
Proliferation
Deformity
Distribution of disease

Advanced imaging, add:

Effusion
Synovial proliferation
- Masslike?
- Low signal?

Cartilage loss
- Focal?
- Diffuse?

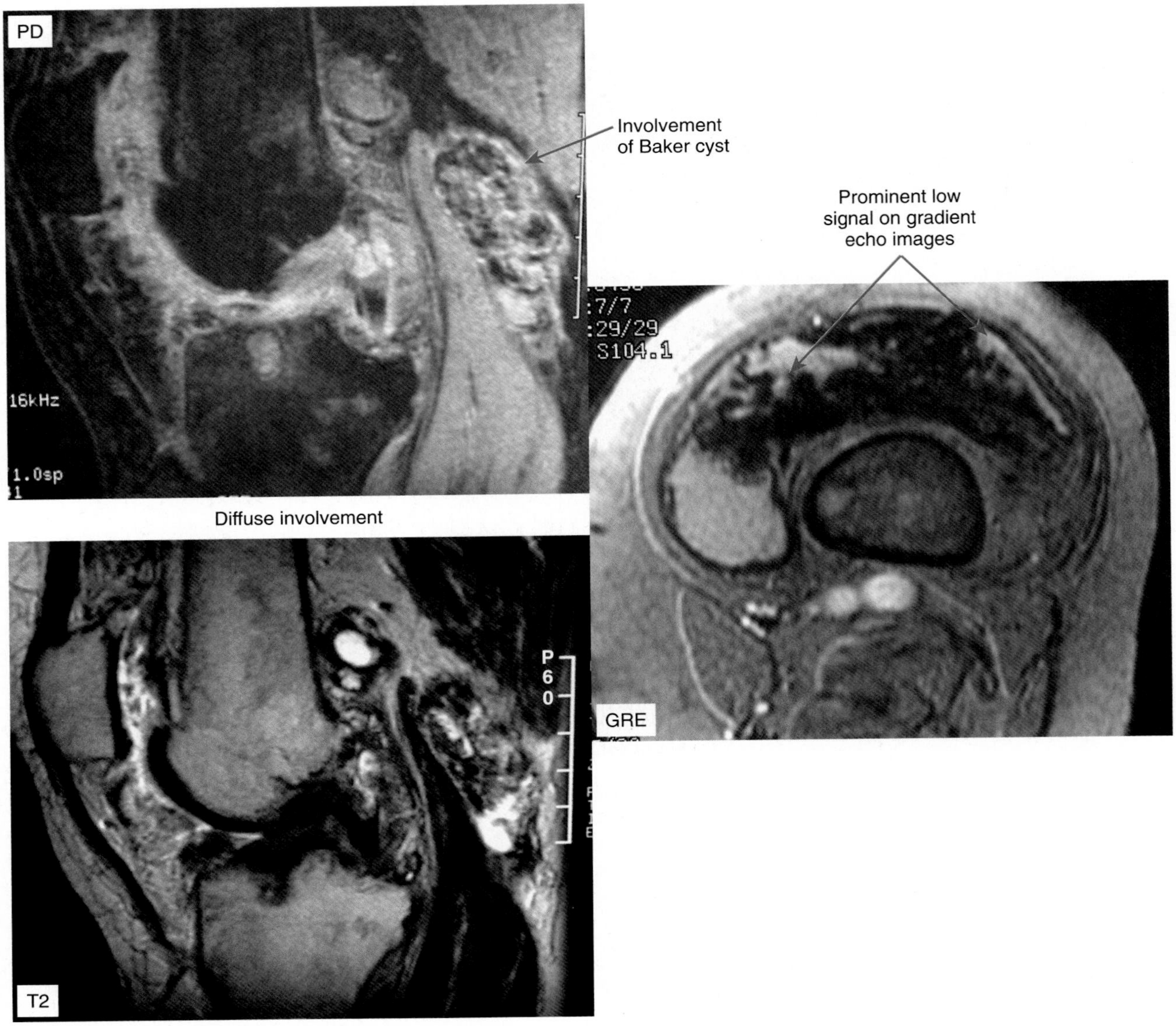
PD
Involvement
of Baker cyst
Prominent low
signal on gradient
echo images
:7/7
:29/29
S104.1
16kHz
1.0sp
Diffuse involvement
P
6
0
GRE
T2

Figure 4-66 Pigmented villonodular synovitis. In later stages with diffuse disease, extensive hemosiderin deposition is observed, which "blooms" with low signal on gradient echo images.

proliferation (and evaluation for masslike synovium or low-signal synovium), and (3) cartilage loss (and determination of diffuse versus focal cartilage loss).

THE SOFT TISSUES

Soft Tissue Swelling

Swelling in the setting of arthritis can be from joint effusion or synovial proliferation, ganglion cyst, soft tissue edema, tenosynovitis, bursitis, or deposition of amyloid, calcium, crystals, or pus (Box 4-8). Effusion is a common but nonspecific finding in the arthropathies. If trauma is excluded, arthritis should be the main consideration. Unexplained effusion involving a single joint without trauma or apparent degeneration should always raise suspicion of septic arthritis. Inflammatory arthropathies tend to have large effusions (Box 4-9).

Osteoarthritis and prior surgery can result in synovial proliferation, which is typically mild. Inflamma-

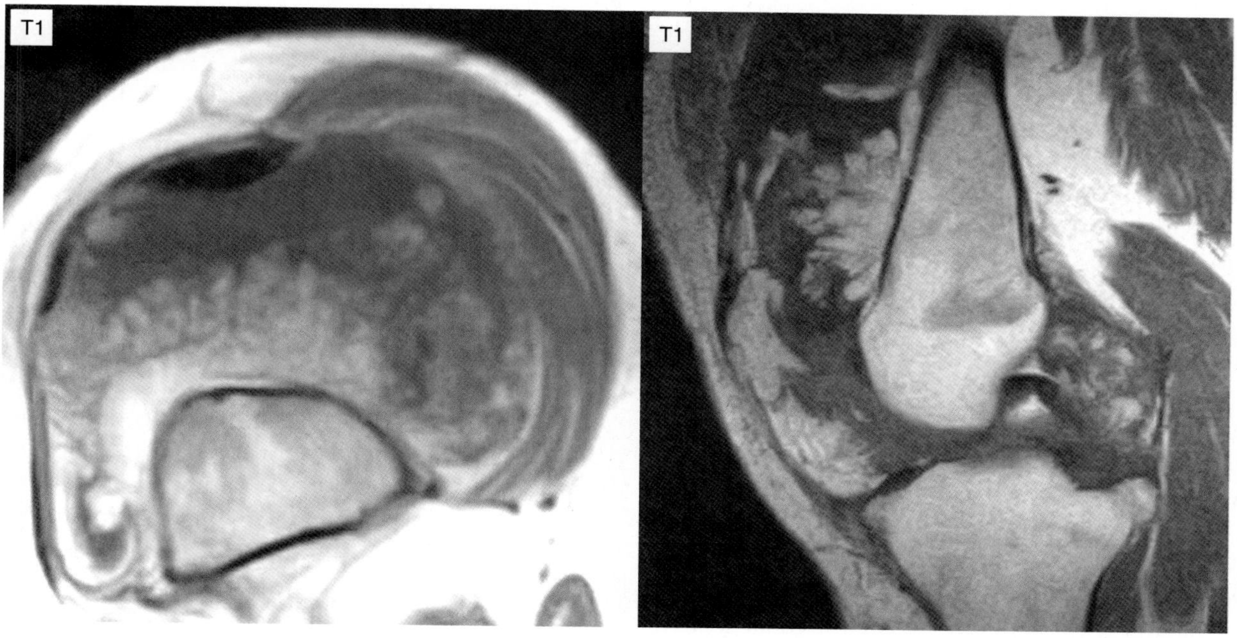
T1
T1

Figure 4-67 Lipoma arborescans. MR imaging shows masslike synovial proliferation with signal corresponding to fat, with numerous frondlike excrescences.

BOX 4-8 SOFT TISSUE SWELLING IN ARTHRITIS: DIFFERENTIAL DIAGNOSIS

Joint effusion
Synovial proliferation
Ganglion cyst
Soft tissue edema
Tenosynovitis
Bursitis
Deposition of amyloid, calcium, crystals, or other material

Unexplained effusion involving a single joint without trauma should first raise suspicion for septic arthritis.

BOX 4-9 SYNOVITIS EXTENT AND ARTHRITIS

Mild: Post-op, osteoarthritis
Moderate/marked: Septic arthritis, inflammatory arthropathies
Masslike: Pigmented villonodular synovitis, synovial osteochondromatosis, rheumatoid arthritis, gout

Ganglion cysts may become complex if they contain synovial proliferation (e.g., in rheumatoid arthritis) or if they are traumatized (e.g., at the foot/ankle); definitively demonstrating communication of a cyst with a joint or tendon sheath can help exclude tumor (in addition to the fact that ganglion cysts are usually lobulated and most tumors are not).

tory arthropathies may show marked synovial proliferation, but the extent is variable. In active rheumatoid arthritis, synovitis is typically masslike, a characteristic also seen with PVNS and occasionally with synovial osteochondromatosis (see Box 4-9). Synovitis is seen on ultrasound as complex fluid; power Doppler ultrasound can also demonstrate degree of synovial vascularity. On T2-weighted MR images synovitis appears as "dirty fluid." Some arthropathies have low-signal synovium on T2-weighted images (see Box 4-6) related to (1) fibrosis (e.g., postop), (2) hemosiderin—PVNS or hemophilia, (3) calcification—synovial osteochondromatosis, (4) gout, (5) rheumatoid arthritis, and (6) amyloid. Intravenous gadolinium is very useful to define extent of synovitis, which enhances dramatically especially if inflammatory.

Synovitis may cause erosions; this depends on the extent and location of synovial proliferation, chronicity of disease, vascularity of the synovium and volume of the joint involved. Small joints such as the digits undergo erosion frequently, whereas erosion at large joints such as the knee are uncommon. Although erosions are common in inflammatory arthropathies, they do not necessarily indicate inflammation; they are seen also in PVNS, synovial osteochondromatosis, and arthropathy of renal failure.

Ganglion cysts arise from synovial compartments (joints or tendon sheaths) and can cause focal soft tissue swelling. These cysts may be seen incidentally but are often associated with osteoarthritis and chronic inflammatory arthropathies, especially those with very prominent synovial proliferation such as rheumatoid arthritis. On ultrasound, these can be documented as cystic lesions without blood flow, but it may be difficult to find the neck leading to the joint or tendon. If communication to a joint or tendon sheath is not seen, cystic neoplasms such as synovial sarcoma or malignant fibrous histiocytoma should be considered. On CT, ganglia show fluid density but can be hard to detect, even with contrast; in addition, the ganglion neck is generally difficult to see. MRI is best for documenting location, size, lobulated cystic nature, and, most important, communication with a synovial structure confirming benign etiology. Gadolinium is generally not necessary and may make the lesion look more aggressive (even tumor-like) because ganglion cysts can contain synovial proliferation, especially if traumatized or connected to an inflamed joint or tendon. Intra-articular contrast may be useful if necessary to document communication with the cyst.

Diffuse soft tissue edema is seen in some arthropathies, especially psoriatic arthritis, Reiter disease (in which there can be diffuse soft tissue swelling of one or more digits, called sausage digits), septic arthritis, and neuropathic arthropathy. Tenosynovitis is common in inflammatory arthropathies such as rheumatoid arthritis, gout, psoriatic arthritis, and Reiter disease, as well as infection. Mechanical and traumatic tenosynovitis is very common. However, when there are multiple tendon sheaths involved, when there is a large amount of complex fluid, or when there is similar disease of a joint or bursa, an inflammatory arthropathy should be considered. Tendons without sheaths obviously are not affected by synovial disease. However, inflammation of the paratenon or adjacent bursae may contribute to tendon pathology. If the tendon is also thickened, it may represent tendinosis, or tendon infiltration.

Table 4-1 Tendon Pathology in the Setting of Arthritis

Degenerative	Diabetes/neuropathic disease, rheumatoid arthritis
Infiltrative	Gout, amyloid
Iatrogenic	Steroid treatment for arthopathy

Some tendons are susceptible to degeneration when there is underlying arthritis. The classic example is posterior tibialis tendinosis in the setting of rheumatoid arthritis, or diabetes with neuropathic disease. Tendon enlargement can also be from tendon infiltration, which can be seen in gout and amyloid. Tendon tears can also be seen in the setting of chronic renal failure or can be due to chronic steroid treatment for inflammatory arthritis (Table 4-1).

Bursitis can be mechanical or inflammatory. Mechanical bursitis occurs in areas of repetitive friction; olecranon bursitis can result from leaning on the elbows (also called "student's elbow"). Mechanical bursitis also occurs in the foot, related to poorly fitting shoes or deformity. Bursae are synovial-lined structures. In rheumatoid arthritis and other arthopathies such as gout, bursae can become enlarged, distended with fluid and with proliferative, inflammatory synovial tissue. Calcific bursitis can be seen in gout and hydroxyapatite deposition disease. The latter most commonly affects the subacromial/subdeltoid bursa of the shoulder, a result of rupture of hydroxyapatite crystal deposits within the rotator cuff tendons into the adjacent bursa with subsequent acute bursal inflammation. Inflammatory or crystalline bursitis can result in erosion of the adjacent bone. Septic bursitis should be considered when a distended bursa is seen on any modality. Infection causes prominent bursal enlargement and synovial proliferation, with complex fluid on ultrasound and MRI, and thick marginal enhancement on contrast-enhanced MRI (Table 4-2). However, bursitis related to inflammatory arthritis can look identical to septic bursitis by imaging; thus aspiration is often indicated.

Soft Tissue Calcification

Calcification in the soft tissues may be a clue to the etiology of an underlying arthropathy (Table 4-3). Calcification in the form of hydroxyapatite deposition disease, presenting as a focus of toothpaste-like calcium on imaging exams, can occur in bursae, but can also be seen within tendons and around joint capsules. Acute inflammatory episodes occur as the crystals extend into the adjacent tissues. These crystals can rarely deposit within joints, causing an acute, destructive arthropathy resembling neuropathic disease or an aggressive infection. Inflammatory episodes are associated with surrounding edema and enhancement on contrast-enhanced MRI with an aggressive pattern that may be mistaken for infection, unless the calcium is detected to indicate the correct diagnosis.

Vascular calcifications are commonly seen in diabetics; when an underlying arthropathy is seen along with this finding, the diagnosis of neuropathic osteoarthropathy should be considered. In chronic renal failure with renal osteodystrophy, large cloud-like, sometimes fluidic periarticular calcium deposits (tumoral calcinosis) may be present in addition to vascular calcification. Dense, coarse deposits of calcium are seen in the soft tissues of the distal extremities in scleroderma (which can be associated with a rheumatoid-like pattern of disease in the hands and wrists, a form of mixed connective tissue disease) and dermatomyositis. Dense soft tissue calcification can also be seen in fibrodysplasia ossificans progressiva (also known as myositis ossificans progressiva or "stone man disease") and can lead to joint ankylosis. Longitudinally oriented linear calcification of peripheral nerves has been described in leprosy, which may result in a mutilating neuropathic pattern in the affected extremity.

Table 4-2 Bursitis: Differential Diagnosis

Underlying Process	Characteristics of Bursitis
Mechanical: Chronic	Noncalcified; focal
Mechanical: Acute	Dense if hemorrhagic; ill-defined (MR: intermediate–high T1)
Gout	Dense or calcified
Hydroxyapatite deposition disease (HADD)	Fluffy calcification
Septic	Noncalcified; ill defined
Rheumatoid arthritis	Noncalcified; ill defined
Reiter/psoriatic	Noncalcified; ill defined
Synovial osteochondromatosis	Small calcifications; foci of low T2 signal on MRI
Pigmented villonodular synovitis	MR: low signal on T2

Mechanical bursitis, bursitis related to inflammatory arthritis, and septic bursitis can look identical on all modalities, including MRI; aspiration may be necessary.

Soft Tissue Masses

Noncalcified soft tissue masses can be seen in association with certain arthropathies (Box 4-10); in rheumatoid arthritis, rheumatoid nodules are occasionally

Table 4-3 Soft Tissue Calcification and Associations

Calcification	Radiographic Appearance	Location	Differential Diagnosis
Calcific tendinosis/bursitis	Cloud-like	Tendons/bursae	HADD gout (bursitis)
Chondrocalcinosis	Faint to sharp	In cartilage	CPPD arthropathy Gout Diabetes Renal failure Hemochromatosis Wilson disease
Tumoral calcinosis	Cloud-like	Around joints	Renal failure
Vascular	Linear	Soft tissues	Diabetes (neuropathic) Renal failure
Connective tissue disease	Sharp	Soft tissues	Scleroderma Dermatomyositis MCTD
Heterotopic ossification	Sharp/denser at periphery	Pelvis/hips Most common	Paralysis Injury Surgery
Neural	Linear	Soft tissues	Leprosy

CPPD, crystalline calcium pyrophosphate dihydrate; HADD, hydroxyapatite deposition disease; MCTD, mixed connective tissue disease.

SECTION III

BOX 4-10 SOFT TISSUE MASSES IN ARTHRITIS

Gouty tophi
Ganglion cysts
Rheumatoid nodules
Bursitis
Amyloid

BOX 4-11 DEMINERALIZATION APPEARANCE

Diffuse

Osteoporosis
Osteomalacia
Radiographic technique (artificial)
Immobilization
Iatrogenic (medications)

Periarticular

Rheumatoid arthritis
Immobilization
Reflex sympathetic dystrophy
Septic arthritis
Miscellaneous inflammatory arthropathies

seen in the hands, arms, and feet (along extensor surfaces or areas exposed to friction). Tophi form in gout, especially in the hands and feet; they uncommonly calcify but appear radiographically dense. Patients with sarcoidosis can also present with focal soft tissue masses in the digits, associated with a "lacy" trabecular pattern of destruction most commonly seen in the middle and distal phalanges. Focal soft tissue prominence associated with arthritis may also be caused by ganglia or synovial cysts, which can extend from joints or tendon sheaths in osteoarthritis or chronic inflammatory arthropathies. Amyloid deposits can also occur around joints (i.e., shoulder) and appear masslike.

MINERALIZATION

Demineralization is a nonspecific finding, which can result from immobilization, hyperemia, reflex sympathetic dystrophy, medication, osteomalacia, or osteoporosis (Box 4-11). Radiographic technique and window/level can also lead to misinterpretation of demineralization. Rheumatoid arthritis classically causes periarticular demineralization. Periarticular demineralization related to immobilization is seen on MRI as subchondral and subcortical high T2 signal.

BOX 4-12 TYPICAL PATTERNS OF JOINT NARROWING AND DIFFERENTIAL DIAGNOSIS

Diffuse versus Focal

Diffuse: Rheumatoid arthritis, septic arthritis, psoriatic/Reiter, gout, hemophilia, neuropathic disease, osteoarthritis (small joints), pigmented villonodular synovitis, synovial osteochondromatosis (late), thermal injury
Asymmetric within joint: Osteoarthritis (large joints)

Symmetry

Unilateral: Injury (fractures, labral tear), septic arthritis
Asymmetric: Psoriatic/Reiter, gout
Symmetric: Ankylosing spondylitis, hemophilia (weight-bearing joints)
Any: Osteoarthritis (depends on cause), neuropathic disease

Preservation of Joint Space

Amyloidosis

A ganglion cyst, like a Baker cyst at the knee, may be a sign of chronic or recurrent effusion and thereby may reflect internal derangement. Look carefully for a thin neck to a fibrocartilage structure that may indicate parameniscal or paralabral cyst and underlying tear of the structure. Presence of a ganglion or Baker cyst in a child should raise concern for juvenile chronic arthritis.

THE JOINT SPACE AND SUBCHONDRAL BONE

Joint Narrowing

The pattern of narrowing of the joint can often result in narrowing of the diagnostic differential (Box 4-12). Joint narrowing equals cartilage loss. Cartilage loss related to osteoarthritis is typically asymmetric (focal) in larger joints (e.g., medial compartment of the knee, superomedial hip), whereas inflammatory arthropathies including infection and other chondrolytic processes such as hemophilia result in diffuse (concentric) narrowing. In small joints such as the hands, both osteoarthritis and inflammatory arthritis cause diffuse narrowing; in this case erosions, hallmarks of osteoarthritis or other clues are needed to generate a differential. Note that in weight-bearing joints (especially the knees) the full extent of joint narrowing may not be seen without standing views.

Chondrocalcinosis

Chondrocalcinosis is defined as mineralization of hyaline cartilage or fibrocartilage related to deposition of calcium pyrophosphate dihydrate (CPPD) crystals and is most commonly observed in the menisci of the knee. Chondrocalcinosis is common in older people and is usually incidental and asymptomatic. Pseudogout, also known as CPPD arthropathy, is seen in a subset of individuals with chondrocalcinosis, who present with goutlike symptoms (recurrent joint swelling and pain) but have no gout crystals on aspiration.

Subchondral Sclerosis

Subchondral sclerosis is one of the hallmarks of osteoarthritis and is generally seen in more advanced or chronic cases. In fact, if subchondral density is seen without other hallmarks of osteoarthritis, one should consider avascular necrosis. One basic principle of bone radiology is that bone "knows" how to react to stress or irritation in only one way—to form more bone. (The converse is also true; that is, when the bone is relieved of stress, it resorbs). Therefore, when the subchondral bone is exposed to additional stresses as the shock-absorbing cartilage is worn away, the underlying bone fortifies itself. The same process is often observed at the metaphyses adjacent to arthritic joints; the cortex thickens owing to slow periosteal apposition called "buttressing." On MRI, subchondral sclerosis is low signal on all sequences, but is often intermixed with cysts and subchondral edema related to overlying cartilage loss.

Subchondral Cysts

Like subchondral sclerosis, cysts (often referred to as "geodes") are seen radiographically in more advanced cases of osteoarthritis. Although subchondral cystic change is a hallmark of osteoarthritis, it is very nonspecific and is seen in a variety of arthropathies, including rheumatoid arthritis, gout, CPPD arthropathy, hemophilia, and neuropathic disease. Cysts can grow to large size and be confused for tumor on radiographs; the classic example is at the acetabulum, where a large cyst (called an Egger's cyst) forms in advanced osteoarthritis. If the lucent lesion has thin sclerotic margins, one can attribute it to a nonaggressive process, and other hallmarks of osteoarthritis at the joint confirm the diagnosis. CT may be helpful if the margins are not clearly benign on radiographs. Another important principle is that not everything lucent on radiographs is a cyst. Subchondral "lucent lesions" are also seen with solid tumors (e.g., giant cell tumor) and with amyloid deposition. MRI with contrast is an excellent way to differentiate a cyst from a solid lesion.

Subchondral cyst formation and progression are important to recognize on MRI, so as not to confuse findings with bone bruise, avascular necrosis, or another process. In the early stages, a flame-shaped focus of subchondral edema is seen extending perpendicular to the articular surface, arising from a focus of cartilage loss. However, this finding can be seen with tiny cartilage fissures as well, which may not be apparent, especially on low-field scanners. Over time, this flame-shaped edema becomes consolidated and rounded; at this point the overlying cartilage loss is usually apparent. Eventually discrete, rounded cysts form, and the cyst may be visible on radiographs.

Intraosseous ganglion cysts can simulate subchondral cysts related to osteoarthritis, but the joint may not have the other hallmarks of osteoarthritis. Intraosseous ganglia are lobulated, which helps document their benign nature. They are common at the knee, often arising from the anterior cruciate or posterior cruciate ligament attachments (associated with anterior cruciate ligament mucoid degeneration or cruciate cyst) or proximal tibiofibular joint and at the calcaneus arising from the subtalar joint. Parameniscal and paralabral cysts may also extend into bone, especially at the glenohumeral joint, the knee, the hip, and the wrist; when a lobulated, cystic lesion is seen arising from a joint margin, a careful search for underlying fibrocartilage tear should be performed.

Intra-articular Bodies

Bodies are commonly seen in osteoarthritis and may be composed of fibrocartilage, hyaline cartilage, fibrosed synovial tissue, or fragments of bone. Bodies may be calcified and visualized on radiographs, but often advanced imaging modalities are needed to

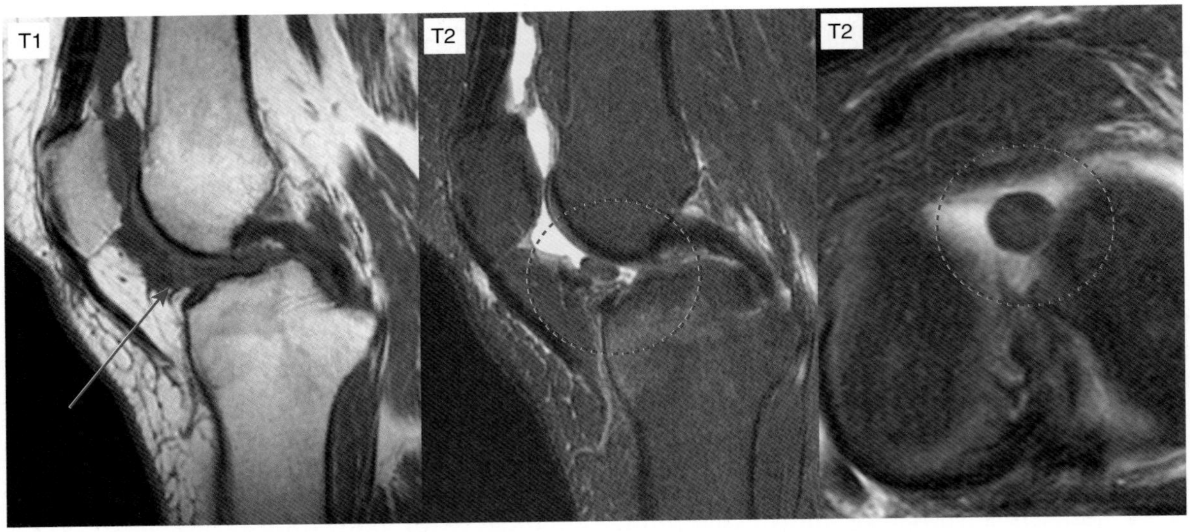
T1
T2
T2

Figure 4-68 **Intra-articular body.** T1-weighted imaging without fat suppression in at least one plane is useful for distinguishing a suspected body from capsular fat.

fully characterize quantity and location of noncalcified bodies, or to distinguish synovial calcification from a true intra-articular body. Because bodies may be composed of a combination of tissues, their MR signal characteristics are variable. They often blend with capsular signal if there is no joint effusion. Intra-articular contrast is especially useful for this purpose, and CT arthrography or MR arthrography may be used; visualization of fluid or contrast completely surrounding an intra-articular focus helps document the presence of a body. However, on MRI it is important to differentiate long, thin spurs and fatty synovial extensions from bodies; on fat-suppressed images these can appear as low signal and surrounded by fluid on one or two planes. It is important to acquire a non–fat-suppressed sequence on one plane and to carefully review all three planes for attachment of the structure to the bone or capsule (Fig. 4-68). Osteochondral lesions may also form intra-articular bodies in the absence of osteoarthritis (Fig. 4-69). The bodies in osteoarthritis are few in number and different in size, which helps distinguish osteoarthritis from synovial osteochondromatosis, in which the bodies are small, numerous, and similar in size.

In rheumatoid arthritis and other chronic inflammatory arthropathies, fibrosed bits of synovial tissue can break off and become intra-articular bodies; these are called "rice bodies" because they are rice-shaped and white at arthroscopy.

Ankylosis

If developmental coalition and prior surgical fusion have been excluded, considerations include end-stage forms of certain arthropathies, such as juvenile chronic arthritis. Adult rheumatoid arthritis rarely causes fusion (ankylosis) except at the wrist and foot. The end stage of psoriatic arthritis and Reiter disease can result in ankylosis or a destructive, "mutilans" pattern. If there is fusion of the sacroiliac joints, the likely cause is ankylosing spondylitis or inflammatory bowel disease, but beware of pitfalls (adolescence, renal failure, and osteoarthritis, in which the sacroiliac joints can appear ill-defined owing to immaturity, bone resorption, and bridging osteophytes, respectively). End-stage erosive osteoarthritis can cause fusion, usually at the distal interphalangeal joints. Severe osteoarthritis resulting in immobility may also result in fusion. Septic arthritis is another cause of ankylosis. Prior trauma, frostbite, burns, and electrical injury can cause fusion across joints. Heterotopic ossification can also bridge joints (Box 4-13).

EROSIONS

Erosions are seen in many arthropathies, and the pattern can suggest the proper diagnosis (Box 4-14). There are three types of erosions: central, marginal, and periarticular.

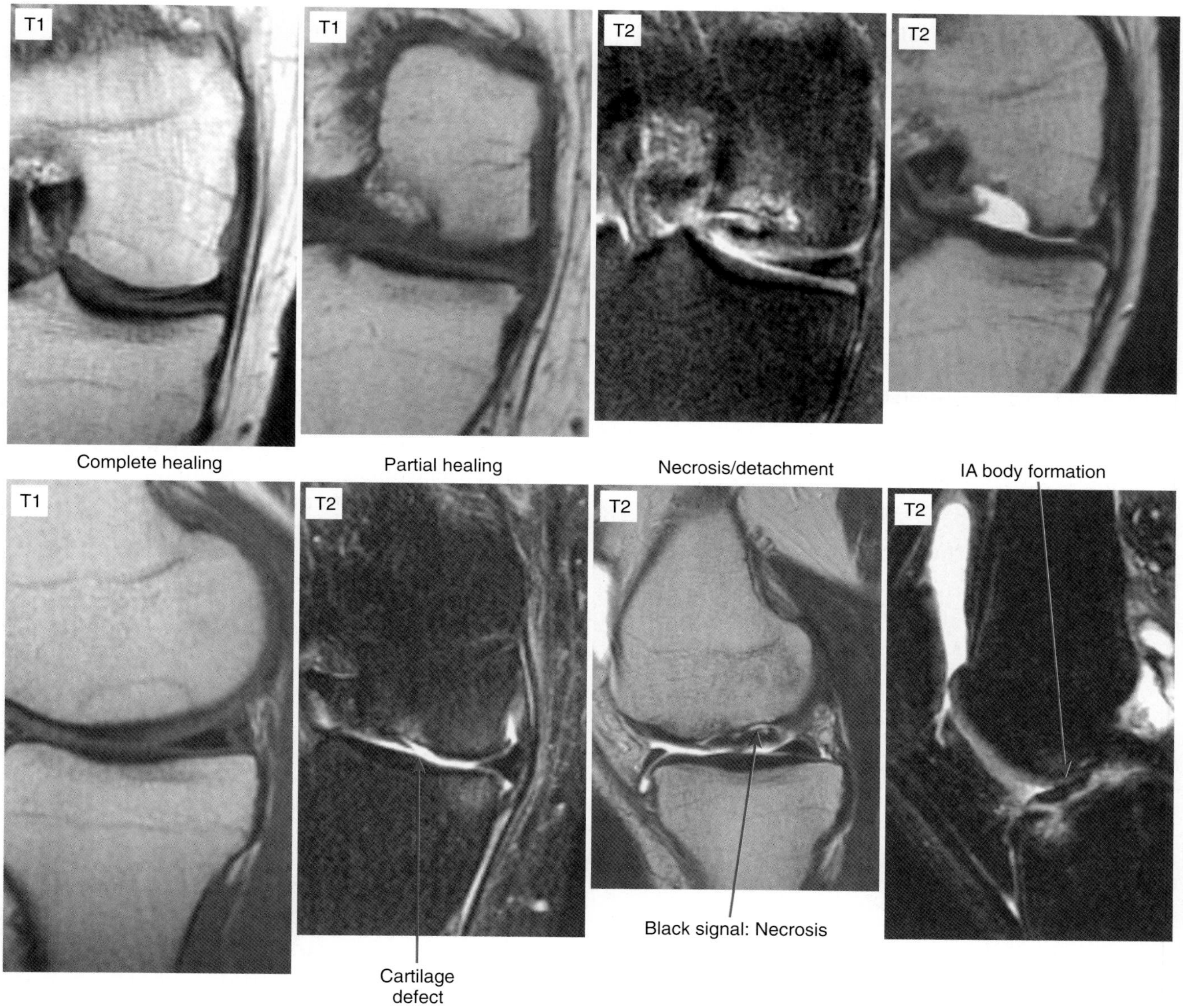
T1
T1
T2
T2
Complete healing
Partial healing
Necrosis/detachment
IA body formation
T1
T2
T2
T2
Cartilage defect
Black signal: Necrosis

Figure 4-69 Fate of an osteochondritis dissecans lesions (OCD). Wherever an OCD occurs, imaging characteristics and course of progression are similar. If the overlying cartilage is intact and the patient is young, the underlying bone can heal with little or no sequelae. More commonly, the overlying cartilage is also injured, leading to extension of fluid into the lesion, necrosis of the underlying bone, cyst formation, and eventual separation of the fragment. Description of findings in the report should discuss the status of the cartilage (e.g., defect) and underlying bone (e.g., necrosis), and give some indication of instability (fluid surrounding fragment, cystic change, separation of fragment). IA, intra-articular.

Central Erosions

Central erosions occur at the central articular surface and are classically seen in erosive osteoarthritis. However, central erosive change may also be seen in severe mutilating forms of inflammatory arthropathies such as psoriatic arthritis, which form a ball-in-cup appearance of the joint. Gouty tophi in the joint may also cause central erosion.

Marginal Erosions

Marginal erosions occur at the unprotected surface of the joint (the bare area) between the edge of articular cartilage and the capsule. Inflammatory synovium at this site causes hyperemia and mass effect, inciting an erosion. Early erosions are ill-defined; old erosions that often have sclerotic margins. Marginal erosions are classically seen in rheumatoid arthritis but

BOX 4-13 CAUSES OF ANKYLOSIS

Developmental fusion (coalition)
Surgical fusion
Ankylosing spondylitis/inflammatory bowel disease (spine, sacroiliac joints)
Juvenile chronic arthritis
Rheumatoid arthritis (uncommon)
Reiter/psoriatic
Erosive osteoarthritis (digits)
Severe degenerative disk disease (spine)
Diffuse idiopathic skeletal hyperostosis (DISH; spine)
Thermal/electrical injury
Septic arthritis (end-stage)
Heterotopic ossification/fibrodysplasia ossificans progressiva

BOX 4-14 EROSION LOCATION AND DIFFERENTIAL DIAGNOSIS

Central
- Erosive osteoarthritis
- Thermal injury
- Psoriasis (late)
- Reiter (late)

Marginal
- Rheumatoid arthritis
- Psoriasis (proliferative)
- Reiter (proliferative)
- Gout

Periarticular
- Gout

are also seen in psoriatic arthritis and Reiter disease (often with a fluffy or whiskered appearance), as well as in septic arthritis and intra-articular gouty crystal deposition.

Periarticular Erosions

Periarticular erosions occur outside the joint capsule and arise from gouty tophi or soft tissue masses. They are often described as having an overhanging edge or "rat bite" appearance with sharp margins.

Extra-articular erosions also occur at attachments of fascia, ligaments, and tendons or adjacent to bursae. These erosions are nonspecific and can happen in gout as well as rheumatoid arthritis, Reiter disease, and psoriatic arthritis. With the latter two conditions, the erosions can have fluffy margins like the proliferative marginal erosions in those diseases. Hydroxyapatite deposition disease involving tendon insertions can also result in erosion (especially at the humeral head and femur). This is often interpreted as a tumor, but if the adjacent calcification is recognized the correct diagnosis can be made without biopsy or advanced imaging. CT can be helpful for documenting subtle tendon calcification.

BOX 4-15 SACROILIAC JOINT DISEASE

Bilateral symmetric
- Anklyosing spondylitis
- Inflammatory bowel disease
- Osteitis condensans ilii (iliac side)

Bilateral asymmetric
- Psoriatic
- Reiter
- Rheumatoid arthritis
- Osteoarthritis

Unilateral
- Infection
- Psoriatic
- Reiter

Mimickers of sacroiliitis
- Adolescence (articular surfaces undeveloped)
- Hyperparathyroidism (bone resorption)
- Osteoarthritis (anterior bridging spurs)
- Post-op (iliac bone graft donor site)

Erosions also occur at the sacroiliac joints in sacroiliitis, seen on radiographs as joint widening and loss of the subchondral white line (and on MRI as loss of the black line of the articular surface) (Box 4-15). In ankylosing spondylitis and inflammatory bowel disease, this may lead to fusion.

PROLIFERATION

Osteophytes are seen in primary and secondary osteoarthritis, as well as erosive osteoarthritis. One must be careful not to exclude an inflammatory arthritis from the differential based on the presence of osteophytes, since secondary osteoarthritis is so common in chronic arthropathies. If the distribution is atypical for osteoarthritis or if other features of prior inflammation (e.g., sclerotic erosions, diffuse joint narrowing) are present, then consider secondary osteoarthritis. The features of the underlying inflammatory arthropathy may be long gone, but the distribution can often suggest the cause (e.g., exuberant osteoarthritis at the great toe and Lisfranc joint should suggest gout).

Osteophytes generally form at joint margins, but may occur at the articular surface related to an overlying cartilage defect. On radiographs they look like buttons ("button osteophytes") and are easily seen on CT. On MRI they are filled with fatty marrow and are best seen on non–fat-suppressed T1-weighted images. Osteophytes fill in the underlying cartilage defect, and often there is little to no distortion of the actual articular contour.

Enthesophytes (spurs at attachment sites of fascia, ligaments and tendons) are not necessarily associated with symptoms; more commonly they are related to repetitive stress, resulting in bone response and growth at the attachment. However, if the enthesophyte is ill-defined and associated with soft tissue swelling, then superimposed tendinopathy, bursitis, or enthesial inflammation should be considered. On MRI, if there is bone marrow edema in or adjacent to an enthesophyte, it is likely to be symptomatic. Psoriatic arthritis and Reiter disease can cause periostitis with fluffy enthesophytes; bursitis from gout or rheumatoid arthritis can erode enthesophytes.

Periosteal reaction is seen in psoriatic arthritis and Reiter disease as well as in infection. Periosteal resorption can be associated with renal osteodystrophy, mainly occurring at the epimetaphysis and along concave cortices. Longstanding osteoarthritis can cause periosteal apposition, in which case altered stresses at the epimetaphyseal zone cause bony buttressing. This is most commonly seen at the medial aspect of the femoral neck in severe osteoarthritis.

Thick bone proliferation is seen in ankylosing spondylitis, with syndesmophyte formation. Spinal bone proliferation is also seen in diffuse idiopathic skeletal hyperostosis (DISH); individuals with this condition are bone formers. They also typically have enthesophytes around the iliac crests and hips. They may have a predisposition for forming heterotopic bone after surgery. DISH involving the spine is easily seen on a lateral radiograph as "flowing" or undulating anterior ossification, most commonly in the thoracic spine (but cervical and lumbar involvement is common in advanced cases) in elderly persons. In contrast, ossification associated with ankylosing spondylitis occurs in younger adults, occurs first in the lumbar spine and progresses superiorly, and is not bulky but rather thin and flat against the vertebral bodies on the lateral view (Table 4-4).

Table 4-4 Comparison of Diffuse Idiopathic Skeletal Hyperostosis (DISH) and Ankylosing Spondylitis (AS)

	DISH	AS
Age	Old	Young
Early distribution	Thoracic spine	Lumbar spine
Lateral view	Wavy	Flat
Pelvic involvement	Iliac enthesophytes	Sacroiliitis
Fractures	Oblique	Oblique

DEFORMITY

Joint deformity can also help characterize an arthropathy (Table 4-5). Subluxations are seen in rheumatoid arthritis (especially at the metacarpophalangeal joints), neuropathic disease, SLE, and severe, destructive arthropathies of various types. However, osteoarthritis may also cause subluxation, especially at the first carpometacarpal joint. Rheumatoid arthritis also causes boutonnière and swan-neck deformities of the digits, lateral deviation of the fingers (the "windswept hand"), ulnar translocation of the carpus (carpal bones shift over the ulna), intercalated segment instability, and carpal collapse. Protrusio acetabuli can occur from bone-softening disorders including osteomalacia and Paget disease, and from joint prosthesis loosening, but it is also seen in the setting of chronic inflammatory arthropathy, especially rheumatoid arthritis. Spinal segmental instability can be caused by rheumatoid arthritis (with atlantoaxial instability, but also with a stair-step pattern of spondylolisthesis at subaxial levels), neuropathic disease, arthropathy of renal failure, and infectious diskitis. Varus and valgus deformities are seen in inflammatory arthropathies and also in osteoarthritis, especially at the knees with asymmetric cartilage loss.

DISTRIBUTION

Determining the distribution of an arthropathy is extremely important in developing a differential diagnosis (Box 4-16). For example, rheumatoid arthritis commonly affects the carpus and metacarpophalangeal/proximal interphalangeal joints of the hand/wrist, whereas primary osteoarthritis typically affects the proximal interphalangeal / distal interphalangeal joints and the base of the thumb. In the foot,

Table 4-5 Joint Deformity and Differential Diagnosis

Windswept digits	Rheumatoid arthritis
Ulnar translocation	Rheumatoid arthritis
Carpal collapse	Rheumatoid arthritis, scapholunate advanced collapse
Boutonnière deformity	Rheumatoid arthritis
Swan neck	Rheumatoid arthritis
Arthritis mutilans	Rheumatoid arthritis, gout, psoriatic, Reiter, neuropathic
Talar (tibial) tilt	Hemophilia
Protrusio acetabuli	Rheumatoid arthritis, particle disease, bone-softening disorders (e.g., osteomalacia, Paget)
Collapse of the arch of the foot (rocker-bottom)	Neuropathic, posterior tibial tendon dysfunction
Atlantoaxial instability	Rheumatoid arthritis, ankylosing spondylitis, spondyloepiphyseal dysplasias, Down syndrome
Segmental instability of the spine	Paralysis, fusion above or below, interspinous ligament injury, annular tear/facet arthropathy, amyloid, prior diskitis, pars defect, neuropathic
Varus/valgus in extremities	Rheumatoid arthritis, severe osteoarthritis
Subluxation in extremities	Rheumatoid arthritis, severe osteoarthritis, systemic lupus erythematosus, miscellaneous inflammatory arthropathies, neuropathic

In the setting of rheumatoid arthritis, ankylosing spondylitis, or other sources of atlantoaxial instability, or if the neutral c-spine lateral view shows questionable widening of the interval, a flexion/extension series (voluntary, to the level of patient comfort—never forced) should be acquired before surgery, in which neck flexion/extension occurs in an obtunded state during intubation.

BOX 4-16 DISTRIBUTION OF COMMON ARTHROPATHIES

Primary osteoarthritis: First carpal metacarpal, scaphoid-trapezium-trapezioid, interphalangeals, weight-bearing joints, first metatarsophalangeal (MTP)

Rheumatoid arthritis: Carpus, metacarpophalangeals (MCPs), MTPs (especially fifth), elbow, shoulders, cervical spine, knees, hips, ankles—bilateral symmetric

Psoriatic arthritis: Interphalangeals, MCPs, MTPs, sacroiliac (SI) joints—bilateral asymmetric

Reiter disease: Interphalangeals (feet), MTPs, SI joints—bilateral asymmetric

Ankylosing spondylitis: L > T > C spine, SI joints, hips—bilateral symmetric

Gout: First interphalangeal (foot), first MTP, Lisfranc, various hand/wrist joints—bilateral asymmetric

Neuropathic osteoarthropathy (related to diabetes; see also Box 4-4): Lisfranc, hindfoot, MTPs—unilateral or bilateral asymmetric

Hemophilia:
- Weight-bearing joints; ankles, knees—bilateral symmetric
- Scattered traumatized upper extremity joints—unilateral or bilateral asymmetric

Juvenile chronic arthritis: Knees, hips, ankles, wrists—bilateral symmetric (if polyarticular)

Typically monarticular: Septic arthritis, secondary osteoarthritis (e.g., post-trauma), synovial osteochondromatosis, pigmented villonodular synovitis

rheumatoid arthritis particularly involves the metatarsophalangeal joints, especially the fifth, and spares the toe phalanges. Rheumatoid arthritis also tends to be symmetric in involvement.

Hemophilic arthritis commonly involves weight-bearing joints and is usually bilateral in the lower extremities and trauma-related in the upper extremities. Gout typically involves the great toe and Lisfranc joint but can also involve scattered peripheral joints in the hand. Arthritis related to frostbite involves the distal extremities but tends to spare the thumb (which is protected by the clenched hand); electrical injury involves one or more rays in distribution of the electrical current propagation. Psoriatic arthritis often involves a whole digit and tends to be asymmetric. Reiter disease appears similar to psoriatic arthritis but classically involves joints in the lower extremity. Polyarticular versus monarticular is another important consideration. Monarticular arthropathies include septic arthritis, PVNS, and synovial osteochondromatosis. If an arthropathy cannot be clearly described on radiographs of the hands, imaging of the feet may be helpful, and vice versa.

GENDER AND AGE

Gender and age are also important when considering a differential diagnosis for an arthropathy (Box 4-17).

BOX 4-17 GENDER AND AGE OF INDIVIDUALS WITH ARTHRITIS

Children: Juvenile chronic arthritis
Young adults: Rheumatoid arthritis, psoriatic, Reiter, pigmented villonodular synovitis, synovial osteochondromatosis
Older adults: Gout, osteoarthritis, erosive osteoarthritis
Male: Ankylosing spondylitis, gout, Reiter
Female: Rheumatoid arthritis, connective tissue disease

For example, rheumatoid arthritis is more common in females, whereas ankylosing spondylitis, hemophilia, and Reiter disease are male-dominated. Most inflammatory arthropathies are active in younger people in their 20s to 40s. In older age, the arthritis often becomes quiescent with superimposed osteoarthritis. PVNS, hemophilia, and synovial osteochondromatosis are also diseases of young people. Osteoarthritis and crystal-associated disorders are generally seen in older persons.

Chapter 5

INFECTION OF THE MUSCULOSKELETAL SYSTEM

CHAPTER OUTLINE

Infection constitutes one of the true musculoskeletal imaging emergencies. Imaging appearance depends on the anatomic location, infecting organism, and modality used. Infection is common, and radiologists should be familiar with its common and atypical manifestations. Infection can mimic other conditions radiologically, so one should always consider the diagnosis as part of the differential for an unknown condition.

Use of different imaging modalities in the setting of clinically suspected infection is somewhat controversial and varies based on the specific situation as well as local expertise and scanner availability. Therefore, imaging modalities are incorporated into each section of this chapter when relevant.

MODES OF SPREAD

The musculoskeletal system can be contaminated by three principal routes: hematogenous spread, contiguous spread, and direct implantation. Overall, hematogenous spread is the most common.

Appendicular Skeleton

Because of rich synovial vascularity, the joints can be hematogenously implanted with infection at any age. The pattern of hematogenous osteomyelitis in the appendicular skeleton varies with age (Fig. 5-1). In the infant, metaphyseal nutrient vessels pass through the growth plate to the epiphysis, and osteomyelitis often involves the epiphysis. In children and adolescents, blood vessels are excluded from the more mature growth plate, and organisms deposit preferentially in the metaphyseal capillaries; this explains the metaphyseal location of Brodie abscesses. After the growth plate closes, vessels again extend to the epiphysis. After hematogenous infection, the process can spread contiguously along fascial planes to adjacent structures. The infectious material can also dissect through to the skin surface, creating a sinus tract and leading to spontaneous drainage.

In the diabetic foot, contiguous spread is far more common than hematogenous spread. Diabetic patients acquire ulcers through which infection (typically multiorganism) spreads to underlying bones and joints. This mode of spread is also very common

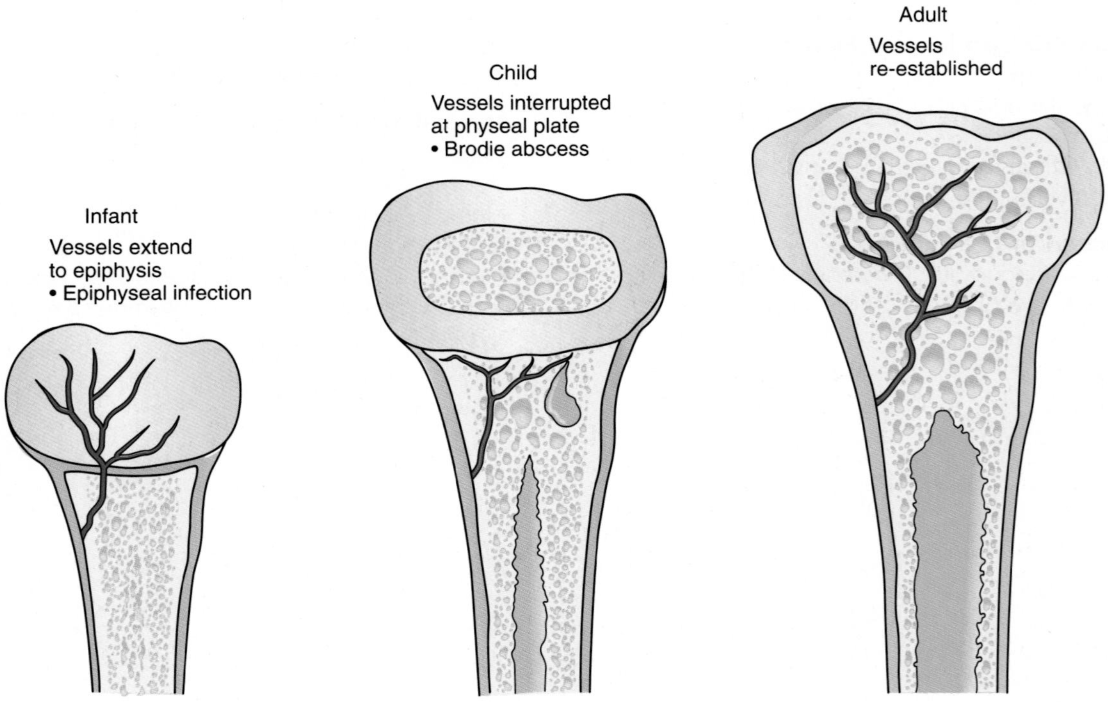
Infant
Vessels extend
to epiphysis
• Epiphyseal infection
Child
Vessels interrupted
at physeal plate
• Brodie abscess
Adult
Vessels
re-established

Figure 5-1 *Vascular distribution during development and influence on sites of hematogenous infection.*

in paralyzed patients, occurring at areas of pressure or friction such as the ischial tuberosities, sacrum, greater trochanters, and posterior calcaneus.

Axial Skeleton

Inoculation of the spine is predominantly hematogenous; this can occur via arterial or venous routes. The venous route occurs via the Batson plexus (a valveless venous complex responsible for draining blood from the pelvis, the lumbar spine, and the lower thoracic spine). Direction of flow is away from the vertebral column in most situations, but with increased intra-abdominal pressure, the direction can reverse and blood from the pelvis can flow in retrograde fashion into the vertebral bodies. The plexus penetrates each vertebra at the central aspect of the posterior vertebral body margin, with a Y-shaped channel within the vertebra that branches out to anastomotic vessels at the periphery. Although spread of infection to the spine through the Batson plexus cannot explain infection of the cervical and upper thoracic spine and is considered less common than arterial spread, it remains an explanation for vertebral infection in patients with pelvic infection and subsequent lumbar vertebral infection, as well as in patients with tuberculosis spondylitis in which involvement of the upper lumbar spine and thoracolumbar junction predominates and genitourinary involvement is common.

Arterial spread occurs via paired arteries that course along the posterior margin of the vertebral bodies. One branch enters the posterior vertebral body and supplies the posterior-central aspect. Another branch passes through the neural foramen and forms an anastomotic network of vessels surrounding the metaphyseal aspect of the vertebral body margin (adjacent to the endplates), with end-arterioles in the periphery of the anterior-lateral vertebral body next to the endplates.

Both arterial and venous patterns of spread result in inoculation of the endplate first. Therefore, the most common source of disk infection is considered to be direct spread from the adjacent endplate. The disk is composed of mucoproteinaceous material that offers a rich supply of nutrients for the infecting organism, and extension of infection through the disk and into the opposite endplate is rapid. This causes the classic pattern of involvement of the disk and adjacent endplates commonly seen in infectious spondylitis.

Although the intervertebral disk is considered avascular, children and some young adults have vessels penetrating into the disks from the endplates, a distribution that has been theorized to explain the incidence of primary diskitis in children. In older adults with degenerative disk disease, the disks may become re-vascularized, which can explain reports of increased incidence of infection in degenerated disks.

Unlike contiguous spread of infection from the endplates to the disk previously described, contiguous spread from an extraspinal source to the vertebral column is considered relatively uncommon. Some of the more common sources for contiguous spread in the axial skeleton include parapharyngeal infection extending to the cervical spine, pulmonary infection extending to the thoracic spine, and extension of pelvic infection or sinus tracts from bowel to the sacrum or lumbar spine. Paralyzed patients with decubitus ulcers can also undergo extension of infection contiguously to the spine more superiorly.

Direct implantation is a potential source of infection for the axial and the appendicular skeleton. This can occur after penetrating trauma or invasive procedures.

DISEASE CATEGORIES AND FINDINGS

Cellulitis

Cellulitis is an acute infection of the subcutaneous tissues; the diagnosis is most often clinical. However, MR imaging is helpful for evaluating the underlying tissues for such findings as myositis, abscess, sinus tract, fasciitis, and osteomyelitis. MRI is also useful for determining the extent of involvement of the infective process. Contrast enhancement is extremely useful for differentiating cellulitis from noninflammatory edema and also for delineating abscesses and sinus tracts that characteristically rim-enhance. Cellulitis results in diffuse regional enhancement, whereas bland or dependent edema demonstrates no more enhancement than the surrounding tissues, even when extensive (Fig. 5-2).

On MRI, infection—whether in soft tissue or bone—results in metabolization of fat. Hence, low T1 signal is observed on MRI in conjunction with the high T2 signal and enhancement that characterize the inflammatory process. Since it takes some time for this resorption to occur, in the very early stages of

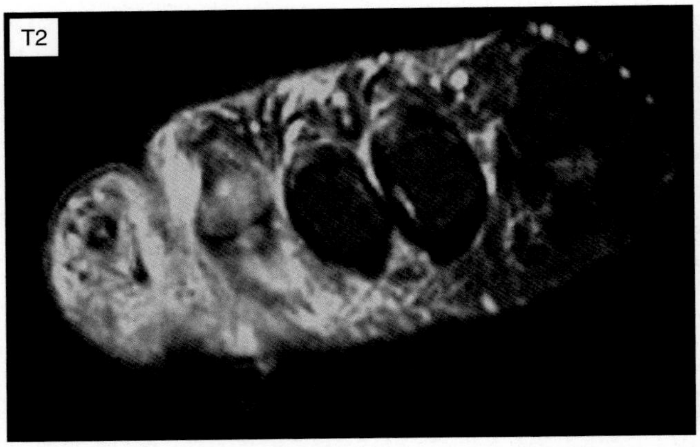
T2

Diffuse edema on T2; inflammatory tissue is obscured

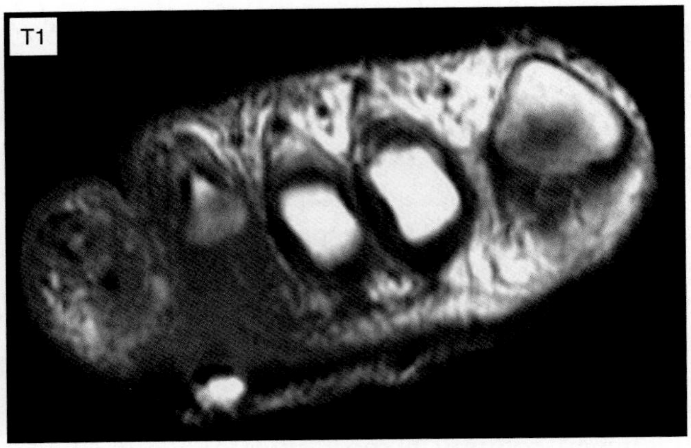
T1

Replacement of subcutaneous fat signal on T1

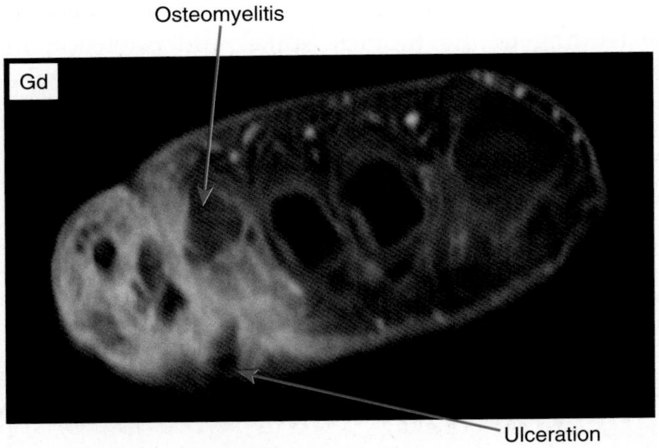
Osteomyelitis
Gd
Ulceration

Gd uptake delineates region of inflammation

Figure 5-2 Cellulitis on MRI: diabetic with plantar ulceration. Diffuse soft tissue edema and enhancement with replacement of fat signal on T1. Intravenous contrast is useful to distinguish inflammation from bland soft tissue edema.

infection (cellulitis and osteomyelitis) fat in the soft tissues or marrow may not be completely replaced, but there may be only slightly lower T1 signal than the surrounding tissues. Therefore, although replacement of fat signal is more specific for infection in the appropriate clinical setting, edema on T2 or short T1 inversion recovery (STIR) or enhancement is more sensitive.

Pyomyositis and Infectious Fasciitis

Muscle infection (pyomyositis) via hematogenous route is uncommon. However, the incidence is increased in the setting of immunosuppression (e.g., AIDS, organ transplantation, bone marrow transplantation, chemotherapy) as well as intravenous drug abuse. Pyomyositis occurs mainly in the lower extremities, particularly the thigh, and is often multifocal. Although hematogenous muscle infection is rare, secondary muscle infection related to contiguous spread is common and is frequently seen in the spine (psoas abscesses), pelvis (gluteal muscles related to ischial decubitus ulcers), and foot (in diabetics with pedal ulceration)

MRI is highly sensitive, with hyperintensity on T2-weighted or STIR images being initially diffuse. On T1-weighted images, the muscle may appear enlarged, but signal may appear relatively normal. Perifascial infiltration may be seen on T1- and T2-weighted sequences. Post-contrast images show diffuse enhancement in the early stages and help to separate this process from other entities such as diabetic myonecrosis. However, in later stages superimposed necrosis may also occur, and abscess formation can result in heterogeneous enhancement. With disease progression, more focal fluid collections are evident. Post-contrast images demonstrate rim enhancement of these small abscesses. Areas of abscess and necrosis often require debridement. Contrast-enhanced sequences can provide the surgeon with a roadmap for treatment. Ultrasound can also be useful to detect abscess formation (Fig. 5-3).

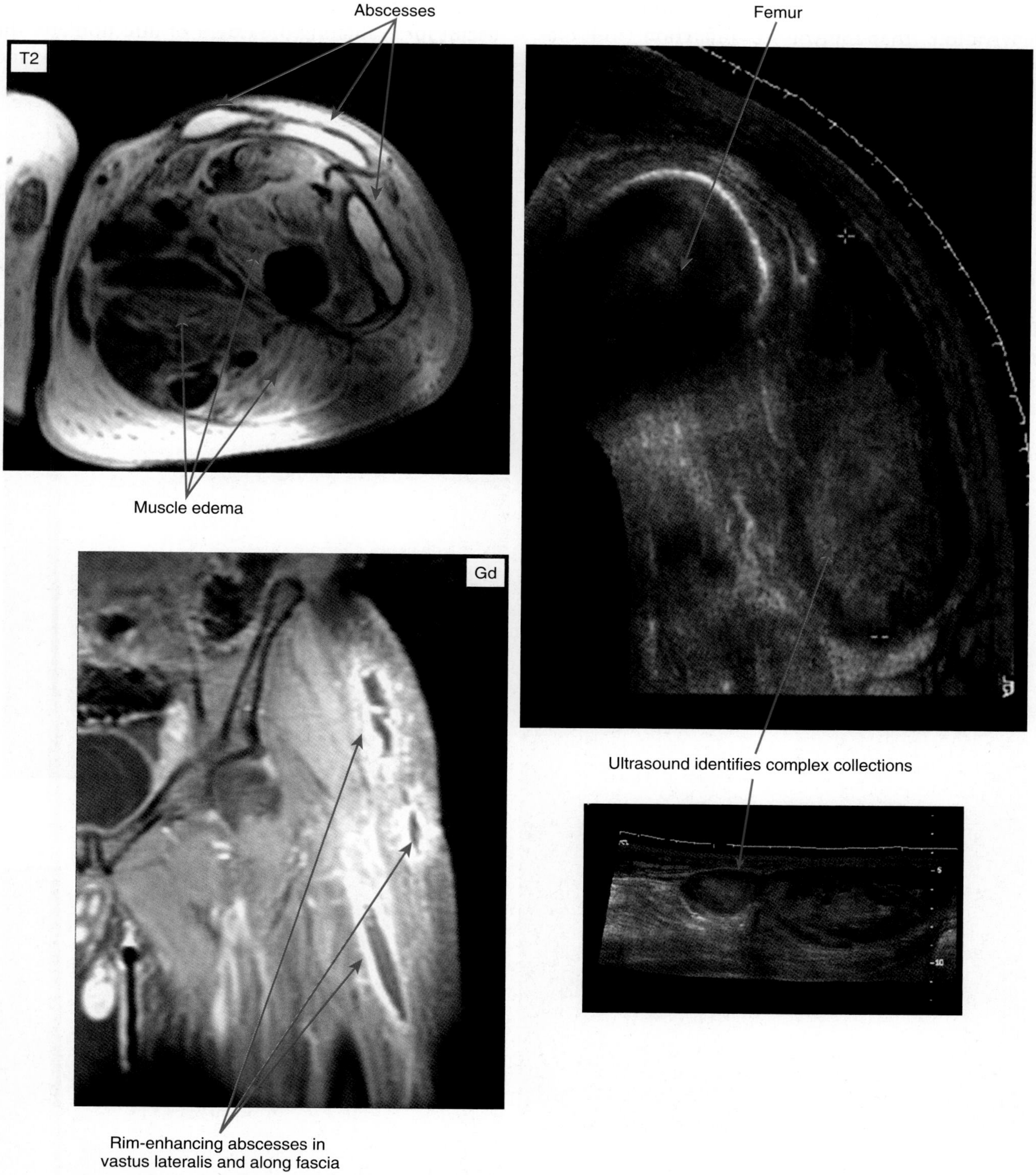
Abscesses
T2
Muscle edema
Femur
Gd
Ultrasound identifies complex collections
Rim-enhancing abscesses in
vastus lateralis and along fascia

Figure 5-3 Pyomyositis and fasciitis. MRI is excellent for identifying extent and underlying bone and joint involvement. However, ultrasound is quick and excellent for identifying soft tissue collections and can be used as a localization modality for drainage.

Muscle edema on MRI is nonspecific, with many differential diagnostic possibilities including injury, denervation, rhabdomyolysis, infarction and diabetic myonecrosis, autoimmune myositis, and tumor. Therefore, clinical correlation is essential (see Chapter 15).

Infectious fasciitis is a true surgical emergency, requiring immediate debridement and decompression as well as aggressive antibiotic therapy. Although MRI is very sensitive for evaluation of fascial inflammation, fascial edema and even enhancement are not specific for clinically aggressive fascial infection. In addition, fascial gas seen in aggressive cases may be difficult to see on routine MRI sequences, and delay in acquisition of the scan may preclude MRI as a sufficient diagnostic tool in this setting. CT or even radiographs may be more useful in this regard, owing to wide availability, rapid acquisition, and high sensitivity for fascial gas (Figs. 5-4 and 5-5). MRI remains useful for evaluating the extent of infection and the presence of underlying abscess, septic arthritis, and osteomyelitis.

Abscess

An abscess is a localized collection of necrotic tissue, inflammatory cells, and neutrophils, walled off by a highly vascular and typically irregular inflammatory pseudocapsule. A variable degree of surrounding soft tissue edema/cellulitis surrounds the process. Before liquefaction, an abscess is referred to as a phlegmon, an ill-defined inflammatory region of the subcutaneous or deep soft tissues without discrete fluid collection. With maturation, the infected tissue undergoes necro-

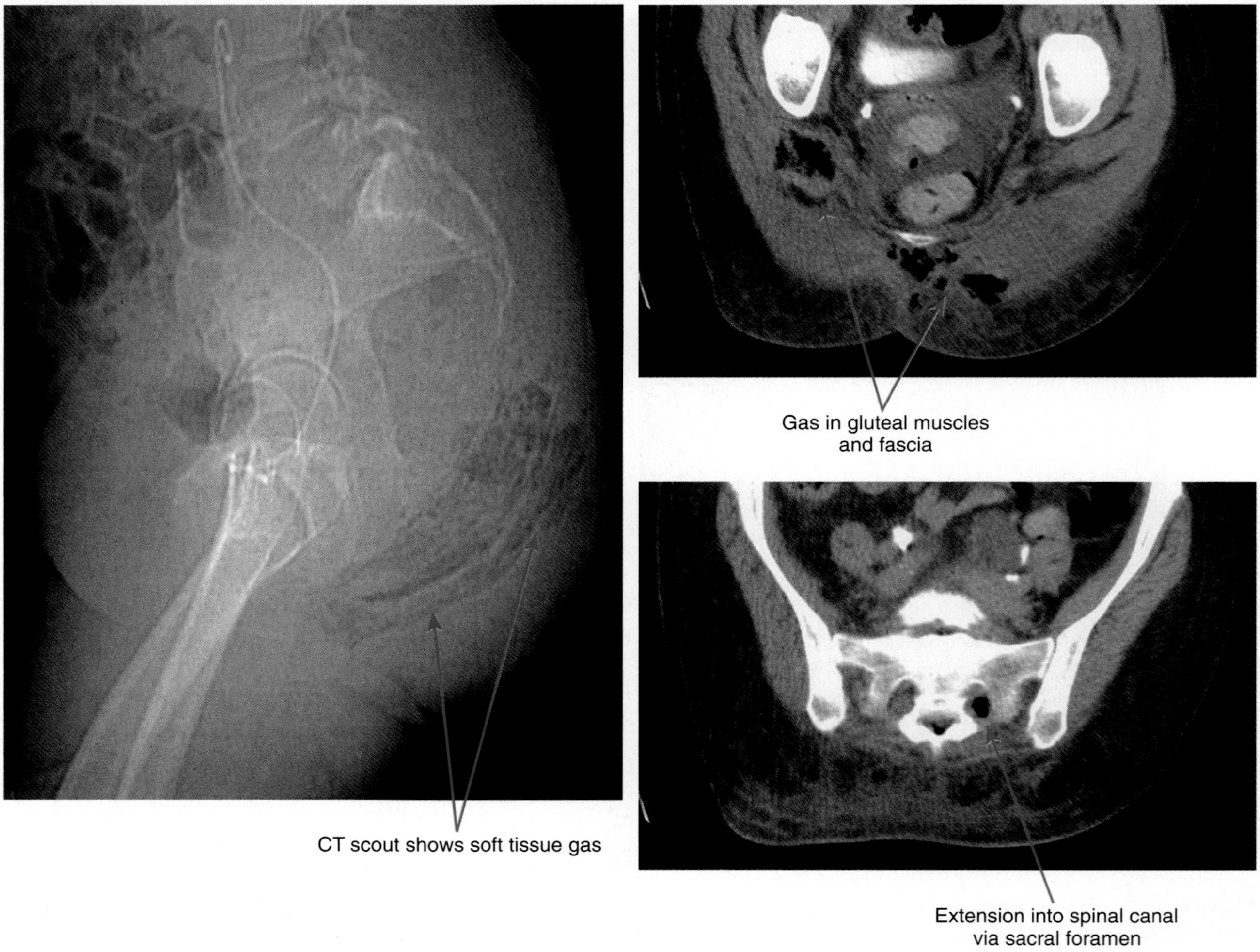
Gas in gluteal muscles and fascia
CT scout shows soft tissue gas
Extension into spinal canal via sacral foramen

Figure 5-4 Necrotizing fasciitis and myositis. Noncontrast CT is optimal for detecting soft tissue gas with high sensitivity if clinically suspected. Gas can be more difficult to detect on MRI, and fascial edema/enhancement is nonspecific.

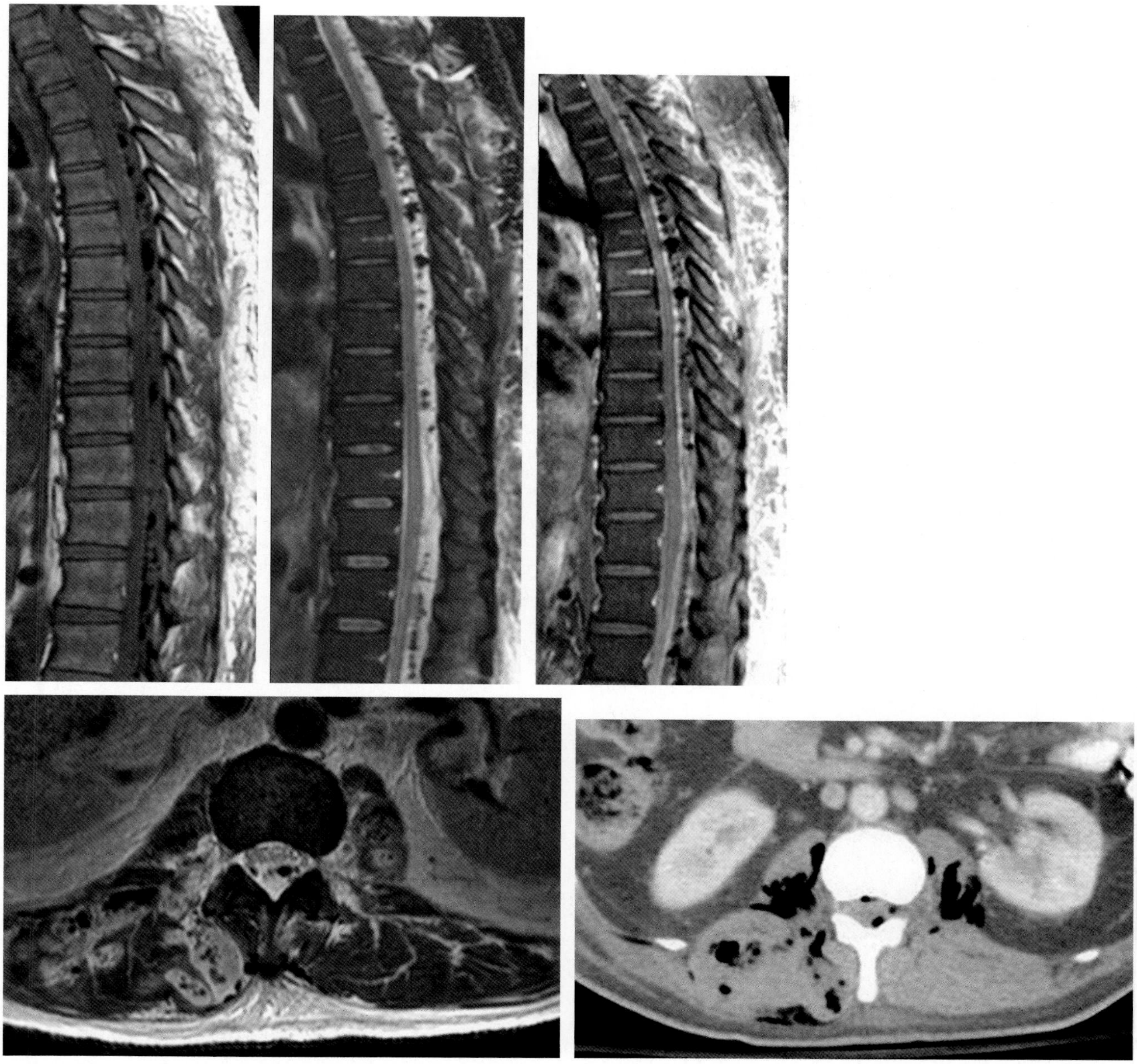

Figure 5-5 Necrotizing fasciitis arising from a wound in the sacral region, with gas extending along the paraspinal muscles and psoas muscles and within the spinal canal. The gas is more readily visualized on CT.

sis and liquefaction, thus becoming an abscess, with a peripheral hypercellular and hypervascular zone, particularly in the acute phase.

On MRI, the central cavity of an abscess is hypointense on T1-weighted images, but apart from asymmetric prominence of the soft tissues the abscess may not be apparent since signal can be similar to that of adjacent muscle. Most abscess collections are hyperintense on T2-weighted or STIR images with a variable degree of surrounding soft tissue edema. This edema may be intense, and, again, the abscess cavity may blend with surrounding tissues. Fluid-sensitive sequences tend to show heterogeneous signal within the abscess, reflecting the necrotic tissue within. The margin, composed of hypervascular inflammatory tissue, demonstrates thick enhancement after contrast administration. The central portion remains hypointense, making the abscess cavity stand out on fat-suppressed post-contrast images (Fig. 5-6). The multiplanar capability of MR and soft tissue contrast make it the ideal modality in planning before surgery or percutaneous drainage.

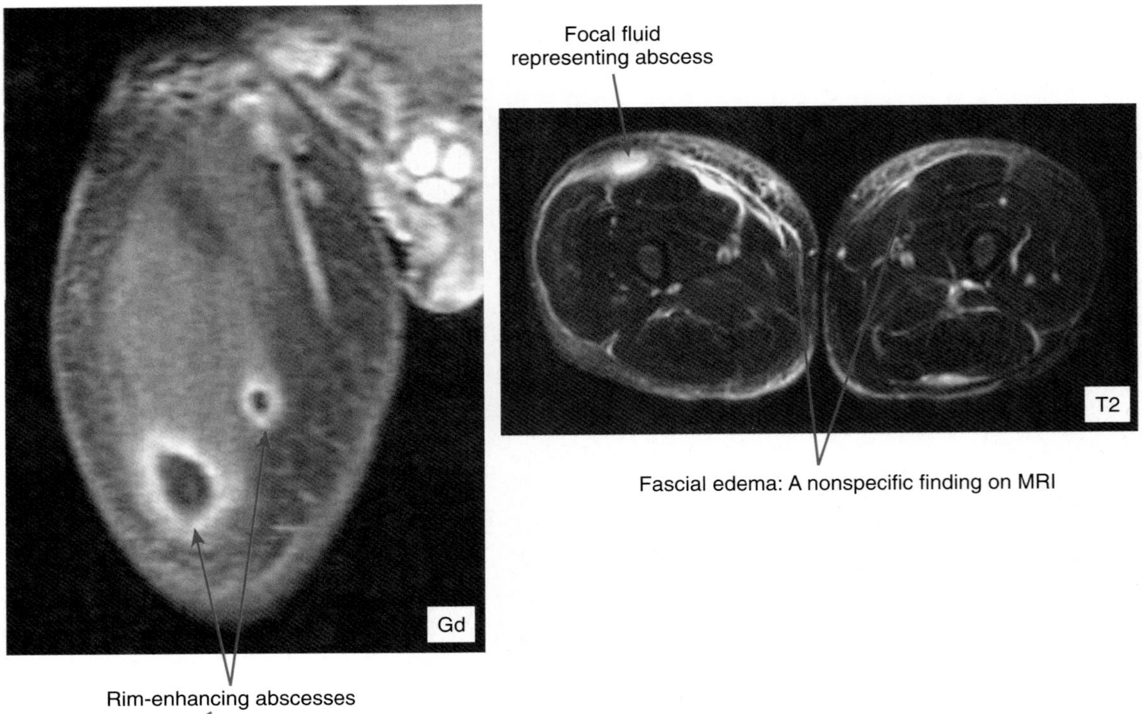
Focal fluid
representing abscess
T2
Fascial edema: A nonspecific finding on MRI
Gd
Rim-enhancing abscesses

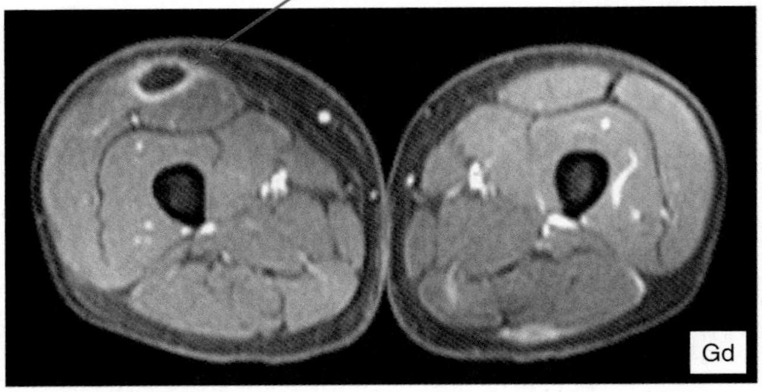
Gd

Figure 5-6 Soft tissue abscess; hematogenous spread in a drug user.

Heterotopic bone formation, as seen in spinal cord injury and following trauma or surgery, may be confused in its early stage of development with abscess formation because these foci are also often T2-hyperintense and rim-enhanced after gadolinium administration. Careful interpretation is warranted in the spinal cord injury patients, who are concomitantly at increased risk of decubitus ulcers and thus abscess formation. Gradient-echo images, demonstrating blooming artifact, may be of assistance in differentiating between these two pathologic processes by MRI. CT is helpful for detecting subtle marginal calcifications seen in early heterotopic ossification (Fig. 5-7).

CT or ultrasound can be obtained alternatively for suspicion of abscess, especially if MRI is contraindicated. CT should be performed for this purpose with contrast to delineate the rim enhancement; this appearance is similar to that on MR images, but much more faint. On CT, fluid is different in density from muscle, but complex fluid seen in abscesses, especially in the presence of hemorrhage, can make small collections of fluid difficult to see. Rim enhancement helps to detect such collections and delineate extent. Sinus tracts and abscesses that communicate with the skin may also fill with air, and portions may be visible based on this finding. Ultrasound is excellent for detection of fluid collections, and power Doppler can identify the hyperemia of the pseudocapsule and surrounding tissues that results in rim enhancement on other modalities. Ultrasound is the modality of choice for aspirating such collections. However, ultrasound is limited compared with contrast-enhanced MR with regard to the overall picture as to extent of the

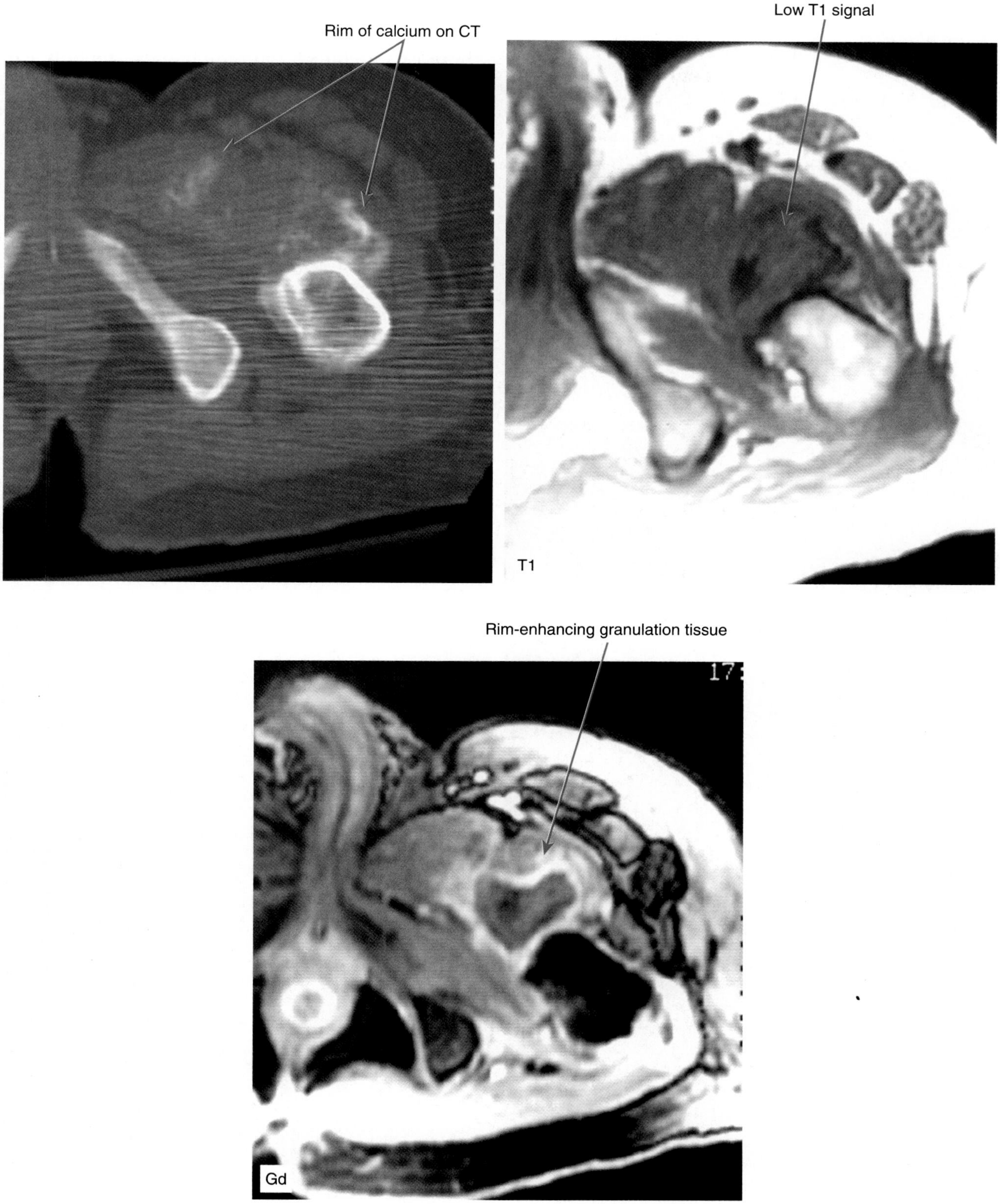
Rim of calcium on CT
Low T1 signal
T1
Rim-enhancing granulation tissue
Gd

Figure 5-7 Heterotopic ossification (HO) in a paralyzed patient. *In the early stages, HO can resemble an abscess on MRI owing to central liquefaction and surrounding granulation tissue. CT can be useful to identify marginal calcification.*

inflammatory process affecting various tissues (see Fig. 5-3).

Septic Arthritis and Septic Bursitis

Joint effusion is a hallmark of septic arthritis, whereas focal soft tissue swelling in the region of an anatomic bursa or over a bony prominence may indicate septic bursitis. In both, fluid is often complex on MRI. Complex fluid is also a characteristic of other noninfectious inflammatory arthropathies such as rheumatoid arthritis, gout, psoriasis, and, to a lesser degree, even osteoarthritis; unless clinical information is available, it may be impossible to tell the difference (see Chapter 4, Arthritis). Conversely, whenever a monarticular arthropathy is encountered, infection should be excluded. On radiographs, the only early sign is an effusion and juxta-articular soft tissue swelling, which, depending on the joint, may be difficult or impossible to detect (Figs. 5-8 through 5-10). Like abscesses, septic arthritis and bursitis on MRI demonstrate thick rim enhancement. Because of hyperemia, rarefaction (decreased density) of the subchondral bone next occurs, seen as subchondral edema on MRI (Figs. 5-11 through 5-13). Erosions begin at the margins of the joint, again as in rheumatoid arthritis, but while the infection progresses frank destruction of the articular surfaces may occur.

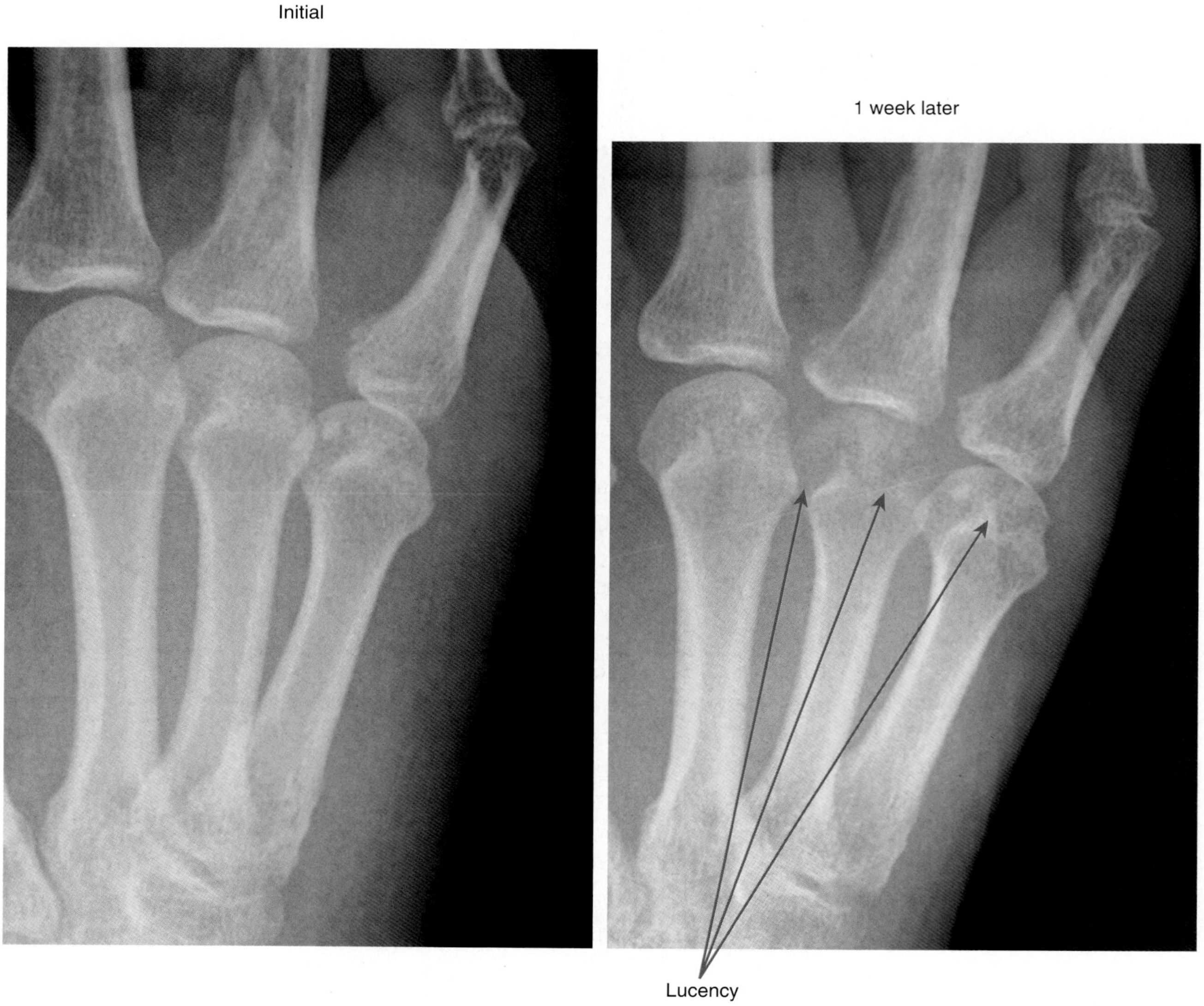
Initial
1 week later
Lucency

Figure 5-8 Septic arthritis of the fourth and fifth MCP joint. Radiograph within days of infection and a week later showing only slight demineralization on follow-up.

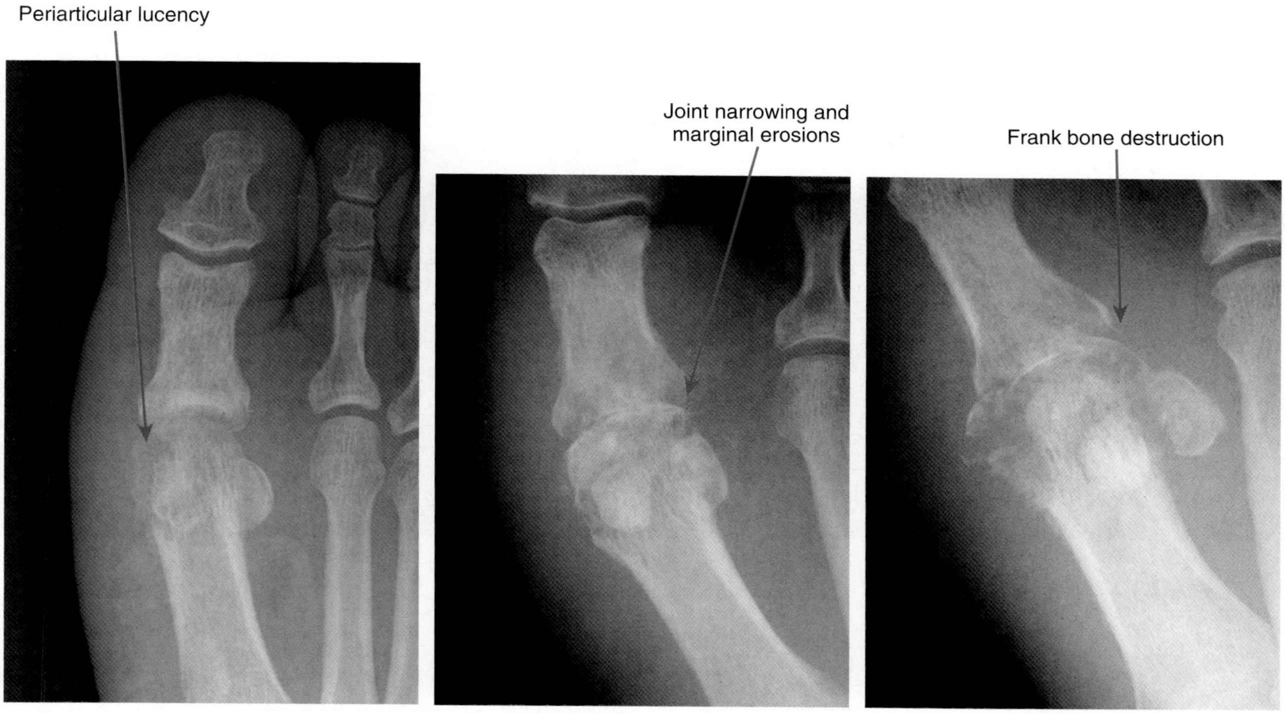
Periarticular lucency
Joint narrowing and marginal erosions
Frank bone destruction

Figure 5-9 Progression of septic arthritis on radiographs.

In some joints, erosions and effusion are difficult to see on radiographs, such as the sacroiliac joint. For the sacroiliac joint look at the inferior aspect of the joint (the synovial portion) and see whether there is loss of the thin white line, which represents the articular surface seen tangentially. This is the characteristic appearance of erosion in this location. Cartilage destruction (inflammatory breakdown products are chondrolytic) eventually results in joint narrowing, radiographically visible in later stages. As above, linear subchondral edema is common on MRI in septic arthritis. However, when the edema or enhancement extends beyond the subchondral bone into the medullary cavity, in the appropriate clinical setting osteomyelitis should be considered.

After surgery, joints may also have joint effusion and synovial proliferation, and shortly after surgery—even arthroscopic surgery—the hyperemic synovium can simulate infection. The soft tissues are often very swollen and periarticular fluid collections can also be seen, depending on the surgical approach and extent. Labeled white blood cell (WBC) nuclear medicine scan can show uptake, but if there is clinical suspicion of infection at this point, aspiration may be the best overall diagnostic option. Nevertheless, MRI can be useful to exclude medullary marrow edema or enhancement associated with osteomyelitis (Figs. 5-14 and 5-15). Unless there has been extensive medullary drilling or exposure, typically the marrow signal abnormality is limited to the immediate surgical zone and signal abnormality in remote areas should be considered suspicious. For example, shortly after anterior cruciate ligament reconstruction there will be edema limited to immediately around the tunnels and in the subchondral bone. Reactive synovitis after surgery can clinically simulate infection and often prompts MRI requests. Some implants, especially bioabsorbable components (e.g., screws, anchors, sutures) can incite an inflammatory response. MRI shows a very complex effusion and subchondral marrow edema. One clue that a bioabsorbable screw was used is a low signal focus without any metallic artifact. The bioabsorbable components are invisible on radiographs, and without provided history, surgical changes are subtle and may be overlooked. Again, it may be necessary to aspirate the joint in this setting if infection is suspected.

Osteomyelitis

Osteomyelitis refers to infection of the medullary portion of the bone marrow, whereas *osteitis* indicates

Text continued on page 198

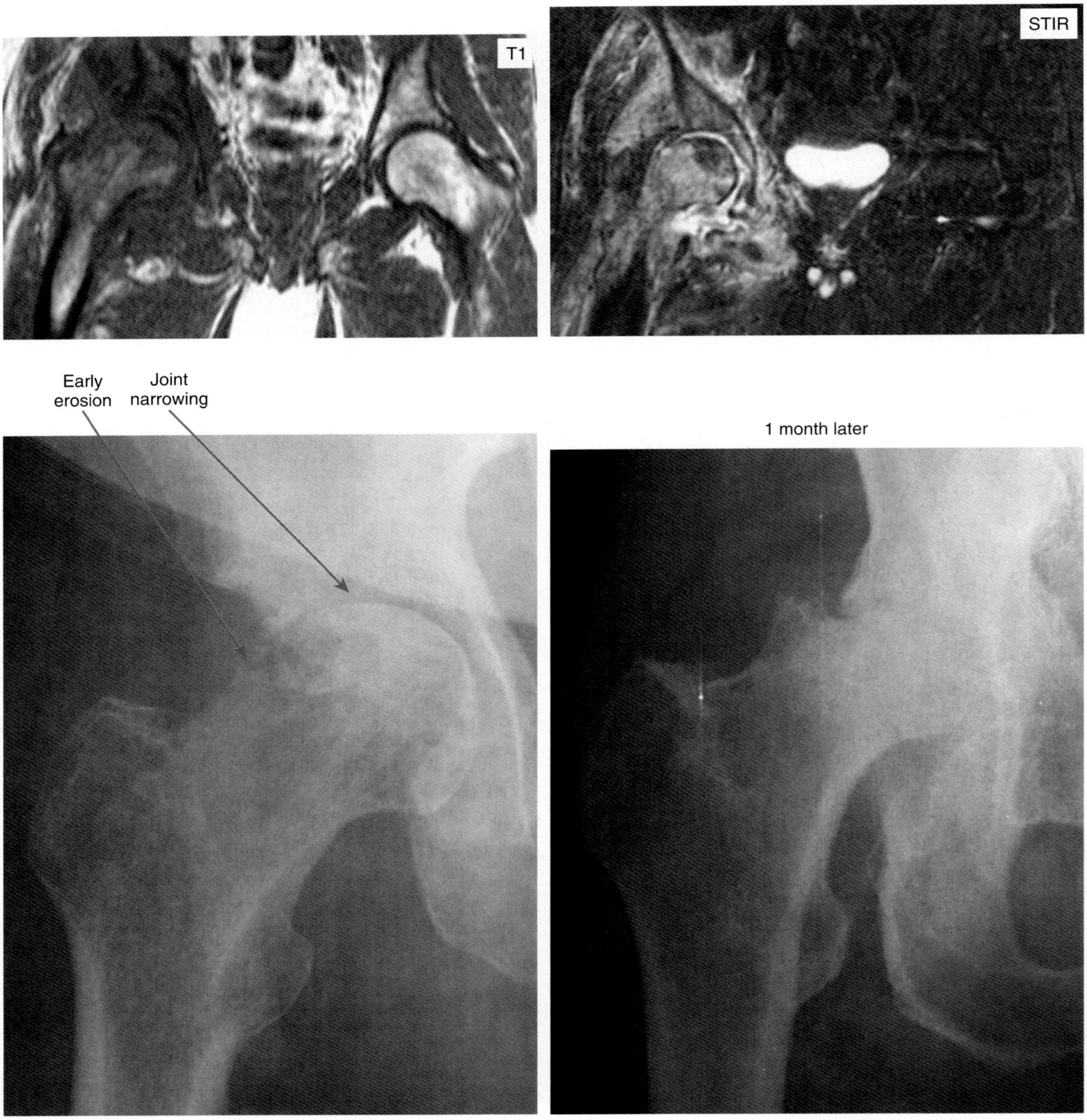
T1
STIR
Early erosion
Joint narrowing
1 month later

Figure 5-10 Septic arthritis and osteomyelitis—late destruction.

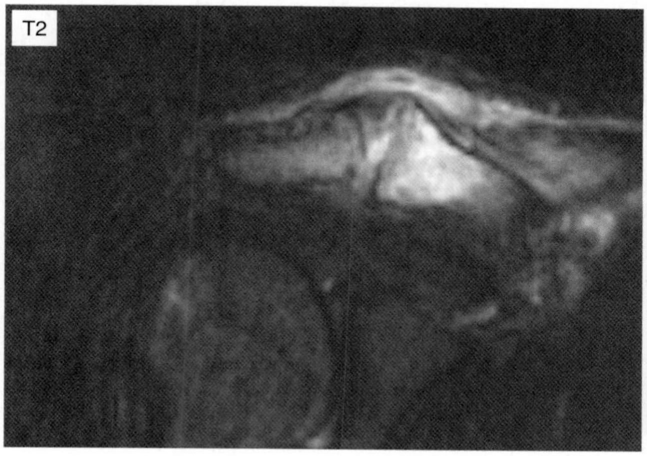
T2

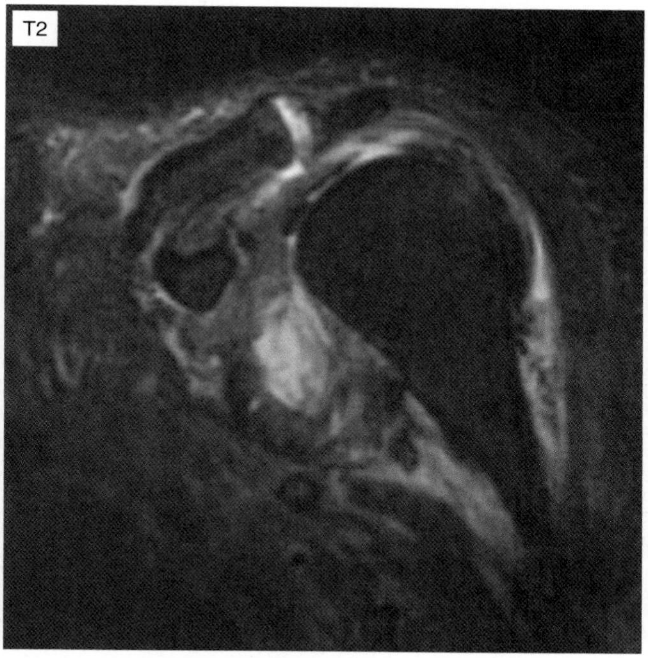
T2

AC joint septic arthritis
• Contiguous spread from glenohumeral joint

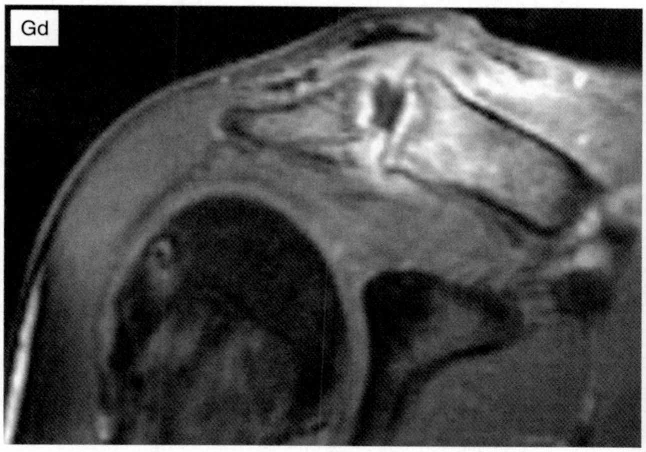
Gd

AC joint septic arthritis
• Hematogenous spread

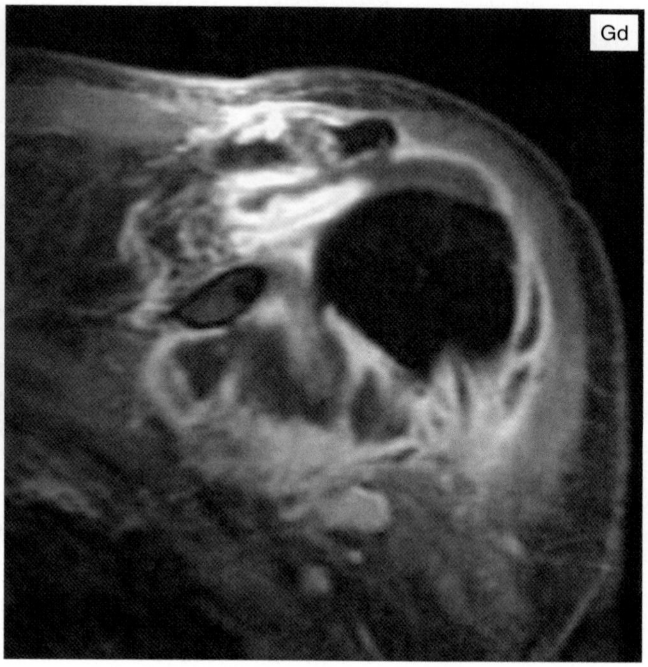
Gd

Figure 5-11 Hematogenous acromioclavicular (AC) joint involvement versus contiguous spread from the glenohumeral joint. Gadolinium contrast helps determine extent of involvement.

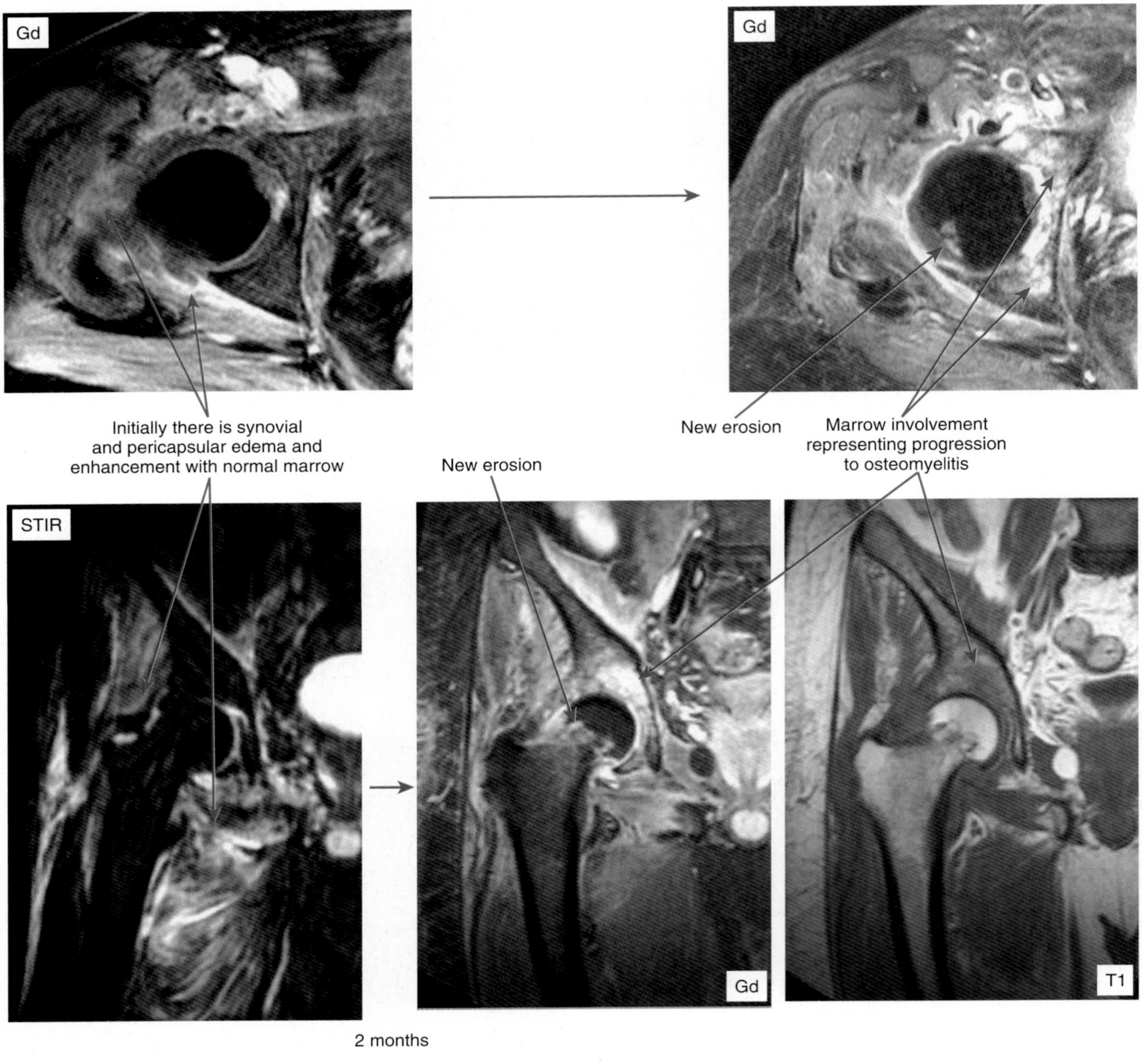
Gd
Gd
Initially there is synovial and pericapsular edema and enhancement with normal marrow
New erosion
Marrow involvement representing progression to osteomyelitis
New erosion
STIR
Gd
T1
2 months

Figure 5-12 Hip septic arthritis despite treatment progressing to osteomyelitis 2 months later.

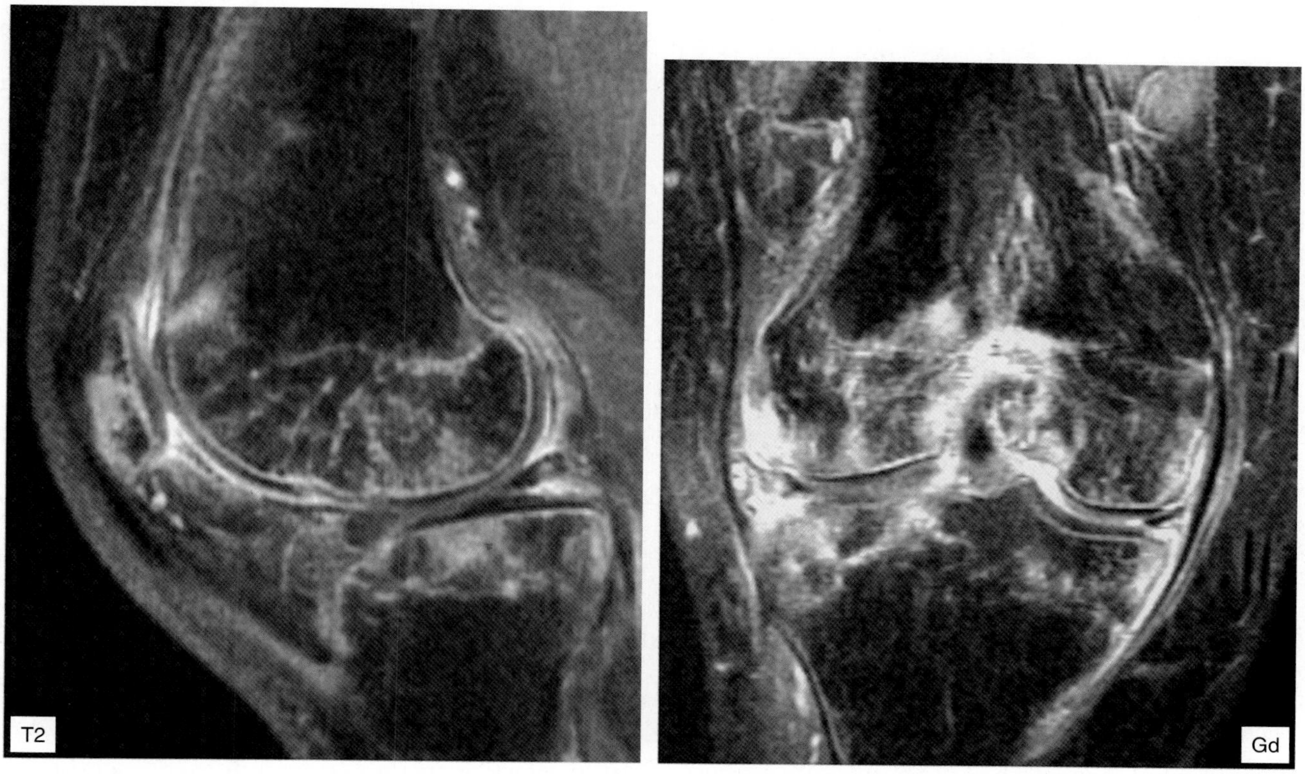
T2
Gd

Figure 5-13 **Septic arthritis on MRI.** Thin subchondral and perivascular edema/enhancement is typical. However, if edema, enhancement or low T1 signal extends into the medullary cavity, secondary osteomyelitis should be considered.

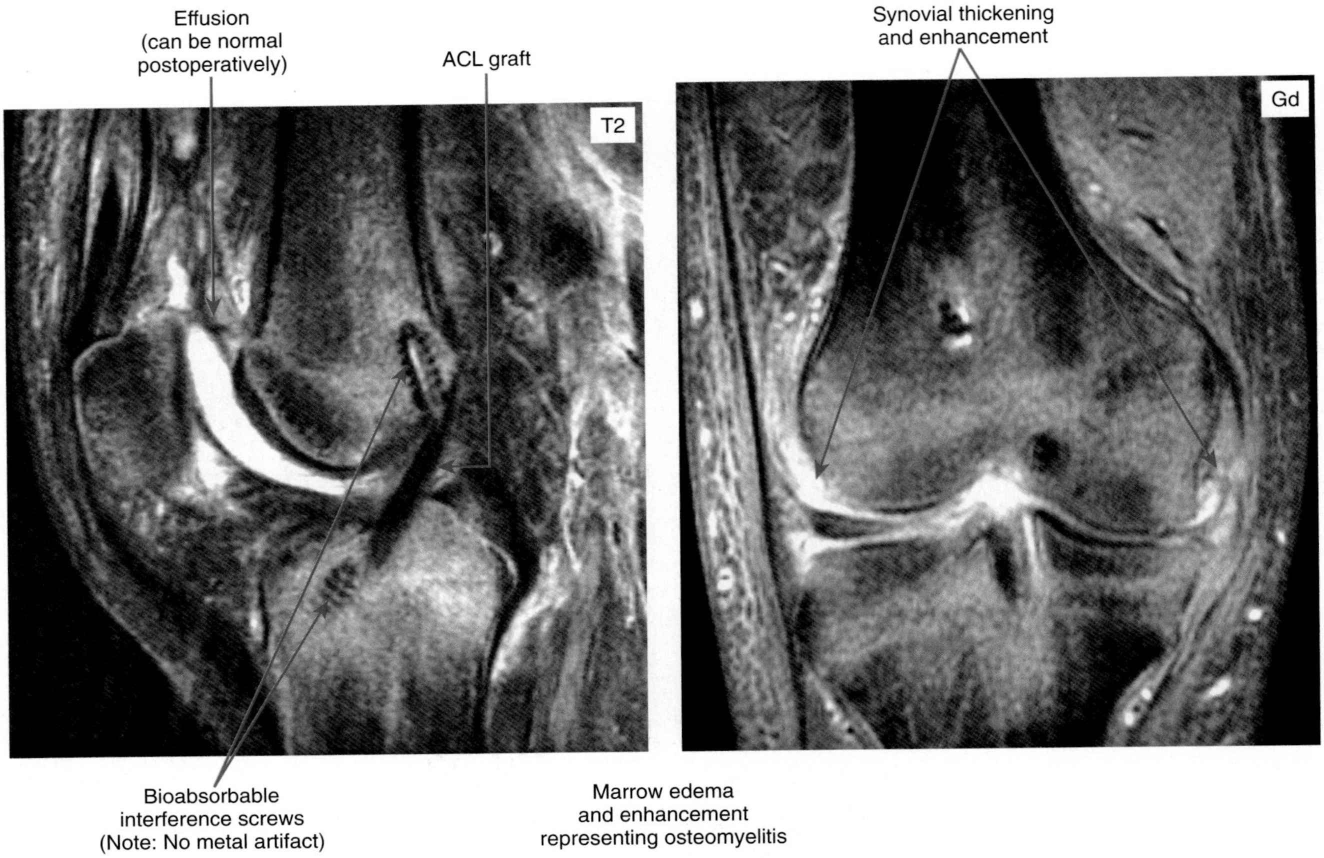
Effusion
(can be normal
postoperatively)
ACL graft
T2
Synovial thickening
and enhancement
Gd
Bioabsorbable
interference screws
(Note: No metal artifact)
Marrow edema
and enhancement
representing osteomyelitis

Figure 5-14 Infection following anterior cruciate ligament (ACL) reconstruction. Few patients are imaged using MRI shortly after surgery, so differentiating postoperative findings from pathology can be confusing. However, unless there was significant marrow alteration (e.g., reaming), most orthopedic surgical procedures, even amputation, leave little to no marrow edema. Therefore, any marrow edema or enhancement should be regarded with suspicion. Ultimately, aspiration is the test of choice, but MRI can be useful to exclude underlying osteomyelitis. One pitfall is that some patients have a reaction to implants (especially bioabsorbable implants, as seen above), which can cause effusion, synovitis, and marrow edema.

involvement of the surface of the bone only. A *sequestrum* represents a segment of necrotic bone that is separated from living bone by granulation tissue. An *involucrum* denotes a layer of living bone that has formed about the dead bone. An opening in the involucrum is termed a *cloaca* (Figs. 5-16 and 5-17). A Brodie abscess is an intraosseous abscess in children usually caused by *Staphylococcus aureus* infection and represents a subacute or chronic infection (Fig. 5-18). Chronic osteomyelitis occurs under areas of chronic ulceration or after trauma or surgery with unsuccessful or inadequate treatment of acute bone infection. The infection may smolder for many years, occasionally presenting with drainage through sinus tracts and acute-on-chronic osteomyelitis. Necrotic bone (e.g., sequestrum) is often colonized with organisms even after effective treatment, and must be debrided to avoid re-emergence of active infection. *Chronic recurrent multifocal osteomyelitis* is a rare disorder primarily involving children and adolescents and characterized by a prolonged, fluctuating course most often involving tubular bones, the clavicle, and less often the spine. No organisms are cultured and it may be a noninfectious condition possibly related to a type of immunocompromised state as yet undefined or an organism such as a virus as yet unidentified.

Acute osteomyelitis is difficult to detect on radiographs in the early stages (Fig. 5-19). Adjacent soft tissue swelling is present but is nonspecific and may not be seen at all in deep structures. Cortical rarefaction or resorption is next seen as a region of decreased cortical density or a permeative pattern in the cortex.

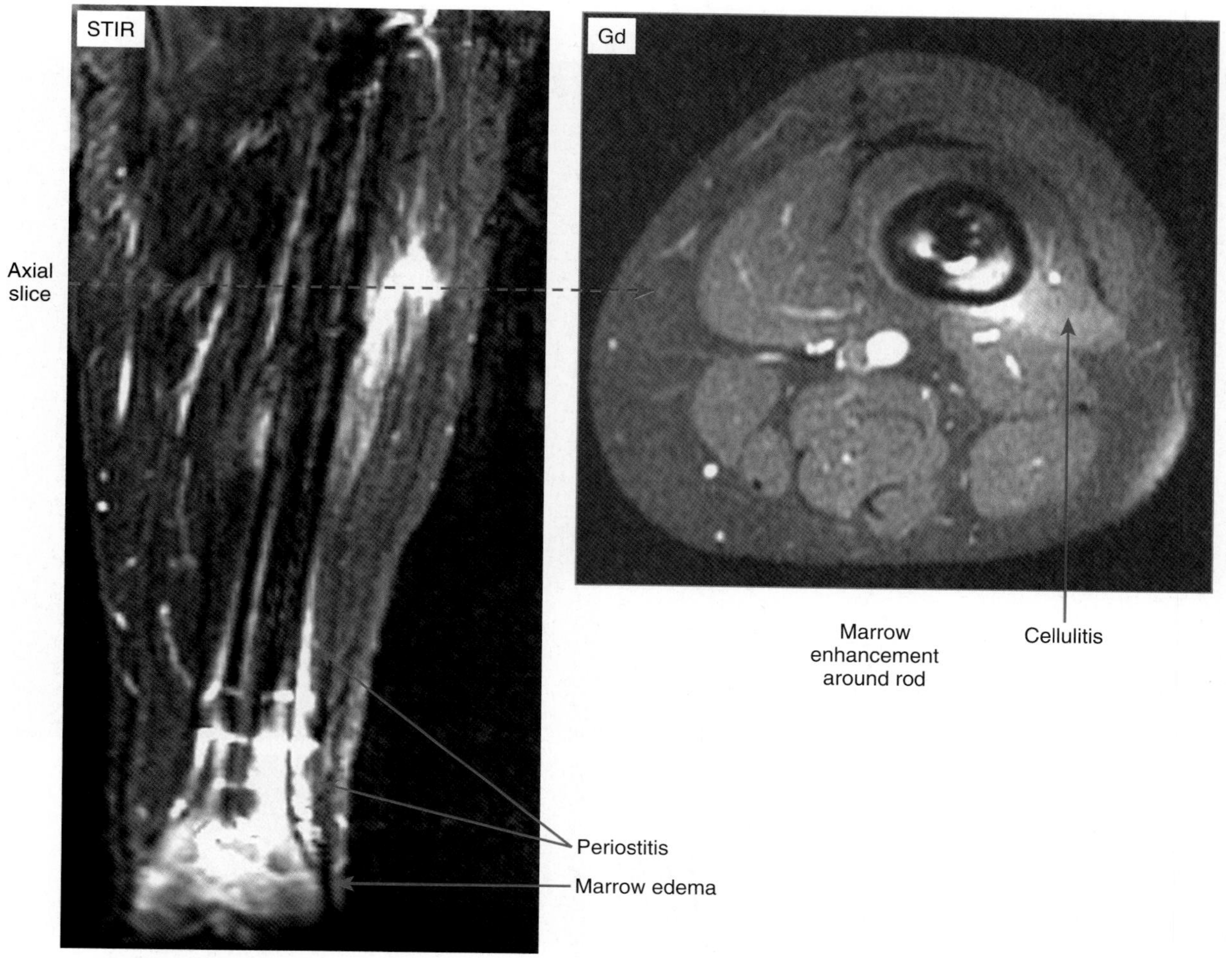
STIR
Gd
Axial
slice
Marrow
enhancement
around rod
Cellulitis
Periostitis
Marrow edema

Figure 5-15 Osteomyelitis around metal rod. Depending on the type and configuration of the metal component, MRI may not be significantly limited. For example, rods and other components with simple surfaces give less artifact than components with complex surfaces (e.g., screws), and titanium components create less artifact than cobalt chrome or stainless steel.

By the time frank cortical destruction is seen, the infectious process is well established and generally extensive. The classic radiologic appearance is a lytic, permeative process, characteristic of "small round cell" lesions. Radiographs are still useful as the first test to exclude other pathology, to obtain a baseline exam, and to evaluate for calcifications.

Tc-99m-MDP (methylene diphosphate) three-phase bone scan has high sensitivity for detection of osteomyelitis if there is adequate blood flow to distribute radiotracer. Classically, osteomyelitis presents as rapid uptake on the early inflow phase due to hyperemia, with persistent activity on the second, blood pool phase, and concentration of activity within bone on the delayed phase acquired hours later, indicating increased bone turnover (Fig. 5-20). Uptake on all phases suggests osteomyelitis in the appropriate clinical setting, but these findings can be seen in other inflammatory, traumatic, and neoplastic conditions, as well as neuropathic osteoarthropathy. Increased specificity has been reported with acquisition of a fourth phase, obtained after 24 hours.

Gallium scan, though commonly used for detection of inflammatory processes around the body, has shown limitations in the musculoskeletal system, particularly in the spine and diabetic foot. Instead, when there is a question of infection versus some

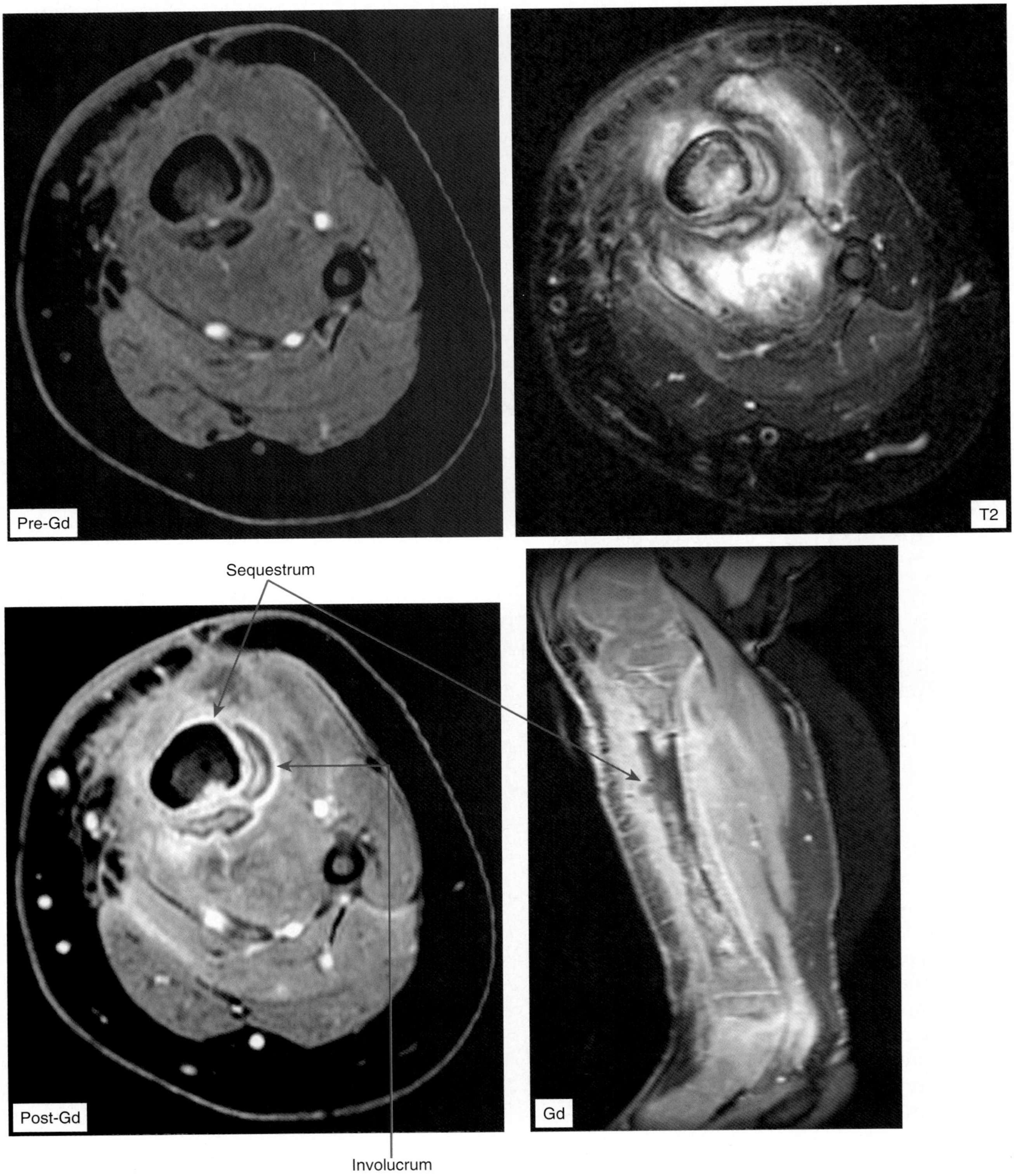
Pre-Gd
T2
Sequestrum
Post-Gd
Gd
Involucrum

Figure 5-16 *Acute-on-chronic osteomyelitis.*

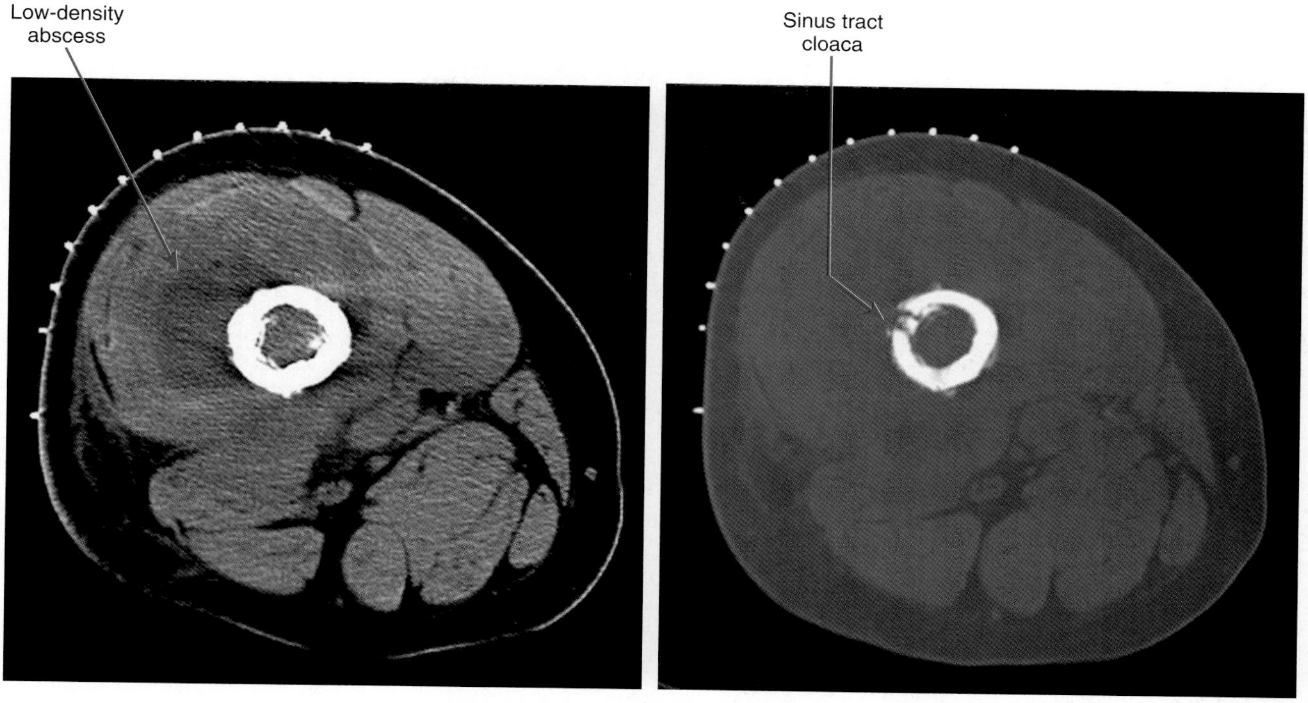
Low-density
abscess
Sinus tract
cloaca

Figure 5-17 Osteomyelitis on CT. Detection of sinus tract and abscess.

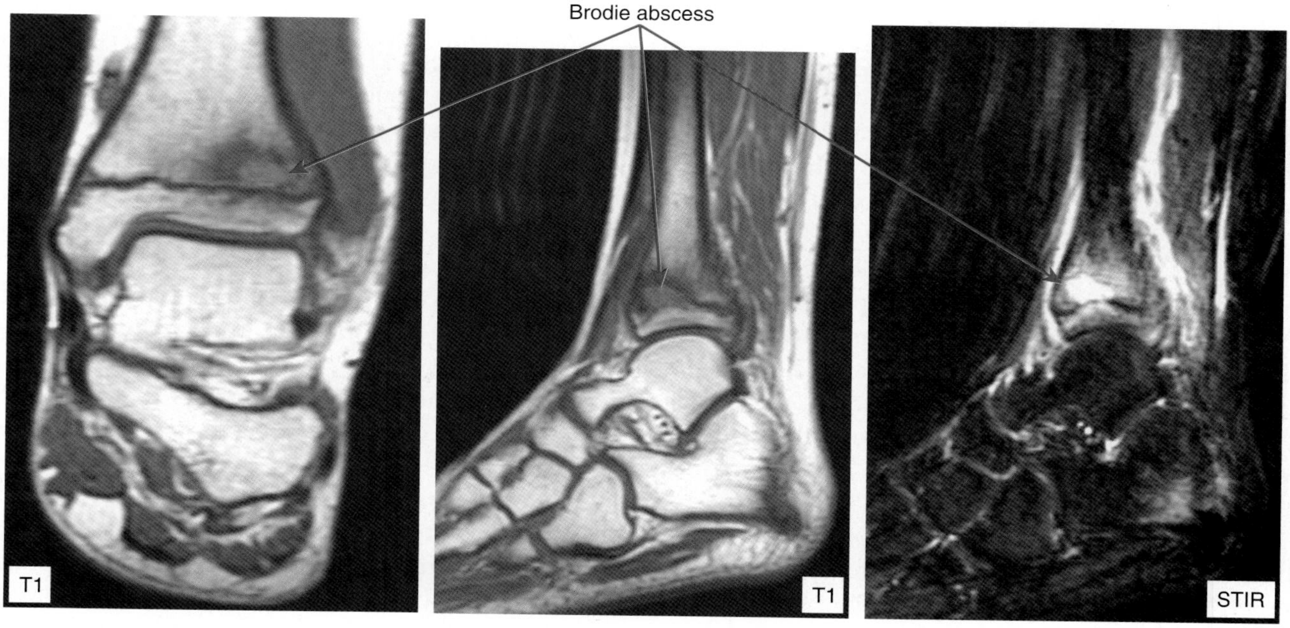
Brodie abscess
T1
T1
STIR

Figure 5-18 A Brodie abscess in an adolescent. Note how the lesion abuts or "drips" toward the physeal plate.

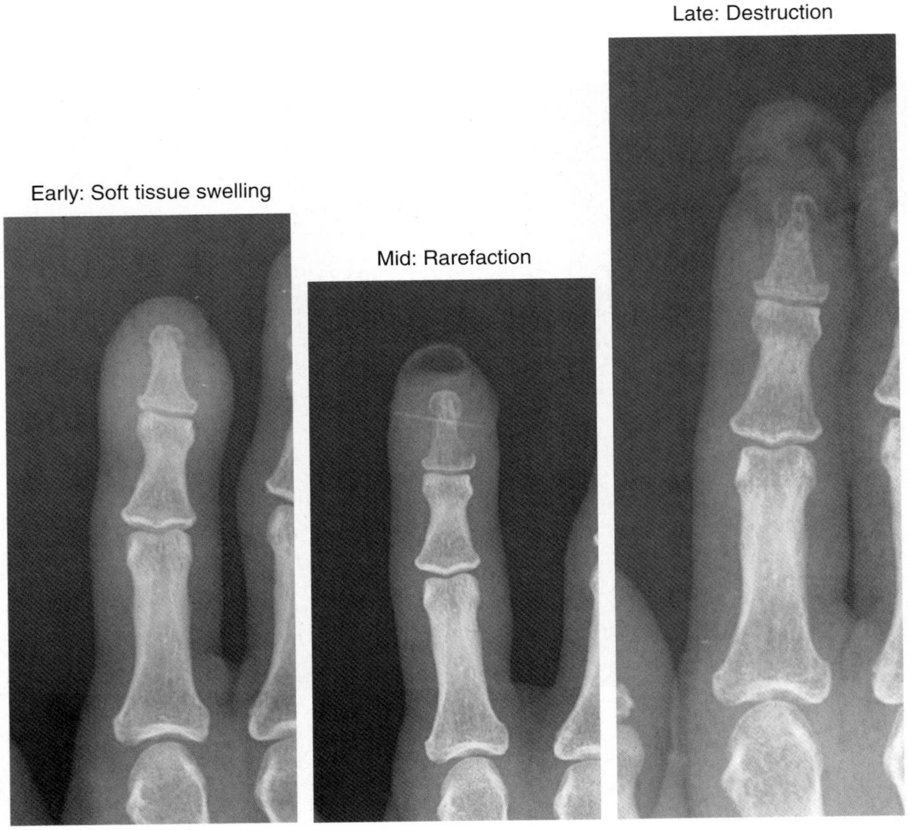
Early: Soft tissue swelling
Mid: Rarefaction
Late: Destruction

Figure 5-19 Osteomyelitis. Radiographic findings at different stages.

other process, imaging using WBCs tagged with indium-111 or technetium-99m is recommended. Labeled WBCs are taken up preferentially by inflammatory tissue; this is nonspecific with regard to involved tissue, and cellulitis or abscess results in abnormal activity similar to osteomyelitis. Therefore, the exam is typically interpreted in conjunction with three-phase bone scan, with corresponding uptake concentrating in bone indicative of osteomyelitis. Although the combination is specific, nuclear medicine exams involve a delay and anatomic resolution is low, making these techniques less useful for urgent evaluation (e.g., spine infection) or as preoperative anatomic roadmaps.

For clinically suspected infection, MRI is the test of choice in most settings. Normal marrow signal on T1 and STIR or fat-suppressed T2-weighted sequences excludes osteomyelitis. Apart from high sensitivity and specificity, MRI facilitates medical and surgical treatment planning by detecting abscesses, septic arthritis and tenosynovitis, and sinus tracts and can accurately define soft tissue and osseous extent of involvement. The MRI report should always describe these characteristics as well as the presence of any nonenhancing tissue representing necrosis, which usually requires debridement.

On MRI, the classic sign of osteomyelitis is replacement of marrow fat on T1-weighted images, with marrow edema and enhancement on fluid-sensitive and post-contrast images (Fig. 5-21). However, it should be obvious that these findings are not specific for infection and can be seen in a variety of diseases and injuries.

There are other factors to consider that may assist in generating a differential diagnosis

1. *Clinical findings:* Often MRI is read in a vacuum, without a clinical reference point. If a case appears to represent infection, every effort should be made to review lab values related to infection (WBC count, sedimentation rate, C-reactive protein) as well as those that may shed light on the underlying disease (glucose: diabetes; creatinine: renal failure). Clinical presentation and exam should be reviewed: Are the symptoms minimal compared with the extent of imaging findings? If

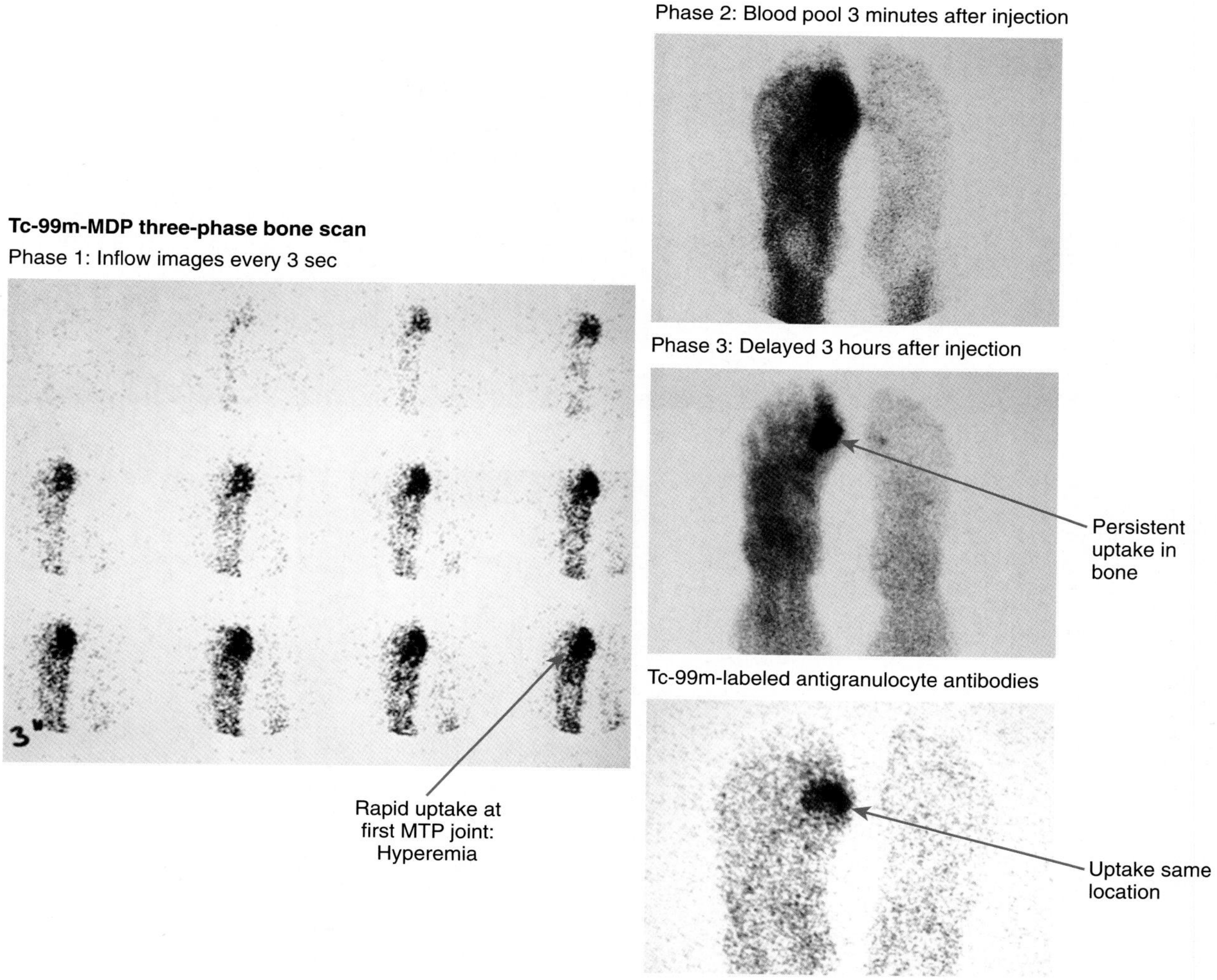
Phase 2: Blood pool 3 minutes after injection
Tc-99m-MDP three-phase bone scan
Phase 1: Inflow images every 3 sec
Phase 3: Delayed 3 hours after injection
Persistent uptake in bone
Tc-99m-labeled antigranulocyte antibodies
Rapid uptake at first MTP joint: Hyperemia
Uptake same location

Figure 5-20 Septic arthritis and osteomyelitis at the first metatarsophalangeal joint diagnosed by nuclear medicine techniques. MDP, methylene diphosphonate; MTP, metatarsophalangeal. (Courtesy of Hans Ledermann, MD, Basel, Switzerland.)

so, maybe neuropathic osteoarthropathy, amyloidosis, or a chronic inflammatory arthropathy should be entertained. Are symptoms greater than the imaging findings? If so, gout may be a consideration.

2. *Appearance on different planes:* Some entities have a particular morphology on different imaging planes. This is especially true with fracture, which may look ill defined in one plane and sharp/linear in the perpendicular plane. Neuropathic fractures in the feet of diabetics are often overcalled as infection unless the fracture line is sought on all imaging planes. Osteomyelitis, despite the often ill-defined permeative, "small round cell" pattern on radiographs, is typically fairly well defined on MRI. On the other hand, traumatic lesions often have ill-defined margins on MRI, depending on their severity and chronicity. Tumors also typically appear well defined on MRI despite having an aggressive appearance on radiographs. This brings up two important issues: MRI should not be used to determine the aggressiveness of a lesion; and tumor should always be considered if infection is the primary diagnosis, especially if the clinical scenario does not fit the imaging findings.

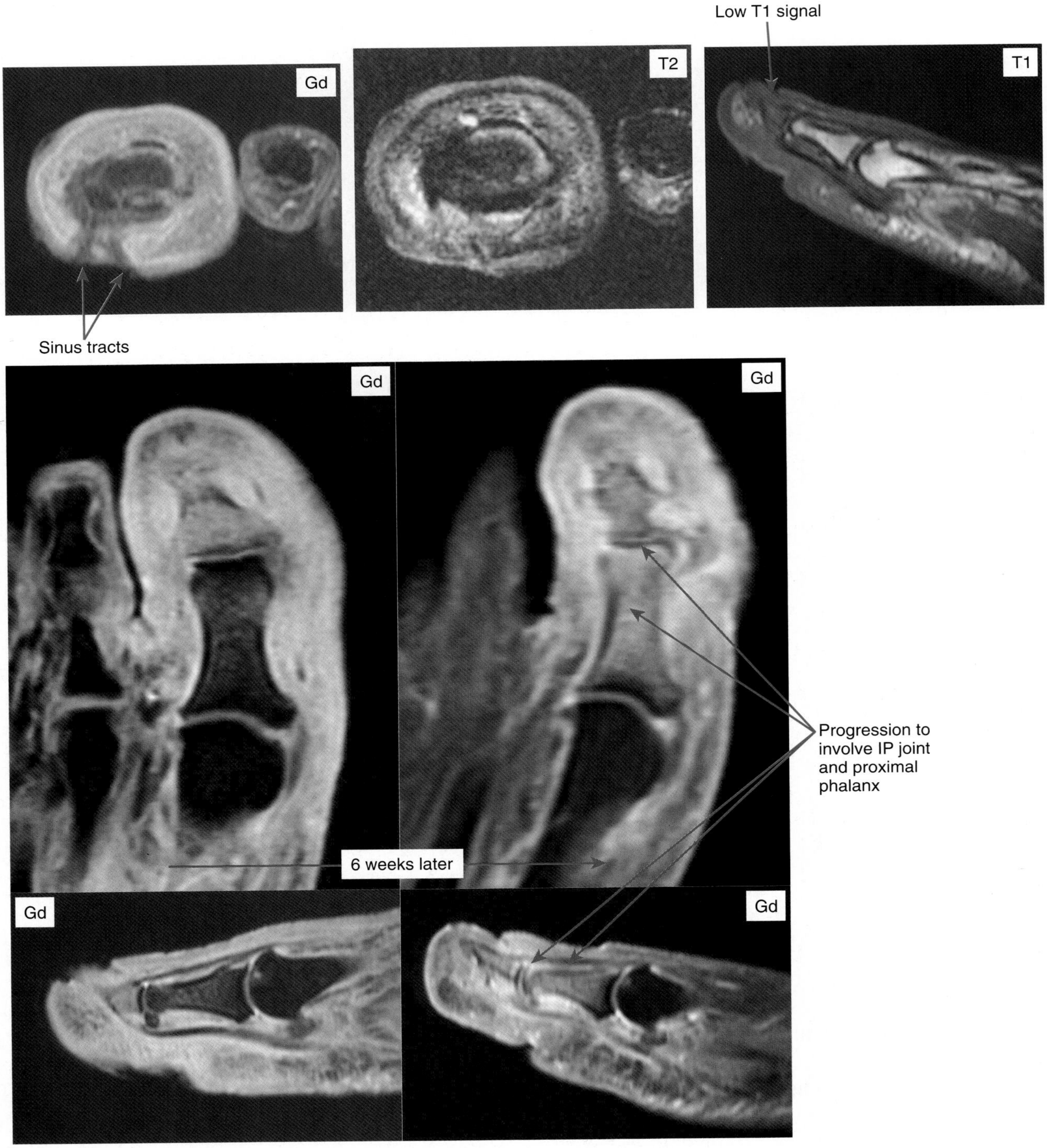
Low T1 signal
Gd
T2
T1
Sinus tracts
Gd
Gd
Progression to involve IP joint and proximal phalanx
6 weeks later
Gd
Gd

Figure 5-21 Typical features of bacterial osteomyelitis on MRI: Diabetic patient with progression on follow-up. Osteomyelitis is characterized on MRI by replacement of marrow fat on T1-weighted images, marrow edema on fluid-sensitive sequences (e.g., T2-weighted or STIR), and medullary contrast enhancement. However, these findings alone are not specific and must be correlated with other imaging findings including cellulitis, periosteal reaction, abscess, sinus tracts, joint effusion, and erosion, as well as clinical features. IP, interphalangeal.

3. *Distribution:* Infection easily crosses synovial joints and disks, but these represent a relative barrier to tumor. Therefore, if an adjacent articular surface is involved, an arthritis is the primary consideration, and if it is monarticular in the appropriate setting, infection may be suggested. However, aggressive tumors can cross joints as well, especially those with extensive ligamentous connections allowing migration of tumor cells.
4. *Periostitis:* Periostitis is a well-known finding in osteomyelitis, especially of long bones. On radiographs, the periostitis associated with infection is typically a thick and undulating nonaggressive pattern (Fig. 5-22). On MRI, periosteal reaction appears as linear edema and enhancement along the outer cortex, wrapping around the bone. Two important issues are that this finding is also not specific for infection and that some bones and parts of bones do not exhibit significant periosteal response. First, other entities such as stress fracture, tumor, and infarction can show periosteal reaction, and the pattern of aggressiveness of the periostitis may not be reliably distinguished on MRI. Second, periosteal reaction associated with various conditions is mainly a characteristic of the long bones. Carpal and tarsal bones, as well as the periarticular region of bones do not have a well-defined periosteum and do not show the same reaction as the metaphyses and diaphyses of long bones. In addition, flat bones such as the pelvis and scapula and small bones such as the phalanges may not show the classic features described in long bones.
5. *Soft tissue findings:* The adjacent soft tissues are very important in the evaluation of possible infection seen on MRI (Figs. 5-23 through 5-25). Hematogenous infection to joints or bone typically creates an inflammatory reaction in the adjacent soft tissues. Sinus tracts and abscesses may arise from the infected bone/joint.

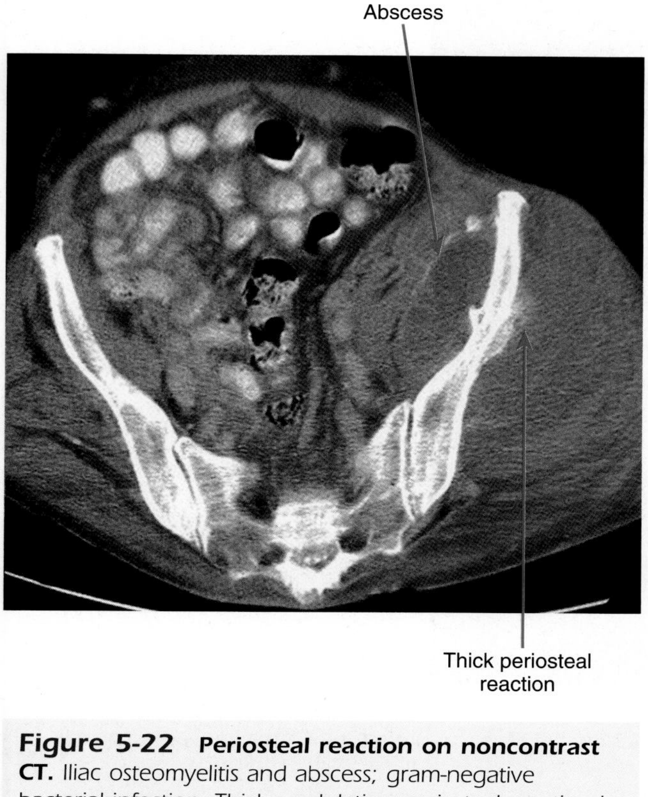
Abscess
Thick periosteal reaction

Figure 5-22 Periosteal reaction on noncontrast CT. Iliac osteomyelitis and abscess; gram-negative bacterial infection. Thick, undulating periosteal reaction is typical of infection. However, the finding is nonspecific and can be seen with other processes with low aggressiveness.

Patterns of spread are predictable, based on location and orientation of fascial planes: Lumbar spine infection spreads along the psoas; sacroiliac infection spreads along the iliacus and into the sciatic notch and glutei (see Fig. 5-25); sternoclavicular infection spreads into the retrosternal space, the lower neck, and the pectoralis major; infections of the hands and feet may spread along tendon sheaths.

Normal or abnormal communications can hasten spread of infection. Septic arthritis can spread along tendon sheaths, especially if the tendon communicates with the joint (long head of the biceps and the glenohumeral joint, flexor hallucis longus and ankle/subtalar joint, and popliteus and knee joint). Joints may communicate (ankle and subtalar joint, wrist joints through ligament tears), and joints and bursae may communicate (the hip joint and the iliopsoas bursa, the glenohumeral joint, and the subacromial-subdeltoid bursa and acromioclavicular joint through a rotator cuff tear). Also, if there is disruption of the cartilaginous surface of a joint, infection may spread more easily into the underlying bone.

For infections that occur as a result of contiguous spread (as in the diabetic foot and pelvis in paralyzed patients), evaluation of the soft tissues is essential. In this setting if there is a marrow abnormality and the adjacent subcutaneous fat is preserved, other etiologies such as neuropathic disease should be considered.

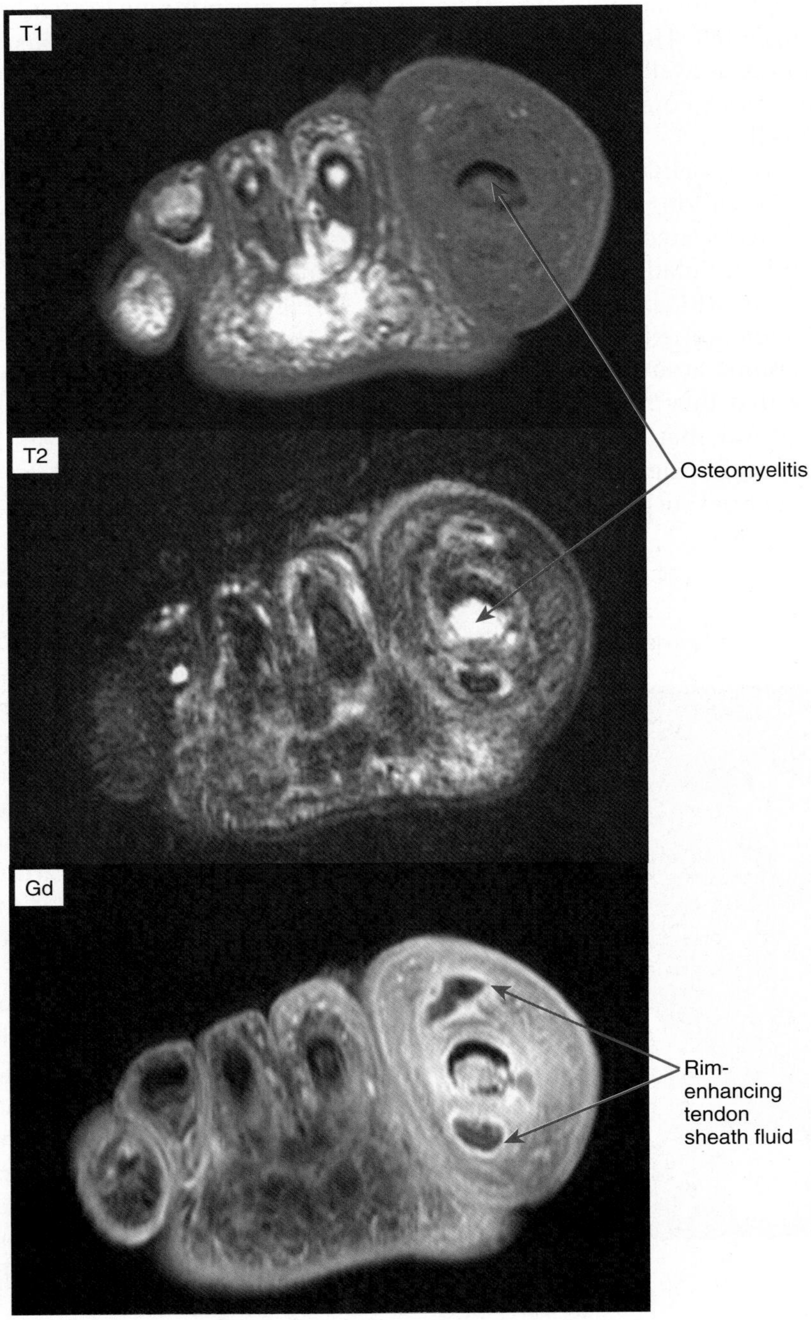
T1
T2
Gd
Osteomyelitis
Rim-
enhancing
tendon
sheath fluid

Figure 5-23 Osteomyelitis and septic tenosynovitis via contiguous spread in the great toe of a patient with diabetes.

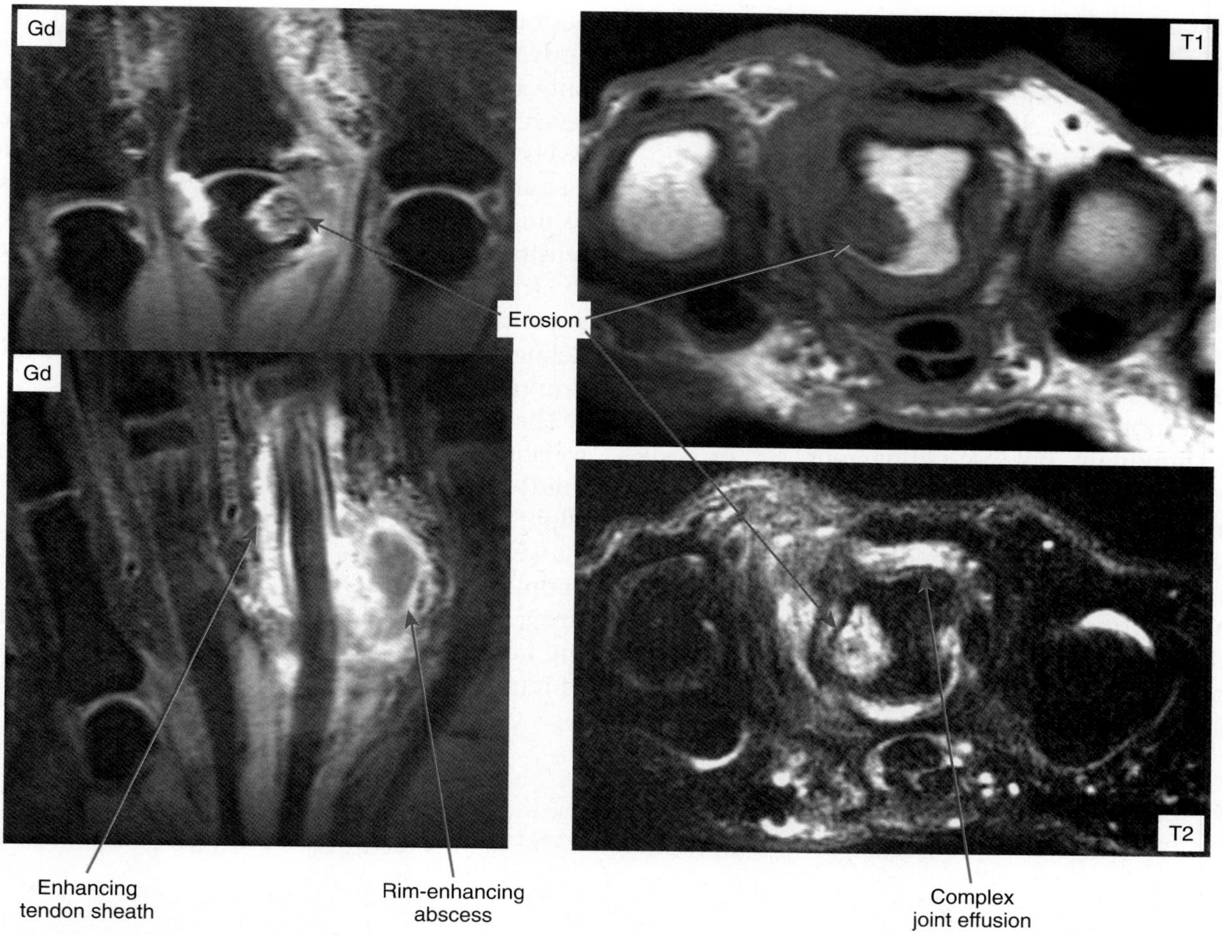
Gd
T1
Erosion
Gd
T2
Enhancing
tendon sheath
Rim-enhancing
abscess
Complex
joint effusion

Figure 5-24 Septic arthritis and tenosynovitis. Direct implantation in a patient with wounds after punching another person in the mouth.

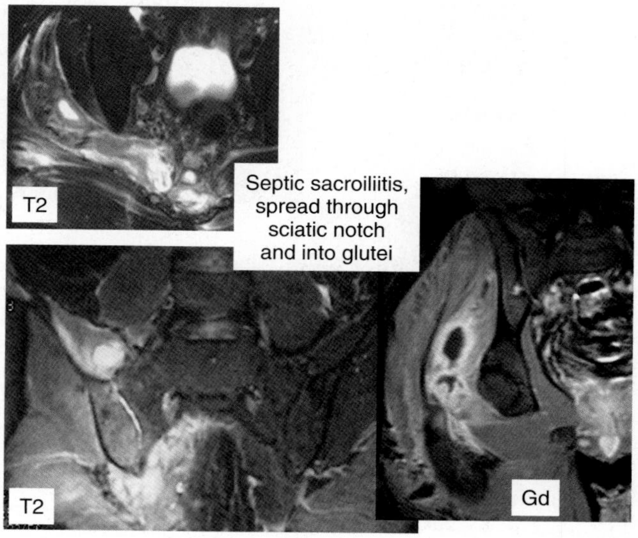
T2
Septic sacroiliitis,
spread through
sciatic notch
and into glutei
T2
Gd

Figure 5-25 Sacroiliac septic arthritis. Infection generally tends to spread in a predictable way along fascial planes. When small joints are involved, infected fluid often leaks into adjacent compartments. Sacroiliac infection spreads anteriorly along the iliopsoas, inferiorly into the sciatic notch, posteriorly into the glutei, and superiorly toward the spine.

INFECTION OF THE SPINE

Spine infection deserves special consideration; it is a relatively common clinical condition that can result in serious morbidity. Recognition of early radiographic and MRI manifestations is extremely important to avoid serious complications.

Radiologic diagnosis of spine infection is best made with MR imaging, which is very sensitive for early detection of infection and accurate for delineation of extent of involvement and identification of paraspinal abscess for operative planning. However, identification of spine infection using other modalities is important, because radiographs, CT, or bone scan are often ordered initially.

Radiographs are typically the first study obtained as part of the radiologic workup of suspected infection. Early manifestations of pyogenic infectious spondylitis on radiographs include disk narrowing, vertebral endplate osteolysis or irregularity, and paraspinal soft tissue mass (Fig. 5-26). Eventually, gross destruction of the endplates, collapse of the vertebral body, deformity, and sclerosis may occur. Generally, only one disk level is involved, although in more severe or chronic cases, spread to adjacent vertebral levels can occur along paravertebral ligaments or fascial planes. MRI is the primary modality for establishing the diagnosis of infectious spondylitis. High sensitivity (ranging from 90% to 100%) and specificity (ranging from 80% to 95%), combined with anatomic detail, allow accurate diagnosis as well as delineation of extent of involvement and identification of paraspinal and epidural abscess.

The infected disk demonstrates low signal on T1-weighted images and high signal (approximating fluid) on T2-weighted images (see Fig. 5-26). Fat-suppression technique is recommended on the T2-weighted images to best demonstrate associated endplate edema. On T1- and T2-weighted sagittal images, the endplates may be irregular, with loss of the normal low-signal cortical line. Administration of intravenous gadolinium in conjunction with a fat-

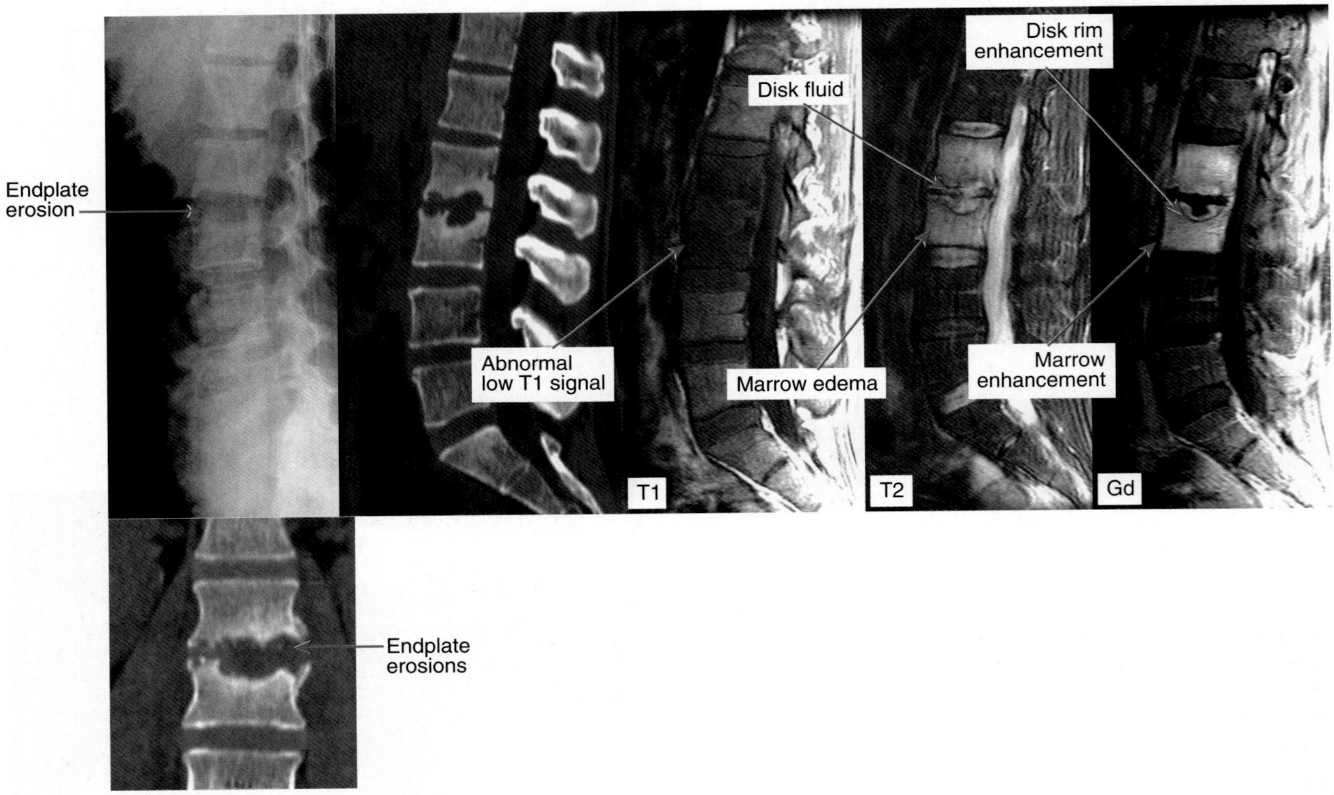

Endplate erosion
Abnormal low T1 signal
Disk fluid
Marrow edema
Disk rim enhancement
Marrow enhancement
T1
T2
Gd
Endplate erosions

Figure 5-26 Classic appearance of diskitis on radiography, CT, and MRI.

suppressed T1-weighted imaging sequence can aid diagnostic confidence; the infected disk demonstrates rim enhancement along the disk margins, with enhancement of the adjacent vertebral endplates. Occasionally, the entire vertebral body above and below the affected disk level enhance diffusely.

T2-weighted images and fat-suppressed T1-weighted gadolinium-enhanced images are particularly useful for identification of paraspinal or epidural abscess. These abscesses are typically longitudinally oriented, extending along paraspinal ligaments or fascial planes, often far from the original site of infection. On T2-weighted images, the abscess shows increased signal intensity, approximating fluid, but often with lobulated margins and internal complexity representing septations, debris, or devitalized tissue. Gadolinium-enhanced images show rim enhancement at the margins of the abscess, which is generally thick and irregular.

Infectious Spondylitis: Differential Diagnosis

Certain noninfectious conditions can result in radiologic findings that can mimic those of infectious spondylitis.

Degenerative Disease

Like infection, degenerative disk disease results in disk narrowing, with associated endplate irregularity and sclerosis. In addition, Schmorl nodes (intravertebral disk herniation) cause the appearance of endplate irregularity and in early stages show marrow edema on MRI (Fig. 5-27). Although soft tissue mass is absent (except for disk bulge), this is not a reliable discriminator on radiographs or CT. However, disk degeneration is commonly associated with a vacuum phenomenon that is nearly 100% specific for absence of infection. As a result, this sign should be sought in cases of suspected infection; lateral radiographs in flexion and extension can aid in identification of vacuum phenomena (Fig. 5-28). CT is quick and can be excellent for detection of small vacuum phenomena at suspected levels. On MRI, modic type 1 endplate changes can mimic infection, with decreased T1 signal and increased T2 signal. However, the associated disk will show low signal on T1- and T2-weighted images if degenerated compared with the high T2 signal seen in infection. MRI can also detect paraspinal edema and mass effect, which are absent in degenerative disk disease. Facet osteoarthritis, like other arthritic joints, can exhibit adjacent bone

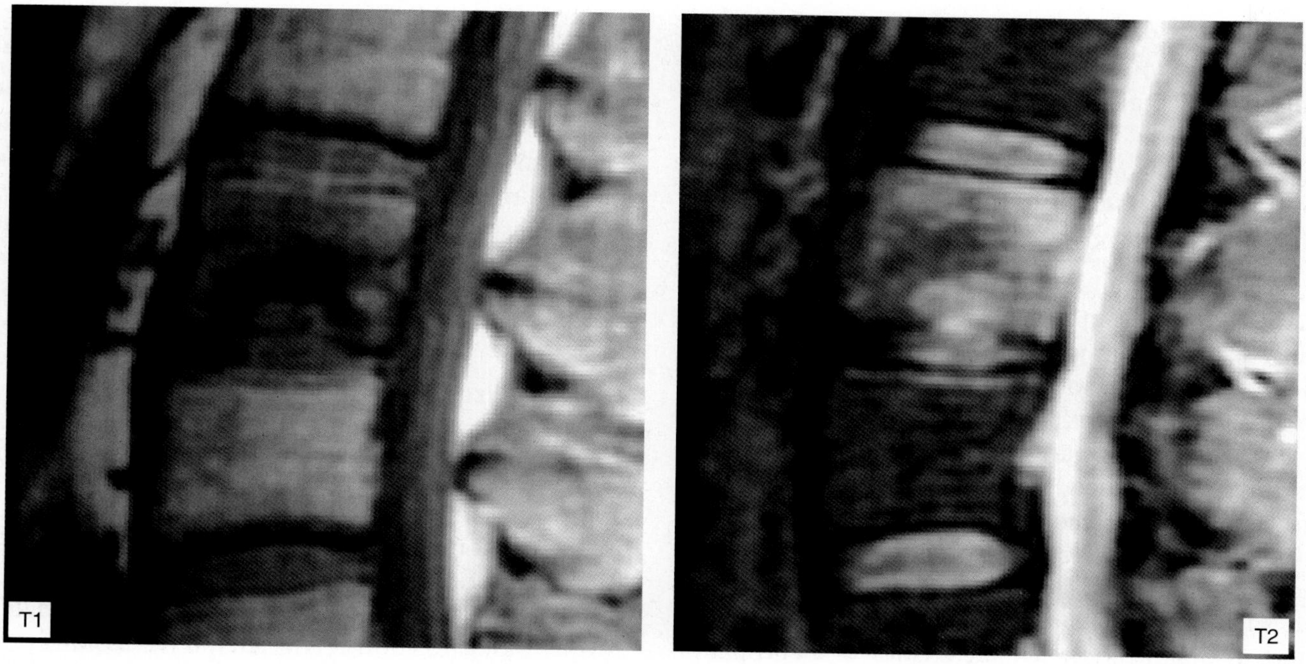
T1
T2

Figure 5-27 Acute Schmorl nodes can be mistaken for infection or tumor. Communication with the disk representing intravertebral herniation of disk material is key. Marrow edema/enhancement may be intense but is generally at one endplate, and the disk is typically lower in signal with some desiccation.

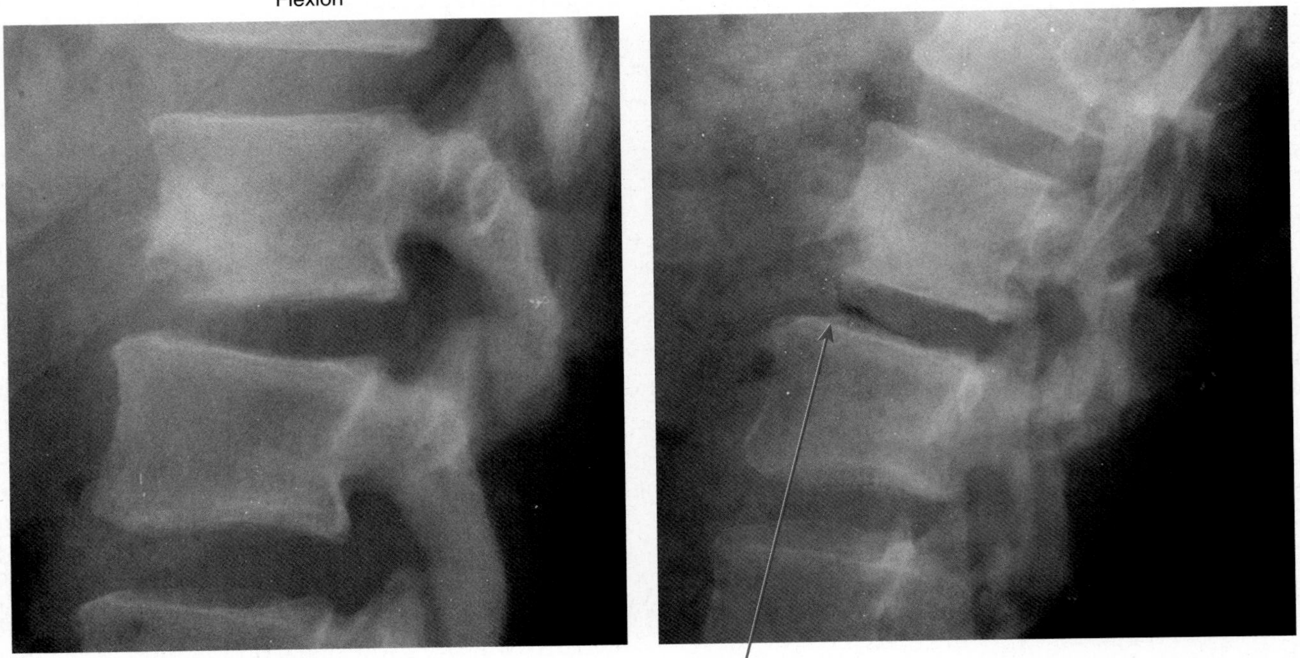
Flexion
Extension
Vacuum
phenomenon

Figure 5-28 Flexion/extension radiographs are a useful and inexpensive method of diagnosing segmental instability and lack of infection. Although not 100% specific, eliciting a vacuum phenomenon on extension is nearly always indicative of absence of infection at that level.

marrow edema and should not be confused with infection.

Segmental Instability/Neuropathic Disease

(Figs. 5-29 and 5-30)

Instability and neuropathic disease of the spine radiographically appear as aggressive degenerative disk disease, often with subluxation (spondylolisthesis), debris and disorganization, and preservation of bone density characteristically seen in other joints with neuropathic osteoarthropathy. Endplate irregularity can be marked, associated with disk narrowing, resembling an infectious etiology. Again, identification of a vacuum phenomenon is the best discriminator; fortunately, vacuum phenomena are common in situations of instability and neuropathy. Debris and disorganization, characteristics of neuropathic joints, can also aid diagnostic confidence. Facet joint involvement is common in segments with instability or neuropathic disease; it is rare in infectious spondylitis. On MR images, neuropathic spine can appear similar to infection. The neuropathic level can demonstrate high T2 signal in the disk, as well as edema in the adjacent vertebral bodies, and paraspinal edema and mass effect. In some cases, it can be difficult to differentiate neuropathic disease from infection, and aspiration/biopsy may be necessary.

Dialysis-Associated Spondyloarthropathy

(Fig. 5-31)

In patients with chronic renal failure, an aggressive-appearing spondylosis with disk narrowing, endplate irregularity or destruction, and sclerosis can occur at one or multiple levels and can resemble infection radiographically. The condition is most likely related to amyloid deposition at affected intervertebral levels. In this situation, radiographic signs of secondary hyperparathyroidism should be sought, including rugger-jersey spine, osteopenia, resorption of bone at

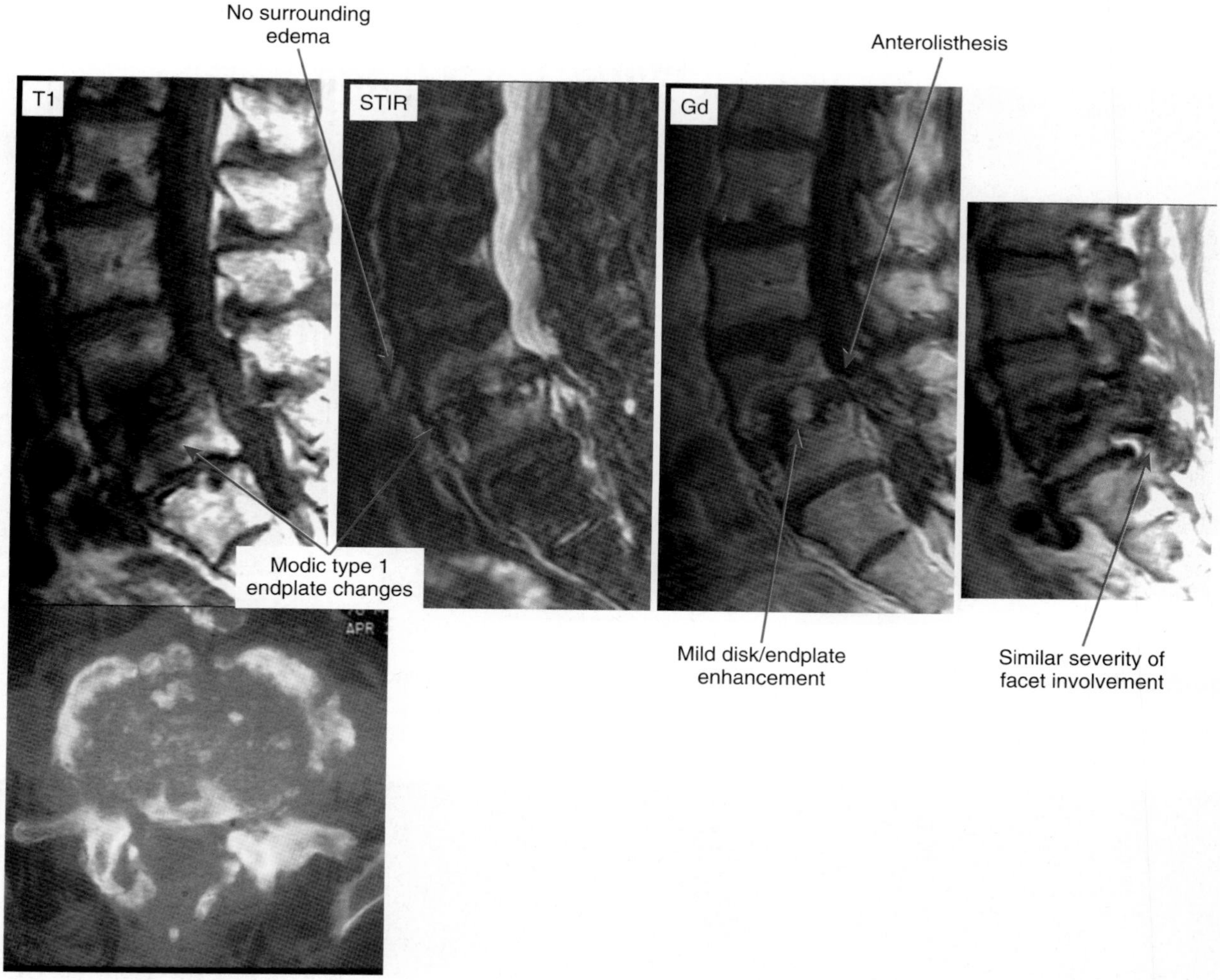
No surrounding edema
Anterolisthesis
T1
STIR
Gd
Modic type 1 endplate changes
Mild disk/endplate enhancement
Similar severity of facet involvement
CT: Bone proliferation

Figure 5-29 Segmental instability can simulate infectious spondylitis. Endplate irregularity can be seen in addition to Modic type 1 endplate changes, T2 hyperintensity in the disk, and endplate enhancement—all suggesting infection. Evidence supporting lack of infection include low T2 signal in the disk, similar facet involvement/spondylolisthesis (suggesting chronic disease and instability), and lack of surrounding soft tissue edema and mass effect. If a vacuum can be demonstrated or induced on radiographs or CT, this strongly supports instability rather than infection.

the sacroiliac joints, terminal tufts and radial aspect of the phalanges, and distal clavicles. Amyloid deposition in other areas can present as para-articular soft tissue masses or juxta-articular lucent lesions. On MRI, amyloid appears as low-signal material on T1- and T2-weighted sequences. However, fluid collections are often present. As a result, in some situations differentiation from infection can be difficult, prompting aspiration and biopsy. If amyloid is suspected, the pathologist should be made aware of this; Congo red stain is used to detect amyloid.

Postoperative Changes

Unfortunately, it can be difficult to differentiate recent postoperative changes from such procedures as diskectomy and fusion from those of superimposed infection. High T2 disk signal, diffuse enhancement, and fluid collections can all be seen in the postoperative period. Follow-up MRI examinations may provide useful information since postoperative changes should gradually subside. MRI can identify suspicious sites of enhancement or fluid collections to

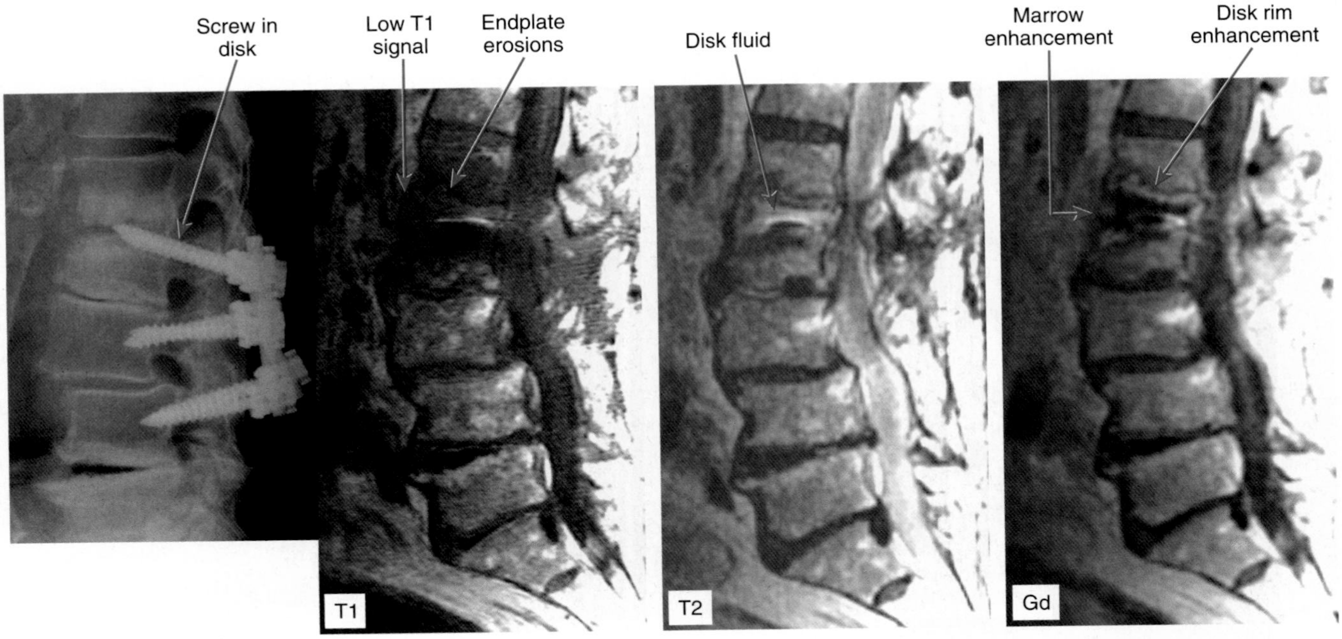
Screw in disk
Low T1 signal
Endplate erosions
Disk fluid
Marrow enhancement
Disk rim enhancement
T1
T2
Gd

Figure 5-30 Instability (with screw in disk) simulating diskitis on MRI. Biopsy showed no evidence of infection.

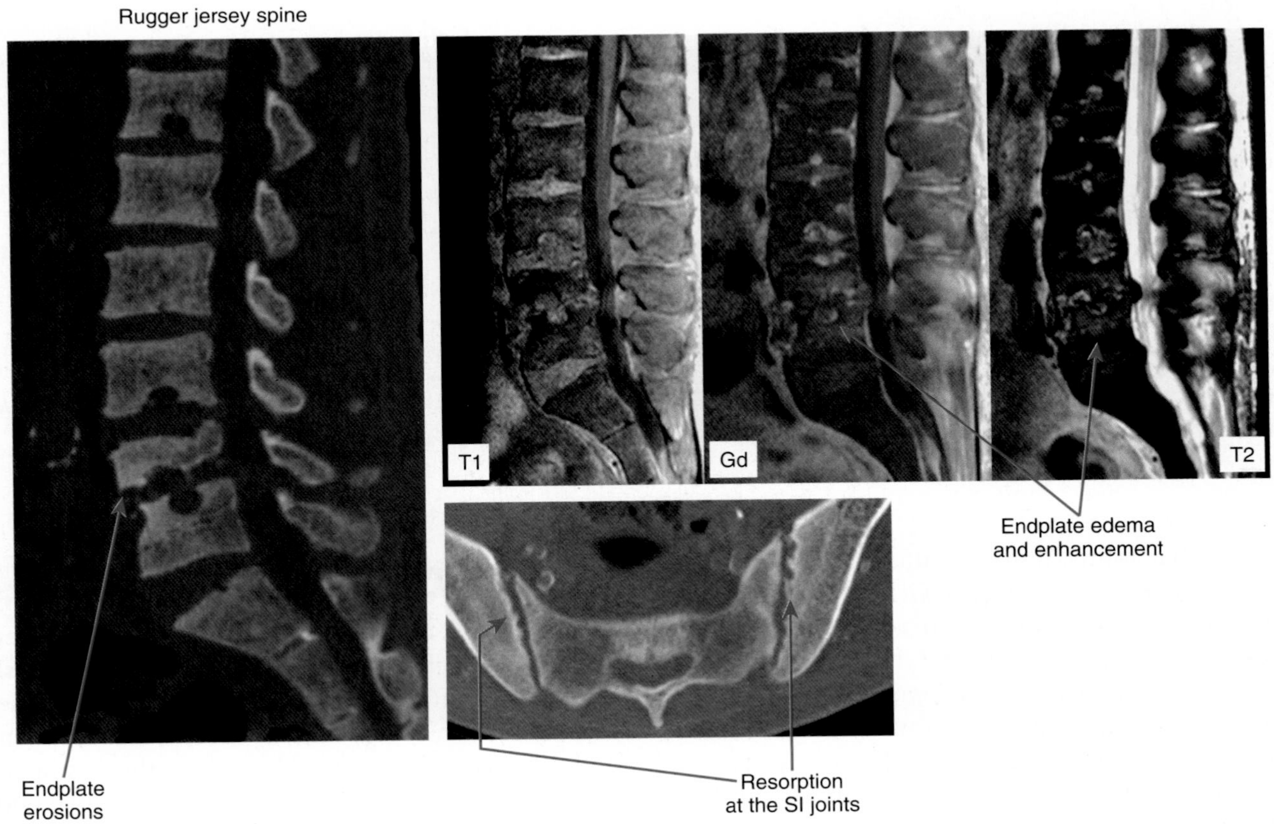
Rugger jersey spine
T1
Gd
T2
Endplate edema and enhancement
Endplate erosions
Resorption at the SI joints

Figure 5-31 Amyloid can mimic diskitis on imaging studies. Disk involvement can result in endplate destruction, with resulting reactive endplate edema making it difficult to exclude infection even if secondary hyperparathyroidism is apparent. Amyloid is low signal on T1- and T2-weighted images, but surrounding fluid collections and marrow edema are common; if biopsy is performed, the pathologist should be alerted to the possibility of amyloid. SI, sacroiliac.

aspirate for culture. In this situation, a scintigraphic scan using labeled WBCs may also be useful.

HISTOLOGY AND CULTURE

Bone biopsy is performed when clinical and radiologic evaluation is not conclusive or when microbial diagnosis is needed for selecting antibiotic coverage. Definitive diagnosis of osteomyelitis relies on positive culture results of causative organisms from a biopsy sample or characteristic histologic findings, including aggregates of inflammatory cells (including neutrophils, lymphocytes, histiocytes, and plasma cells), erosions of trabecular bone, and marrow changes that range from loss of normal marrow fat in acute osteomyelitis to fibrosis and reactive bone formation in chronic disease. Limitations of percutaneous and surgical bone biopsy include sampling error, false-negative cultures (especially in patients receiving antibiotics), difficulties in distinguishing other osteopathy from osteomyelitis histologically, and the risk of introducing contaminating uninfected bone after passing the needle through a soft tissue infection. Culture results of percutaneous bone biopsy specimens in pedal infection may be unreliable because of contamination from underlying infected soft tissue; also, in diabetic feet, multiorganism infections predominate. Bone biopsy cultures in osteomyelitis in general may be falsely negative in up to 50% to 70% of cases (if antibiotics have been used, the negative result can be as high as 80% and a patient on antibiotics should be taken off medication for at least 48 hours before sampling). Sensitivity of histopathologic diagnosis is higher. Therefore, bone biopsy should always include a histology evaluation as well as culture.

Staphylococcus aureus is the most common bacterium cultured in cases of septic arthritis and osteomyelitis. Less common are *Streptococcus, Klebsiella, Pseudomonas* species, and others. When chronic ulceration is the source of infection, multiple organisms are often cultured. Mycobacterial infections are becoming more common in the general population as resistant strains emerge. Parasitic and fungal infections are relatively rare, but prevalence depends on the region and travel history as well as clinical factors. For instance, travel to the southwestern United States should raise suspicion of coccidioidomycosis; an immunocompromised state increases the incidence of opportunistic infections such as fungi. Seasonal variations can also occur. For instance, a child from the northeastern United States presenting with a monarticular inflammatory arthritis in the spring should make one think of Lyme disease as reflecting the presence of deer ticks, which constitute the vector.

OTHER CLINICAL ISSUES

Infection of the Diabetic Foot

Recurrent Infection After Amputation

Decades ago the treatment for osteomyelitis of the foot in diabetic patients included aggressive debridement—basically amputation, leaving a functional stump (transmetatarsal, Lisfranc, Chopart, Symes, or below-knee amputation). However, owing to improvement in revascularization procedures and realization that amputation results in acceleration of disease in the contralateral extremity because of the shift in weight-bearing, the surgical goal over the past decade has been to preserve as much foot as possible and resect only the infected bone. The new postoperative challenge, therefore, has been to heal the surgical site in an ischemic foot and to leave no infected bone that would result in recurrent disease.

As described previously, mere diagnosis of osteomyelitis is no longer adequate in many cases. The radiologist must precisely characterize the extent of infection in bone and describe any other conditions relevant to surgical planning (septic arthritis, septic tenosynovitis, abscesses, devitalized tissue). For this reason, MRI has emerged as the imaging modality of choice.

Limb-sparing surgery results in a new imaging challenge. That is, after amputation for osteomyelitis, patients often return for follow-up imaging if the wound breaks down or if the swelling and erythema are unexpectedly prominent or fail to resolve. Wound breakdown can be from residual or recurrent infection, but can also be seen with ischemia. Fortunately, the findings on MRI associated with residual or recurrent osteomyelitis are straightforward. After amputation, regardless of time course, the marrow should have no edema or enhancement. There are exceptions, of course. For example, if the patient is stressing the stump with an ill-fitting prosthesis or is experiencing lack of sensation, edema may be seen. However, as a rule, any bone marrow edema at the amputation site should be considered suggestive for

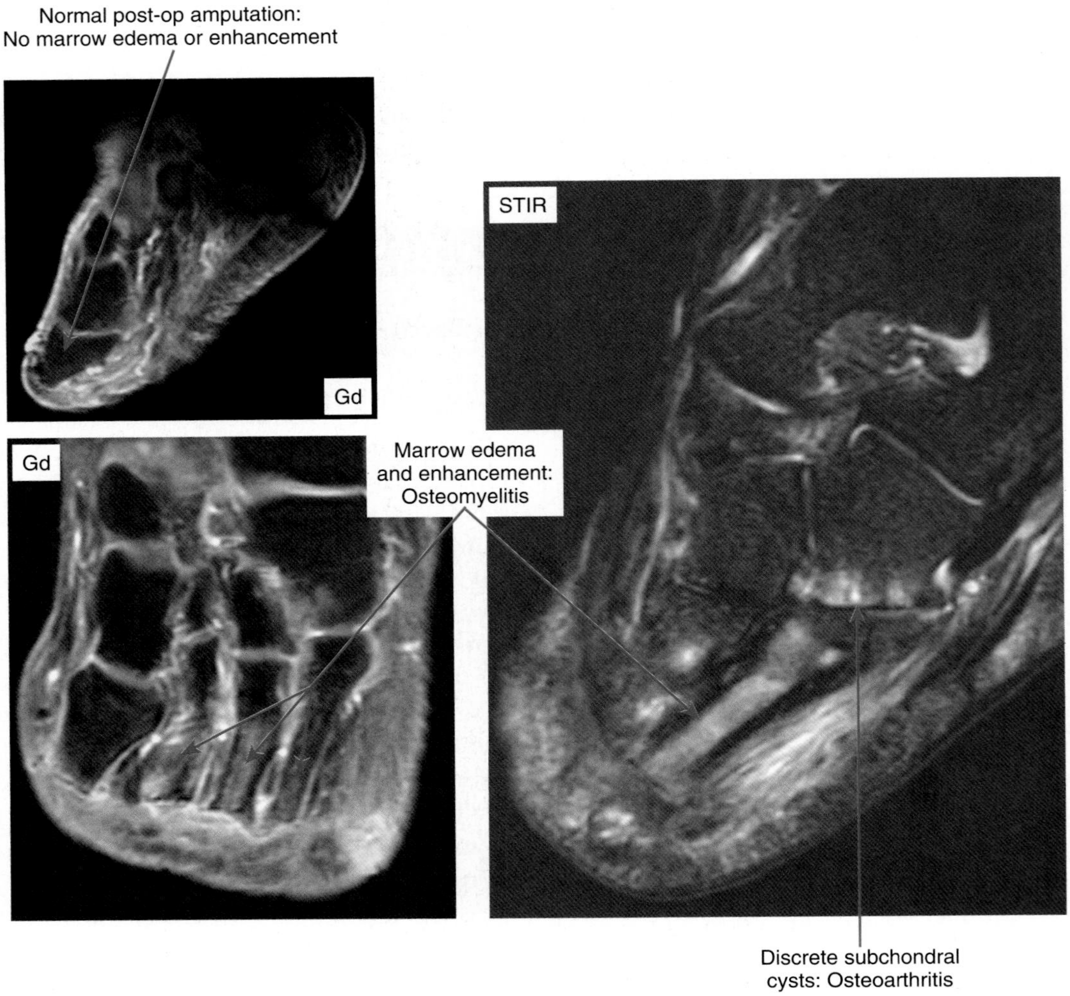
Normal post-op amputation:
No marrow edema or enhancement
Gd
STIR
Gd
Marrow edema
and enhancement:
Osteomyelitis
Discrete subchondral
cysts: Osteoarthritis

Figure 5-32 Transmetatarsal amputation in a diabetic patient with recurrent infection. Normally, minimal to no alteration of marrow signal is seen around the amputation site, even shortly after surgery.

infection (Fig. 5-32). It can also be helpful to review the preoperative MRI to see whether all infected bone was removed. Obviously, rim-enhancing fluid collections and sinus tracts are useful secondary signs (Fig. 5-33). Also, consider that increased soft tissue enhancement at the wound site means that hypervascularity is present and ischemic wound breakdown is less likely than infection.

Neuropathic Osteoarthropathy versus Infection

Evaluation of diabetic patients with clinically suspected pedal infection is common in some practices; the imaging algorithm is not defined because the quality and availability of imaging equipment and reader expertise vary. There are two basic clinical scenarios resulting in referral for imaging: (1) a patient with early neuropathic arthropathy (e.g., little to no deformity) who presents with a warm, swollen erythematous foot (the question being whether the condition is an infection or a noninfectious manifestation of neuropathy); (2) a patient with chronic neuropathic disease and deformity presenting with ulceration or swelling (the question being whether superimposed infection is present). These scenarios create different imaging appearances as outlined in the next two sections. Another characteristic of diabetic feet is diffuse soft tissue edema, as well as muscle atrophy (seen in early phases on MRI as T2 hyperin-

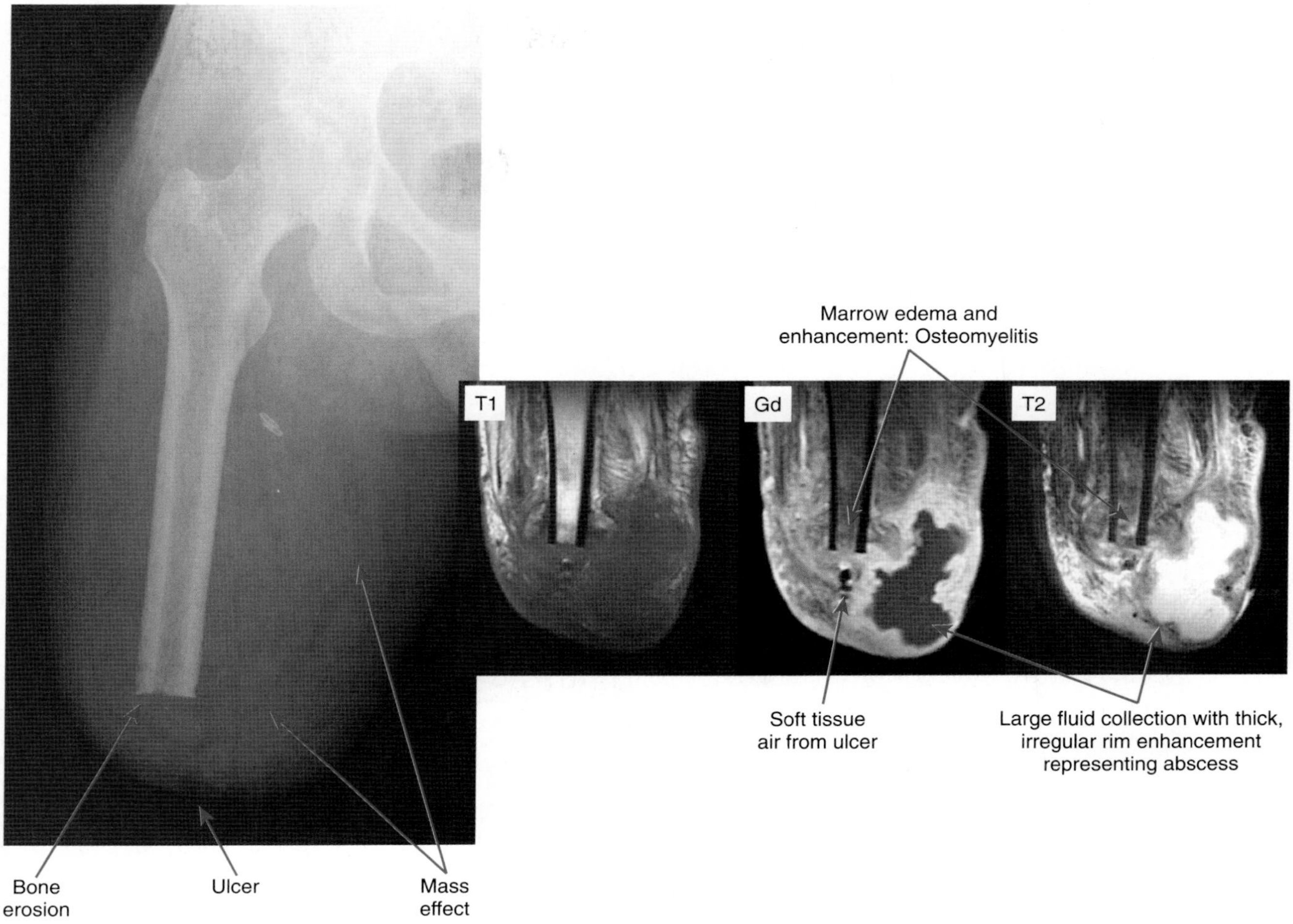
Marrow edema and
enhancement: Osteomyelitis
T1
Gd
T2
Soft tissue
air from ulcer
Large fluid collection with thick,
irregular rim enhancement
representing abscess
Bone
erosion
Ulcer
Mass
effect

Figure 5-33 *Signs of infected amputation site with ulceration, cellulitis, abscess, and osteomyelitis.*

tensity). This can be confusing when interpreting MR images for infection. This is another reason (in addition to improved detection of sinus tracts, abscesses, and synovitis) for using intravenous contrast dye in the routine protocol for evaluation of the diabetic foot (Fig. 5-34).

Early Neuropathic Arthropathy: Infection versus Neuropathic Disease (Figs. 5-35 and 5-36)

In early neuropathic arthropathy, there may be little radiographic evidence of underlying disease. On radiographs the soft tissues appear swollen, but the underlying bones show few findings. There may be a subtle malalignment at an involved joint; at the tarsometatarsal (Lisfranc) joint, which is most commonly affected by neuropathic disease in diabetics, the second metatarsal base migrates dorsally and laterally. CT can document the malalignment. However, although subluxation is the hallmark of early neuropathic disease, it is not specific. At this stage, three-phase bone scan is typically hot on all phases owing to the marked hyperemia and reactive bone formation resulting from the joint injury and instability. A labeled WBC scan can be useful; lack of uptake in an area hot on the delayed phase of a bone scan is strong evidence that no infection is present. However, the labeled WBC scan must be interpreted in conjunction with the bone scan, since lack of uptake could alternatively imply lack of blood flow. Also, uptake can be seen with cellulitis or abscess, so the finding must correlate with focal bone uptake on the three-phase bone scan to support osseous involvement. The presence of inflammatory cells in noninfected

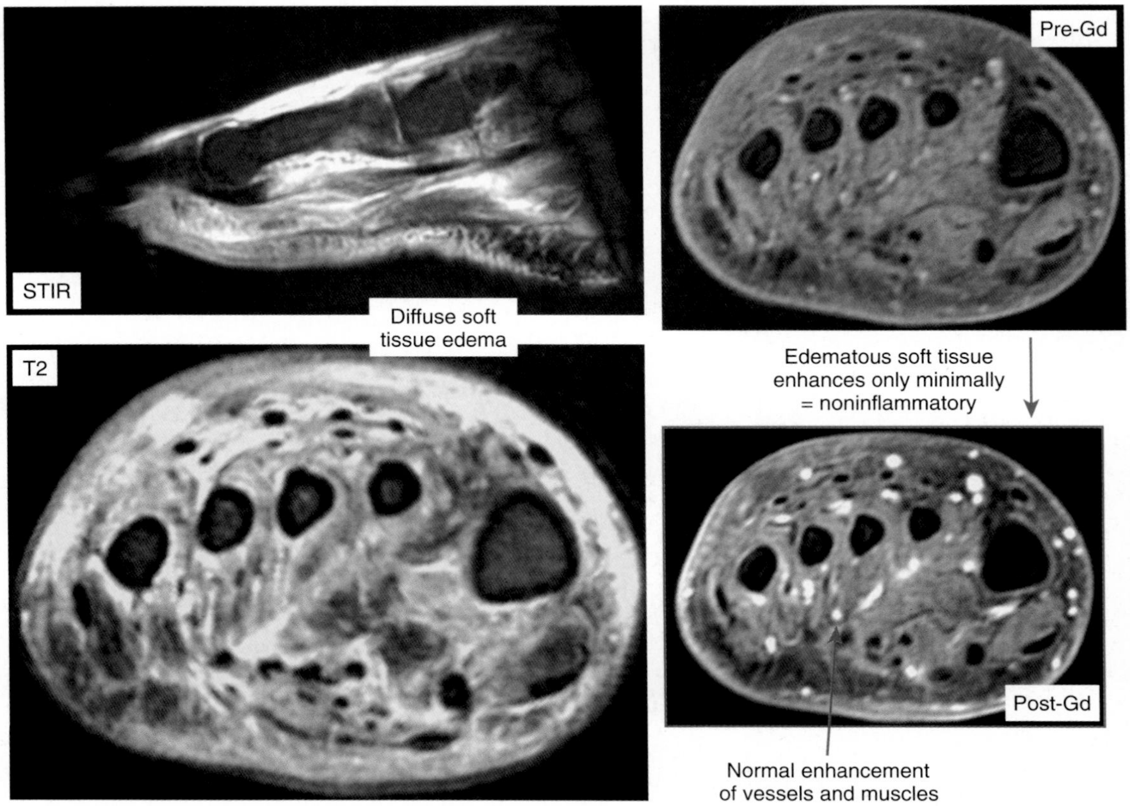

Pre-Gd
STIR
Diffuse soft tissue edema
T2
Edematous soft tissue enhances only minimally = noninflammatory
Post-Gd
Normal enhancement of vessels and muscles

Figure 5-34 The diabetic foot commonly exhibits soft tissue edema on MRI. This noninflammatory edema may be mistaken for cellulitis. Intravenous contrast can distinguish these.

neuropathic joints can result in occasional false-positive exams in patients with early neuropathic disease. This is especially true with gallium scan; labeled WBC scan is more specific. MRI in noninfected early neuropathic arthropathy shows diffuse soft tissue edema, which generally shows little enhancement, reflecting lack of inflammation. Bone marrow edema/enhancement is pronounced and is often diffuse; effusions are common. The presence of a fracture in the setting of neuropathic disease causes intense, diffuse marrow edema and enhancement (Fig. 5-37). Marrow edema and enhancement at this stage are pitfalls and are often misinterpreted as infection. However, such extensive marrow involvement, if infectious, should have signs of corresponding soft tissue infection (e.g., replacement of subcutaneous fat signal, focal enhancement, rim-enhancing abscess, sinus tract, ulcer), since contiguous spread is the rule in diabetic pedal infection.

Chronic Neuropathic Disease and Superimposed Infection (Figs. 5-38 through 5-42)

Chronic neuropathic disease/deformity presenting clinically with ulceration or swelling is another common situation prompting imaging evaluation. Chronic neuropathic osteoarthropathy in the foot/ankle is evident on radiographs as the five "Ds": deformity, debris, disorganization, dislocation, density of bone preserved. Bone destruction or dissolution may also occur. Progression of dorsal subluxation of the metatarsal bases results in a rocker-bottom deformity, reversing the curvature of the arch of the foot. The cuboid becomes weight bearing, which is a nidus for ulcer formation. Deformity at the metatarsophalangeal joints can also result in ulceration under the metatarsal heads. Radiographic signs of superimposed infection include bone lysis, periostitis, and joint erosions, although these

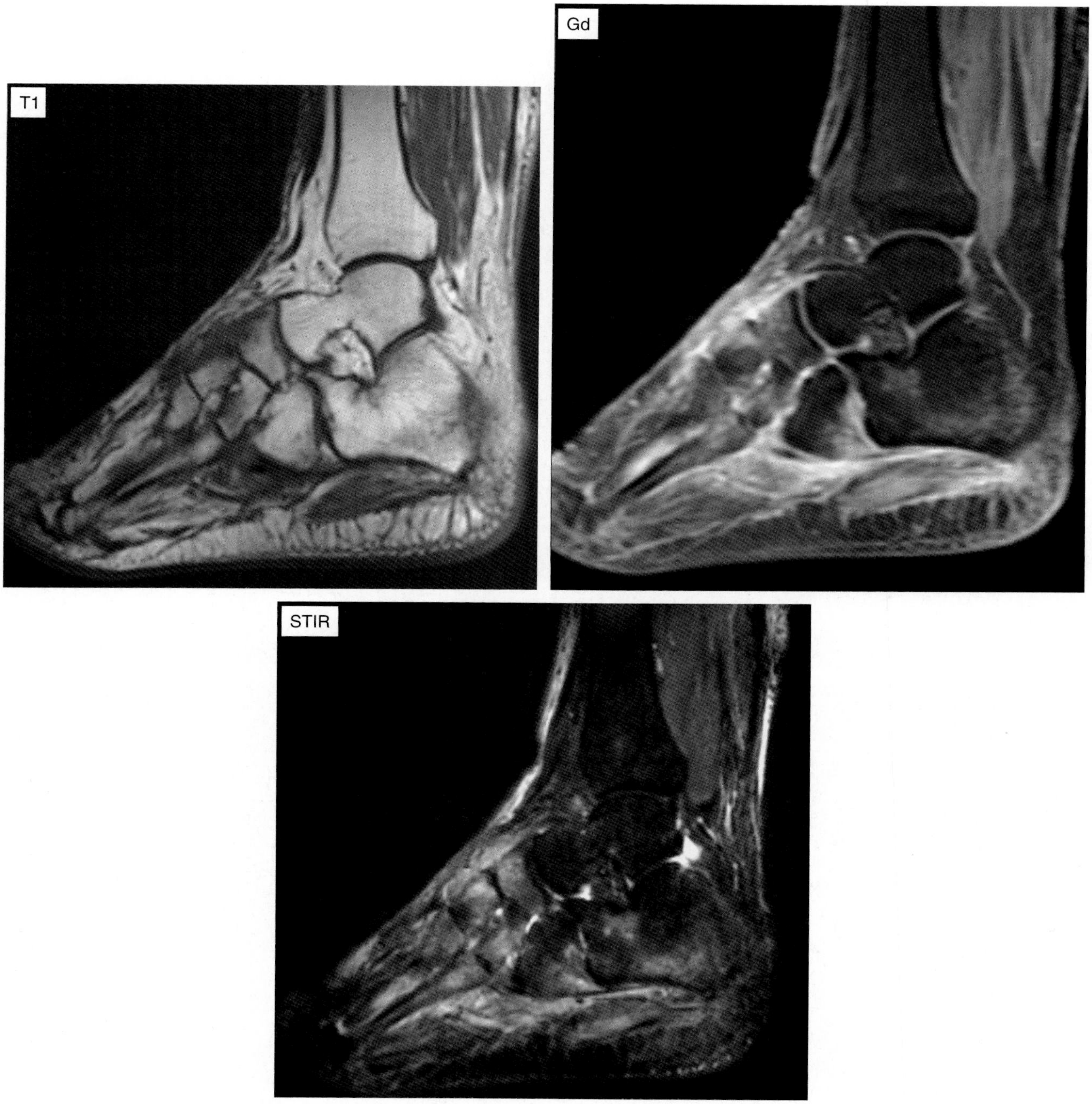
T1
Gd
STIR

Figure 5-35 Acute neuropathic osteoarthropathy of the midfoot without infection. Note lack of malalignment seen with more chronic disease. Intense bone marrow edema is seen, along with enhancement of bone, synovium and periarticular tissues. However, marrow fat is mostly preserved, and the subcutaneous fat signal is also intact. If this finding represented extensive infection, the surrounding subcutaneous tissues would almost inevitably be involved, reflecting contiguous spread in the diabetic foot.

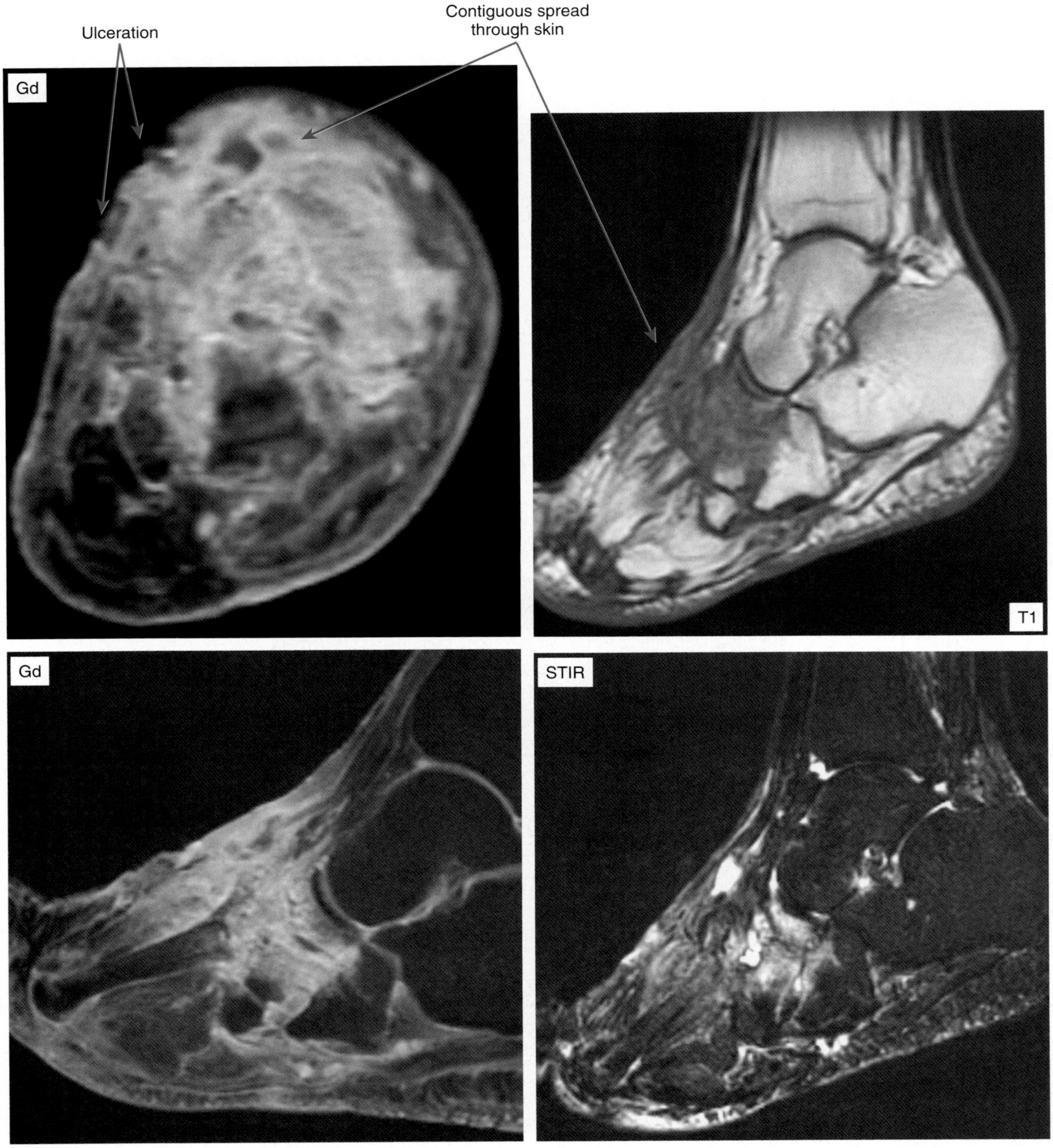
Ulceration
Contiguous spread through skin
Gd
T1
Gd
STIR

Figure 5-36 Early neuropathic arthropathy with superimposed osteomyelitis.

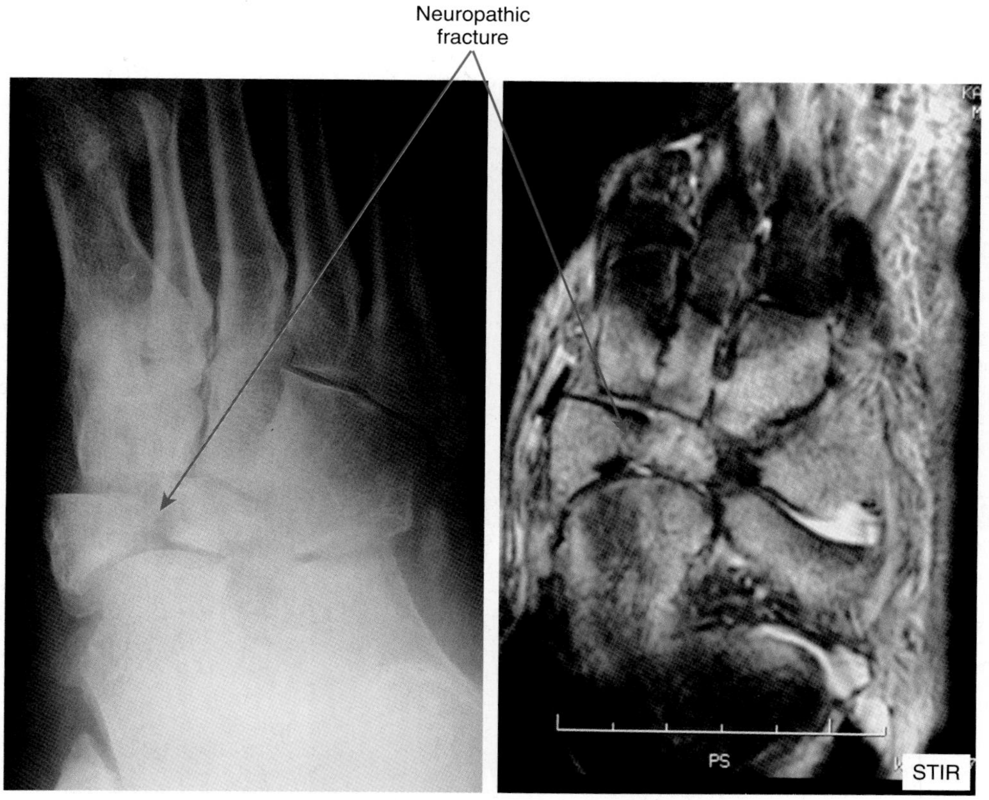
Neuropathic
fracture
PS
STIR

Figure 5-37 Neuropathic fracture. This results in intense surrounding bone marrow edema, which can simulate infection clinically and on MRI.

findings can be seen with chronic neuropathic disease as well; also, change from recent prior exams is suggestive. CT rarely provides additional useful information.

A three-phase bone scan can be misleading; false-negative exams can be seen in the setting of ischemia, which is common in this population. False-positive exams are seen, since ulceration and cellulitis cause early-phase uptake whereas chronic joint disease leads to delayed uptake. Gallium scan is nonspecific. Labeled WBC scan is more specific and remains useful in differentiating severe noninfected neuropathic disease from superimposed infection.

MRI remains the best single test for evaluation of pedal infection in diabetic patients. However, differentiation of osteomyelitis and neuropathic osteoarthropathy—acute or chronic—can be difficult because both can demonstrate marrow edema and enhancement, joint effusion, and surrounding soft tissue edema. There are some rules of thumb to use to help differentiate these entities on MR images (Table 5-1). These guidelines are based on the fact that osteomyelitis of the foot and ankle is by far most commonly related to contiguous spread from the skin. Infection spreads in all directions from the soft tissue origin. Therefore, a bone marrow abnormality without adjacent skin ulceration, sinus tract, or soft tissue inflammation is less likely to represent infection. This concept is especially useful when there are extensive bone marrow signal abnormalities; in this setting, infection is unlikely if the subcutaneous tissues are uninvolved. Diffuse soft tissue edema on T2-weighted or STIR images is nonspecific, seen in many patients related to vascular insufficiency, friction from shoes, trauma, and especially in diabetic patients. However, if the edema is associated with replacement of fat signal and enhancement, it is more likely to represent cellulitis, which, next to a marrow signal abnormality, would suggest infection.

Another consideration is that neuropathic osteoarthropathy is a predominantly articular process. Because it is a manifestation of instability, often

Text continued on page 225

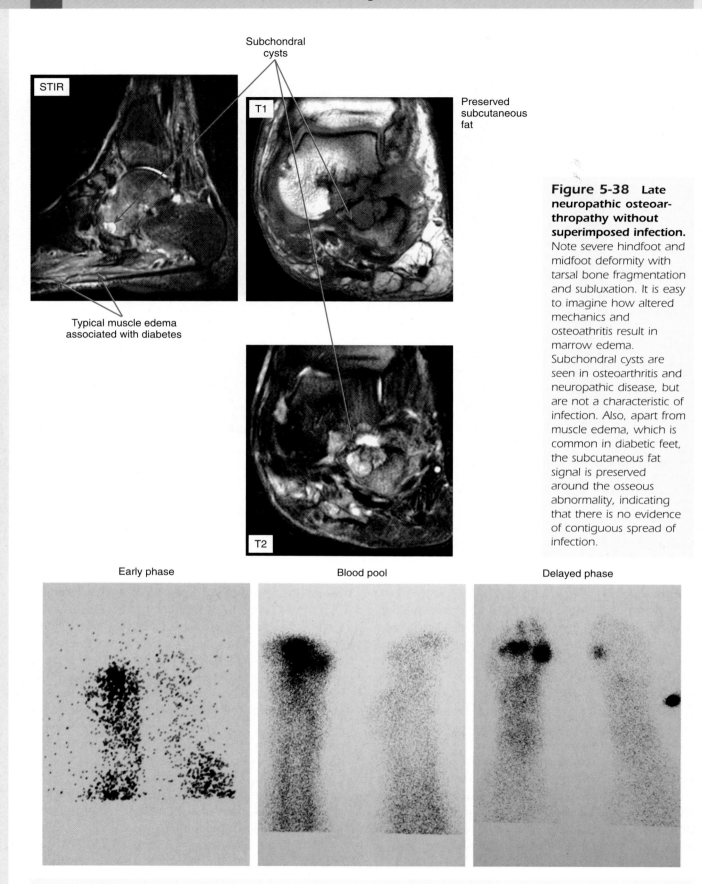

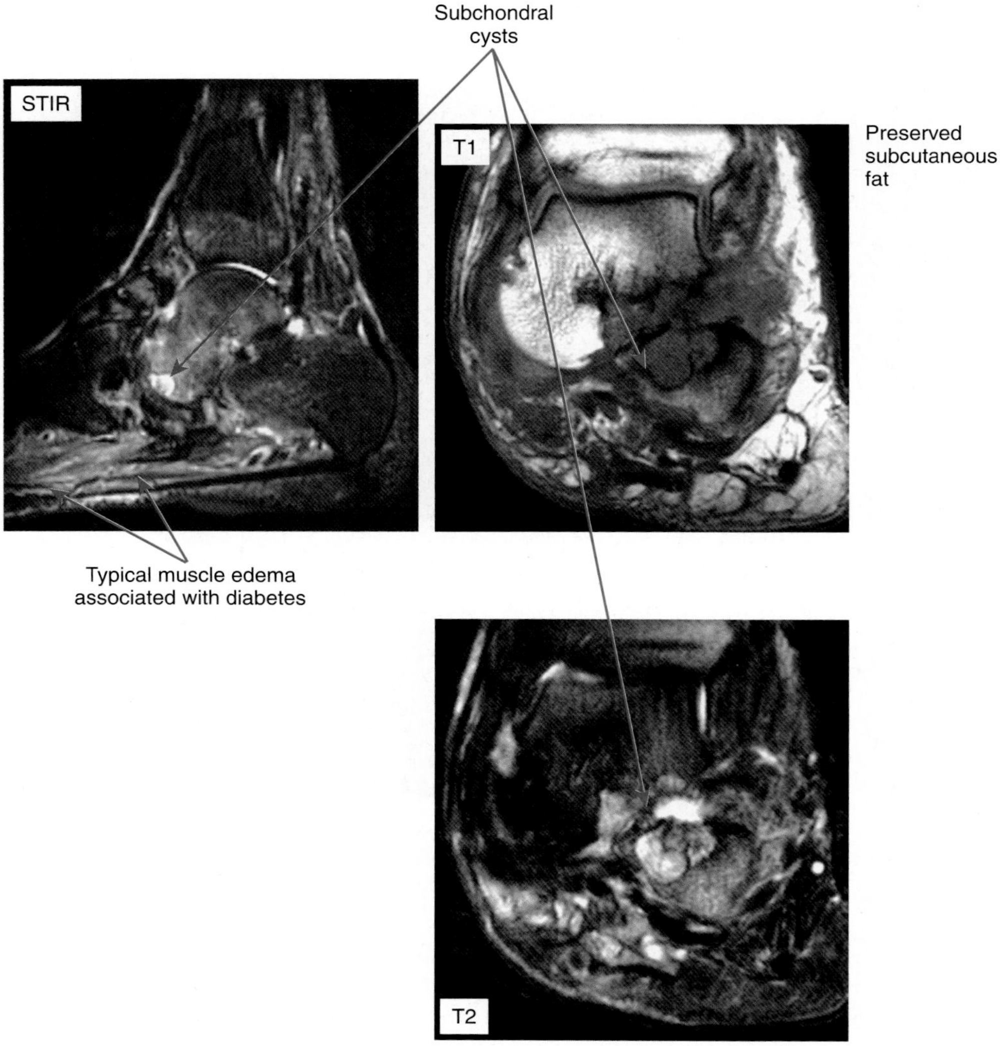
Subchondral
cysts
STIR
T1
Preserved
subcutaneous
fat
Typical muscle edema
associated with diabetes
T2

Figure 5-38 Late neuropathic osteoarthropathy without superimposed infection. Note severe hindfoot and midfoot deformity with tarsal bone fragmentation and subluxation. It is easy to imagine how altered mechanics and osteoathritis result in marrow edema. Subchondral cysts are seen in osteoarthritis and neuropathic disease, but are not a characteristic of infection. Also, apart from muscle edema, which is common in diabetic feet, the subcutaneous fat signal is preserved around the osseous abnormality, indicating that there is no evidence of contiguous spread of infection.

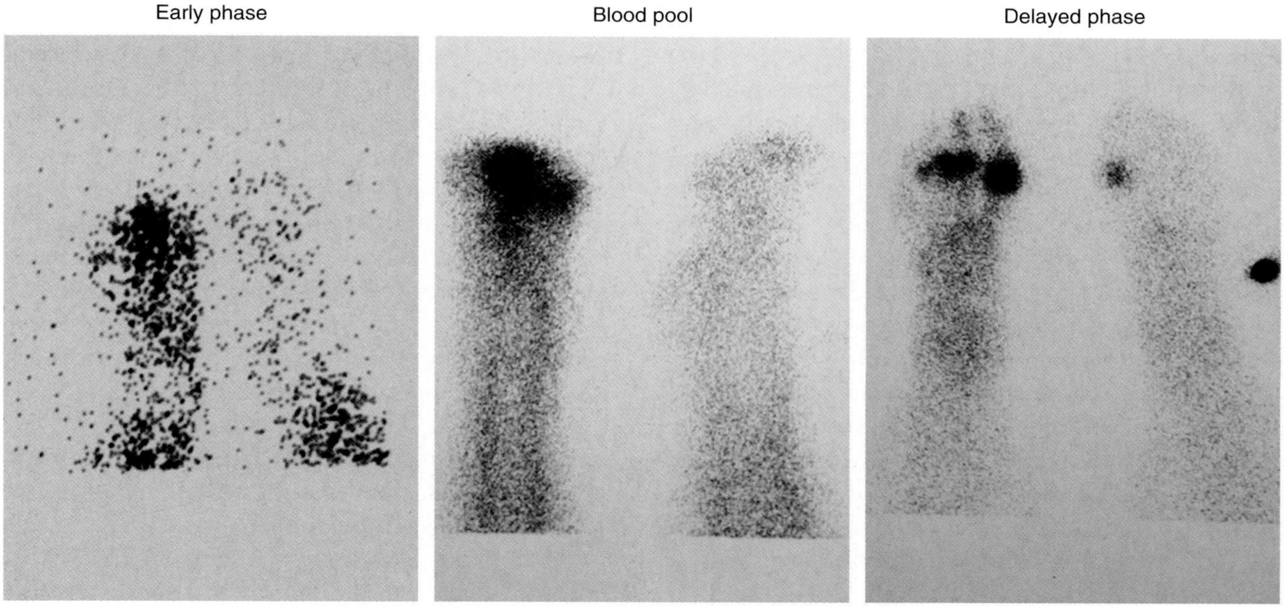
Early phase
Blood pool
Delayed phase

Figure 5-39 Neuropathic disease of the metatarsophalangeal joints on three-phase bone scan. (Courtesy of Hans Ledermann, MD, Basel, Switzerland.)

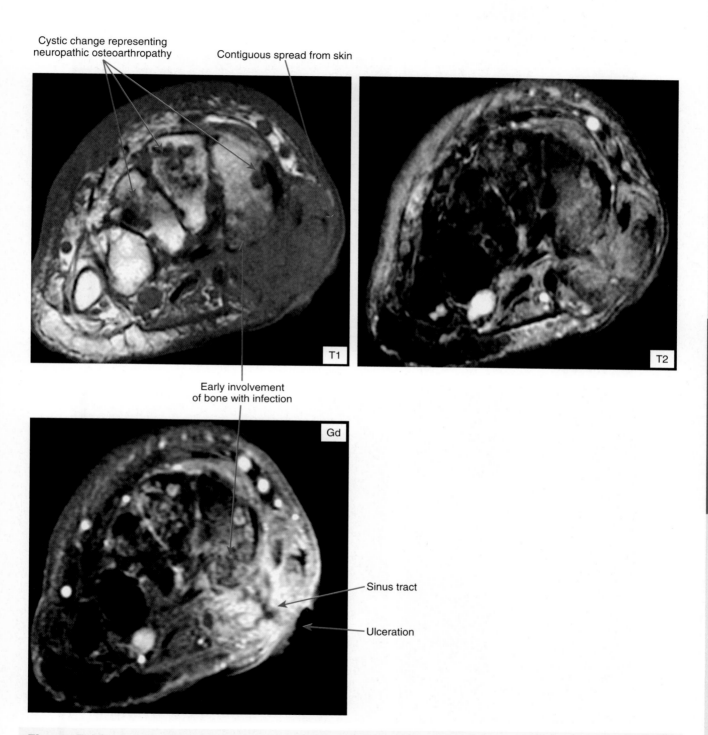

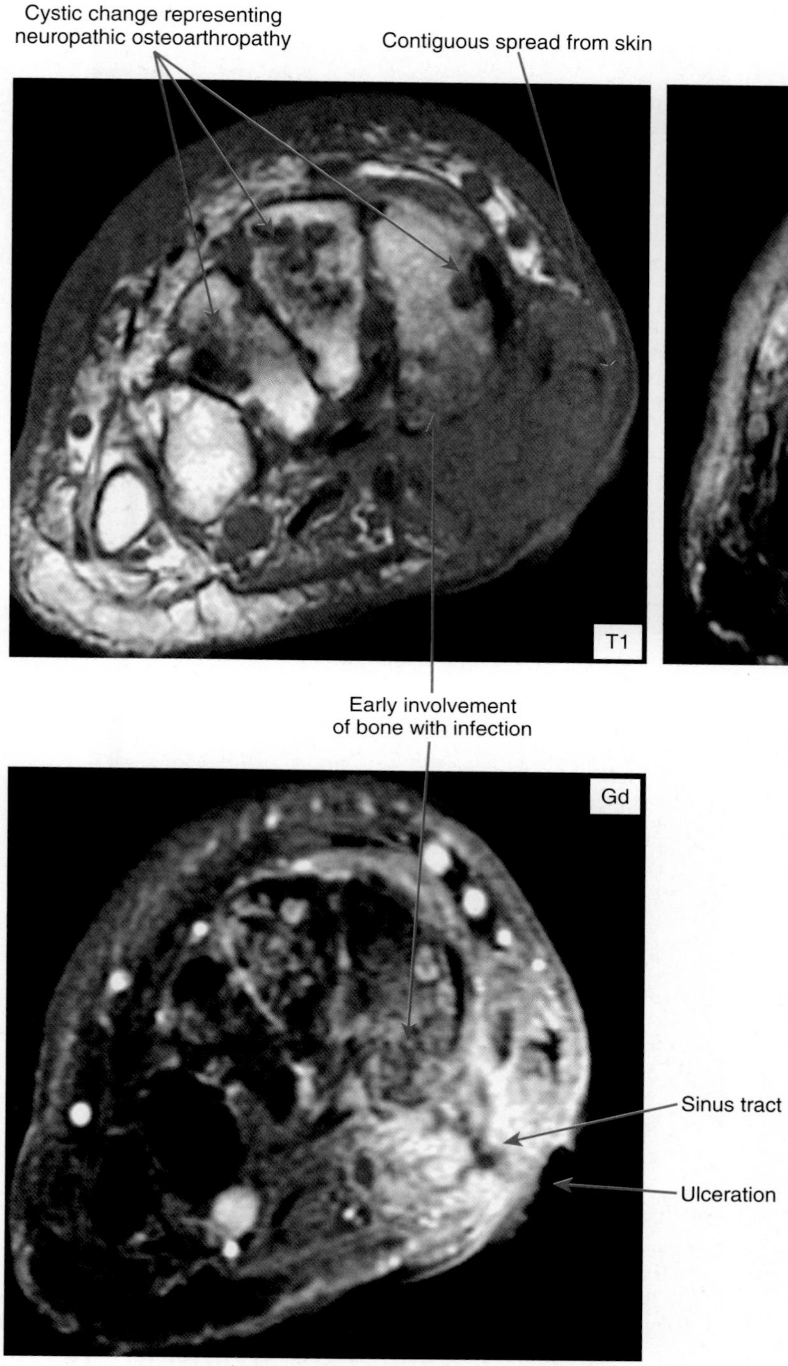
Cystic change representing neuropathic osteoarthropathy
Contiguous spread from skin
T1
T2
Early involvement of bone with infection
Gd
Sinus tract
Ulceration

Figure 5-40 Chronic neuropathic disease with early osteomyelitis.

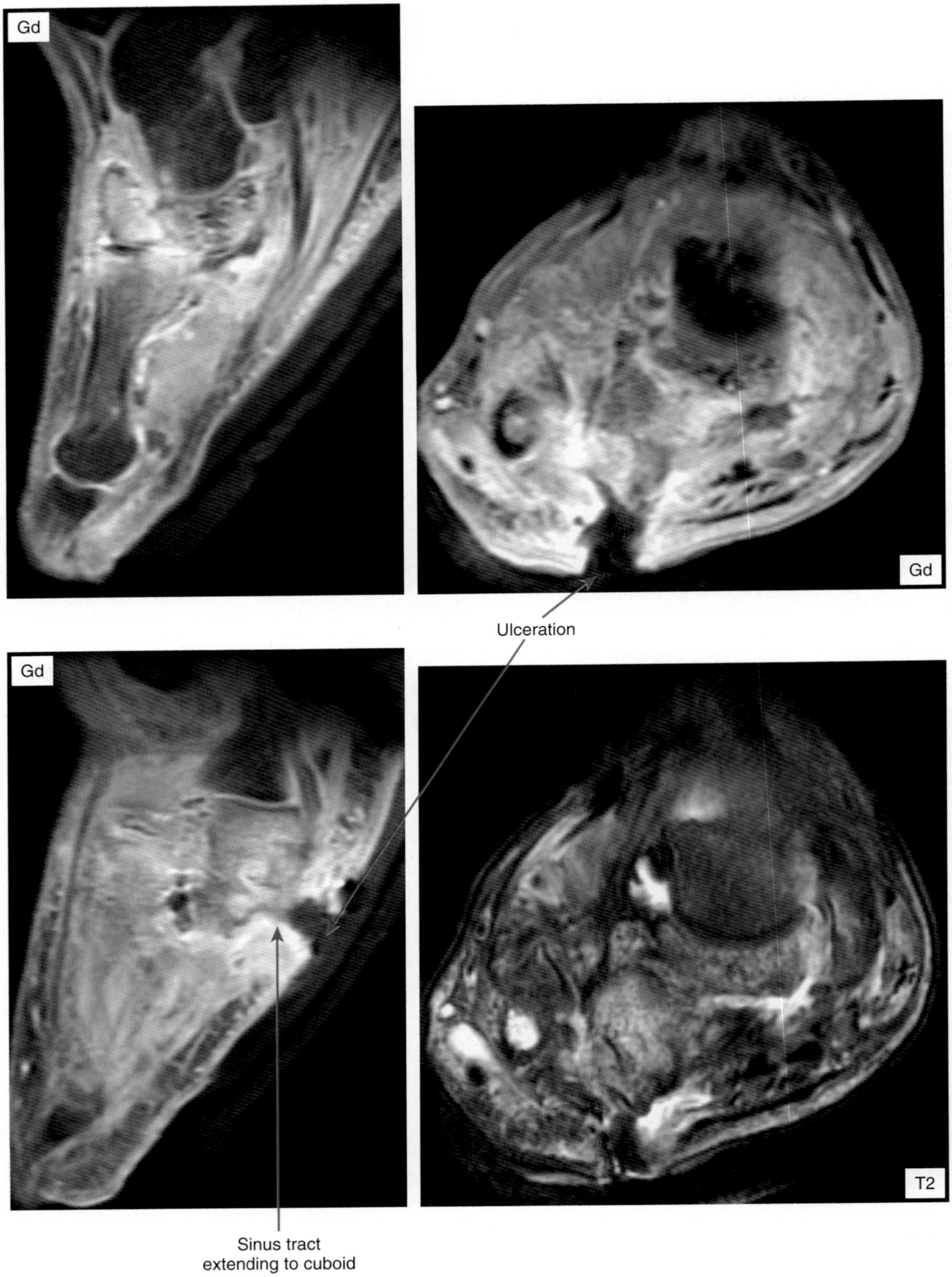
Gd
Gd
Ulceration
Gd
T2
Sinus tract
extending to cuboid

Figure 5-41 *Chronic neuropathic disease with superimposed osteomyelitis.*

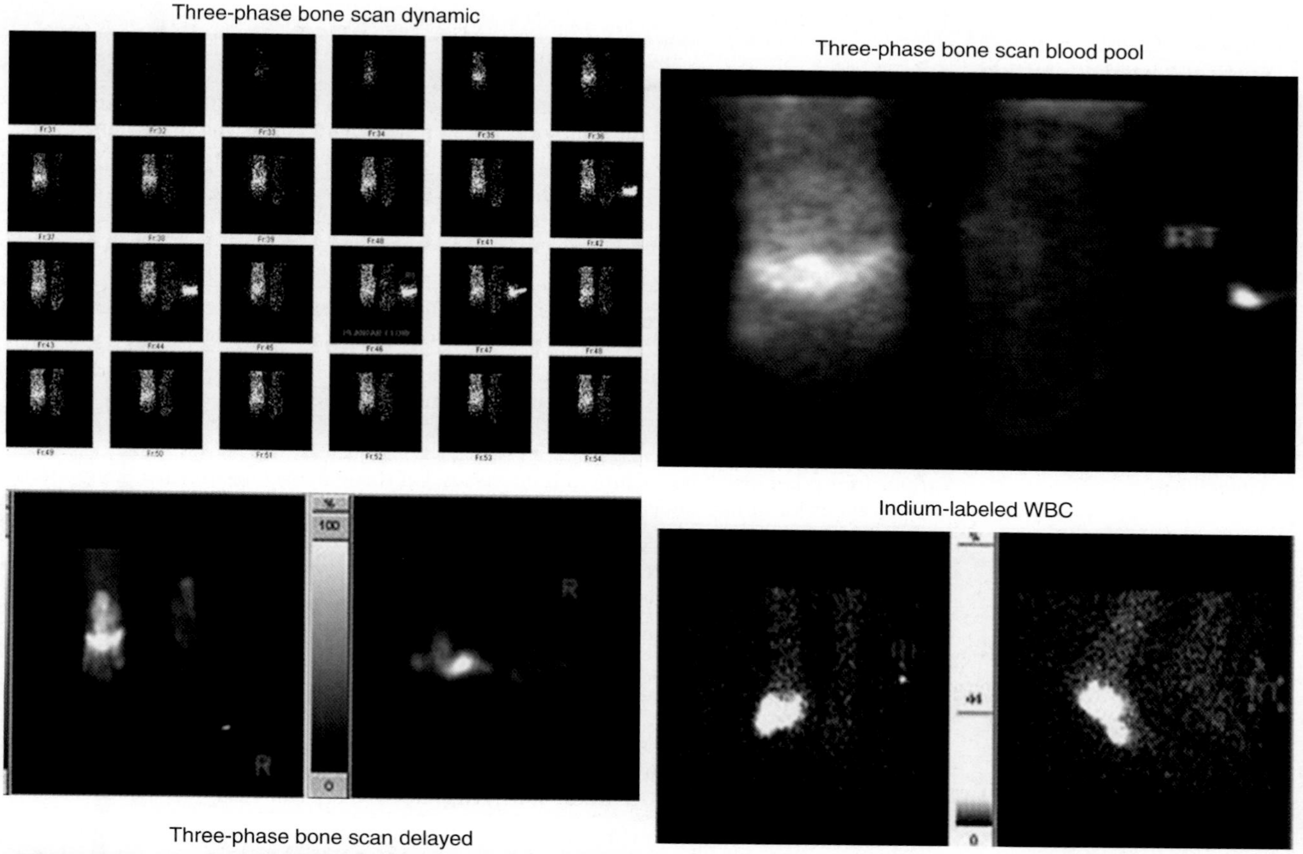
Three-phase bone scan dynamic
Three-phase bone scan blood pool
Indium-labeled WBC
Three-phase bone scan delayed

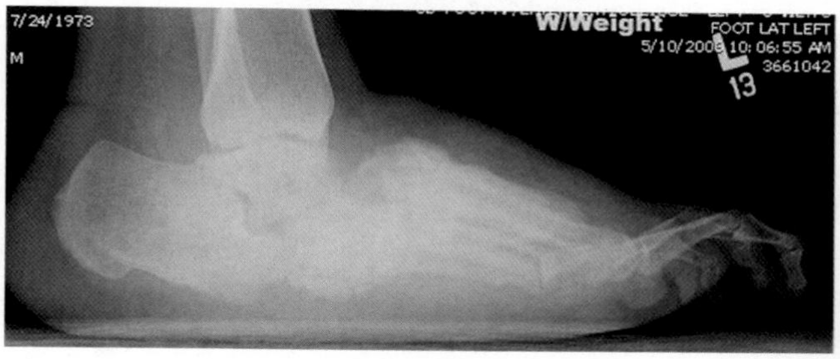
7/24/1973
M
W/Weight
FOOT LAT LEFT
3661042

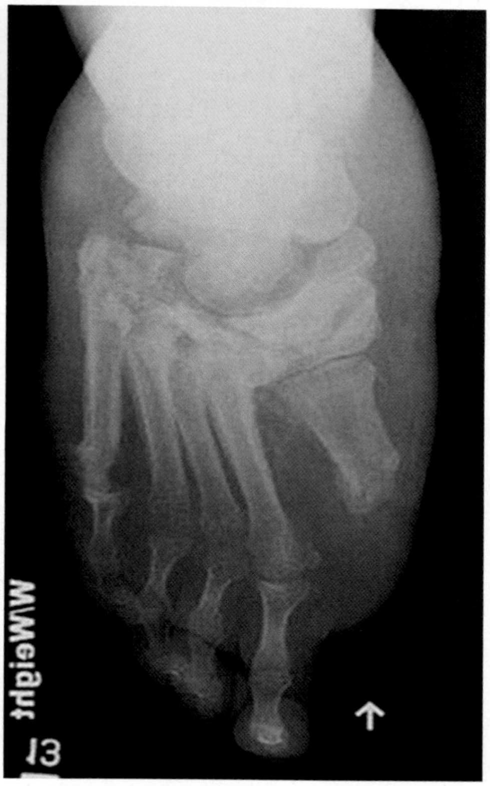
W/Weight

Figure 5-42 Neuropathic osteoarthropathy and osteomyelitis diagnosed by comparing findings on three-phase bone scan and labeled WBC scan. Uptake in bone on three-phase bone scan could be related to neuropathic osteoarthropathy alone. Intense uptake in the same location on the labeled WBC scan increases the likelihood of superimposed infection. (Courtesy of Hans Ledermann, M.D., Basel, Switzerland.)

Table 5-1 Differentiation of Disease Entities on Imaging Examinations

Atypical Bacterial Infection	
Lyme disease	Tick-borne organism common in the spring in the northeastern United States. In addition to classic skin lesions and systemic symptoms, it can result in arthralgias and unexplained joint effusion
Brucellosis	Endemic in midwestern United States, Saudi Arabia, South America, southern Europe, from infected milk/meat ingestion; causes septic arthritis, osteomyelitis, and diskitis; spine involvement relatively common; may appear atypical on imaging, like TB; however, no specific manifestations
Actinomycosis	Most common sites: Mandible, spine, ribs, pelvis; often begins as lung infection that grows through the rib cage ("necessitates"; also called "necessitating pneumonia")
Bacillary angiomatosis	Infection with rickettsial organisms can result in a skin lesion with prominent vascularity; underlying bone can become involved with a permeative pattern
Fungal Infection	
Aspergillosis	Various forms: Localized destruction of bone versus soft tissue mass, disseminated. Lung involvement common; underlying immunosuppression common
Coccidioidomycosis	Endemic in southwest United States. Travel history common. Localized destructive lesion versus soft tissue mass. Disseminated form with multiple masses. Simulates bone metastases or soft tissue sarcoma
Candidiasis	Typically associated with immunosuppression; may appear as disseminated abscesses
Sporotrichosis (rose thorn disease)	Saprophyte on vegetation, enters body through cut; enters lymphatic system; extremity infection with lymph node involvement. Presents as nodal mass on imaging (especially epitrochlear)
Mucormycosis	Sinus involvement; bone destruction on imaging
Histoplasmosis	*Histoplasma capsulatum* endemic in United States; lung/mediastinal involvement; bone involvement rare. *H. dubosii* in Africa, bone involvement more common
Mycetoma	Various organisms; tropical climates, India, Africa, South America; chronic granulomatous infection, invasive, foot most common (Madura foot)
Parasitic Infection	
Echinococcus	*E. granulosus* versus *E. multilocularis;* parasitic cysts can look like abscesses on CT and MRI, with calcification; involvement of bone rare but can result in lytic, "blow-out" lesions
Cysticercosis	Involvement of muscles with small multifocal calcifications
Filariasis	Involvement of lymphatic channels, resulting in obstruction/valvular incompetence and extremity swelling (elephantiasis)
Syphillis	Spirochete infection; congenital infection with diffuse sclerosis/periostitis. Adult infection with destructive lesions in tertiary form
Viral Infection	
HIV	Musculoskeletal manifestations—mostly related to opportunistic infections—which often become disseminated because of immunocompromised state. Also susceptible to neoplasia including lymphoma and Kaposi sarcoma
Unknown	
Chronic recurrent multifocal osteomyelitis	Rare condition seen in adolescents and children characterized by a prolonged or fluctuating course of infectious-like processes involving various bones. Although imaging appearance and symptoms suggest infection, no causative organism has been identified. Etiology may stem from an immunocompromised state or viral organism. Involved bones have radiologic findings typical of osteomyelitis and/or Brodie abscess. However, multiple foci around the body are often seen at presentation, with spontaneous remission and recurrence or onset at new locations subsequently (see Fig. 5-66)

multiple joints in a region are similarly affected (e.g., the entire Lisfranc joint, Chopart joint, or multiple adjacent metatarsophalangeal joints). This finding and other articular manifestations of neuropathic disease (subluxation, cysts, necrotic debris) are not as common in infection. Also, marrow changes associated with neuropathic osteoarthropathy can be extensive (especially at the midfoot), but tend to be centered at a joint and subarticular bone and are present on both sides of the joint fairly equally. Osteomyelitis shows more diffuse marrow involvement and unless there is primary septic arthritis, the marrow changes are generally greater on one side of the joint.

Location of disease is also important. Osteomyelitis occurs predominantly at the metatarsal heads, the toes, the calcaneus, and the malleoli, a distribution that mirrors that of friction, callus, and ulceration. Neuropathic osteoarthropathy is by far most common at the Lisfranc and Chopart joints. However, in a patient with foot deformity, contiguous spread of infection can occur at atypical sites (e.g., the cuboid in cases of rocker-bottom deformity).

In patients with underlying neuropathic osteoarthropathy, superimposed ulceration and soft tissue infection can create a significant diagnostic dilemma. In this setting, to diagnose osteomyelitis look for focal marrow signal abnormalities adjacent to the site of soft tissue infection that are different from the other areas of neuropathic involvement. Aspiration or biopsy of suspicious areas may be required. If percutaneous biopsy is performed, the needle route should be planned away from the area of soft tissue infection. If there is no osteomyelitis, a sample obtained via infected soft tissue could inoculate the bone. Culture results of percutaneous bone biopsy specimens in pedal infection may be unreliable owing to contamination from underlying infected soft tissue.

Infection in Paralyzed Patients (Figs. 5-43 through 5-45)

Paralyzed and bedridden patients are prone to pressure ulceration and contiguous spread of infection. This is most commonly seen at the pelvis (at the ischial tuberosities, the greater trochanters, and the sacrum/coccyx), the posterior calcanei, and the knees over the condylar prominences. Typically, a deep ulcer is seen extending to the bone, with underlying acute or chronic osteomyelitis. The ulcer and associated wide sinus tract are thick-walled, with marked surrounding enhancement representing chronic granulation tissue and acute inflammation. Chronic osteomyelitis and hyperemia often result in bone resorption, especially at the ischia, which can appear diminutive or whittled radiographically. In acute infection, septic arthritis of an adjacent joint is common, and the joint may contain air extending through the tract from the skin; abscess formation occurs in the adjacent soft tissues and can extend far from the site of inoculation, spreading along fascial planes. For example, it is common in acute infections arising from ischial decubitus ulcers to see inflammation and abscess extending into the obturator region and pubis anteriorly, through the sciatic notch to the gluteus region, and superiorly to the sacrum and lumbar spine.

Infection Around Metal Implants (Figs. 5-46 through 5-48)

Assessment of the postoperative patient, especially after arthroplasty, is difficult. Radiographs may show signs of loosening such as lucency at the bone-cement or bone-implant interface, subsidence (component "sinking into" the underlying bone), and periosteal reaction. However, these findings appear late in the course of infection and are relatively insensitive (see Fig. 5-15). Metal artifact may preclude evaluation on MR or CT. Metal reduction techniques on MR can be helpful, such as increasing bandwidth (refer to the metal protocol on the accompanying CD) and acquiring pre-contrast and post-contrast sequences. Marrow edema and enhancement in the surrounding bone can be detected occasionally, but more commonly thick rim-enhancing fluid collections around the components are seen, which suggest infection. Multidetector CT, with its capability to reduce metal artifact, is also helpful for diagnosing infection in this setting. Focal lucency around the implants and fluid collections can be observed on CT. Bone scan can show increased uptake in the areas of infection, and labeled white cell scanning is also useful. Ultimately, however, aspiration with culture and fluid analysis should be performed to document presence or absence of infection (see Chapter 2). Contrast arthrography is useful for detecting communicating soft tissue collections. MRI can serve an adjunctive role, diagnosing fluid collections far from the implants that may need to be drained during surgery.

Text continued on page 231

SECTION III

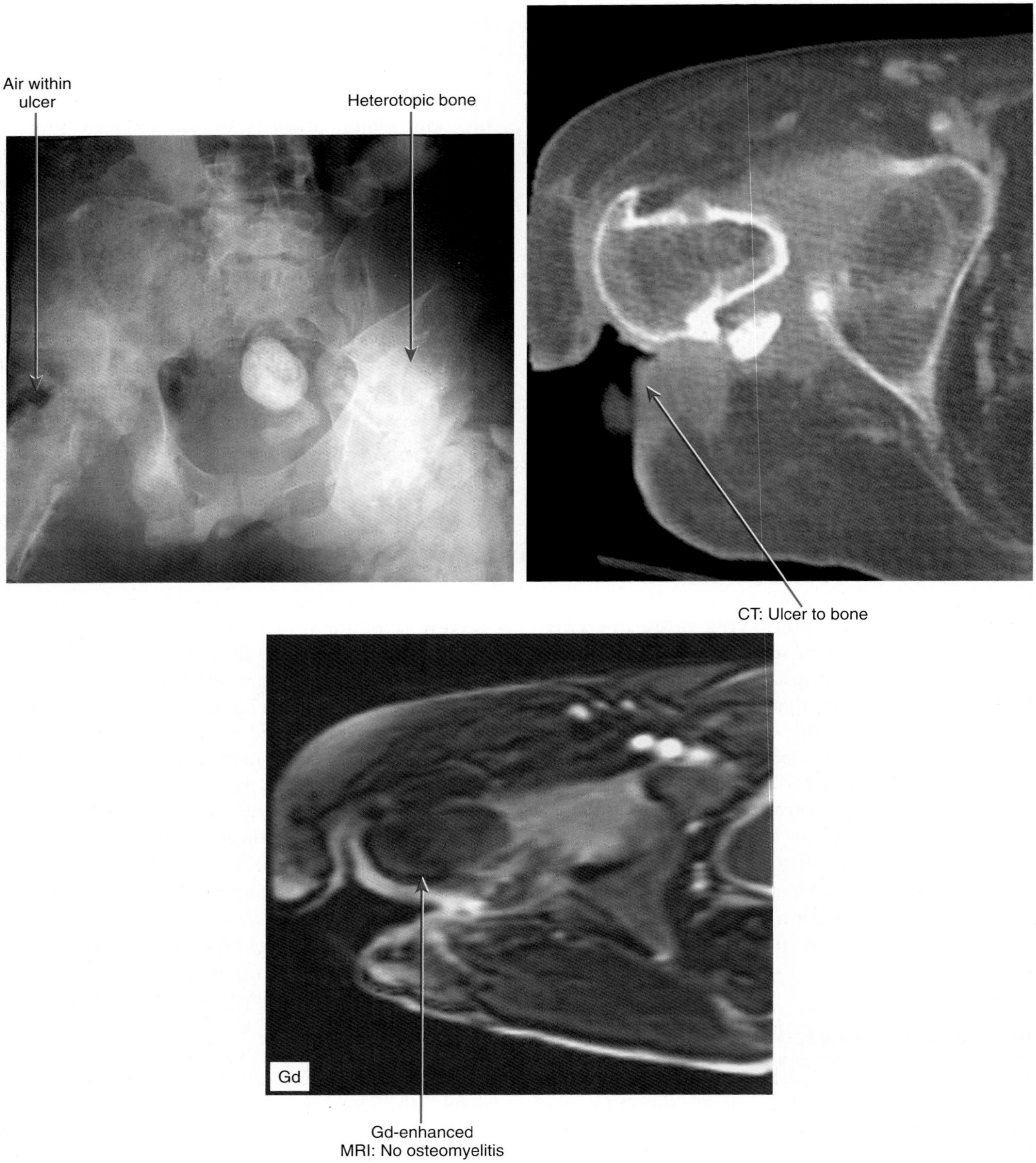
Air within
ulcer
Heterotopic bone
CT: Ulcer to bone
Gd
Gd-enhanced
MRI: No osteomyelitis

Figure 5-43 Paralyzed patient with heterotopic bone formation around the left hip and decubitus ulcer at the right hip. MRI is ideal for evaluating underlying osteomyelitis and extent of soft tissue disease.

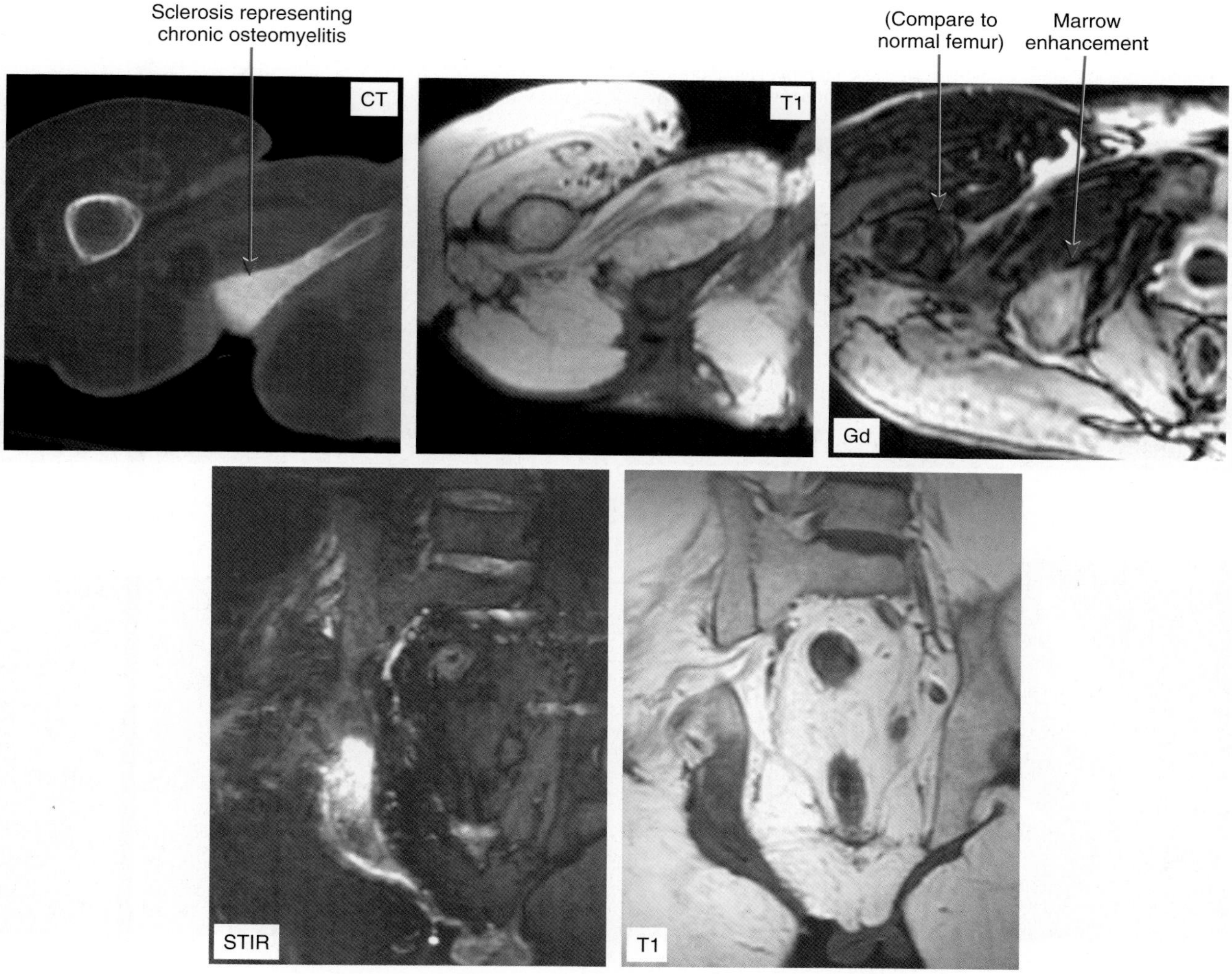
Sclerosis representing chronic osteomyelitis
CT
T1
(Compare to normal femur)
Marrow enhancement
Gd
STIR
T1

Figure 5-44 Chronic osteomyelitis in a paralyzed patient, characterized by bone sclerosis on CT. Active infection is seen on MRI as marrow edema on STIR and marrow enhancement.

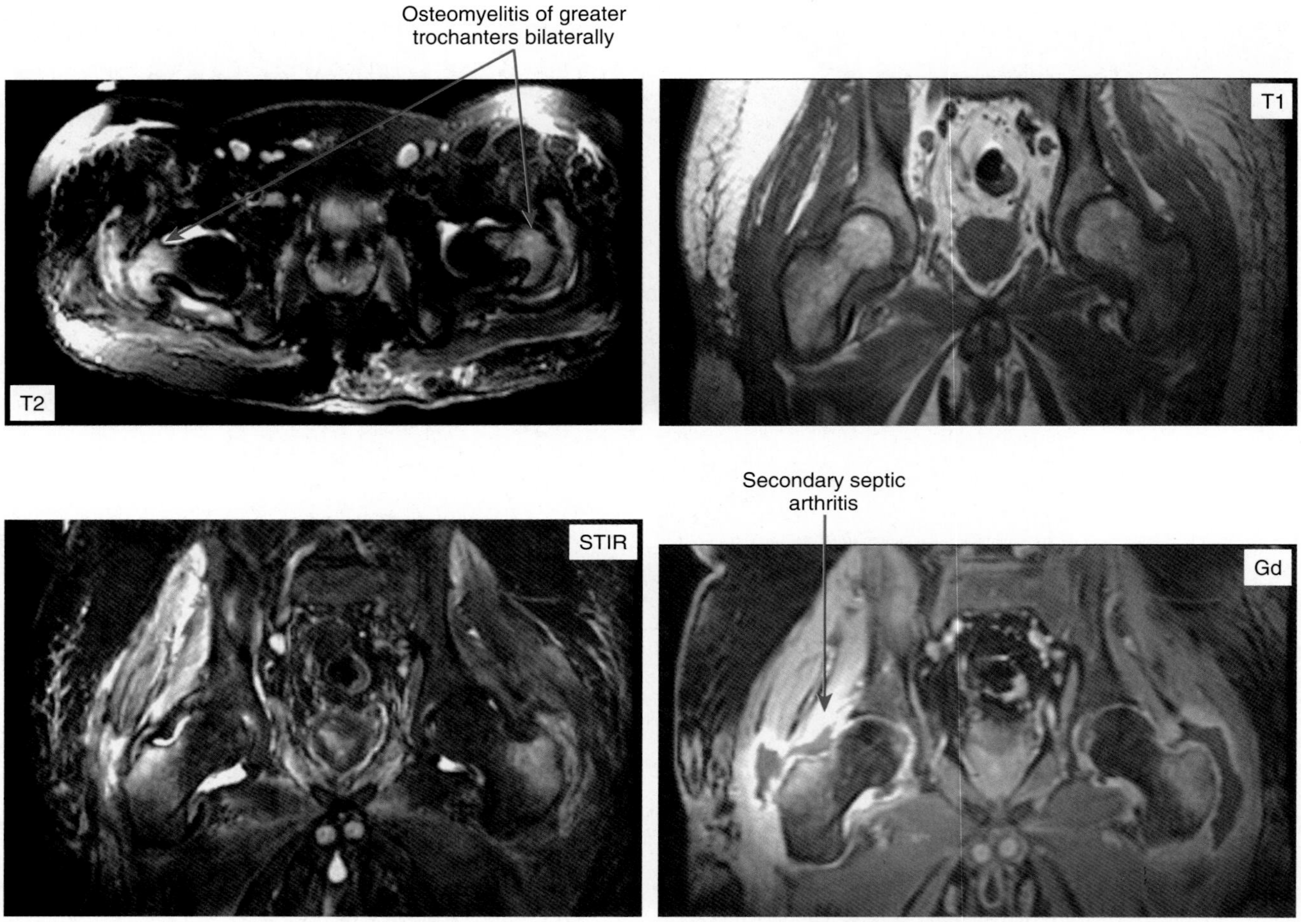
Osteomyelitis of greater trochanters bilaterally
T2
T1
STIR
Secondary septic arthritis
Gd

Figure 5-45 Paralyzed patient with septic bursitis of greater trochanteric and osteomyelitis bilaterally.

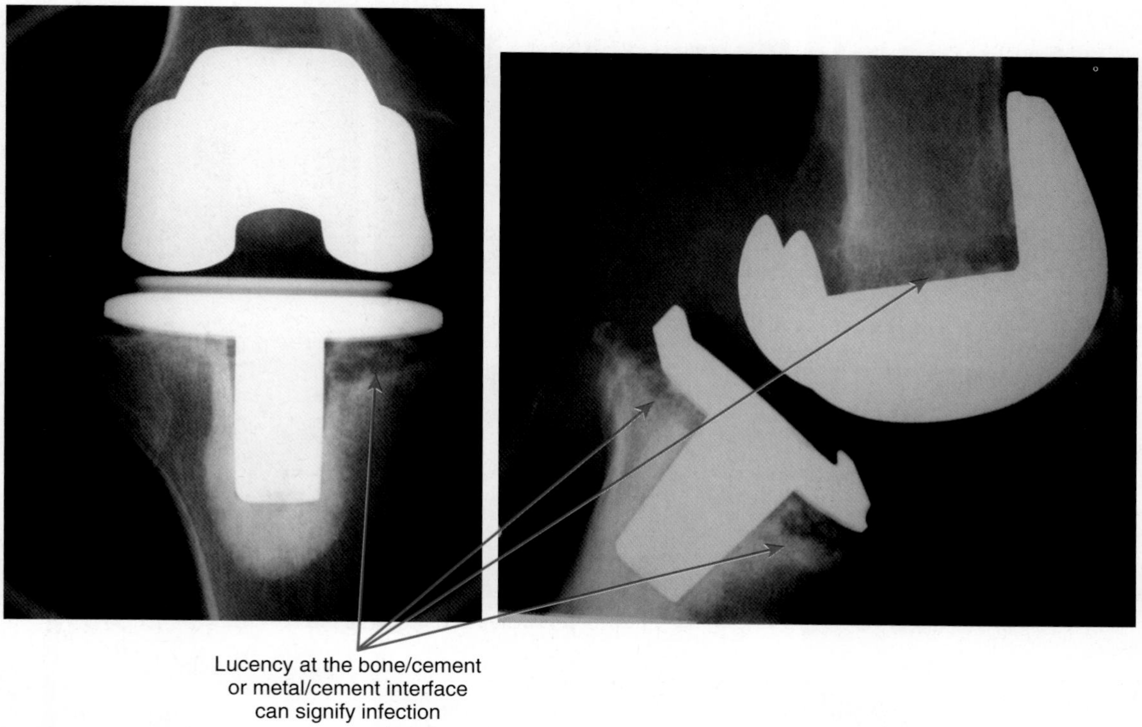
Lucency at the bone/cement
or metal/cement interface
can signify infection

Figure 5-46 Total knee arthroplasty with infection. It is important to compare with the post-op exam as well as interval exams to look for changes, since some areas of lucency can occur normally especially at the edges of the components. Purulent fluid was aspirated. Particle disease can result in a similar radiographic appearance.

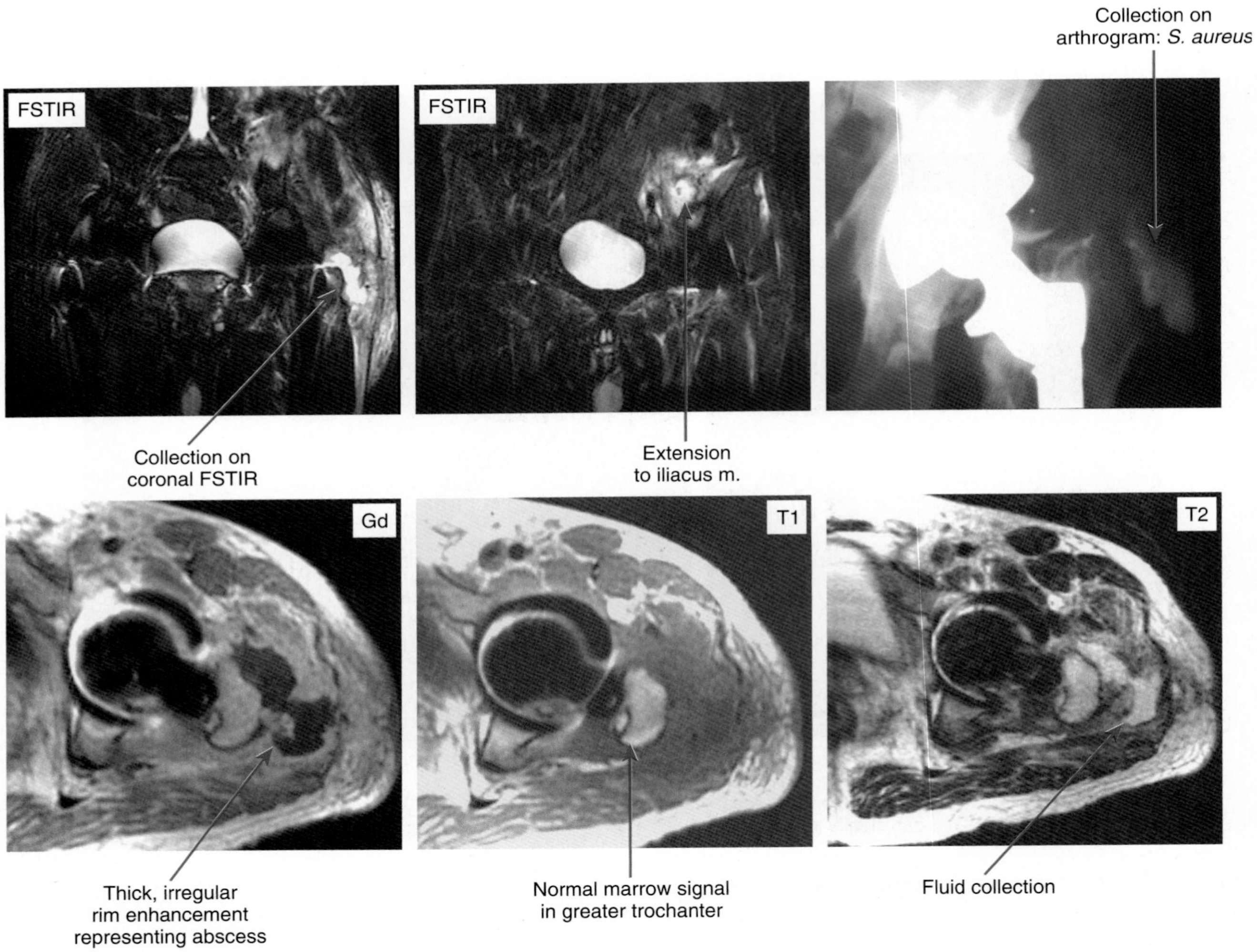
Collection on
arthrogram: S. aureus
FSTIR
FSTIR
Collection on
coronal FSTIR
Extension
to iliacus m.
Gd
T1
T2
Thick, irregular
rim enhancement
representing abscess
Normal marrow signal
in greater trochanter
Fluid collection

Figure 5-47 Hip prosthesis infection: evaluation with MRI. Using a metal protocol, good visualization of the surrounding tissues can be achieved. MRI shows location and extent of periprosthetic fluid collections and (depending on composition of the prosthesis) abnormalities in the adjacent marrow.

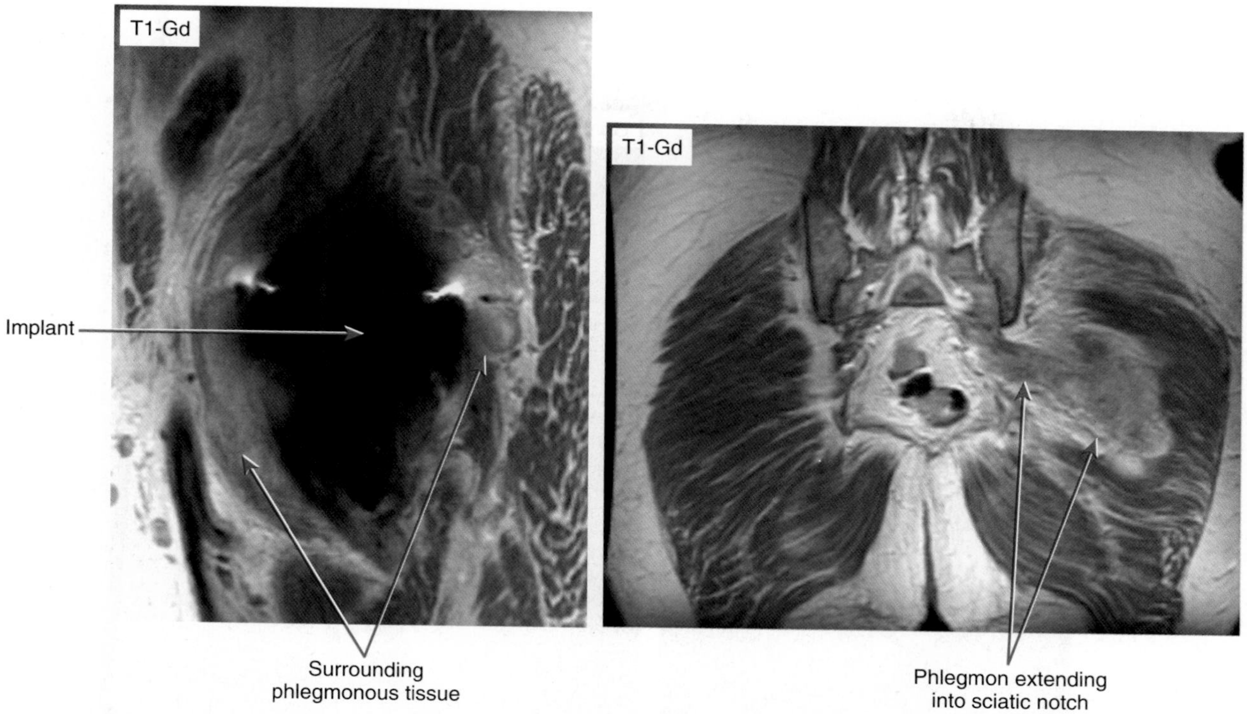
T1-Gd
Implant
Surrounding phlegmonous tissue
T1-Gd
Phlegmon extending into sciatic notch

Figure 5-48 Following total hip arthroplasty, this patient developed fever and symptoms of sciatic nerve irritation. MRI shows phlegmonous tissue extending from the hip into the sciatic notch. Significant metal artifact is due to presence of a cobalt-chrome implant, which is more prone to artifact than titanium. Noncontrast T1-weighted images are useful to distinguish hematoma (usually exhibits some high signal) from phlegmon (low T1 signal). Contrast is useful to depict areas of inflammation.

ATYPICAL MANIFESTATIONS OF INFECTION

"Classic"/Advanced Osteomyelitis

In most civilized areas, musculoskeletal infection is diagnosed in the early stages, on clinical grounds and by imaging, before reaching the advanced stages that yield "classic" findings. Therefore, we are entering an era in which the traditional radiologic appearance of osteomyelitis can be considered "atypical." Nevertheless, it persists in isolated cases as well as in rural and disadvantaged populations; associated imaging findings should be recognized by radiologists for their uncommon yet important presentation.

As infection sets in, areas of bone become necrotic, and a sequestrum, a fragment of dead bone seen on imaging as a sclerotic, nonenhancing focus of calcification, may be seen. The sequestrum is often surrounded by abscess or granulation tissue. The sequestrum acts as a persistent nidus of infection. Because of this devitalization, antibiotics cannot penetrate this tissue, and bacteria can remain incorporated for long periods in a dormant state, periodically reactivating infection. Therefore, successful treatment depends on debridement of necrotic bone. In the advanced untreated state, the body attempts to wall off the infection by forming reactive bone around the site. This shell of active bone formation surrounding the necrotic bone is an involucrum; on imaging it resembles a thick shell of periostitis. The bone actually tries to expel the sequestra, forming a hole in the living bone (a cloaca). A sinus tract extends from the cloaca to the skin, eventually decompressing pus and fragments of dead bone (see Fig. 5-16).

Chronic Osteomyelitis
(Figs. 5-49 through 5-51)

Chronic osteomyelitis is commonly seen in paralyzed patients, in feet of diabetics, and occasionally

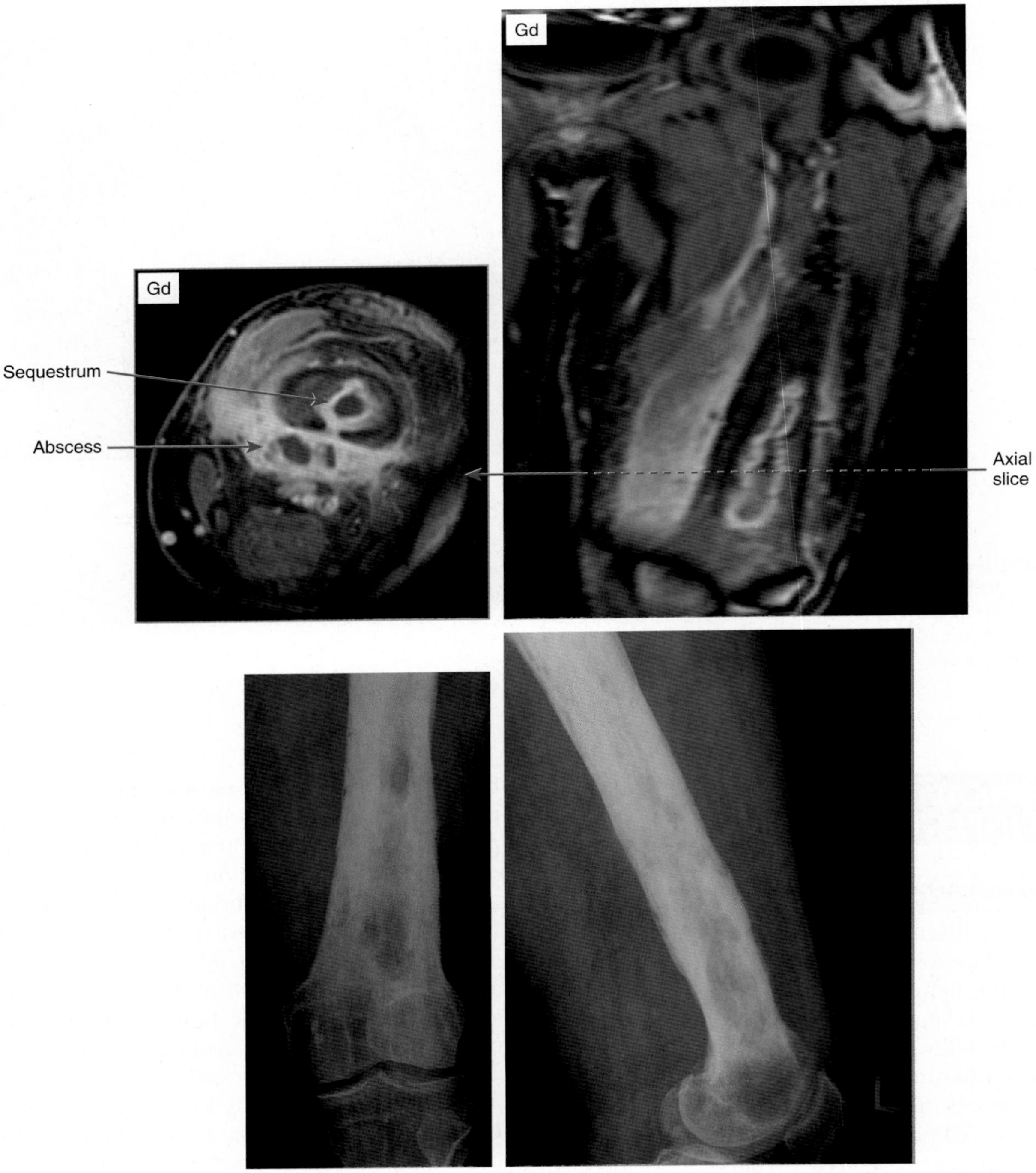
Gd
Gd
Sequestrum
Abscess
Axial slice
L

Figure 5-49 Acute on chronic osteomyelitis. Sclerosis and periosteal thickening are compatible with a longstanding process. Active nature is suggested by areas of enhancement in the bone and adjacent soft tissue. Central medullary infarct serves as a sequestrum resulting in persistent infection.

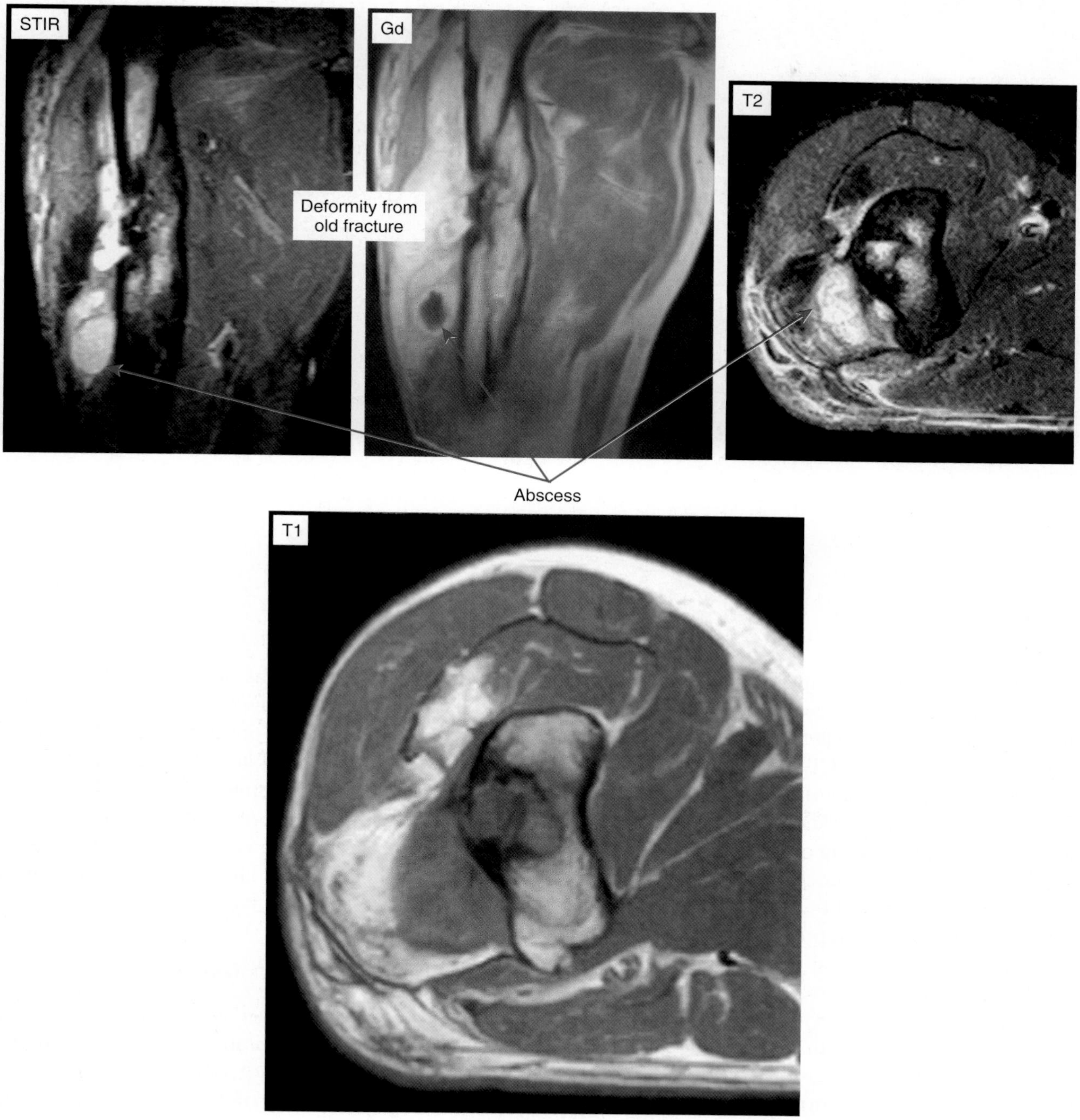
STIR
Gd
T2
Deformity from old fracture
Abscess
T1

Figure 5-50 Acute-on-chronic osteomyelitis following fracture.

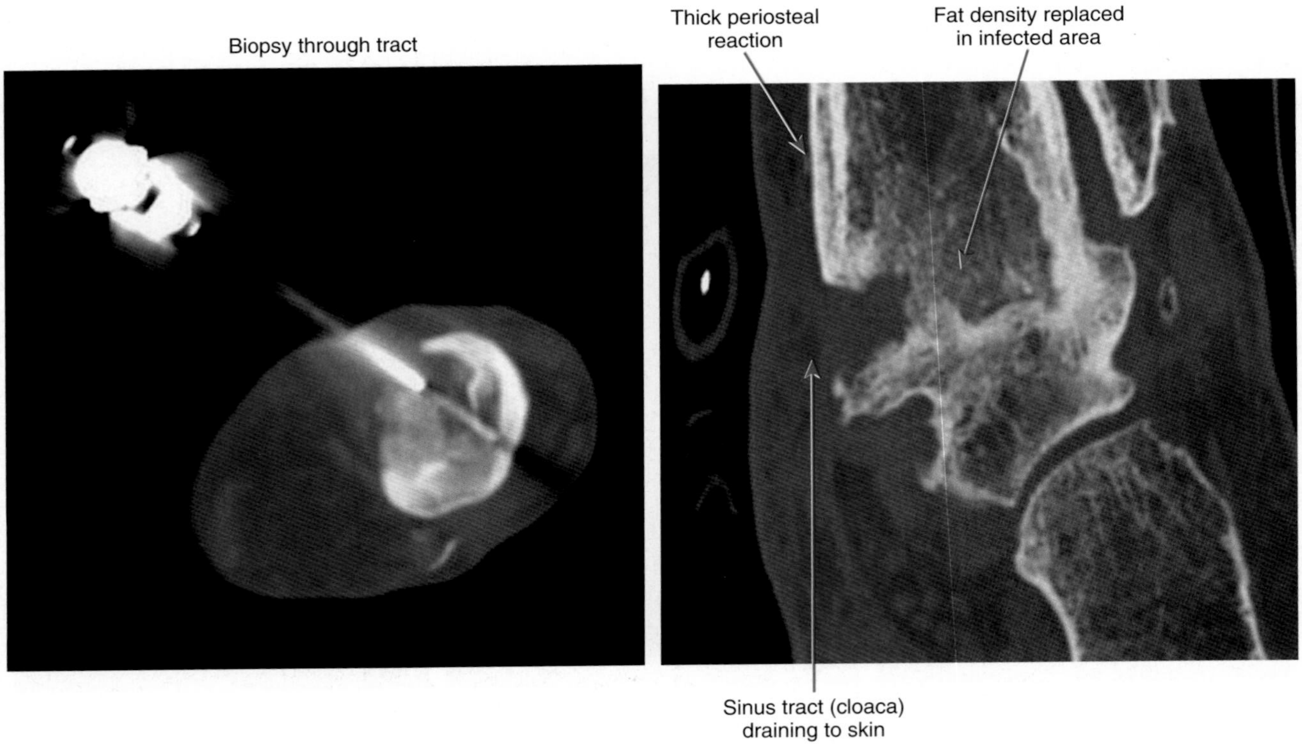
Biopsy through tract
Thick periosteal reaction
Fat density replaced in infected area
Sinus tract (cloaca) draining to skin

Figure 5-51 Biopsy for chronic osteomyelitis.

following an open fracture; it can also occur in immunocompromised patients with atypical organisms, and in chronically untreated/mistreated infections. Radiographically and on CT, chronic osteomyelitis is often characterized by a mixed pattern of lysis and sclerosis with cortical thickening or thick, wavy periosteal reaction. "Sclerosing osteomyelitis of Garre" is a manifestation of this process. The sclerosis is typically low signal on both T1- and T2-weighted images, with granulation tissue representing active infection demonstrating hyperintensity on T2-weighted images and enhancement on contrast-enhanced images. Necrotic bone (sequestrum) may be seen on CT as a focus of dense bone surrounded by lytic granulation tissue, and on MRI as a focus or region of hypointensity on all sequences, surrounded by edematous inflammatory tissue. It is very important in this setting to use intravenous contrast so that necrotic areas will stand out, much like abscesses, with central nonenhancement and intense surrounding contrast uptake. These avascular regions of necrotic bone serve as a nidus for continuing infection and require debridement.

Other features, such as cortical thickening, may also be present, with a low signal intensity rim being frequent. A sinus tract, if present, is usually T2-hyperintense with tram track–like enhancement. Abscesses may also be present in active infection. MRI serves as a useful preoperative tool before surgical debridement. Sclerosis may raise concern for tumor, such as lymphoma; history and laboratory information are important to evaluate as well.

Infected Devitalized Tissue (Figs. 5-52 and 5-53)

Devitalized or ischemic tissue can cause a number of problems in the setting of infection. First, as previously mentioned, a focus of devitalized bone (sequestrum) can be a source of persistent or recurrent active infection. Second, ischemic tissue heals poorly if debridement is incomplete, often leading to wound breakdown and recurrent infection; optimally debridement is coupled with revascularization if the option is available. Third, this devitalized tissue can be a source of misdiagnosis; on bone scan, regional

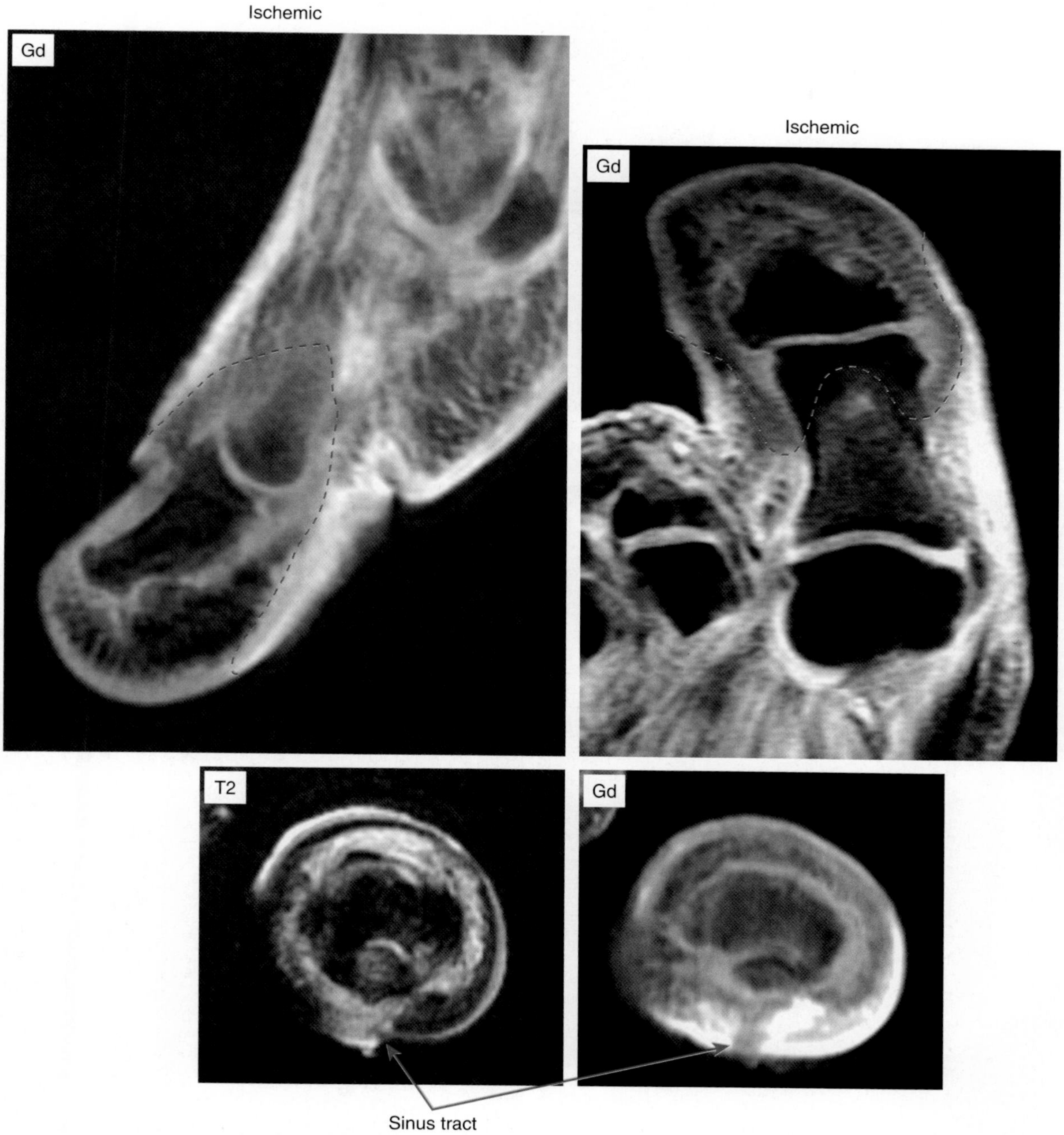
Ischemic
Gd
Ischemic
Gd
T2
Gd
Sinus tract

Figure 5-52 Soft tissue devitalization seen on contrast-enhanced MRI of the foot of a diabetic patient. Normal vascularized tissue enhances slightly; in ischemic or necrotic tissue enhancement is absent or minimal. Typically, there is hyperemic tissue at the margins (or in the case of cellulitis, inflammatory tissue), which demonstrates increased enhancement, making the ischemic region more obvious. This pattern is similar to infarction of other organs. Preoperative identification of devitalized areas is useful to surgeons to guide debridement.

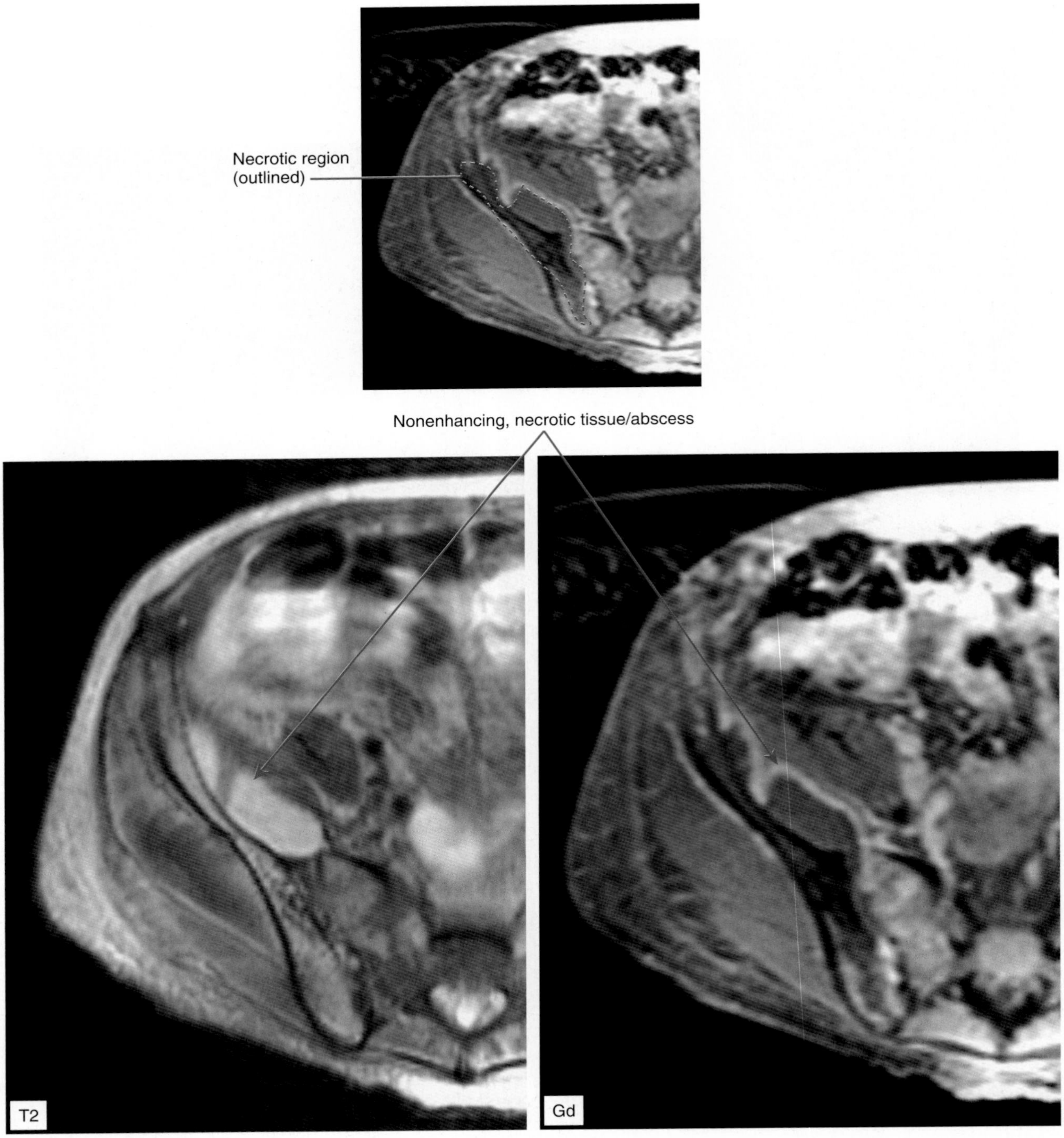
Necrotic region (outlined)
Nonenhancing, necrotic tissue/abscess
T2
Gd

Figure 5-53 Osteomyelitis of the iliac bone with abscess and devitalization. Devitalized areas are not effectively treated with intravenous antibiotics and generally require debridement or drainage.

ischemia can mask areas of osteomyelitis. On contrast-enhanced MRI, infected, devitalized tissue will not enhance.

On post-contrast MR images, devitalized tissue shows lack of enhancement and usually a zone of surrounding hyperemic tissue with more enhancement than normal tissue beyond, outlining the dead tissue. Ischemic tissue can be more difficult to detect, with relatively less enhancement than surrounding tissues; there may not be a rim of increased enhancement. Regions of interest (ROIs) can be performed pre-contrast and post-contrast and compared with normal muscle. Dynamic contrast enhancement using a rapid T1-weighted fat suppressed spoiled GRE sequence can be useful to evaluate this process.

Early Osteomyelitis (Fig. 5-54)

Detecting a marrow abnormality on T1-weighted images is very useful for diagnosing osteomyelitis in the appropriate clinical setting; however, preservation of marrow fat can occasionally be misleading. If the infection is caught early, marrow fat may not be metabolized yet and T1 signal can look almost normal. If the image is windowed carefully, or if the ROI of the marrow is compared with adjacent bones, a difference may be observed, suggesting the correct diagnosis when there is surrounding soft tissue infection. With this in mind, beware of volume averaging in small bones, which can make marrow signal artifactually look lower; confirm the finding on the short axis plane, and/or use a slice thickness smaller than the width of the bone being imaged in that plane. If there is still a question of the diagnosis, a three-phase bone scan, short-term follow-up MRI, or biopsy can provide the answer.

Infection Superimposed on Underlying Disorders

Underlying metabolic disorders can alter marrow signal on MRI and uptake on bone scan, leading to errors in interpretation. Such conditions include marrow-packing disorders such as Gaucher disease or marrow hyperplasia as from severe anemia or colony-stimulating factor treatment (both of which can result in diffusely increased T2 signal), as well as hemosiderin deposition (e.g., numerous blood transfusions or hemochromatosis) and marrow fibrosis (resulting in diffusely low signal on MRI). Bone infarction also causes a diagnostic dilemma (Fig. 5-55). Acute infarction can cause an appearance of periosteal reaction on radiographs, marrow edema on MRI, and reactive bone turnover as well as migration of inflammatory cells with abnormal uptake on nuclear medicine scans. Chronic infarction is less of a dilemma, with a fairly characteristic appearance on various modalities. However, in the setting of clinical deterioration it can be difficult to differentiate superimposed acute infarction from infection. Secondary signs of infection on MRI such as fluid collections, sinus tracts, and overlying cellulitis can be helpful, as well as gadolinium enhancement, which would not be expected in infarcted tissue. Occasionally, imaging cannot distinguish infection from these underlying disorders, and biopsy is indicated.

Bone Reaction to Soft Tissue Inflammation

In response to chronic ulceration and/or cellulitis the periostium can lay down new bone, forming what has been termed an "ulcer osteoma," or inflammatory exostosis (Fig. 5-56). Adjacent to soft tissue inflammation, the cortex may become hyperemic and demonstrate edema and enhancement on MR images. If the abnormality does not extend into the medullary space, it is termed "osteitis" (Fig. 5-57). This does not represent osteomyelitis but could be a sign of pending bone involvement and may warrant follow-up.

Atypical Organisms

Imaging appearance of the so-called "atypical infections," that is, with fungal, mycobacterial, or parasitic etiologies, can differ from those of routine bacterial infections previously described. In addition, unlike bacterial infections, clinical systemic manifestations and laboratory values may not immediately suggest infection. Radiologic manifestations of bacterial infections stem from common characteristics such as rapid course, metabolization and destruction of cartilage and fat, immune response resulting in generation of debris (pus), and reactive bone response. Atypical organisms often proceed slowly and survive on different materials, altering the imaging appearance. For example, infective bacteria in synovial joints or intervertebral disks rapidly metabolize

Text continued on page 242

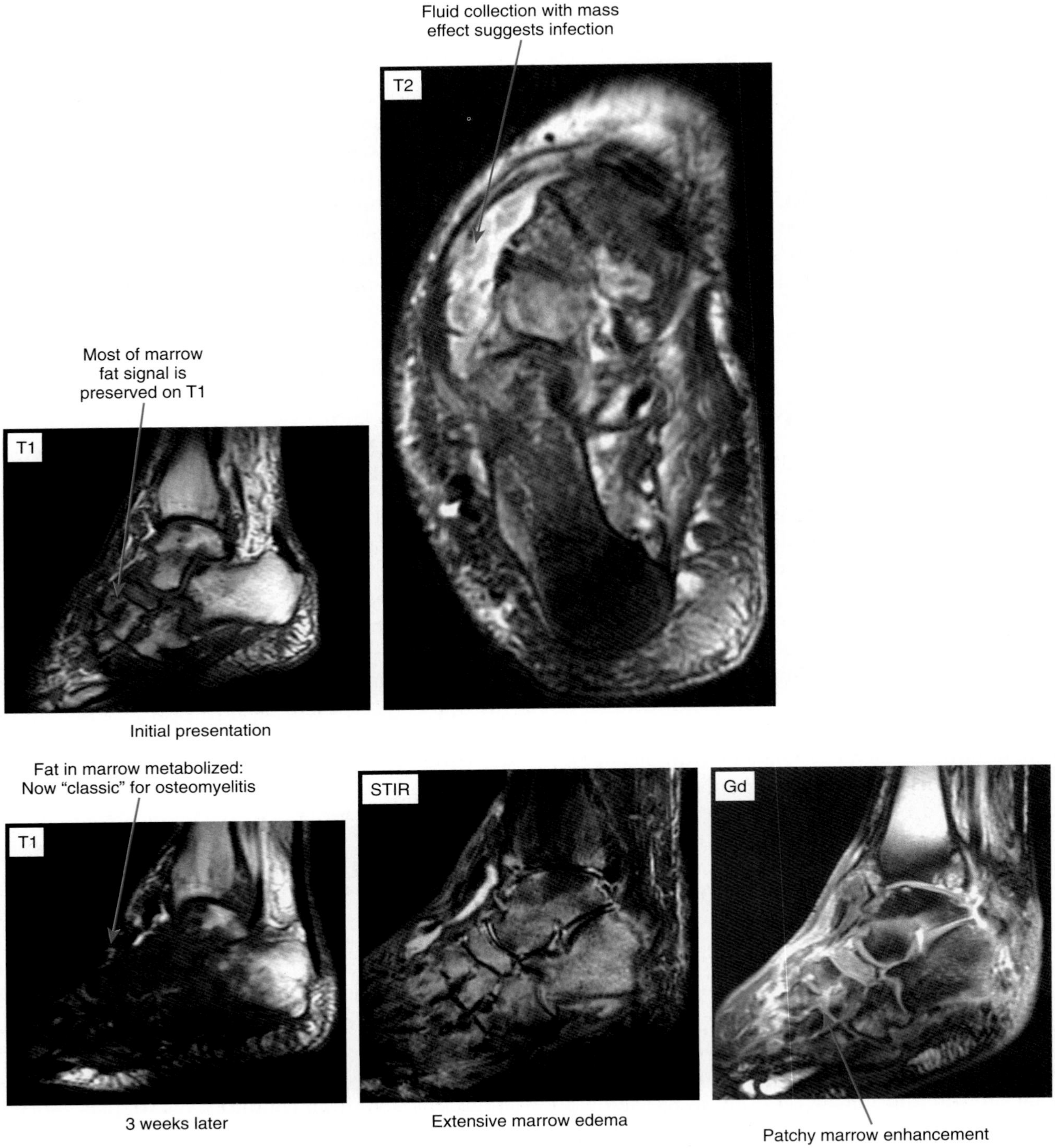
Fluid collection with mass effect suggests infection
T2
Most of marrow fat signal is preserved on T1
T1
Initial presentation
Fat in marrow metabolized: Now "classic" for osteomyelitis
T1
3 weeks later
STIR
Extensive marrow edema
Gd
Patchy marrow enhancement

Figure 5-54 Early osteomyelitis. Fat signal on T1 may be preserved early in the course of disease.

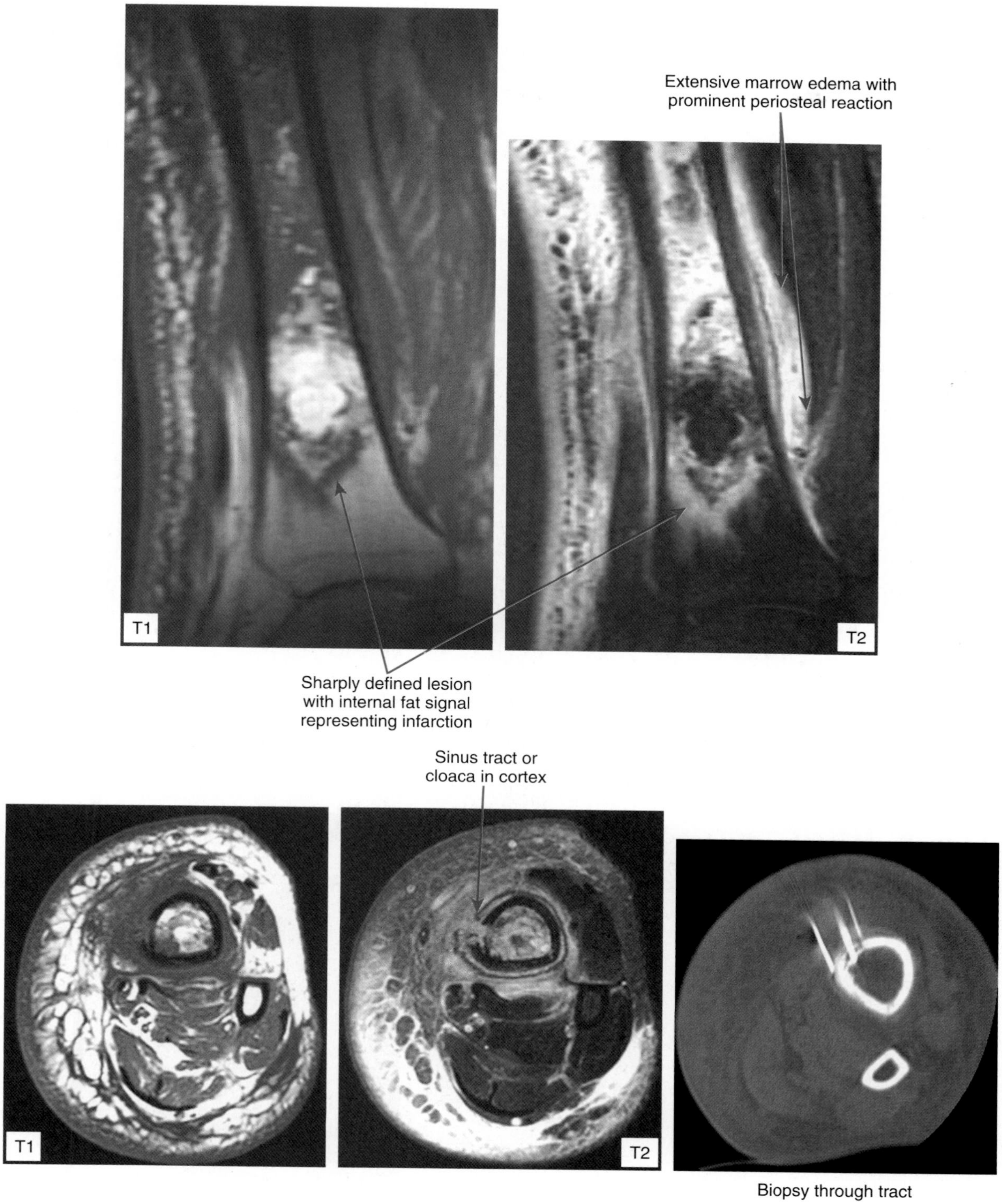
Extensive marrow edema with prominent periosteal reaction
T1
T2
Sharply defined lesion with internal fat signal representing infarction
Sinus tract or cloaca in cortex
T1
T2
Biopsy through tract

Figure 5-55 Osteomyelitis superimposed on infarction in sickle cell disease. Acute infarction can resemble infection on radiographs and CT (with periosteal reaction), MRI (with diffuse edema), and bone scan (with areas of hyperemia and increased uptake). Some differentiating features include sinus tract, rim-enhancing fluid collection, and diffuse marrow enhancement. This patient refused contrast; infarction was suspected because of sharply marginated signal abnormality in the distal tibia with internal fat. More proximally, the fat is replaced and the marrow edema is ill defined; there is intense periosteal reaction. Superimposed infection was suspected for these reasons as well as a hole in the cortex with adjacent edema suggestive of a sinus tract. Biopsy revealed osteomyelitis.

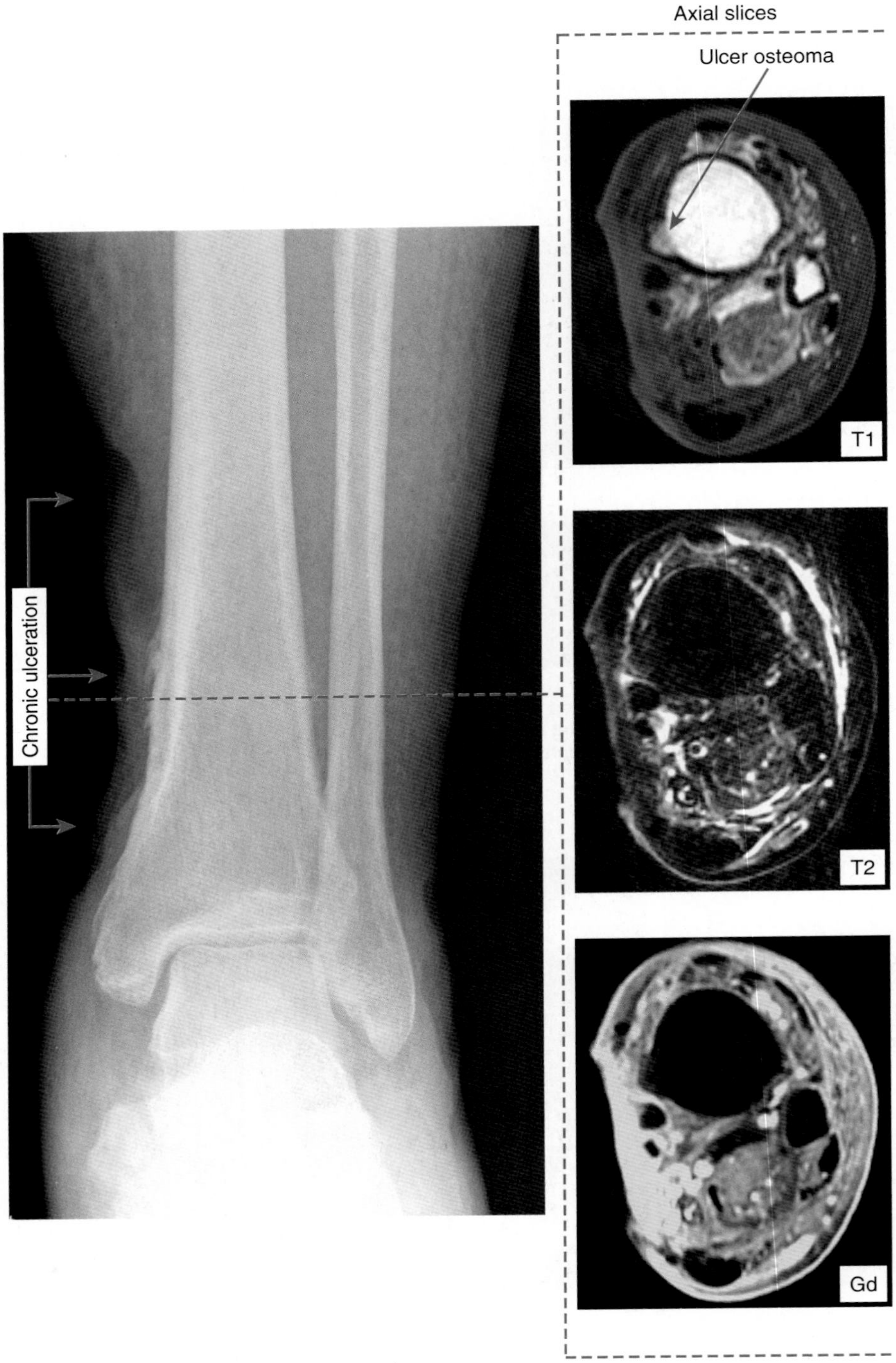
Axial slices
Ulcer osteoma
T1
T2
Gd
Chronic ulceration

Figure 5-56 Ulcer osteoma. Reactive edema and bone formation adjacent to chronic soft tissue inflammation.

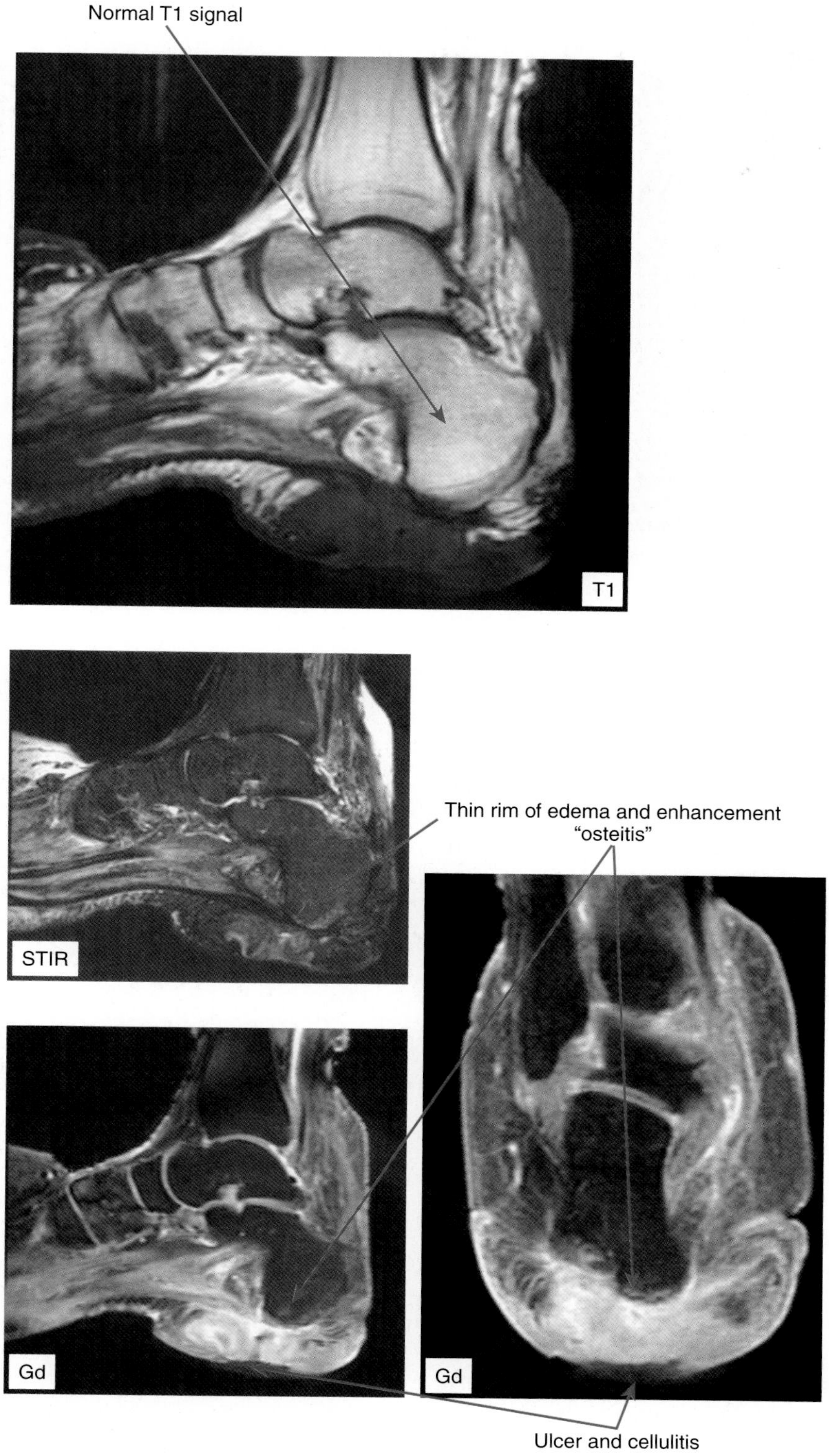
Normal T1 signal
T1
STIR
Thin rim of edema and enhancement
"osteitis"
Gd
Gd
Ulcer and cellulitis

Figure 5-57 **Osteitis.** Reactive hyperemia due to overlying inflammation.

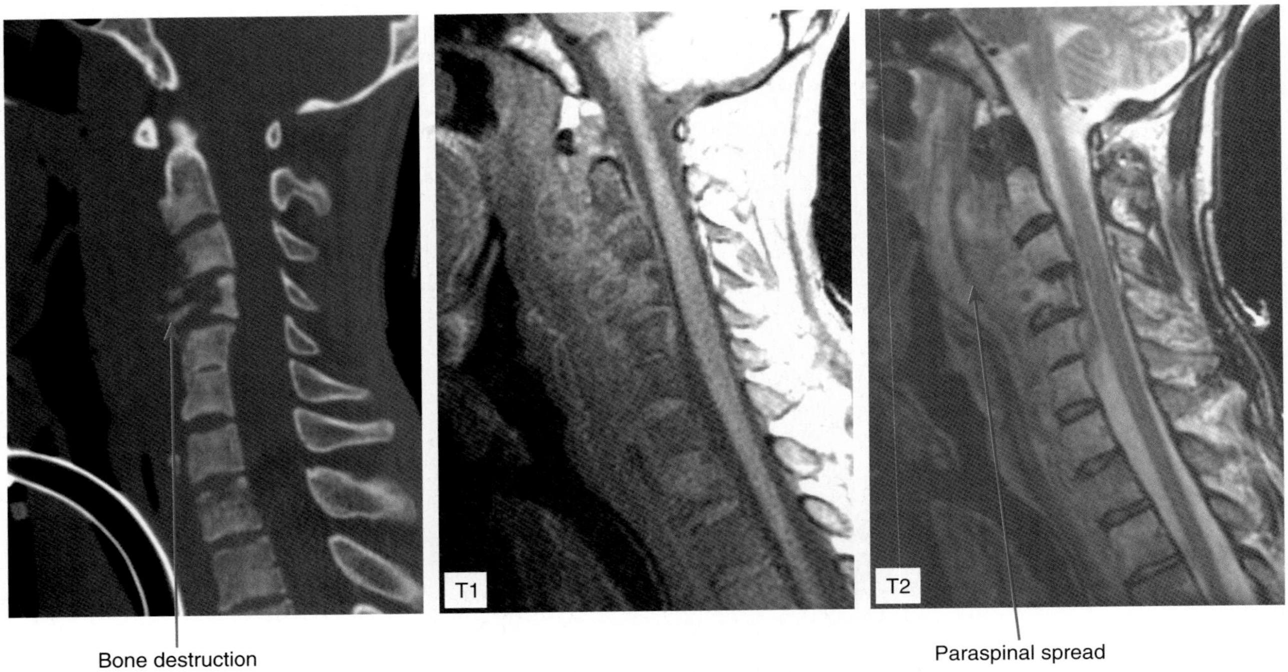
T1
T2
Bone destruction
Paraspinal spread

Figure 5-58 Spinal involvement by tuberculosis may spare the disk until late, spreading to other vertebral levels via paraspinous ligaments rather than through disks like typical bacterial infection.

proteoglycan matrix that composes hyaline cartilage and disk material, resulting in rapid joint/disk narrowing and destruction. Mycobacteria have different nutritional preferences and therefore tend to spare articular cartilage and disk material early on, setting up indolent joint infections and preferring to spread along paraspinal fascial planes along multiple levels rather than through the disk at one level. This results in the "classic" appearance of mycobacterial infections. However, in real life it is usually very difficult to use these differences as discriminators of bacterial versus mycobacterial infections, since mycobacterial infections more typically look exactly like routine bacterial infections.

Mycobacterial Infections
(Figs. 5-58 through 5-61)

Mycobacterial infections, especially *Mycobacterium tuberculosis*, most commonly affect the spine. Early descriptions were made by Pott in 1779, but the changes of tuberculous spondylitis have been observed in skeletons of prehistoric humans. The advent of modern antibiotic therapy initially made the disease relatively rare. In more recent years, there has been a resurgence of tuberculosis cases caused by drug-resistant strains and an increasing prevalence

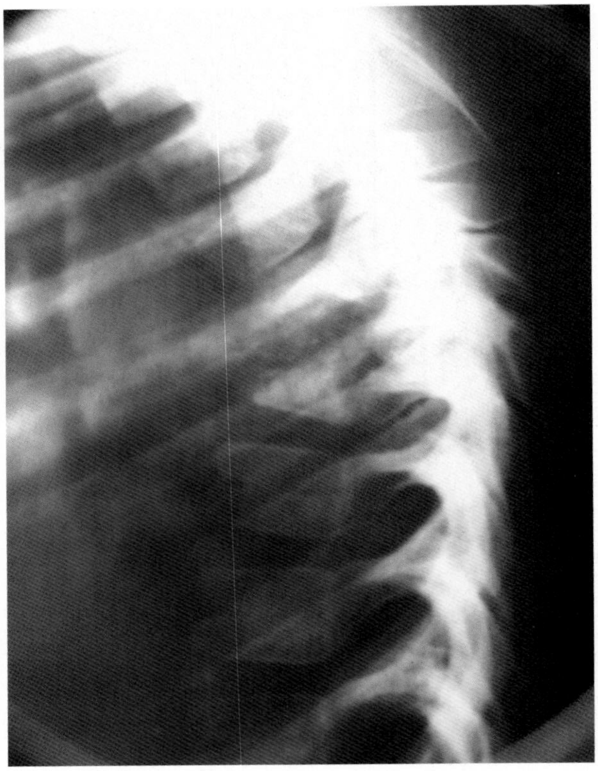

Figure 5-59 Chronic spinal tuberculous infection resulting in kyphotic ("gibbus") deformity.

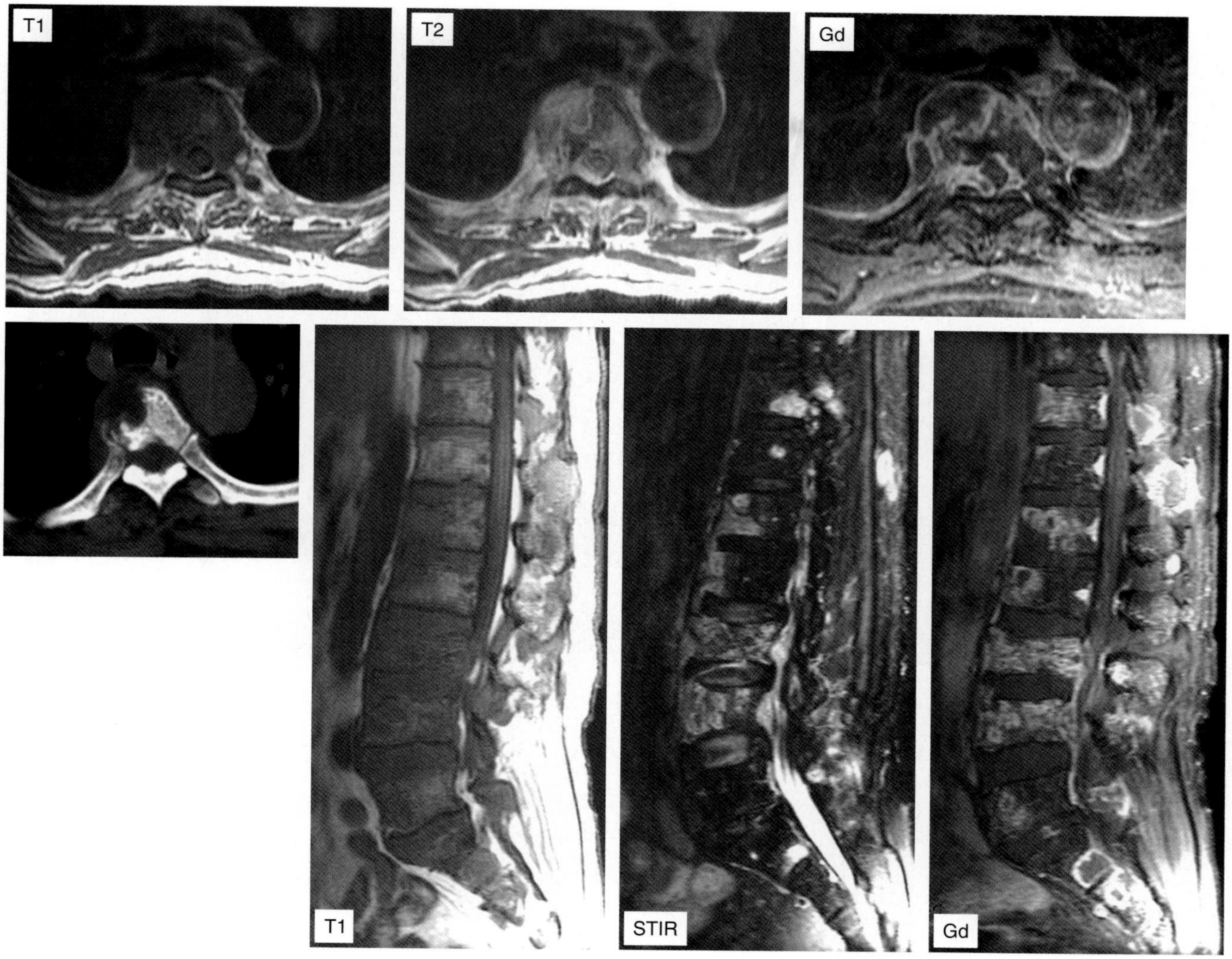
T1
T2
Gd
T1
STIR
Gd

Figure 5-60 Disseminated tuberculous infection. Masslike destruction can occur in TB; multifocal disease can resemble metastases.

of immunocompromised individuals. Tuberculosis is typically spread via a hematogenous route, although some cases in the thoracic spine have been related to contiguous spread from pulmonary parenchymal and pleural disease. Most patients with skeletal involvement have primary involvement of other organ systems, especially pulmonary or genitourinary.

Clinically, tuberculous spondylitis can present insidiously, with progressive back pain, occasionally with neurologic symptoms. Fever may be low grade or not present, and the WBC count may be mildly elevated or normal. Involvement of other organ systems may not be readily apparent clinically. A PPD skin test is generally positive, although it can be negative during overwhelming infection. The most common imaging presentation in the spine and appendicular skeleton is the same as in routine bacterial infection. However, occasionally "classic" features are seen including preservation of the disk or articular cartilage, paraspinal spread, extensive bone destruction, or adjacent soft tissue calcification. The Phemister triad represents the "classic" appearance of tuberculous arthritis and consists of juxta-articular osteopenia, preservation of the joint space, and erosions.

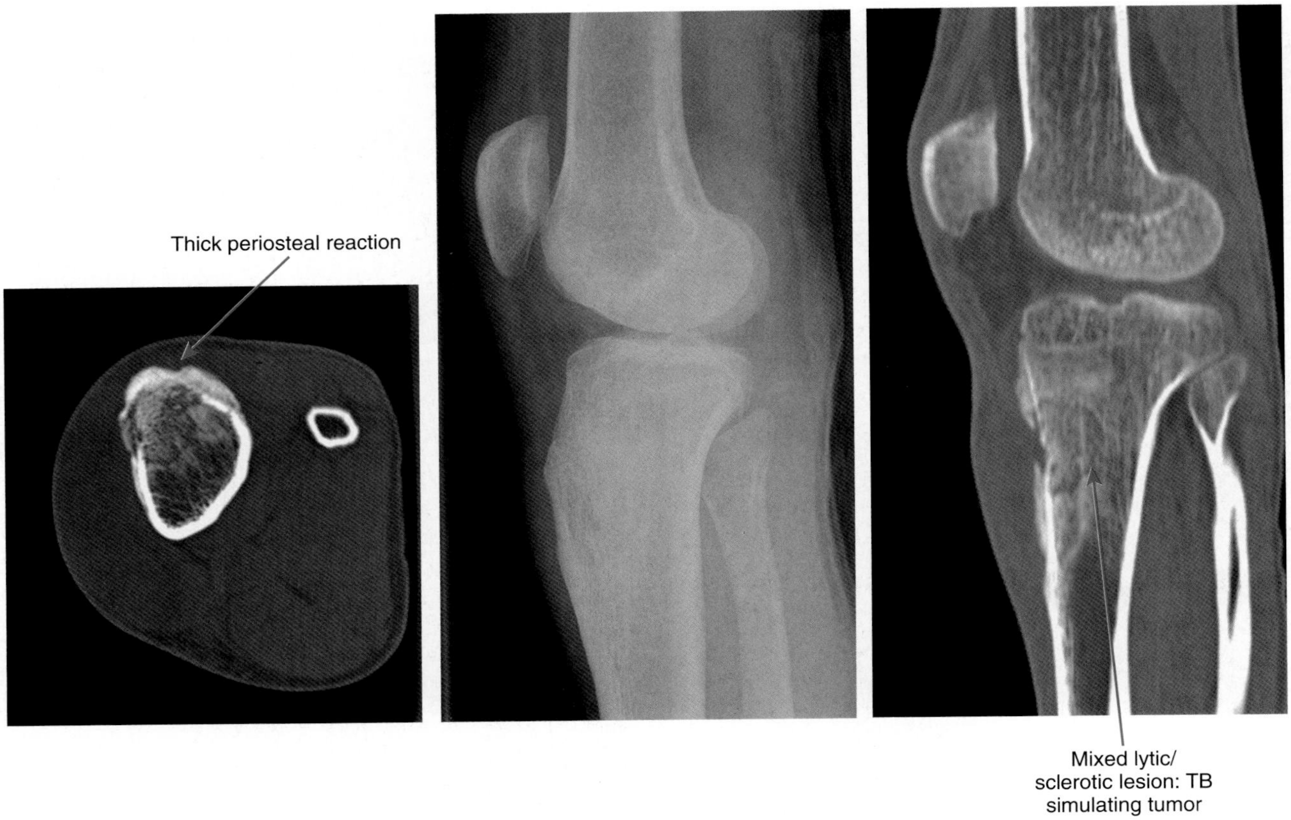
Thick periosteal reaction
Mixed lytic/
sclerotic lesion: TB
simulating tumor

Figure 5-61 Tuberculous and other atypical infections can involve the appendicular skeleton, creating unusual patterns that may simulate tumor. Bone sclerosis, lysis (with masslike destruction or a permeative pattern) or mixed patterns can be seen. Periosteal reaction varies but with more chronic processes tends to be thick and wavy like chronic bacterial infection.

Other Mycobacterial Infections

Other atypical mycobacterial infections may also involve the musculoskeletal system, including *Mycobacterium kansasii, Mycobacterium scrofulaceum,* and *Mycobacterium avium-intracellulare.* There are no specific musculoskeletal imaging features, but the diagnosis can be suspected based on typical involvement of other organs (e.g., lung with *M avium-intracellulare* infection, lymph nodes with scrofula).

Mycobacterium leprae is the causative agent in leprosy; it is seen in Africa, South America, and Asia. The organism exhibits a long incubation period, which may be over many years. Direct involvement of the musculoskeletal system can result in bone destruction; peripheral nerve involvement (visible occasionally as nerve calcification) results in atrophic neuropathic disease. Ultimately, this may result in a mutilating condition of the distal extremities and face.

Other Atypical Infections
(Figs. 5-62 through 5-66)

These atypical infections are rare and for most practicing radiologists are seen only in textbooks. However, if the patient population is prone to certain infections (e.g., immigrants from countries where these organisms are commonplace), it is important for the radiologist to be aware of the manifestations of atypical infections prevalent in their population.

One characteristic appearance that suggests an atypical infection is presence of one or more destructive masses. This finding is seen in some mycobacterial, fungal, and parasitic infections, and, although

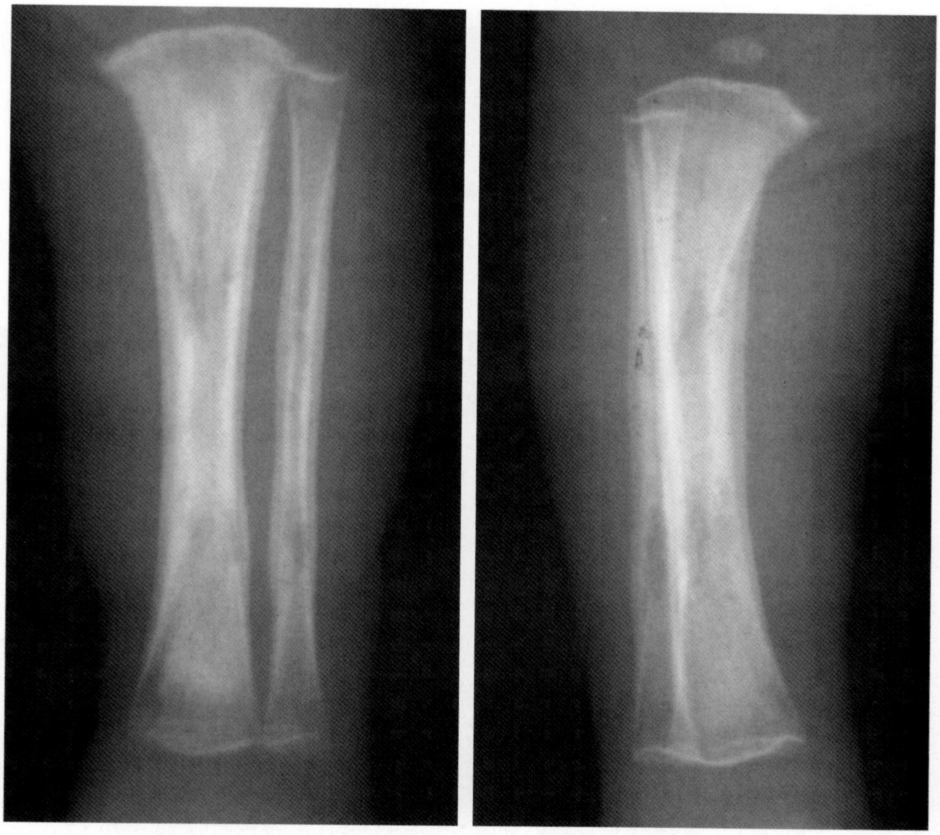

Figure 5-62
Congenital syphilis.
Mixed lytic/sclerotic pattern is seen diffusely, with thick periosteal reaction.

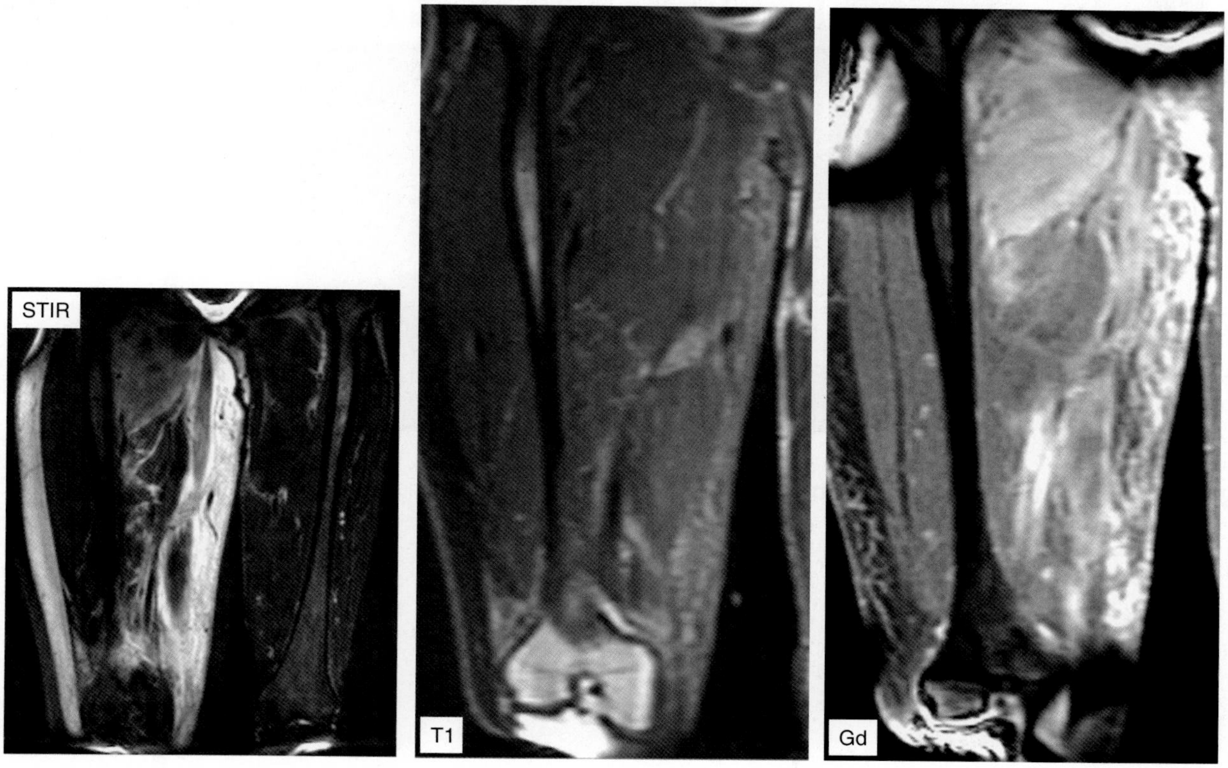
STIR
T1
Gd

Figure 5-63 ***Candida*** **myositis in the thigh of an AIDS patient.** Many fungal infections involving the musculoskeletal system are seen in patients with an immunocompromised state and/or travel history to endemic areas.

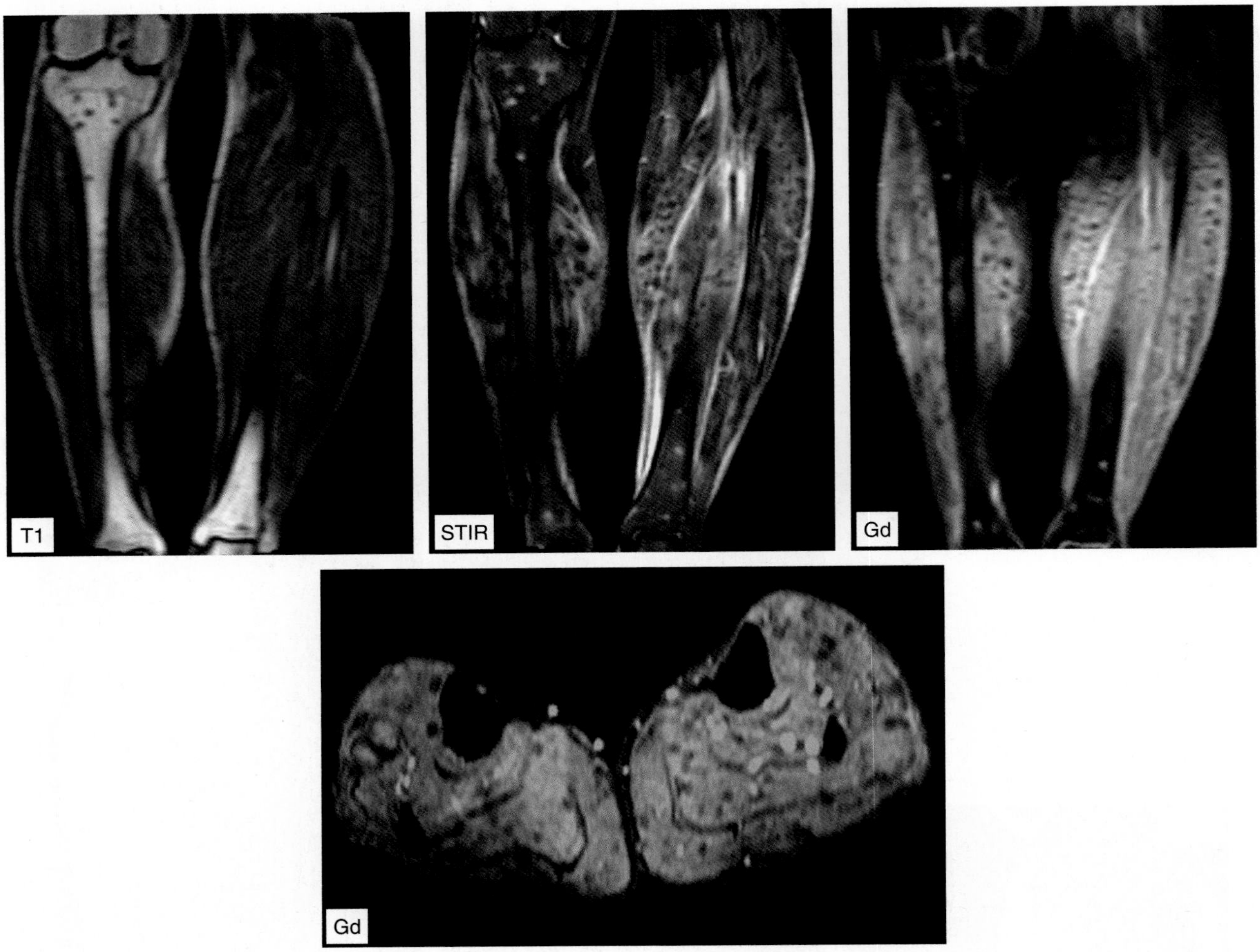
T1
STIR
Gd
Gd

Figure 5-64 Disseminated fungal infection. Note innumerable foci in bone and muscle.

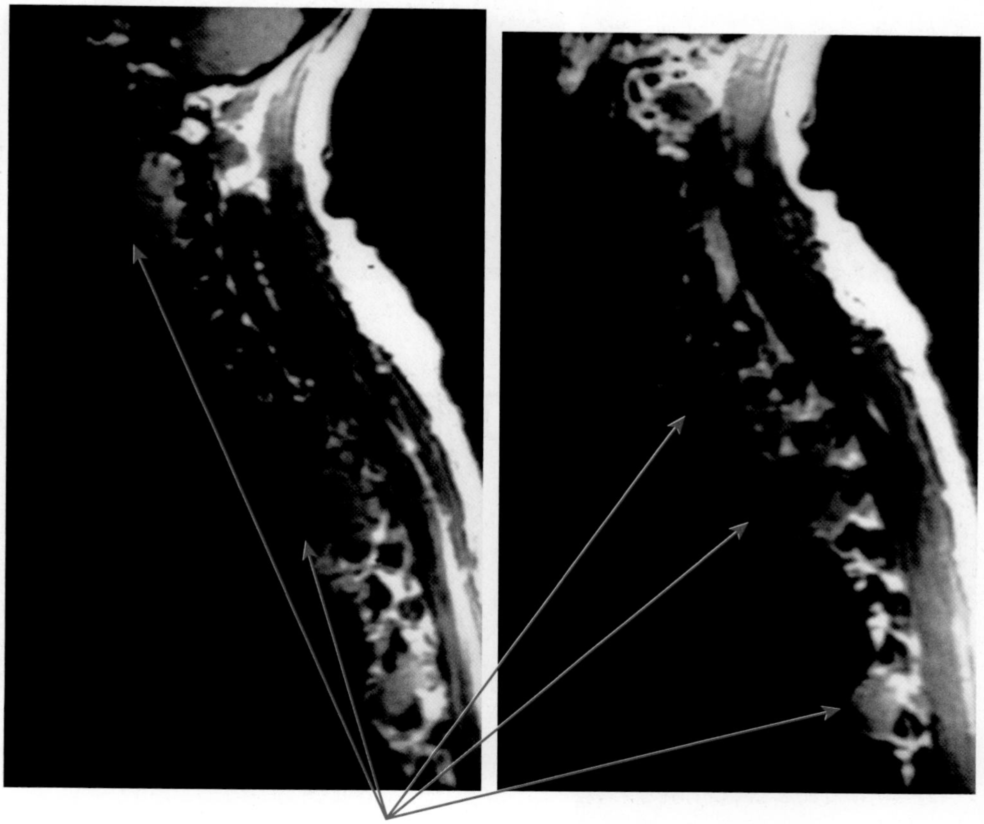
Multiple masses characterize many disseminated atypical infections and are easily confused with metastatic disease

Figure 5-65 Disseminated coccidioidomycosis presenting on MRI as multiple masses.

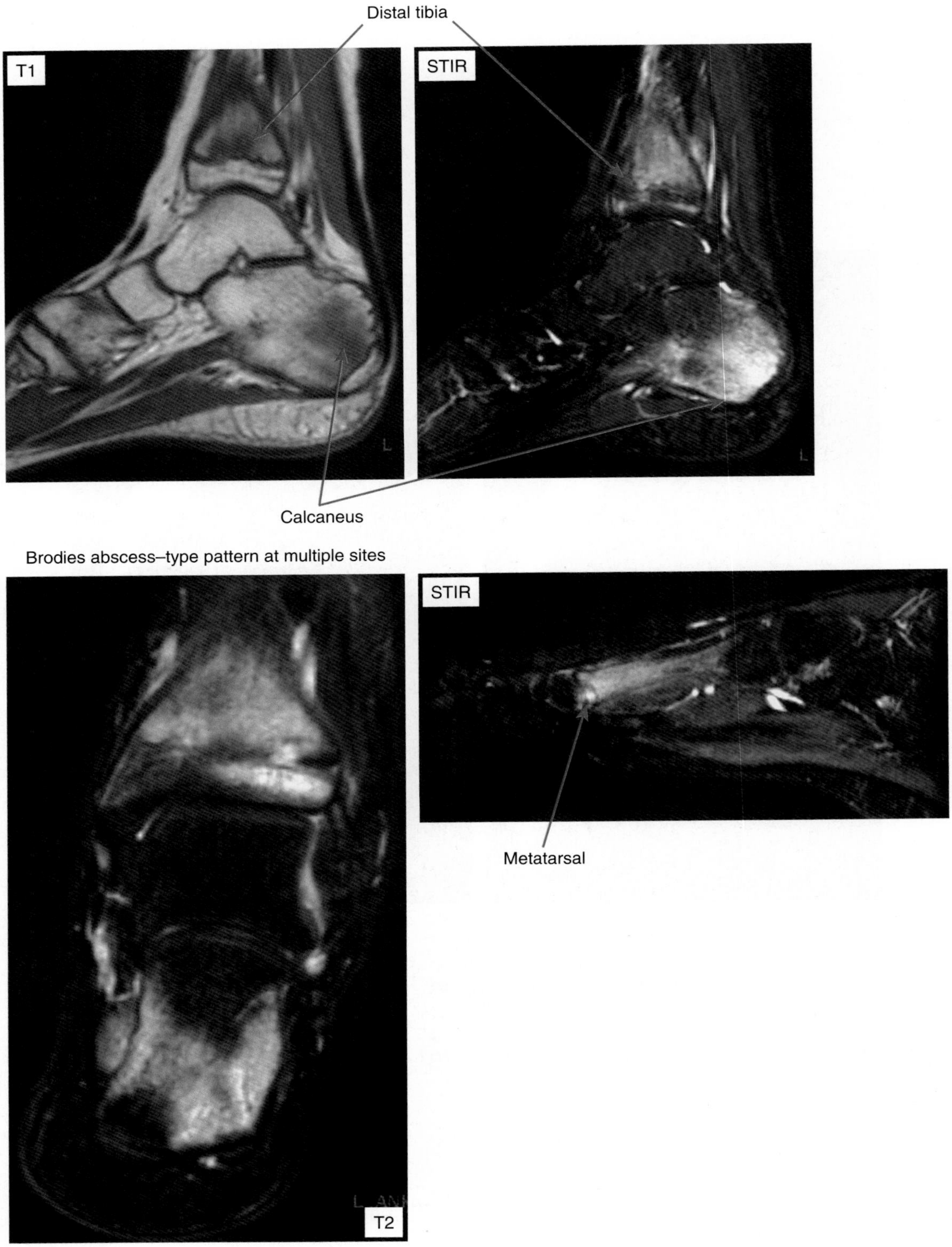
Distal tibia
T1
STIR
Calcaneus
Brodies abscess–type pattern at multiple sites
STIR
Metatarsal
T2

Figure 5-66 Chronic recurrent multifocal osteomyelitis (CRMO). Relapsing/multifocal infection, possibly viral. Immunosuppression likely.

not specific, suggests something other than routine bacterial infection. More commonly unless there are systemic findings or history suggesting infection, these lesions masquerade as primary bone tumors or metastatic lesions. Therefore, whenever a bone biopsy is performed, one must keep in mind the possibility of atypical infection. An immunocompromised state may also alter the imaging appearance of an infection or result in infection with atypical organisms. Those that may be seen along with distinguishing imaging features, if any, are listed in Table 5-1.

Chapter 6

APPROACH TO BONE AND SOFT TISSUE TUMORS AND TUMOR-LIKE CONDITIONS

CHAPTER OUTLINE

Evaluating bone and soft tissue tumors requires a multi-modality approach. Each modality has advantages and disadvantages, and a rational, tailored algorithm should be used. Reflexive, simultaneous ordering of all modalities when a lesion is found or clinically suspected should be discouraged.

Imaging techniques for patients with suspected soft tissue masses may be requested because of soft tissue abnormality palpated by the patient or physician or because of symptoms such as pain or other complaints with no detectable mass on physical examination. The type of imaging technique initially selected varies depending on the history and physical findings as well as the suspected location of the lesion.

MODALITIES

Radiography

Radiography remains the primary initial imaging study for detection and characterization of bone tumors. When a classically benign-appearing lesion is detected on routine radiographs, additional studies may not be required unless surgical intervention is contemplated and further anatomic information is needed. In this setting, either CT or MRI may be most appropriate for preoperative evaluation.

For soft tissue masses, certain radiographic features may provide valuable insight into the diagnosis or may guide additional examinations that may be required. For example, a well-defined lucency in the soft tissues may indicate a lipoma, which could be evaluated for either CT or MRI. Patients with subtle bone change or soft tissue calcification may be more appropriately studied with CT. Also, lesions projecting from bone as in osteochondroma can present as deep soft tissue masses clinically.

Arthrography is rarely if at all indicated for evaluation of soft tissue masses. Synovial cysts or ganglion cysts can be documented as benign by demonstrating communication with the joint after intra-articular injection of contrast material. However, this technique is rarely necessary. Similarly, with few exceptions such as arteriovenous malformations and hemangiomas, angiography is also not frequently performed for the detection or staging of soft tissue lesions.

Computed Tomography

For bone lesions, CT is very useful for evaluation of margins, matrix mineralization, and cortical breakthrough. If an osteoid osteoma is suspected, thin-cut CT is helpful in finding the lucent nidus. CT is also useful for visualizing soft tissue masses, defining compartmental involvement, and detecting mineralization and bone involvement. However, since the introduction of MRI, CT has largely been replaced as the technique of choice for evaluation of soft tissue masses. CT may still be appropriate for evaluation of some soft tissue lesions, such as lipomas, calcified lesions, and myositis ossificans. In addition, patient size or location of the lesion may dictate that CT would be the preferred technique. Such locations include the abdominal or chest wall, where motion artifact can create suboptimal imaging with MRI. A report by the Radiology Diagnostic Oncology Group on 133 soft tissue tumors suggested that MRI and contrast-enhanced CT are comparable with reference to determining tumor size and involvement of surrounding structures. Nevertheless, the American College of Radiology expert panel lists MRI as the most appropriate initial imaging examination for evaluation of a suspected soft tissue mass.

Ultrasound

Ultrasound is valuable in differentiating cystic from solid soft tissue lesions and has also been used to study vascularity of lesions (Figs. 6-1 and 6-2). For soft tissue prominence at a joint, ultrasound may offer a specific diagnosis (e.g., ganglion cyst and paralabral or parameniscal cyst; Fig. 6-3). However, ultrasound is not as useful for characterizing pathology or defining the extent of true soft tissue masses, except in situations in which lesion echogenicity (e.g., lipoma; Fig. 6-4) or morphology (e.g., nerve sheath tumor, Fig. 6-5) is specific.

Magnetic Resonance Imaging

When routine radiographic features of a bone lesion are indeterminate or when the lesion is more aggressive and considered to be potentially malignant, MRI is frequently required and is useful for characterization as well as staging. Soft tissue masses always require evaluation with CT or MRI. More commonly MRI is used unless there is calcification that CT could better characterize. Gadolinium contrast is useful for distinguishing cystic, myxoid, or necrotic components from solid regions; it is also useful when scanned in dynamic fashion rapidly after a bolus to characterize tumor vascularity. Although certain fea-

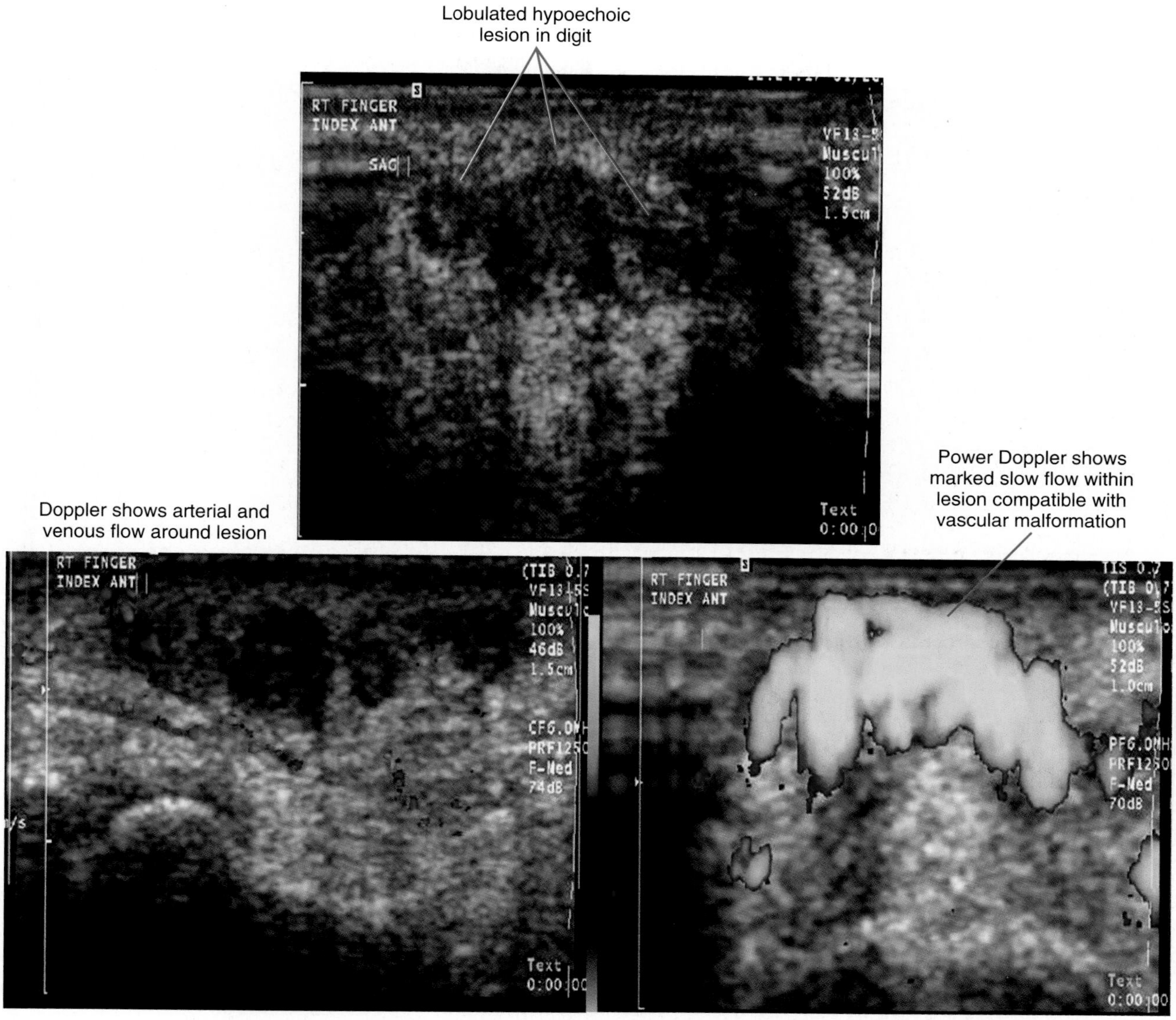
Lobulated hypoechoic lesion in digit
Doppler shows arterial and venous flow around lesion
Power Doppler shows marked slow flow within lesion compatible with vascular malformation
RT FINGER
INDEX ANT

Figure 6-1 Hemangioma of the finger.

tures on MRI can often be used to narrow the differential diagnosis for bone and soft tissue, it is unreliable for characterizing tissue type and is not even specific for distinguishing many benign from malignant lesions. Therefore, the radiologist should not become overconfident and should always keep in mind the limitations of each modality as well as the broad range of nontumors and tumor-like lesions that can simulate true neoplasms.

Even when MRI cannot characterize the type of lesion, it remains very useful for percutaneous biopsy and surgical planning. MRI is the technique of choice for evaluating and staging primary bone sarcomas, including neurovascular involvement. It is useful for determining tissue characteristics of a bone lesion, such as fat, hemorrhage, fibrous tissue, and fluid–fluid levels. Of course, patient size and clinical status as well as the presence of certain metallic or electrical implants may preclude the use of MRI.

Nuclear Medicine

Bone scan is predominantly useful for evaluation of multiplicity of lesions. However, if the primary lesion

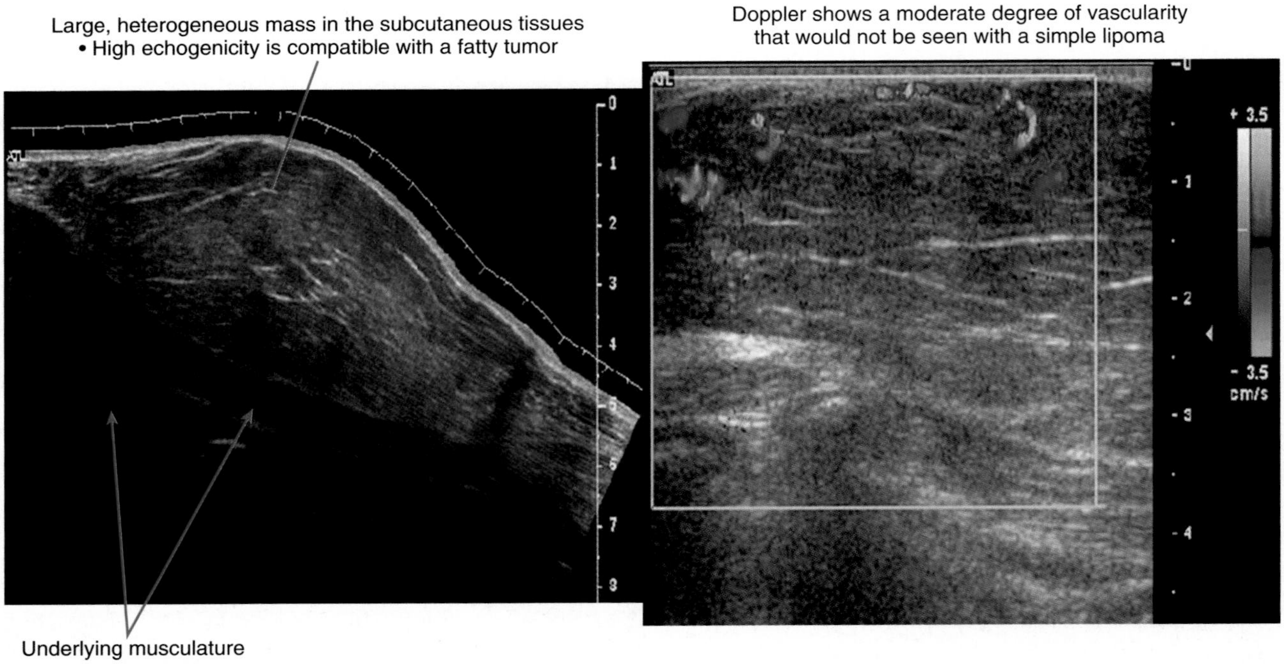
Large, heterogeneous mass in the subcutaneous tissues
• High echogenicity is compatible with a fatty tumor
Doppler shows a moderate degree of vascularity that would not be seen with a simple lipoma
Underlying musculature

Figure 6-2 Liposarcoma of the abdominal wall: flow and complexity.

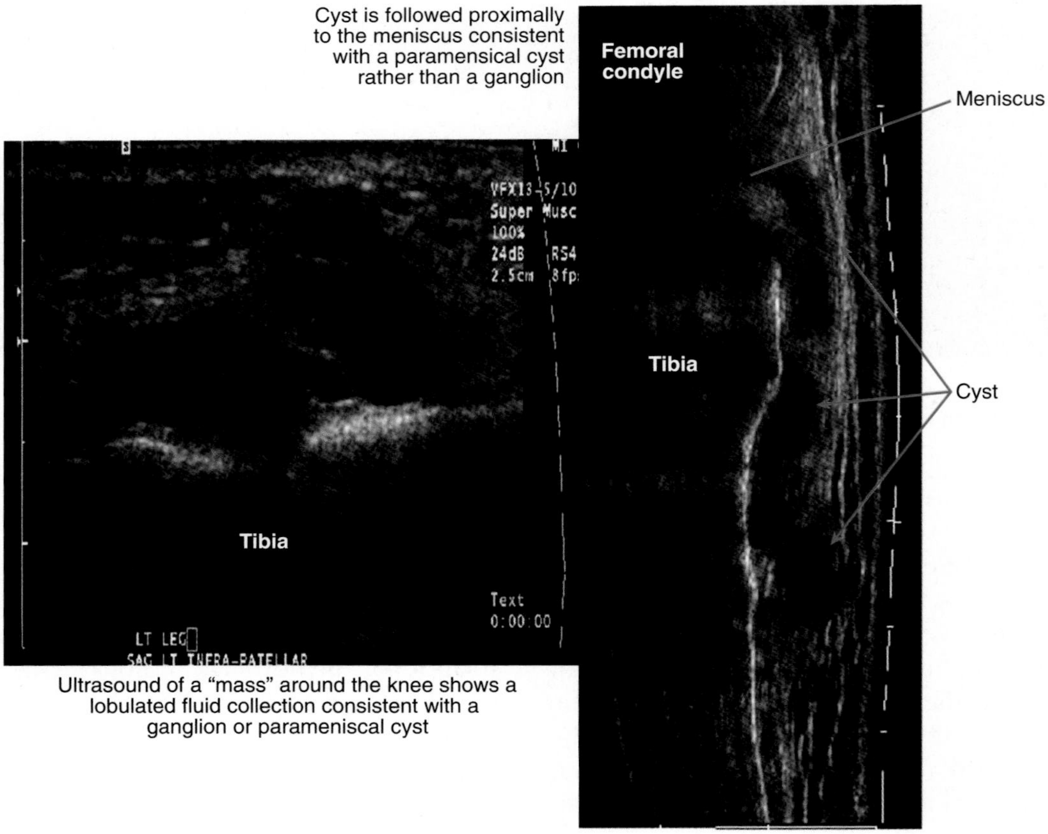
Cyst is followed proximally to the meniscus consistent with a paramensical cyst rather than a ganglion
Femoral condyle
Meniscus
Tibia
Cyst
Tibia
Ultrasound of a "mass" around the knee shows a lobulated fluid collection consistent with a ganglion or parameniscal cyst

Figure 6-3 Mass inferior to the knee joint. Ultrasound shows a lobulated fluid collection with a neck to the meniscus, consistent with a parameniscal cyst.

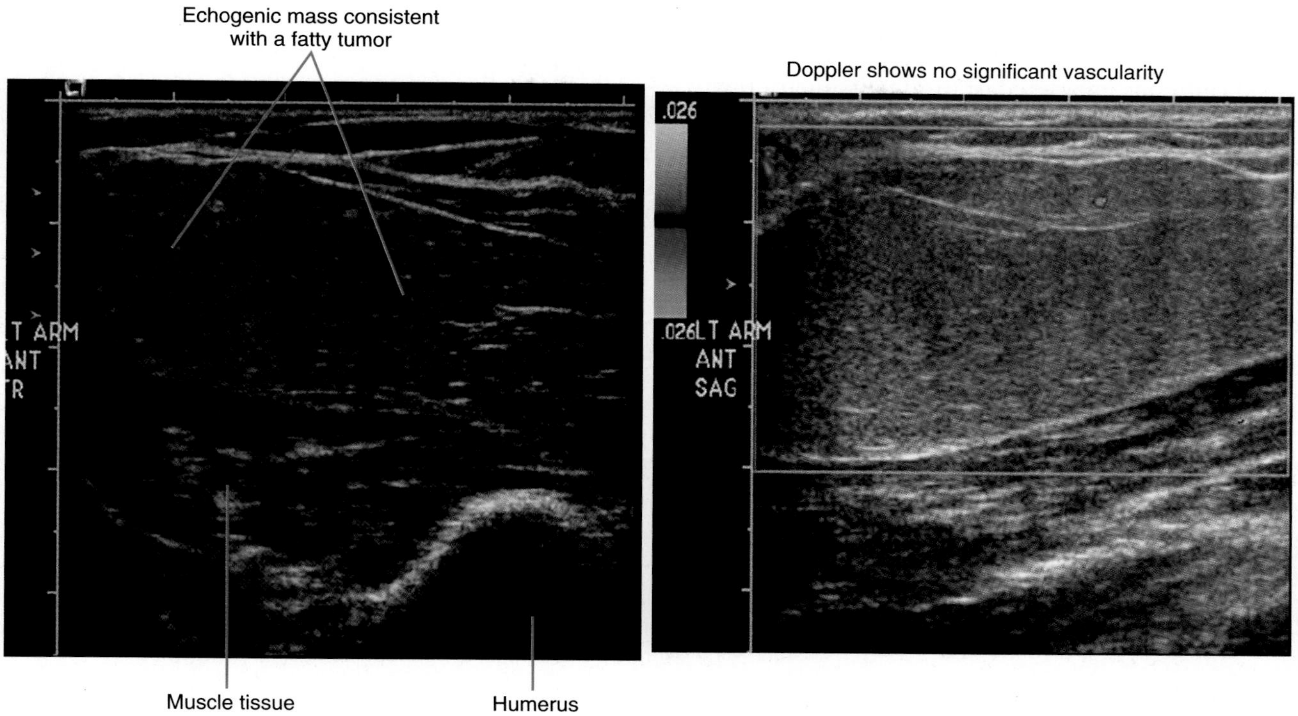
Echogenic mass consistent with a fatty tumor
Doppler shows no significant vascularity
.026
.026LT ARM
ANT
SAG
Muscle tissue
Humerus

Figure 6-4 **Lipoma of the arm.**

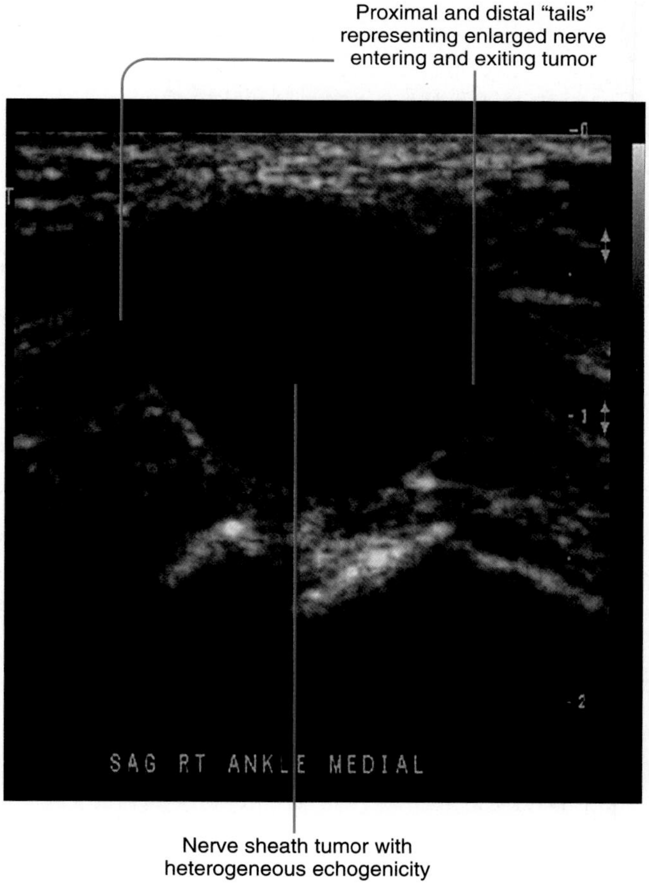
Proximal and distal "tails" representing enlarged nerve entering and exiting tumor
SAG RT ANKLE MEDIAL
Nerve sheath tumor with heterogeneous echogenicity

Figure 6-5 **Nerve sheath tumor: posterior tibial nerve.**

in question (or lesion detected with another modality) shows no increased uptake on bone scan, the scan should be considered of limited value for detecting other deposits. This is often the case with purely lytic metastases and myeloma (Fig. 6-6). On the other end of the spectrum, diffuse involvement (skeletal carcinomatosis), as seen in cases of metastatic prostate or breast carcinoma, can produce such generalized uptake that the bone scan looks relatively normal except for lack of uptake by the kidneys (described as a "superscan"). Bone scan is also very useful for detecting the metastatic lesions of osteosarcoma, which avidly concentrate radiotracer. Osteosarcoma tends to metastasize to lung, and bone scan can be helpful for surveillance of recurrence as well as distant metastases.

Another situation in which bone scan can be useful is the differentiation of a benign sclerotic focus, such as a bone island or fibrous dysplasia with little to no increased uptake, from a blastic metastasis, which has

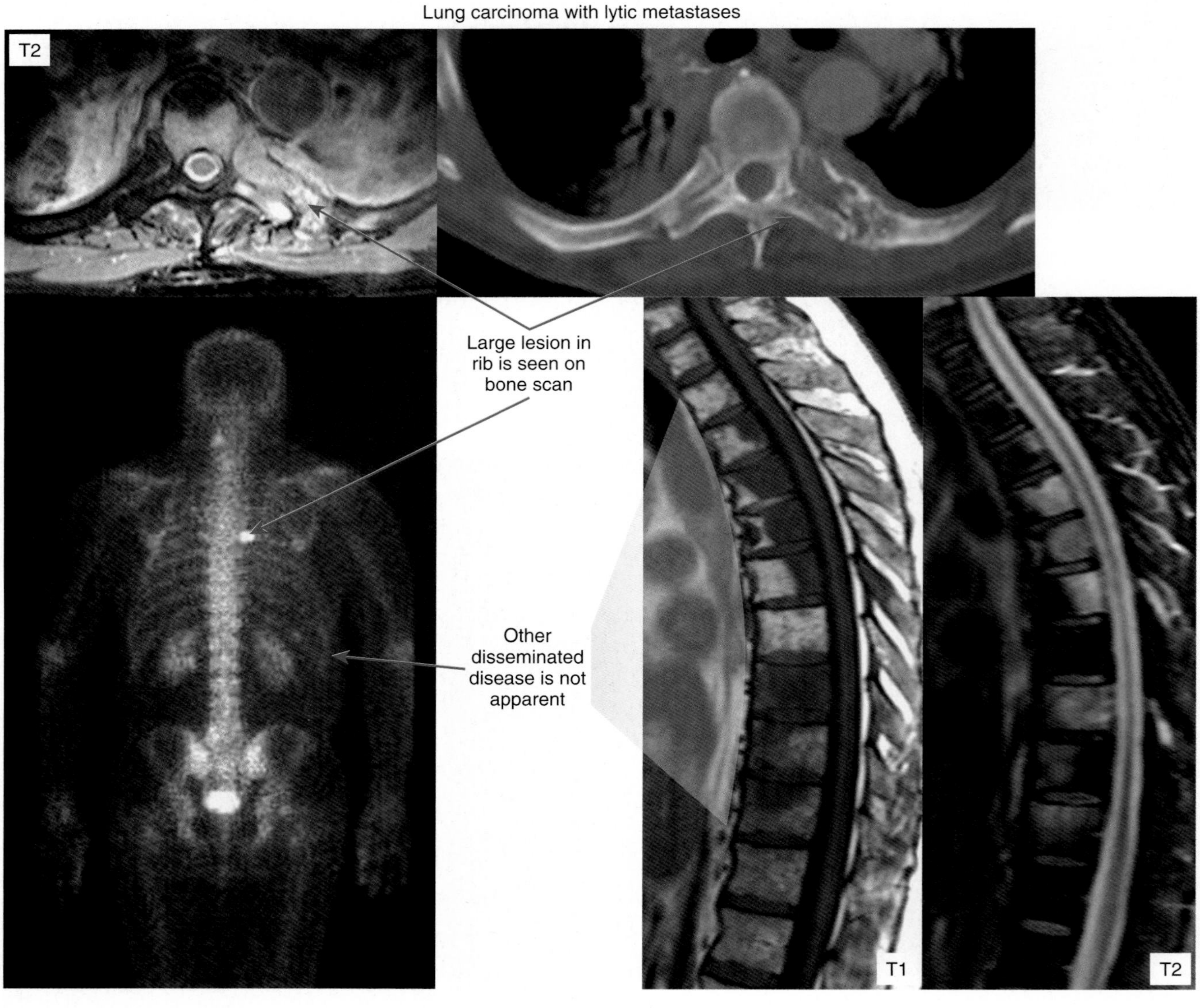
Lung carcinoma with lytic metastases
T2
Large lesion in rib is seen on bone scan
Other disseminated disease is not apparent
T1
T2

Figure 6-6 Bone scan can be insensitive to lytic metastases. In this case of metastatic lung carcinoma, purely lytic metastases are not well seen on bone scan. Regardless, bone scan is an essential part of any metastatic workup, since it provides global information; but it must be seen as a complementary examination, interpreted in conjunction with other modalities.

a high degree of uptake. For patients with ill-defined symptoms and normal radiographs, a radionuclide bone scan may be used to localize the abnormality. Following a positive bone scan, either MRI or CT may be selected to better define the nature of the lesion. Radionuclide studies are not indicated in most situations for evaluation of soft tissue masses. Techniques such as positron-emission tomography (PET) scanning have been used mainly for evaluation of metastatic disease and follow-up of treated lesions but show promise for identifying active areas of a tumor before biopsy (Fig. 6-7).

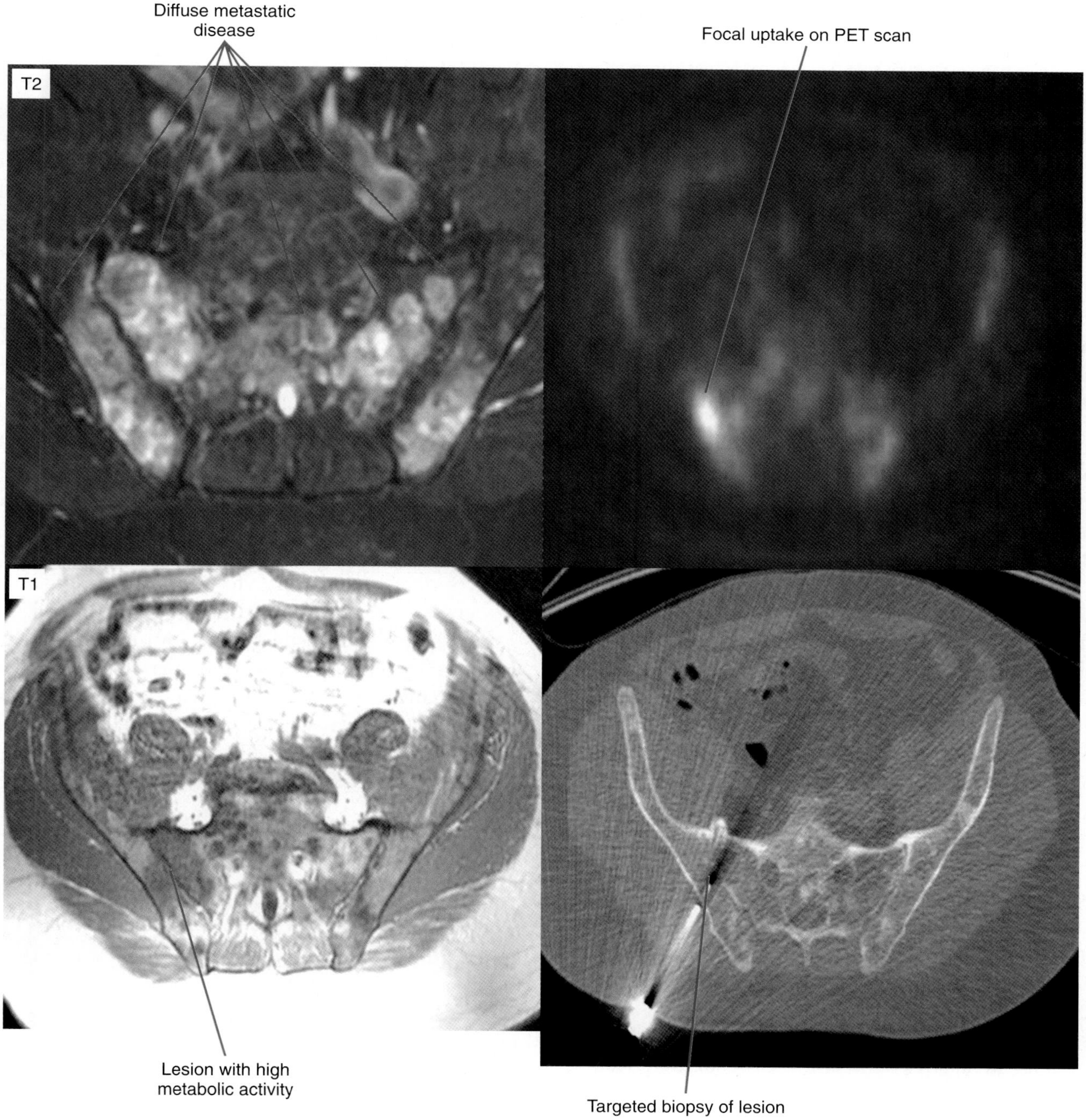
Diffuse metastatic disease
Focal uptake on PET scan
T2
T1
Lesion with high metabolic activity
Targeted biopsy of lesion

Figure 6-7 Selection of site to biopsy using PET (positron-emission tomography) scan. The area of maximal metabolic uptake could potentially provide the highest diagnostic yield. PET, positron-emission tomography.

Summary of Modalities

Radiography remains the optimal initial examination for a clinically suspected musculoskeletal tumor. When lesions are characteristically benign, imaging workup may cease, but additional imaging may still be useful for preoperative planning. Further characterization of an indeterminate lesion usually requires CT and/or MRI. CT is preferred for patients with suspected osteoid osteoma and subtle cortical abnormalities, and for evaluating lesion calcification or tumor matrix. Bone scan is predominantly useful for evaluation of multiplicity of lesions. MRI is the preferred technique for staging of musculoskeletal neoplasms in soft tissue and bone. PET scanning is useful for evaluation of metastases and tumor recurrence.

IMAGING OF TUMORS: GENERAL COMMENTS

For bone and soft tissue masses, regardless of the modality, the radiologist must first ensure that the entire lesion is imaged. If the borders are poorly defined, an MRI is the best test to define lesion margins.

For preoperative evaluation of a primary tumor, it is helpful to the surgeon to include a scout or single large field-of-view sequence of the bone (or adjacent bone in the case of soft tissue tumor) in a longitudinal plane, with the end of the bone visualized. Because only fluoroscopy is available in most operating rooms, this assists the surgeon in localizing the expected lesion margins during definitive resection.

Primary bone and soft tissue malignancies are rare compared with metastatic disease. Benign lesions of bone and soft tissue are far more common than sarcomas. Yet the radiologist must be cautious not to assign a benign differential diagnosis to a lesion that does not show specific features. Biopsy should be considered for equivocal cases. The exception is when biopsy may create a false impression of aggressiveness, as in a stress fracture. Some benign lesions evolve quickly and develop classically benign features or they regress, providing support for benignity. Suspected stress fracture or myositisossificans can be followed up over a short period of time (i.e., 1 month). History is important!

TUMOR-LIKE LESIONS (BONE OR SOFT TISSUE) ON IMAGING EXAMINATIONS

Some lesions can classically resemble tumors and should be considered before assigning a differential diagnosis. Alternate modalities may be needed to exclude these benign non-neoplastic entities. These entities include

Infection: Occasionally infection can present with a masslike quality on MRI, CT, or radiography. This is especially true with atypical organisms such as mycobacterial species and fungal infections, such as coccidioidomycosis. Appropriate history (e.g., travel) and clinical scenario (e.g., fever, immunocompromised state) should always be considered.

Hemophilic pseudotumor: Intraosseous hemorrhage can occur, resulting in a large lytic blowout lesion that heals with sclerotic margins; the differential diagnosis early on includes an aggressive metastatic lesion or plasmacytoma. Age and gender should be considered if history is not available. Hemophilia has a predilection for young males, as well as acute blood products in the lesion on CT or MRI and associated arthritis.

Amyloid: Amyloid deposits can occur in primary or secondary forms of amyloidosis (secondary form seen in chronic renal failure), but both look the same, with soft tissue masses around joints, periarticular lytic lesions, and vertebral endplate destruction. Appropriate history is important (renal failure) as well as other signs of secondary hyperparathyroidism. On MRI, amyloid deposits are low signal on T1- and T2-weighted sequences.

GENERAL TIPS: BONE OR SOFT TISSUE TUMORS

Appearance of Lesions Recently Biopsied

Biopsy makes a lesion look more aggressive on CT and MRI, resulting in surrounding edema and enhancement that makes it difficult or impossible to define the lesion's true margins. If a biopsy is near a neurovascular bundle, this can change a planned surgery from a limb salvage to an amputation. It is very important to obtain all imaging before biopsy.

Appearance of Treated Lesions

The appearance of bone and soft tissue can change after treatment. Considering the lesions themselves, lytic, metastatic lesions can become more sclerotic, especially breast metastases. Bone scan may demonstrate a paradoxic increase in activity because of bone healing (flare phenomenon). The pattern of red marrow can change on MRI. For example, rebound following chemotherapy or treatment with colony-stimulating factor can result in an increase in hematopoietic marrow, which is often more cellular and thereby brighter in T2 and STIR signal than typical red marrow. Radiation therapy results in replacement of red marrow with fatty yellow marrow (Fig. 6-8). Treatment can also affect the soft tissues. For example, radiation therapy causes soft tissue edema, especially of the underlying muscles within the port. This edema may last for years and can simulate a number of pathologic conditions from trauma to infection to neurologic disease; no mass effect is seen. In later follow-up, the muscles may exhibit fatty atrophy.

Staging of Primary Musculoskeletal Tumors

Description of the imaging appearance of a bone or soft tissue tumor should include a description

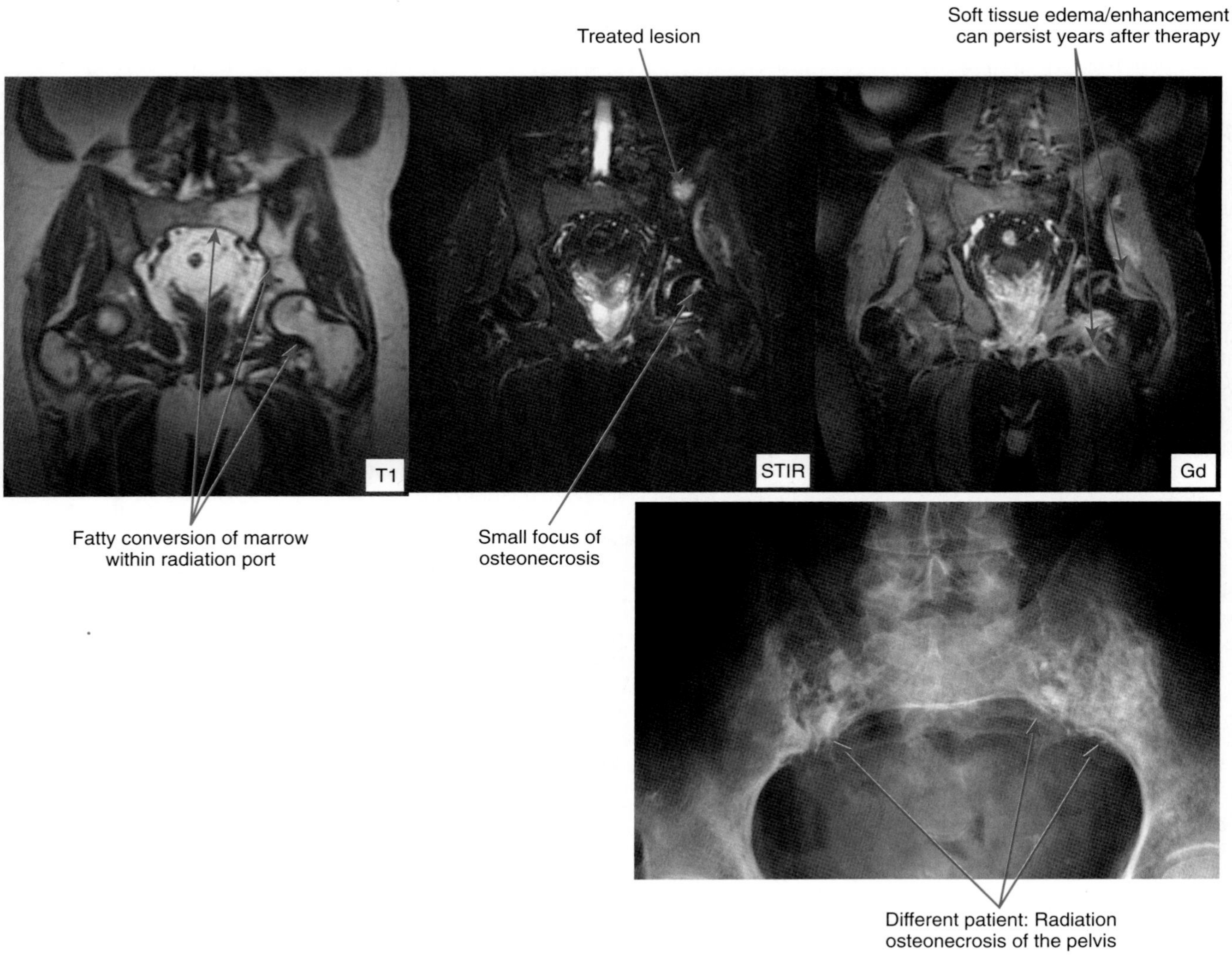
Treated lesion
Soft tissue edema/enhancement can persist years after therapy
T1
STIR
Gd
Fatty conversion of marrow within radiation port
Small focus of osteonecrosis
Different patient: Radiation osteonecrosis of the pelvis

Figure 6-8 Radiation therapy-related bone marrow changes and osteonecrosis.

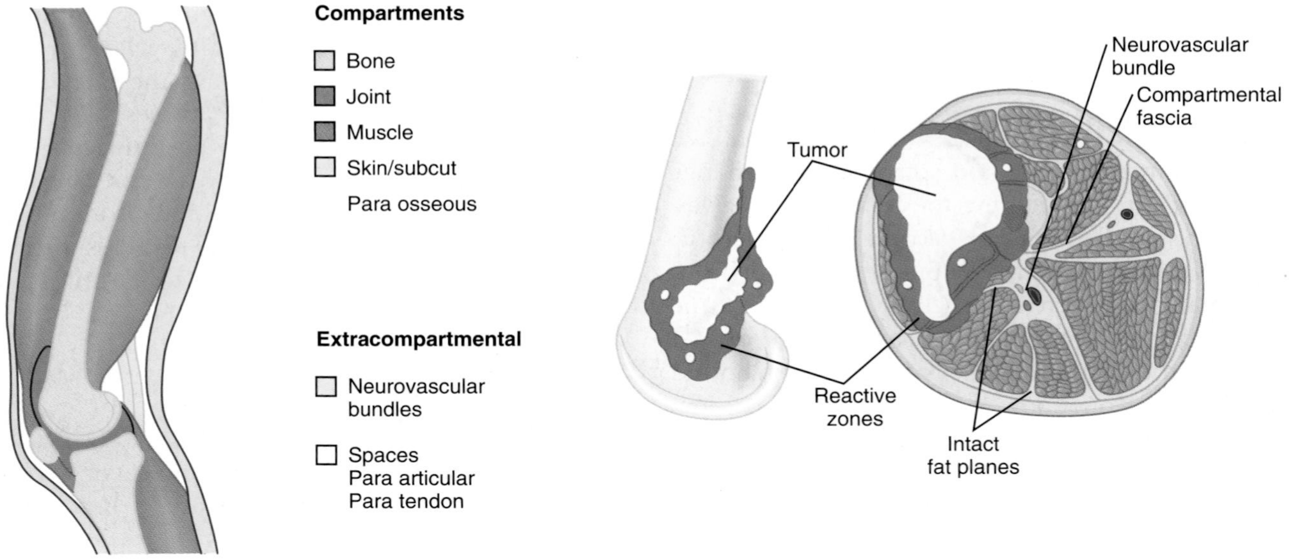
Compartments
Bone
Joint
Muscle
Skin/subcut
Para osseous
Extracompartmental
Neurovascular bundles
Spaces
Para articular
Para tendon
Neurovascular bundle
Compartmental fascia
Tumor
Reactive zones
Intact fat planes

Figure 6-9 Definition of tissue compartments. Aggressive bone lesion with extracompartmental spread to anterior compartment. (Courtesy of W.F. Enneking, MD.)

of local aggressiveness and extension into other compartments, such as from bone to adjacent muscles, from one fascial compartment to another, from anywhere into a neurovascular compartment, and distant metastases (Fig. 6-9 and Table 6-1). This information is combined with histologic aggressiveness (Grade 0: G0 = benign; Grade 1: G1 = low-grade malignant; Grade 2: G2 = high-grade malignant) to determine the overall stage (Table 6-2).

Table 6-1 Anatomic Compartments

Intracompartmental (A)	Extracompartmental (B)
Intraosseous	Soft tissue extension
Intra-articular	Soft tissue extension
Superficial to deep fascia	Deep fascial extension
Paraosseous	Intraosseous or extrafascial
Intrafascial compartments	Extrafascial planes or spaces
Ray of hand or foot	Midfoot and hindfoot
Posterior calf	Popliteal space
Anterolateral leg	Groin—femoral triangle
Anterior thigh	Intrapelvic
Medial thigh	Midhand
Posterior thigh	Antecubital fossae
Buttocks	Axilla
Volar forearm	Periclavicular
Dorsal forearm	Paraspinal
Anterior arm	Head and neck
Posterior arm	
Periscapular	

From Enneking WF, Spanier SS, Goodman MA. A system for the surgical staging of musculoskeletal sarcoma. Clin Orthop 1980; 153:106–120.

GENERAL APPROACH TO BONE TUMORS

The following text provides the radiologist with a formula for determining whether a lesion is truly a tumor, whether the tumor is aggressive or nonaggressive, and basic principles for determining tissue type when possible.

PITFALLS AND PSEUDOTUMORS

Stress Fracture

It is not common for stress fractures to be confused with tumor, since the clinical context usually guides

Table 6-2 Surgical Stages of Sarcomas

Stage	Grade	Site
1A	Low (G1)	Intracompartmental (T1)
IB	Low (G1)	Extracompartmental (T2)
IIA	High (G2)	Intracompartmental (T1)
IIB	High (G2)	Extracompartmental (T2)
III	Any (G) Regional or distant metastasis	Any (T)

From Enneking WF, Spanier SS, Goodman MA. A system for the surgical staging of musculoskeletal sarcomata. Clin Orthop 1980; 153:106–120.

the referring doctor to request specifically to "rule out stress fracture." Yet it continues to occur, as evidenced by fractures referred for biopsy. There are clearly situations in which the radiologist is more likely to confuse stress fracture with tumor. Biopsy of such a lesion can have devastating results, as in an erroneous pathologic diagnosis of osteosarcoma (due to mitoses and osteoid formation), so it is important to be aware of the following situations.

1. *Elderly patient with an insufficiency fracture.* Fracture should be considered in elderly osteoporotic patients who present with chronic pelvic/sacral pain (Fig. 6-10). Sacral stress fracture appears as sclerosis on radiographs and ill-defined edema on MRI, usually bilateral, often with abnormal T1 signal due to chronicity at presentation. CT is very useful for confirming subtle linear sclerosis or interruption of the sacral neural foramina at multiple sites in a vertical pattern. However, this can also be confirmed on MRI as a low-signal vertical line on T2-weighted images. Insufficiency fractures can occur in other locations in the pelvis and lower extremity (e.g., the supra-acetabular region), often incited by altered weight-bearing due to knee or hip arthroplasty or a painful condition. Resorption at the fracture site can also simulate a lytic metastasis.
2. *Atypical location/orientation.* Stress fractures can occur in unexpected locations (Fig. 6-11) related to particular activities (e.g., spine—ballet, gymnastics; distal humerus—pitching; distal radius—gymnastics, basketball; femur—gymnastics, jumping-planting leg; tarsal bones—running). The radiologist may not think of stress injury in these locations, and in some instances (tarsal bones, flat bones, spine) because of the small size of the bone or the lack of periosteum, the appearance may be atypical. Stress fractures in subchondral locations are often confused with avascular necrosis, such as spontaneous necrosis of the knee (SONK) or with transient osteoporosis of the hip, and can also be seen at the ankle. Occasionally, the orientation of the stress fracture causes confusion, such as in the tibia, where vertically oriented stress fractures are not uncommon (Fig. 6-12). Following axial images, the linear nature of the subcortical dark signal is evident.
3. *Early stress fracture/stress response.* On radiographs of children, subtle sclerosis or periosteal response can prompt concern for malignancy. In this case, history of change in activity should be sought, with short-term follow-up radiographs (after 2 to 4 weeks) usually adequate for documenting expected evolution of findings. Nowadays, parents are often unwilling to wait, and MRI is useful to confirm the diagnosis.
4. *"Reading in a vacuum"—incomplete clinical information.* Whenever tumor enters the differential diagnosis, the history and clinical presentation should be evaluated because of the overlap of imaging findings of tumor with fracture, infection, and other non-neoplastic entities.

Radiographs and CT may early reveal indeterminate or confusing findings, such as subtle periosteal reaction or an area of bone sclerosis. Given the clinical context, look closely for sclerosis to be primarily subcortical in location, with the fracture oriented perpendicular to the trabecular pattern. Bone scan shows a focus of markedly increased uptake, usually eccentric, but the pattern is nonspecific. MRI can confirm a suspected diagnosis, with a characteristic dark line on T1- and T2-weighted images extending from the cortex into the medullary cavity, surrounded by edema (see Fig. 6-12). Tumors, on the other hand, show a discrete lesion on MRI without the dark line.

Schmorl's Node and Hemispheric Spondylosclerosis

Schmorl's nodes are often associated with reactive sclerosis, or hemispheric spondylosclerosis. When

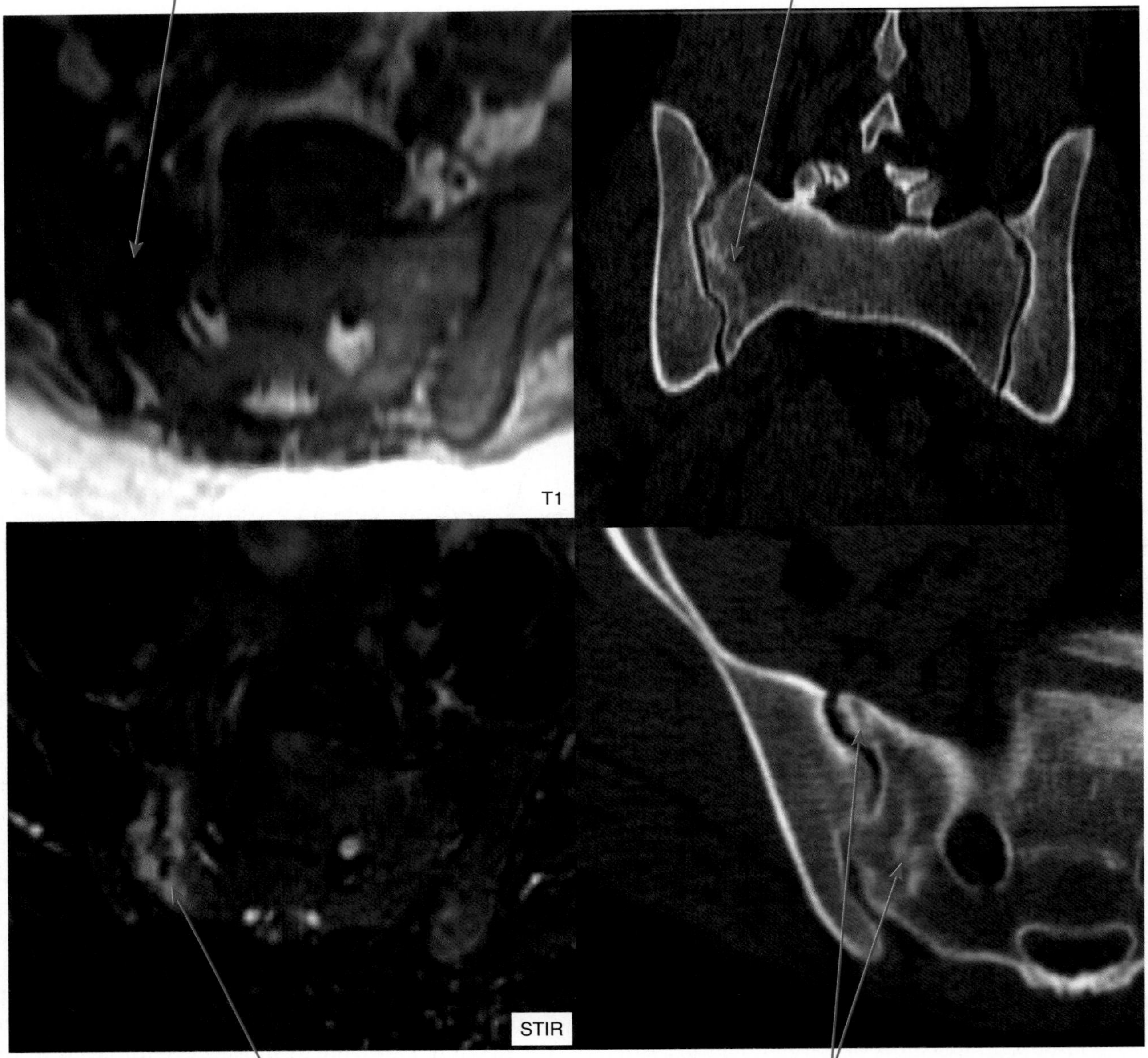

Stress fracture can be confused for tumor
Fracture line
T1
STIR
Fracture line
Fracture line

Figure 6-10 Ill-defined edema in the sacral ala should raise suspicion of stress fracture, especially in the elderly or in those who have recently had pelvic radiation therapy. The vertically oriented fracture line can usually be seen on coronal images but is characteristic on the axial plane as well. In chronic fractures, T2-weighted images typically show a well-defined fracture line surrounded by ill-defined marrow edema. However, depending on acuity the imaging features can vary, so the fracture line should be sought on all imaging planes/sequences. On CT, ill-defined sclerosis can simulate tumor, but close inspection reveals linear nature and/or vertical interruption of the sacral foraminal lines. The fracture is often bilateral and passes across a sacral vertebral body (responsible for the H sign on bone scan).

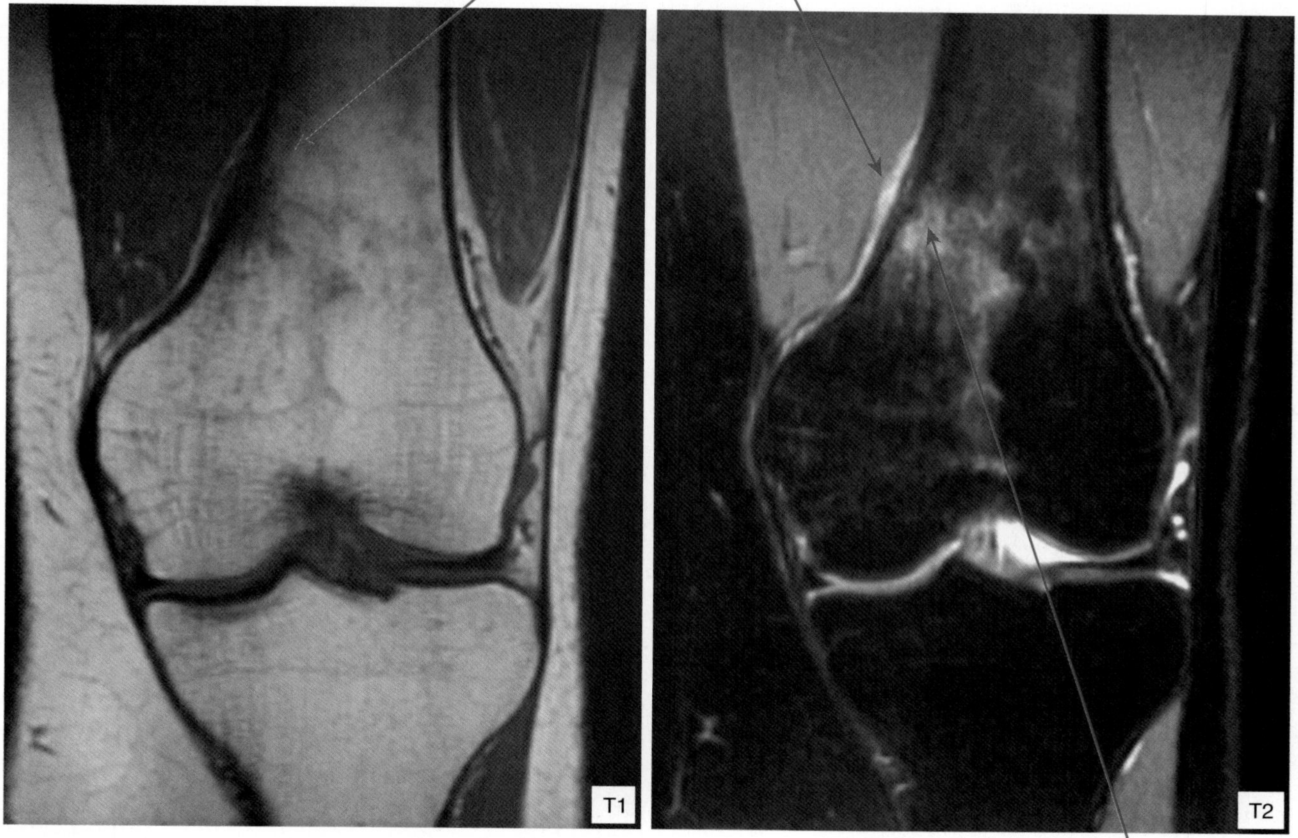
Bone tumors typically show a discrete mass on MRI, even if infiltrative on radiographs
Stress fracture
• Edema without discrete lesion
Periostitis on MRI
T1
T2
A subcortical dark line, even if small, is highly specific for stress fracture– best seen on fat-suppressed T2-weighted images

Figure 6-11 Stress fractures in atypical locations may simulate tumor. History is important, but visualization of a low-signal subcortical line is highly specific; biopsy can be misleading, showing osteoid matrix and mitoses similar to osteosarcoma. Therefore, if stress fracture is a possibility, MRI (to look for the subcortical line) or short-term radiographic follow-up (stress fractures evolve quickly—usually over a few weeks, developing smooth, thick periosteal reaction) is preferred.

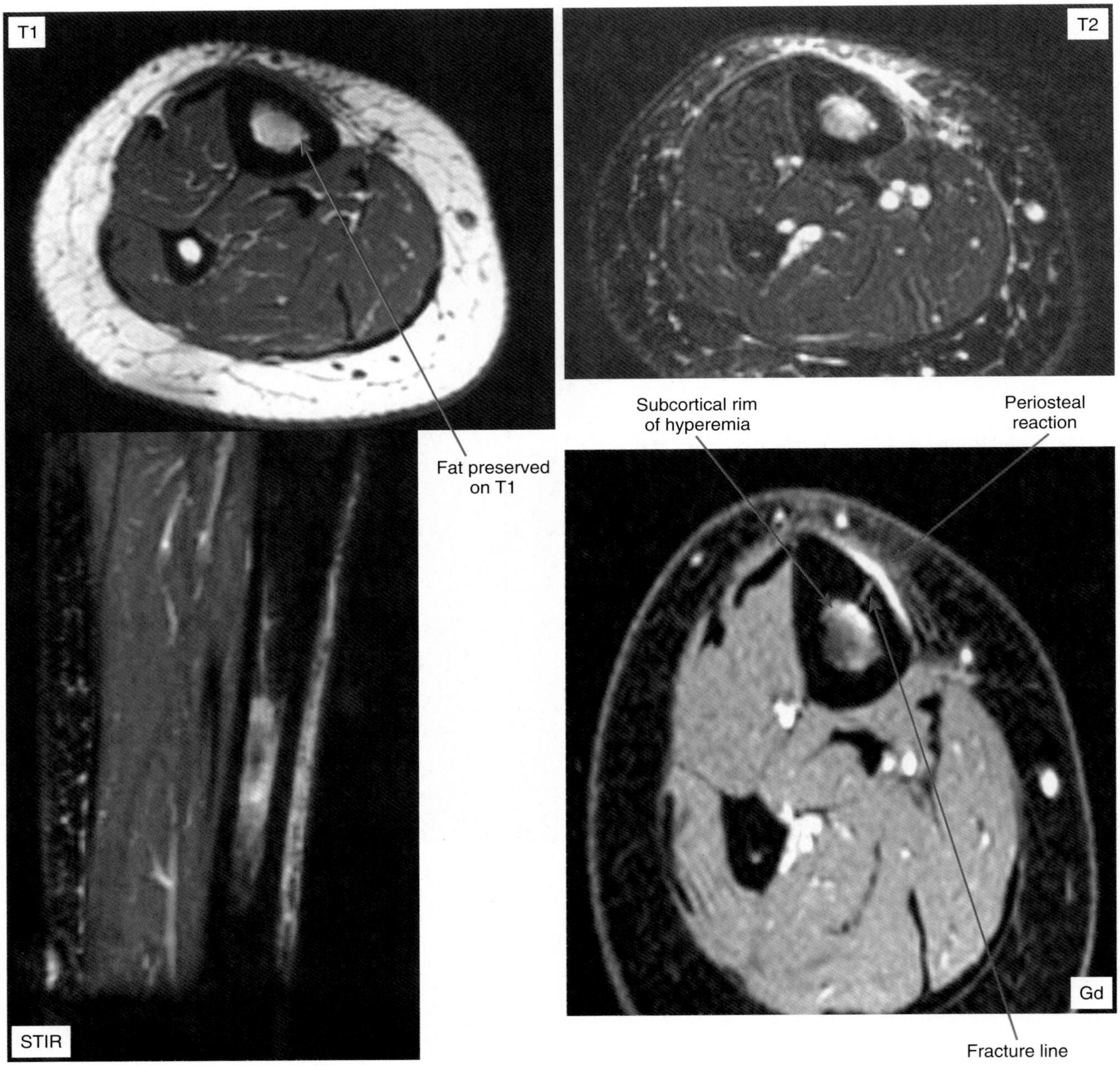
T1
T2
Subcortical rim of hyperemia
Periosteal reaction
Fat preserved on T1
STIR
Gd
Fracture line

Figure 6-12 Longitudinal stress fracture. Atypical locations and appearances of stress on various modalities can simulate tumor. In the tibia, stress fractures can be longitudinally oriented. The key is to look for the fracture line and the subcortical rim of edema/enhancement characteristic of stress.

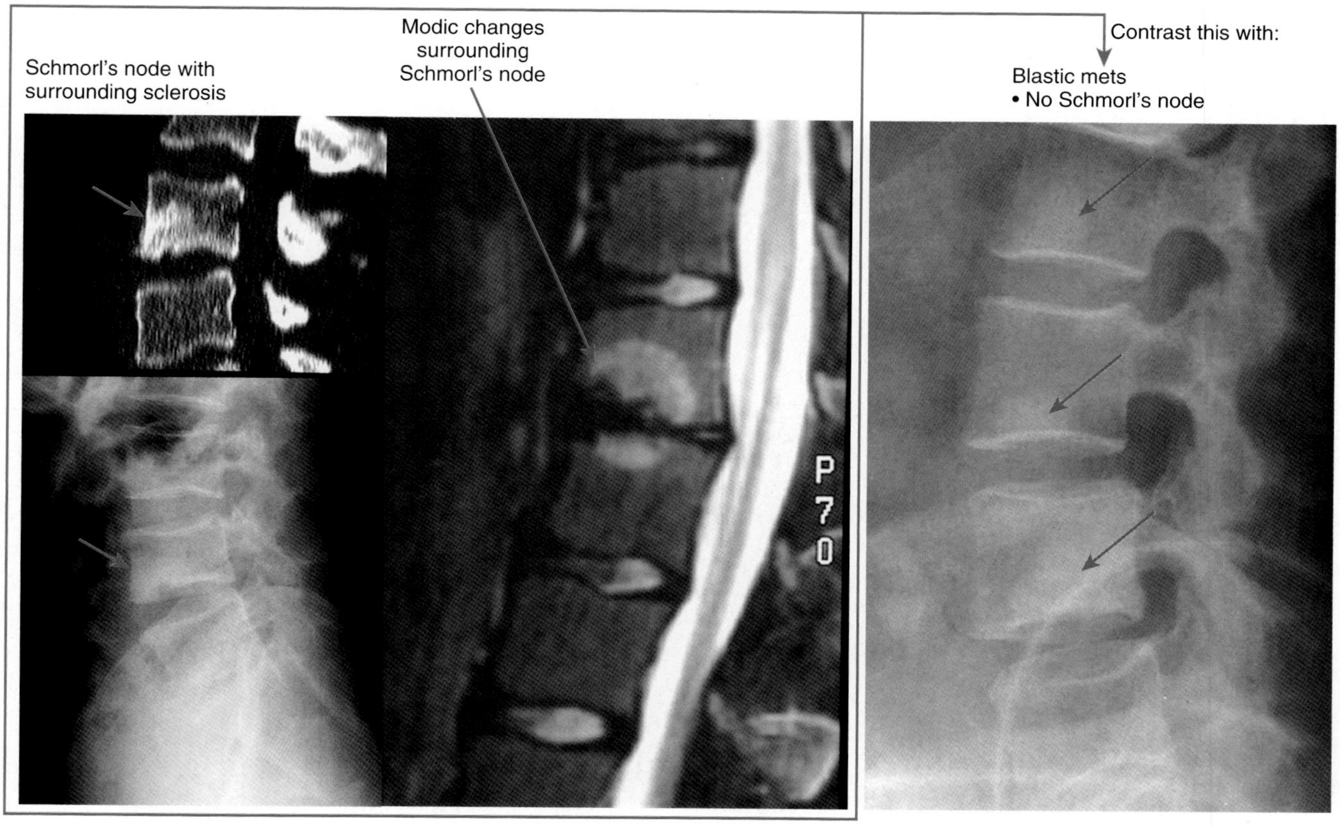
Schmorl's node with surrounding sclerosis
Modic changes surrounding Schmorl's node
P 7 0
Contrast this with:
Blastic mets
• No Schmorl's node

Figure 6-13 Schmorl's node and hemispherical spondylosclerosis. Modic-type degenerative changes occur around the node, which represents intraosseous extension of disk material. In later stages, Modic type 3 changes can ensue with rounded sclerosis (hemispherical spondylosclerosis). This can simulate a blastic metastasis. Associated endplate invagination can help differentiate these.

extensive, this can simulate a sclerotic metastasis (Fig. 6-13). On radiographs, communication with the adjacent disk and associated degeneration may not be apparent, but this can be confirmed with CT or MRI.

Bone Island (Enostosis) Versus Blastic Tumor

Bone islands are essentially benign hamartomas consisting of a focus of cortical bone within medullary bone. They can simulate a solitary metastasis on radiographs. Bone islands are usually seen as solitary or scattered foci but are seen in greater numbers in tuberous sclerosis and sclerosing bone dysplasias. There are a few imaging features suggesting their benign etiology. First, the margins of bone islands classically "blend" with the adjacent trabeculae. Also, bone islands tend to be ovoid in shape; metastases tend *not* to be round (Fig. 6-14). These characteristics are not as comforting when reviewing an examination of a patient with a history of cancer. In this setting, a bone scan is very useful. Bone islands show minimal to no increased uptake, whereas, if large enough, a blastic metastasis should show intense uptake. In addition, bone scan can detect other lesions. CT may detect the trabecular blending better than bone scan, but it is not usually very useful. MRI can be useful because bone islands are typically monotonous black signal on all sequences, whereas metastatic lesions often contain some T2 hyperintensity and enhancement, even if blastic. PET scan could be useful, again, only if the lesion is large enough to detect. Like bone scan, if the PET scan is negative and the lesion is less than 1 cm, further workup (such as biopsy) may still be necessary.

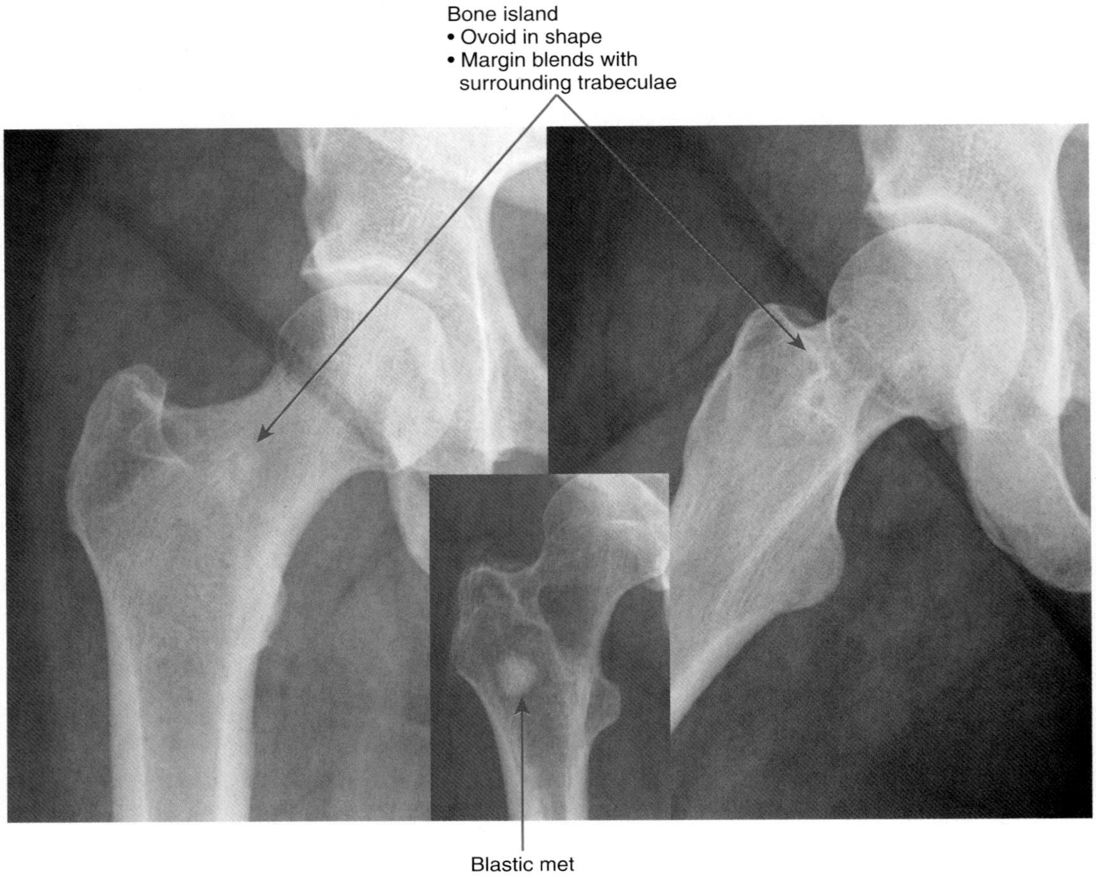
Bone island
• Ovoid in shape
• Margin blends with surrounding trabeculae
Blastic met

Figure 6-14 Bone islands may simulate blastic metastases. Bone islands are generally ovoid in shape with fuzzy margins that blend with surrounding trabeculae. Blastic metastases are typically rounded and have sharper margins. However, there is considerable overlap in appearance. If there is concern, a bone scan can differentiate a blastic metastasis (high degree of uptake) from a bone island (no increased uptake or slightly "warm").

Paget Disease

Paget disease deserves special mention in this chapter, not only because it can simulate tumor, but also because of its association with certain tumors. The disease usually affects people over age 50, but it can be seen in those in their late 30s. It can affect virtually any bone in the body but it favors the pelvis, proximal femur, sacrum, and spine. The disease passes through an early lytic phase and a late reparative phase. The early phase is characterized by well-defined regions of osteolysis. This has been described on radiographs as osteolysis circumscripta in the skull and a "blade of grass" appearance in long bones, the latter referring to a sharp, dagger-shaped lucency. The margin of osteolysis represents the advancing front of the process, which characteristically begins at the end of a bone with the exception of the tibia, where it may start at the tibial tuberosity. Eventually, the margin extends over a large area. If not recognized as such, early pagetoid bone can simulate a lytic tumor. MRI is very useful as a second modality because the involved bone does not show findings typical of tumor. Various MRI appearances have been described in part reflecting the phasic nature of the disease, but often the marrow shows some retained fat signal and/or mild diffuse edema. Bone scan is especially helpful for establishing the diagnosis because involved bone shows intense, geographic uptake of radiotracer along an entire bone or an extensive portion of the bone.

In the healing, or reparative, phase, bone is laid down appositionally (i.e., along the cortex) and within the medullary cavity, causing the bone to

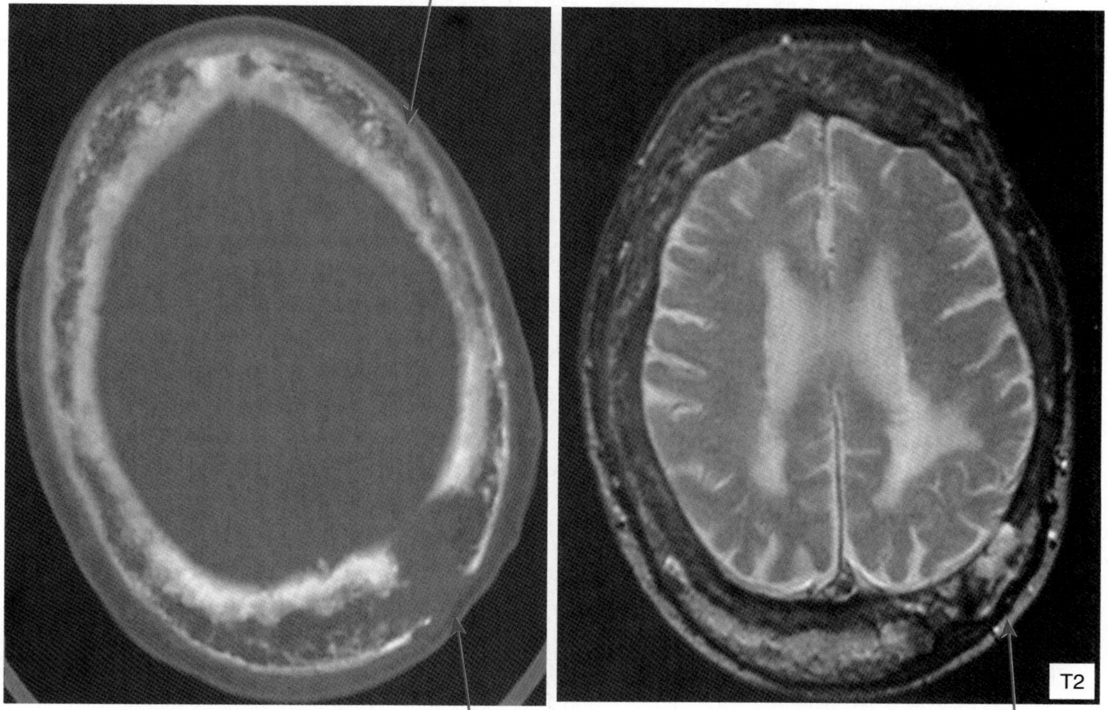
Pagetoid bone
• Cortical thickening
• Expansion
• Coarse trabeculae
T2
Lytic lesion
T2 hyperintensity

Figure 6-15 Lytic area in pagetoid bone—secondary sarcoma (osteosarcoma, fibrosarcoma, or chondrosarcoma) until proven otherwise. Giant cell tumors can also occur and present as a lytic lesion, as in this case.

appear denser and forming the characteristic hallmarks of Paget disease: cortical thickening, trabecular coarsening, and an appearance of bone expansion. In its softened state, the deformities of Paget disease occur in affected bones owing to stresses from weight-bearing. This includes protrusio acetabuli and bowing of long bones, with a "shepherd's crook deformity" of the proximal femur. Deformity at joints can cause osteoarthritis, and expansion of bone can result in narrowing of vascular and neural foramina.

Late involvement of Paget disease is characteristic on radiographs, with the hallmarks as above. However, in unclear cases, CT is useful to confirm the presence of cortical thickening and fat density in the marrow. Bone scan is quite specific, with geographic uptake as previously discussed. MRI often shows some fat in the underlying marrow. Secondary tumors can occur, and any focal lytic areas, cortical destruction, or soft tissue mass associated with pagetoid bone should be pursued (Fig. 6-15). Sarcomas, including osteosarcomas, chondrosarcomas, and fibrosarcomas can occur and are very aggressive with a poor prognosis. Giant cell tumors can also occur and appear very similar, but usually without a significant soft tissue mass. Biopsy is needed to document histology of suspicious areas.

Sclerosing Bone Dysplasias

Osteopoikilosis, osteopathia striata, and melorheostosis are sclerosing bone dysplasias, which are benign conditions resulting in areas of bone formation. This dysplasia occurs either within the medullary cavity, as with osteopoikilosis and osteopathia striata, or along the cortex and adjacent soft tissues, as with melorheostosis. Osteopoikilosis is the one most often confused with tumor. In this condition, numerous small foci of sclerotic bone representing bone islands

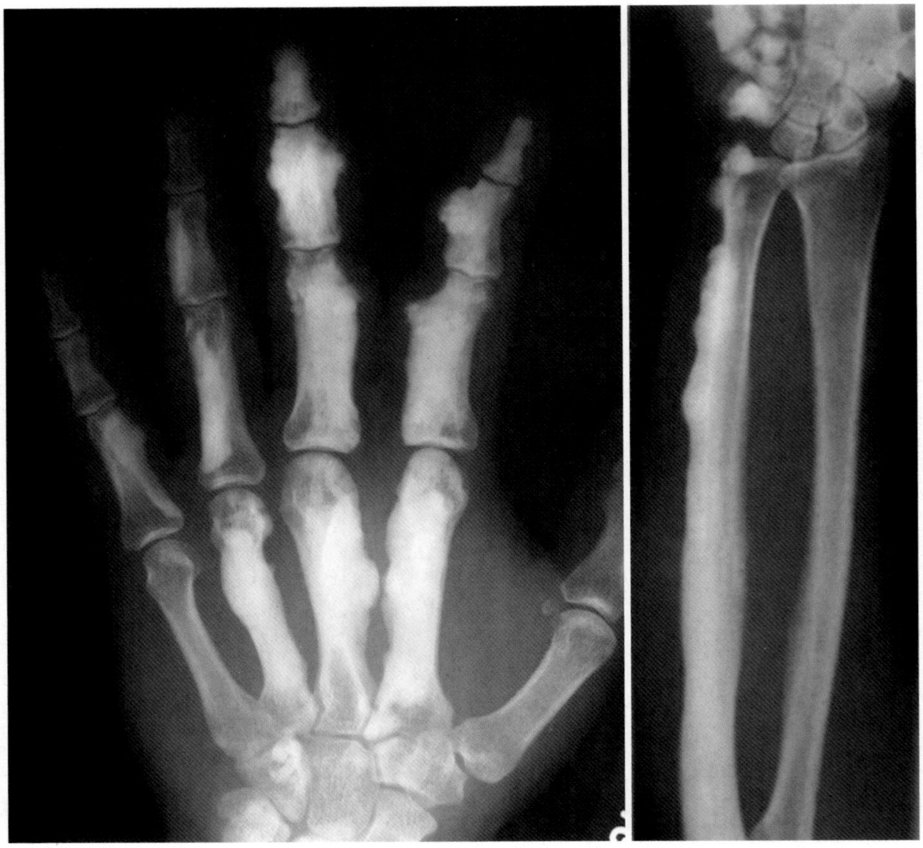

Figure 6-16 Melorheostosis with characteristic "dripping wax" pattern of sclerosis.

are seen in the epiphyses and apophyses. The correct diagnosis is usually suggested by the fact that this distribution is the opposite of typical metastatic disease, which usually spares the growth centers. Osteopathia striata (Voorhaave disease) has a linear pattern of medullary sclerosis and is not usually confused with malignancy. In melorheostosis (Fig. 6-16), the bone formation is along the cortex and/or adjacent soft tissues (dripping wax pattern) in a sclerotomal distribution along the neural supply of the affected bones. Because of this, multiple bones may be involved along the nerve distribution. These dysplasias can also appear together in mixed patterns.

Sarcoidosis

Sarcoid is most common in the middle and distal phalanges of the hands and feet but can involve any bone. The classic lacy destruction and lack of periosteal reaction are usually recognized in the phalanges, but in other bones the pattern may mimic an aggressive neoplasm. The bone lesions are usually painful. When seen in young adults, these lacy lesions should prompt correlation with history or chest radiographs. If imaged with MRI alone, the findings may not appear characteristic, and the lesion can be misinterpreted as an aggressive one (Fig. 6-17).

Pseudolesion/Red Marrow

Areas of normally sparce trabeculae can simulate a lytic lesion on radiographs and sometimes on CT (Fig. 6-18). Common locations are the greater tuberosity of the proximal humerus, the proximal femur (called Ward triangle), and the body of the calcaneus. If unclear, MRI can confirm the presence of fat or hematopoietic marrow within these regions.

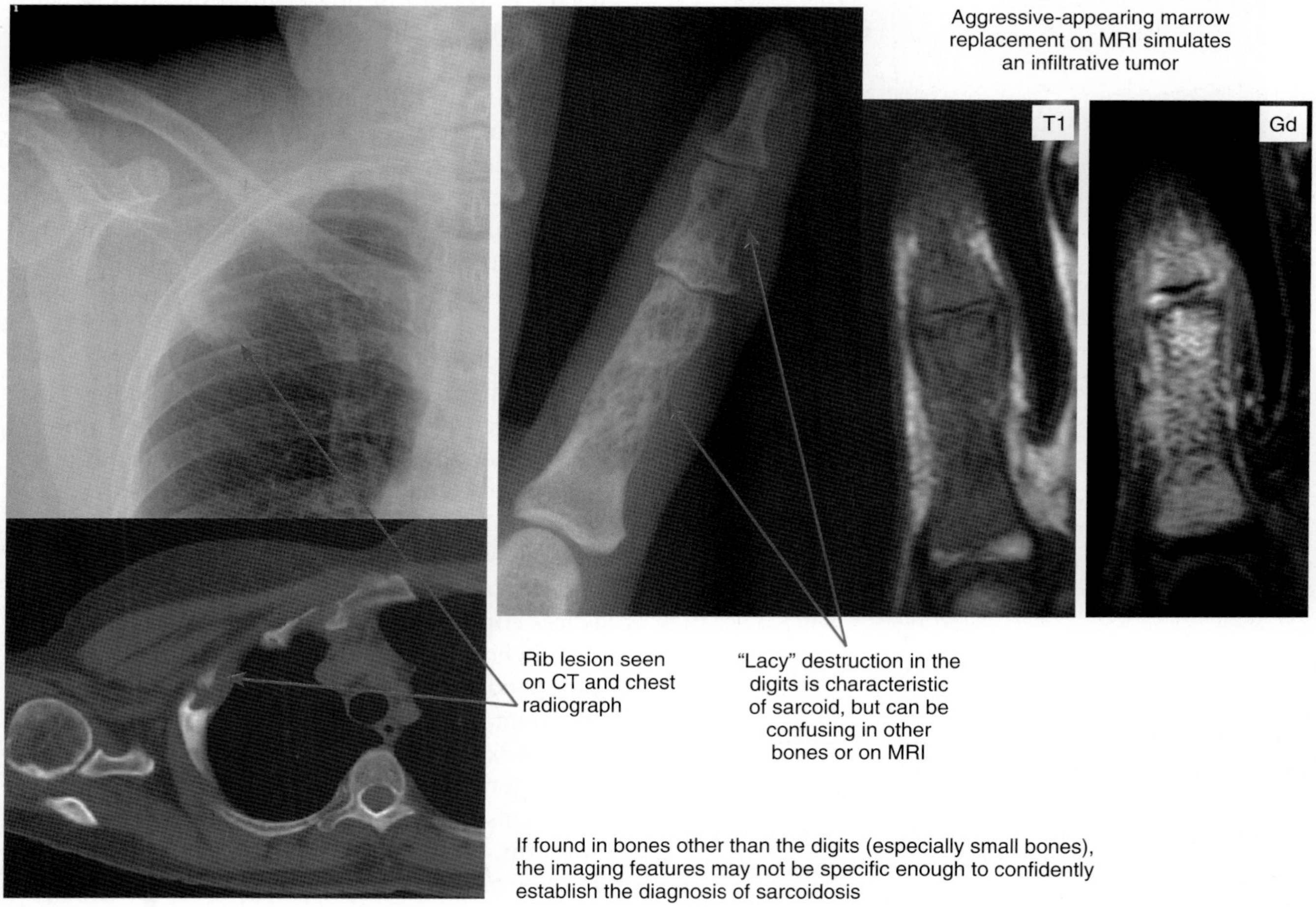
Aggressive-appearing marrow replacement on MRI simulates an infiltrative tumor
T1
Gd
Rib lesion seen on CT and chest radiograph
"Lacy" destruction in the digits is characteristic of sarcoid, but can be confusing in other bones or on MRI
If found in bones other than the digits (especially small bones), the imaging features may not be specific enough to confidently establish the diagnosis of sarcoidosis

Figure 6-17 Sarcoid can affect any bone and may require biopsy even with the appropriate history or corresponding pulmonary findings. The pathologist should be alerted to the possibility of sarcoid of bone, and an adequate specimen should be obtained to evaluate for noncaseating granulomas that are characteristic of the disease.

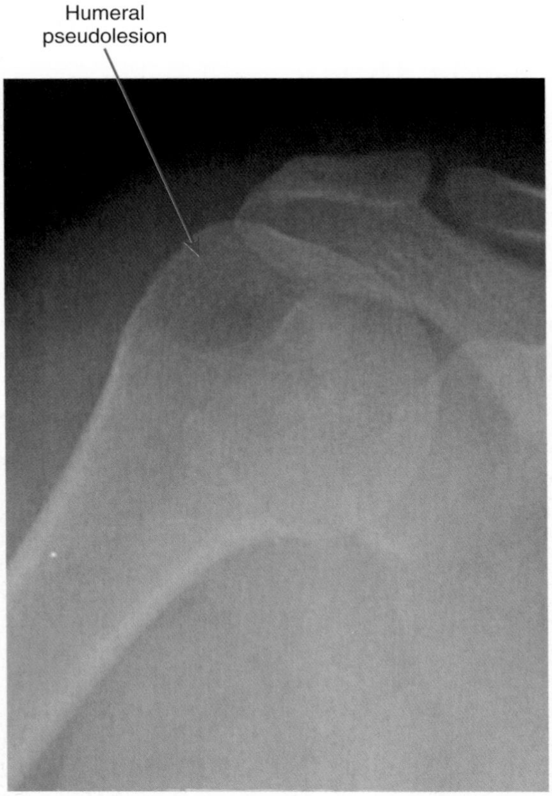
Humeral pseudolesion

Figure 6-18 Humeral pseudolesion. Relative lack of trabeculation and projection results in focal lucency of the greater tuberosity. This is also common at the proximal femur and the calcaneal body.

On MRI, hematopoietic marrow is usually overlooked except when it is perceived on images from a certain sequence (e.g., STIR), when it is in an atypical location (as in the proximal radius), or when it is seen in older persons with heterogeneous replacement with fatty marrow. The key to recognizing hematopoietic marrow is signal and location.

Signal. Red marrow is intermediate on T2-weighted images, bright on STIR, and intermediate on T1-weighted images. The T1-weighted images are key. Since red marrow contains fat, it will be brighter than muscle (Fig. 6-19). A process such as tumor that replaces marrow would be expected to be relatively isointense to muscle (Fig. 6-20). This is the same principle as in MRI of the spine in which, if the marrow on T1-weighted images is darker than that of the disk, there should be concern for tumor infiltration. If there is a question, comparison of sequences acquired in-phase and out-of-phase can be very useful (Fig. 6-21). Similar to imaging of adrenal masses, this technique has the ability to detect small amounts of fat within a suspicious area of bone. Red marrow contains about half fat and half cellular hematopoietic components, which contain a large amount of water. On in-phase images, the signal from fat and water is additive; on out-of-phase images, the signal subtracts. If a voxel contains both fat and water, the signal decreases on out-of-phase images compared with in-phase images. Therefore, hematopoietic marrow drops in signal, usually more than 50%. Like tumor, purely fatty marrow does not drop in signal, so the other sequences must be taken into account. Severe anemias and treatment with marrow-stimulating agents can produce red marrow with a highly cellular nature (Fig. 6-22), but interspersed fat cells should still lead to the correct diagnosis on T1-weighted sequences and in-phase and out-of-phase imaging.

Location. Radiologists should be aware of the distribution of hematopoietic marrow and appearance in children and adults (Fig. 6-23). Distribution follows certain principles. Epiphyses and apophyses should contain fatty marrow once they are ossified (Fig. 6-24). Two exceptions are the humeral head, in which subchondral red marrow is common and can be extensive, and the femoral head, which is less common and usually limited to a thin rim of subchondral signal (see Fig. 6-21). This signal can persist into adulthood. Diaphyses typically lose their red marrow in childhood, but not always. The proximal metaphyses of the humerus and femur tend to maintain red marrow into old age. This is also seen in the pelvis, spine, ribs, clavicles, sternum, and skull. More hematopoietic marrow is seen in females, especially if obese (Box 6-1).

BOX 6-1 DIFFERENTIAL DIAGNOSIS: PROMINENT HEMATOPOIETIC MARROW

- Young age
- Obesity
- Female
- Smoker
- Anemia
  - Sickle cell disease
  - Thalassemia
- Altitude
- Colony-stimulating factor
- Chemotherapy recovery

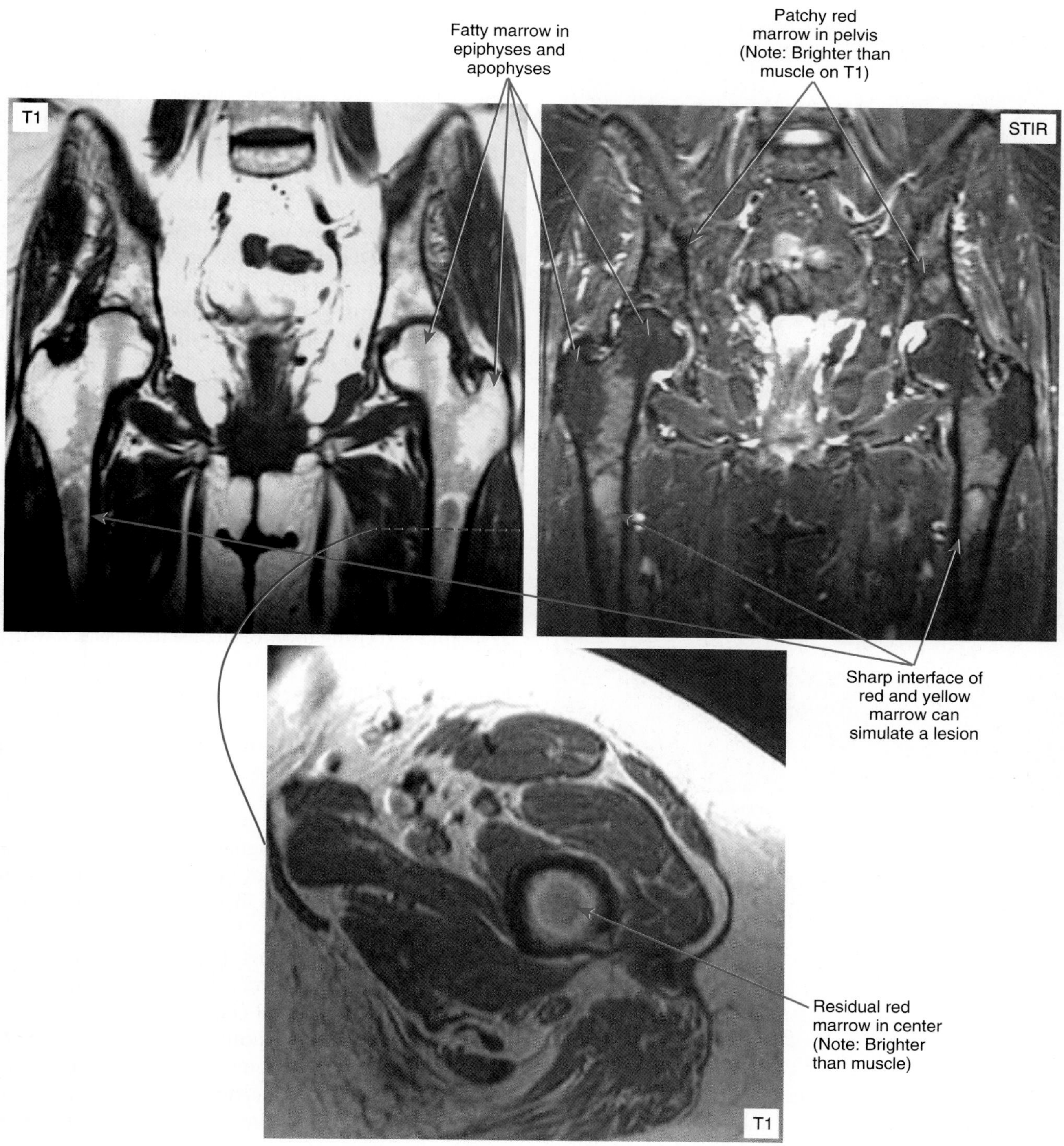
Fatty marrow in epiphyses and apophyses
Patchy red marrow in pelvis (Note: Brighter than muscle on T1)
T1
STIR
Sharp interface of red and yellow marrow can simulate a lesion
Residual red marrow in center (Note: Brighter than muscle)
T1

Figure 6-19 **Normal red and yellow marrow distribution in the pelvis and hips of an adult.**

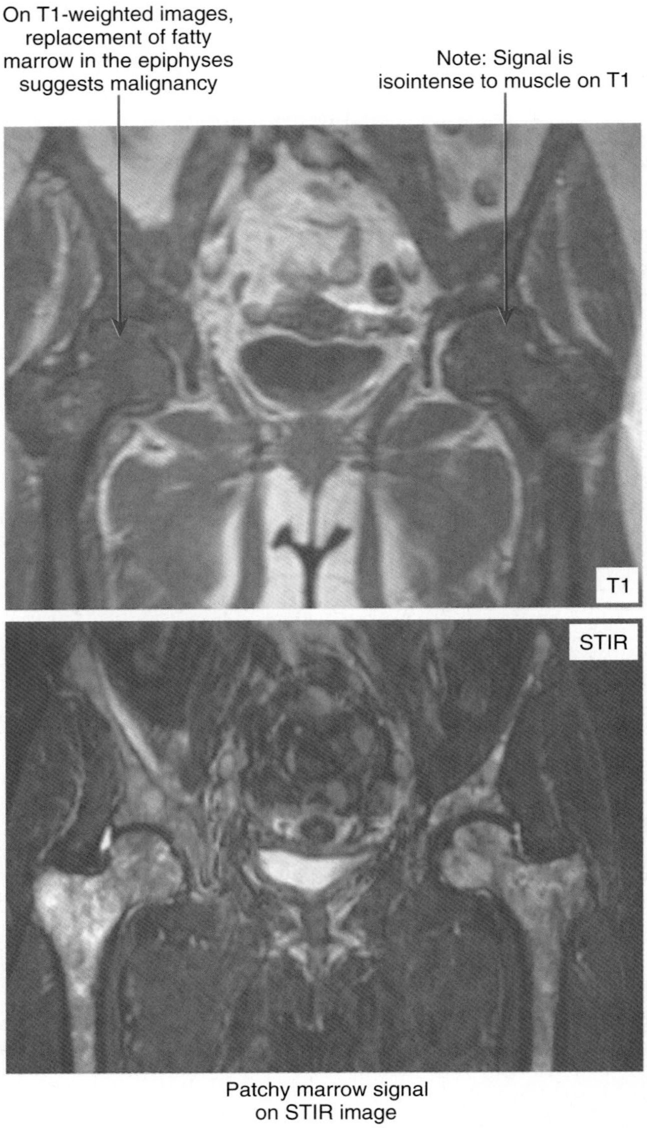
On T1-weighted images, replacement of fatty marrow in the epiphyses suggests malignancy
Note: Signal is isointense to muscle on T1
T1
STIR
Patchy marrow signal on STIR image

Figure 6-20 Breast metastases with diffuse marrow involvement.

Obviously, more red marrow will be seen in young patients, recognized as normal in the axial skeleton but often causing confusion in the peripheral extremities, where they are seen as small foci of hyperintensity at the wrist and ankle (Fig. 6-25). Prominent hematopoietic marrow can be seen in anemias and following certain treatments. Radiation therapy causes regression of red marrow in the field, with geographic fatty marrow distribution.

Interpreting a Pair of In-Phase and Out-of-Phase Sequences

First, one must perform quality assurance (Fig. 6-26). All parameters except echo time (TE) must be constant. The patient should not move or be rescouted in between. The best way to accomplish this is to acquire both echoes in the same series, performed as a double echo—out-of-phase and in-phase. A two-point Dixon fat-water separation sequence, available as an option on many machines, incorporates this automatically. Next, make sure the TEs are optimized for the field strength and that an adequate out-of-phase effect is achieved (Fig. 6-27). The out-of-phase images should show a dark line at fat/muscle interfaces. Since muscle contains a large amount of water, its signal will cancel when fat is in the same voxel. Next, perform regions of interest (ROIs) on an area of water signal (e.g., cerebrospinal fluid, bladder, joint fluid); there should be little or no change. ROIs of tissue must be performed the same in terms of size and location. Decrease in signal can be expressed as a percentile. The out-of-phase sequence is also useful as a rapid screening tool for metastatic lesions, which generally stand out dramatically against a dark background. Subsequent comparison with T1-weighted images and measurement of ROIs narrow the diagnostic differential, excluding hemangiomas and focal fat.

Pitfalls

- Little or no drop in signal also occurs in lesions composed entirely of fat (avascular necrosis, hemangioma, fatty marrow, lipoma Fig. 6-28), or fluid (cysts).
- Very infiltrative lesions (e.g., myeloma). These lesions can preserve microscopic areas of fat and result in drop in signal (Fig. 6-29).
- Hemosiderin (transfusions, hemochromatosis) or densely calcified lesions. Blooming artifact can occur, since gradient-echo (GRE) sequences are usually used, altering the intended effect (Fig. 6-30).
- Change in other parameters resulting in change in overall signal characteristics.
- Different size or location of ROIs used for in-phase versus out-of-phase.

Text continued on page 281

Tissue	Composition	Out- versus In-Phase
Fatty marrow	fat >>H_2O	No noticeable decrease
Red marrow	H_2O = fat	Marked decrease
Tumor	No fat	No change

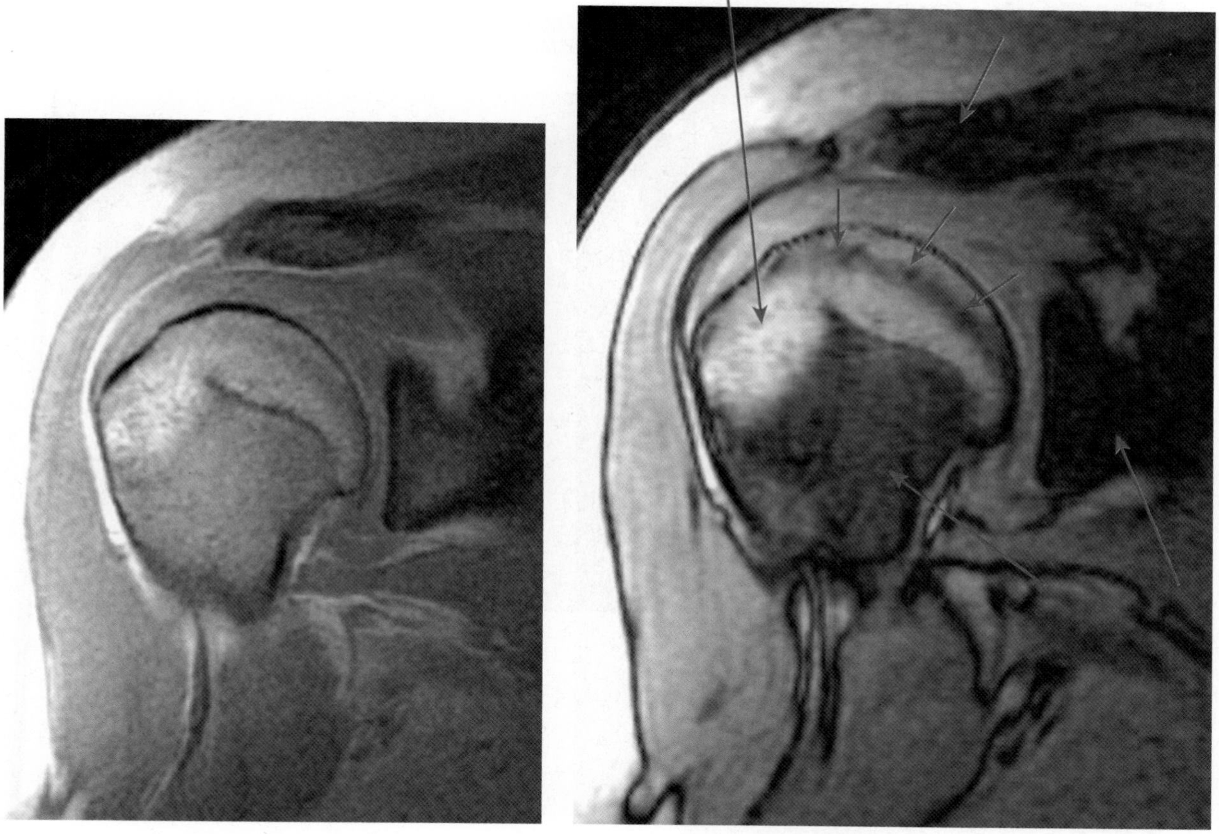
Fatty marrow remains bright
In-phase
Fat and fluid signal adds
Out-of-phase
Fat and fluid signal subtracts
Red marrow drops in signal

Figure 6-21 **Principle for use of in-phase and out-of-phase imaging for differentiation of red marrow from tumor.**

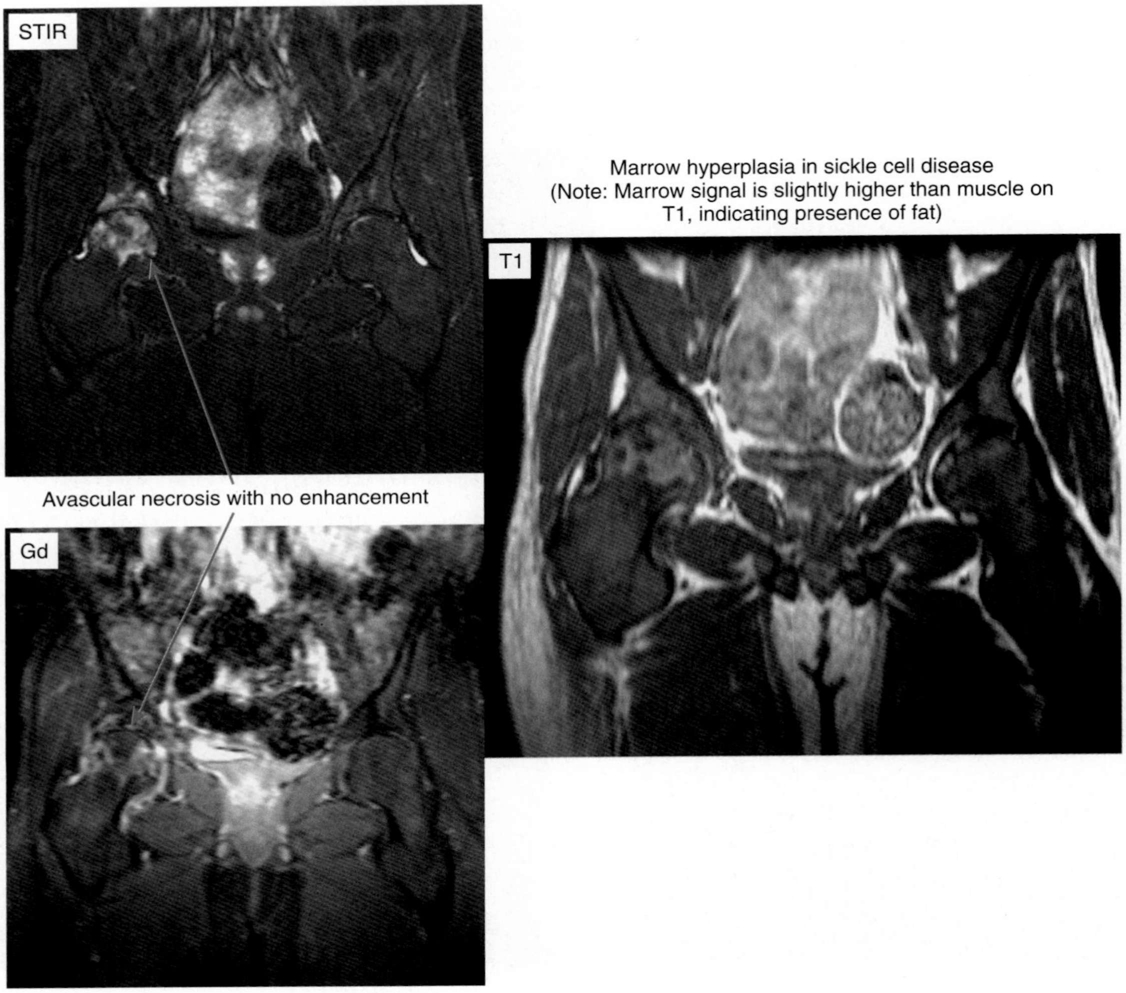
STIR
Marrow hyperplasia in sickle cell disease
(Note: Marrow signal is slightly higher than muscle on T1, indicating presence of fat)
T1
Avascular necrosis with no enhancement
Gd

Figure 6-22 Marrow in sickle cell disease. Severe anemias can result in red marrow hyperplasia with prominent distribution, lower T1 signal due to higher cellularity, and persistence or repopulation of epiphyses and apophyses. Multiple transfusions can also result in hemosiderin deposition in the marrow and lower signal on all sequences.

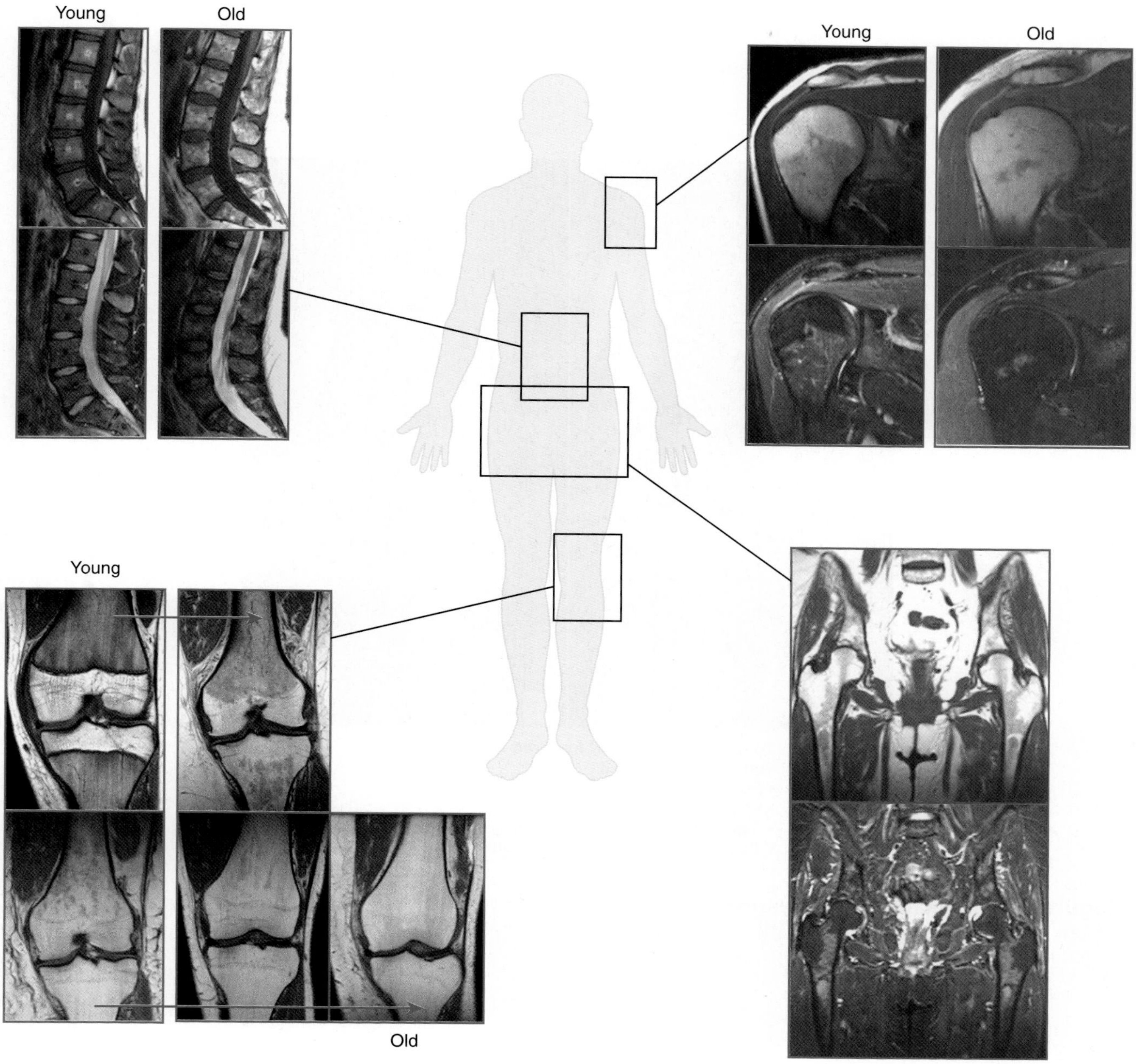
Young
Old
Young
Old
Young
Old

Figure 6-23 Hematopoietic marrow and appearance in adults.

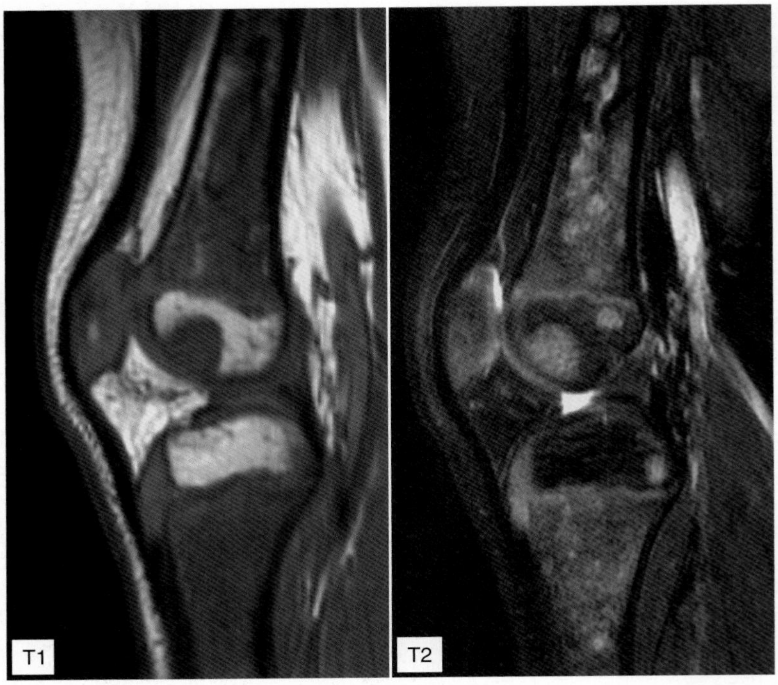
T1
T2

To differentiate tumor from red marrow
Tumor is more likely if
- Epiphysis is involved
- Focal rounded appearance
- Signal approximates muscle on T1

If there is doubt, perform in- and out-of-phase sequence

Figure 6-24 Metastatic neuroblastoma in a child. The ossified portion of the epiphysis should always be composed of fatty marrow, the exception being the humeral head and occasionally the femoral head, both of which can have a strip of red marrow in the subchondral bone even in adulthood.

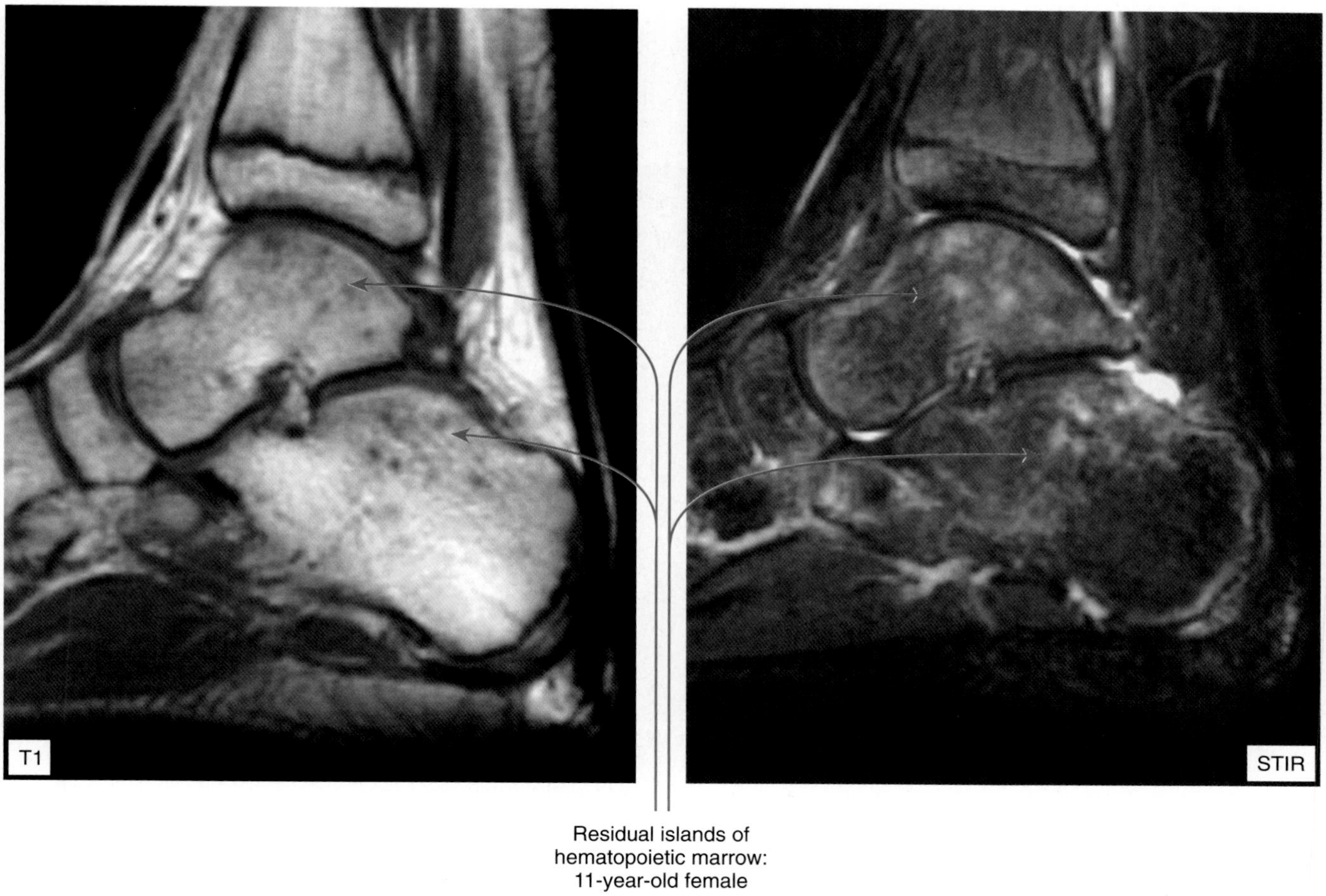
T1
STIR
Residual islands of
hematopoietic marrow:
11-year-old female

Figure 6-25 Adolescents often exhibit residual hematopoietic marrow in the hands and feet on MRI. Distribution is patchy or spotty.

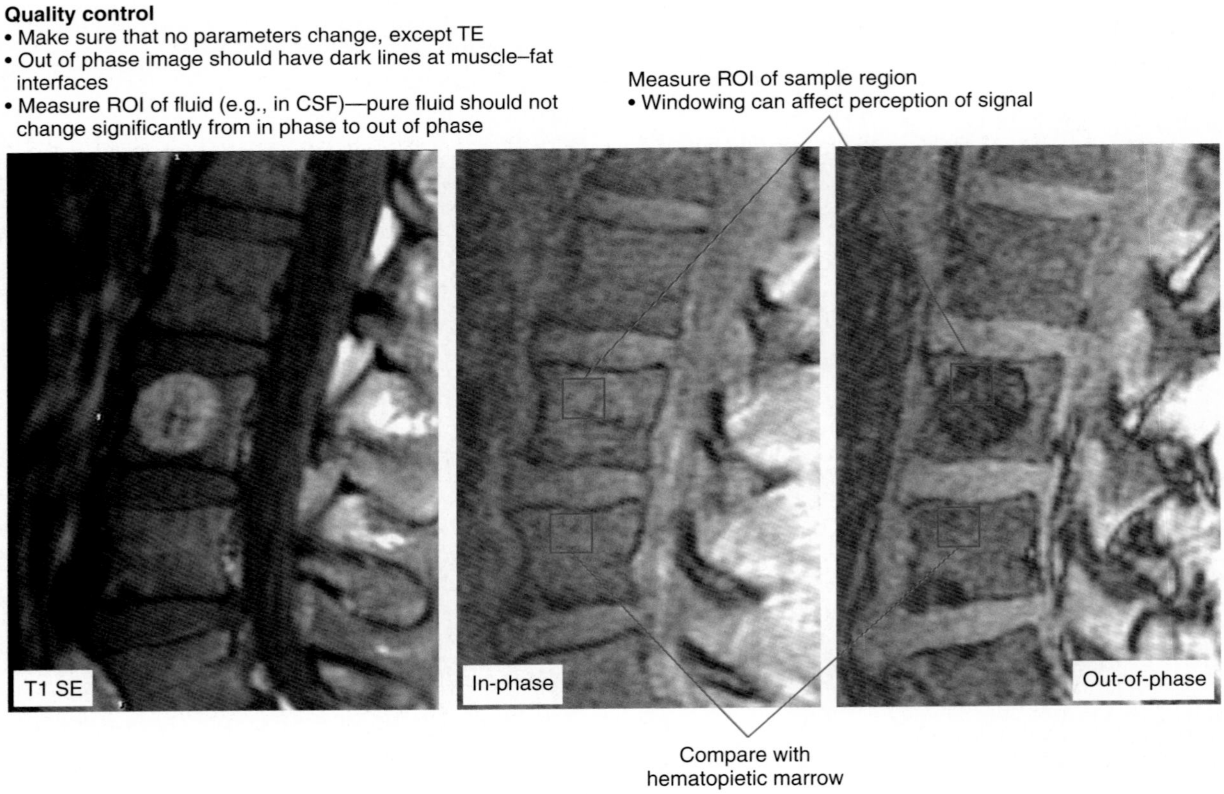
Quality control
• Make sure that no parameters change, except TE
• Out of phase image should have dark lines at muscle–fat interfaces
• Measure ROI of fluid (e.g., in CSF)—pure fluid should not change significantly from in phase to out of phase
Measure ROI of sample region
• Windowing can affect perception of signal
T1 SE
In-phase
Out-of-phase
Compare with hematopietic marrow

Figure 6-26 In this case the predominantly fatty hemangioma drops in signal on the out-of-phase image compared with the in-phase image, indicating presence of a small amount of water. The technique has a similar effect for lesions that contain a small amount of fat, which are more difficult to distinguish from malignancy on routine sequences. Intravenous contrast is not very useful in these cases (and may be misleading), since many benign lesions including hemangiomas enhance. CSF, cerebrospinal fluid; ROI, region of interest; TE, echo time.

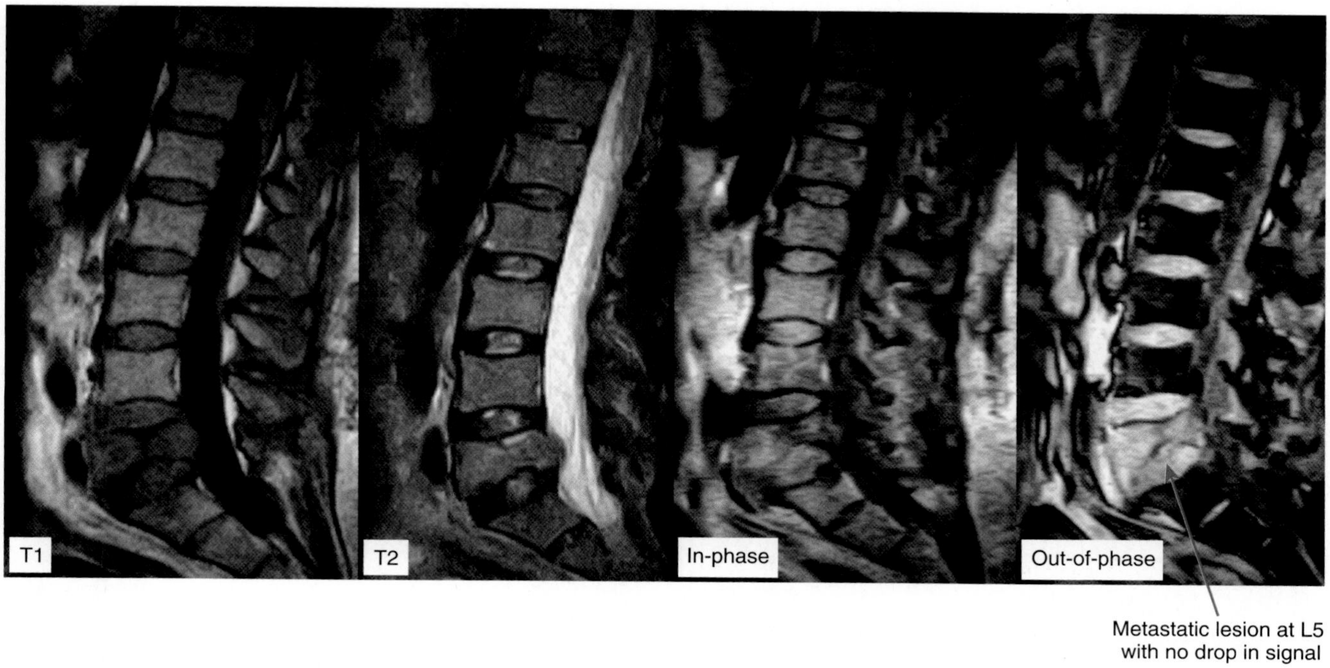
T1
T2
In-phase
Out-of-phase
Metastatic lesion at L5 with no drop in signal

Figure 6-27 In-phase and out-of-phase imaging can also be performed at low field strength using longer echo times. Here on a 0.3 T scanner, a metastatic lesion at L5 shows no drop in signal on out-of-phase compared with in-phase, consistent with lack of internal fat.

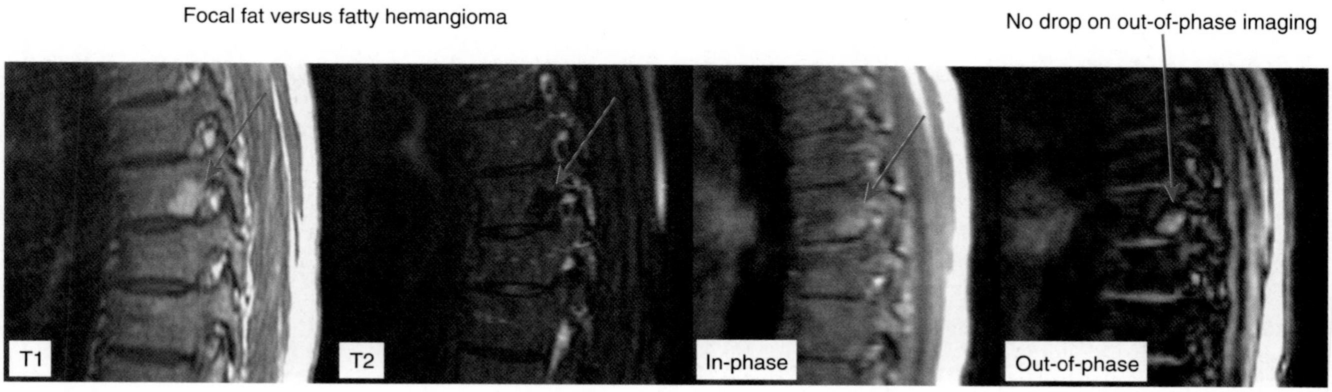
Focal fat versus fatty hemangioma
No drop on out-of-phase imaging
T1
T2
In-phase
Out-of-phase

Figure 6-28 Areas of focal fatty marrow—as well as lesions composed of all fat, including some hemangiomas and degenerative endplates—do not drop on out-of-phase images. Sclerotic lesions may appear to drop because of magnetic susceptibility artifact. In-phase and out-of-phase images must be read in conjunction with routine T1- and T2-weighted sequences as well as other available modalities.

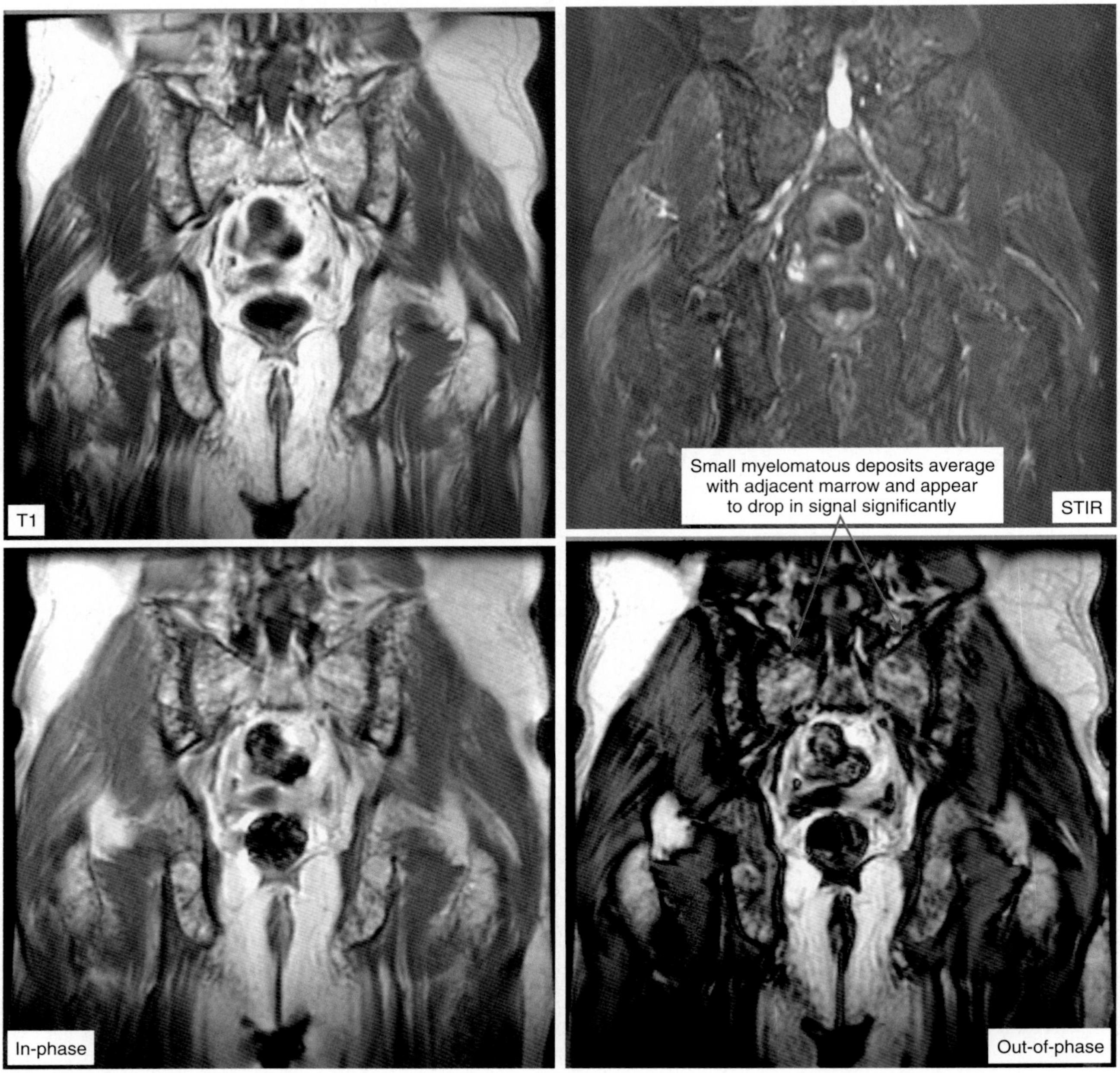
T1
STIR
Small myelomatous deposits average
with adjacent marrow and appear
to drop in signal significantly
In-phase
Out-of-phase

Figure 6-29 Pitfall of in-phase and out-of-phase imaging: multiple myeloma. Large tumors replace marrow fat. Small deposits of tumor can result in volume averaging with adjacent fatty or hematopoietic marrow resulting in a drop in signal on out-of-phase images.

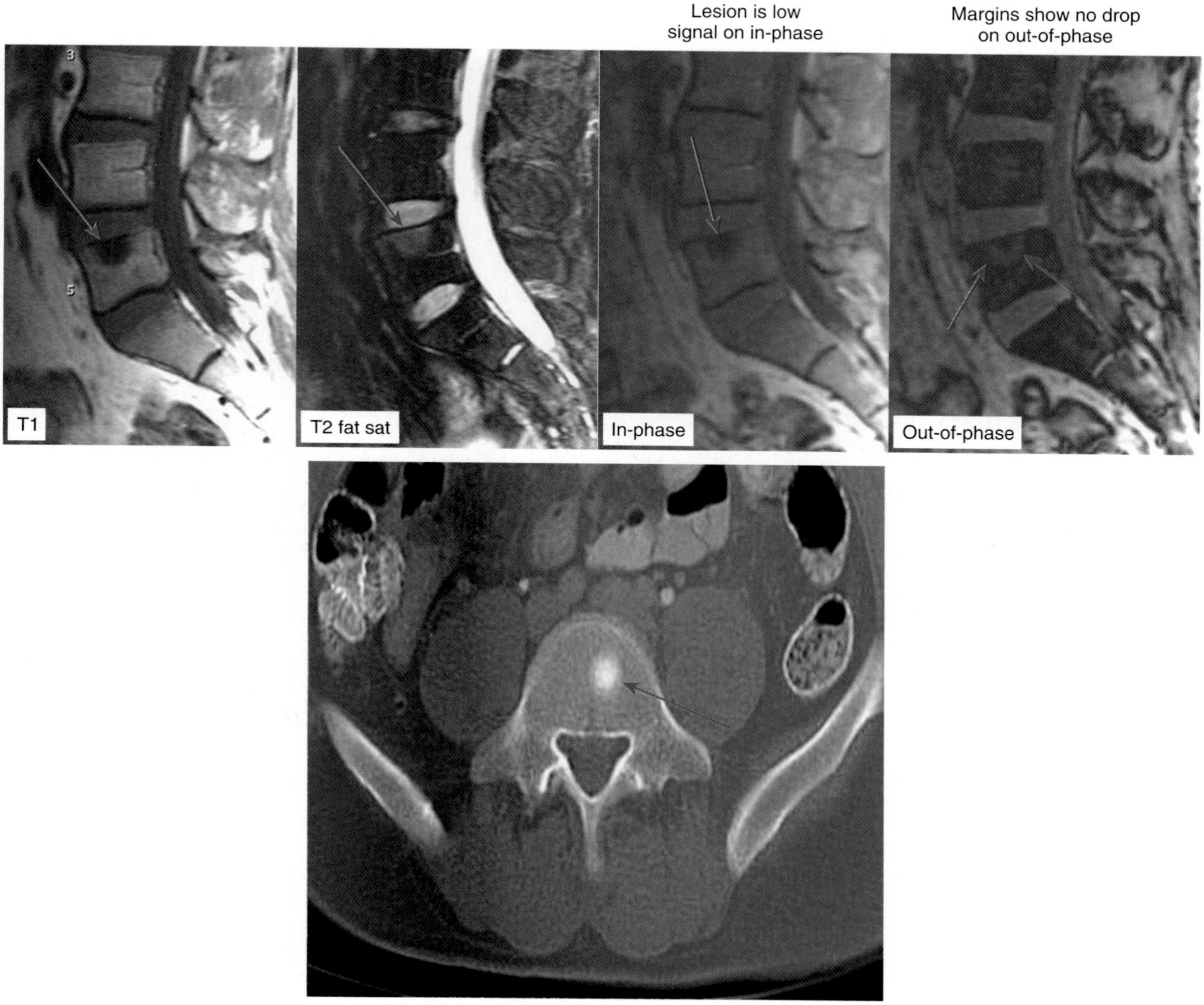
Lesion is low
signal on in-phase
Margins show no drop
on out-of-phase
T1
T2 fat sat
In-phase
Out-of-phase

Figure 6-30 Sclerotic lesion: neuroendocrine metastasis. Sclerotic lesions are typically dark on in-phase gradient-echo (GRE) images due to susceptibility artifact, and signal change may not have the same range or significance as with nonsclerotic lesions.

Normal and Abnormal Values In a 1.5 T study of normal spinal hematopoietic marrow in 569 adult vertebral bodies, drop in signal averaged 58.5% ± 15.9% and ranged from 11% to 93%. Age did not significantly affect results but weight did. Heavier individuals have more hematopoietic marrow. Two hundred-fifteen benign and 51 malignant lesions were also evaluated. Fifty-one metastatic lesions averaged 2.8% ± 21.3% drop; 8 osteoporotic fractures averaged 49.3% ± 18.4% drop in signal. There was overlap in signal drop between benign and malignant lesions, so a hard cutoff value is difficult to determine. In our practice, if a lesion is indeterminate for malignancy on conventional sequences, a drop in signal of more than 50% is considered benign. Less than 30% drop generally causes more concern and incites further workup. A drop in signal of less than 20% in a lesion that is also suspicious on conventional sequences is definitely a concern for the presence of malignancy.

Aggressive Osteoporosis

Areas of aggressive osteoporosis related to sudden immobilization can simulate myeloma on

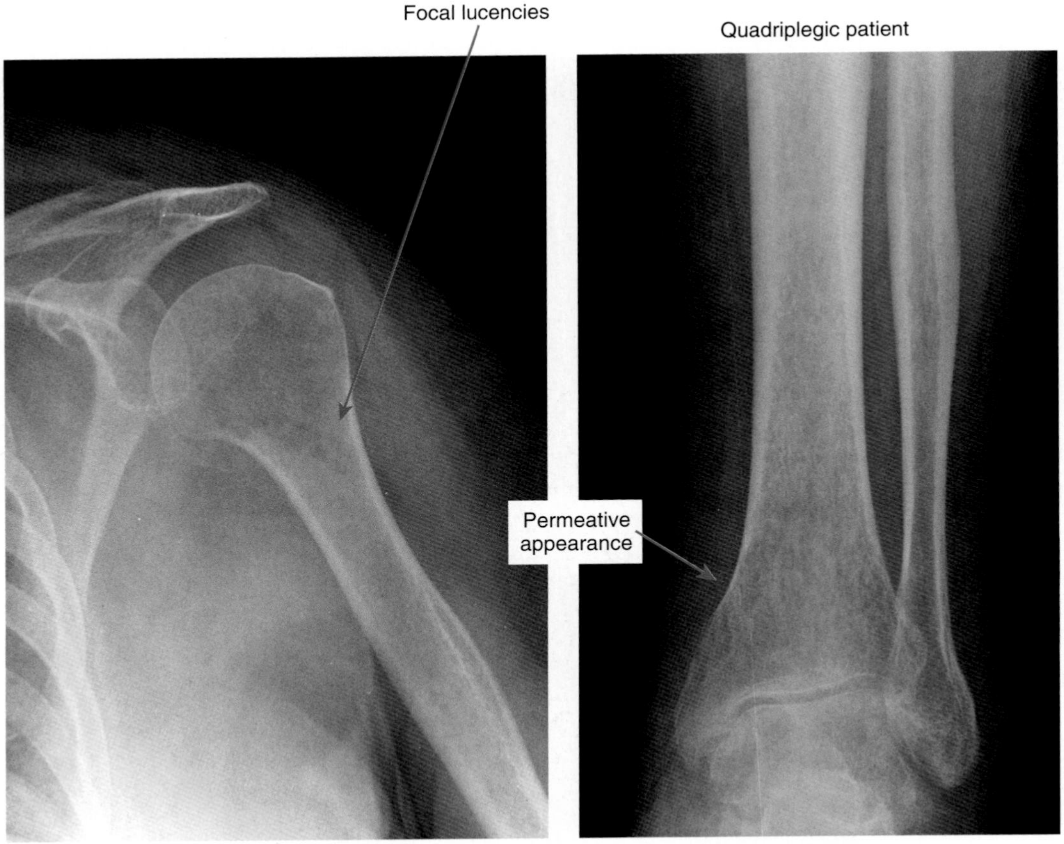
Focal lucencies
Quadriplegic patient
Permeative appearance
Osteopenia with focal lucencies in the proximal humerus following a stroke and sudden immobilization

Figure 6-31 Immobilization, especially occurring suddenly (i.e., following a stroke, or casting) can result in a permeative pattern simulating malignancy. Appropriate history should be sought, but occasionally MRI is needed to exclude tumor. On MRI immobilization can present as hyperintensity on fat-suppressed, fluid-sensitive sequences distributed predominantly in a subcortical/subchondral location and adjacent to attachment sites of tendons, ligaments, and fascia.

radiographs (Fig. 6-31). This is especially common in patients after a stroke on the paralyzed side and is seen as multiple small radiolucencies. When this is observed, especially unilaterally, the associated history should be sought.

Aggressive demineralization related to immobilization of the extremities (e.g., related to fracture) is usually obvious on radiographs but can cause confusion on MRI. Disuse osteopenia can be seen on MRI as bone marrow edema, which has a characteristic pattern, distributed in the subchondral bone and at attachment sites of tendons, ligaments, and fascia (Fig. 6-32). Edema may also be seen around intraosseous blood vessels. This is a normal finding and should not be confused with pathology.

Osteoporotic Spinal Compression Fracture

Osteoporotic compression fractures are common, and imaging can often document the process as benign, thereby avoiding unnecessary biopsy and associated complications. Some rules of thumb have been described with findings increasing or decreasing the likelihood of underlying tumor. MRI is the best modality overall for differentiating a benign from a malignant compression fracture, and research is currently being performed to establish prediction models based on MRI findings. However, other examinations have advantages, and all the information available should be used before resorting to biopsy. For example, a whole body bone scan can establish

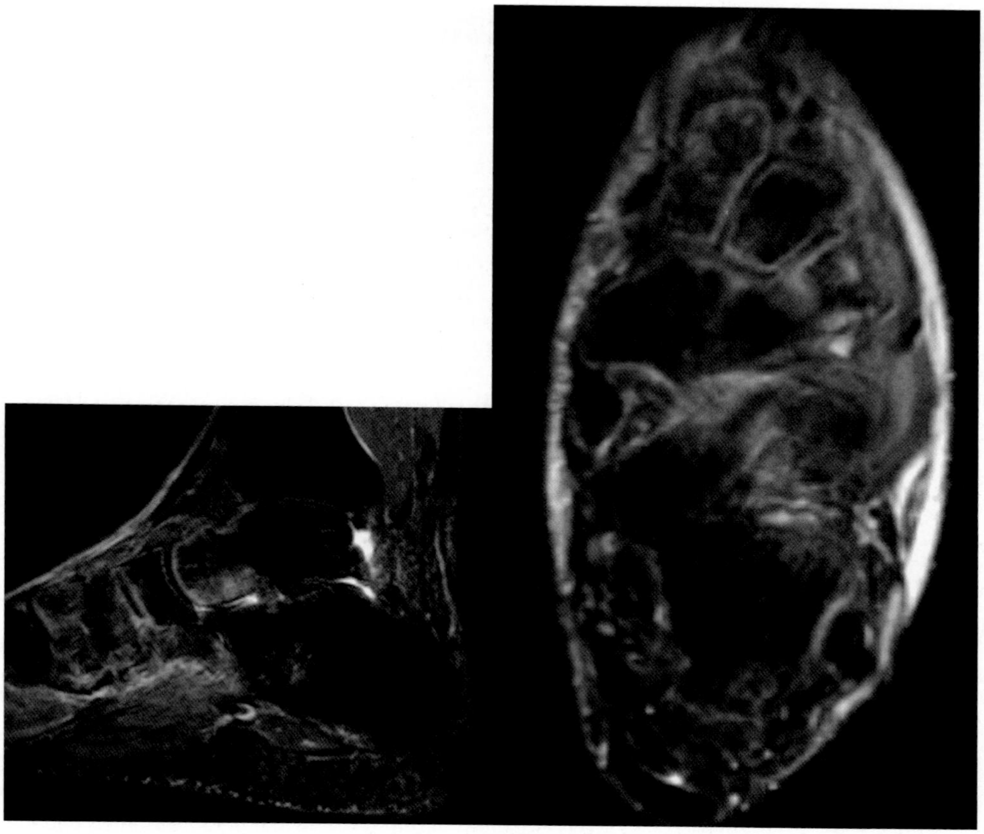

Figure 6-32 Marrow edema-like signal associated with immobilization. Pattern is similar to disuse osteopenia seen on radiographs.

multiplicity. Laboratory findings, such as serum protein electrophoresis/urine protein electrophoresis, can establish the presence of myeloma, but marrow sampling is often needed. DEXA (dual-energy x-ray absorptiometry) scan or other modalities can establish severity of osteoporosis (Table 6-3).

If a fracture is suspicious for tumor based on the imaging findings, biopsy is indicated. However, a bone scan can be used to find other lesions (e.g., in the pelvis) that may be safer to sample. In the case of a solitary fracture with low suspicion in a position that is either unsafe to biopsy or in a patient who cannot tolerate biopsy, a short-term follow-up MRI may be indicated. Fat should begin to be restored within the vertebral body within 1 to 2 months.

Over the past decade, with proliferation of the use of vertebroplasty, differentiation of benign from malignant compression fractures by noninvasive means has become less of an issue. Because vertebroplasty is an indicated treatment for malignant compression fracture and does not preclude subsequent radiation therapy or stabilization surgery, samples of the bone can be acquired at the time of vertebroplasty. The etiology can thereby be established at the same time the fracture is treated.

LESION FOUND ON AN IMAGING EXAM: WHAT TO DO NEXT?

Bone Lesion Found on Radiographs

Some lesions are characteristic on radiographs, and with experience and pattern recognition the specific diagnosis can be made. In other cases, the primary role of the radiologist is multifactorial, including:

Determining whether the lesion may be a tumor
Determining the aggressiveness of the lesion
Assisting the clinician with regard to the next step in the workup

Table 6-3 Differential Features of Benign versus Malignant Vertebral Compression Fracture

Category	Importance	Relevance
Age/gender	Low	Male/younger patients less likely to have osteoporosis (unless there is underlying metabolic disease)
Underlying discrete bone lesion	High	Osteoporotic compression fractures usually display diffuse marrow edema, not a discrete lesion
Multiplicity	High	Multiple compression fractures can be seen with tumor or osteoporosis; however, acute compression fractures with focal bone lesions elsewhere strongly imply metastasis or myeloma
Presence of new and old fracture	Moderate	Healed compression fractures imply underlying osteoporosis severe enough to cause fracture; recurrent fractures are common in this population
Fracture line	High	Visible fracture line on MRI is more likely to occur in benign osteoporotic fracture
Soft tissue mass	High	Although hematoma can be seen with fracture, it is less common with osteoporotic compression fracture. Soft tissue mass (especially with diffuse enhancement) implies malignancy
Smooth versus lumpy-bumpy soft tissue swelling	Low	Lumpy-bumpy soft tissue swelling around a compression fracture is seen more commonly in malignancy
Superior versus inferior endplate	Low	Osteoporotic fractures most commonly involve the superior endplate; inferior endplate involvement is seen slightly more commonly in malignant fractures
Less than 20% drop in signal on in/out of phase (not fat on T1)	High	Tumor excludes fat, which is at least partially preserved in fractures. Less than 20% drop in signal from in-phase to out-of-phase (meaning little to no fat) in an acute fracture that is low signal on T1 strongly implies malignancy
Gas within vertebral body	High	Gas (vacuum) within the vertebral body (Kümmell phenomenon) implies osteonecrosis or unstable fracture (i.e., pseudarthrosis) and virtually excludes tumor. This finding can occasionally be induced by acquiring radiographs or CT in extension

Ensuring that findings are reported accurately and communicated to the referring clinician with an appropriate level of urgency

Certain radiographic features have been described that can characterize bone lesions as aggressive or nonaggressive. However, an important concept is that aggressiveness does not equal malignancy. For example, some benign lesions have an aggressive appearance such as eosinophilic granuloma and infection. Features that should be evaluated for each lesion include:

Periosteal reaction
Margin of the lesion
Expansion/endosteal scalloping
Cortical breakthrough/soft tissue mass

Periosteal Reaction

The periosteum is a layer of cells overlying the metaphysis and diaphysis of long bones. Flat bones also have a periosteum, but some bones such as the vertebrae, carpal bones, and tarsal bones do not have a mature periosteum and will not mount a significant periosteal reaction to similar irritation. The periosteum is responsible for appositional growth and repair of bone; that is, it lays down new bone along the cortex. When a bone undergoes stress chronically, it thickens the cortex in response. In fact, the periosteum reacts in only one way—by forming more bone. Different patterns of periosteal reaction reflect the degree of irritation of the periosteum and how fast the periosteum is pushed away from the bone by the growth of the lesion (Fig. 6-33).

Types of Periosteal Reaction

Thick, undulating—implies slow growth; the periosteum has time to lay down new bone (low aggressiveness). Examples: infection, osteoid osteoma, and stress fracture.

Lamellated (onion skin)—implies periodic rapid growth; periosteum periodically pushed away, lays

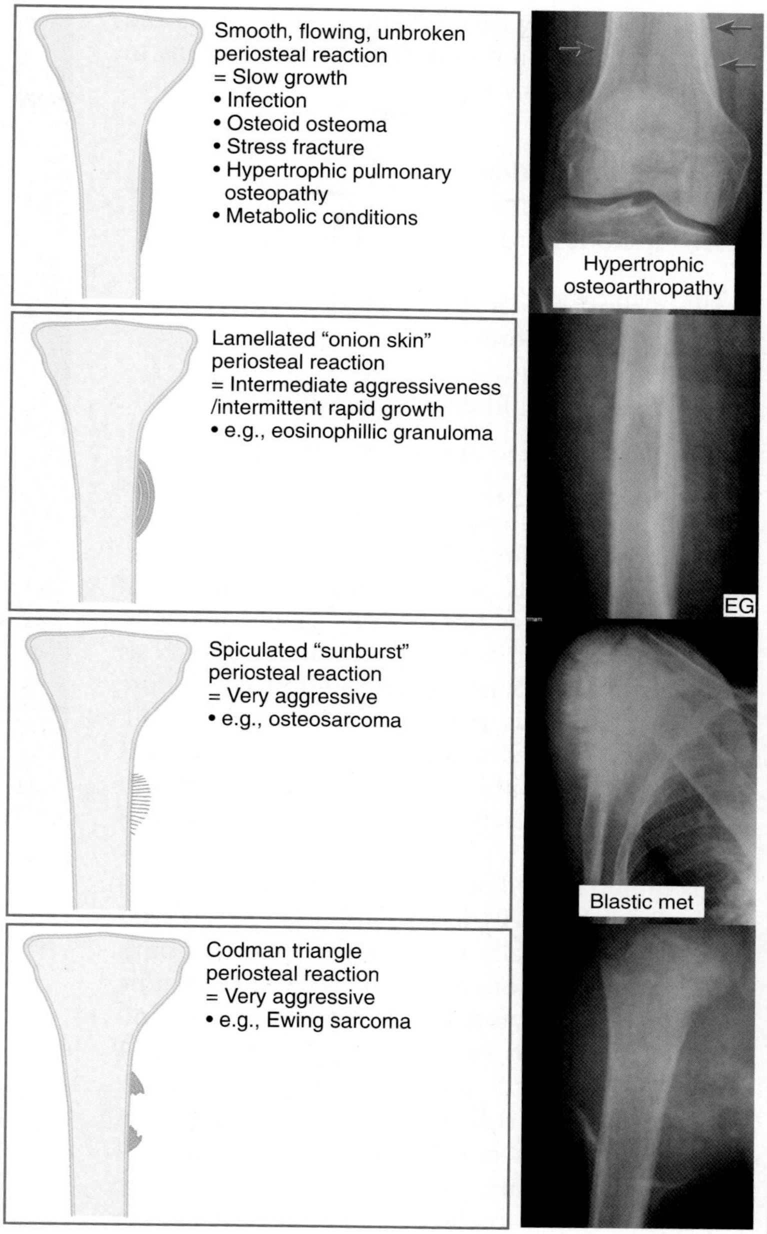
Smooth, flowing, unbroken periosteal reaction
= Slow growth
• Infection
• Osteoid osteoma
• Stress fracture
• Hypertrophic pulmonary osteopathy
• Metabolic conditions
Hypertrophic osteoarthropathy
Lamellated "onion skin" periosteal reaction
= Intermediate aggressiveness /intermittent rapid growth
• e.g., eosinophillic granuloma
EG
Spiculated "sunburst" periosteal reaction
= Very aggressive
• e.g., osteosarcoma
Blastic met
Codman triangle periosteal reaction
= Very aggressive
• e.g., Ewing sarcoma

Figure 6-33 Types of periosteal reaction.

down layer of calcium, etc. (intermediate aggressiveness). Example: eosinophilic granuloma.

Sunburst—implies very rapid growth; periosteum forms bone as it is pushed away, creating streaks of calcium perpendicular to cortex (very aggressive). Example: osteosarcoma.

Codman triangle—indicates very rapid growth; at the midpoint of the mass, growth is so rapid that periosteum cannot respond. At the margins where growth is slower, the periosteum lays down bone in a triangular configuration (very aggressive). Examples: osteosarcoma, Ewing sarcoma, and aggressive infections.

Some tumors grow so rapidly that no periosteal reaction is observed, such as fibrosarcoma, lymphoma, and Ewing sarcoma. Often a soft tissue mass is seen as the tumor rapidly "percolates" through the cortex.

Margins

Evaluation of the margins of a lesion is extremely important when generating a differential diagnosis, and for determining aggressiveness. Radiologists and tumor surgeons commonly classify bone lesions in terms of the Lodwick system.

Lodwick Classification

Type 1: Geographic
- 1A—sclerotic border: Classic thin, sclerotic margin
- 1B—distinct border: Not sclerotic
- 1C—indistinct border

Type 2: Moth-eaten

Type 3: Permeative; ill-defined transition

Only type 1A can be attributed to a benign process. A thin, sclerotic margin is a sign that the lesion has been present for a long time without growth, allowing the bone to form a shell around it. This is commonly seen in cysts, such as simple or unicameral bone cysts as well as intraosseous ganglia and subchondral cysts, and other benign lesions, such as nonossifying fibromas (fibroxanthomas) before healing and fibrous dysplasia. A potential pitfall, however, is a treated malignancy, as in a metastasis treated with chemotherapy. In this case, as growth slows the bone reacts and forms a sclerotic rim (Fig. 6-34).

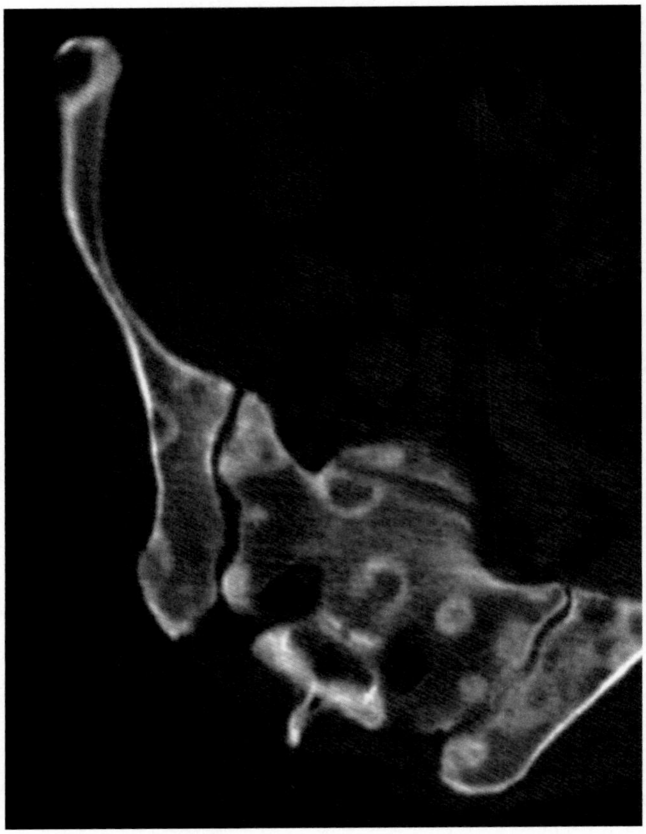

Figure 6-34 Healing metastatic lesions after treatment can exhibit sclerotic margins similar to lesions with low aggressiveness. History is important.

It is important to know that well-defined nonsclerotic margins (type 1B) do not imply a benign process! Myeloma is classically well defined (punched out). Also, metastatic lesions are often 1B. Type 1C is more aggressive than 1A and 1B; giant cell tumor is typically 1C, with areas of cortical interruption on CT (Fig. 6-35). Types 2 and 3 are clearly aggressive. However, they may still be benign. The classic benign type 2 or 3 lesion is infection, which is often ill defined. In this case, periosteal reaction may be helpful, since infection tends to have a more mature reaction (smooth, thick). Eosinophilic granuloma can also appear aggressive, that is, ill defined and often permeative in early phases. The type 3 permeative pattern is typically seen with small round cell lesions, with the differential diagnosis including Ewing sarcoma, lymphoma/leukemia, eosinophilic granuloma, and infection.

Marginal patterns can be confusing if they are mixed; for example, part of the lesion has thin sclerotic margins and another area is ill defined. There are certain situations in which this occurs. If a part of a benign lesion is obliquely oriented in the medullary cavity, it may falsely appear ill defined on a radiograph acquired en face. This emphasizes the importance of multiple views. If the lesion is truly partially aggressive, it may represent transformation of a benign lesion into malignancy. This may occur in chondroid lesions and has been reported to occur rarely in other situations, such as infarct transforming into malignant fibrous histiocytoma. A surface lesion (centered at the cortex) can also have mixed features. For instance, a sessile osteochondroma, or juxtacortical chondroma, can have a benign appearance at its interface with the medullary cavity but an aggressive, irregular appearance of the outer cortex.

Expansion/Endosteal Scalloping

Expansion of bone, in which the cortex is deflected or remodeled outward, can be a sign of aggressiveness, but this sign is also a characteristic of many benign lesions (Fig. 6-36). Expansion is typically included in the list of periosteal reactions, since it occurs as a result of solid new bone formation at the

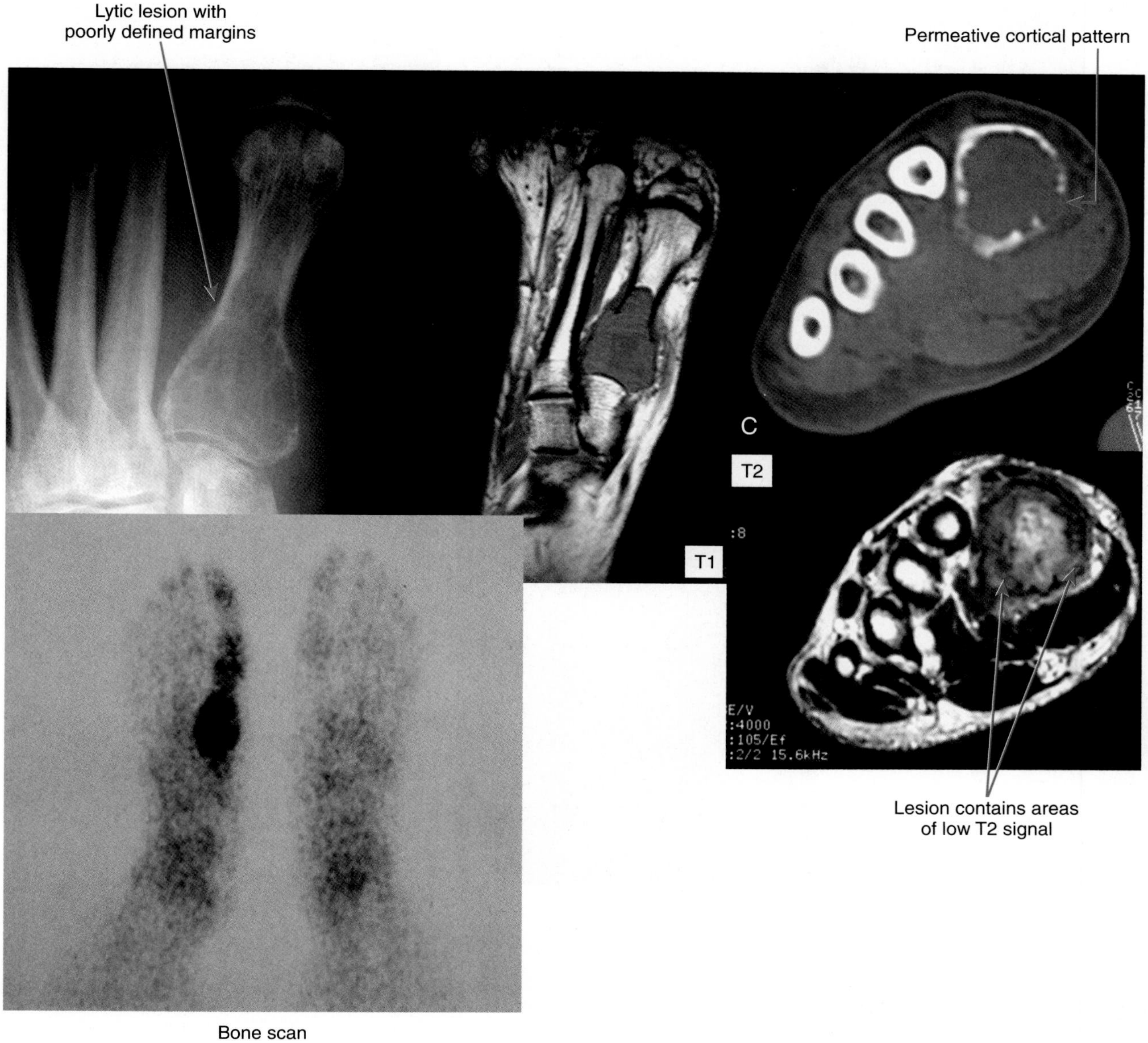
Lytic lesion with poorly defined margins
Permeative cortical pattern
C
T2
T1
Lesion contains areas of low T2 signal
Bone scan

Figure 6-35 Giant cell tumors (GCT) classically have an aggressive appearance, with sharp (or slightly indistinct) but nonsclerotic margins on radiographs and a "dot-dash" pattern of cortical interruption on CT. Pattern on CT can suggest a malignancy. Biopsy is necessary, but the diagnosis of GCT can be suggested by relatively low signal on T2-weighted MRI.

periosteum secondary to intramedullary lesion growth. Slight focal expansion is seen in lesions such as nonossifying fibroma and fibrous dysplasia. Diffuse expansion of bone can be seen in Paget disease and in marrow-packing disorders such as thalassemia and Gaucher disease. A large degree of expansion can be seen in aggressive lesions such as hemorrhagic metastases (e.g., lung, renal, thyroid carcinoma) and plasmacytoma/myeloma. However, some benign lesions such as simple bone cyst cause expansion, and aneurysmal bone cyst and hemophilic pseudotumor can also cause significant expansion, or a so-called "blowout lesion." Therefore, unless other signs point to an aggressive or a nonaggressive lesion, expansion itself is not specific for malignancy.

Endosteal scalloping occurs when an intramedullary lesion grows or expands and thins the inner cortex. The classic lesion causing scalloping is enchon-

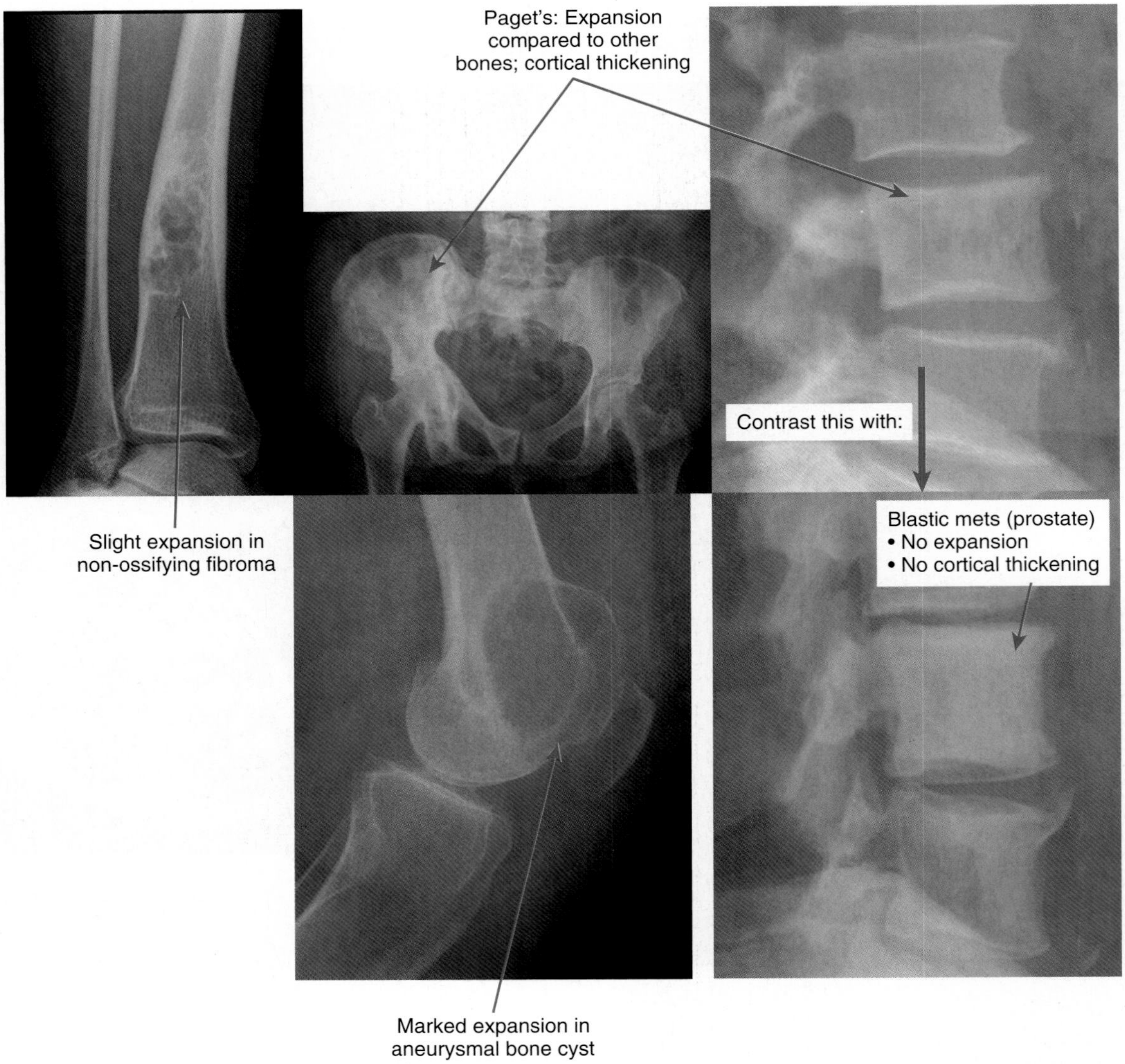
Paget's: Expansion compared to other bones; cortical thickening
Contrast this with:
Blastic mets (prostate)
• No expansion
• No cortical thickening
Slight expansion in non-ossifying fibroma
Marked expansion in aneurysmal bone cyst

Figure 6-36 Expansion of bone can be seen in both benign and malignant conditions. Some fast-growing processes (i.e., intraosseous hemorrhage in hemophilia) can result in blowout lesions, as well as aneurysmal bone cyst and malignant conditions such as myeloma and metastatic disease (especially aggressive/hemorrhagic lesions such as renal, lung, and thyroid lesions).

droma. However, this finding is also nonspecific and relates more to lesion rate of growth than to histology (Fig. 6-37). When prominent, or involving over half the cortical thickness, endosteal scalloping has been suggested as a sign of aggressiveness with regard to chondroid lesions.

Scalloping of Outer Cortex Scalloping of the outer cortex, in which the bone is focally bowed inward with a thin sclerotic margin, is seen with slow-growing lesions outside the bone. Because this implies slow growth, it is typically seen with benign lesions, such as giant cell tumor of tendon sheath, nerve sheath tumors, and ganglia.

Cortical Breakthrough and Soft Tissue Mass

Cortical breakthrough and soft tissue mass constitute a sign of aggressiveness. Sometimes a benign lesion, such as an aneurysmal bone cyst, can appear to break through, but on CT a thin shell of cortex is seen. Soft tissue mass is seen in many bone malig-

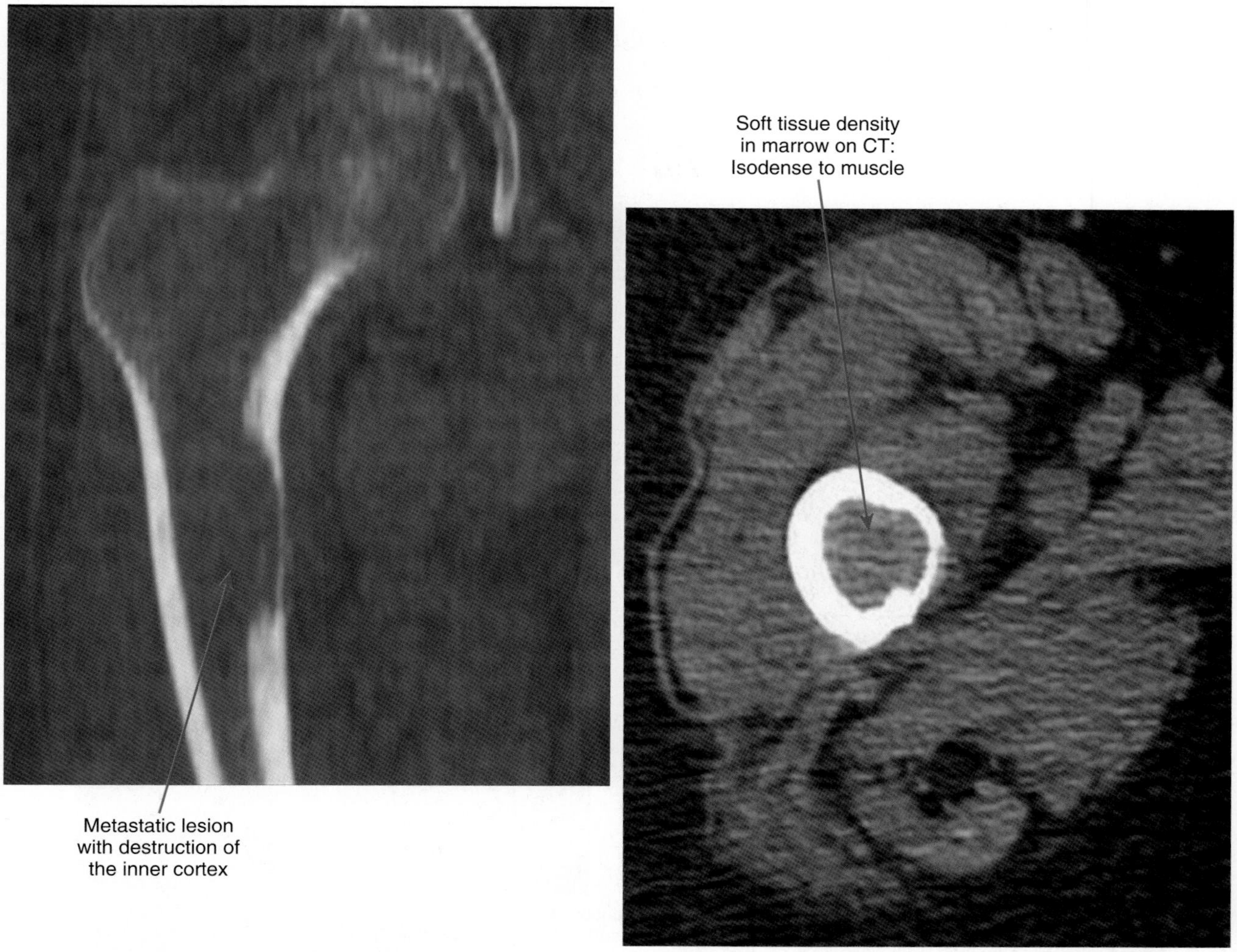
Soft tissue density
in marrow on CT:
Isodense to muscle
Metastatic lesion
with destruction of
the inner cortex

Figure 6-37 Endosteal scalloping is seen with both slow-growing lesions such as enchondromas, as well as early involvement from malignancies—in this case a metastatic lesion from lung carcinoma. Note that here instead of expanding and remodeling the cortex, the inner cortex is being destroyed, a sign of the aggressive nature of the lesion.

nancies but is especially common in Ewing sarcoma (Fig. 6-38).

Matrix Mineralization If a lesion contains mineralization (calcification), there are a number of possibilities:

- The lesion is blastic or mixed lytic-blastic.
- The lesion is lytic, and there is dystrophic calcification.
- The lesion is forming chondroid, osteoid, or fibrous matrix that is calcifying.

Types of matrix include osteoid, chondroid, and fibrous. Determining the type of matrix mineralization can be very useful in narrowing the differential diagnosis. If unclear on radiographs, CT is an excellent modality for characterizing matrix.

Osteoid Matrix and Differential Diagnosis Osteoid matrix has a cloudlike appearance on radiographs and CT (Fig. 6-39). This should not be confused with ossification, which has a zonal phenomenon (denser at the periphery on radiographs because of rim calcification) and a structure. Osteoid matrix has no discernible internal architecture. Ossification has a nonaggressive implication, whereas calcification representing osteoid matrix can be seen in osteosarcoma.

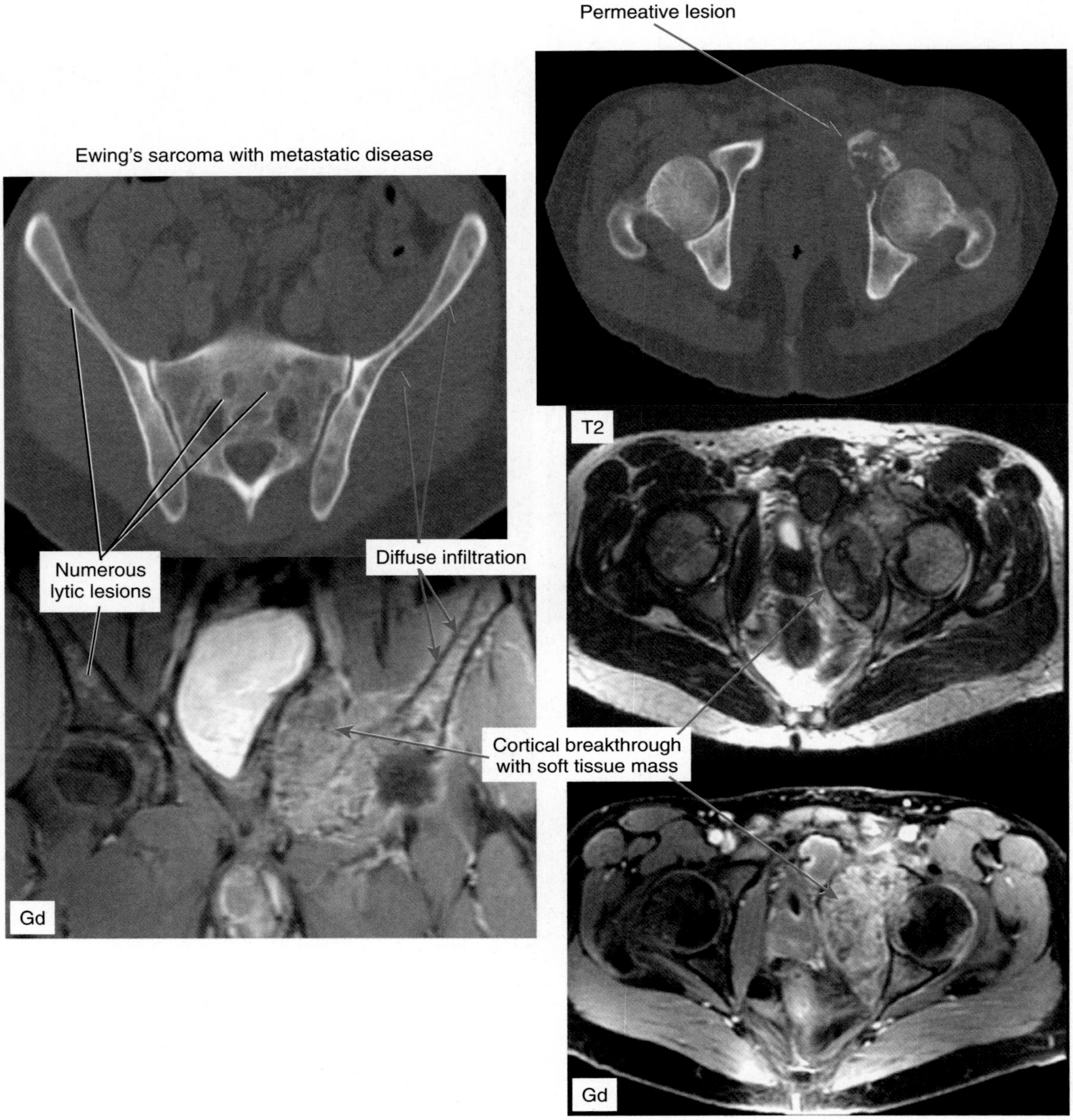

Permeative lesion
Ewing's sarcoma with metastatic disease
T2
Numerous lytic lesions
Diffuse infiltration
Cortical breakthrough with soft tissue mass
Gd
Gd

Figure 6-38 Cortical breakthrough and soft tissue mass. This indicates a more aggressive process. Ewing's sarcoma classically presents with a soft tissue component that is often large. Lymphoma, metastases, and other lesions can also exhibit soft tissue extension, and this finding is not specific. Some benign conditions can also show cortical breakthrough and soft tissue mass effect such as infection and fracture through a benign lesion with associated hematoma.

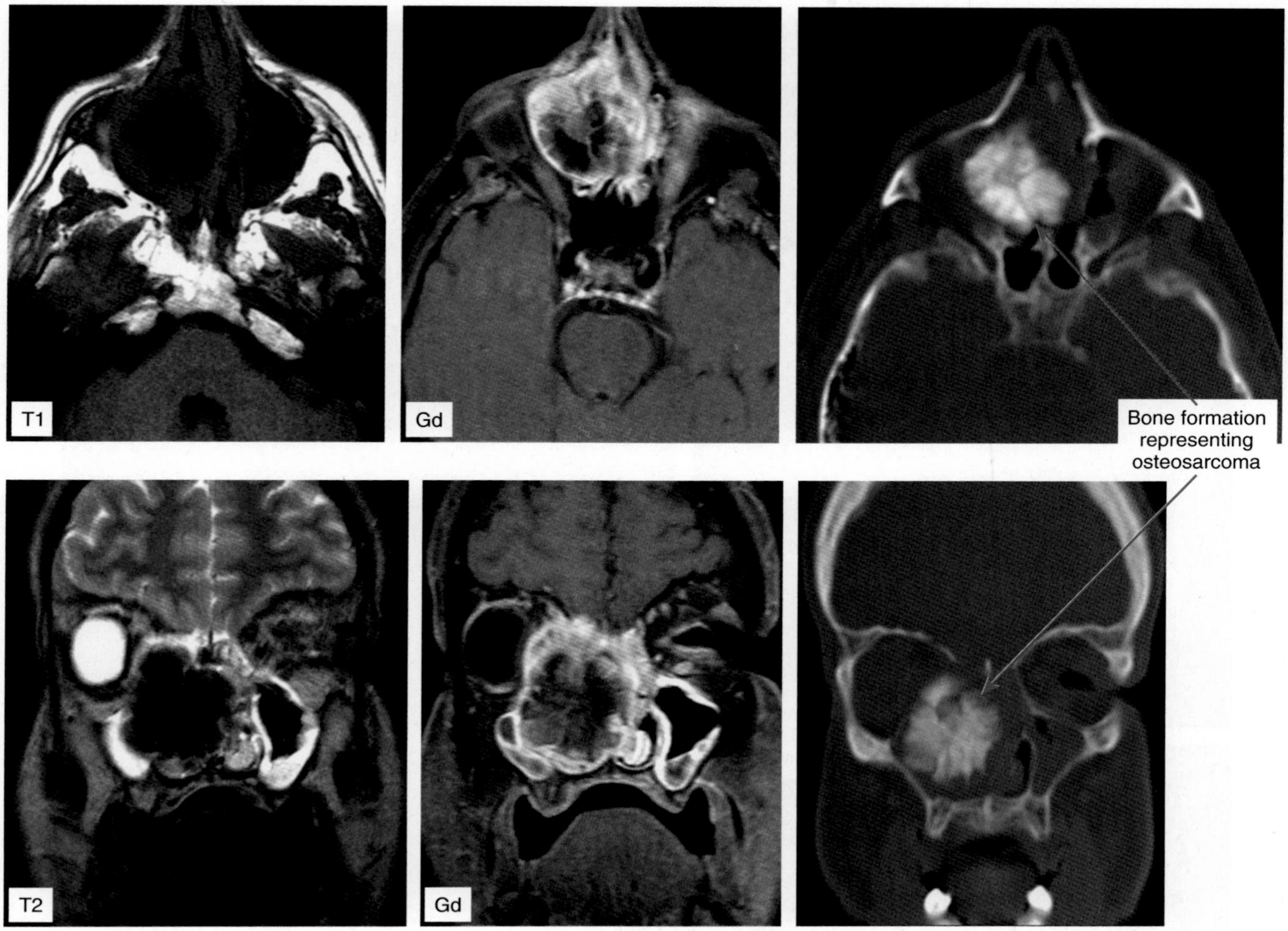
T1
Gd
Bone formation representing osteosarcoma
T2
Gd

Figure 6-39 Forty-three-year-old man with a history of enucleation and radiation therapy for retinoblastoma as a child. He now presents with secondary osteosarcoma developing at the margin of the radiation port.

A mimicker of osteoid matrix is tumoral calcinosis, which is deposition of calcium salts in the soft tissues (Fig. 6-40). It is most commonly associated with chronic renal failure and secondary hyperparathyroidism, although an idiopathic form is seen in adolescents. The finding typically occurs around joints, but important differences from osteoid matrix in bone lesions is that it remains in the soft tissues and often exhibits fluidic calcium (milk of calcium with dependent levels on CT). Also, of course, there may be findings of secondary hyperparathyroidism around the body.

Hydroxyapatite deposition disease (HADD) can mimic osteoid matrix on a smaller scale. It also looks cloudlike but is limited to a small focus within a tendon or bursa. Rarely, a bone erosion containing a focus of calcification can be seen with calcific tendinosis (Fig. 6-41).

True osteoid matrix is seen in bone-forming lesions, especially osteosarcoma. Osteoid matrix can also be seen in osteoblastomas.

Chondroid Matrix and Differential Diagnosis Chondroid matrix is characterized by "arcs and rings" of calcification (Fig. 6-42). These curvilinear calcifications correspond to the lobulated pattern of architecture seen on MRI and at histology. A common mimicker of chondroid matrix on radiographs is the calcification associated with bone infarction (Fig. 6-43). Some differences can help distinguish these

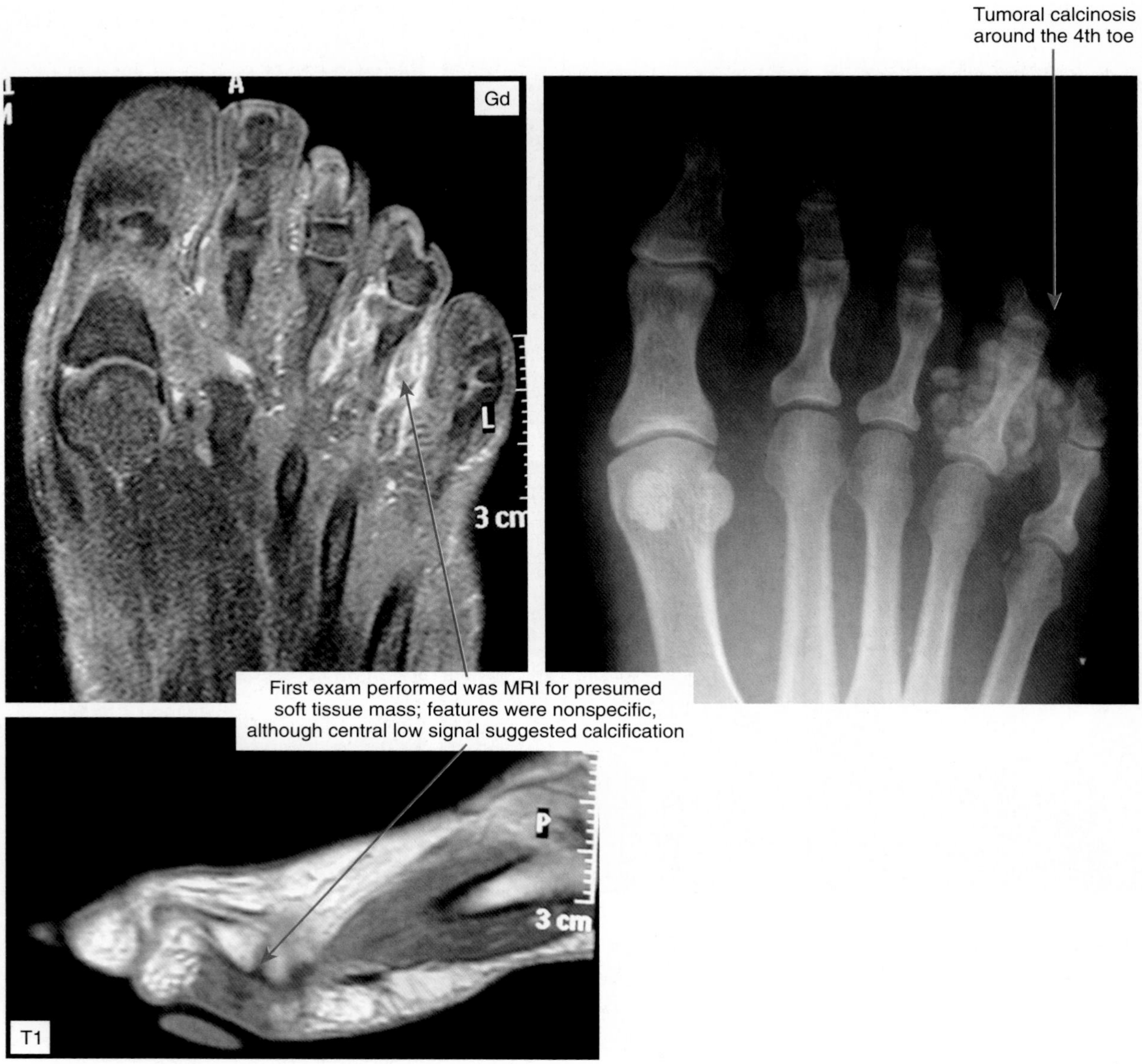
Tumoral calcinosis around the 4th toe
Gd
A
L
3 cm
First exam performed was MRI for presumed soft tissue mass; features were nonspecific, although central low signal suggested calcification
P
3 cm
T1

Figure 6-40 Tumoral calcinosis. The calcification is cloudlike and on radiographs can be confused with hydroxyapatite deposition disease or even a mass with osteoid matrix (i.e., osteosarcoma). Features can be confusing on MRI if not correlated with radiographs. A history of metabolic disease (especially renal failure) should be sought.

entities. First, the calcification in infarcts is more sharp, well defined, and serpentine. Second, whereas enchondroma calcification is rounded with soft-appearing margins, infarcts are more linear and sharply defined, often paralleling the periosteum. On MRI, chondroid lesions are rounded and show lobulation with T2 hyperintensity and rim/septal enhancement, whereas infarcts show a dark and bright line (double-line sign) at the margin, often containing internal fat signal (mummified fat).

CHONDROID LESIONS: IMAGING AND MANAGEMENT

Chondroid lesions—such as enchondroma, juxtacortical/periosteal chondroma, osteochondroma, chondromyxoid fibroma, chondroblastoma, and chondrosarcoma—deserve special consideration because they often generate questions regarding diagnosis and management.

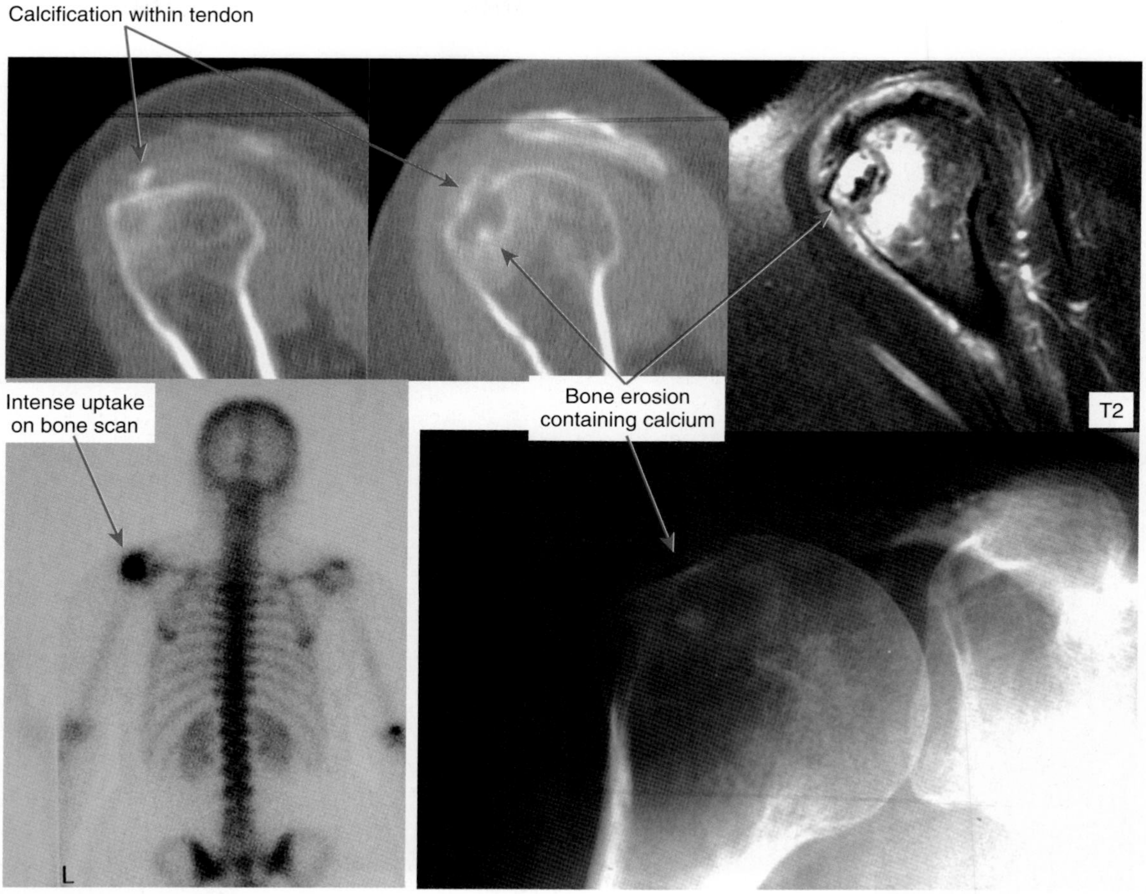
Calcification within tendon
Intense uptake on bone scan
Bone erosion containing calcium
T2
L

Figure 6-41 Calcific tendinosis can cause erosion of bone at the tendon attachment and lead to concern for tumor.

Common Imaging Characteristics

Chondroid lesions of different types have some common imaging features based on the presence of chondroid tissue. On radiographs and CT, chondroid matrix calcifies in a characteristic arcs and rings pattern. On MRI, this chondroid tissue is "bright as a light bulb" on T2-weighted images owing to the high water content of the cartilage elements. A lobulated appearance with septal and rim enhancement also reflects the underlying cartilaginous lobules. Calcification shows up as regions of low signal and susceptibility artifact.

Differentiating large enchondroma from low-grade chondrosarcoma is a fairly common and complex issue. Unfortunately, there are no hard and fast rules. Although histology is the gold standard, the pathologist may also have difficulty. Sampling bias of a percutaneously acquired specimen, along with histologic criteria—such as the number of mitoses per high-power field, which reflect the ill-defined spectrum of benign to malignant—often causes the pathologist to seek out the radiologist to make the final call. Percutaneous biopsy can potentially result in seeding of the biopsy tract with tumor cells. Complete resection can yield a definitive diagnosis, but may cause significant morbidity depending on the location. Radiologic studies also fail to identify specific findings for differentiating benign from low-grade malignant lesions. Radiographically, besides the obvious signs of cortical breakthrough, soft tissue mass, and periostitis, signs that suggest malignancy include size larger than 5 cm and significant endosteal scalloping. Of course, any change over time is suspicious, including increase in size, scalloping, or change in internal mineralization pattern.

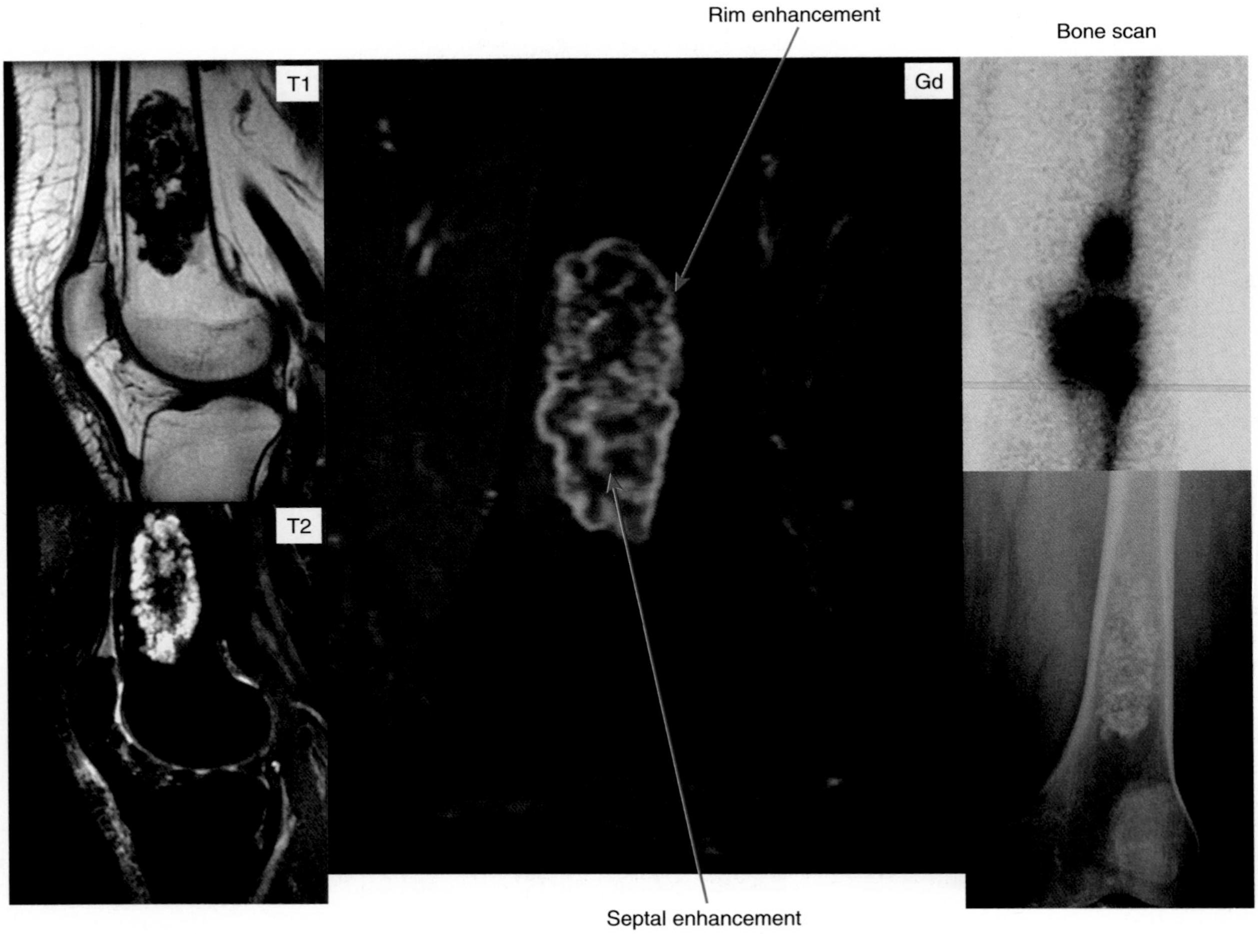
Rim enhancement
Bone scan
T1
Gd
T2
Septal enhancement

Figure 6-42 Chondroid lesion characteristics on MRI. Note marked hyperintensity on T2-weighted images representing the prominent hydration state of the cartilage tissue. Lobulation corresponds to histologic rings of chondrocytes. Calcifications create low-signal foci. Intravenous contrast results in rim and septal enhancement around the lobules. Degree of uptake on bone scan does not correlate well with histologic aggressiveness.

If the lesion is indeterminate by imaging and pain is unexplained by adjacent pathology, biopsy is generally advised. Because of potential sampling bias, these lesions typically proceed to open biopsy. However, location may prompt an initial effort at percutaneous needle sampling. As with any primary tumor, if percutaneous needle biopsy is requested, the approach should be discussed with the bone tumor surgeon to ensure that no potential flaps are compromised and that the tract is along the potential incision line.

If a lesion is classic for enchondroma, but pain cannot be easily attributed to other musculoskeletal pathology (e.g., adjacent internal derangement), follow-up is also prudent. The same is true for a large but otherwise non–aggressive-appearing lesion without pain. Incidentally found clearly benign-appearing enchondromas without symptoms are not generally monitored. Lesions of the distal appendicular skeleton tend to be less aggressive and are not usually followed up.

Osteochondromas may also cause a management dilemma. Sessile (without a stalk) osteochondromas can appear aggressive and prompt inappropriately aggressive intervention. Any osteochondroma with pain should raise concern of malignant degeneration; but there are other causes of pain, such as overlying bursitis, mass effect on adjacent nerves and other structures, pseudoaneurysm formation, and fractured stalk. If the cause of pain is not apparent on radio-

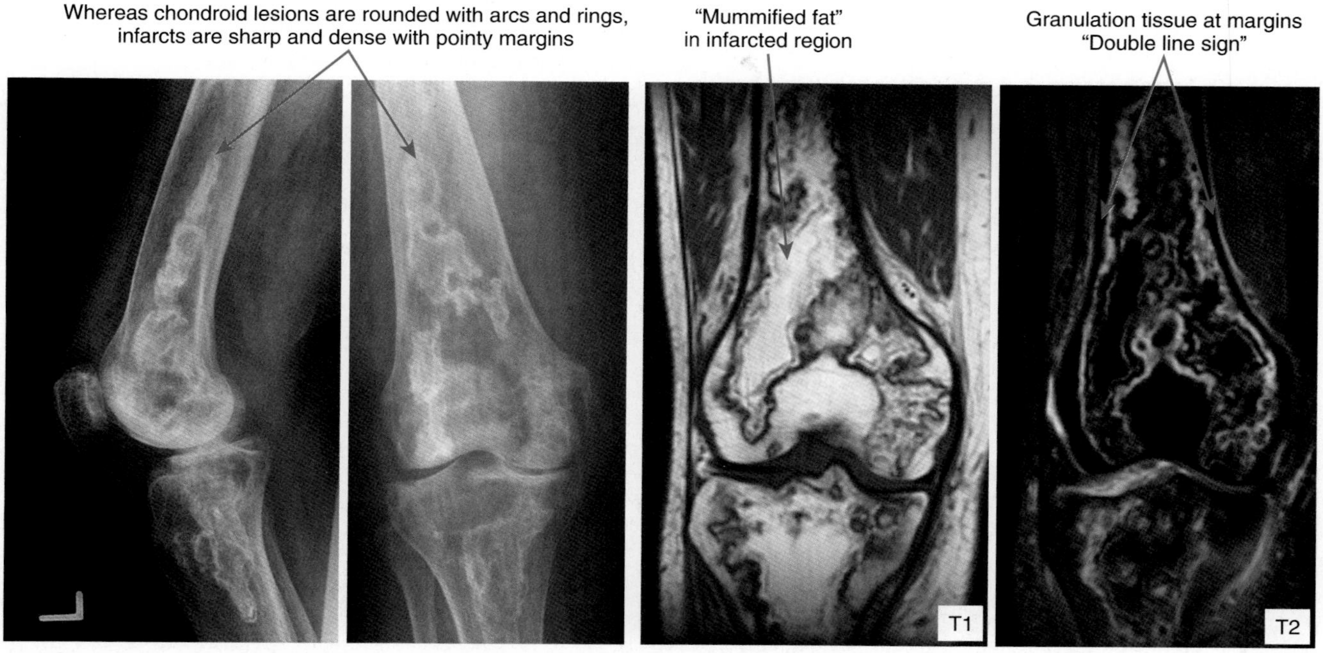
Whereas chondroid lesions are rounded with arcs and rings, infarcts are sharp and dense with pointy margins
"Mummified fat" in infarcted region
Granulation tissue at margins "Double line sign"
T1
T2

Figure 6-43 Large infarcts in sickle cell disease. Well-defined sclerosis on radiographs, with geographic pattern on MRI.

graphs, MRI is the best single test for differentiating these other painful entities. MRI can also evaluate the thickness of the cartilage cap (more than 2 cm is more concerning), as well as soft tissue extension and stalk/intramedullary invasion of an aggressive lesion. The protocol should be designed to visualize fluid from overlying bursitis separate from the hyperintense cartilage cap; the best type of sequence for this purpose is a T1-weighted spin-echo or GRE sequence with fat suppression (Fig. 6-44). On this sequence, cartilage is hyperintense and fluid is low in signal. Comparison with a fat-suppressed fluid-sensitive sequence in the same plane can then be used to detect bursal fluid. Ultrasound is useful but fails to provide an assessment of the cartilage cap itself. Contrast can be useful, since bursitis, neuromas, and vessels all show enhancement. The cartilage cap shows rim and septal enhancement typical of chondroid tissue.

Of course, if prior radiographs are available for comparison, diagnosis may be facilitated; any change over time after skeletal maturity should be cause for concern.

Unfortunately there are no good data on time interval for follow-up imaging of a chondroid lesion and on when it is safe to stop. The interval can also be based on level of concern. Since low-grade lesions are slow growing, it is probably reasonable to reimage after 3 months initially, increasing to every 6 months for 2 years or so, and then annually. Most of the time radiographs are adequate, but if the imaging finding that generated the concern is visualized best on CT or MRI, then that modality is preferred as a follow-up examination.

Fibrous Matrix and Differential Diagnosis

Fibrous matrix has been described as a ground-glass appearance on radiographs and CT (Fig. 6-45), a description that many people have a difficult time conceptualizing. A better description is that fibrous matrix has density without trabeculation. The main differential diagnosis for this appearance radiographically is that of a cystic or lytic lesion, in which trabeculae are replaced or destroyed and the cortex in front and in back of the lesion gives the impression of calcified matrix. The presence of fibrous matrix can be confirmed by CT. On MRI, the appearance is variable but is often intermediate in signal and

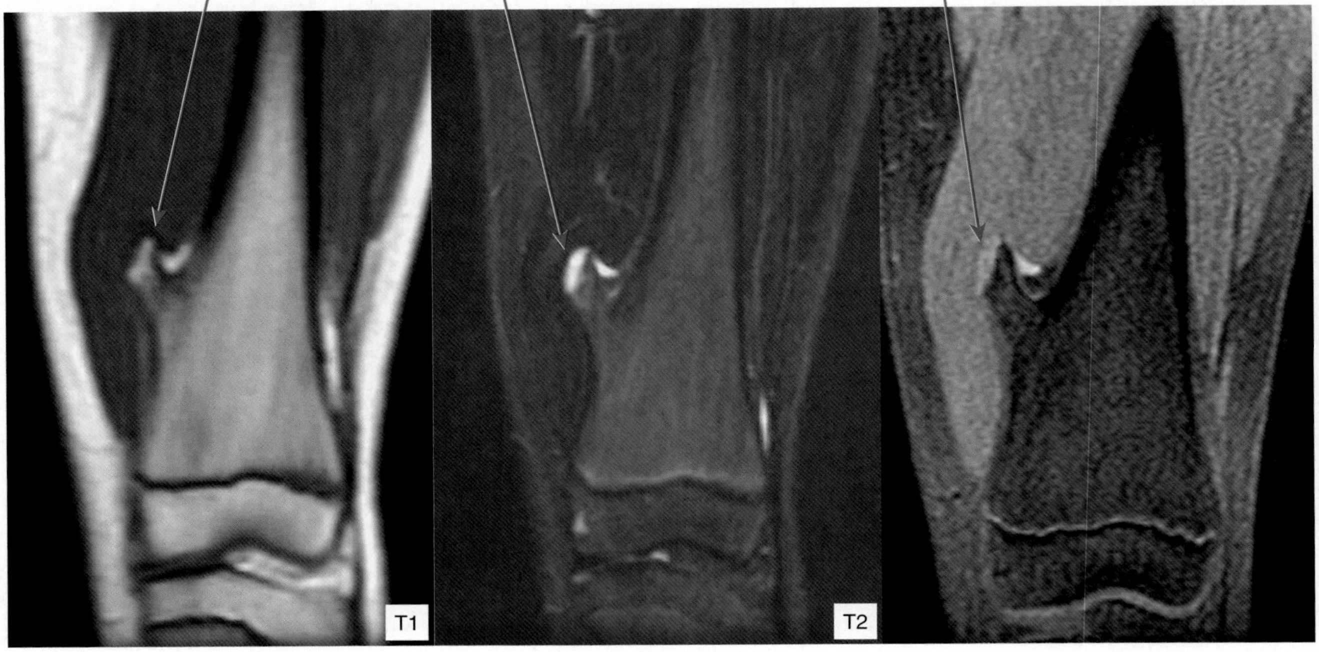

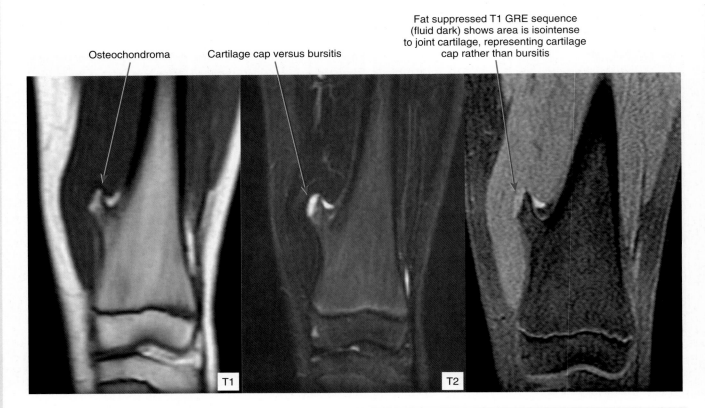

Osteochondroma
Cartilage cap versus bursitis
Fat suppressed T1 GRE sequence (fluid dark) shows area is isointense to joint cartilage, representing cartilage cap rather than bursitis
T1
T2

Figure 6-44 Osteochondromas can present with pain, which may be arising from one of a multitude of causes (including fracture, bursitis, neuroma, pseudoaneurysm, and malignant degeneration). MRI is the single best test for evaluating the source of the pain, if not obvious on radiographs (e.g., fracture through the stalk). Incorporation of a T1-weighted fat-suppressed gradient echo sequence can be used to differentiate cartilage cap from overlying bursitis. On this sequence, fluid is dark and cartilage is intermediate-to-bright. Comparison can be made with joint fluid and hyaline cartilage. Addition of intravenous contrast can evaluate for neuroma or vascular compression/pseudoaneurysm formation. Ultrasound can also be used for this purpose. CT is useful to evaluate for subtle fracture of the stalk as well as erosion of the stalk due to malignant transformation.

homogeneously enhancing. Fibrous lesions that contain matrix such as fibrous dysplasia and chondromyxoid fibroma, however, are often heterogeneous, containing other elements (such as cysts in fibrous dysplasia) and chondroid tissue in chondromyxoid fibroma.

Skeletal/Long Bone Survey

Skeletal and long bone surveys are radiographic studies often ordered to evaluate for metastatic extension of tumor, and it is important to realize their limitations. Areas of trabecular rarefaction, osteoporosis, and vascular channels, which are considered nonlesions, may be mistaken for tumor, leading to low specificity. Also, because a significant amount of bone loss must be present (approximately 30% to 50%) before a lesion is seen on radiographs, the examination has low sensitivity as well. Similar to the once utilized trauma skull radiographic examination, a negative skeletal survey can give patients and clinicians a false sense of security and delay the correct diagnosis. Today, the skeletal survey remains complementary to other examinations such as MRI and bone scan and still has a role in follow-up of metastases and myeloma in patients with established radiographically visible disease. In the future, the radiographic survey may be replaced by a wholebody MRI.

Pathologic Fracture

Pathologic fracture can occur through a benign or malignant lesion (Fig. 6-46). However, if there is no imaging prior to fracture it can be difficult to distin-

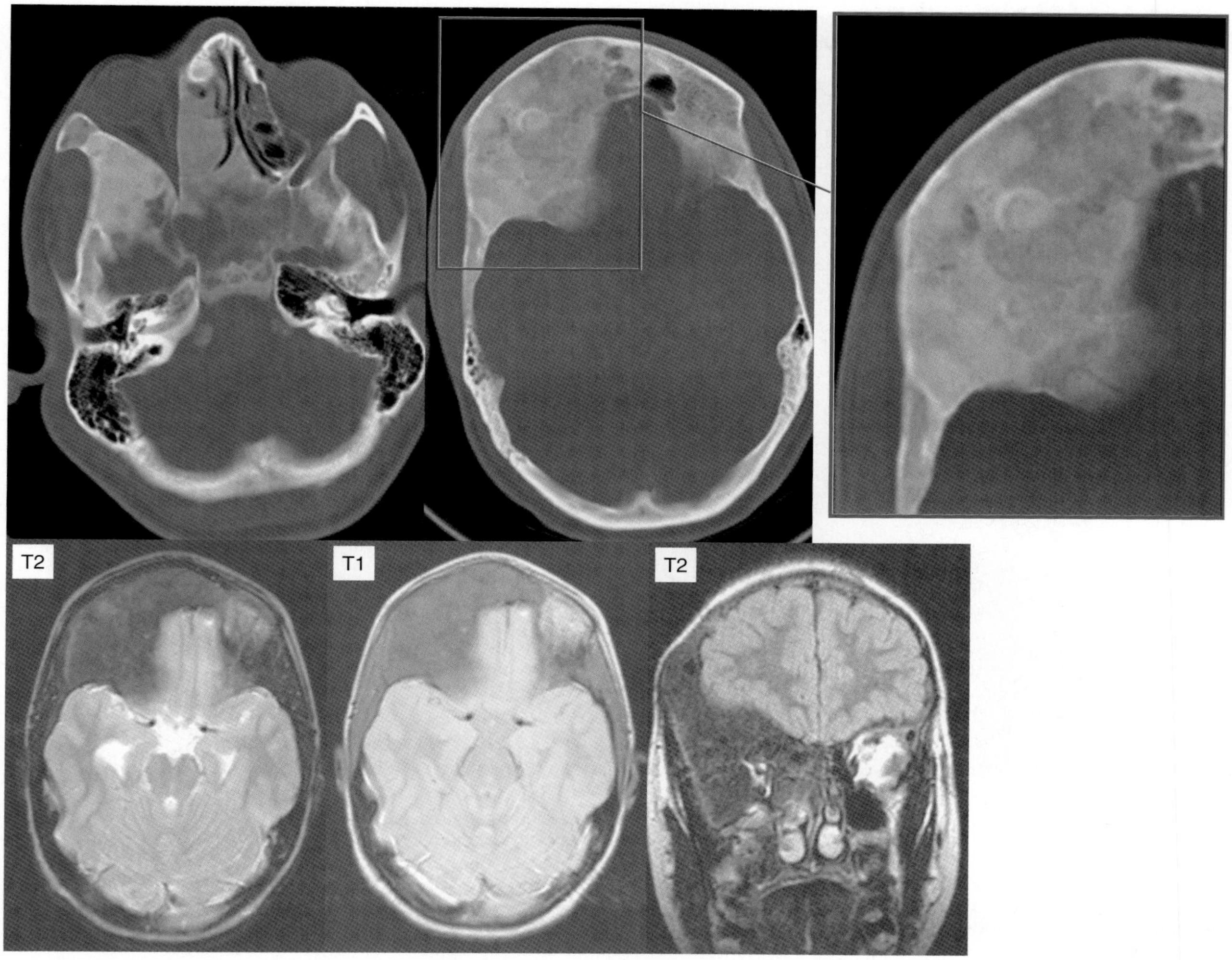
T2
T1
T2

Figure 6-45 Fibroid matrix is characterized by a ground-glass appearance (diffuse density without trabeculation) as seen in this case of fibrous dysplasia.

guish these fractures because hematoma, hyperemia, periosteal reaction, and bone resorption can make the lesion look more aggressive on any modality. Biopsy may be required. The classic radiographic sign of a fallen fragment is helpful but rarely seen. A fallen fragment is a fracture fragment in a dependent portion of a benign cystic bone lesion. If a fracture occurs in an unexpected location or occurs as a result of minimal trauma, an underlying mass may be suspected. If radiographs are noncontributory, MRI with contrast carried out shortly after the injury can visualize the underlying tumor. If it is delayed, hematoma at the fracture site can vascularize and simulate tumor. Bone scan or spine/pelvis or marrow survey on MRI may be useful to exclude other lesions.

Intra-articular Lesions

Intra-articular masslike lesions are rarely malignant. Rather, they are nearly always related to an arthritis (Box 6-2). Masslike synovial proliferation is especially common in rheumatoid arthritis, but this is usually diffusely distributed. Gout can cause focal intra-articular masses, as can focal forms of pigmented villonodular synovitis and synovial chondromatosis.

Possible Tumor Found on CT

This situation encompasses two issues: (1) Is there a lesion at all? (2) Is there a definite lesion in which

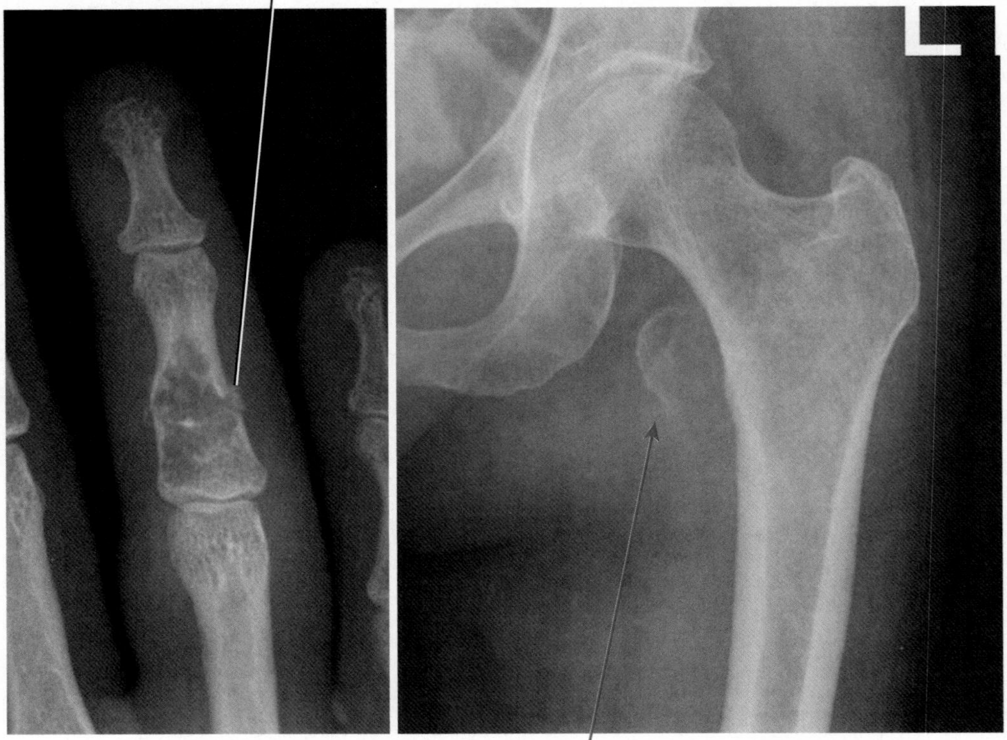
Enchondroma of the phalanx with fracture
Lung adenocarcinoma metastasis: Pathological avulsion fracture of the lesser trochanter

Figure 6-46 Pathologic fracture can occur through benign or malignant lesions. Fracture can make the lesion appear more aggressive on all modalities. Avulsion of the lesser trochanter typically indicates underlying pathology.

BOX 6-2 DIFFERENTIAL DIAGNOSIS FOR SYNOVIAL MASSES

Pigmented villonodular synovitis
Synovial osteochondromatosis/intracapsular chondroma
Rheumatoid arthritis
Gout
Complex ganglion/synovial cyst

the question is malignancy versus benign lesion, or some other pathology requiring further attention (such as infection)?

First, in trying to decide whether a finding is actually a lesion, one should look at the underlying trabecular pattern. True focal lesions alter the trabeculae, destroying or remodeling them. Measure region of interest values; if the Hounsfield units follow fat, the lesion may represent a region of sparse trabeculae simulating a lesion. It can be useful to compare sides. If still indeterminate, typically the best next test is MRI or bone scan. Bone scan is helpful if multiple lesions are seen suggesting metastatic disease. However, if the lesion is solitary and hot on bone scan, the differential is still wide. MRI can not only document presence of a lesion but also narrow the differential.

If a true lesion is seen on CT, it should be evaluated for periosteal reaction, matrix mineralization, margins, cortical breakthrough, and soft tissue mass (Table 6-4).

Lesion Found on MRI

It is a common problem to find a lesion on MRI, and as in many other similar situations, there is no clear

Table 6-4 Common Benign Lesions on CT That Prompt Further Workup

Lesion	Finding on CT	Suggestion of Diagnosis	Best F/U if Necessary
Subchondral cyst/ intraosseous ganglion	Focal lucency adjacent to joint	Sclerotic margins/adjacent to joint/lobulated	X-ray/reformat CT/MRI
Schmorl's node	Focal lucency in vertebra	Sclerotic margins/adjacent to endplate	Reformat CT; MRI: contiguous w disk
Bone island	Focal sclerotic lesion	Ovoid shape/blending w trabecular pattern	Bone scan—not hot, no other lesion
Sparse trabeculae	Ill-defined lucency	Fat density	MRI—fat signal
Vascular channel/ hemangioma	Lobulated/serpentine lucency	Near vascular channels	MRI—vessels w fat, prominent trabeculae
Fibrous dysplasia	Mixed lytic/sclerotic	Geographic/pelvis-proximal femur/young age	Bone scan—warm/not increased
Infarct	Focal sclerosis	Geographic/irregular shape/ sclerotic margin/fat density	MRI—double-line sign/fat internally
Osteoporotic compression fracture	Sclerotic vertebra/+/− ST edema	Osteopenia/loss of height/no mass/vacuum	X-ray/reformat CT/MRI (see Table 6-3)
Paget disease	Sclerosis*	Cortical thick/coarse trabeculae/expansion	X-ray/MRI/bone scan

*If destructive area or soft tissue mass is seen, consider secondary sarcoma.

consensus in the literature to guide management. Imaging should be geared toward detecting specific features of benign lesions, at which point the workup can stop. If no specific features are elucidated, follow-up imaging or biopsy may be indicated, depending on the degree of concern (e.g., a history of malignancy). If aggressive features are detected on MRI, biopsy is generally indicated unless potentially explained by a benign process such as stress fracture.

One of the first questions to ask is, "Does any fat, even a small amount, reside within the lesion?" If so, the lesion most likely represents either hemangioma or a focus of hematopoietic marrow. This situation is especially common in the spine, since hemangiomas are particularly common and heterogeneous distribution of hematopoietic marrow is commonly seen in older patients. Small amounts of fat can be detected on MRI by performing in-phase and out-of-phase sequences, as previously described.

Should the Patient Receive Contrast?

For an osseous spinal lesion, this is usually not helpful. Hemangiomas enhance—variably, some strongly, some not at all—as will hematopoietic marrow (slightly). Many benign lesions enhance, as do benign fractures and infection. In general, contrast distributes in areas with marrow edema (Box 6-3). Contrast can be helpful in distinguishing solid from cystic/myxoid/necrotic lesions and to scout more active areas to biopsy. Dynamic contrast can be used to determine the vascularity of a lesion for anticipated biopsy or open surgery. If the differential diagnosis includes infarction, contrast can also be useful to demonstrate lack of enhancement.

METASTATIC LESIONS AND MYELOMA

Frequency of certain lesions should always be taken into account. Primary bone sarcomas in young patients are very rare, so when a lesion looks aggres-

BOX 6-3 DIFFERENTIAL DIAGNOSIS: BONE LESION WITH SURROUNDING MARROW EDEMA/ENHANCEMENT ON MRI

Infection
Stress fracture/trauma
Giant cell tumor
Osteoid osteoma/osteoblastoma
Chondroblastoma
Pathologic fracture through lesion

sive in this population, always consider more common entities such as infection or trauma. On the other hand, in patients over 50 years of age metastatic disease and myeloma are common. Therefore, even if a lesion appears well defined, always consider the possibility of malignancy.

The presence of multiple lesions should increase the suspicion of metastatic disease, regardless of the imaging modality, the likelihood increasing with age. For patients over 50 years, metastases should also be high on the differential when a solitary tumor or indeterminate lesion is found on a small field-of-view examination. A skeletal survey, bone scan, MRI marrow survey, or PET scan can help define the extent of disease. Of these, skeletal survey is the least sensitive but probably the most frequently ordered. Bone scan can also be insensitive, especially for lytic metastases and myeloma, and a false increase in tracer uptake (a flare phenomenon) can be seen after treatment owing to increased bone repair. With diffuse involvement, as in skeletal carcinomatosis, especially from breast or prostate metastases, a "superscan" can be seen, with intense diffuse skeletal uptake and lack of renal tracer concentration. MRI marrow survey can be as simple as sagittal spine and coronal pelvis imaging with large field-of-view T1 and fluid-sensitive sequences or with use of a moving table scan a true whole-body examination can be acquired. PET scan has potential application for follow-up of treated tumor, but could potentially also be used to evaluate foci of metabolically active metastases.

Regarding location, both metastases and myeloma tend to occur most commonly in the same distribution as that of red marrow. This includes the spine; flat bones (such as ribs), clavicles, sternum, pelvis, and skull; and proximal femurs and humeri (Fig. 6-47). Myeloma occasionally manifests in the distal extremities. Metastatic lesions can also occur distally ("acral mets"), but these are usually seen in very aggressive neoplasms (e.g., breast, thyroid, renal carcinoma) or lesions with access to the pulmonary venous system, resulting in diffuse arterial seeding (e.g., lung carcinoma, tumors with lung metastases).

Metastases and myeloma tend not to occur in epiphyses or apophyses. However, advanced marrow infiltration by tumor can involve the growth centers, whereas red marrow almost always spares epiphyses and apophyses. As mentioned earlier, growth centers, once ossified, should contain only fatty marrow. Red marrow repopulation or hyperplasia from stimulation or severe anemia also usually spares these areas. Therefore, if an epiphysis or an apophysis shows replacement of fatty marrow on MRI, diffuse metastases or myelomatous involvement should be suspected (see Fig. 6-20).

Although multiplicity suggests metastases or myeloma, occasionally primary sarcomas, especially osteosarcoma and Ewing sarcoma, present with "skip lesions" in the same bone (synchronous) or in other bones at the same or different times (metachronous). Therefore, imaging characterization of a primary tumor should always include visualization of the entire involved bone.

Myeloma can present in three radiographic forms, which often overlap: diffuse osteoporosis, small punched-out lesions, and large, blow-out lesions. As mentioned earlier, for a lesion to be detected radiographically a large proportion of trabeculae must be destroyed or replaced or the cortex must be breached. Most metastases and myelomatous lesions begin in the medullary cavity, eventually penetrating the cortex. On CT and MRI, this is evident based on the relatively large marrow component, which is nearly always underestimated on radiographs. Some lesions arise eccentrically at the periosteum or subcortical bone and destroy the cortex early ("cortical mets"). This is seen in breast, renal, thyroid, and lung metastases. A punched-out lesion is seen on radiographs, and on MRI, a prominent mass is seen centered at the cortex. Some lesions are characteristically lytic or blastic, whereas others may be lytic, blastic, or mixed (Box 6-4).

Burned-out Lesions

Some benign lesions as a course of their natural history or because of underlying hemorrhage heal with fatty marrow, leaving a ghost of the lesion margins that remains for a long period of time. Bone heals with fatty marrow, as can be seen after fracture, orthopedic pin removal, or healing after a drilling procedure, and after regression of a marrow lesion (Fig. 6-48). Lipoma of bone or fibromyxoma in many cases may be the sequela of a previous lesion. Although calcaneal cysts have been postulated to form out of cystic degeneration of a lipoma, it seems more likely that a calcaneal cyst, which arises as an intraosseous ganglion from the subtalar joint, regresses or hemorrhages and heals with fat replacement.

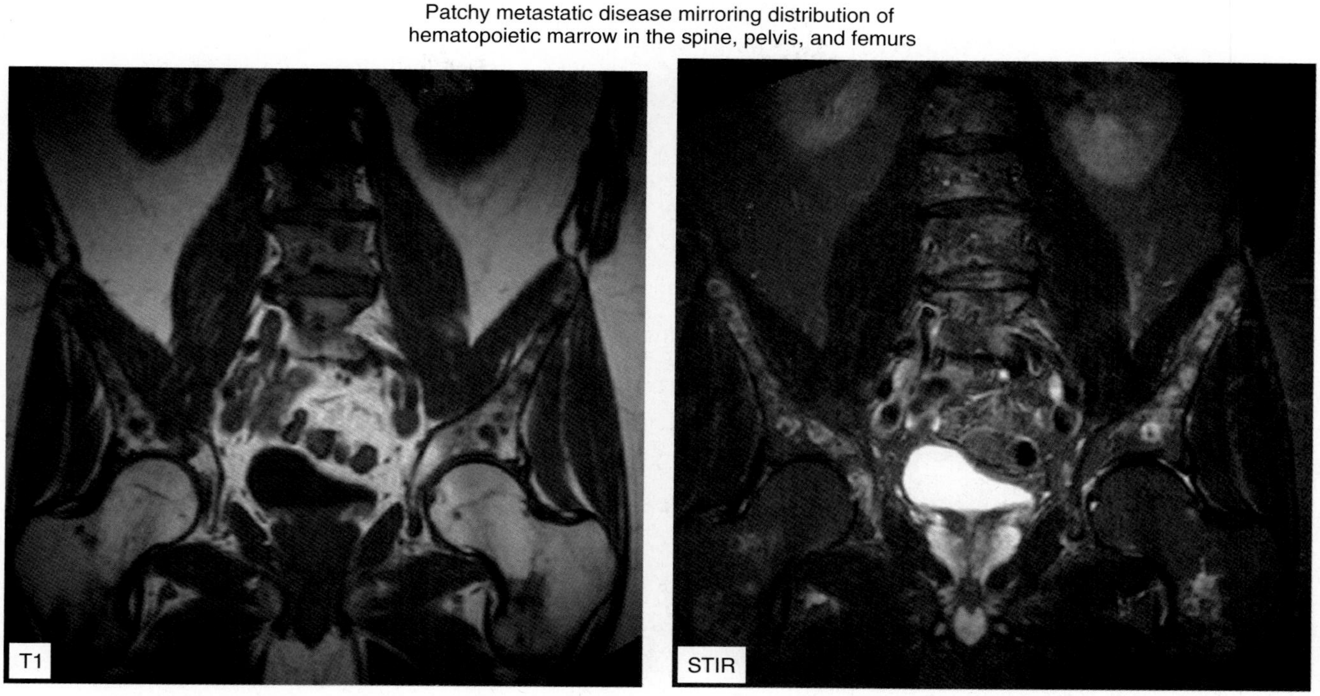
Patchy metastatic disease mirroring distribution of hematopoietic marrow in the spine, pelvis, and femurs
T1
STIR

Figure 6-47 Distribution of metastatic disease mirrors that of hematopoietic marrow. Note that tumor deposits are isointense to muscle on T1-weighted images. Both metastases and hematopoietic marrow can be relatively bright on fluid-sensitive sequences (e.g., STIR and fat-suppressed T2-weighted images), and therefore T1-weighted noncontrast images are key.

BOX 6-4 RADIOGRAPHIC APPEARANCE OF BONE METASTASES AND MYELOMA: REPRESENTATIVE EXAMPLES

Lytic
Myeloma
Lung
Renal
Thyroid
Breast
Lymphoma

Blastic
Prostate
Breast
Carcinoid
Lymphoma
Treated lesion

Mixed
GI/adenocarcinoma
Lymphoma
Breast

Radiation Osteonecrosis

Radiation-induced osteonecrosis can occur in any body part exposed to therapeutic levels of radiation, but it is especially common in the pelvic bones (see Fig. 6-8). The necrotic bone is sclerotic and can appear irregular, often inciting concern on radiographs for recurrent tumor or local tumor spread. The first step is to document that the lesion is in a prior radiation port. Surgical clips from tumor or nodal dissection are often a clue. Search for findings more typical of infarction, such as sharp serpentine sclerosis oriented along the medullary cavity of a long bone; subchondral crescentic sclerosis at a joint may be seen in the area. Bone lysis or destruction seen on radiographs or CT should raise concern of the presence of tumor. Osteonecrosis does not cause mass effect, so the presence of a soft tissue mass on CT or MRI should prompt biopsy. MRI can show variable internal signal, but sharp margination with a double-line sign can help document infarction rather than tumor.

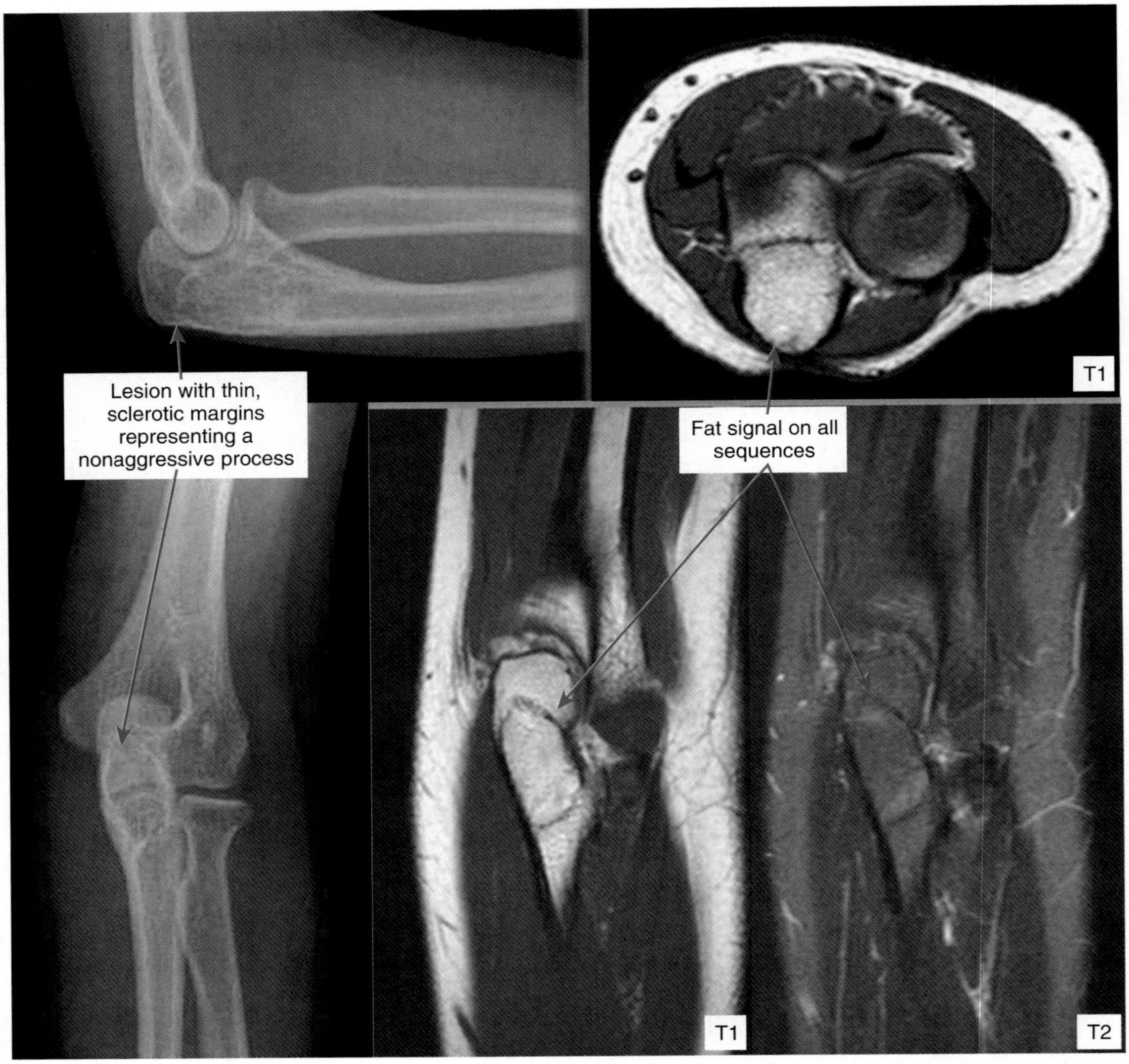
T1
Lesion with thin, sclerotic margins representing a nonaggressive process
Fat signal on all sequences
T1
T2

Figure 6-48 Burned-out lesions—those that resemble some primary lesion on radiographs but show internal fat signal on MRI—most likely represent involuted benign lesions, although the differential includes intraosseous lipoma. Regardless, monotonous fat signal in a lesion on MRI is compatible with a benign process. Since primary bone tumors and metastatic lesions exclude, push away, or destroy marrow fat, any fat within an intraosseous lesion suggests benign etiology.

Bone scan is not specific owing to uptake of tracer in the surrounding reactive bone. However, PET scan may prove to be useful, with lack of uptake indicating low metabolic activity. Comparison with prior examinations is helpful, but necrosis can progress over time. Ultimately, biopsy of suspicious or changing areas may be needed. Pathologic fracture can occur through necrotic bone, further complicating evaluation. Healing response is slow or absent.

Radiation during development can result in growth disturbance in the radiation field. For example, radiation of a Wilms' tumor in the kidney of a child can result in vertebral anomalies and scoliosis due to asymmetric growth disturbance (Fig. 6-49).

Radiation-Induced Sarcomas

Sarcomas can arise in delayed fashion within a radiation field. This is seen 10 to 15 years or longer after treatment and classically occurs at the margin of the port, where the dose was lower. Various types

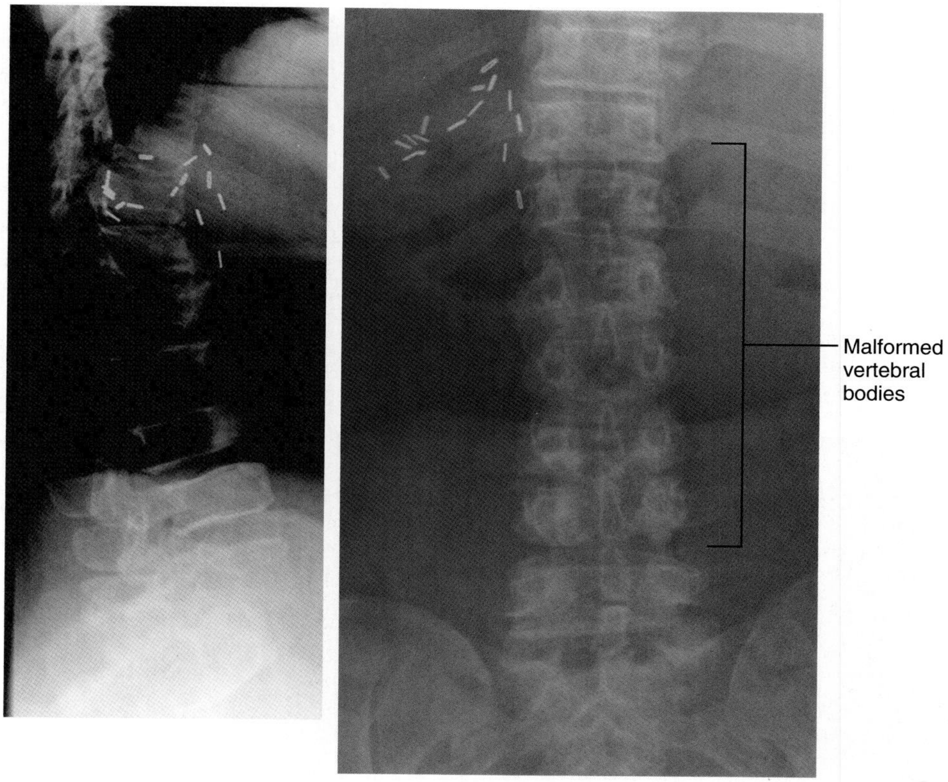
Malformed
vertebral
bodies

Figure 6-49 Growth disturbance and early disk degeneration in a 30-year-old patient with radiation treatment for Wilms' tumor as a child.

of sarcomas can occur, such as osteosarcoma, fibrosarcoma, and chondrosarcoma. Tumors are usually very aggressive with poor prognosis. Destruction of bone is seen, with osteoid or chondroid matrix corresponding to histologic type (Fig. 6-50; see also Fig. 6-39).

GENERAL APPROACH TO SOFT TISSUE TUMORS

There are many benign and malignant soft tissue tumors, but only a minority has features that are characteristic enough to make a specific imaging diagnosis. This is facilitated by MRI, which is the modality of choice for imaging a suspected soft tissue mass. Fortunately, these few entities make up a large proportion of all soft tissue masses that present for imaging, and most of these are benign. Also, a variety of nontumor lesions present as masses.

Therefore, the role of the radiologist is first to determine whether the lesion is a true tumor or a pseudolesion. Often on MRI, the cause of a pseudolesion can be determined. If the lesion is determined to most likely be a tumor, the next question is, "Is the lesion unquestionably benign?" If not, the radiologist's function switches from analytical to descriptive, detailing the margins, location, fascial and bone compartments involved, proximity to neurovascular structures, and vascularity or presence of feeding vessels, giving the referring surgeon valuable information to plan biopsy and definitive treatment (Fig. 6-51). Note that a histologic diagnosis is not essential; most malignant soft tissue tumors have no specific features on imaging. Biopsy and histologic analysis is generally required for definitive diagnosis. If the lesion is indeterminate for tumor, the radiologist may recommend alternate imaging modalities or short-term follow-up rather than biopsy, depending on the level of clinical and imaging suspicion.

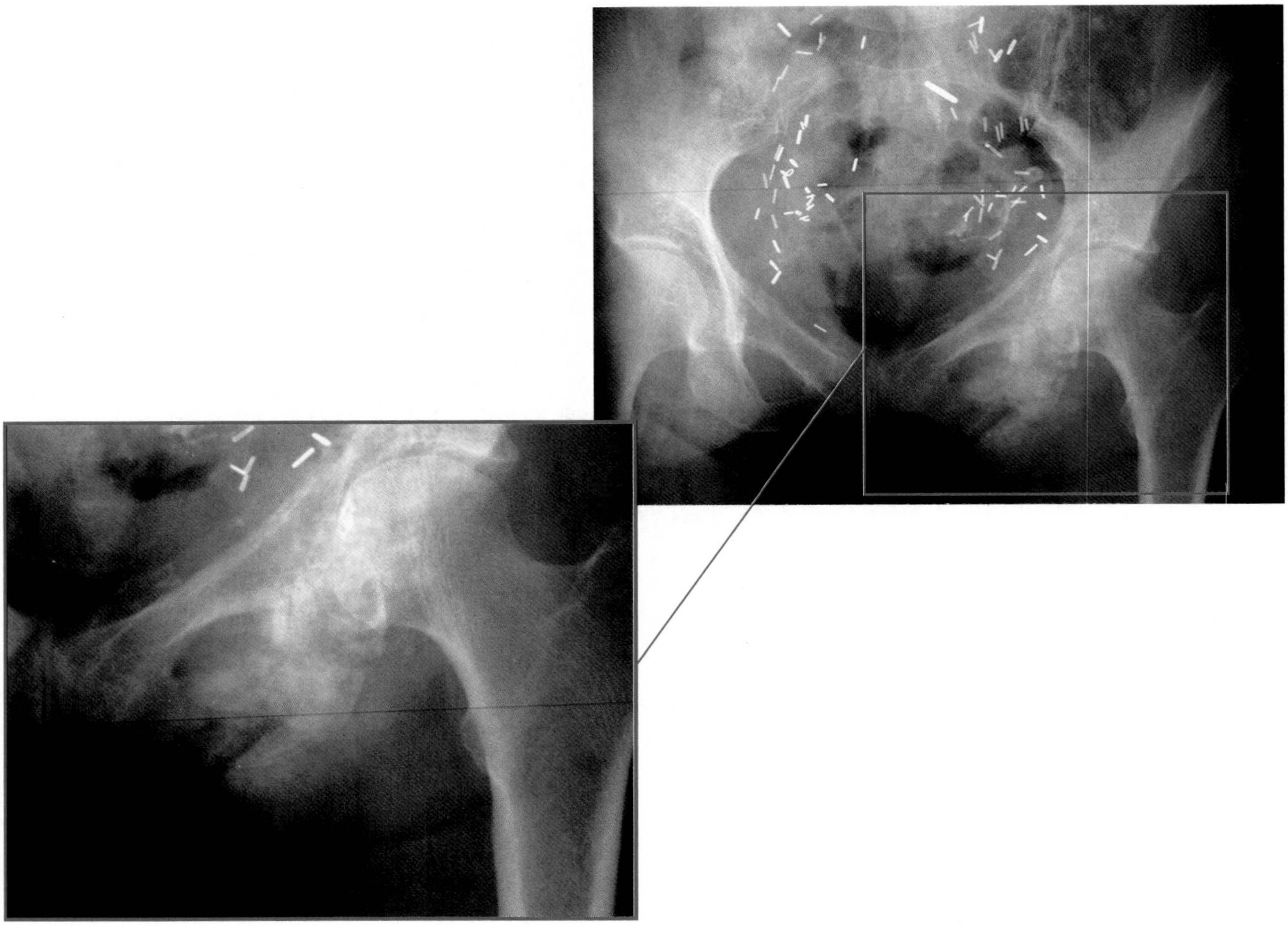

Figure 6-50 Osteoid matrix and bone destruction representing secondary osteosarcoma forming at the margin of a radiation port for rhabdomyosarcoma, treated when the patient was a child.

PITFALLS AND PSEUDOTUMORS

Accessory Muscle

An accessory muscle can hypertrophy in response to alteration in activity and can be perceived as a mass. Ultrasound of the area shows no mass. MRI confirms that the focus corresponds to muscle signal and is longitudinally oriented (Fig. 6-52).

Fascial Defect

Fascial defects are usually caused by trauma or surgery, leaving a rent in the fascia that allows muscle to herniate through. On MRI, this is seen as a bump at the fascial margin with muscle signal. However, the herniation is usually intermittent, occurring only in various positions or stresses. MRI can be performed with the patient making the mass pop out, but ultrasound offers more flexibility in evaluating the dynamic nature of these lesions.

Nonencapsulated Lipoma

This term is a euphemism for obesity with asymmetric distribution of fat. Often in obese patients, a mass is perceived, but on MRI there is no lesion beneath the skin markers. This term can be used to avoid a potentially insulting report. It is true that nonencapsulated lipomas exist and are often seen on imaging as a region of fat density or signal with fewer septations than the surrounding subcutaneous fat as well as deflection of fascial planes reflecting mass effect.

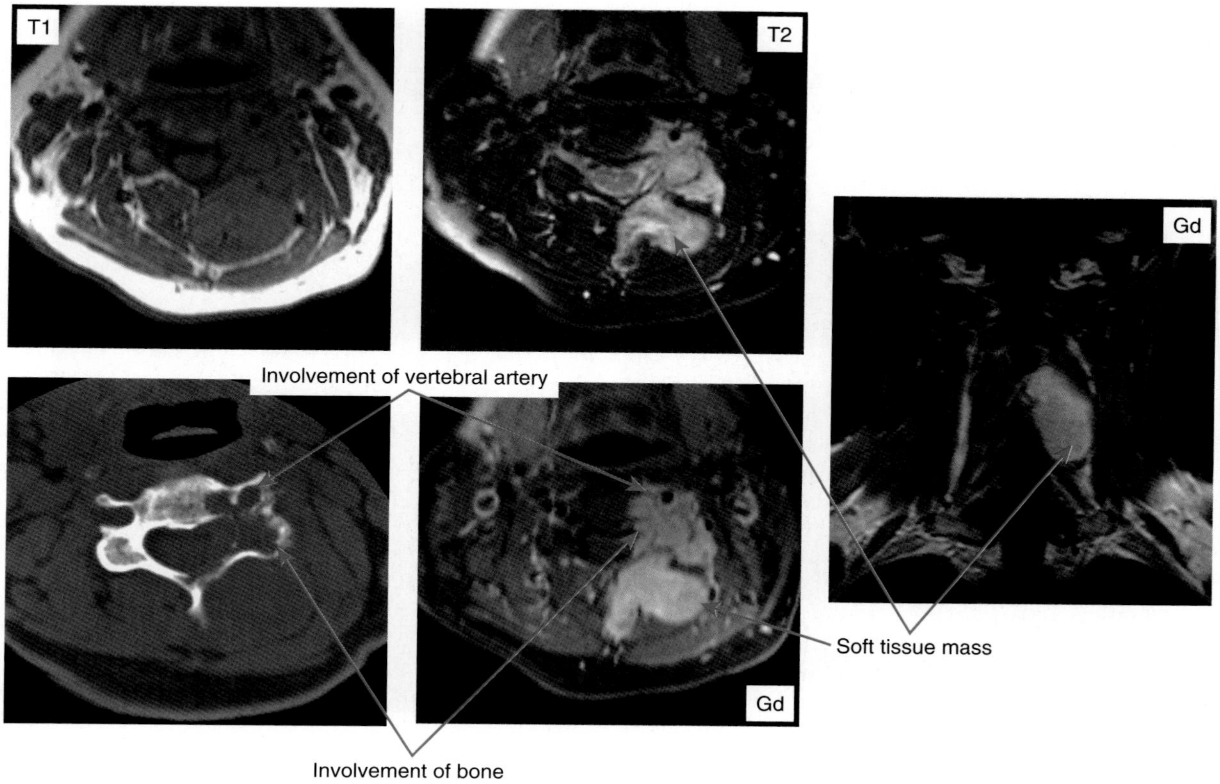
T1
T2
Gd
Involvement of vertebral artery
Soft tissue mass
Gd
Involvement of bone

Figure 6-51 Soft tissue mass secondarily involving bone: synovial sarcoma of the cervical spine. Despite its name, synovial sarcoma does not originate from joints, but rather arises in soft tissues, usually near joints, especially in the lower extremity. Synovial sarcoma, like other soft tissue malignancies, may invade the adjacent bone, representing a form of extracompartmental spread and worsening the prognosis. Involvement of neurovascular structures also alters treatment options and should be noted.

Complex Ganglion Cysts

Ganglion cysts can occasionally simulate tumors. In areas prone to trauma they may become complex and heterogeneous, containing synovial proliferation or chronic blood products. Baker cysts, which are really synovial cysts, are a prime example, often appearing complex. Around the foot and ankle, cysts are also commonly complex. Two principles help distinguish cysts from tumors.

The first principle is that ganglion cysts are very common, whereas malignant tumors arising from joints or tendon sheaths are very rare. Therefore, if the cystic lesion connects via a neck to an adjacent joint or tendon sheath, it is extremely unlikely to be malignant. Also, in this case there is often concurrent internal derangement of the joint, adjacent ligament tear, or tendon abnormality that incited the process, which increases the confidence of the radiologist. Occasionally, when unclear, injection of contrast into the joint with demonstration of communication is enough to stop further workup. Second, lobulation is a characteristic of ganglion cysts that is uncommonly seen in malignant tumors; however, lobulation cannot be used as a specific feature for benignity, and if the cystic lesion is not connected to a synovial compartment, biopsy may be necessary. After all, malignant fibrous histiocytoma (MFH), the most common soft tissue malignancy seen in older individuals, often occurs around the knee and can simulate a Baker cyst. In young patients, synovial sarcomas can be cystic mimicking a ganglion cyst, and they tend to occur in the lower extremity near joints. Intravenous contrast-enhanced MRI can occasionally distinguish a ganglion (thin rim enhancement is typical) from tumor (complex or nodular enhancement), but

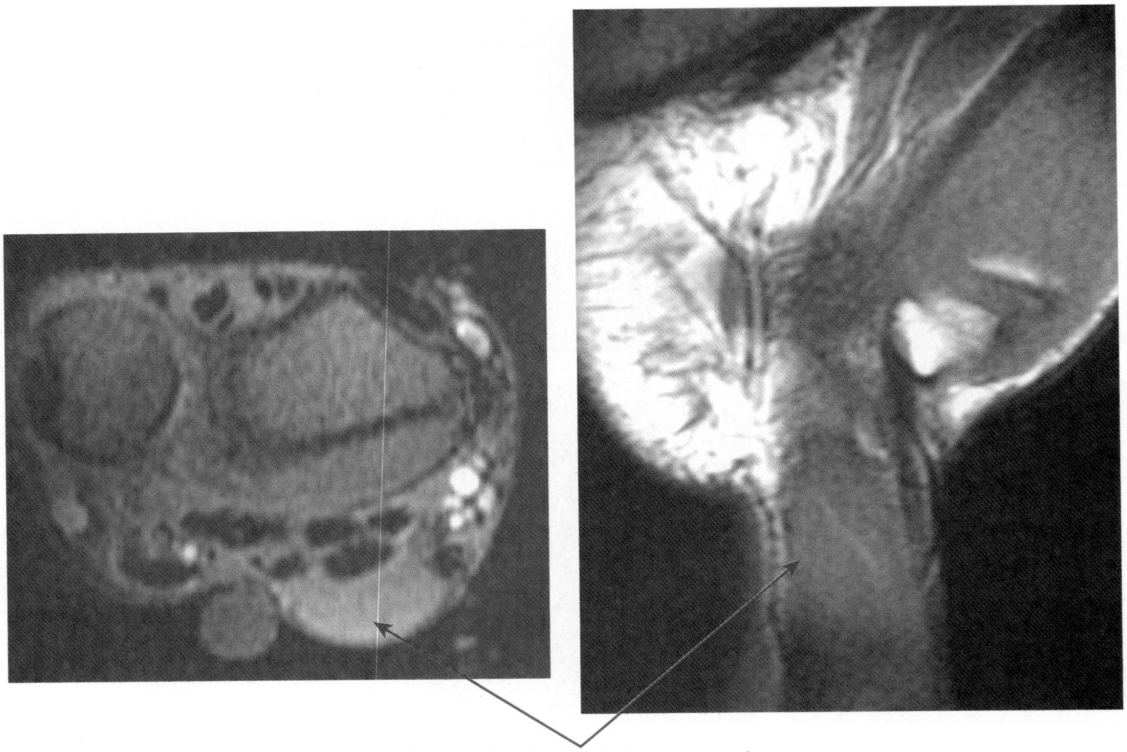
Hypertrophied palmaris longus muscle

Figure 6-52 Anomalous muscles can present as masses. Look for longitudinal orientation and signal isointense with other muscles.

if the cyst contains synovial proliferation this may not be a useful discriminator. Ultrasound also has limited use, since it can be hard to depict the communication, and many tumors are cystic. A classic pitfall is a myxoid liposarcoma, which can simulate a cyst on MRI and even ultrasound. When gadolinium contrast is administered, the true solid nature can be appreciated (Fig. 6-53).

There is a high prevalence of ganglion cysts around joints presenting as soft tissue masses clinically. In fact, an MRI request for "rule out soft tissue mass" around a joint can be evaluated with a routine joint protocol. In the unlikely event that the lesion is indeterminate or a true mass, the patient can be brought back for contrast-enhanced images (Fig. 6-54).

Lymph Node

Lymph nodes in typical locations are usually easily distinguished from soft tissue masses. However, in locations not commonly recognized as part of the lymphatic system, normal and inflammatory nodes can be confused for masses. Two such locations are the popliteal fossa (the popliteal node) and the medial elbow (the epitrochlear node, Fig. 6-55). Nodes can be recognized as such by their bean-shaped morphology and fatty hilum, looking like a mini-kidney. The presence of a fatty hilum and typical morphology is consistent with a benign etiology. Nodes in these and other locations can become enlarged as a reaction to acute or chronic inflammation in the extremity more distally. The classic inflammatory epitrochlear lymph node is associated with rose thorn disease (*Sporothrix schenkii*), a fungal infection of the hand and arm. At the posterior knee, a prominent lymph node around the vascular structures of the popliteal fossa, the popliteal node, is often seen and is usually normal, although it could reflect more distal inflammation.

Inflammatory Pseudomasses/Deposition

Patients with inflammatory arthropathies, especially gout and rheumatoid arthritis, can present with a

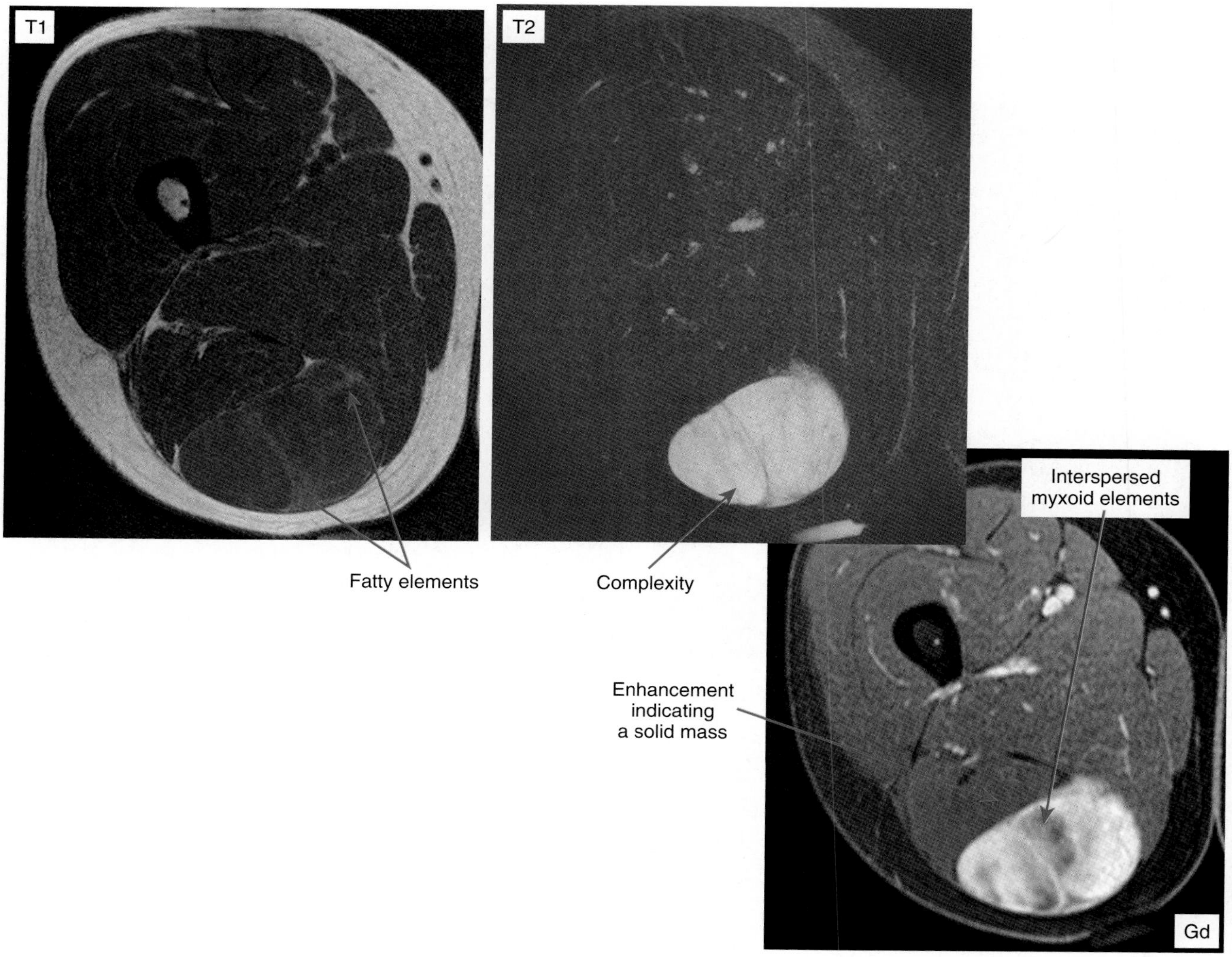
T1
T2
Gd
Fatty elements
Complexity
Interspersed myxoid elements
Enhancement indicating a solid mass

Figure 6-53 Some soft tissue malignancies can simulate cysts on MRI and ultrasound, especially those with prominent cystic or myxomatous elements. In this case, complexity and lack of communication with a joint or sheath raise suspicion. Also, areas of T1 hyperintensity are compatible with fatty or hemorrhagic elements. Contrast enhancement indicates solid, vascular tissue—in this case a myxoid liposarcoma.

soft tissue mass. Tendons, bursae, and periarticular locations are susceptible; search for appropriate history or articular findings of those conditions. Other noninflammatory arthropathies can present as masses around joints or tendon sheaths, such as pigmented villonodular synovitis and synovial osteochondromatosis. The former contains hemosiderin, seen on low signal on T2-weighted and GRE MRI sequences, and does not calcify, and the latter usually shows numerous calcified bodies. Amyloid deposits can also manifest with mass effect, usually around joints. This is generally associated with renal failure and secondary hyperparathyroidism, so history and associated radiographic findings are useful. If the mass is densely calcified on radiographs, tumoral calcinosis is in the differential but care must be taken to exclude a bone-forming tumor with osteoid matrix, such as parosteal osteosarcoma.

Myositis Ossificans/Spontaneous Hematoma

If a lesion found on MRI is hyperintense on T1-weighted images and if no gadolinium contrast was given, it contains fat or blood. The differential diagnosis for fat-containing lesions is listed in Box 6-5.

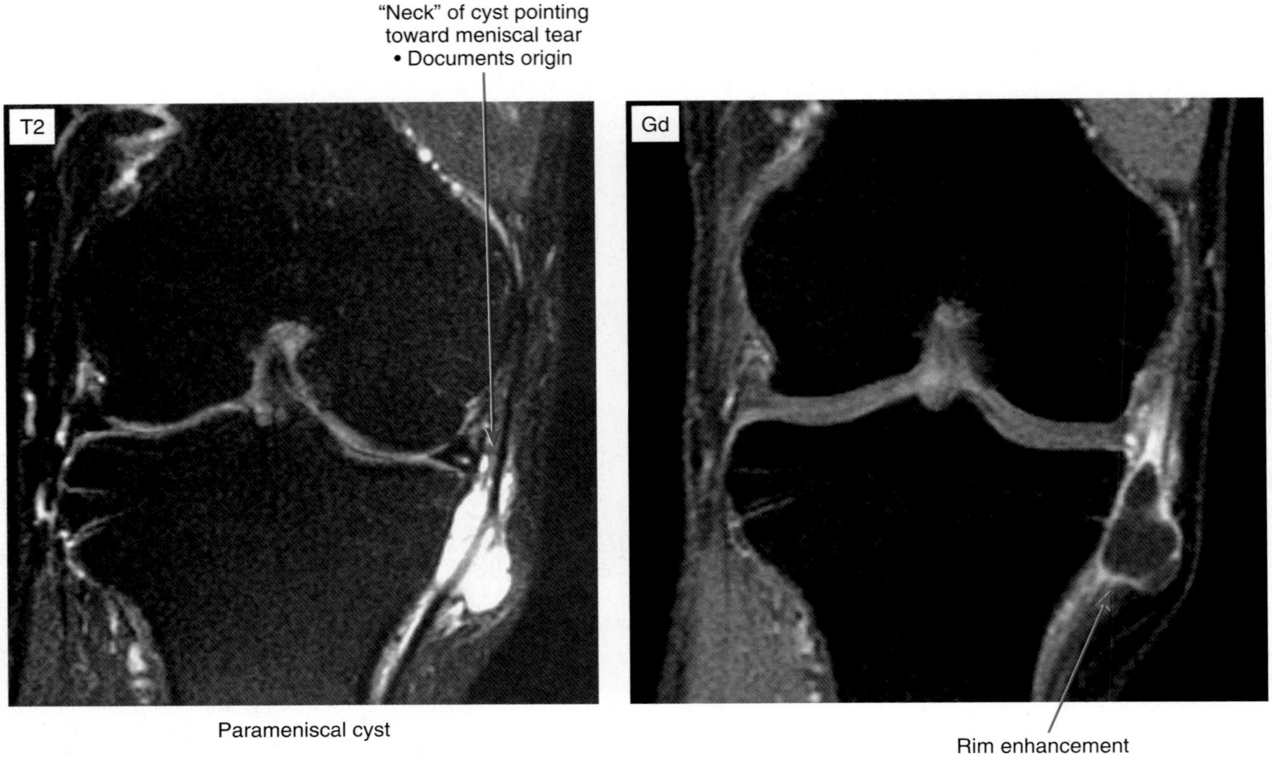
"Neck" of cyst pointing
toward meniscal tear
• Documents origin
T2
Gd
Paramensical cyst
Rim enhancement

Figure 6-54 For masses palpated around joints, especially the knee and wrist, cysts (ganglion cysts, parameniscal/paralabral cysts, Baker cysts) are very common, much more common than true masses. Therefore, intravenous contrast is less beneficial in these situations, and it may be more prudent to perform a routine noncontrast examination, looking for communication of the structure with a joint, meniscus, labrum, or tendon sheath documenting its etiology. If no communication can be seen, contrast may be added to evaluate solid areas for potential biopsy.

BOX 6-5 FAT-CONTAINING LESIONS

Fatty tumor
- Lipoma
- Liposarcoma

Fatty mature marrow
- Soft tissue: Myositis ossificans; extramedullary hematopoiesis

Hemangioma/vascular malformation

Fat suppression is very useful for differentiating fat from blood, since fat suppresses and blood does not. In fact, a very useful sequence if blood is suspected is a fat-suppressed, noncontrast T1-weighted sequence. Blood will be hyperintense. Of course, in later stages with methemoglobin or hemosiderin, blood transforms to low signal on T2 and low to intermediate on T1. Unlike neuroimaging, in the musculoskeletal system there is a less tightly regulated oxygen supply, so time course of changes in blood signal seen in the brain cannot be applied to the peripheral soft tissues. Blood can last for days or weeks with signal characteristics of acute blood, and areas of hyper- and hypointensity are often mixed. When a hematoma in the soft tissues begins to "organize," it becomes vascularized and enhances heterogeneously. At this stage, the lesion often simulates a soft tissue tumor. Even if organizing hematoma is suspected, follow-up may be required unless the history or clinical picture is crystal clear, as in clearly inciting trauma in a young person, a history of anticoagulant therapy or hemophilia, and a mass progressively decreasing in size. Keep in mind, though, that many soft tissue sarcomas present after minor trauma, when they become noticed or hemorrhage, so even in a young patient, the risk of underlying sarcoma (e.g., synovial sarcoma) should be

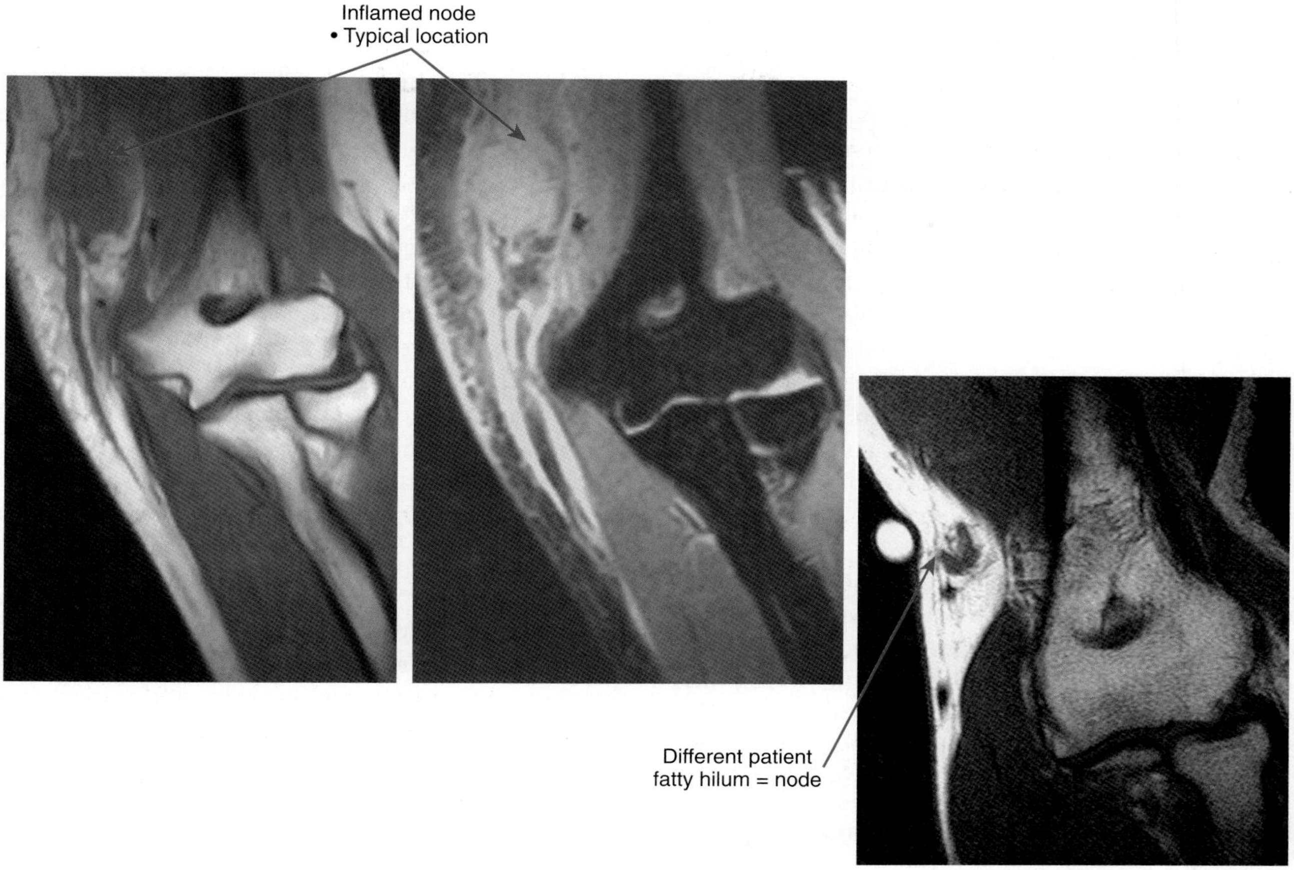
Inflamed node
• Typical location
Different patient
fatty hilum = node

Figure 6-55 Epitrochlear lymph node. Enlarged or inflamed lymph nodes can simulate a tumor clinically and on imaging. Location and kidney shape with a fatty hilum can suggest the diagnosis. However, enlargement can be a sign of tumor (especially lymphoma) or nearby infection.

considered. In older patients who present with a spontaneous hematoma, the same is true. Follow-up is prudent.

What kind of follow-up is recommended? Unfortunately, there is little to no research to guide recommendations. Also, as the latter examples illustrate, a wide variety of patient scenarios and degrees of clinical and imaging suspicion exists. Time course is based mainly on degree of suspicion. Modality for follow-up is also debatable. An MRI pre- and post-contrast is very useful for evaluation of soft tissue masses, but it is somewhat nonspecific regarding benign versus malignant diagnosis. However, if MRI was acquired as a baseline examination, a follow-up MRI can be directly compared to look for regression of aggressive features. Follow-up MRI can be performed after 1 to 2 months, depending on the degree of suspicion. Lack of enhancement or minimal thin rim enhancement supports a benign diagnosis. Lack of regression, increased mass effect, or increased focal enhancement should prompt consideration of biopsy. If MRI is acquired as follow-up, a non–fat-suppressed GRE sequence can be useful to look for circumferential low signal representing peripheral rim calcification seen with hematomas. The zonal phenomenon typically seen radiographically in myositis ossificans is seen as a rim of dark signal on MRI from either hemosiderin or calcification, both of which bloom on GRE sequences. Be sure not to fat suppress, however, because blooming artifact may blend with low signal from suppressed fat.

In the same light, radiographs can occasionally be useful as follow-up examinations to look for the zonal phenomenon, a rimlike calcification resulting in a dense mass where the margin is denser than the center. This rim calcification can form relatively quickly, often within 2 to 3 weeks. CT can be useful for detecting subtle calcification. Rapid formation of a zonal phenomenon supports a benign diagnosis. However, although the zonal phenomenon has been classically touted as specific for a benign diagnosis, rare cases of malignancy, especially slow-growing low-grade varieties of synovial sarcoma, can rarely demonstrate rimlike calcification. However, the architecture of a lesion can be used to confidently identify a lesion as benign. Calcification in the soft tissues has a wide differential including benign (e.g., tumoral calcinosis) and malignant entities, such as synovial sarcoma, whereas ossification (i.e., corticomedullary differentiation) has a limited and benign differential (e.g., myositis ossificans).

PET scan and PET-CT can also be useful if the lesion is large enough. Lack of uptake on PET corresponding to a hemorrhagic lesion should support a benign diagnosis. However, there is little information on the use of this modality to monitor hemorrhagic lesions.

True Soft Tissue Mass Found on Imaging

MRI is the test of choice for evaluation of soft tissue masses, and for excluding pseudomasses. However, it is not reliable for differentiation of benign from malignant, except for certain lesion types. Malignant soft tissue tumors are not always infiltrative. In fact, most appear well defined. A lesion can be classified as benign only if it displays certain specific features for particular benign processes.

Examples of Specific Diagnoses for Soft Tissue Masses on MRI

Lipoma. Monotonous fat signal on MRI; no septations or few, thin septations; no enhancement.

Hemangioma. Mass composed of blood vessels/vascular spaces with interspaced fat; phleboliths (Fig. 6-56).

Ganglion/Parameniscal/Labral Cyst. Lobulated fluid signal structure connected to a joint, tendon sheath, or fibrocartilage structure (see Fig. 6-54).

Fibroma. Soft tissue lesion associated with fascia; low signal on MRI (Fig. 6-57).

Giant cell tumor of tendon sheath (GCTTS). Soft tissue lesion associated with tendon sheaths in hands or feet; low signal on MRI due to hemosiderin deposition (Fig. 6-58).

Glomus tumor. Small, round lesion in the digit (usually nailbed), very bright T2, enhances brightly (Fig. 6-59).

Elastofibroma. Ill-defined triangular or ovoid shaped lesion deep to the serratus anterior, interspersed with fat (Fig. 6-60).

Myxoma. Ovoid focus of fluid signal, usually intramuscular; no enhancement or thin rim-enhancement (Fig. 6-61).

Nerve sheath tumor. Ovoid lesion with "tails" associated with neurovascular bundle; low-signal bulls-eye center (Fig. 6-62).

Morton neuroma (perineural fibrosis). Low-signal focus with enhancement inferior and just distal to space between metatarsal heads.

Fibrolipomatous hamartoma. Enlarged nerve containing fat (Fig. 6-63).

Dermal and subcutaneous lesions are typically small and notoriously difficult to differentiate by imaging. Diagnoses are protean and range from benign/inflammatory (e.g., sebaceous cyst, foreign body granuloma) to malignant (melanoma, dermatofibrosarcoma protuberans). Generally, clinical examination, course, and biopsy are primary management tools, with ultrasound or MRI used to evaluate deep extension for surgical management. Those found incidentally on MRI usually generate a fairly useless differential and request for clinical inspection. A mass lesion on the fascia should raise the possibility of nodular fasciitis, a reactive nontumor lesion presenting clinically as a rapidly growing mass in an extremity. These lesions have a variable appearance and may arise in subcutaneous or intramuscular locations, but usually enhance brightly with fascial tails (Fig. 6-64).

Mass Not Definitively Benign

What should one do when there is a lesion that cannot be classified as benign, even after MRI? The lesion should be described in terms of the location, size, and extent, the fascial compartment involved, and whether the lesion extends beyond the fascial margins into another compartment. Attention should be paid to the neurovascular bundles, since involvement can change management from a limb salvage surgery to an amputation. T1-weighted images are considered by most to be essential for evaluation of fascial compartments and neurovascular bundles. If

Text continued on page 317

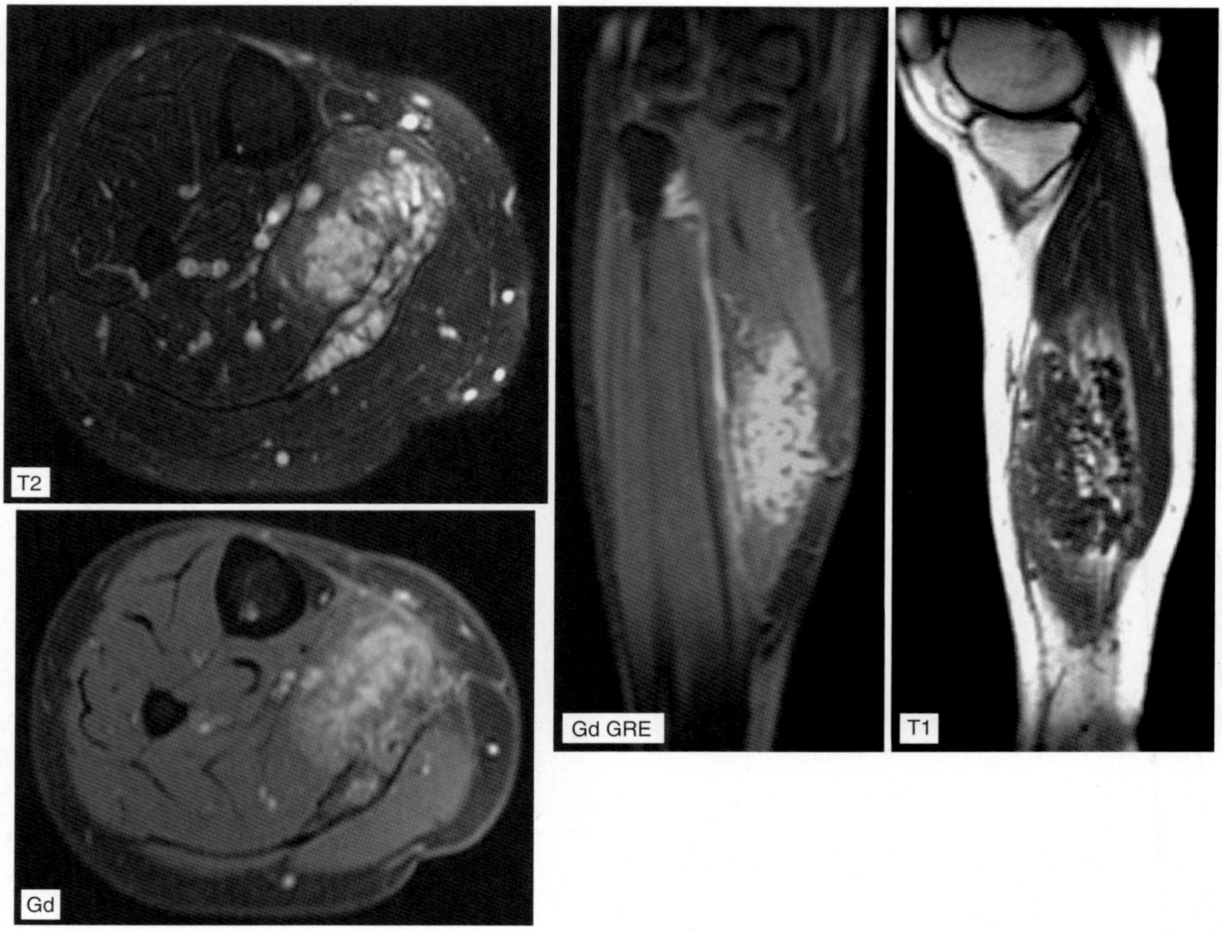
T2
Gd
Gd GRE
T1

Figure 6-56 Hemangiomas and vascular malformations are very common in soft tissues. They also have a fairly pathognomonic appearance on MRI, with interspersed fat signal and prominent vascular channels. They often create little mass effect for their size and in fact may be associated with adjacent muscle atrophy. Other vascular malformations causing hyperemia during development can cause localized hypertrophy. Vascular malformations of soft tissue can cross fascial planes and even involve adjacent bone causing cortical holes from engorged vascular channels reminiscent of more aggressive permeative lesions.

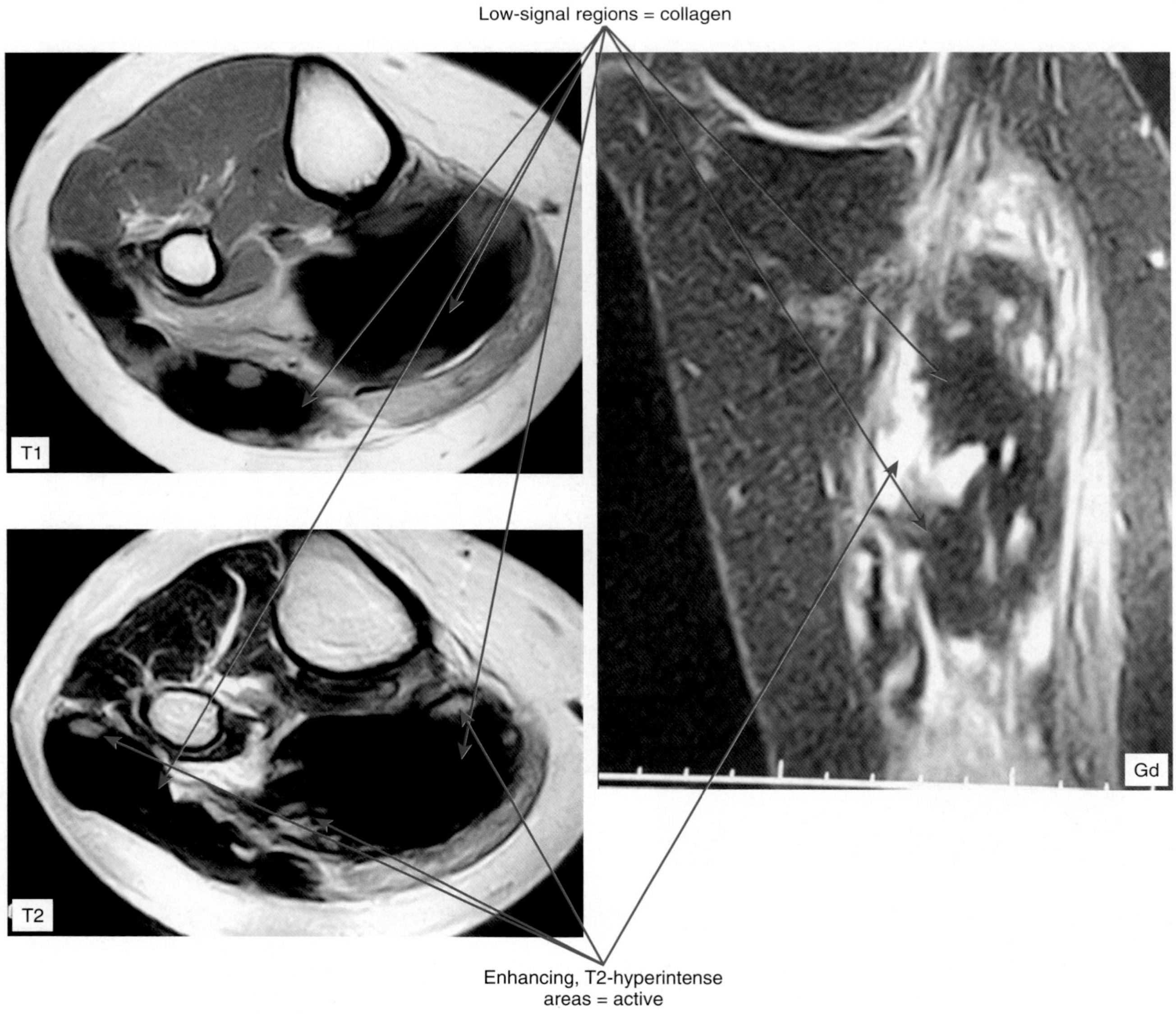
Low-signal regions = collagen
T1
T2
Gd
Enhancing, T2-hyperintense areas = active

Figure 6-57 Deep fibromatosis. Lesions are invasive and often cross fascial barriers. Low signal is characteristic and represents mature collagen deposition. Enhancing or T2-hyperintense regions are more fibroblastic and metabolically active.

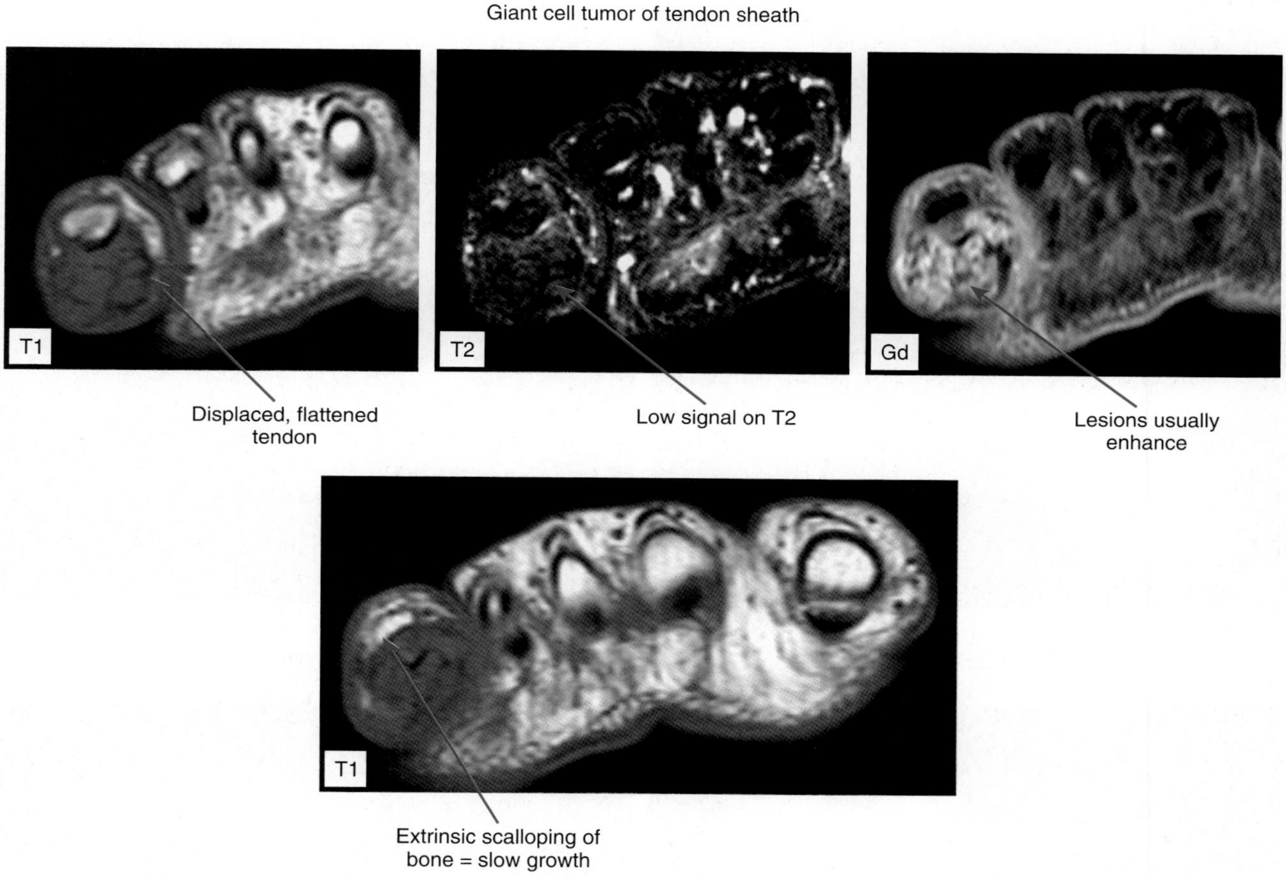
Giant cell tumor of tendon sheath
T1
T2
Gd
Displaced, flattened tendon
Low signal on T2
Lesions usually enhance
T1
Extrinsic scalloping of bone = slow growth

Figure 6-58 Giant cell tumor of tendon sheath. This lesion can be identified with some confidence when in a characteristic location (associated with a tendon sheath, usually of a digit) and with a characteristic signal pattern (low signal on T2-weighted images). Extrinsic scalloping of bone is not uncommon.

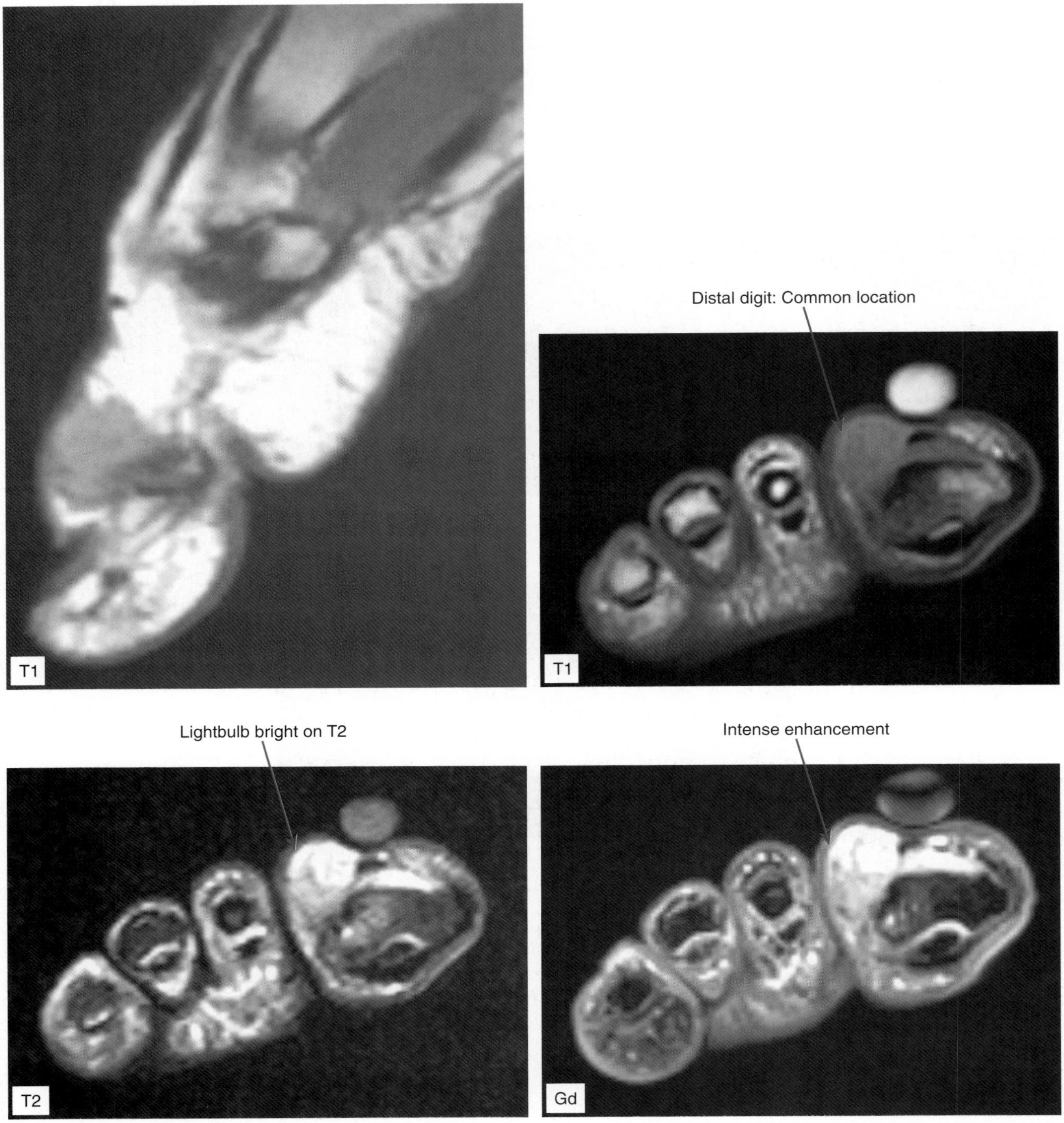
T1
Distal digit: Common location
T1
Lightbulb bright on T2
T2
Intense enhancement
Gd

Figure 6-59 Glomus tumor also has a characteristic appearance on MRI—a small, round lesion of a digit, usually distal, "bright as a light bulb" on T2, enhances brightly; exquisitely tender on examination.

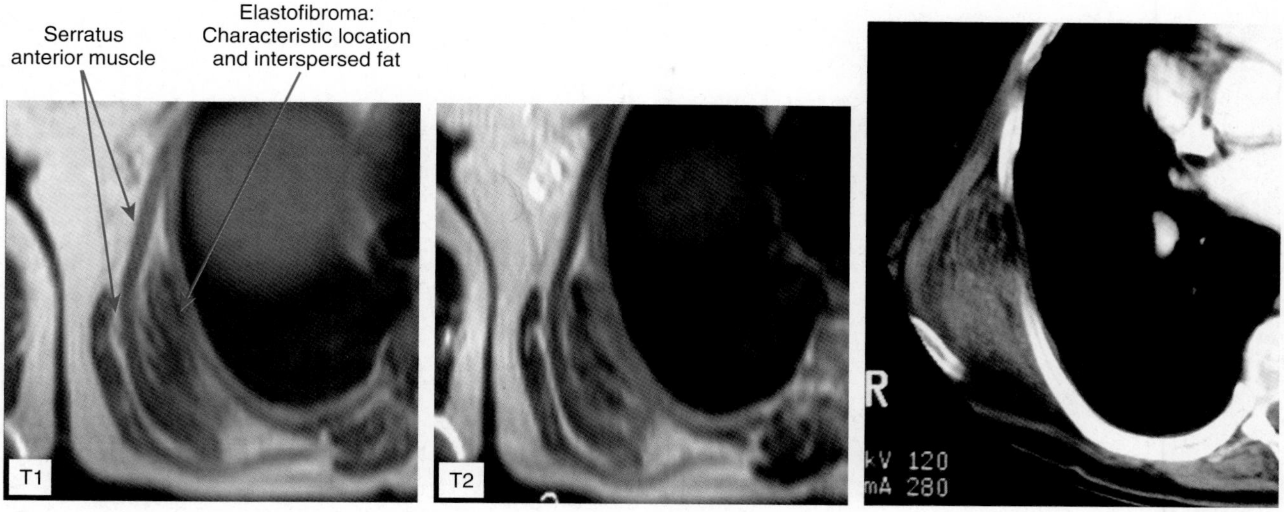
Serratus anterior muscle
Elastofibroma: Characteristic location and interspersed fat
T1
T2
R
kV 120
mA 280

Figure 6-60 Elastofibroma is a non-neoplastic process presenting with inferior scapular mass effect clinically; MRI features are characteristic, with an ill-defined lesion between the rib cage and the serratus anterior muscle at the inferior scapular margin, interspersed with fat signal. CT scan is also specific with a lesion in the characteristic location with streaks of fat density. The finding is often bilateral. Biopsy is not required.

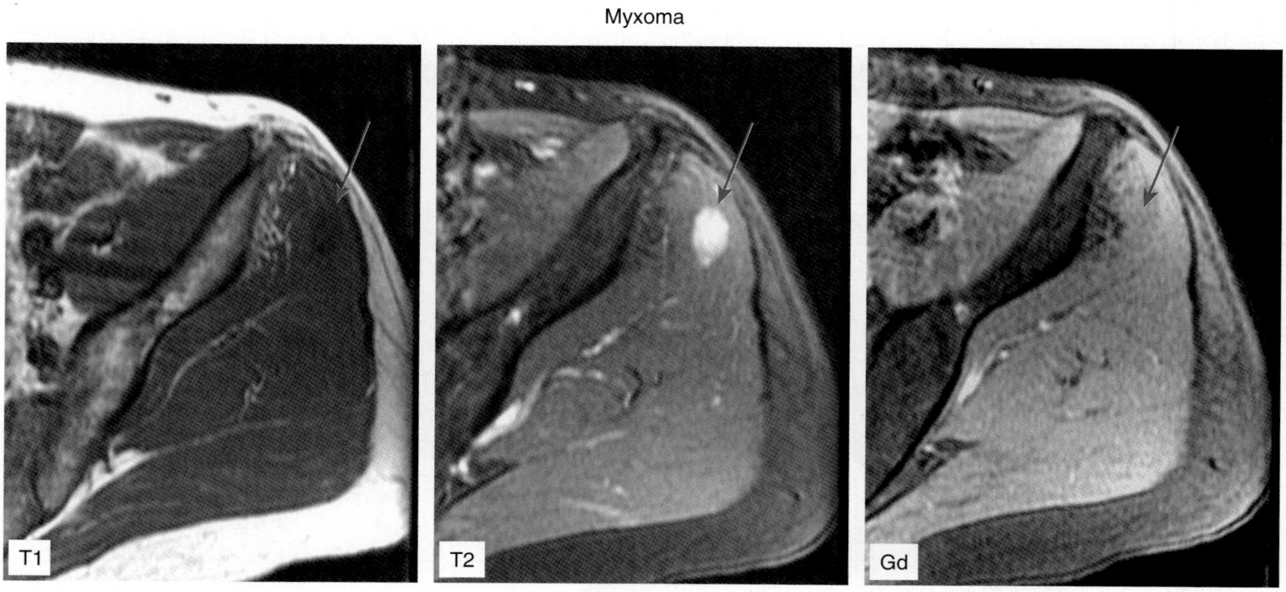
Myxoma
T1
T2
Gd

Figure 6-61 **Myxoma.** Fluid signal on T1, T2; no enhancement or thin rim enhancement.

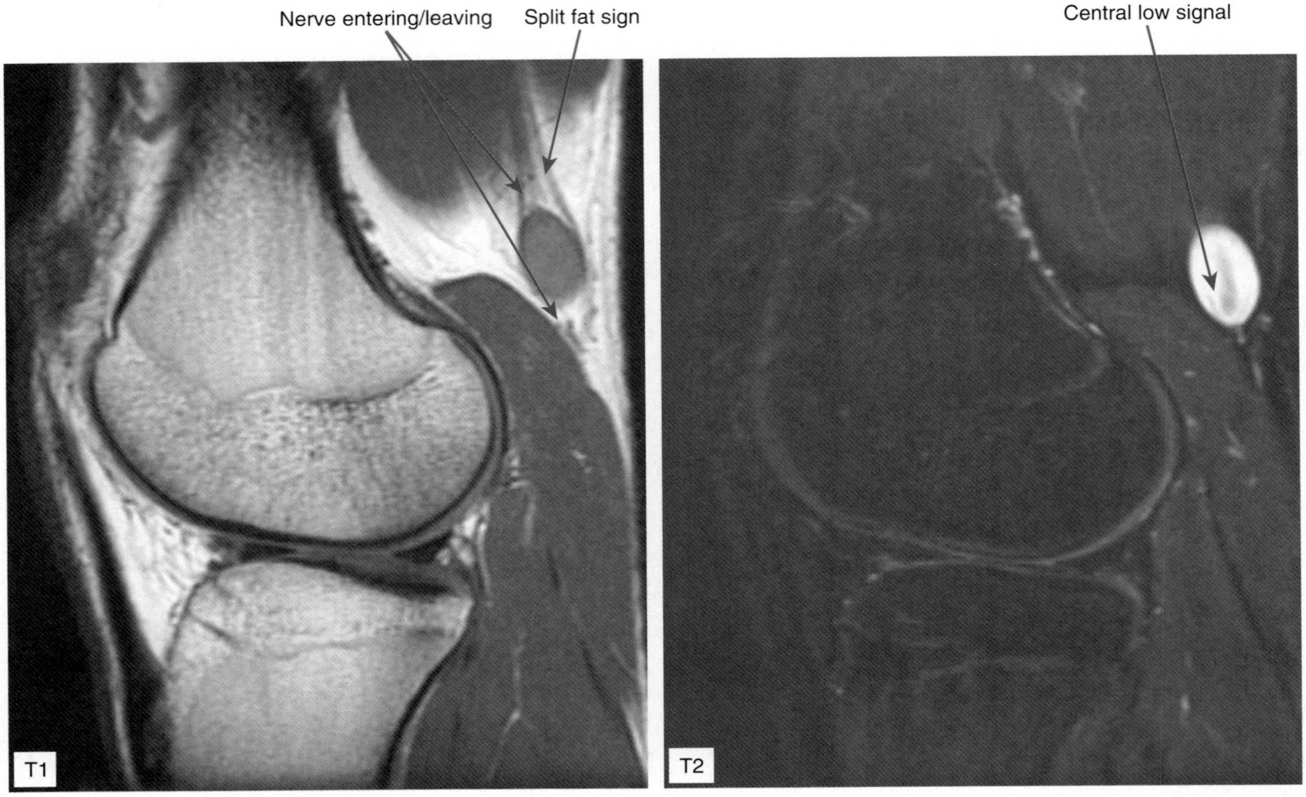
Nerve entering/leaving
Split fat sign
Central low signal
T1
T2

Figure 6-62 Nerve sheath tumor can be suggested based on location and imaging characteristics. An ovoid mass along the neurovascular bundle is suggestive but not pathognomonic. Visualization of a nerve entering and leaving, a target sign with a central low signal focus, as well as the split-fat sign with muscle fibers pushed away and leaving a tract of fat signal, is more specific. Differentiation of neurofibroma from schwannoma is difficult. The larger and more complex the lesion, the higher the risk of neurofibrosarcoma.

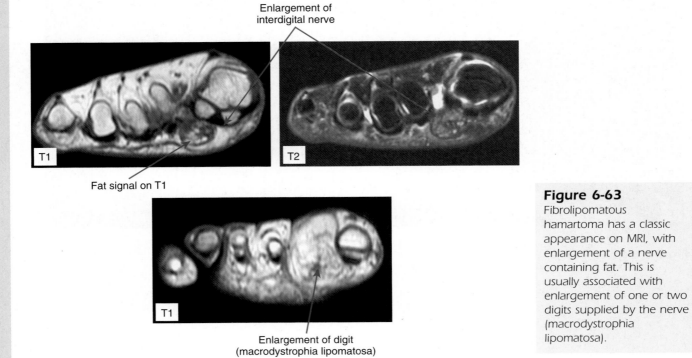

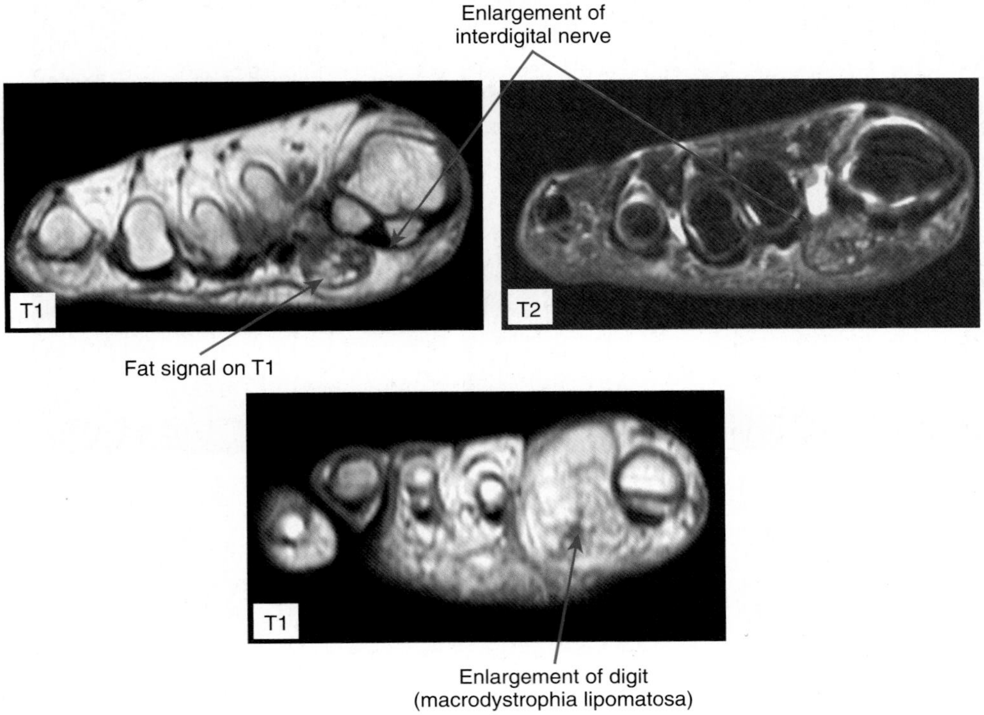
Enlargement of interdigital nerve
T1
T2
Fat signal on T1
T1
Enlargement of digit (macrodystrophia lipomatosa)

Figure 6-63 Fibrolipomatous hamartoma has a classic appearance on MRI, with enlargement of a nerve containing fat. This is usually associated with enlargement of one or two digits supplied by the nerve (macrodystrophia lipomatosa).

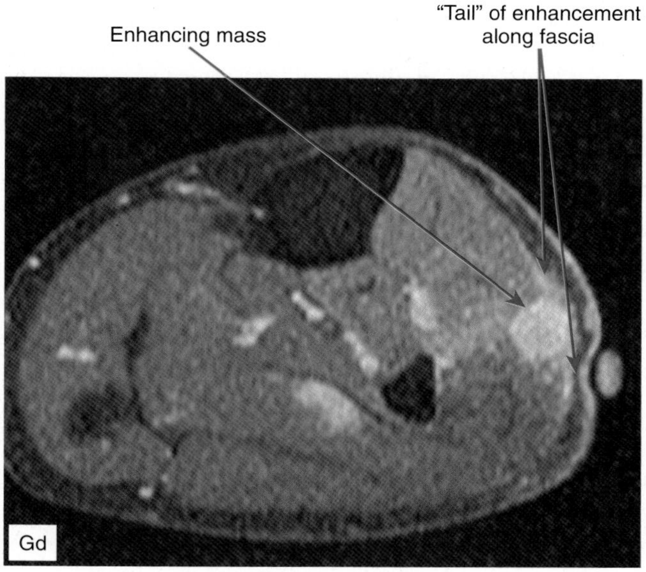
Enhancing mass
"Tail" of enhancement along fascia
Gd

Figure 6-64 Nodular fasciitis is an inflammatory, non-neoplastic condition. It is more common in the upper extremities and usually exhibits rapid onset of swelling. A mass (focal or ill defined) is seen on MRI, which may appear in the subcutaneous fat along the fascia or in muscle. One clue to the diagnosis can be a "tail" of enhancement along the fascia. Diagnosis can be suggested on MRI, but biopsy is generally required to exclude malignancy.

no fat plane separates the mass from these structures, this should be described.

Typically, unless there is some history that sheds additional light on the cause, biopsy is indicated. Intravenous contrast is useful to determine optimal areas for biopsy, since enhancing areas provide better yield. Nonenhancing areas can be cystic or myxoid components or may represent necrotic areas. If the biopsy is being acquired percutaneously, care must be taken to discuss the approach with the tumor surgeon who is performing the definitive surgery. If the lesion is a primary soft tissue malignancy, passage of the needle can contaminate a compartment that could have been used as a flap. Also, the surgeon generally requests that the biopsy tract or tracts be positioned along the line of the intended surgical incision.

Role of Contrast

Intravenous contrast rarely leads to narrowing of the differential in the case of soft tissue lesions. However, as above, it can be very useful for detecting myxoid or necrotic areas within a lesion. Dynamic contrast enhancement can also be useful for evaluation of the vascularity of a lesion.

Specific Tumor Types: Differential Diagnosis

Soft tissue malignancies of various histologies look similar on MRI. As previously mentioned, the radiologist generally need not be specific about the lesion type. However, an educated guess regarding histology can occasionally be made using age, location, and imaging features.

Age, Localization, and Imaging Features: Influence on Lesion Type Some tumors have a clear predilection for certain age groups:

Child: rhabdomyosarcoma
Adolescent /young adult: synovial sarcoma
Older adult: malignant fibrous histiocytoma

Other lesions have a tendency to occur in particular locations, such as the following:

- Retroperitoneum
  - Liposarcoma
  - Leiomyosarcoma
- Digits of hands and feet, nailbed
  - Glomus
  - Epidermoid inclusion
- Tendon
  - Giant cell tumor of tendon sheath (see Fig. 6-58)
  - Ganglion
  - Rheumatoid arthritis/gout/inflammatory arthropathy
- Neurovascular bundle
  - Nerve sheath tumor
- Foot
  - Plantar fascia
    - Plantar fibroma
  - Interdigital nerve
    - Morton neuroma
  - Malignancy
    - Synovial sarcoma
    - Clear cell sarcoma

Imaging appearance can often be a clue to the diagnosis:

- Calcification
  - Synovial sarcoma
  - Lipoma/liposarcoma
  - Angiomatous lesion
  - Soft tissue osteosarcoma/chondrosarcoma

SECTION III

High signal on T1: differential diagnosis—fat or blood (fat-suppressed MRI sequence can differentiate)
Low signal on T2: differential diagnosis—calcium, fibrous tissue, hemosiderin, air, metallic artifact (e.g., postoperative)

Associations of Soft Tissue Tumor/Tumor-like Conditions Some soft tissue tumors are associated with other conditions:

Mastectomy/lymph node dissection *and* lymphangiosarcoma (Fig. 6-65)
Fibrous dysplasia *and* myxoma (Mazabraud syndrome)
AIDS *and* Kaposi sarcoma
Macrodystrophia lipomatosa *and* fibrolipomatous hamartoma
Melorheostosis *and* vascular malformations
Multiple enchondromas *and* vascular malformations (Ollier disease)

MRI Signal Characteristics of Hemorrhagic Lesions Unlike in the central nervous system, blood in the musculoskeletal tissues does not follow a predictable time-specific course. Acute blood products may last for days or weeks, and acute and chronic blood products commonly coexist (Table 6-5).

Soft Tissue Metastases Lymph node involvement along the course of lymph drainage from a tumor-laden region may be seen with any malignancy. Metastases to extranodal soft tissues are uncommon, but can be seen with certain entities. For example, in

Table 6-5 MRI Signal of Blood at Different Stages

	Hgb	T1	T2
Hyperacute	Oxyhemoglobin	High	High
Acute	Deoxyhemoglobin	Low	Low
Subacute	Methemoglobin	High	Variable
Chronic	Hemosiderin	Low	Low

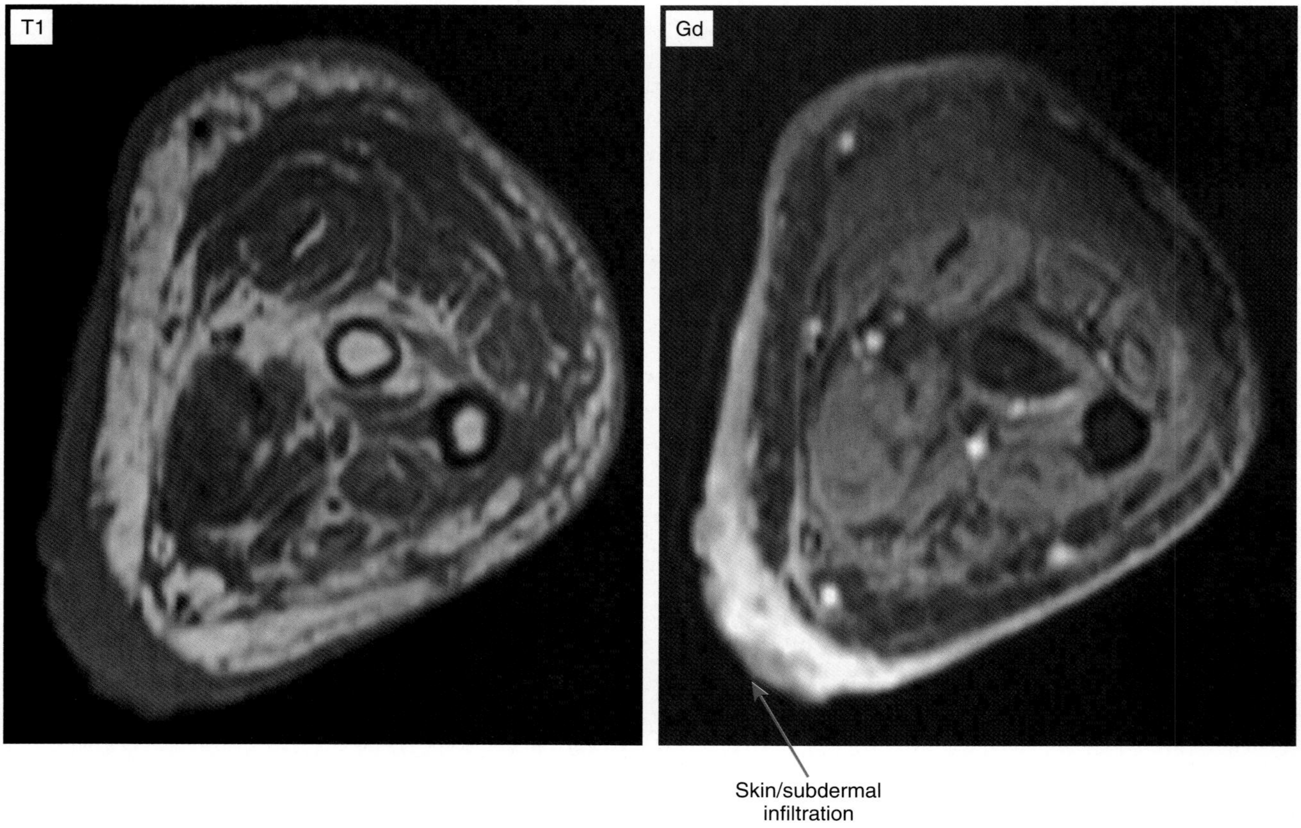
T1
Gd
Skin/subdermal infiltration

Figure 6-65 Infiltration of the skin and subdermal tissues in lymphangiosarcoma. Patient had a history of axillary lymph node dissection for breast cancer.

melanoma, metastases may have some hyperintensity on T1-weighted images owing to the paramagnetic properties of melanin (Fig. 6-66). In lymphoma, diffuse soft tissue infiltration simulating cellulitis may be seen. Various other aggressive malignancies may metastasize to soft tissues, but rarely. Multiplicity should raise concern for soft tissue metastatic disease.

Tumor Recurrence One challenge presented to radiologists is to evaluate MRI of a tumor that has been resected and/or treated with chemotherapy or radiation. It is important to acquire the baseline MRI, which should be performed a month or so after surgery—enough time for the surgical edema to diminish, but too soon for the tumor to return. It is also helpful to review the pretreatment MRI to see what the original tumor looked like. Was it discrete? Was it infiltrative? How extensive was it? Did it involve muscle/neurovascular bundle/bone? If no baseline was acquired, assessment may be difficult. If there is no edema, enhancement, or mass effect in the surgical bed or regional soft tissues, recurrence is unlikely, and routine surveillance should continue. Usually follow-up examinations are performed every 6 months for a few years to ensure stability.

Edema and/or enhancement alone do not necessarily constitute a sign of recurrence if the finding is not masslike, because the effects of treatment—such as surgical scarring and radiation therapy—can result in edema and enhancement. However, this finding is expected to progressively diminish or remain stable on subsequent follow-up examinations. If edema or enhancement increases, there may be cause for concern.

Signs of prior radiation therapy include regional muscle atrophy, muscle and subcutaneous edema, and fat replacement of bone marrow within the radiation port. Fatty atrophy of muscle and fat replacement of the bone marrow is likely to be permanent, and the soft tissue edema can persist for years. Scar tissue can result in focal enhancement, but scarring is associated with a lack of mass effect and often with cicatrization (fascial tenting toward the finding). Mass effect with enhancement should suggest recurrence (Figs. 6-67 and Fig. 6-68). However, mass effect may also be seen with a seroma, a walled-off postoperative fluid collection. Seromas generally only have thin rim enhancement and appear shortly after surgery on the baseline examination (Fig. 6-69). A neuroma also may occur after amputation (Fig. 6-70). However, this can be correctly identified because it follows the nerve distribution. PET scanning can also be useful for monitoring patients for tumor recurrence and differentiation from scar tissue (Fig. 6-71).

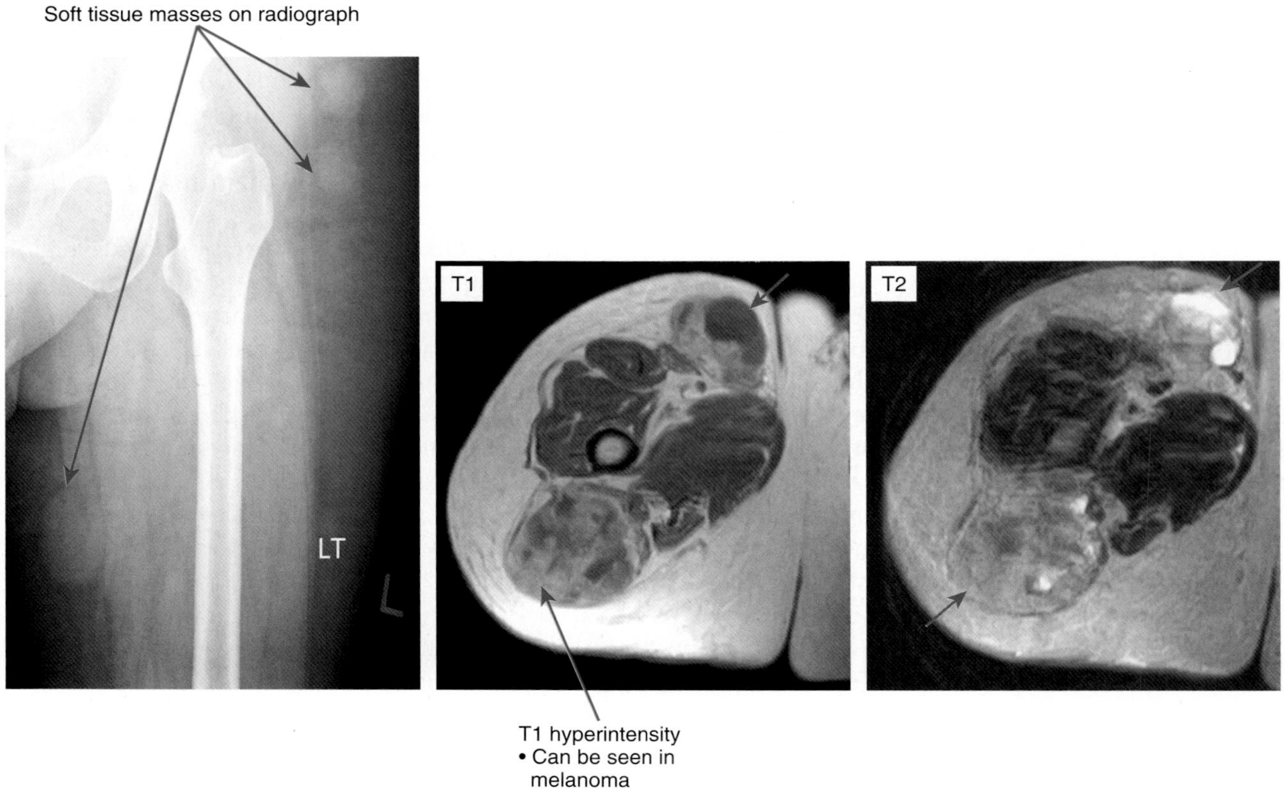
Soft tissue masses on radiograph
LT
T1
T2
T1 hyperintensity
• Can be seen in melanoma

Figure 6-66 Melanoma may metastasize to soft tissues. Other tumors can metastasize to soft tissues but much more rarely. Melanoma can exhibit some T1 hyperintensity, simulating hemorrhage or fat.

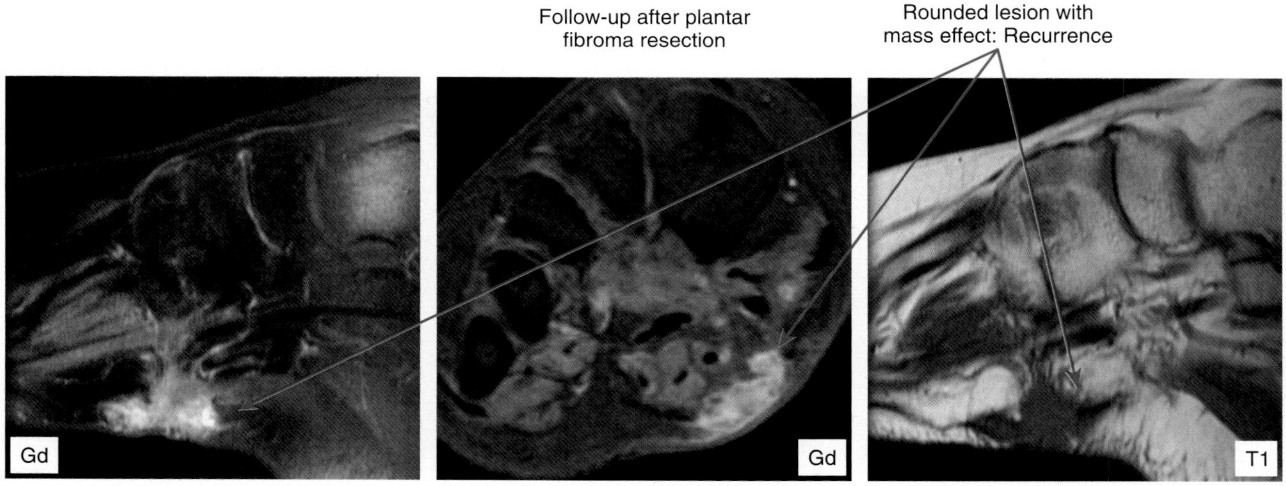
Follow-up after plantar fibroma resection
Rounded lesion with mass effect: Recurrence
Gd
Gd
T1

Figure 6-67 **Plantar fibroma recurrence.** After a tumor is treated, a baseline MRI is very useful for comparison with subsequent surveillance examinations. Scar tissue enhances but is flat and shows no mass effect, often with cicatrization (negative mass effect). Recurrence is signified by a rounded appearance with mass effect on adjacent structures and increase in prominence over time.

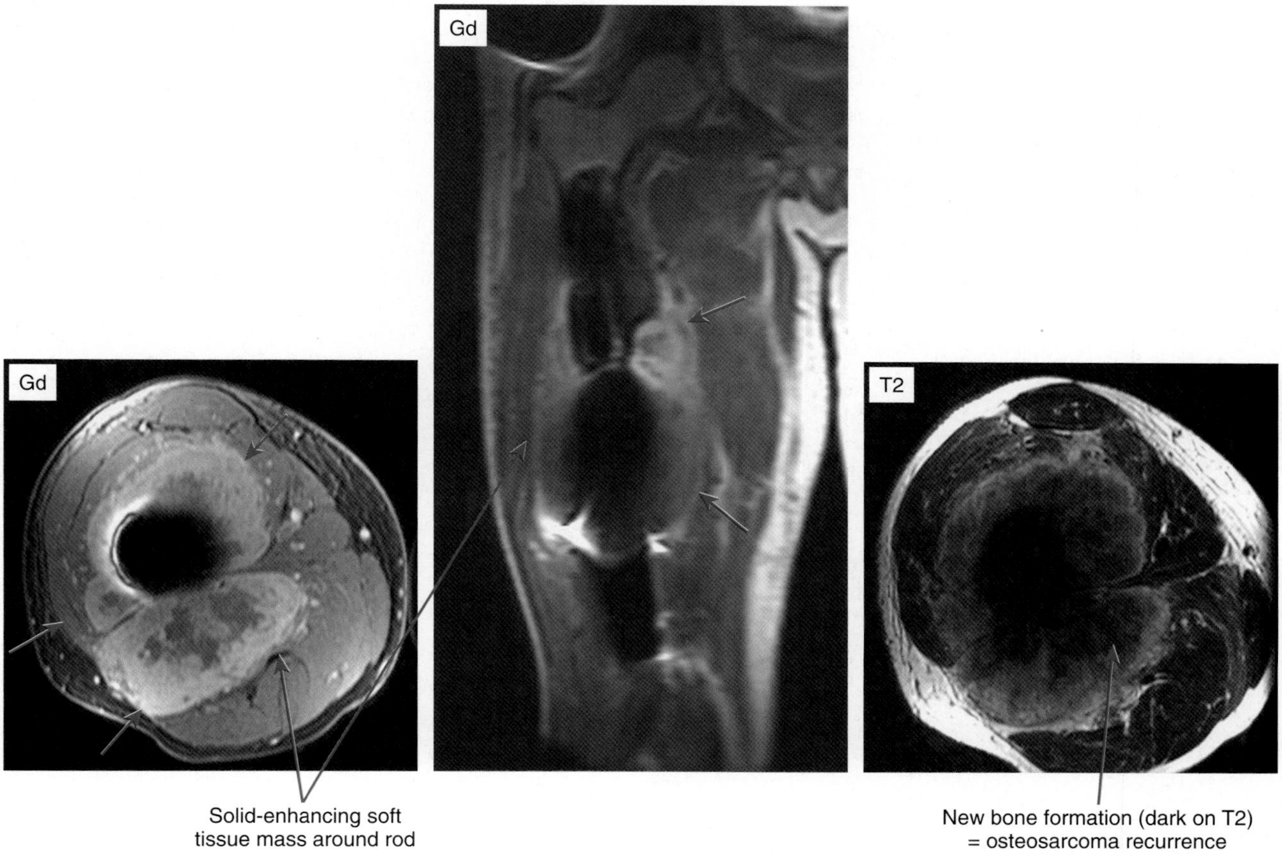
Gd
Gd
T2
Solid-enhancing soft tissue mass around rod
New bone formation (dark on T2) = osteosarcoma recurrence

Figure 6-68 Recurrent osteosarcoma in limb-salvage surgery. Following limb-salvage surgery for malignancy, surveillance is essential to detect early recurrence. Modality used for surveillance depends on a number of factors including the modality used for baseline imaging (it is useful to compare), the presence of metal (may reduce effectiveness of MRI), the body part, and the characteristics of the tumor. For example, for osteosarcoma, radiographs or CT may be useful to detect small calcifications representing new bone formation in a recurrence.

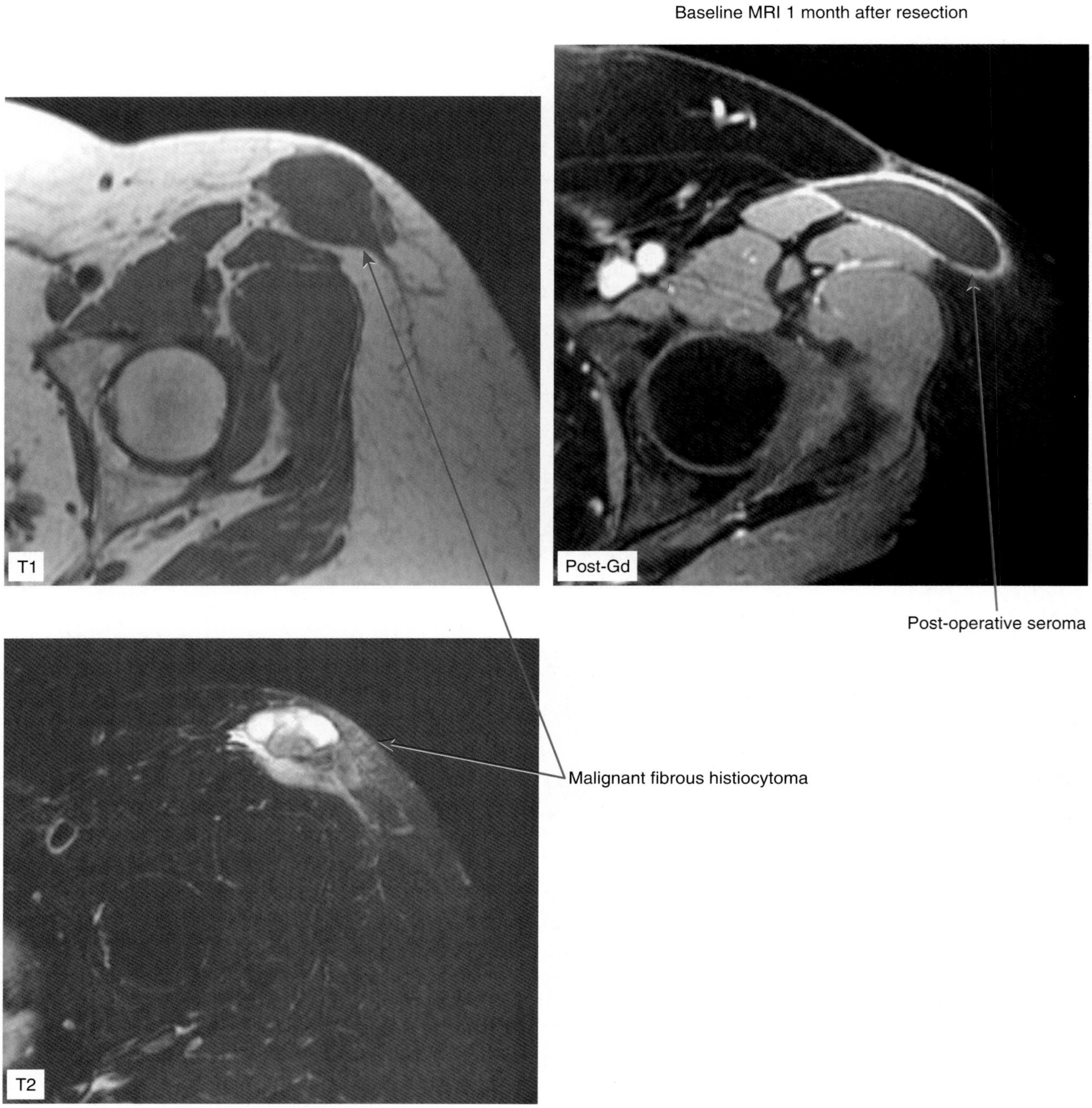
Baseline MRI 1 month after resection
T1
Post-Gd
Post-operative seroma
T2
Malignant fibrous histiocytoma

Figure 6-69 Example of a baseline MRI examination 1 month after resection of malignant fibrous histiocytoma, showing a seroma with thin rim enhancement. Any increase in size, nodularity, or solid enhancing areas should be considered suspicious for recurrence.

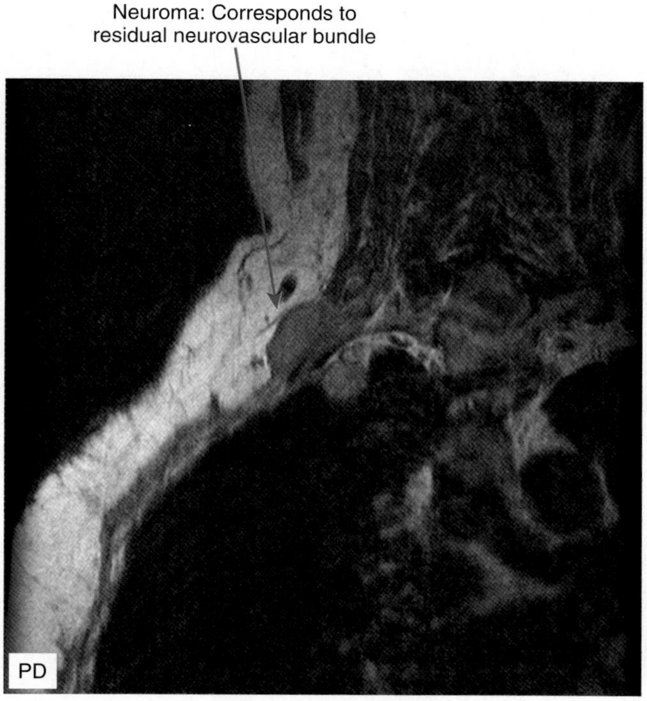
Neuroma: Corresponds to
residual neurovascular bundle
PD

Figure 6-70 **Postamputation neuroma.** Not all masses following tumor resection represent recurrence. Seromas can persist in the surgical bed but generally do not enlarge on follow-up. Neuromas can arise at the end of resected nerves, as in this case of a follow-up examination after four-quarter amputation for malignancy. (Courtesy of Douglas Mintz, MD, New York.)

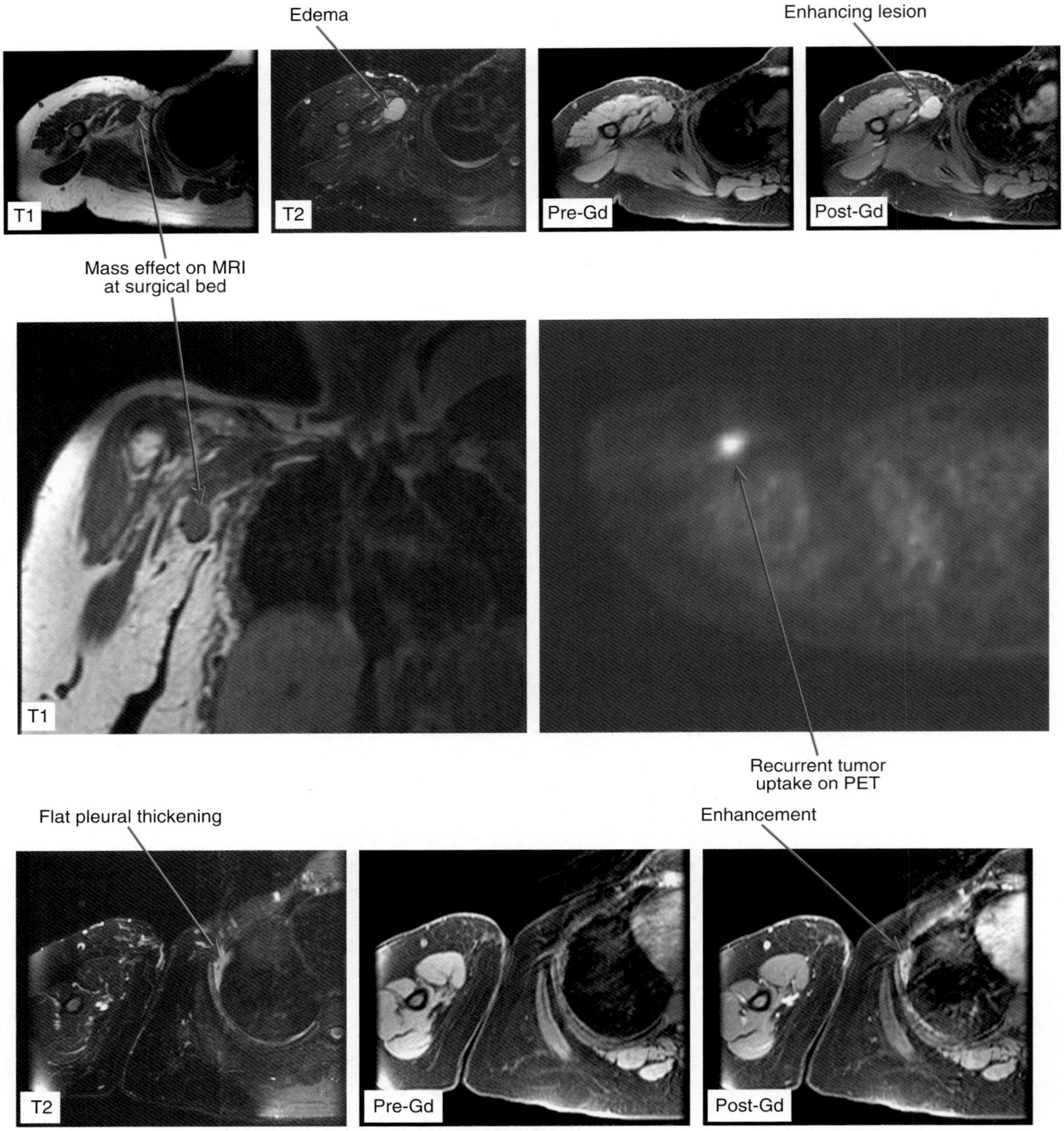
Edema
Enhancing lesion
T1
T2
Pre-Gd
Post-Gd
Mass effect on MRI at surgical bed
T1
Recurrent tumor uptake on PET
Flat pleural thickening
Enhancement
T2
Pre-Gd
Post-Gd

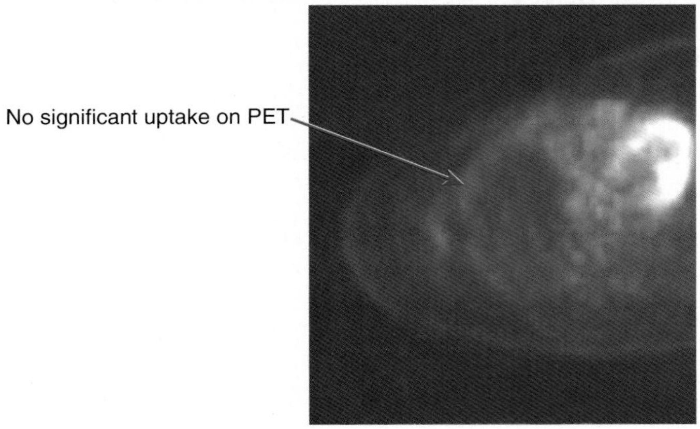
No significant uptake on PET

Figure 6-71 Usefulness of positron-emission tomography (PET) for differentiation of recurrent tumor from scar. This patient had a history of breast carcinoma in her 20s. Follow-up MRI and PET now show axillary radiation-induced sarcoma with standardized uptake value (SUV) over 2.0 on PET. More inferiorly, pleural scar enhances on MRI but is negative on PET. For follow-up tumor PET imaging, the generally agreed-upon cutoff is an SUV greater than 2.0, although there is significant overlap of benign and malignant postoperative tissue. For primary musculoskeletal soft tissue tumors, PET is not routinely used because there is broad overlap in SUV, based on degree of aggressiveness and metabolic activity.

SECTION IV

PROBLEM SOLVING: Anatomic Regions

Chapter 7

IMAGING OF THE SHOULDER

CHAPTER OUTLINE

The shoulder girdle is a complex anatomic unit that is designed to maximize the position on the hand and opposing thumb in three-dimensional space. The shoulder is often thought of as synonymous with the glenohumeral joint, but is actually composed of four separate joints (sternoclavicular, scapulothoracic, acromioclavicular, and the glenohumeral). These four joints work synergistically with numerous muscles and ligaments to optimize motion of the upper extremity and to balance range of motion and stability. Shoulder pain is a very common complaint and is most often seen in association with acute trauma or repetitive overuse. Recent advances in cross-sectional imaging, including CT and MRI, have revolutionized the evaluation of the shoulder, particularly with regard to the soft tissue structures. Conventional radiography, however, remains a mainstay of imaging and is often the first examination ordered for a patient with complaints of shoulder pain.

MODALITIES

Radiography

Radiographs are often the first imaging study obtained in the patient presenting with the chief complaint of shoulder pain. The complex anatomy of the shoulder girdle has led to the development of numerous radiographic views, each designed to optimize the evaluation of a specific part of the shoulder girdle. Familiarity with the standard views as well as the specialized projections aid in optimizing the radiographic evaluation of the shoulder based on the clinical presentation and suspected abnormality.

The standard anteroposterior (AP) view is obtained in an anteroposterior direction relative to the body rather than the glenohumeral joint, which is tilted anteriorly 40 degrees in relation to the body, and, as a result, this view shows overlap of the humeral head and the glenoid rim. This view can be obtained in neutral, internal or external rotation and provides the best overall survey of the shoulder girdle. The glenohumeral "true" anteroposterior (Grashey) view is obtained by rotating the patient 35 to 40 degrees posteriorly so that the plane of the beam is directed parallel to the glenohumeral joint rather than the body, thus eliminating the overlap of the glenohumeral joint. This view is particularly helpful for evaluation of glenohumeral joint space and demonstrates loss of articular cartilage and subtle subluxation indicating possible glenohumeral instability.

The axial view provides a lateral view of the glenohumeral joint and is helpful in the evaluation of possible dislocation of the glenohumeral joint, but it requires the patient to abduct the arm, which can be difficult after acute trauma. The scapula "Y" view, on the other hand, provides a lateral view of the glenohumeral joint and can be obtained with the arm down by the side requiring no movement of the upper extremity and is thus more useful in the setting of acute trauma.

Numerous variations of the axillary view have been developed to minimize movement of the arm or to optimize visualization of a particular portion of the glenohumeral joint. One such projection, the *West Point View,* is obtained by placing the patient in the prone position with the arm abducted 90 degrees from the long axis of the body with the elbow and forearm hanging off the side of the table. This view was developed to optimize detection of a Bankart fracture of the anterior glenoid rim and is frequently requested by orthopedic surgeons in patients who have experienced anterior dislocation of the glenohumeral joint. Specialized views are also available to evaluate the scapula, the acromioclavicular joint, and the sternoclavicular joints.

Computed Tomography

Computed tomography (CT) is most commonly used after trauma to the shoulder to evaluate the full extent of osseous abnormalities. Multidetector CT examination with sagittal and coronal reconstructions is often used to evaluate the extent of humeral head and neck fractures. The precise number of fracture fragments, the amount of articular surface step-off, displacement, and the angulation of fracture fragments can accurately be determined with CT examination. Each of these variables is important in relation to the treatment choice and in determining the prognosis for recovery. CT examination is also the study of choice in suspected sternoclavicular joint injuries and accurately depicts subtle fractures and dislocations. The scapula is a complex anatomic structure composed of the body, coracoid and acromion processes, and the glenohumeral articular surface. Suspected scapular fractures are typically evaluated with CT examination, which shows the full extent of injury. Fractures limited to the body of the scapula are usually treated conservatively, whereas fractures of the coracoid or acromion processes or the glenohumeral articular surface may require surgical intervention. After glenohumeral dislocation, CT examination is the study of choice to show the size and position of a glenoid rim fracture fragment, which is important in presurgical planning.

Ultrasound

For musculoskeletal imaging, ultrasound is most extensively studied and more frequently used in the evaluation of the shoulder than of any other joint. Ultrasound accurately depicts rotator cuff pathology and in experienced hands can accurately detect and differentiate a normal cuff from tendinosis, partial- or full-thickness tear. Ultrasound can also be used to dynamically assess for tendon or muscle pathology. The major disadvantages of ultrasound, however, include its limited field of view and its inability to assess the deep soft tissue structures and bones. Ultrasound provides only a very limited evaluation of labrum and articular surfaces. Finally, if the physician assessing the patient did not personally perform the study, it may be difficult to determine whether a complete evaluation has been accomplished.

Magnetic Resonance Imaging

Magnetic resonance imaging (MRI) is particularly well suited for evaluation of the glenohumeral joint, and in most instances it is the study of choice when complex cross-sectional imaging is required. It accurately depicts abnormalities of the rotator cuff and can demonstrate very subtle abnormalities of the capsule and labrum that are associated with glenohumeral instability. The use of intravenous or intra-articular gadolinium often increases the conspicuity of these subtle labral lesions. The osseous structures are nicely depicted, including osseous Bankart and Hill-Sachs lesions.

Imaging protocols vary based on the field strength of the magnet and on personal preferences. However, standard shoulder imaging protocols typically include T2-weighted sequences with fat saturation in the oblique sagittal, oblique coronal, and axial imaging planes. Proton density or gradient-echo axial sequences are also often performed in the axial imaging plane. Finally, T1-weighted images are obtained in the oblique coronal and oblique sagittal imaging planes to aid in the evaluation of marrow abnormalities and to evaluate for fatty atrophy of the cuff musculature. If either intravenous or intra-articular gadolinium is administered, then the T1-weighted sequences are performed with fat saturation to increase conspicuity of enhancing structures.

IMPINGEMENT: ROLE OF OSSEOUS OUTLET AND ACROMION

Painful impingement of the shoulder is a clinical entity that results from compression of the rotator cuff and subacromial-subdeltoid bursa between the greater tuberosity of the humeral head and the protective overriding osseous outlet and acromion. Clinical impingement includes symptomatic subacromial-subdeltoid bursitis and tendinopathy resulting from the compressive forces of the adjacent osseous structures. Over time, this process may lead to a partial- or full-thickness tear of the cuff. The diagnosis of impingement cannot be established on the basis of imaging findings alone, but rather on the basis of the physical examination, which elicits pain during abduction and elevation of the arm. Certain anatomic configurations or abnormalities of the osseous outlet and acromion may result in mass effect on the underlying soft tissue structures during abduction and elevation of the arm, thus placing an individual at an increased risk for developing the clinical syndrome of impingement. This has been referred to as *extrinsic impingement.* Alternatively, impingement may result from glenohumeral instability, which allows subtle subluxation of the humeral head during overhead activities, thus leading to compression of the cuff and bursa. This form of impingement is *internal impingement.*

To be successful, surgical management must not only repair the injured soft tissue structures (cuff repair and debridement of the bursa), but also address the underlying cause of impingement (osseous outlet morphology or glenohumeral instability). It is important to understand the specific osseous configurations associated with impingement and to accurately describe them on each shoulder MR examination to ensure that the surgeon correctly addresses the underlying cause of impingement.

Numerous radiographic and MR findings have been described that are associated with the clinical syndrome of impingement. The acromion, the acromioclavicular (AC) joint, and the coracoacromial ligament should be thoroughly evaluated for these

Table 7-1 MR Evaluation of the Osseous Outlet and Acromion

Anatomic Part	Abnormality	Preferred MR Imaging Plane
Acromion	Type or configuration of undersurface (Types I, II, III, IV)	Sagittal; 1–2 images peripheral to AC joint
	Anterior down-sloping	Sagittal
	Lateral down-sloping	Coronal
	Enthesiophyte formation	Sagittal/coronal
	Os acromiale "double AC joint" sign	Axial—primary Sagittal/coronal—secondary
Acromioclavicular (AC) joint	Osteoarthritis (mass effect on underlying cuff)	Coronal/sagittal
	AC joint separation (grades I, II, III)	Coronal
	Osteolysis of distal clavicle	Coronal
Coracoacromial ligament	Thickening	Sagittal
	Calcification	Sagittal

specific configurations, anatomic variants, and abnormalities (Table 7-1).

Acromion

The anterolateral aspect of the acromion plays the most crucial role in extrinsic compression of the rotator cuff; therefore, any acromial configuration that narrows the subacromial space anterolaterally places a person at risk for the clinical syndrome of impingement. Five aspects of the acromial shape and morphology should be evaluated on each shoulder MR examination.

1. The morphology of the undersurface of the acromion should be described as follows: a type I acromion demonstrates a flat undersurface; type II acromion, a gentle undersurface curvature; type III acromion, an anterior hook; and type IV acromion, a convex undersurface (Fig. 7-1). Acromial types II and III are associated with an increased risk of impingement, and this association was first demonstrated using the scapular Y radiograph (Fig. 7-2). To accurately type the undersurface of the acromion on MRI, evaluate the first or second image lateral to the AC joint on the oblique sagittal imaging plane (Fig. 7-3). The major pitfall with regard to typing the acromion on MRI is the use of the incorrect image or imaging plane. Evaluation of the acromion on a sagittal image that is too far central or peripheral or use of the coronal imaging plane results in an inaccurate typing of the acromion. Currently, there is decreased emphasis in the orthopedic community on the role of acromial morphology (acromial type) with regard to the clinical syndrome of impingement. The other acromial variations listed in the following text are thought to play a more significant role with regard to impingement.

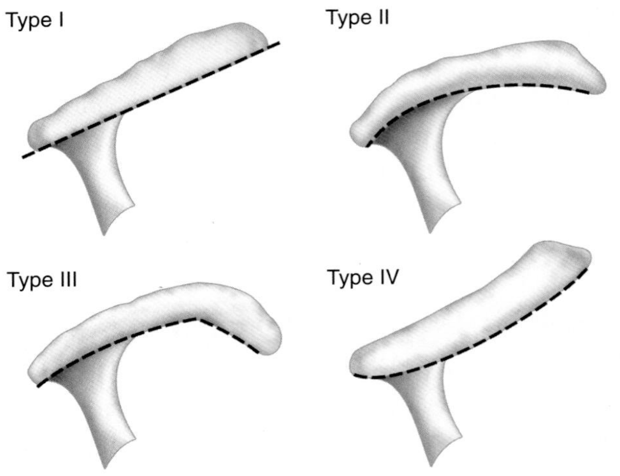
Type I
Type II
Type III
Type IV

Figure 7-1 Acromial configuration. The acromial type is determined by the configuration of the undersurface of the acromion. Acromial types II (gentle undersurface curvature) and III (anterior hook) place an individual at an increased risk for the clinical syndrome of impingement.

2. Anterior down-sloping (Fig. 7-4). Anterior tilt (down-sloping) of the scapula is associated with kyphosis and can result in narrowing of the clinical syndrome of impingement.

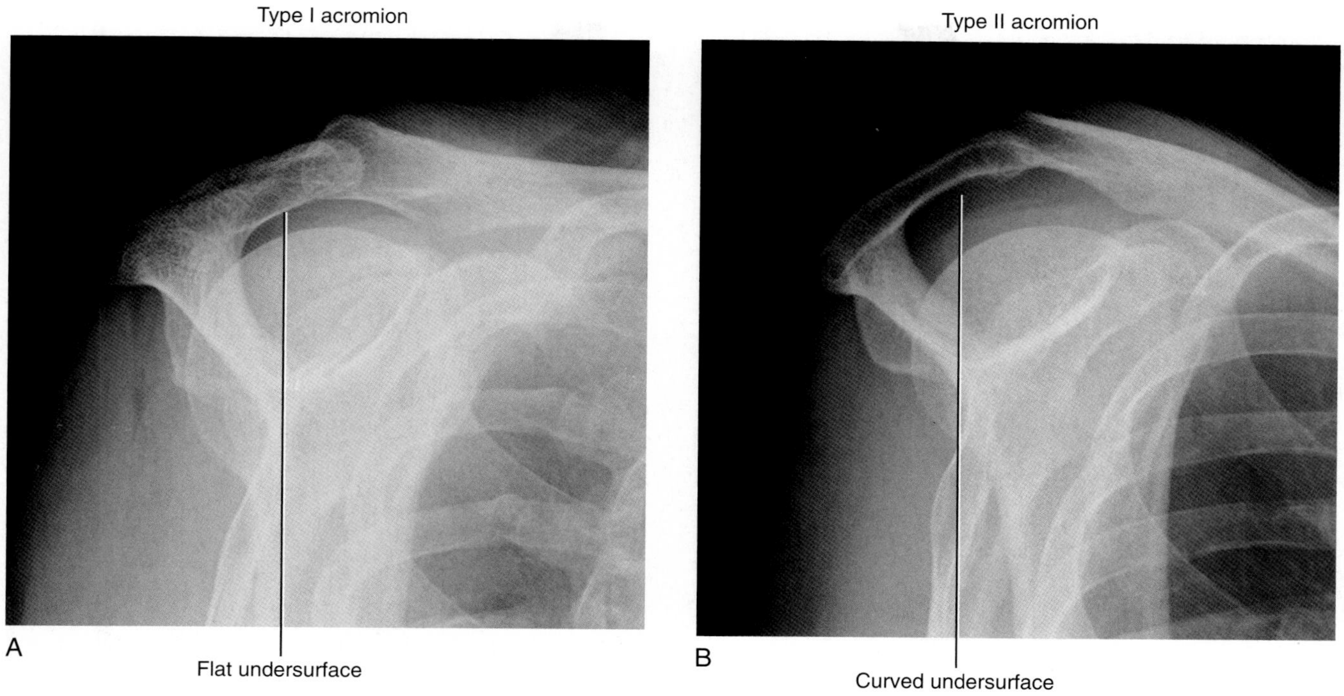
Type I acromion
Type II acromion
A
Flat undersurface
B
Curved undersurface

Figure 7-2 Acromial typing using radiography. *A,* Type I acromion. Scapular Y view of the shoulder demonstrates the undersurface of the acromion to be flat. ***B,*** Type II acromion. Scapular Y view of the shoulder demonstrates a curved undersurface of the acromion.

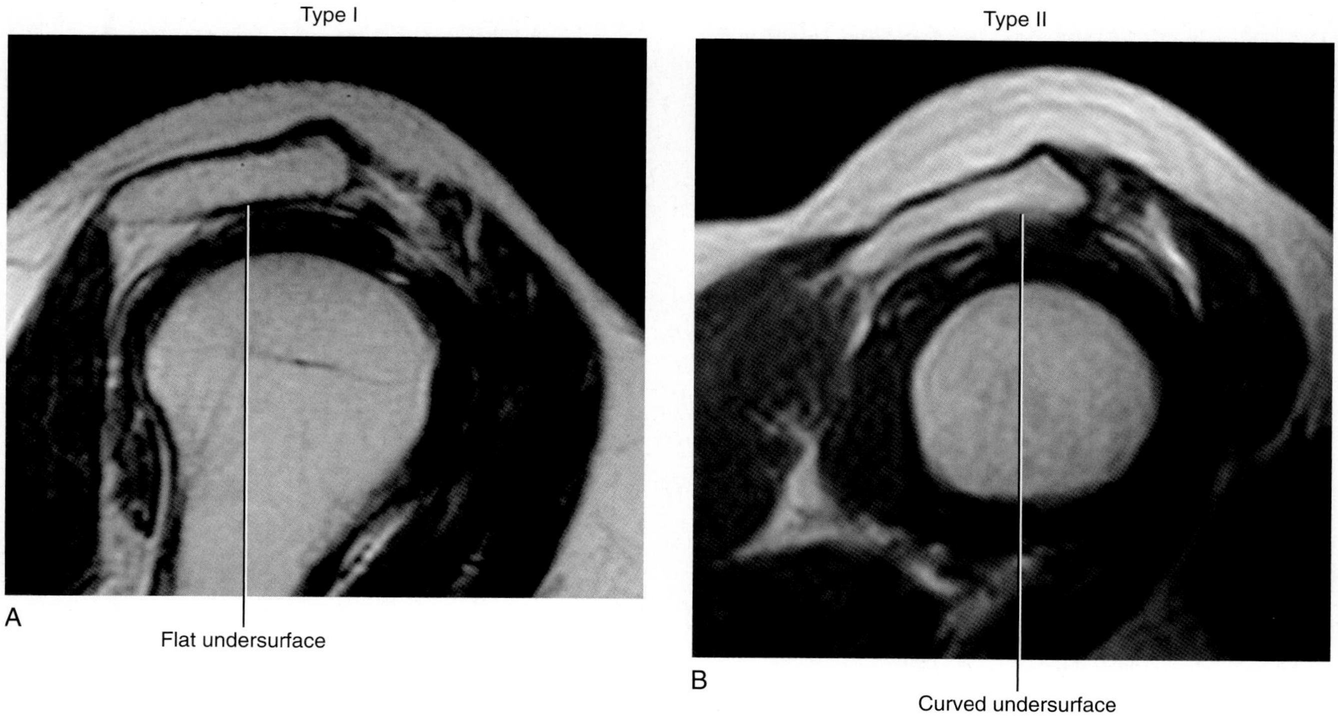
Type I
Type II
A
Flat undersurface
B
Curved undersurface

Figure 7-3 Acromial typing using MRI. *A,* Type I acromion, flat undersurface. ***B,*** Type II acromion, curved undersurface.

Continued

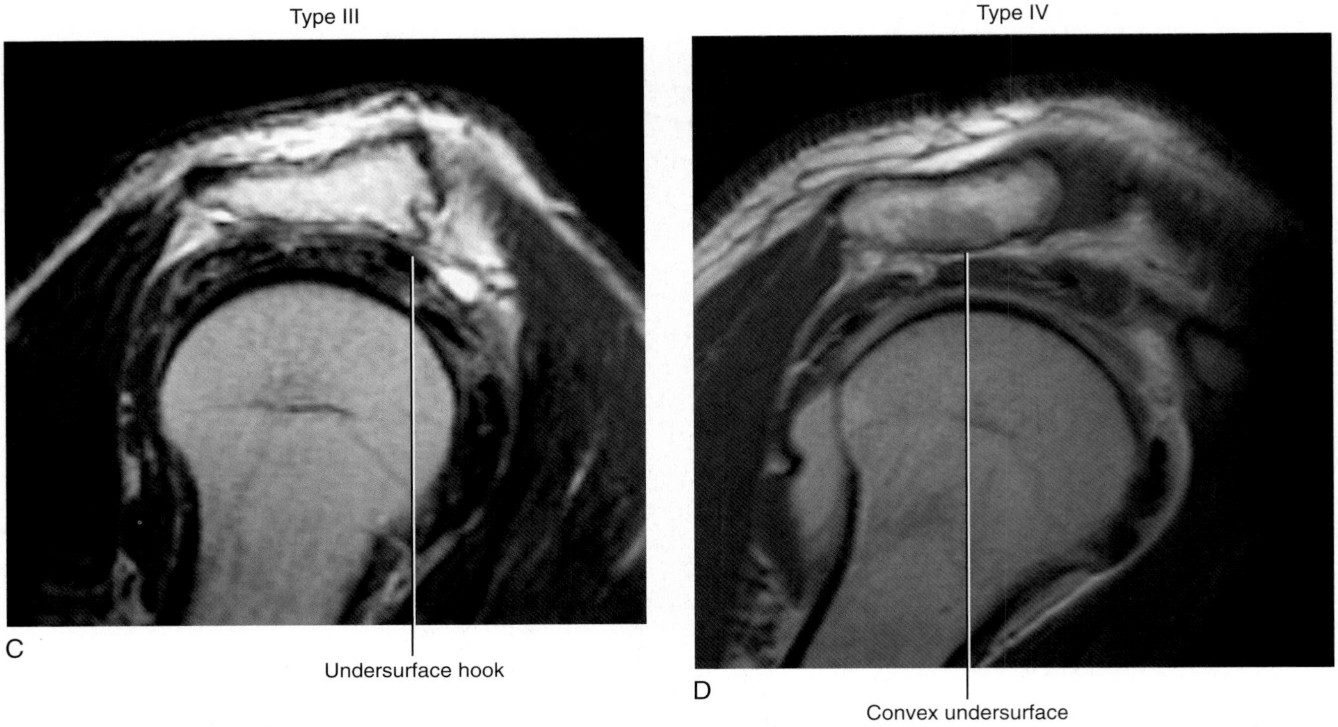
Type III
Type IV
C
Undersurface hook
D
Convex undersurface

Figure 7-3, cont'd **C,** Type III acromion, hooked acromion. **D,** Type IV acromion, convex undersurface.

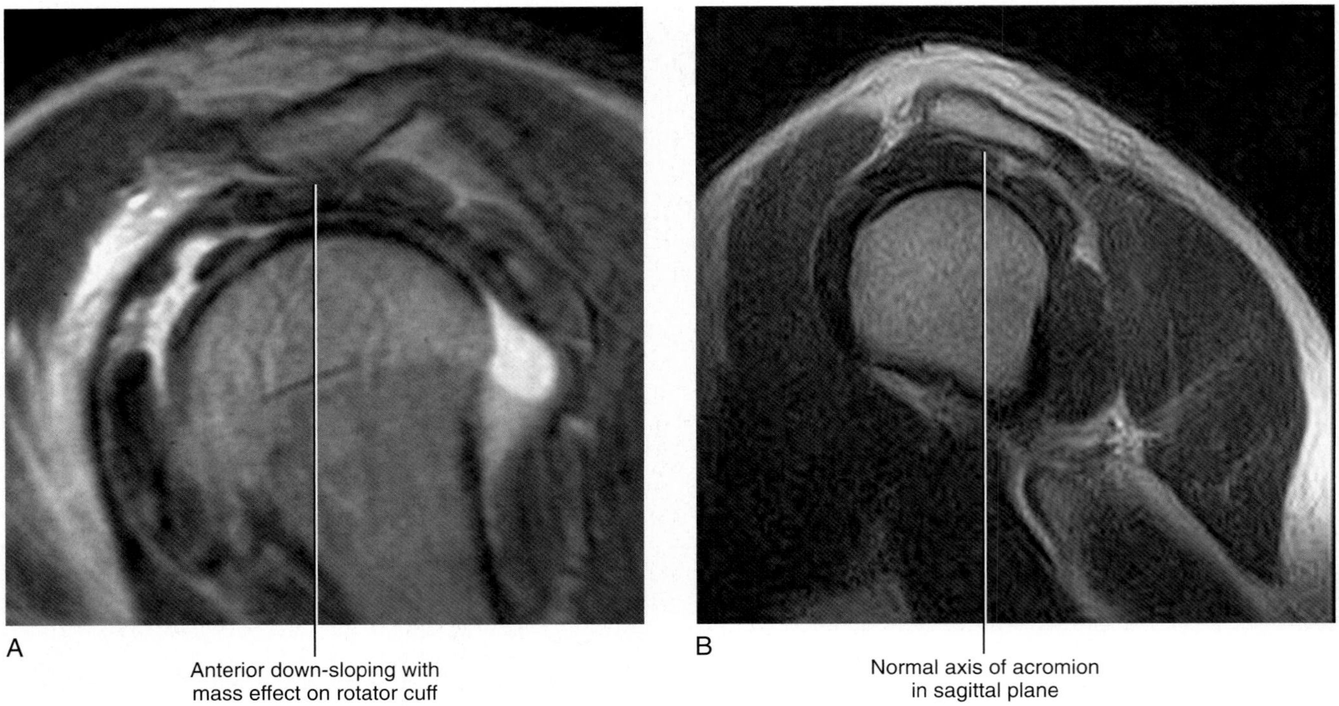
A
Anterior down-sloping with mass effect on rotator cuff
B
Normal axis of acromion in sagittal plane

Figure 7-4 **Anterior down-sloping of the acromion. A,** Anterior down-sloping narrows the acromial-humeral distance and can be a cause of rotator cuff impingement. Evaluation for anterior down-sloping is performed using the sagittal MRI plane. Anterior down-sloping describes the axis of the acromion in the sagittal plane and is independent of the configuration of the undersurface of the acromion as described in Figures 7-1 and 7-2. **B,** Normal acromial axis in the sagittal imaging plane.

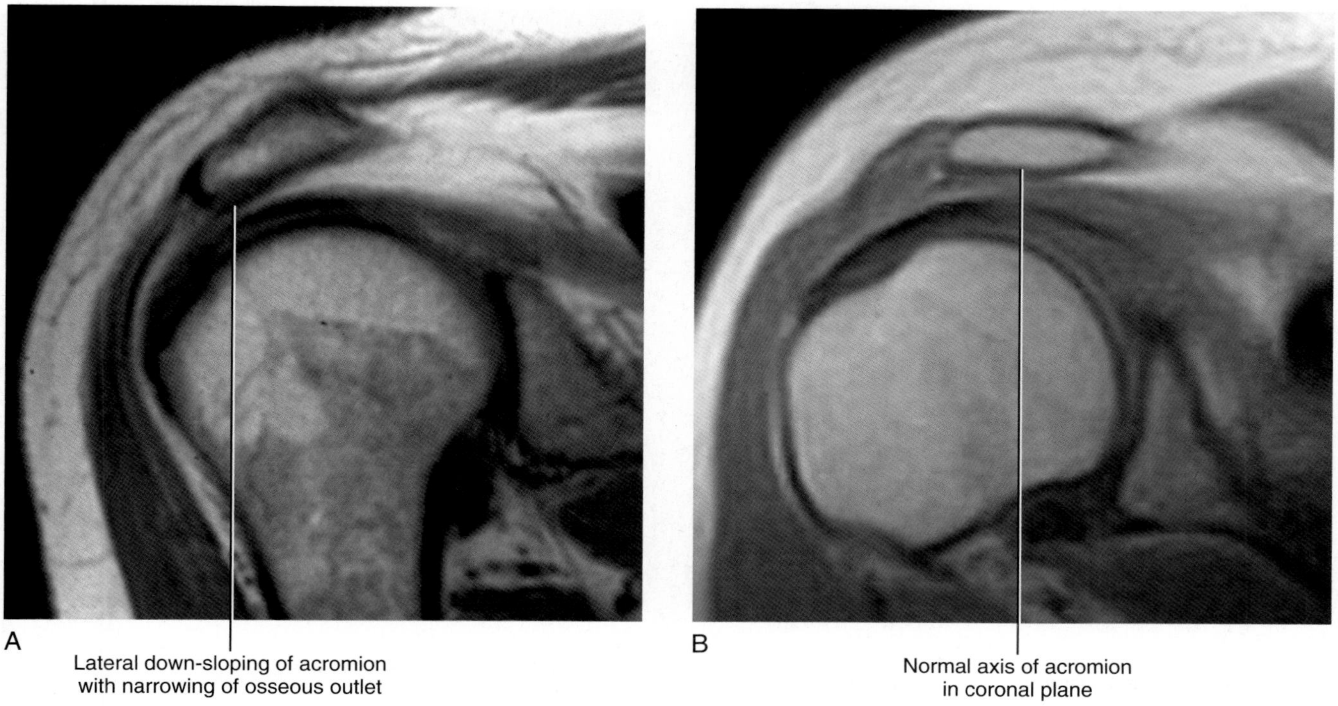
A
Lateral down-sloping of acromion
with narrowing of osseous outlet
B
Normal axis of acromion
in coronal plane

Figure 7-5 Lateral down-sloping of the acromion. A, Lateral down-sloping narrows the acromial-humeral distance and can be a cause of impingement. Evaluation for lateral down-sloping is performed using the coronal imaging plane. Lateral down-sloping of the acromion describes the axis of the acromion in the coronal plane and is independent of the configuration of the undersurface of the acromion. **B,** Normal acromial axis in the coronal imaging plane.

3. Lateral down-sloping (Fig. 7-5).
4. Spur formation off of the undersurface of the acromion (Fig. 7-6A). The deltoid tendon slip attaches to the lateral aspect of the acromion. A common pitfall is to misinterpret the deltoid tendon slip as an acromial spur on MRI. The two can be easily differentiated because the deltoid tendon slip (Fig. 7-6B) appears dark on all pulse sequences, whereas a spur contains fatty marrow elements and demonstrates fat signal intensity on all pulse sequences (bright on T1).
5. Unfused os acromiale (Fig. 7-7).

The acromion develops from several separate ossification centers, which typically fuse by 22 to 25 years of age. Failure of one of these ossification centers to fuse can lead to an unstable os acromiale with osteophytic lipping at the level of the synchondrosis. An unstable, unfused ossification center can act as a fulcrum or hinge and can displace in a downward direction during contraction of the deltoid muscle, narrowing the subacromial distance and leading to impingement of the rotator cuff. Failure to recognize and address an unfused os acromiale at the time of subacromial decompression and rotator cuff repair is a known cause of failed cuff repair. Arthroscopic removal of small fragments (less than 4 mm) is recommended because it does not disrupt the attachment of the deltoid muscle or alter its function. Larger fragments are surgically fused rather than resected to prevent weakness of the shoulder during abduction.

The MR appearance of an unfused os acromiale is variable depending on which ossification center fails to fuse. The unfused os acromiale is best depicted on axial images (Fig. 7-8). However, the most superior axial image obtained on MRI of the shoulder often begins below the level of the acromion; as a result, if one relies solely on the axial images, an unfused os acromiale may be overlooked. Therefore, the oblique sagittal and oblique coronal images should also be evaluated for an unfused os acromiale. An unfused

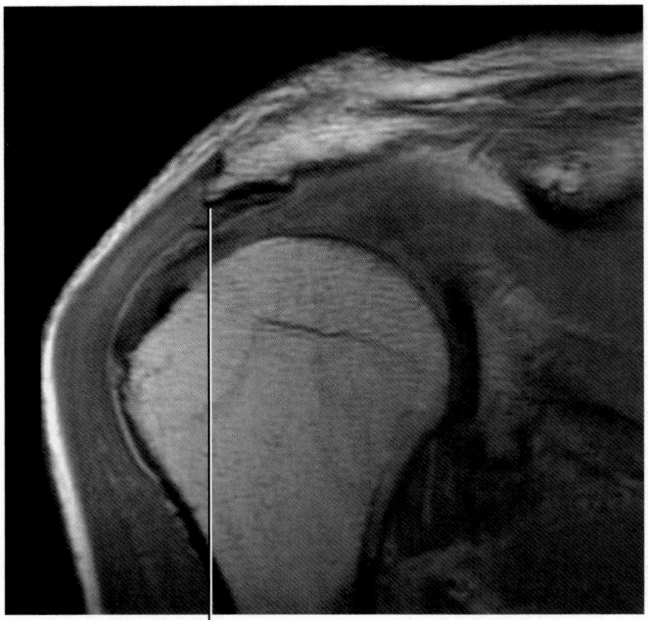
A
Marrow signal within
acromial enthesiophyte

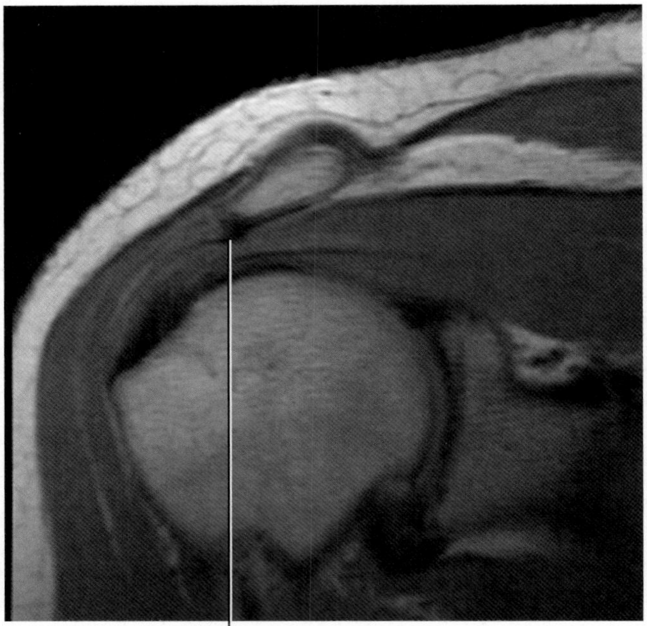
B
Deltoid tendon slip mimicking a spur;
notice the lack of marrow signal

Figure 7-6 Acromial enthesiophyte. A, Coronal T1-weighted image demonstrates an enthesiophyte extending off of the undersurface of the lateral aspect of the acromion, which can be a source of impingement. Note that an enthesiophyte contains fatty marrow elements and follows marrow signal intensity on MRI. **B,** The Deltoid tendon slip can mimic an acromial enthesiophyte on MRI, but can be easily differentiated from an enthesiophyte because it contains no marrow elements and appears dark on all pulse sequences.

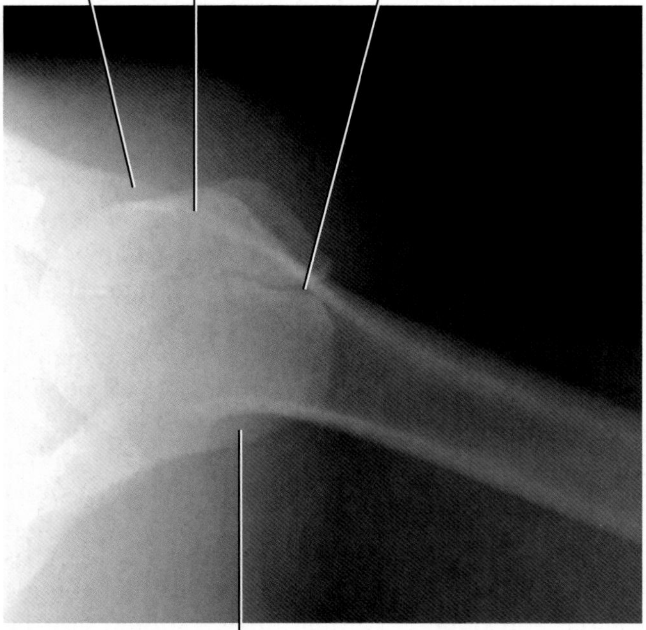
Distal
clavicle
AC joint
Synchondrosis of
the unfused os acromiale
A
Posterior acromion

Figure 7-7 Os acromiale. Unfused os acromiale on axillary view radiograph (**A**) axial CT slice (**B**). The synchondrosis of the unfused os acromiale is best seen on axial images and is depicted as a linear lucency extending across the short axis of the acromion. Sclerosis is often seen on both sides of the unfused synchondrosis. AC, acromioclavicular.

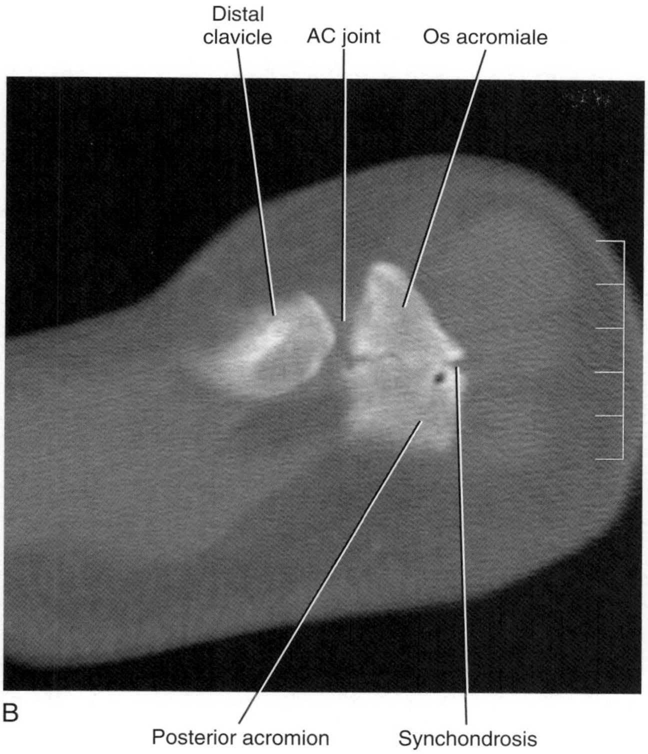
Distal clavicle
AC joint
Os acromiale
B
Posterior acromion
Synchondrosis

Figure 7-7, cont'd

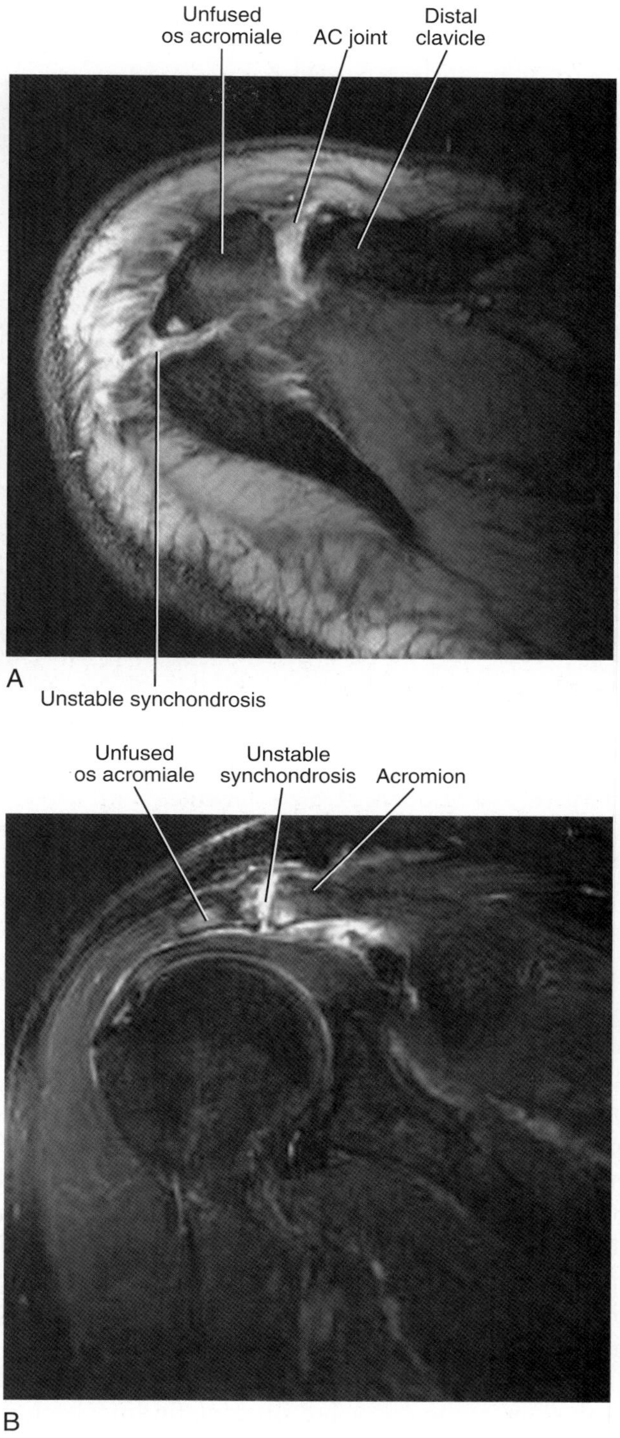
Unfused os acromiale
AC joint
Distal clavicle
A
Unstable synchondrosis
Unfused os acromiale
Unstable synchondrosis
Acromion
B

Figure 7-8 Os acromiale on MR imaging. Unfused os acromiale on axial (**A**) and coronal (**B**) MR images. The presence of fluid signal within the synchondrosis and subcortical cysts on either side of the synchondrosis suggests that the unfused ossification center is unstable and may act as a "hinge" resulting in shoulder impingement. AC, acromioclavicular.

os acromiale on sagittal or coronal images often demonstrates an appearance similar to that of the AC joint and may be misinterpreted as the AC joint. Simultaneous visualization of the AC joint and the unfused os acromiale on the same image gives the appearance of a "double AC joint," and has been referred to as the double AC joint sign. More often, the unfused os acromiale appears as a second AC joint (Fig. 7-9) on an image two to three slices posterior to the true AC joint. The presence of fluid within the synchondrosis or edema surrounding the synchondrosis seen on MR imaging usually indicates pseudarthrosis or fibrous union and is an indication of probable instability.

An unfused os acromiale can occasionally mimic an acromial fracture. The two entities can be differentiated because the accessory ossicle usually appears triangular with sclerotic margins and forms a synchondrosis that is always oriented perpendicular to the long axis of the acromion. An acute fracture, on the other hand, is usually oriented at an oblique angle relative to the long axis of the acromion and demonstrates nonsclerotic irregular margins (Fig. 7-10).

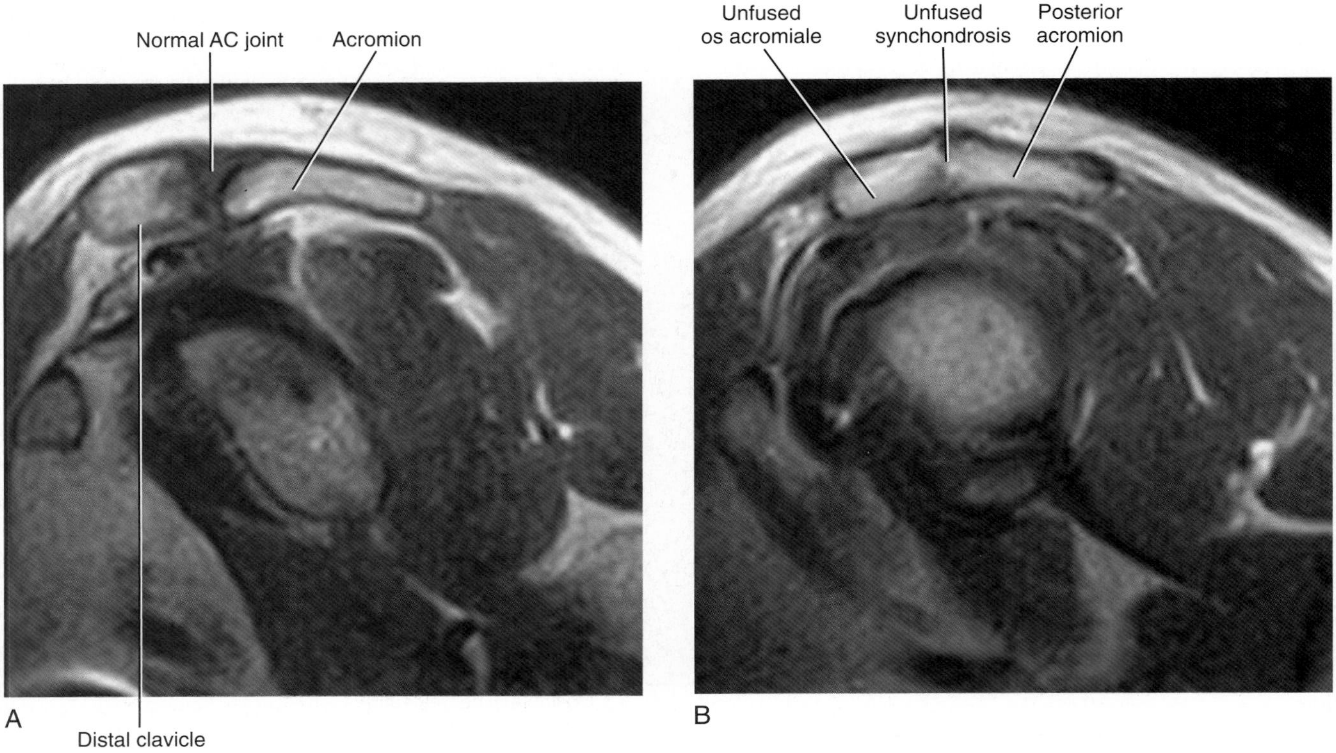
Normal AC joint
Acromion
A
Distal clavicle
Unfused os acromiale
Unfused synchondrosis
Posterior acromion
B

Figure 7-9 Double acromioclavicular-joint. Oblique sagittal images (**A**) through the level of the normal acromioclavicular (AC) joint. The unfused os acromiale appears as a second or double AC joint on a more peripheral image (**B**) and can easily be mistaken for the true AC joint.

Acromioclavicular Joint

Abnormalities of the AC joint are common and are often detected while imaging the shoulder. Osteoarthritis is a very common entity in patients over 40 years of age, whereas in the young athletic individual, post-traumatic AC joint separation and osteolysis of the distal clavicle are common entities. These conditions occasionally mimic one another, but can usually be differentiated on the basis of history and imaging findings (Table 7-2).

Osteoarthritis of the AC joint typically involves both sides of the joint, and imaging findings include capsular hypertrophy, joint effusion, and adjacent soft tissue edema. Osteophyte formation, subchondral marrow signal change, and subchondral cyst formation can also occur on both sides of the joint. The differential diagnosis for marrow edema on both sides of the AC joint includes recent AC joint separation, osteoarthritis, and inflammatory arthritis. Osteoarthritis of the AC joint is often asymptomatic or minimally symptomatic when compared with post-traumatic osteolysis of the distal clavicle, which can be quite painful. Osteoarthritis of the AC joint can be a source of extrinsic impingement on the rotator cuff; however, the AC joint does not play as crucial a role as does the anterior acromion with regard to impingement. The portion of the cuff immediately underlying the AC joint is less rigidly confined than the portion of the cuff underlying the anterior acromion, and degenerative osteoarthritis of the AC joint may result in the appearance of mass effect on the underlying cuff on MRI when there are no clinical symptoms of impingement. Degenerative changes of the AC joint with its associated mass effect on the underlying cuff are best appreciated on sagittal and coronal MR images (Fig. 7-11). Large joint effusion and pericapsular edema are signs that are often associated with synovitis of the AC joint and are associated with an increased incidence of symptomatic AC joint osteoarthritis.

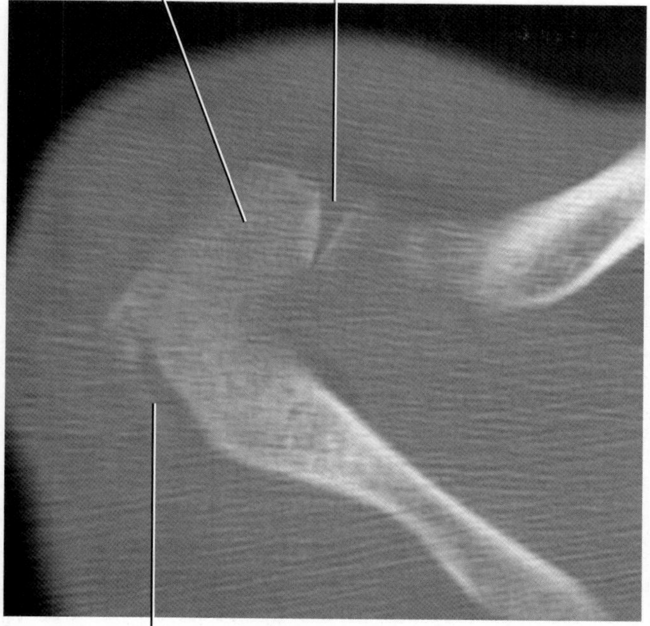
Acromion
AC joint
Fracture

Figure 7-10 Acromiale fracture. Axial CT image demonstrates a minimally displaced fracture of the posterior acromion. The fracture shows an oblique orientation relative to the long axis of the acromion, and the margins of the fracture fragments are nonsclerotic and slightly irregular when compared with an unfused os acromiale (see Figs. 7-7A and B).

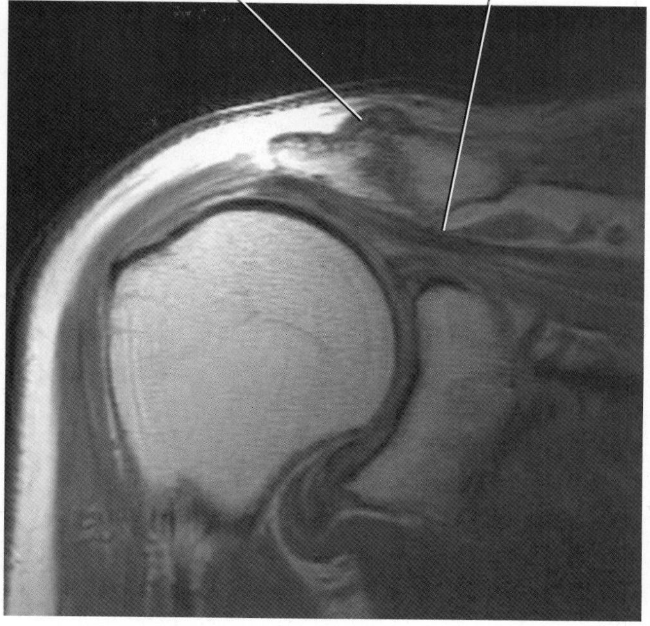
Capsular hypertrophy of the AC joint
Osteophyte causing mass effect on the underlying rotator cuff

Figure 7-11 Osteoarthritis of the acromioclavicular (AC) joint. Osteoarthritis of the AC joint is usually best detected on coronal MR images. On this coronal T1-weighted image, there is capsular hypertrophy, loss of the normal cortex of the distal clavicle and adjacent acromion, and an inferiorly directed osteophyte that results in mass effect on the underlying rotator cuff.

Table 7-2 Acromioclavicular (AC) Joint Osteoarthritis versus Osteolysis Distal Clavicle

	Osteoarthritis	Post-traumatic Osteolysis
Patient	Typically > 40	Young athlete
Symptoms	Minimally symptomatic or asymptomatic	Painful
Etiology	No history of trauma	Acute trauma: Repetitive microtrauma (weight-lifters)
Location of involvement	Both sides of joint	Isolated to distal clavicle
Radiographic findings	Joint space narrowing Osteophyte formation Subchondral cyst/sclerosis	Acute Soft tissue swelling Demineralization distal clavicle Loss cortical margin distal clavicle AC joint appears widened Chronic Reconstitution distal clavicle Subchondral sclerosis/cysts
MR findings	Joint space narrowing Osteophyte formation Subchondral cyst/sclerosis Capsular hypertrophy Joint effusion	Marrow edema distal clavicle Capsular hypertrophy Adjacent soft tissue edema Loss of dark cortical line AC joint widening

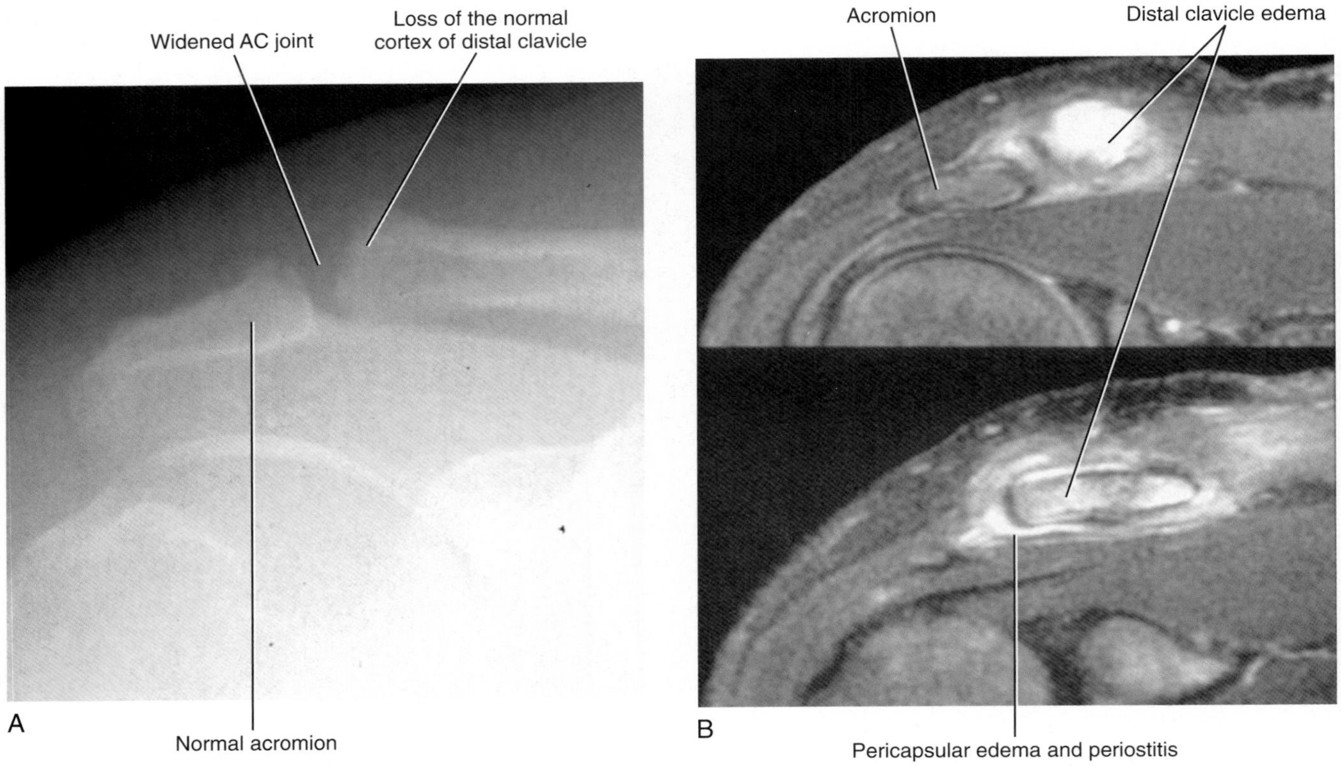
Widened AC joint
Loss of the normal cortex of distal clavicle
A
Normal acromion
Acromion
Distal clavicle edema
B
Pericapsular edema and periostitis

Figure 7-12 Osteolysis of the distal clavicle. Radiograph of the acromioclavicular (AC) joint (**A**) demonstrates mild soft tissue swelling superiorly. There is slight widening of the AC joint, loss of the normal cortical white line of the distal clavicle and mild subchondral cyst formation. The changes are much more pronounced on the clavicular side of the joint. Sequential coronal T2-weighted images (**B**) through the AC joint reveal marked marrow edema isolated to the distal aspect of the clavicle with surrounding soft tissue edema, mild periostitis, and a small joint effusion. Note that the signal intensity within the adjacent acromion is normal.

Post-traumatic *osteolysis of the distal clavicle* is a painful condition that typically occurs after mild to moderate acute trauma to the AC joint or after repetitive microtrauma, as seen in weight lifters and other athletes who experience repetitive stress to the AC joint. Clinically, osteolysis differs from osteoarthritis in that it usually occurs in the young athlete and results in moderate to severe pain, whereas osteoarthritis occurs in the older patient population with no history of trauma or repetitive stress and is minimally painful or asymptomatic.

Initial radiographs in post-traumatic osteolysis demonstrate soft tissue swelling of the AC joint, demineralization, and loss of the cortical margin of the distal clavicle (Fig. 7-12A). The AC joint may appear widened during the acute phase, but over time the distal clavicle usually reconstitutes, at least in part. Chronic changes of subchondral sclerosis and subchondral cystic change isolated to the distal clavicle are common. Early in post-traumatic osteolysis, MRI demonstrates marrow edema isolated to the distal 1 to 3 cm of the clavicle and may demonstrate loss of the normal cortical black line. Findings of a small joint effusion, capsular hypertrophy, and pericapsular edema of the AC joint are often present. Late findings may include widening of the AC joint, mild capsular hypertrophy, and cortical irregularity or subchondral sclerosis involving the distal tip of the clavicle (Fig. 7-12B).

After trauma to the shoulder, the AC joint should also be evaluated for evidence of fracture and AC joint separation. A fracture is seen on MRI as a dark line on both T1- and T2-weighted images with surrounding marrow edema. Separation of the AC joint is graded on a three-point scale (Fig. 7-13).

Grade I injury: Mild strain of the AC joint; the AC and coracoclavicular (CC) ligaments remain intact.

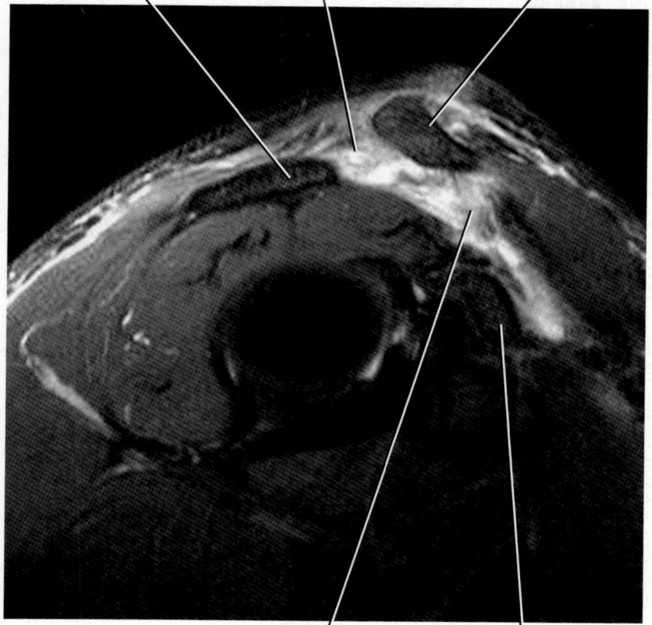
Acromion
Complete disruption of the AC joint capsule
Distal clavicle
Complete disruption of the coracoclavicular ligaments
Coracoid

Figure 7-13 Grade III acromioclavicular (AC) joint separation. There is complete disruption of the AC joint capsule and the coracoclavicular ligaments and elevation of the distal clavicle.

Radiographs of the shoulder are normal, and MRI shows only mild pericapsular edema of the AC joint. The symptoms are mild, treatment is conservative, and the patient usually recovers spontaneously.

Grade II injury: Moderate strain of the AC joint: it is associated with disruption of the AC joint capsule; the CC ligaments remain intact. Radiographs demonstrate slight elevation of the distal clavicle, whereas MRI demonstrates pericapsular AC joint edema in addition to distal elevation of the clavicle. With a grade II injury, the AC joint capsule is disrupted whereas the CC ligaments remain intact. Treatment is conservative and recovery is usually spontaneous.

Grade III injury: Severe injury of the AC joint; both the AC capsule and the CC ligaments are disrupted. Radiographs show complete dislocation of the AC joint with marked elevation of the distal clavicle, and MRI also shows pericapsular edema and disruption of the AC joint capsule and the CC ligaments. Complete AC joint separation (grade III injury) may result in scapular droop and may be a source of extrinsic impingement of the rotator cuff.

Coracoacromial Ligament

The coracoacromial ligament is a stout and sturdy ligament that forms a portion of the osseous outlet and acromion, covering the anterior fibers of the supraspinatus tendon and the rotator interval as it extends from the coracoid process anteriorly to the acromion posteriorly. The ligament is best visualized on oblique sagittal MR images and is usually no more than 2 to 3 mm-thickness (Fig. 7-14A). Thickening, hypertrophy, or calcification of the coracoacromial ligament can result in extrinsic impingement on the anterior portion of the rotator cuff (Fig. 7-14B). A thickened ligament is usually treated with either debridement or release at the time of subacromial decompression. In the younger patient, partial debridement of the ligament is preferable because this helps to prevent superior migration of the humeral head, whereas in the older patient the ligament is usually completely released.

Coracohumeral Impingement (Subcoracoid Impingement)

Coracohumeral impingement is an uncommon cause of rotator cuff impingement that results from the entrapment of the subscapularis tendon within a narrowed coracohumeral space. The normal coracohumeral distance is approximately 11 mm as depicted on axial MR images. A coracohumeral distance of less than 7 mm may result in entrapment of the subscapularis tendon between the humeral head and the coracoid process, eventually leading to a tear of the tendon (Fig. 7-15). In the case of coracohumeral impingement, successful surgical management requires not only repair of the subscapularis tendon but also correction of the narrowed coracohumeral distance. An isolated tear of the subscapularis tendon should prompt an evaluation of the coracohumeral distance to avoid missing this underlying cause of impingement.

ROTATOR CUFF

The rotator cuff is composed of four separate muscles and their tendons. Each muscle originates along either the anterior or posterior margin of the scapula and then extends toward and completely covers the humeral head with tendons inserting onto either

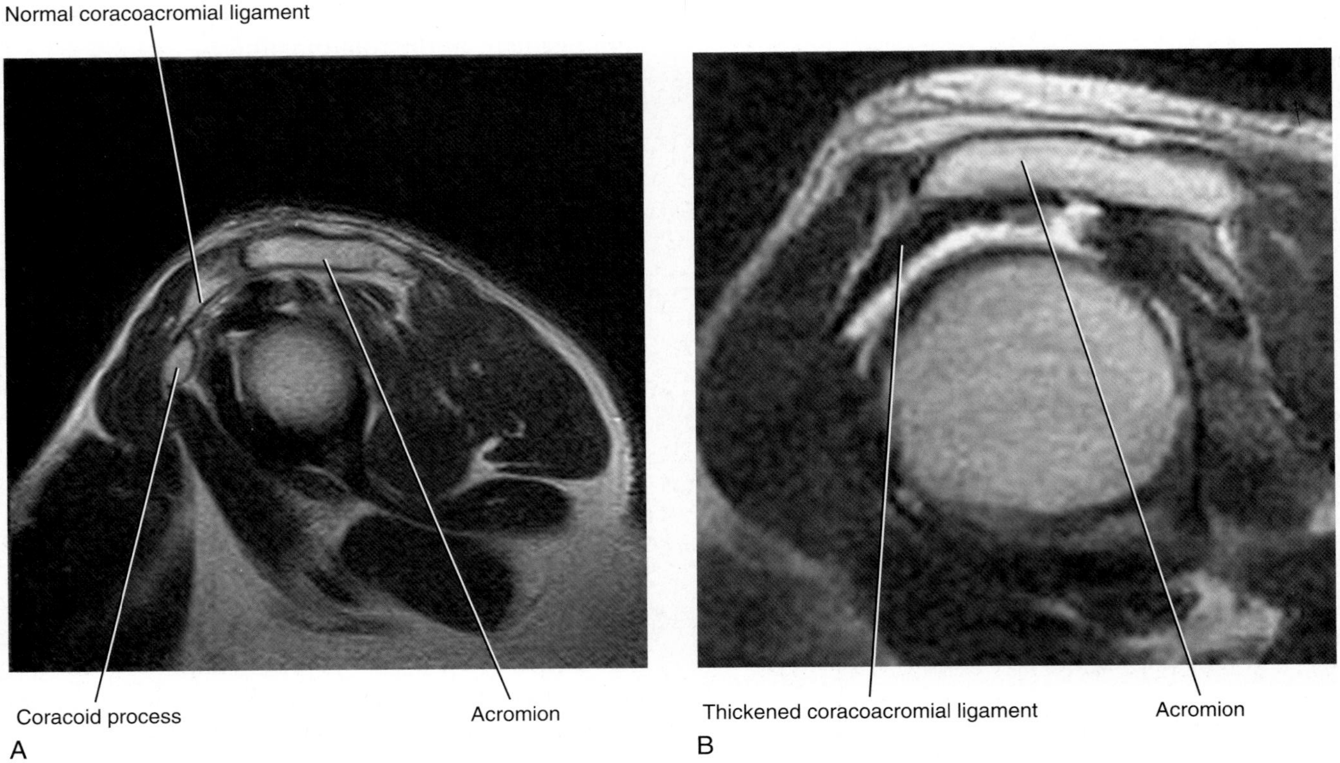
Normal coracoacromial ligament
Coracoid process
Acromion
A
Thickened coracoacromial ligament
Acromion
B

Figure 7-14 Coracoacromial ligament. The normal coracoacromial ligament is smooth-appearing and less than 2 to 3 mm thick and is best visualized on oblique sagittal MR images (**A**) as it extends from the coracoid process to the acromion. **B,** Note marked thickening of the coracoacromial ligament near its acromial attachment. Thickening or nodularity of the ligament can result in impingement of the anterior rotator cuff and treatment is debridement or surgical release at the time of subacromial decompression.

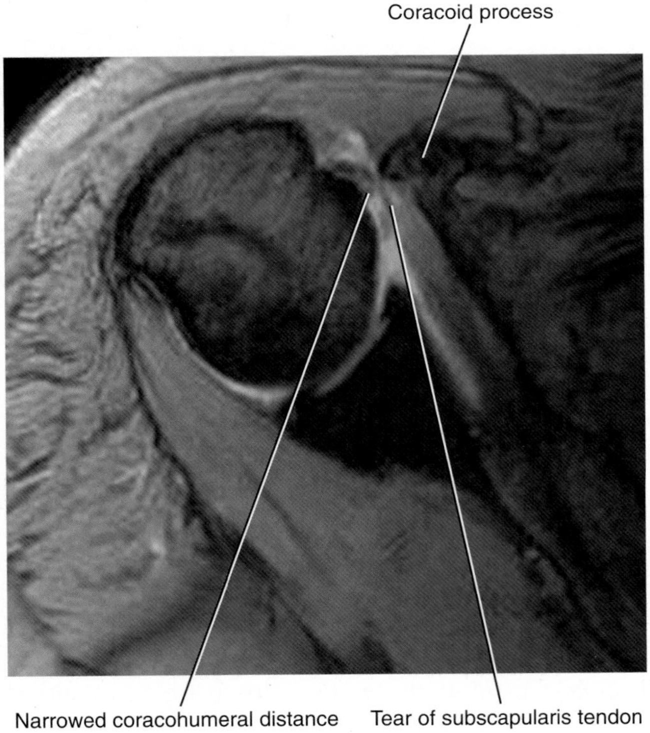
Coracoid process
Narrowed coracohumeral distance
Tear of subscapularis tendon

Figure 7-15 Coracohumeral impingement. Axial T2-weighted MRI shows a narrowed coracohumeral distance resulting in entrapment of the subscapularis tendon and partial-thickness tearing of the tendon near its attachment to the lesser tuberosity.

the greater or lesser tuberosities of the humeral head. The rotator cuff contributes to the motion of the upper extremity and also plays an important role in stabilizing the humeral head within the glenoid fossa during movement of the glenohumeral joint. The rotator cuff is often referred to as an *active* stabilizer of the rotator cuff.

Rotator Cuff Anatomy

The supraspinatus muscle is the most superior of the muscles; it originates from the medial two thirds of the supraspinatus fossa along the dorsal aspect of the scapula. Its tendon inserts onto the highest facet of the greater tuberosity of the humeral head. The infraspinatus muscle is located posterior and inferior to the supraspinatus muscle arising from the middle two thirds of the infraspinatus fossa. The tendon crosses the glenohumeral joint posteriorly to insert onto the middle facet of the greater tuberosity of the humeral head. The supraspinatus and infraspinatus muscles are both innervated by branches of the suprascapular nerve. The teres minor makes up the most inferior portion of the rotator cuff posteriorly. The muscle originates along the dorsal aspect of the lateral margin of the scapula and courses upward and laterally to insert onto the lowest facet of the greater tuberosity. The teres minor is innervated by the axillary nerve. The subscapularis muscle is a broad triangular-shaped muscle that arises from the ventral aspect of the scapula. Its fibers converge to form a broad multislip tendon that inserts onto the lesser tuberosity located on the anterior aspect of the humeral head. The subscapularis muscle is innervated by the upper and lower subscapular nerves.

MR Appearance of the Normal Rotator Cuff

The normal rotator cuff, as just described, is a complex structure, and an accurate assessment of the cuff on MRI requires a thorough understanding of the normal MR appearance of the cuff in all three imaging planes, as well as some knowledge of the common variations and imaging pitfalls that can occur.

The supraspinatus muscle and tendon are best evaluated on the oblique coronal and sagittal imaging planes (Fig. 7-16); the axial images, however, also

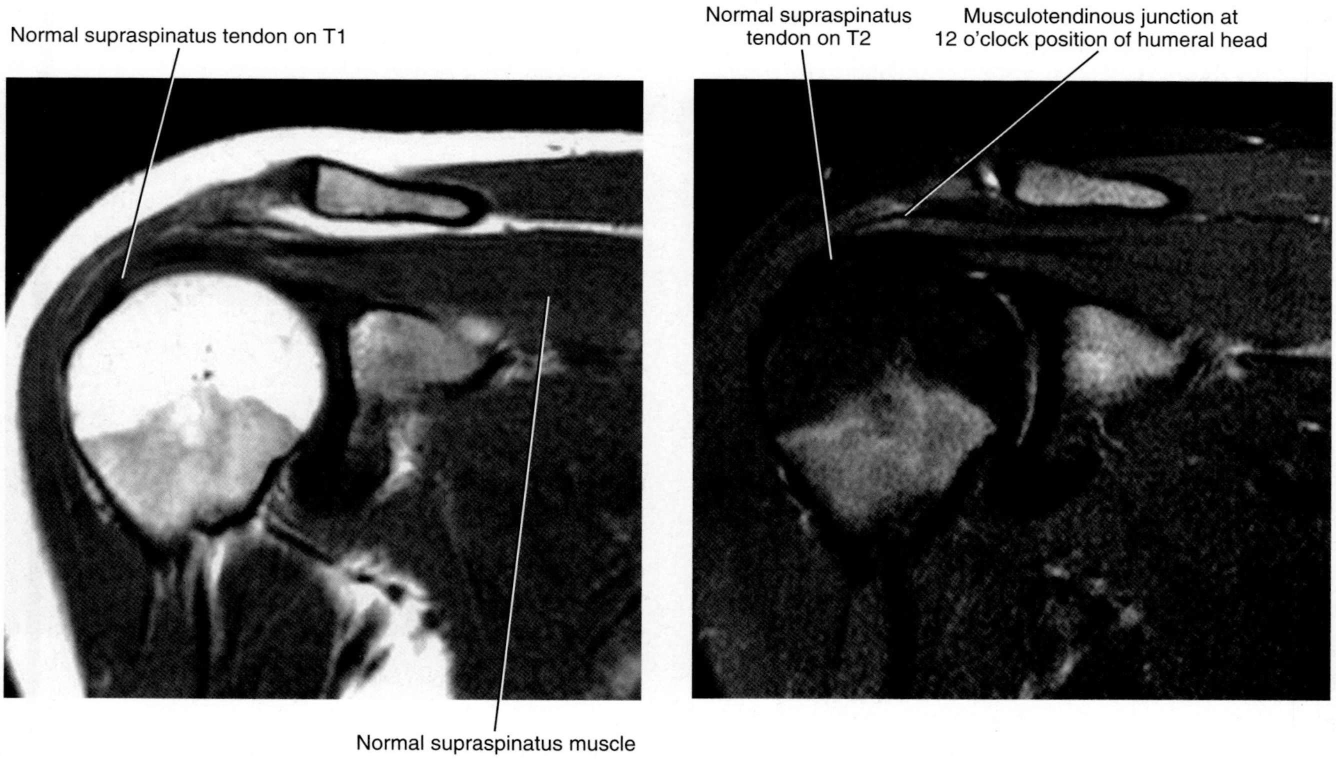

Normal supraspinatus tendon on T1
Normal supraspinatus tendon on T2
Musculotendinous junction at 12 o'clock position of humeral head
Normal supraspinatus muscle

Figure 7-16 Normal MRI appearance of the supraspinatus tendon. The normal supraspinatus tendon demonstrates low T1 and T2 signal and is oriented in the horizontal plane. The normal musculotendinous junction is located in the 12 o'clock position of the humeral head. Muscle is intermediate signal intensity on both T1 and T2-weighted images.

provide important information regarding the status of the supraspinatus. The normal muscle should completely fill the supraspinatus fossa and should demonstrate intermediate T1 and T2 signal. Without fatty atrophy, the muscle should demonstrate a bulk that is relatively similar to that of the infraspinatus and teres minor muscles, as seen on the oblique sagittal images. The supraspinatus muscle tapers from central to peripheral with the normal musculotendinous junction situated at approximately the 12 o'clock position of the humeral head. The infraspinatus and teres minor muscles are also best evaluated on the oblique sagittal and oblique coronal images, and these two muscles should completely fill the infraspinatus fossa. They also taper peripherally with their musculotendinous junctions located at a level similar to that of the supraspinatus muscle. On coronal images, the supraspinatus tendon can easily be differentiated from the infraspinatus because the supraspinatus tendon is oriented horizontally, whereas the infraspinatus tendon is oblique in orientation.

The subscapularis muscle has a broad origin along the anterior border of the scapula and is best evaluated on the axial MR images. However, the oblique sagittal and oblique coronal sequences are important secondary imaging planes. Unlike the other three muscles, the subscapularis musculoskeletal junction is broad with multiple tendon slips arising out of the muscle and extending peripherally to insert in a broad fashion onto the lesser tuberosity of the humeral head.

Tendons arise out of the four separate muscles and then broaden and flatten peripherally, merging to form a single water-tight unit that inserts onto the tuberosities of the humeral head. The normal tendon demonstrates low signal intensity on all MR pulse sequences. Tendon pathology is usually manifested as increased signal or as a focal area of thickening, thinning, or attenuation, surface irregularity or as an area of discontinuity of the cuff.

Ultrasound Appearance of the Rotator Cuff

A complete description of the technique for ultrasound examination of the rotator cuff is beyond the scope of this chapter. However, knowledge of the normal MR appearance of the cuff can aid in the understanding the normal ultrasound appearance of the cuff. The examination often begins by scanning in the transverse imaging plane along the anterior surface of the shoulder to identify the key landmark of the long head of the biceps tendon within the intertubercular groove covered by the subscapularis tendon. Imaging then proceeds in a systematic manner to evaluate the musculotendinous units of each rotator cuff muscle in both the transverse and longitudinal planes. The normal rotator cuff tendon demonstrates a typical bandlike appearance of medium-level echoes located deep to the deltoid muscle. A thin stripe of bright echoes just superficial to the rotator cuff tendon represents the normal subacromial subdeltoid bursa. Muscle is hypoechoic in appearance. The biceps tendon is seen as an oval-appearing area of bright echoes located within the intertubercular groove. The bony surface of the humerus results in a rim of bright echoes (Fig. 7-17).

Sonographic signs of a rotator cuff tear include:

- Nonvisualization of the cuff
- Focal defect or absence of the cuff
- Discontinuity of the cuff

Tendinosis may manifest as focal or diffuse areas of tendon thickening with altered echogenicity, either increased or decreased. A secondary sign of rotator cuff pathology may include fluid within the subdeltoid bursa (Fig. 7-18).

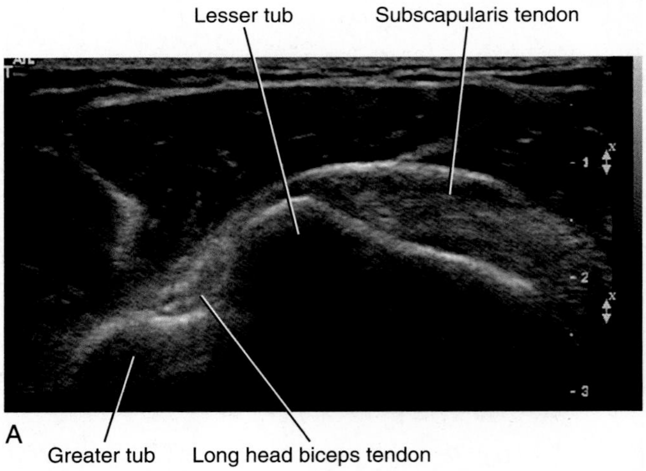
Lesser tub
Subscapularis tendon
A
Greater tub
Long head biceps tendon

Figure 7-17 Normal sonographic appearance of the rotator cuff. A, Transverse scan shows the normal appearance of the biceps tendon within the intertubercular groove covered by the overlying subscapularis muscle.

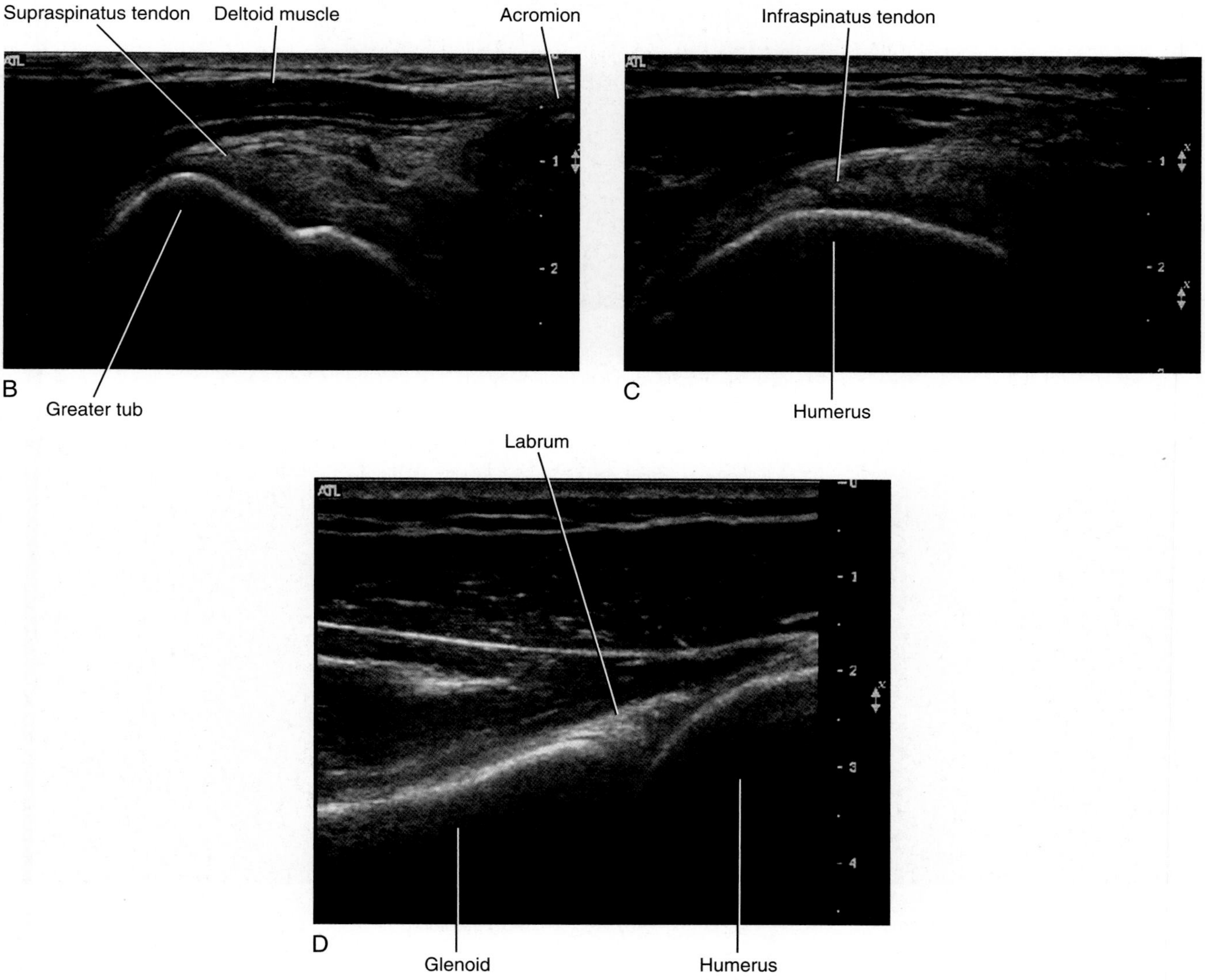
Supraspinatus tendon
Deltoid muscle
Acromion
B
Greater tub
Infraspinatus tendon
C
Humerus
Labrum
D
Glenoid
Humerus

Figure 7-17, cont'd **B** and **C** show the normal appearance of the supraspinatus and infraspinatus tendons. **D,** Longitudinal scan shows the normal appearance of the superior labrum.

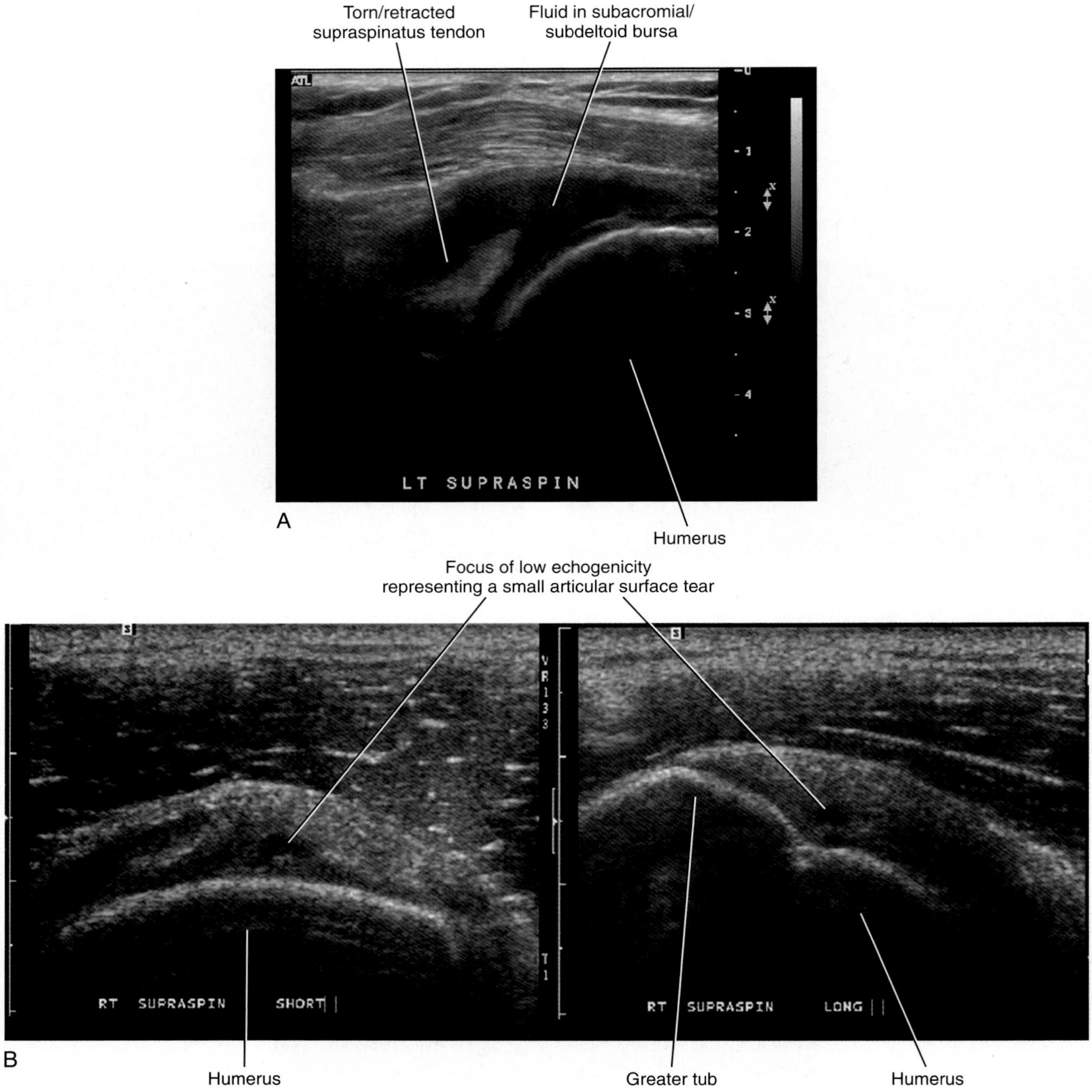
Torn/retracted supraspinatus tendon
Fluid in subacromial/subdeltoid bursa
LT SUPRASPIN
A
Humerus
Focus of low echogenicity representing a small articular surface tear
RT SUPRASPIN SHORT
RT SUPRASPIN LONG
B
Humerus
Greater tub
Humerus

Figure 7-18 Sonographic appearance of rotator cuff pathology. *A,* Large tear of the rotator cuff with retraction. ***B,*** Small interstitial tear of the supraspinatus tendon.

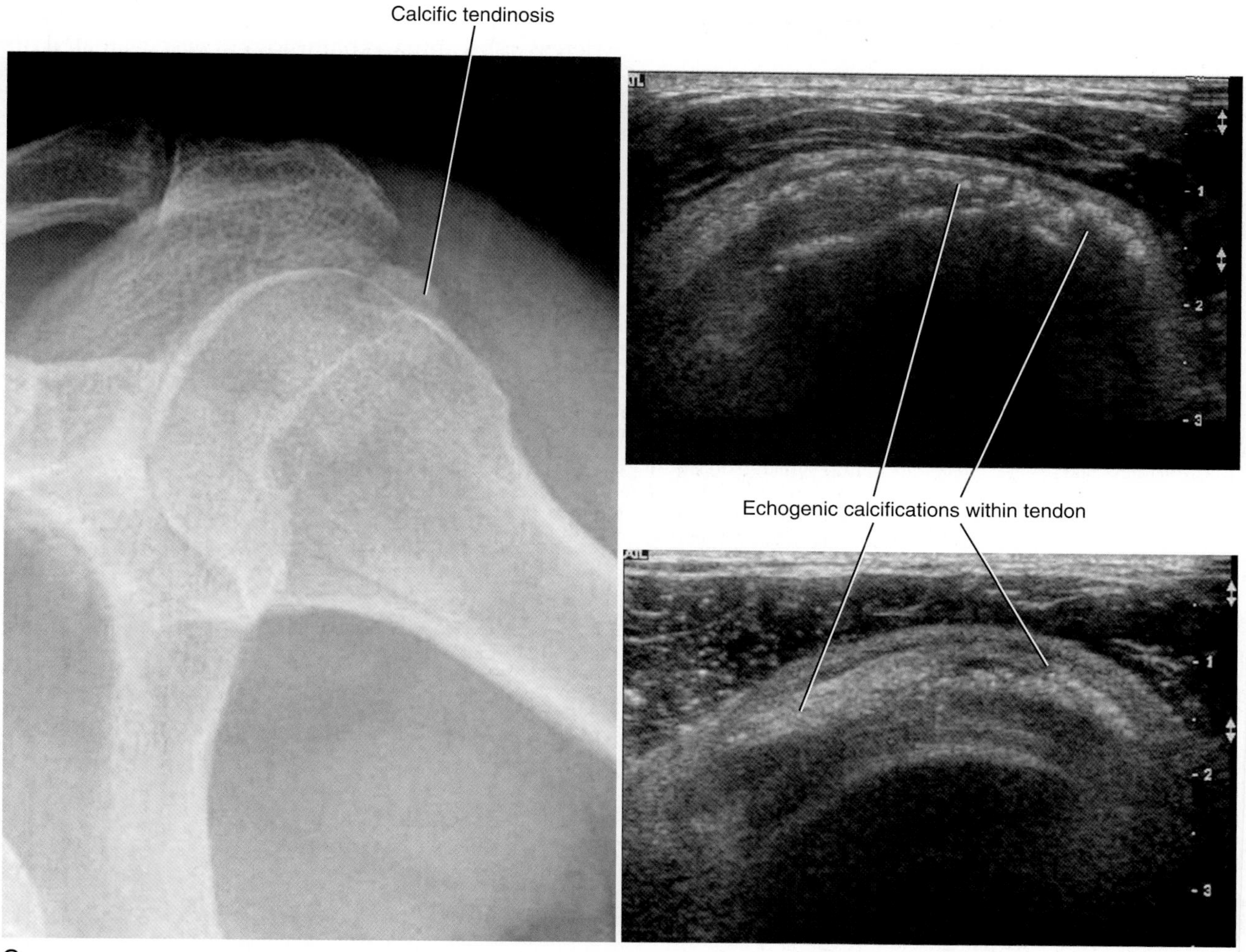
Calcific tendinosis
Echogenic calcifications within tendon

C

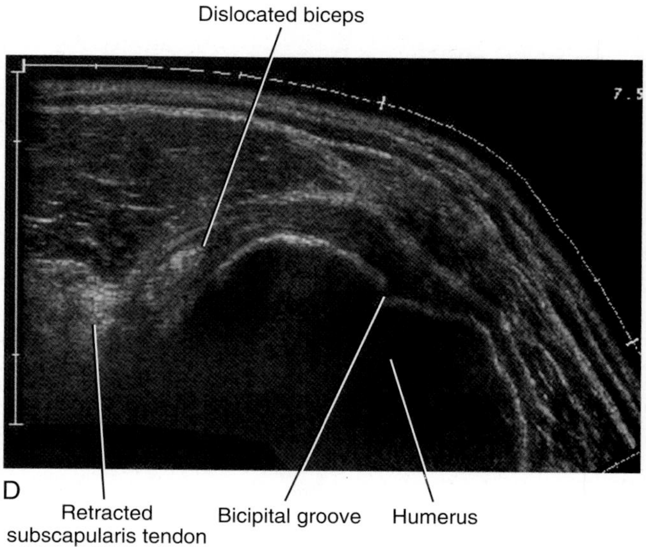
Dislocated biceps
Retracted subscapularis tendon
Bicipital groove
Humerus

D

Figure 7-18, cont'd ***C,*** Calcific tendinosis of the infraspinatus tendon. ***D,*** Subscapularis tear with medial dislocation of the long head of the biceps tendon.

MR Appearance of Rotator Cuff Pathology

The sensitivity and specificity of MRI in the detection of rotator cuff tears range from 88% to 100%. Supraspinatus and infraspinatus pathology is best demonstrated on T2-weighted coronal and sagittal images, whereas subscapularis pathology is best evaluated on axial T2-weighted sequences. Rotator cuff pathology can be classified as discussed in the following text (Table 7-3 and Fig. 7-19).

Table 7-3 MR Appearance of Rotator Cuff Pathology

Cuff Pathology	Appearance on MRI
Normal tendon	Dark on T1 and T2
Tendonopathy	Thickening of tendon Intermediate signal T1/T2
Calcific tendinitis	Globular decreased signal T1/T2 within tendon; often with surrounding soft tissue edema Thickened tendon; intermediate signal T1/T2 "Blooming" artifact on gradient echo
Partial-thickness tear	Fluid signal/gadolinium extending partially through tendon superior to inferior Bursal/articular/interstitial Associated intramuscular cyst No retraction of tendon
Full-thickness tear	Fluid extending completely through tendon top to bottom Retraction of tendon Gap/discontinuity in tendon
Musculotendinous retraction	Measured as the length of the medial-to-lateral tendon gap
Fatty atrophy	Grade—mild/moderate/severe Streaks of high signal on T1—irreversible Loss of muscle bulk relative to other rotator cuff muscles on sagittal imaging—reversible

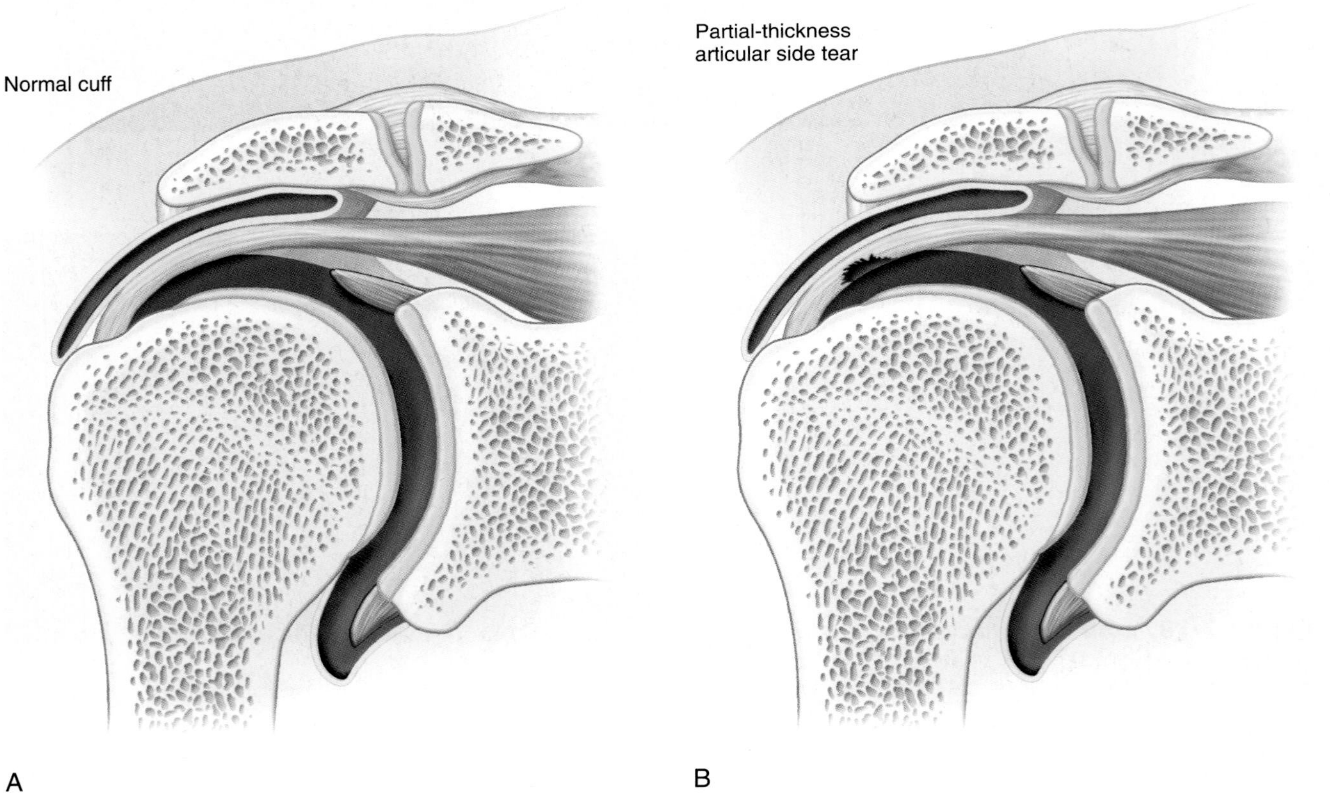
Normal cuff
Partial-thickness
articular side tear
A
B

Figure 7-19 Patterns of rotator cuff tear. A, Normal rotator cuff. **B,** Partial thickness articular sided tear.

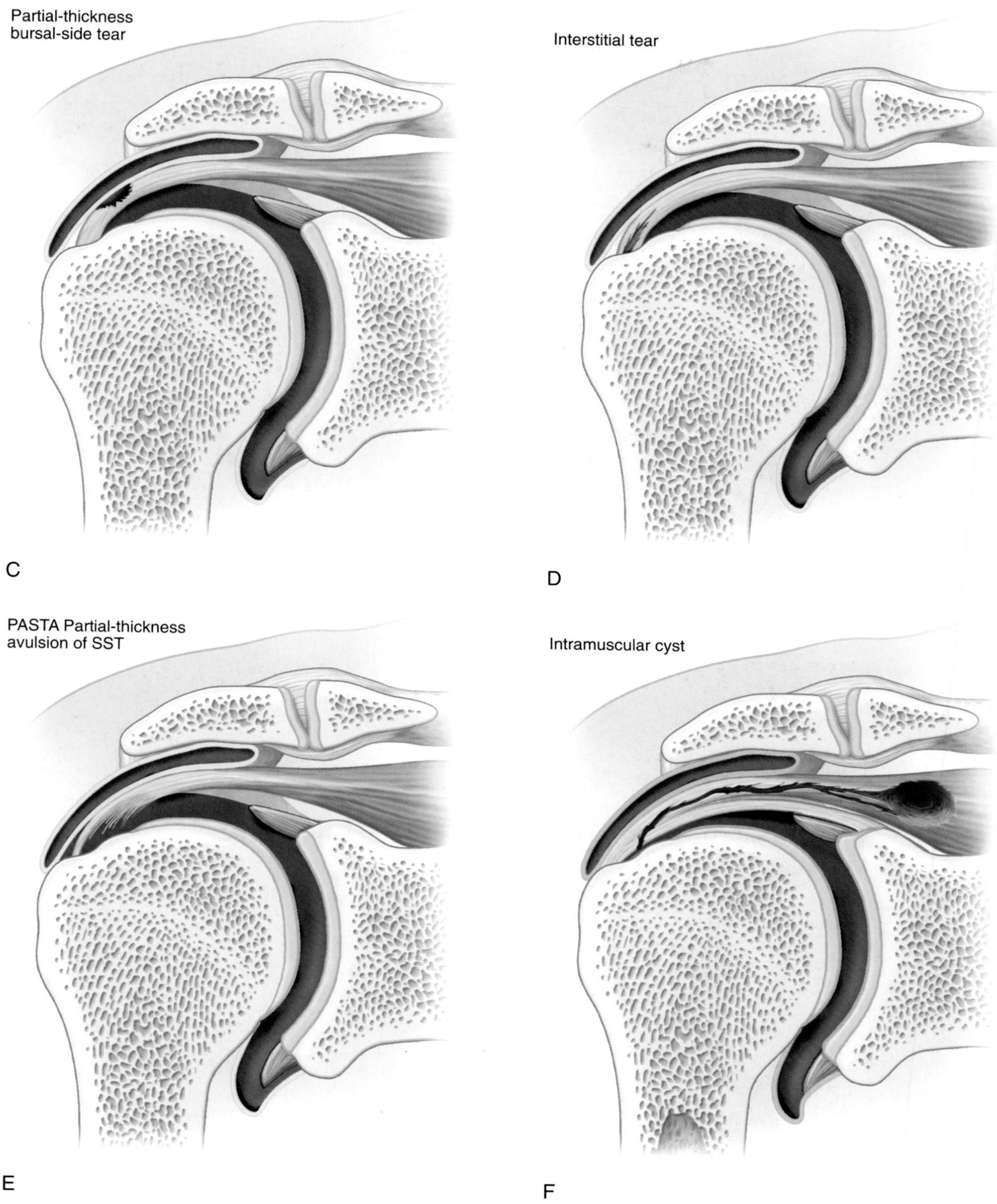

Partial-thickness
bursal-side tear
C
Interstitial tear
D
PASTA Partial-thickness
avulsion of SST
E
Intramuscular cyst
F

Figure 7-19, cont'd **C,** Partial thickness bursal-side tear. **D,** Partial thickness interstitial tear. **E,** Partial-thickness articular surface supraspinatus avulsion (PASTA lesion). **F,** Partial thickness articular-side tear with intramuscular cyst.

Continued

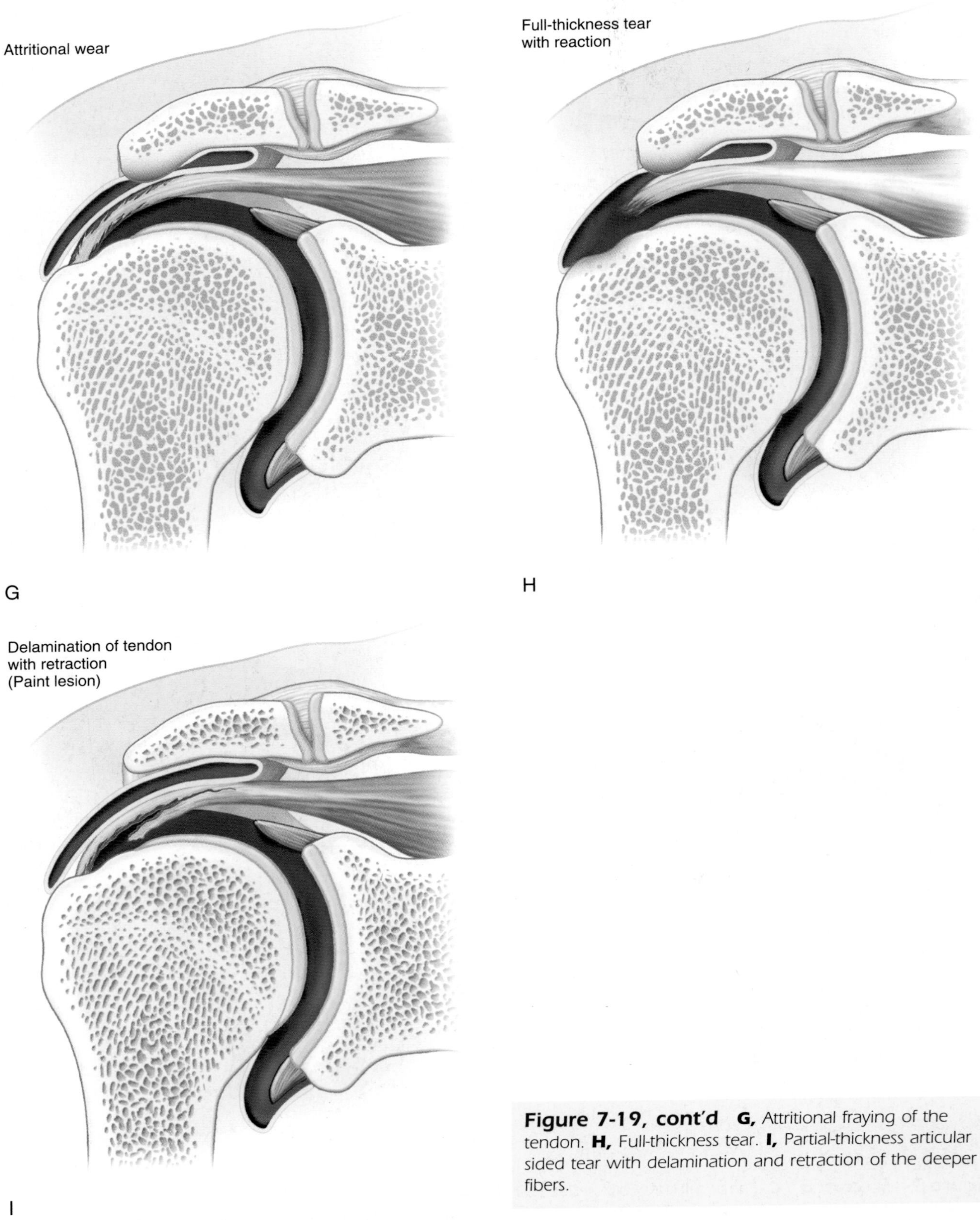
Attritional wear
G
Full-thickness tear
with reaction
H
Delamination of tendon
with retraction
(Paint lesion)
I

Figure 7-19, cont'd **G,** Attritional fraying of the tendon. **H,** Full-thickness tear. **I,** Partial-thickness articular sided tear with delamination and retraction of the deeper fibers.

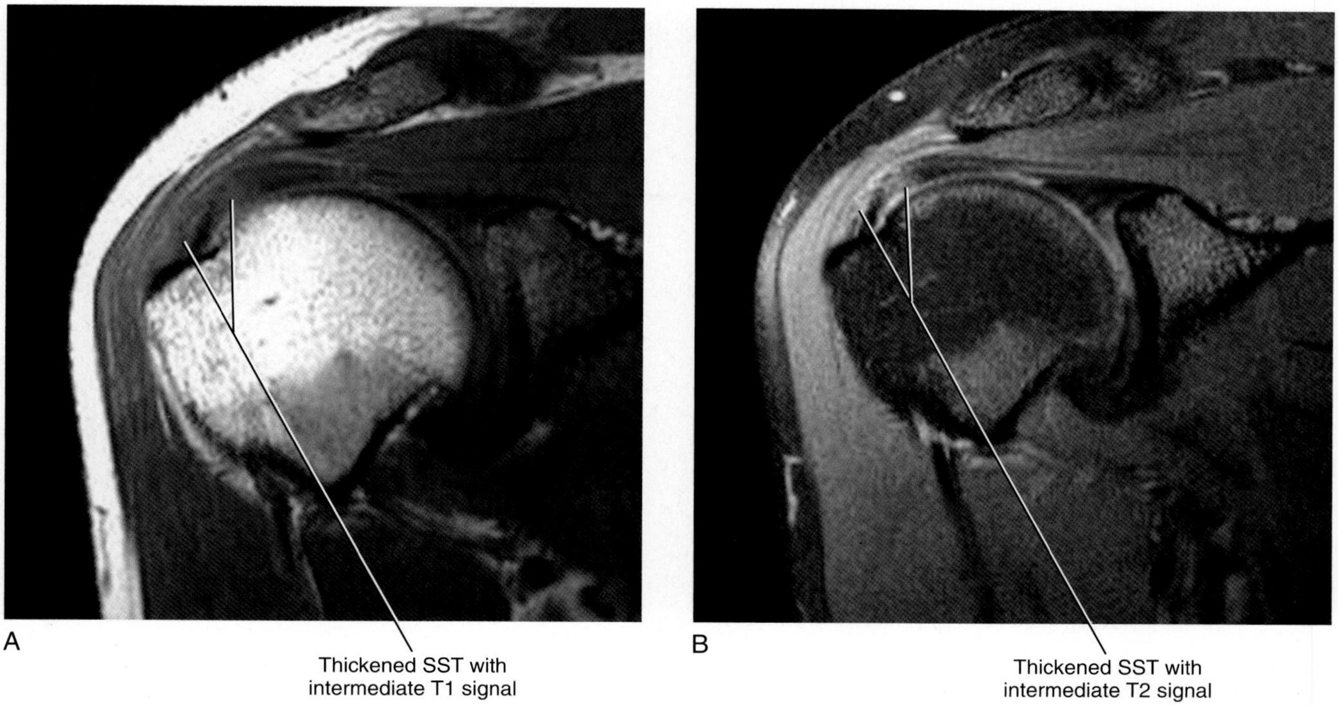
A
Thickened SST with
intermediate T1 signal
B
Thickened SST with
intermediate T2 signal

Figure 7-20 Tendinopathy. T1- (**A**) and T2-weighted (**B**) coronal images demonstrate mild thickening and intermediate signal intensity within the substance of the supraspinatus tendon, but no fluid signal intensity on the T2-weighted image. This is consistent with tendinopathy, but no tear. SST, supraspinatus tendon.

On MRI, *tendinopathy* appears as intermediate signal intensity within the substance of the tendon on both T1- and T2-weighted images (slightly less bright than water on T2 images). The tendon may also demonstrate mild to moderate thickening (Fig. 7-20). Histologically, the increased signal represents mucoid degeneration of the tendon.

Hydroxyapatite deposition disease can occur within the rotator cuff tendon, *calcific tendinitis,* or within other periarticular soft tissues including the glenohumeral ligaments and adjacent bursa, *calcific bursitis* (Fig. 7-21). These calcifications are best detected on radiographs but may also be identified on MRI as focal areas of globular decreased signal on both T1- and T2-weighted images. Calcific tendinitis is often associated with intense inflammatory changes of the adjacent soft tissues, resulting in surrounding increased signal on T2-weighted images. On MRI, it may be difficult in some cases to detect the calcification and to distinguish calcific tendinitis from noncalcific tendinitis. Gradient-echo imaging can be helpful in this regard, since "blooming" artifact seen on gradient-echo images exaggerates the size and appearance of the calcification.

A *partial-thickness tear* of the rotator cuff is defined as a tear that extends partially through the thickness of the tendon from superior to inferior. MR imaging demonstrates fluid signal intensity on T2-weighted images extending partially through the thickness of the tendon. The tear may involve the *bursal* or *articular* surface, or the *interstitial* portions of the tendon (Fig. 7-22). A partial-thickness tear may occasionally be difficult to differentiate from tendinopathy, especially when partial healing has occurred with granulation tissue filling the tendon defect. The granulation tissue may demonstrate intermediate signal intensity on T2-weighted images, mimicking tendinopathy.

One helpful indirect MRI sign that can help in establishing the diagnosis of a partial-thickness rotator cuff tear is the presence of an intramuscular cyst. Joint fluid can track through the defect of a partial-thickness articular surface tear of the rotator

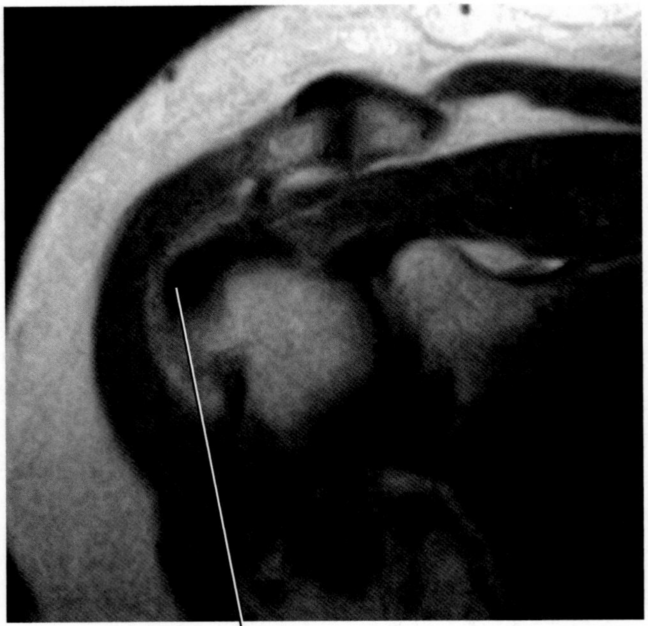
Globular low signal within the SST representing
subtle calcific bursitis on MR imaging

A

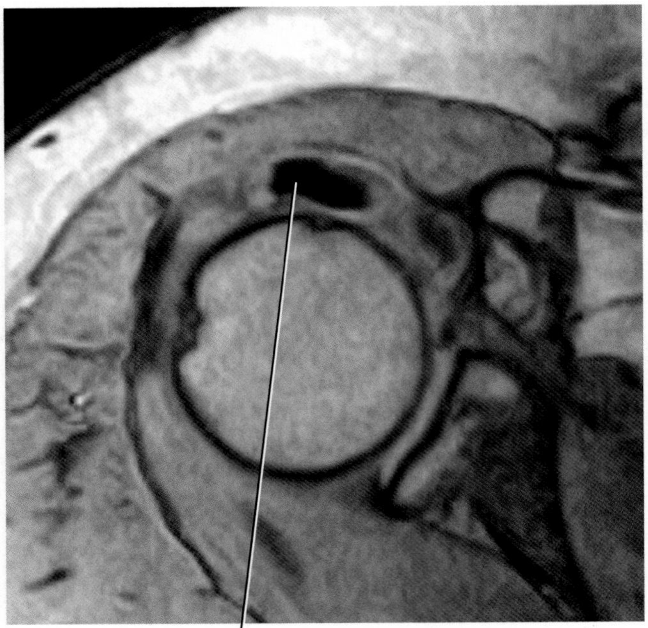
"Blooming" artifact on gradient-echo imaging
increases conspicuity of calcific tendinosis

B

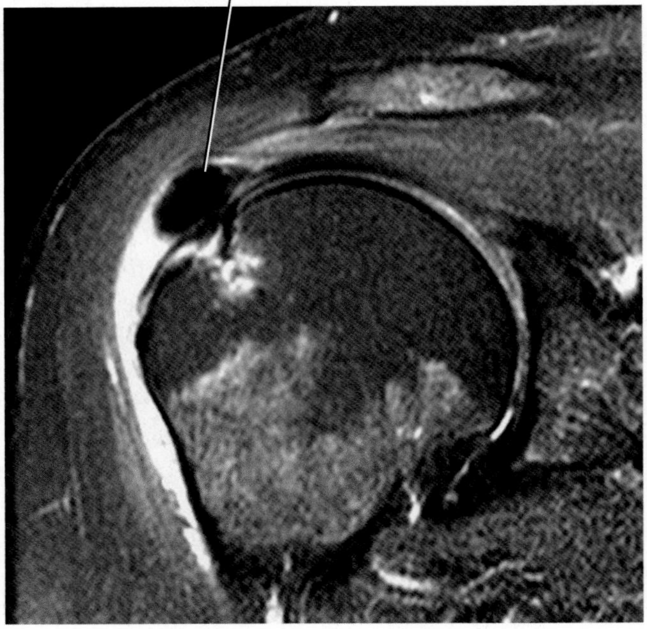
Globular area of low T2-signal within SASD
bursa representing calcific bursitis

C

Figure 7-21 Calcific tendinitis and bursitis. A, T1-weighted coronal image demonstrates a globular area of low signal intensity within the anterior aspect of the supraspinatus tendon (SST) representing calcific tendinosis. **B,** Gradient-echo axial image shows "blooming" artifact, or apparent enlargement of the area of calcific tendinosis increasing the conspicuity of the calcific deposition. SST, supraspinatus tendon. **C,** Coronal T2-weighted image with fat saturation shows a large globular area of low signal surrounded by fluid within the subacromial subdeltoid bursa. SASD, subacromial subdeltoid; SST, supraspinatus tendon.

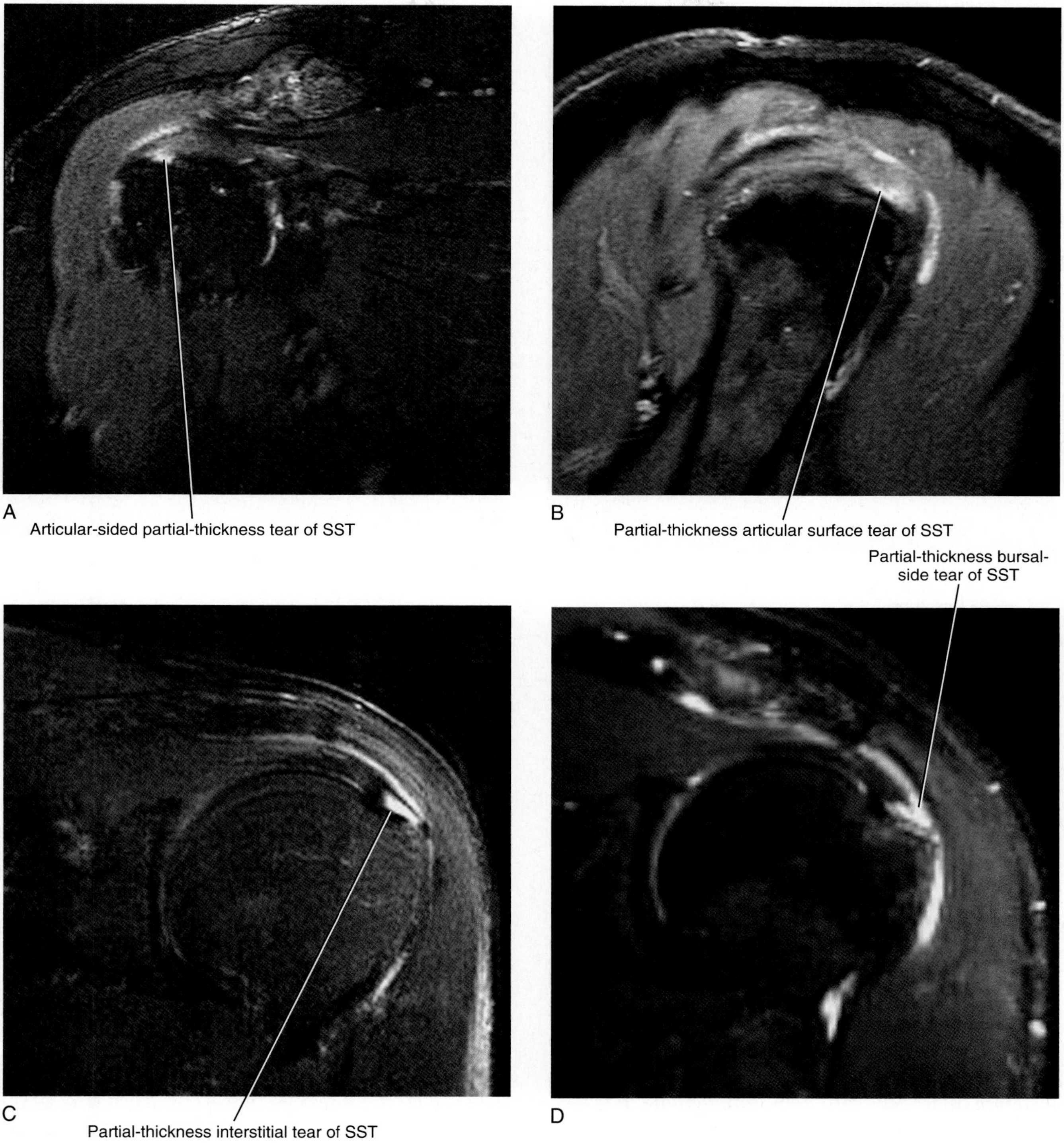
A
Articular-sided partial-thickness tear of SST
B
Partial-thickness articular surface tear of SST
Partial-thickness bursal-side tear of SST
C
Partial-thickness interstitial tear of SST
D

Figure 7-22 Types of partial-thickness rotator cuff tears. Partial-thickness articular surface tear coronal (**A**) and sagittal (**B**) T2-weighted images show fluid signal extending into the articular surface of the supraspinatus tendon (SST). Partial-thickness interstitial tear (**C**), fluid signal is present within the substance of the tendon but does not extend to either the articular or bursal surfaces. Partial-thickness bursal surface tear (**D**), fluid signal extends into the bursal surface of the SST but does not extend completely through to involve the articular surface. *Continued*

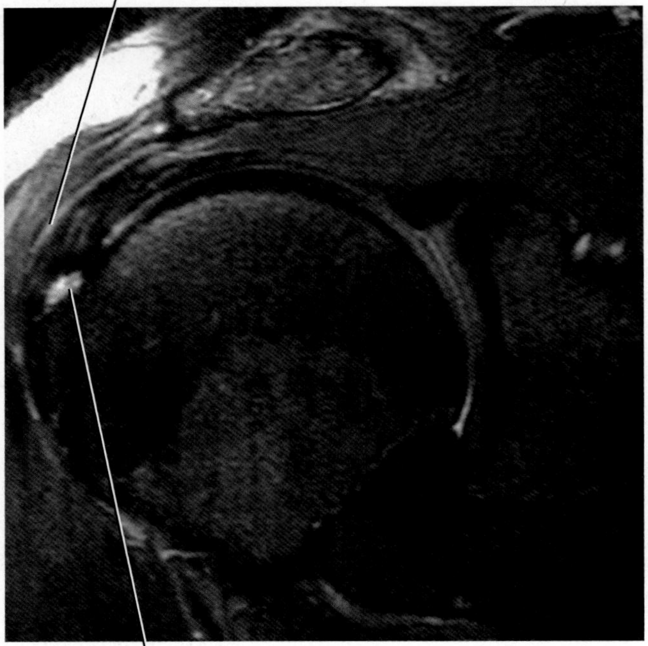
Intact bursal surface of SST
Partial articular-side
SST avulsion
E

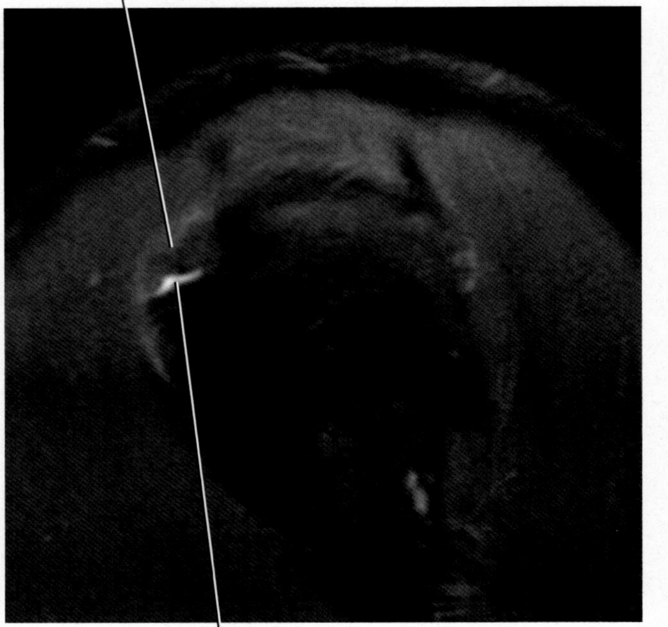
Intact bursal surface of SST
Partial articular-side
SST avulsion
F

Figure 7-22, cont'd Coronal (**E**) and sagittal (**F**) T2-weighted images demonstrate a partial articular-side SST avulsion or PASTA lesion. The undersurface of the SST is avulsed from the greater tuberosity, but the bursal surface remains intact.

cuff tendon and then dissect in a laminar fashion through the tendon and form a cyst within the substance of the rotator cuff muscle. These intramuscular cysts can easily be differentiated from paralabral cysts because they are contained within the fascia of the rotator cuff muscle, best demonstrated on sagittal T2-weighted images. An intramuscular cyst has a high association with partial-thickness tearing of the rotator cuff, just as a paralabral cyst has a high association with a labral tear. The presence of an intramuscular cyst can help differentiate between tendinopathy and a partial-thickness tear of the rotator cuff (Fig. 7-23). Two other imaging tips that can help differentiate between tendinopathy and a partial-thickness articular surface tears of the rotator cuff are the use of direct MR arthrography and ABER (abducted and externally rotated) imaging (with or without intra-articular contrast). Both techniques improve the conspicuity of partial-thickness articular surface tears of the rotator cuff (Fig. 7-24).

It is important to provide an accurate description of the extent and location of a partial-thickness tear because this information can have an impact on the decision to operate and can also influence the surgical approach and the type of surgery. A tear that extends more than 70% through the thickness of the tendon from superior to inferior is usually completed by the surgeon and then treated as a full-thickness tear. A tear that extends less than 30% through the thickness of the tendon is usually treated conservatively or by debridement alone (similar to the surgical treatment of tendinopathy). A tear that extends 30% to 70% through the thickness of the tendon is treated with debridement followed by suturing to shorten the "bridge" that is created by the debridement. In all cases, the cause of impingement must be addressed surgically to prevent recurrence of the rotator cuff pathology.

A *partial articular-side supraspinatus tendon avulsion* or "PASTA" lesion is a subset of partial-thickness tears

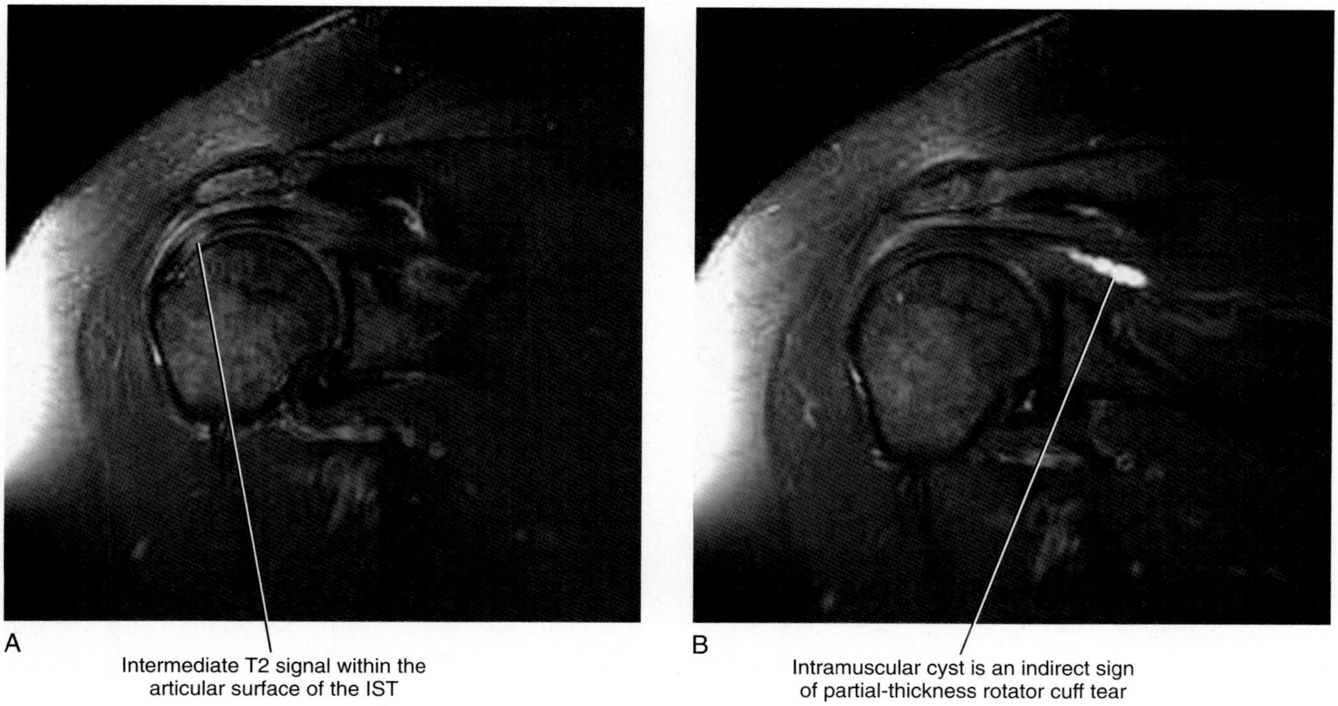
A
Intermediate T2 signal within the articular surface of the IST
B
Intramuscular cyst is an indirect sign of partial-thickness rotator cuff tear

Figure 7-23 **Partial-thickness tear: intramuscular cyst. A,** T2-weighted oblique coronal image demonstrates intermediate signal involving the articular surface of the infraspinatus tendon (IST). By strict MR criteria, this represents tendinopathy and not a tear. **B,** The next most posterior image in the same series demonstrates a cyst within the infraspinatus muscle. This indicates that fluid is tracking into the muscle through a defect or partial-thickness undersurface tear of the IST and confirms the presence of a tear rather than tendinopathy. This was interpreted as a partial-thickness articular surface tear of the IST and was later confirmed at arthroscopy.

that has been recently described in the orthopedic literature. The tear represents a partial-thickness articular-side avulsion of the supraspinatus tendon at its most anterior attachment site. This type of tear deserves special attention and should be accurately described on MRI because the recommended treatment for this subset of tendon tears differs from the standard partial-thickness tears previously described. A transtendon suture technique is performed to preserve the intact portion of the tendon while firmly reattaching the torn portion of the tendon to the humeral footprint. On MRI, a small articular-side avulsion is seen as fluid signal extending into the articular surface of the supraspinatus tendon at its anterior attachment site with partial avulsion of the tendon at this level and represents a subset of the articular surface partial-thickness tears (see Fig. 7-22E and F).

A *full-thickness tear* of the rotator cuff is defined as a tear that extends completely through the thickness of the tendon from superior to inferior. MR demonstrates bright fluid on T2-weighted images extending through the entire thickness of the tendon (Fig. 7-25). There may be retraction of the torn tendon end. Sagittal and axial images can be very helpful in differentiating a partial-thickness from a full-thickness tear, especially when the tear is located at the level of attachment to the humeral head. Small full-thickness tears often involve the most anterior aspect of the supraspinatus tendon immediately adjacent to its attachment to the greater tuberosity. It is important to evaluate the supraspinatus tendon on the most anterior coronal image to avoid missing a small full-thickness tear at the most anterior bone-tendon interface (Fig. 7-26). The extent of tear should be measured and reported in both the anteroposterior and medial-lateral directions. A tear that is larger in the anteroposterior direction is often repaired using a tendon-to-bone suture technique, whereas a tear that is greater in the medial-lateral direction may

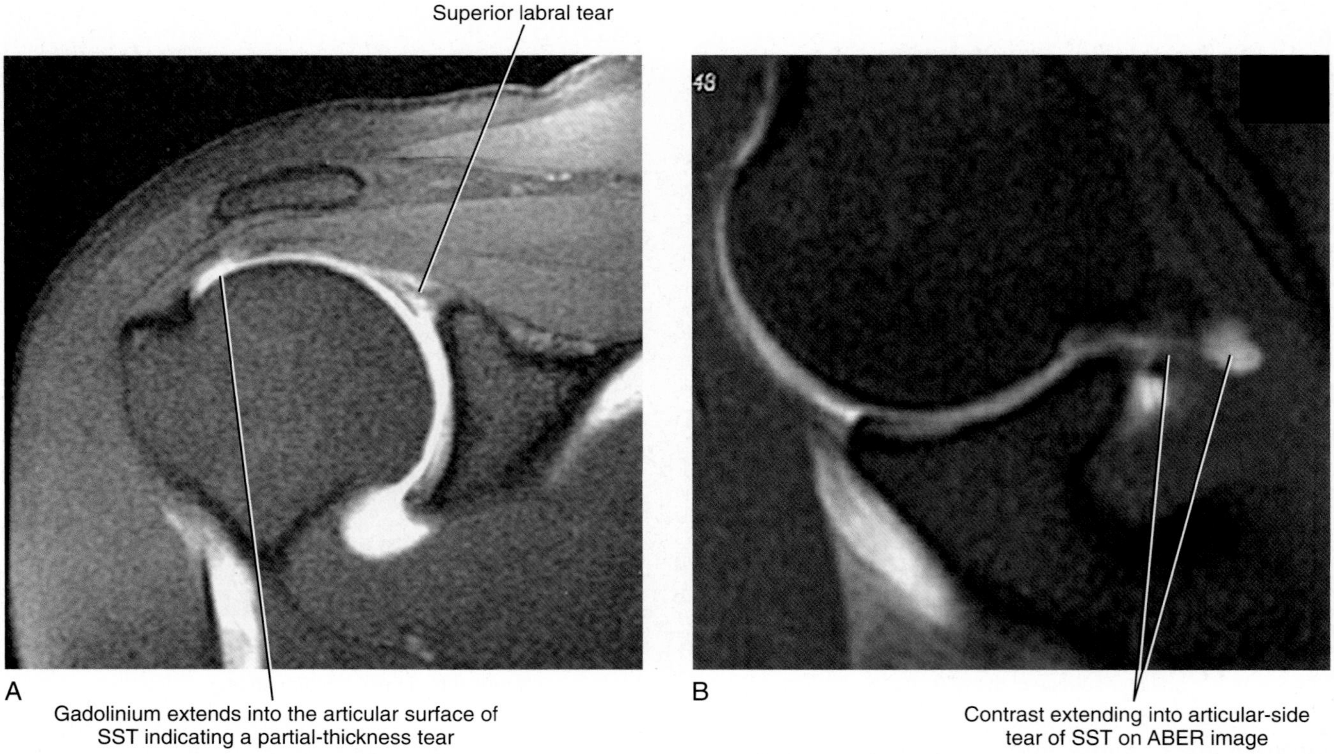
Superior labral tear
A
Gadolinium extends into the articular surface of SST indicating a partial-thickness tear
43
B
Contrast extending into articular-side tear of SST on ABER image

Figure 7-24 Partial-thickness tear: MR arthrography and ABER imaging. A, The presence of intra-articular contrast on this direct MR arthrogram helps to confirm the presence of a subtle articular surface tear of the supraspinatus tendon (SST) on a coronal T1-weighted image. **B,** The abduction external rotation (ABER) image demonstrates contrast extending into the substance of the muscle and is very helpful in confirming the presence of a subtle partial-thickness articular surface tear.

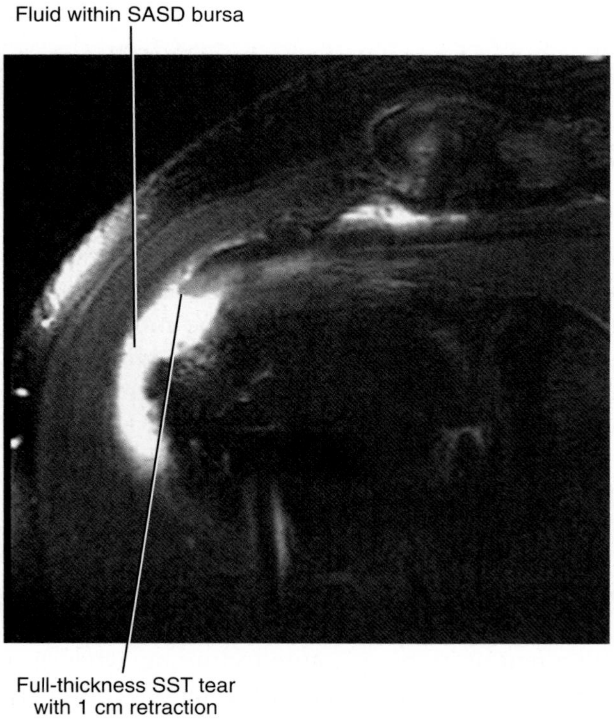
Fluid within SASD bursa
Full-thickness SST tear with 1 cm retraction

Figure 7-25 Full-thickness rotator cuff tear. Coronal T2-weighted image demonstrates fluid extending completely through the thickness of the tendon from superior to inferior, representing a full-thickness tear of the supraspinatus tendon (SST). There is approximately 1 cm of retraction of the torn tendon end and moderate fluid within the subacromial subdeltoid (SASD) bursa.

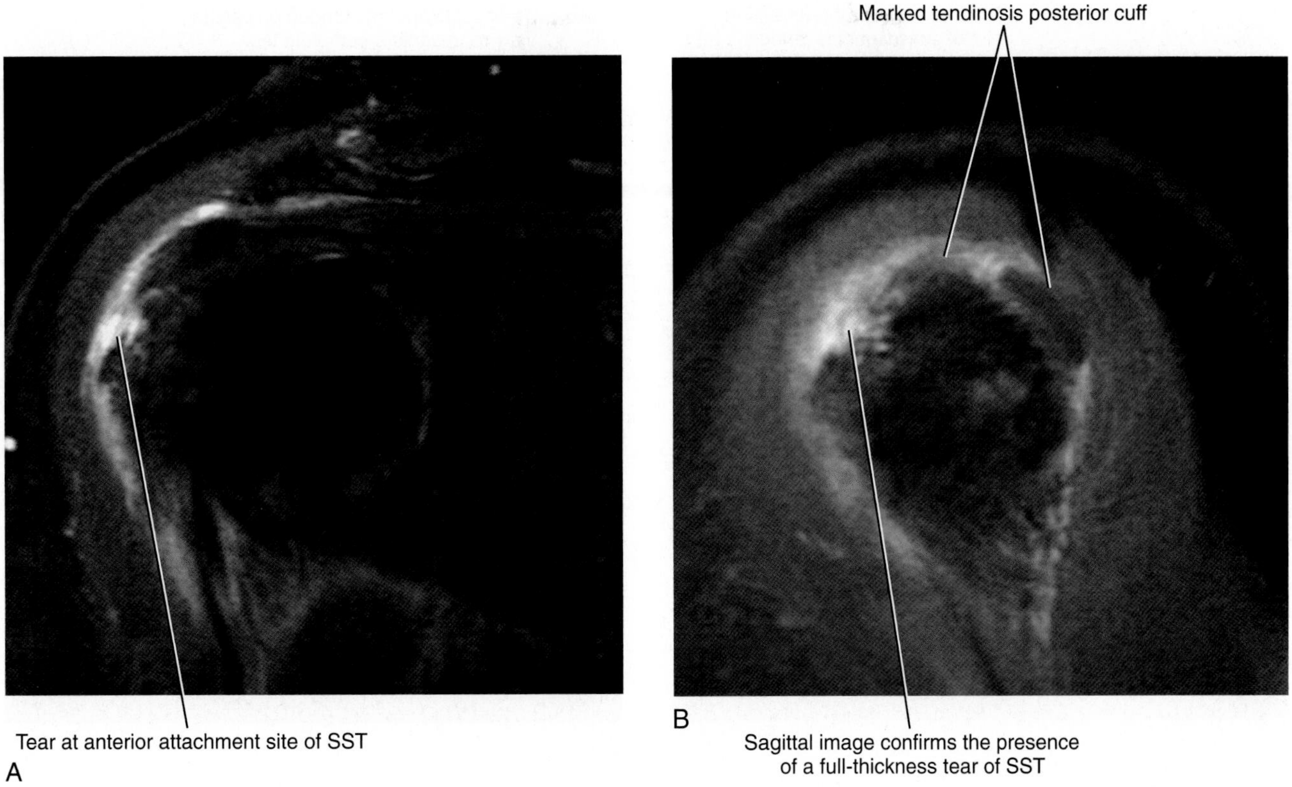
Marked tendinosis posterior cuff
Tear at anterior attachment site of SST
A
B
Sagittal image confirms the presence of a full-thickness tear of SST

Figure 7-26 Full-thickness tear of the anterior supraspinatus tendon (SST). A full-thickness tear often begins at the anterior supraspinatus bone-tendon interface and can only be seen on the most anterior coronal image (**A**) or on the sagittal images (**B**). It is critical to evaluate the most anterior coronal image to avoid missing these small full-thickness supraspinatus tendon tears. At this level, the sagittal and axial images can be very helpful in differentiating a partial- from a full-thickness tear.

be amenable to repair using a mattress type tendon-to-tendon repair technique.

Tears of the subscapularis tendon are best depicted on axial and sagittal images and are often associated with subluxation or dislocation of the biceps tendon out of the intertubercular groove (Fig. 7-27). The subscapularis tendon is typically seen covering the anterior portion of the humeral head on the sagittal imaging plane. Fluid within the expected location of the subscapularis tendon anterior to the humeral head indicates a complete tear with retraction of the torn tendon end.

A *complete tear* of a rotator cuff tendon is defined as a tear that disrupts the entire thickness of the tendon from anterior to posterior, usually resulting in significant musculotendinous retraction. MR images demonstrate complete discontinuity of the tendon, resulting in retraction of the musculotendinous junction. A high-riding humeral head is usually associated with an extensive tear of the rotator cuff, involving at least the supraspinatus and infraspinatus tendons, and in many cases a tear of the subscapularis tendon is also present. The high-riding humeral head is best depicted on coronal images and may be seen abutting the undersurface of the acromion on coronal or sagittal images.

After evaluation of the type and extent of rotator cuff tear, the cuff should also be evaluated for the presence of musculotendinous retraction and fatty atrophy.

The extent of musculotendinous retraction should be described in all patients with a full-thickness rotator cuff tear. The musculotendinous junction of the rotator cuff is normally positioned at the 12 o'clock position of the humeral head. The extent of retraction is best described as the medial-to-lateral gap between the torn ends of the tendon (Fig. 7-28). More than 3 cm of musculotendinous retraction

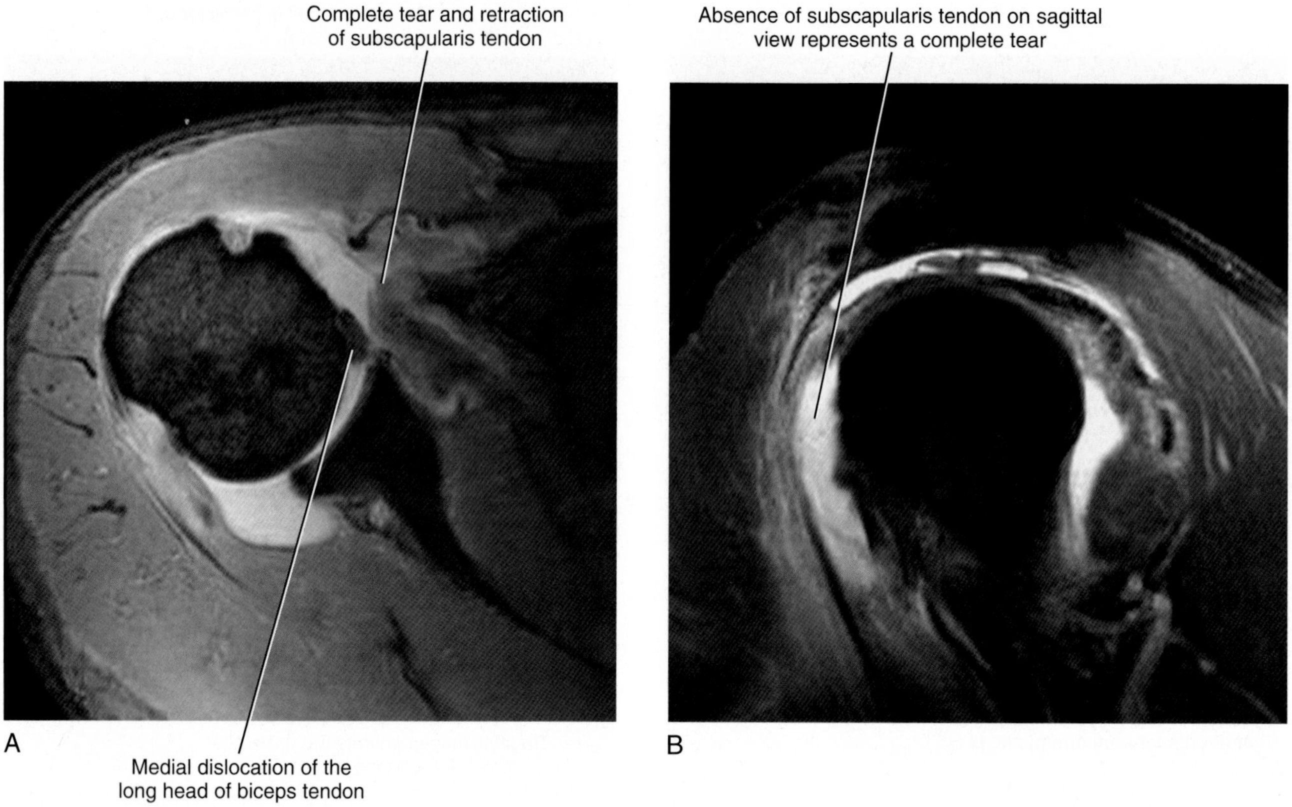
Complete tear and retraction of subscapularis tendon
Absence of subscapularis tendon on sagittal view represents a complete tear
A
B
Medial dislocation of the long head of biceps tendon

Figure 7-27 Subscapularis tendon tear. A, Axial T2-weighted image demonstrates complete avulsion and retraction of the subscapularis tendon with fluid signal present in the expected location of the distal subscapularis tendon. There is also medial dislocation of the long head of the biceps tendon. **B,** Oblique sagittal T2-weighted image demonstrates a tear area on the anterior portion of the humeral head consistent with a torn subscapularis tendon. Normally, the subscapularis tendon covers the anterior portion of the humeral head.

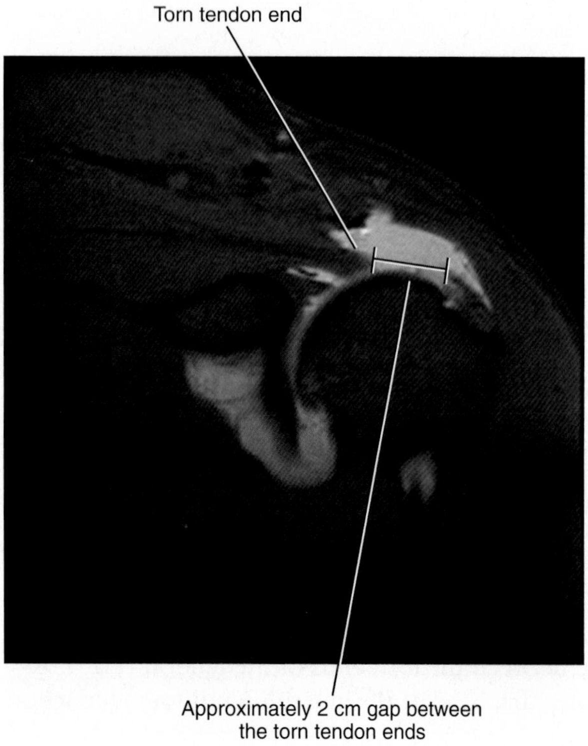
Torn tendon end
Approximately 2 cm gap between the torn tendon ends

Figure 7-28 Musculotendinous retraction. Coronal T2-weighted image demonstrates approximately 2 cm of retraction of the musculotendinous junction. A 2-cm gap between the torn tendon ends indicates the extent of musculotendinous retraction.

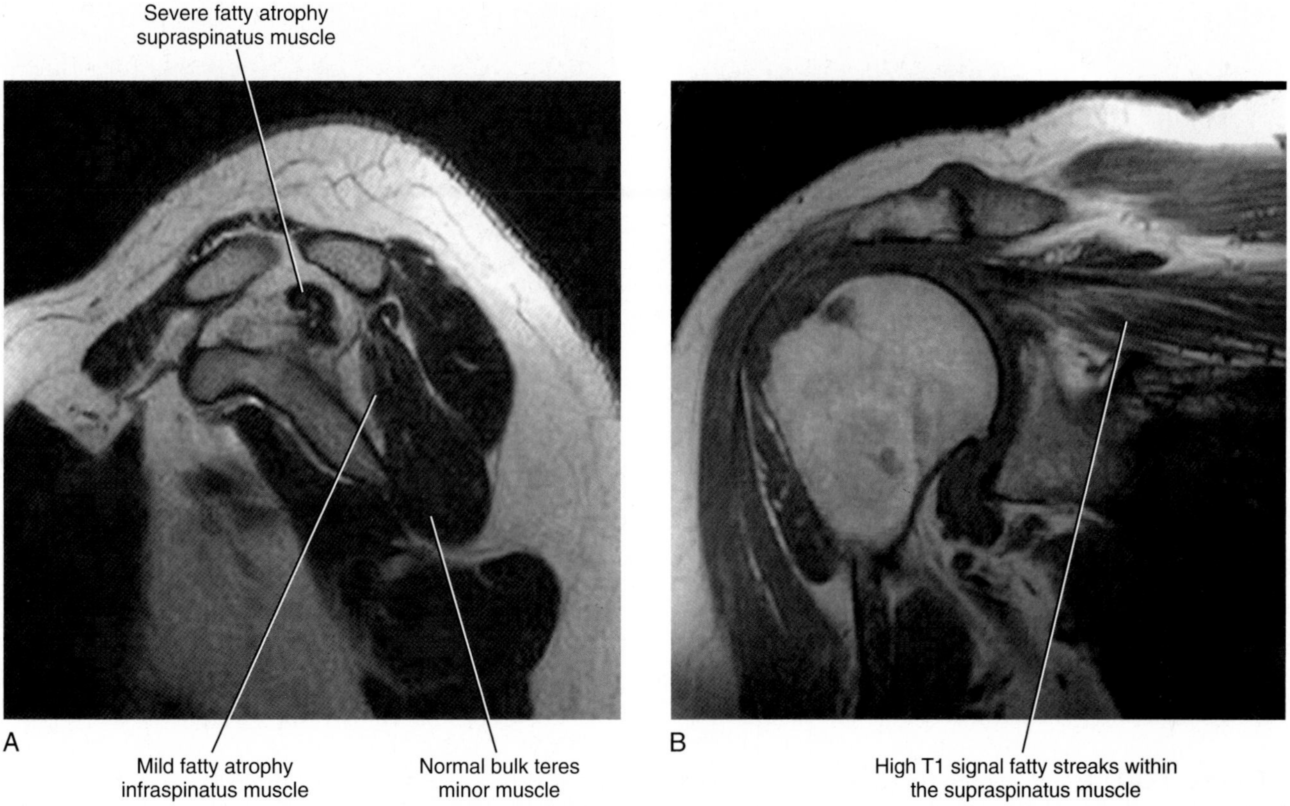
Severe fatty atrophy supraspinatus muscle
A
Mild fatty atrophy infraspinatus muscle
Normal bulk teres minor muscle
B
High T1 signal fatty streaks within the supraspinatus muscle

Figure 7-29 Fatty atrophy of the rotator cuff musculature. A, Oblique sagittal T1-weighted image demonstrates severe fatty atrophy of the supraspinatus muscle and mild fatty atrophy of the infraspinatus muscle. The supraspinatus muscle demonstrates a significant decrease of bulk when compared to the adjacent infraspinatus and teres minor muscles and there is extensive fat surrounding the supraspinatus muscle within the suprascapular fossa. **B,** T1-weighted oblique coronal image demonstrates high T1 signal streaking throughout the supraspinatus muscle representing mild fatty atrophy.

indicates a poor prognosis for cuff repair and is useful information for the surgeon during treatment planning.

Fatty atrophy of the rotator cuff musculature should be graded as mild, moderate, or severe. Fatty atrophy appears in one of two patterns on MRI. The most common MR appearance of fatty atrophy is loss of the normal muscle bulk. The supraspinatus muscle should completely fill the suprascapular fossa, and the circumference of each of the four rotator cuff muscles should be similar. Asymmetric loss of bulk of one or more of the cuff muscles is described as "decreased size" or as a "deconditioned" muscle, and this type of loss of normal bulk is reversible. Comparison among the four muscles is best made on the sagittal imaging plane using the most medial images, and the other rotator cuff muscles can act as an internal standard in depicting asymmetric muscle loss (Fig. 7-29A). A less common appearance of fatty atrophy is that of high T1 signal streaks (fatty streaks) within the substance of the muscle. This appearance is best seen on sagittal or coronal T1-weighted images and represents fat within the muscle (Fig. 7-29B). It also indicates fatty replacement of the muscle and represents irreversible fatty atrophy. Increasing grades of fatty atrophy worsen the prognosis for repair and is useful information for the surgeon during surgical planning.

There are several potential pitfalls with regard to MR evaluation of the rotator cuff tendons (Box 7-1). *Magic angle phenomenon* is a well-described MR artifact that results in increased signal intensity within a tendon that is oriented at a 55-degree angle relative to the main magnetic field. This artifact is primarily a short echo time (TE) phenomenon and is commonly seen when viewing the rotator cuff on short

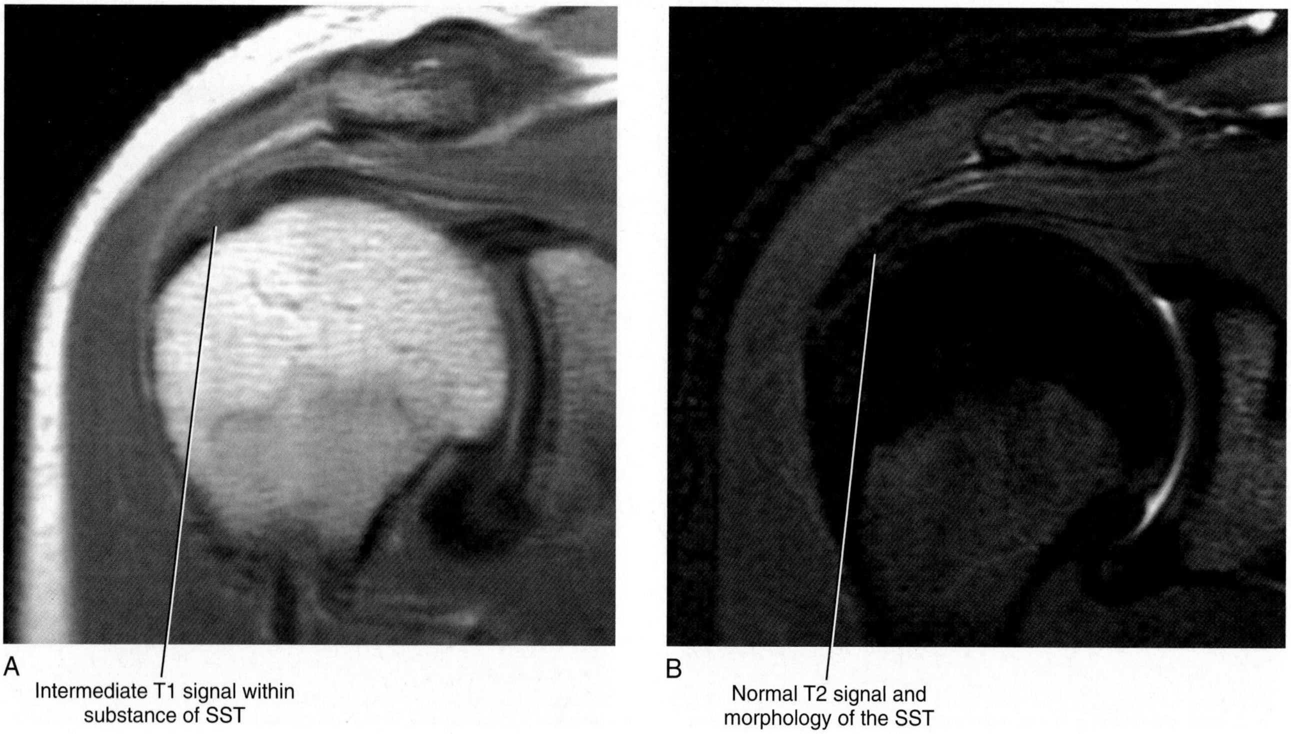
A
Intermediate T1 signal within substance of SST
B
Normal T2 signal and morphology of the SST

Figure 7-30 **Magic angle artifact. A,** Oblique coronal T1-weighted image demonstrates intermediate signal intensity within the supraspinatus tendon (SST) approximately 1 cm from its distal attachment. **B,** The tendon demonstrates normal morphology (no thickening) and appears dark on the T2-weighted image at the same level and these findings are consistent with magic angle phenomenon and should not be misinterpreted as rotator cuff pathology.

BOX 7-1 ROTATOR CUFF EVALUATION: COMMON MR PITFALLS

Magic angle phenomenon
Rotator interval
Overlap of the supraspinatus and infraspinatus tendons
Striated appearance of the normal tendon layers

TE sequences (T1-weighted or proton density). Magic angle phenomenon, when present in the rotator cuff, occurs in the curved portion of the tendon approximately 1 cm from its insertion onto the humeral head and mimics tendinopathy or tear. Magic angle can easily be differentiated from tendon pathology by comparing the T1-weighted images with the T2-weighted images (Fig. 7-30). If the increased T1-weighted signal is a result of magic angle, the tendon morphology will be normal and the area of increased signal on T1-weighted images will appear dark on the T2-weighted images at the same level. The presence of tendinopathy demonstrates intermediate T2-weighted signal and possibly thickening of the tendon, and tear demonstrates high T2-signal (fluid) within the tendon. The upshot is that tendon pathology should be read off of the T2 images.

The MR appearance of the rotator interval (described in greater detail in the next section) is another potential pitfall with regard to rotator cuff imaging. The rotator interval appears as a triangular-shaped defect in the region of the anterior cuff between the anterior margin of the supraspinatus muscle and the superior margin of the subscapularis muscle. The rotator interval is best seen on the oblique sagittal images (Fig. 7-31A and B). The interval contains the long head of the biceps tendon and is covered by the coracohumeral ligament. The defect created by the interval tapers peripherally and should not be misinterpreted as a tear of the rotator cuff.

Overlap of the separate tendon slips of the supraspinatus and infraspinatus tendons can create a zone of increased signal in the region of the posterior cuff that mimics pathology (Fig. 7-31C). This pitfall is

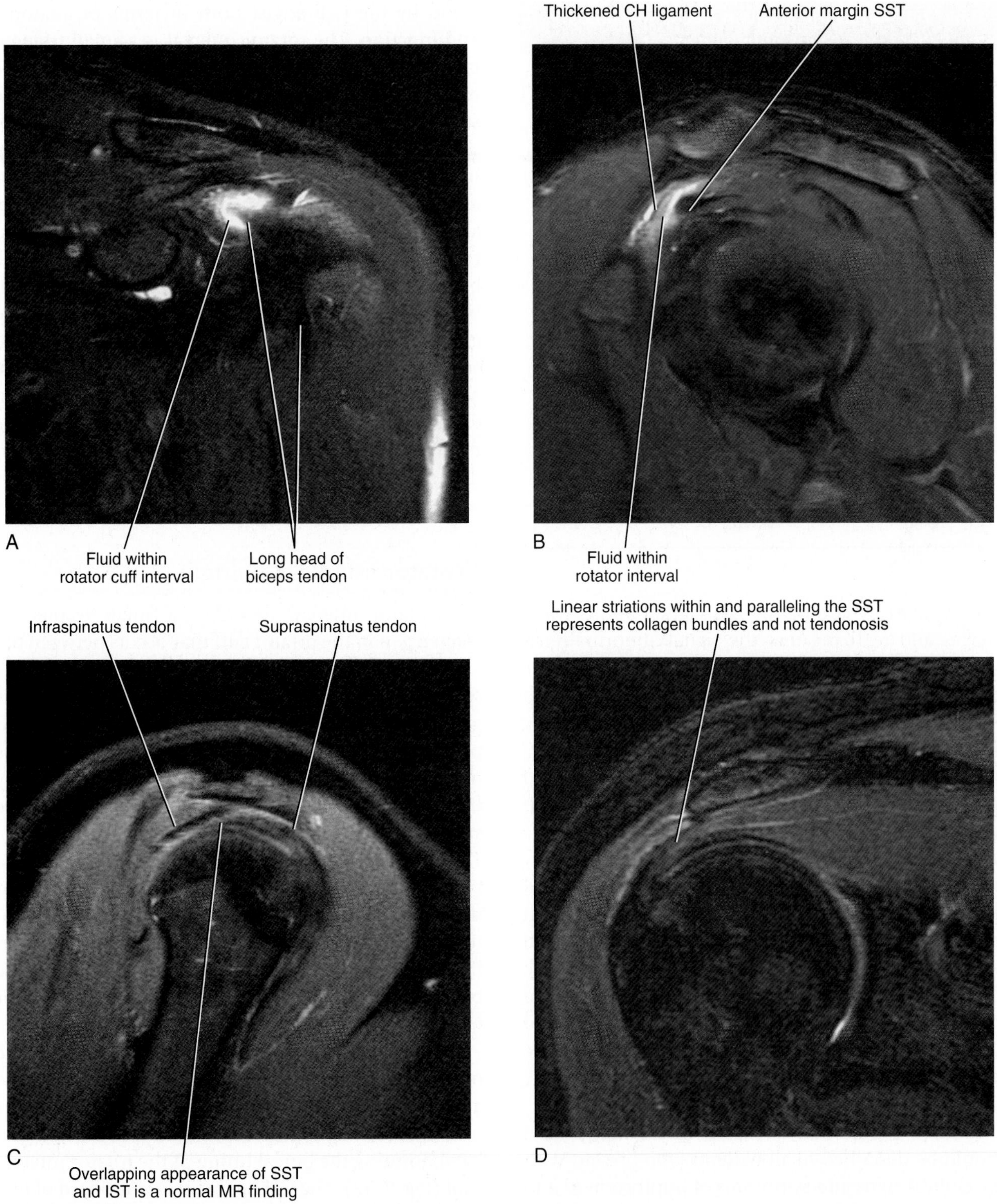
Thickened CH ligament
Anterior margin SST
A
Fluid within rotator cuff interval
Long head of biceps tendon
B
Fluid within rotator interval
Infraspinatus tendon
Supraspinatus tendon
Linear striations within and paralleling the SST represents collagen bundles and not tendonosis
C
Overlapping appearance of SST and IST is a normal MR finding
D

Figure 7-31 Mimics of rotator cuff pathology. Oblique coronal (**A**) and oblique sagittal (**B**) T2-weighted images show fluid within the rotator interval and edema within the coracohumeral (CH) ligament mimicking cuff pathology. **C,** Oblique sagittal T2-weighted image demonstrates overlap of the supraspinatus (SST) and infraspinatus (IST) tendons. This normal appearance should not be misinterpreted as a defect within the cuff. **D,** Oblique coronal T2-weighted image demonstrates linear areas of signal alteration within the SST that parallel the course of the tendon. This striated appearance represents the separate bundles or layers of collagen within the cuff and not cuff pathology.

Table 7-4 What the Surgeon Needs to Know in the Patient with Signs of Impingement

Ariatomic Structure	Potential Abnormalites
Acromion	Types I–IV Anterior or lateral down-sloping Inferiorly directed osteophyte Unfused os acromiale
Acromioclavicular joint	Osteoarthritis Mass effect on underlying cuff
Coracoacromial ligament	Thickening, nodularity, calcification
Subacromial subdeltoid bursa	Fluid, surrounding edema Calcification
Rotator cuff	Tendinopathy (mild, moderate, severe) Partial-thickness tear (articular, interstitial, bursal) Full-thickness tear (size, location) Musculotendinous retraction (size of tendon gap) Fatty atrophy (mild, moderate, severe)

best avoided by comparing the sagittal and coronal images and realizing that the signal abnormality is occurring at the junction of the two tendons. The signal abnormality should be intermediate on both T1 and T2 sequences with no fluid signal extending into or through the substance of the tendon.

One last potential pitfall with regard to rotator cuff imaging is related histologically to the rotator cuff tendons. Each tendon is composed of five separate collagen bundles, which run at angles slightly oblique to one another. On high-resolution MR images these separate bundles can occasionally result in a striated appearance of the tendon and should not be misinterpreted as tendinosis (see Fig. 7-31D). The normal appearance is that of thin linear areas of intermediate signal intensity seen on both T1- and T2-weighted images, which parallels the course of the tendon. Again, the presence of fluid signal within the substance of the tendon is abnormal.

Table 7-4 summarizes those MR findings that should be described in all patients who present with the clinical signs and symptoms of impingement and rotator cuff pathology.

ROTATOR INTERVAL

The rotator interval is an anatomically complex area of the glenohumeral joint that is often misunderstood by the radiologist both in terms of anatomy and function. The rotator interval is a small triangular-shaped gap in the anterosuperior aspect of the rotator cuff, bordered by the anterior margin of the supraspinatus and the superior margin of the subscapularis muscle, which allows passage of the long head of the biceps tendon from an intra-articular to an extra-articular location. The rotator interval plays an important role in glenohumeral stability and ensures normal function of the long head of the biceps tendon. Injury or pathology of the interval can be associated with altered range of motion of the glenohumeral joint, adhesive capsulitis, and progressive signs of impingement and/or degenerative arthropathy. Although isolated injuries of the interval can occur, they are often associated with tears of the most anterior aspect of the supraspinatus tendon and the superior leading edge of the subscapularis tendon.

Rotator Interval Anatomy

The rotator interval describes a small triangular-shaped gap in the rotator cuff that occurs between the anterior margin of the supraspinatus tendon and the superior margin of the subscapularis tendon. This gap is formed by the interposition of the coracoid process between the supraspinatus and subscapularis muscles. The roof of the rotator interval is formed by the coracohumeral ligament (bursal surface) and the superior glenohumeral ligament (articular surface). The intra-articular portion of the long head of the biceps tendon sits within the rotator interval. Together, the coracohumeral and superior glenohumeral ligaments form the biceps tendon "sling" and are primarily responsible for stability of the long head of the biceps tendon as it transitions from its intra-articular to its extra-articular position.

The coracohumeral (CH) ligament arises from the base of the coracoid process and then crosses the anterior aspect of the glenohumeral joint to insert onto the lesser and greater tuberosities of the humeral head, forming the bursal lining of the rotator interval roof (Fig. 7-32). The CH ligament is composed of two separate limbs (medial and lateral). The medial limb courses inferiorly from its origin on the coracoid process to insert onto the superior margin of the subscapularis tendon and the lesser tuberosity. It is the medial limb of the CH ligament that is primarily responsible for preventing medial subluxation of the long head of the biceps tendon. The lateral limb of

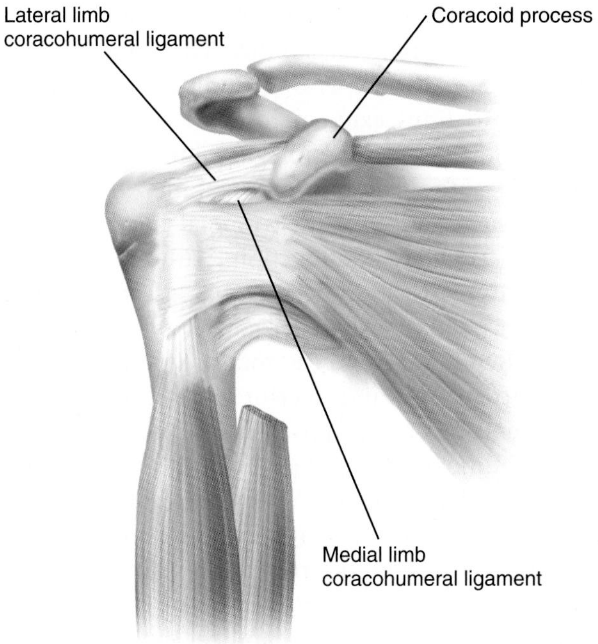
Lateral limb
coracohumeral ligament
Coracoid process
Medial limb
coracohumeral ligament

Figure 7-32 Coracohumeral ligament. Diagram shows the medial and lateral limbs of the coracohumeral ligament.

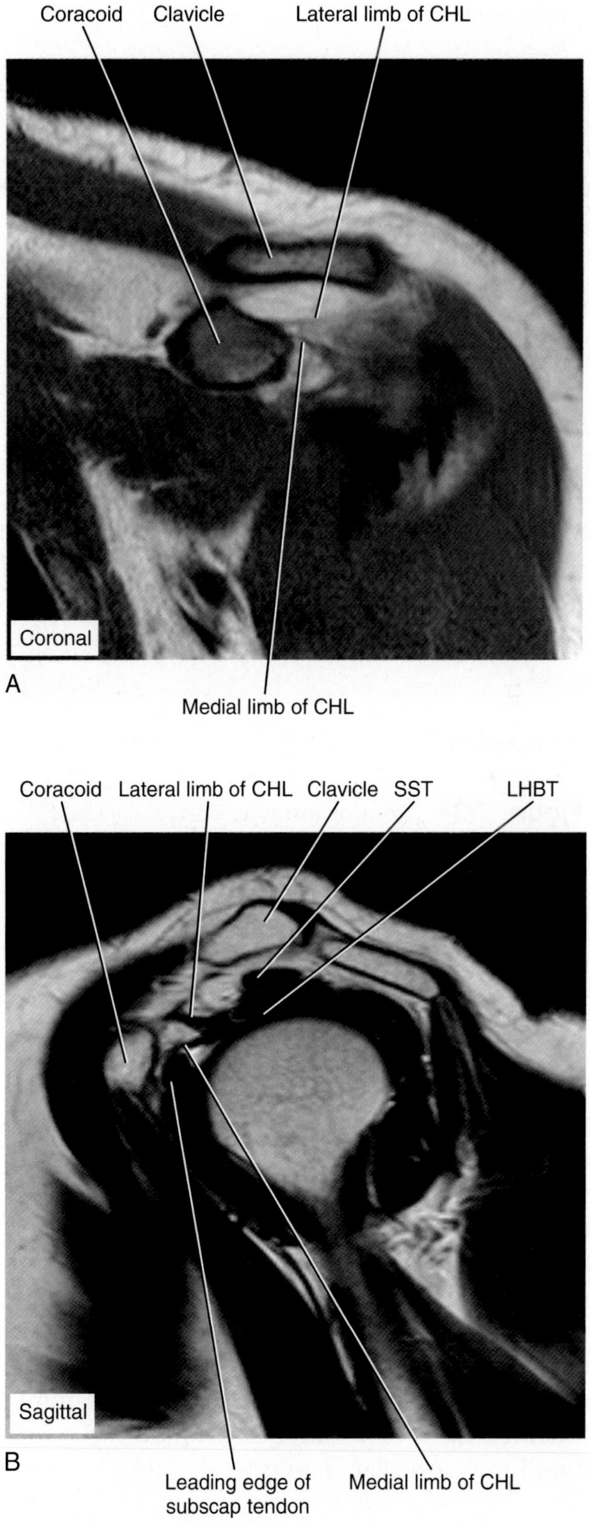
Coracoid
Clavicle
Lateral limb of CHL
Coronal
A
Medial limb of CHL
Coracoid
Lateral limb of CHL
Clavicle
SST
LHBT
Sagittal
B
Leading edge of
subscap tendon
Medial limb of CHL

Figure 7-33 Coracohumeral ligament. Oblique coronal (**A**) and oblique sagittal (**B**) MR images show the medial and lateral limbs of the coracohumeral ligament (CHL) and the relationship of the adjacent subscapularis (subscap) tendon, supraspinatus tendon (SST) and the long head of the biceps tendon (LHBT).

the CH ligament courses in a more horizontal fashion from its origin on the coracoid process to its insertion on the anterior edge of the supraspinatus tendon and the adjacent greater tuberosity (Fig. 7-33).

The superior glenohumeral ligament arises from the superior glenoid tubercle adjacent to the origin of the long head of the biceps tendon. It courses deep to the coracoid process and deep to the coracohumeral ligament to insert onto the lesser tuberosity of the humeral head and makes up the articular lining of the roof of the rotator interval. Together, the CH ligament and the superior glenohumeral ligament surround the intra-articular portion of the long head of the biceps tendon functioning as the primary stabilizer of the tendon. The long head of the biceps tendon originates from the superior glenoid tubercle and then crosses the joint in an oblique fashion sitting within the rotator interval and covered by the coracohumeral and superior glenohumeral ligaments. The long head of the biceps tendon exits the joint at the level of the intertubercular groove, where it is completely covered and stabilized by these two ligaments. At this point, the combination of the medial limb of the CH ligament and superior glenohumeral ligament act as a sling to prevent medial subluxation

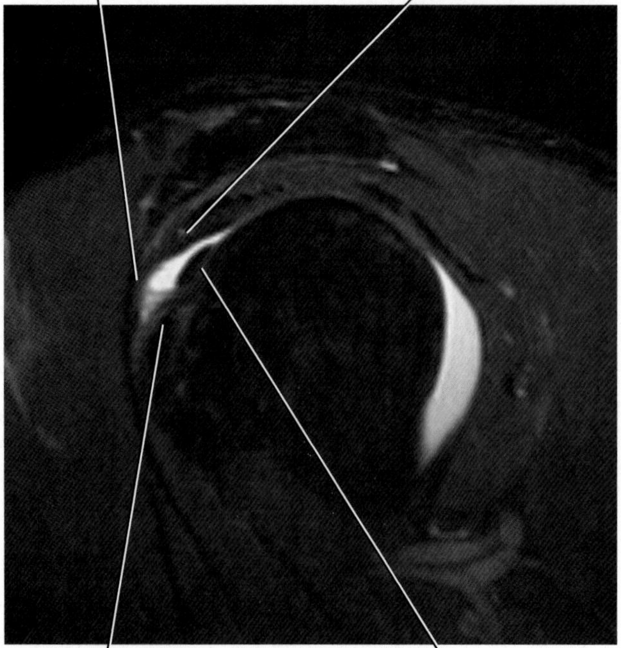
CH ligament
SST
Subscap tendon
LHBT

Figure 7-34 Rotator interval. Oblique sagittal T1-weighted image with intra-articular gadolinium shows the rotator interval located between the anterior margin of the supraspinatus tendon (SST) and the superior margin of the subscapularis (subscap) tendon. The coracohumeral (CH) ligament forms the roof of the interval, and the long head of the biceps tendon (LHBT) sits within the interval.

of the long head of the biceps tendon as it exits the joint.

On MRI, the superior glenohumeral ligament is best visualized as a separate structure in the axial plane, whereas the coracohumeral ligament is best seen in the oblique sagittal or oblique coronal planes (see Fig. 7-33). The rotator interval, as a unit, however, is best visualized and evaluated for pathology in the oblique sagittal plane, especially when the joint is distended either by a native effusion or by the injection of intra-articular contrast (Fig. 7-34).

Rotator Interval Function and Pathology

The rotator interval describes a small area of the anterosuperior glenohumeral joint capsule that lacks reinforcement by the overlying rotator cuff tendon, which at first glance seems rather insignificant with regard to shoulder function and stability. The rotator interval, however, does play an important role with regard to glenohumeral stability. The coracohumeral ligament and the superior glenohumeral ligament combine to limit external rotation of the humeral head, whereas the superior glenohumeral ligament contributes to glenohumeral stability by limiting inferior subluxation of the humeral head while the arm is in 0 degrees of abduction (with the arm down by the side). Disease processes that affect the rotator interval can limit external rotation of the humeral head, whereas injury to the rotator interval can contribute to anterior and inferior instability of the glenohumeral joint and can also allow superior migration of the humeral head, thus leading to progressive degenerative arthropathy. The rotator interval also plays an important role with regard to the stability of the long head of the biceps tendon (Table 7-5).

It is a common misperception that the subscapularis muscle is the primary stabilizer of the long head of the biceps tendon and that disruption or avulsion of the subscapularis tendon results in medial subluxation of the long head of the biceps tendon. In fact, the coracohumeral ligament in combination with the superior glenohumeral ligament provides the primary stabilizing force for the long head of the biceps tendon. An intact rotator interval and coracohumeral ligament prevent medial subluxation of the long head of the biceps tendon even in the presence of a complete tear of the subscapularis tendon. An isolated tear of the coracohumeral ligament at the level of the pulley mechanism, however, allows medial subluxation of the long head of the biceps tendon even with an intact subscapularis tendon. Medial subluxation of the long head of the biceps tendon on the basis of an isolated tear of the coracohumeral

Table 7-5	Rotator Interval
Anatomy	Superior border—leading edge of supraspinatus tendon Inferior border—superior margin of subscapularis tendon Roof Coracohumeral ligament (medial/lateral limbs) Superior glenohumeral ligament Contents—Long head of biceps tendon
Function	Prevents excessive external rotation of humeral head Prevents superior migration of humeral head
Pathologic conditions	Traumatic disruption Inflammatory arthritis Synovitis (adhesive capsulitis)

ligament may actually be the precipitating event that results in interstitial tearing of the subscapularis tendon.

A tear of the rotator interval can result from an acute traumatic event or secondary to repetitive microtrauma, and although isolated tears of the rotator interval have been reported, it is much more common for them to occur in conjunction with a tear of the anterior aspect of the supraspinatus tendon. Disruption of the rotator interval results in shoulder pain and allows superior migration of the humeral head (micro-instability). Isolated tears of the rotator interval can be corrected arthroscopically by suturing the defect closed. MR findings of an isolated rotator interval tear include high T2 signal isolated to the rotator interval or disruption of the capsule of the rotator interval (Fig. 7-35). Direct MR arthrography improves detection of the disrupted capsule at the level of the interval and may actually demonstrate leakage of contrast through the defect into the subacromial subdeltoid bursa.

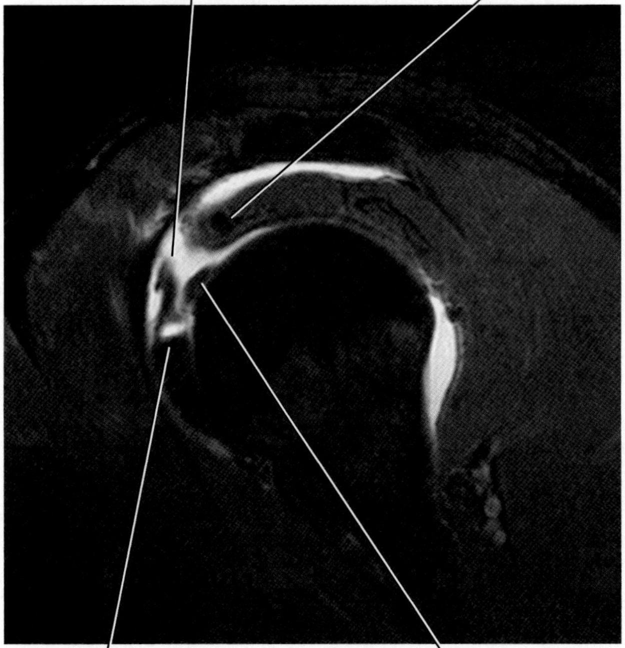
Disrupted CH ligament with
contrast leaking into SASD bursa
SST intact
Subscap tendon
LHBT

Figure 7-35 Isolated rotator interval tear. A 20-year-old man injured his shoulder while throwing. Oblique sagittal T1-weighted image with intra-articular gadolinium shows complete disruption of the coracohumeral (CH) ligament and contrast leaking through the defect into the overlying subacromial subdeltoid (SASD) bursa. The adjacent supraspinatus and subscapularis tendons were normal in appearance in all imaging planes with no adjacent rotator cuff tear.

The rotator interval as an unsupported part of the capsule is also prone to disorders that affect the synovium, including inflammatory arthritides and adhesive capsulitis. Evaluation of the rotator interval in these disorders is best performed with either direct or indirect MR arthrography using the oblique sagittal images.

Adhesive Capsulitis (Frozen Shoulder)

Adhesive capsulitis is a pathologic entity, unique to the shoulder that is characterized by inflammation and thickening of the synovium. The inflammatory changes are especially prominent in those areas of the shoulder that lack reinforcement by the rotator cuff tendons, primarily the rotator interval and axillary recess. The patients most often affected are women 40 to 70 years of age. They present clinically with the complaint of insidious onset of shoulder pain followed by progressive stiffness and weakness of the joint. The onset of symptoms is often related to a previous episode of minor trauma; however, it may be associated with preexisting rheumatologic disorders or diabetes or may be idiopathic in nature. At the time of clinical presentation, the patient is often initially misdiagnosed with impingement syndrome or rotator cuff pathology because the signs and symptoms broadly overlap with those of adhesive capsulitis. Physical examination demonstrates a painful restriction of motion of the shoulder in all directions, but the most pronounced restriction of motion usually involves the external rotation of the humeral head. Treatment of adhesive capsulitis initially involves physical therapy combined with an oral anti-inflammatory drug, whereas refractory cases may require a selective arthroscopic capsular release (Table 7-6).

The clinical presentation and age distribution of patients with adhesive capsulitis overlap with those of rotator cuff pathology. The radiologist must therefore be cognizant of this entity and must be capable of differentiating between rotator cuff pathology and adhesive capsulitis on the basis of imaging findings. No conventional radiographic signs are diagnostic of adhesive capsulitis, although radiographs may be helpful in excluding other sources of pain and decreased range of motion. Conventional

Table 7-6 Adhesive Capsulitis

Risk factors	Female 40–70 yr Preceding minor trauma Rheumatologic disorders Diabetes
Clinical presentation	Insidious onset of pain and stiffness Decreased range of motion Misinterpreted as rotator cuff pathology
Arthrography	Decrease joint volume (<10 mL) Small contracted axillary pouch Lack of contrast in long head of biceps tendon sheath
MRI	Thickened axillary capsule (>4 mm) Pericapsular edema/enhancement Synovitis in rotator interval Thickened coracohumeral ligament

arthrography demonstrates a small contracted joint capsule with a decreased joint volume of less than 10 mL. The axillary pouch appears small and contracted, and there is a lack of contrast filling the long head of the biceps tendon sheath.

Findings on MRI can be subtle and include abnormal soft tissue in the rotator interval, obliteration of the subcoracoid fat triangle, and thickening of the coracohumeral ligament (Fig. 7-36A). There may also be thickening of the joint capsule of more than 4 mm in the region of the axillary pouch (Fig. 7-36B). Inflammatory changes of the capsule may also be seen as increased T2 signal surrounding the capsule of the axillary pouch. Direct MR arthrography may be helpful in establishing the correct diagnosis in two ways. First, there will be a decreased joint volume of less than 10 mL, similar to conventional arthrography. Second, the contrast helps to outline and define the abnormal soft tissue in the rotator interval. Indirect MR arthrography, however, appears to be most specific for establishing the diagnosis of adhesive capsulitis on the basis of imaging. Findings specific for the diagnosis include enhancement of the abnormal soft tissues within the rotator interval combined with enhancement of the capsule and adjacent soft tissues in the region of the axillary pouch (Fig. 7-36C and D).

GLENOHUMERAL INSTABILITY

The topic of glenohumeral instability is complex, and our knowledge and understanding of the synergistic role that the various anatomic structures play in maintaining normal shoulder mobility continue to evolve. In establishing an accurate diagnosis and in developing a successful treatment plan, the surgeon must be familiar with the anatomy and biomechanics of the shoulder and must understand the various patterns of instability. For the radiologist, the challenge is to develop a thorough understanding of the normal anatomy of the glenohumeral joint and its many normal variations and to be able to distinguish these variants from the numerous lesions of instability on the basis of imaging. This section provides a brief overview of the normal imaging anatomy of the shoulder as it pertains to glenohumeral instability. The various lesions of instability are described, and helpful hints and imaging strategies are provided to aid in differentiating labral pathology from the normal labrum and its many anatomic variants.

The configuration of the glenohumeral joint, with a shallow glenoid fossa and the large articular surface of the humeral head, allows for an extensive range of motion of the upper extremity, but this configuration also places the shoulder at high risk for instability. Numerous soft tissue structures contribute to the stability of the glenohumeral joint. These include the static stabilizers (glenoid labrum, joint capsule, and glenohumeral ligaments) and the dynamic stabilizers (rotator cuff and long head of the biceps tendon).

Glenohumeral instability is defined clinically as the symptomatic displacement of the humeral head out of the glenoid fossa. This may range from mild subluxation to complete dislocation. Various descriptors can be used to further categorize shoulder instability. These include the temporal relationship of the instability to the antecedent trauma (first-time versus recurrent), the degree (subluxation versus dislocation), and the direction of instability (anterior, posterior, inferior, or multidirectional). The orthopedic community uses a classification system that places glenohumeral instability into one of two broad categories. The first group of patients gives a history of antecedent trauma followed by unidirectional subluxation or dislocation. The traumatic event results in a Bankart lesion or one of its variants and typically requires surgery to correct the instability. This group of patients is referred to by the acronym TUBS (trauma, unidirectional, Bankart, surgery). The second group of patients gives no history of antecedent trauma, and they typically display bilateral multidirectional glenohumeral instability. The instability is on the basis of capsular laxity rather than on the

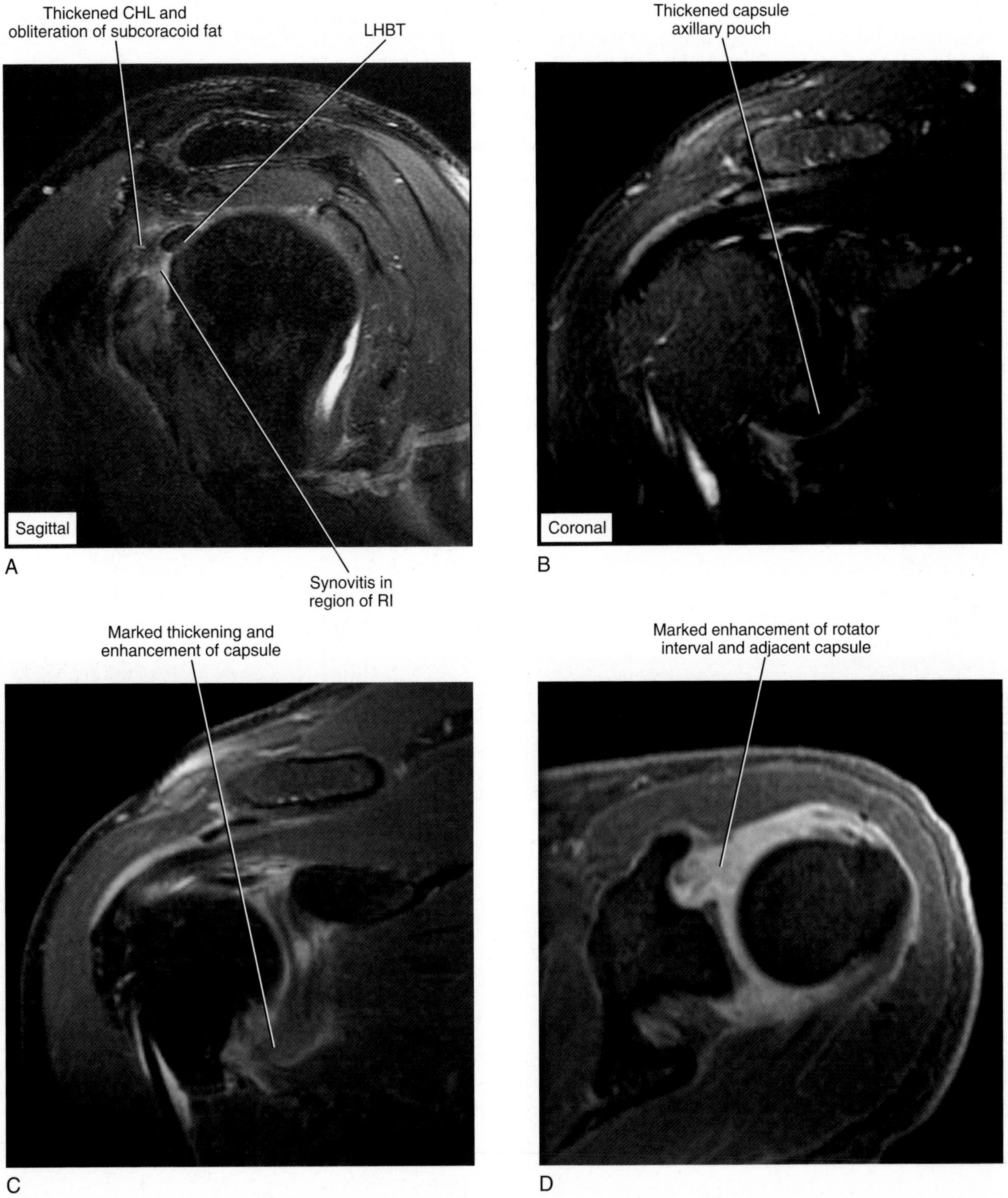
Thickened CHL and
obliteration of subcoracoid fat
LHBT
Sagittal
A
Synovitis in
region of RI
Thickened capsule
axillary pouch
Coronal
B
Marked thickening and
enhancement of capsule
C
Marked enhancement of rotator
interval and adjacent capsule
D

Figure 7-36 Adhesive capsulitis (frozen shoulder). A, Sagittal T2-weighted image demonstrates extensive soft tissue within the rotator interval and obliteration of the subcoracoid fat triangle. **B,** Coronal T2-weighted image demonstrates marked thickening of the anterior capsule as well as mild adjacent soft tissue edema. Coronal (**C**) and axial (**D**) T1-weighted images with fat saturation following administration of intravenous gadolinium demonstrate marked enhancement of the soft tissues surrounding the capsule. CHL, coracohumeral ligament, LHBT, long head of biceps tendon.

basis of labral pathology. These patients are treated first with rehabilitation (strengthening of the rotator cuff musculature) and only after therapeutic failure are offered a capsular-tightening procedure. This group of patients is referred to by the acronym AMBRI (atraumatic, multidirectional, bilateral, rehabilitation, and occasionally requiring an inferior capsular shift). The AMBRI type of instability can usually be diagnosed solely on the basis of history and clinical examination. MR imaging is of little value in the evaluation of these patients because no specific MR finding is diagnostic of multidirectional atraumatic shoulder instability. MR imaging can be very helpful, however, in evaluating patients with a post-traumatic unidirectional instability or patients with unexplained shoulder pain.

Normal Labrum and Capsular Anatomy

The glenoid labrum is a fibrocartilaginous structure that encircles the glenoid rim and serves to deepen the glenoid fossa. On MRI, the normal labrum should appear dark on all pulse sequences. It is usually triangular in appearance, but it may also demonstrate a rounded or blunted appearance. Even when blunted or rounded, the labrum should demonstrate a smooth contour with no irregularity of the surface and no intrinsic signal abnormality. The anterior and posterior labrum is best evaluated on axial imaging, whereas the superior labrum is best seen on the oblique coronal images (Fig. 7-37).

The glenohumeral ligaments represent bandlike areas of capsular thickening that are best visualized

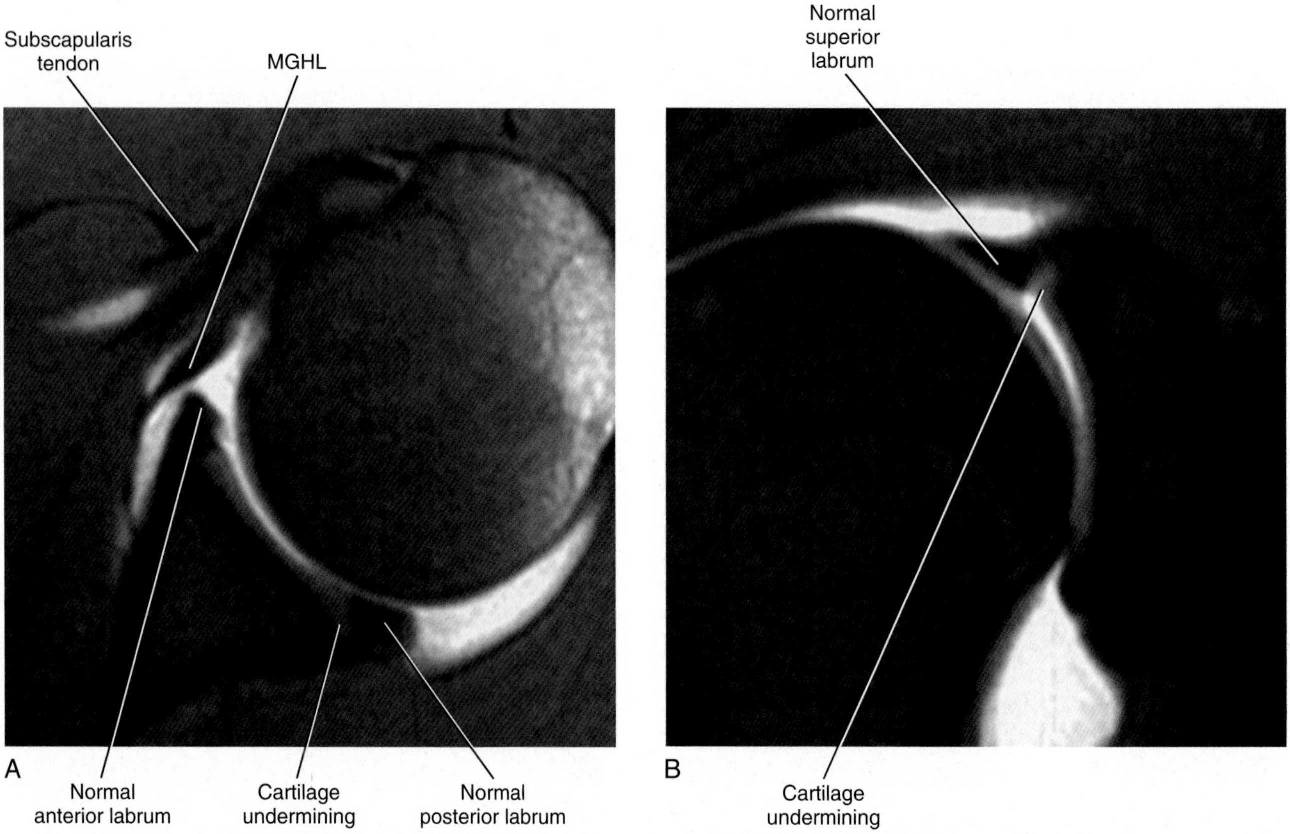
Subscapularis tendon
MGHL
A
Normal anterior labrum
Cartilage undermining
Normal posterior labrum
Normal superior labrum
B
Cartilage undermining

Figure 7-37 Normal labrum. A, Axial image shows the normal anterior and posterior labrum to be triangular in appearance with homogeneous low signal intensity. The middle glenohumeral ligament (MGHL) is located superficial to the anterior labrum and deep to the subscapularis tendon. **B,** Oblique coronal image shows the normal appearance of the superior labrum. It is dark on all pulse sequences and demonstrates a triangular appearance with normal undermining of intermediate signal intensity hyaline articular cartilage.

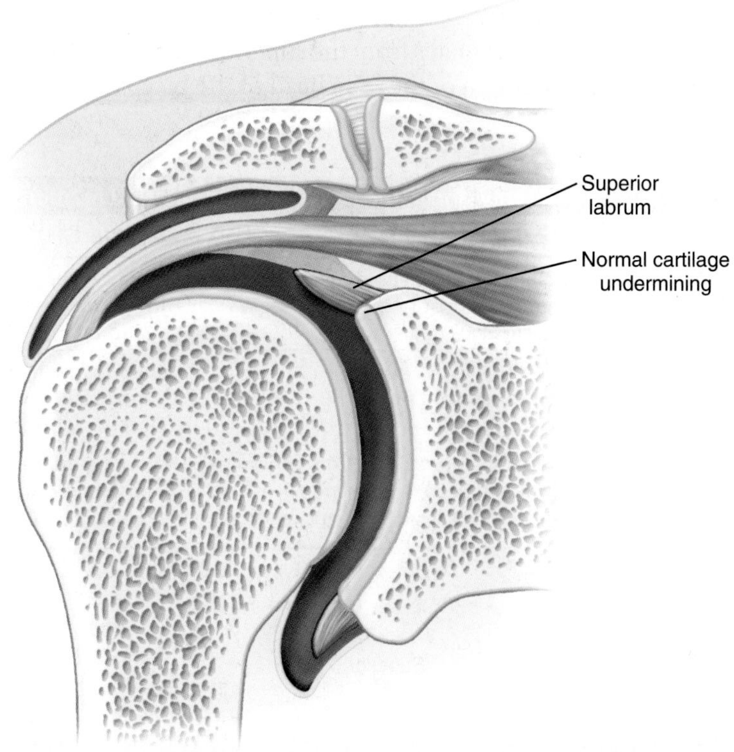
Superior
labrum
Normal cartilage
undermining

C

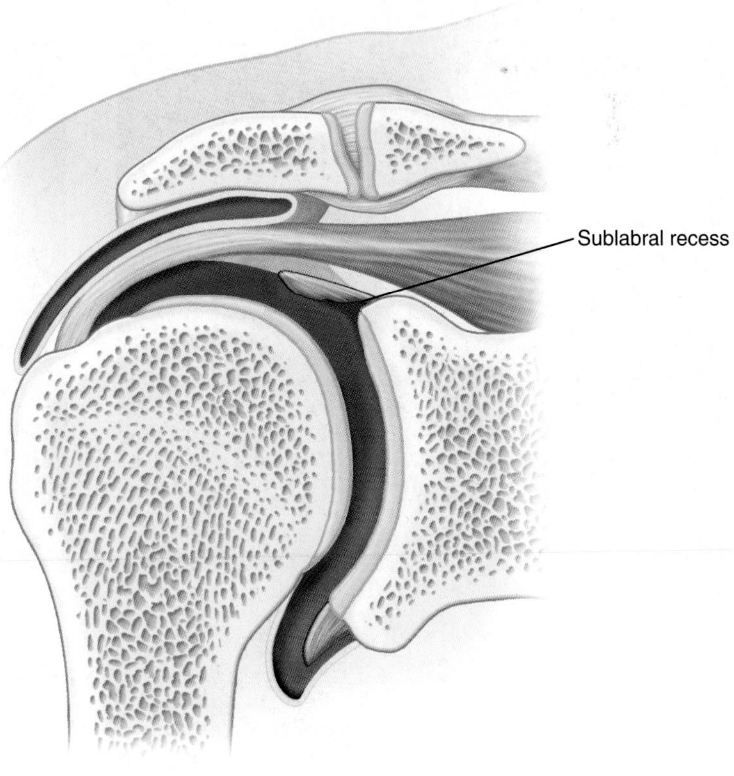
Sublabral recess

D

Figure 7-37, cont'd **C,** Normal cartilage undermining. **D,** Normal sublabral recess.

from inside the joint capsule. There are three glenohumeral ligaments (superior, middle, and inferior), and they play varying roles in stabilizing the glenohumeral joint (Table 7-7). The superior glenohumeral ligament (SGHL) originates from the superior glenoid tubercle near the origin of the long head of the biceps tendon. It is best observed on axial MR images since it parallels the coracoid process and then swings laterally to insert onto the superior aspect of the lesser tuberosity at the level where the long head of the biceps tendon exits the joint (Fig. 7-38A). The SGHL helps prevent inferior subluxation of the humeral

Table 7-7 Anatomy and Function of Glenohumeral Ligaments (GHL)

	Superior GHL	Middle GHL	Inferior GHL
Anatomy	Origin: Superior glenoid tubercle Insertion: Superior aspect of lesser tuberosity	Origin: Superior glenoid tubercle Insertion: Deep fibers subscapular and inferior lesser tuberosity	Origin: Inferior glenoid rim Insertion: Cuff-like insertion along medial humeral neck
MRI	Axial Parallels coracoid process	Axial (variable in size) Superficial to anterior labrum Deep to subscapularis tendon	Axial, coronal, ABER Anterior band, posterior band, axillary pouch
Function	Prevents inferior subluxation of humeral head at 0 degrees abduction Stabilizes long head of biceps tendon	Prevents external rotation of humeral head between 45 and 60 degrees of external abduction	Prevents anterior subluxation of humeral head during full abduction/external rotation

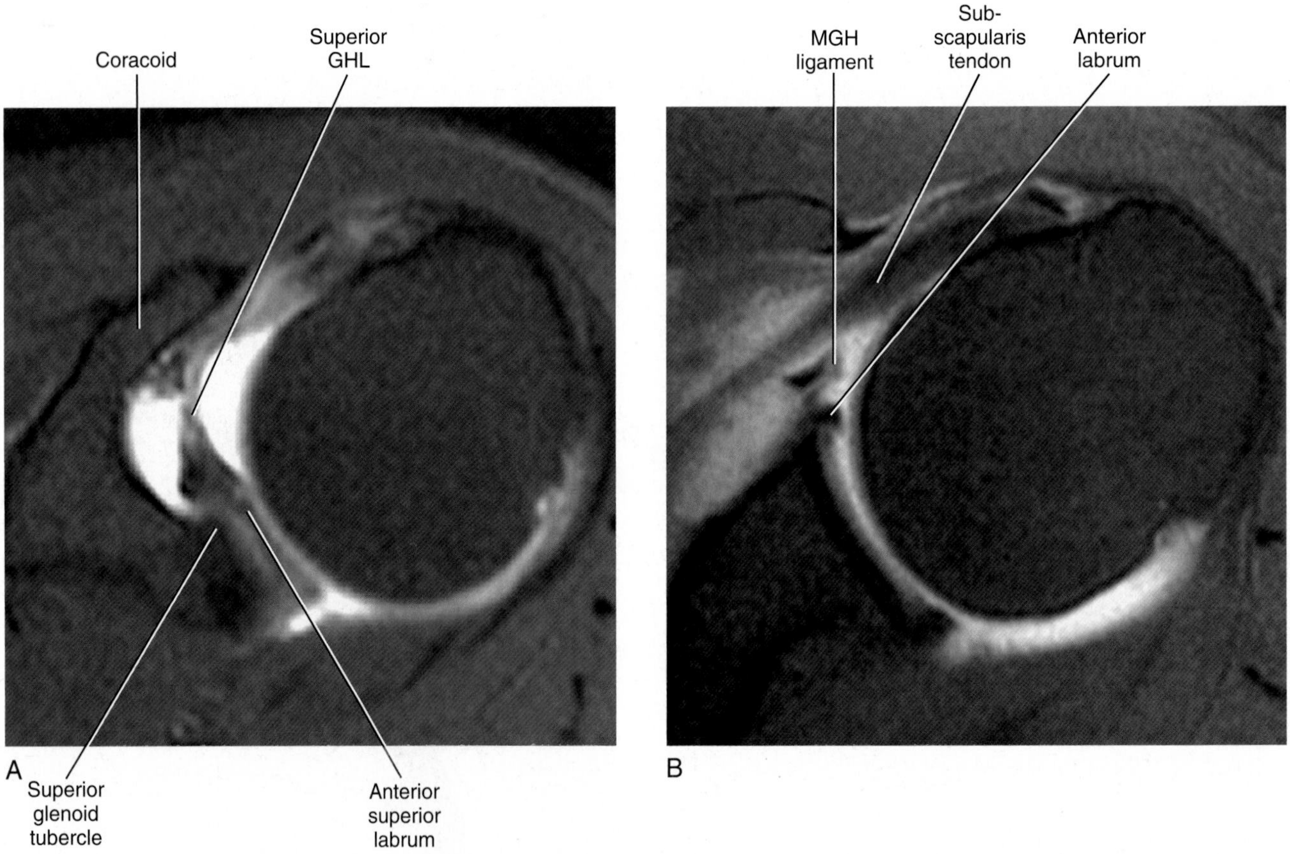
Coracoid
Superior GHL
Superior glenoid tubercle
Anterior superior labrum
A
MGH ligament
Sub-scapularis tendon
Anterior labrum
B

Figure 7-38 Glenohumeral ligaments. A, Axial image shows the normal appearance of the superior glenohumeral (GHL) ligament. It originates on the superior glenoid tubercle and then parallels the coracoid process, finally blending with the deep fibers of the superior aspect of the subscapularis tendon. **B,** Axial image shows the middle glenohumeral (MGH) ligament superficial to the anterior labrum and deep to the subscapularis tendon.

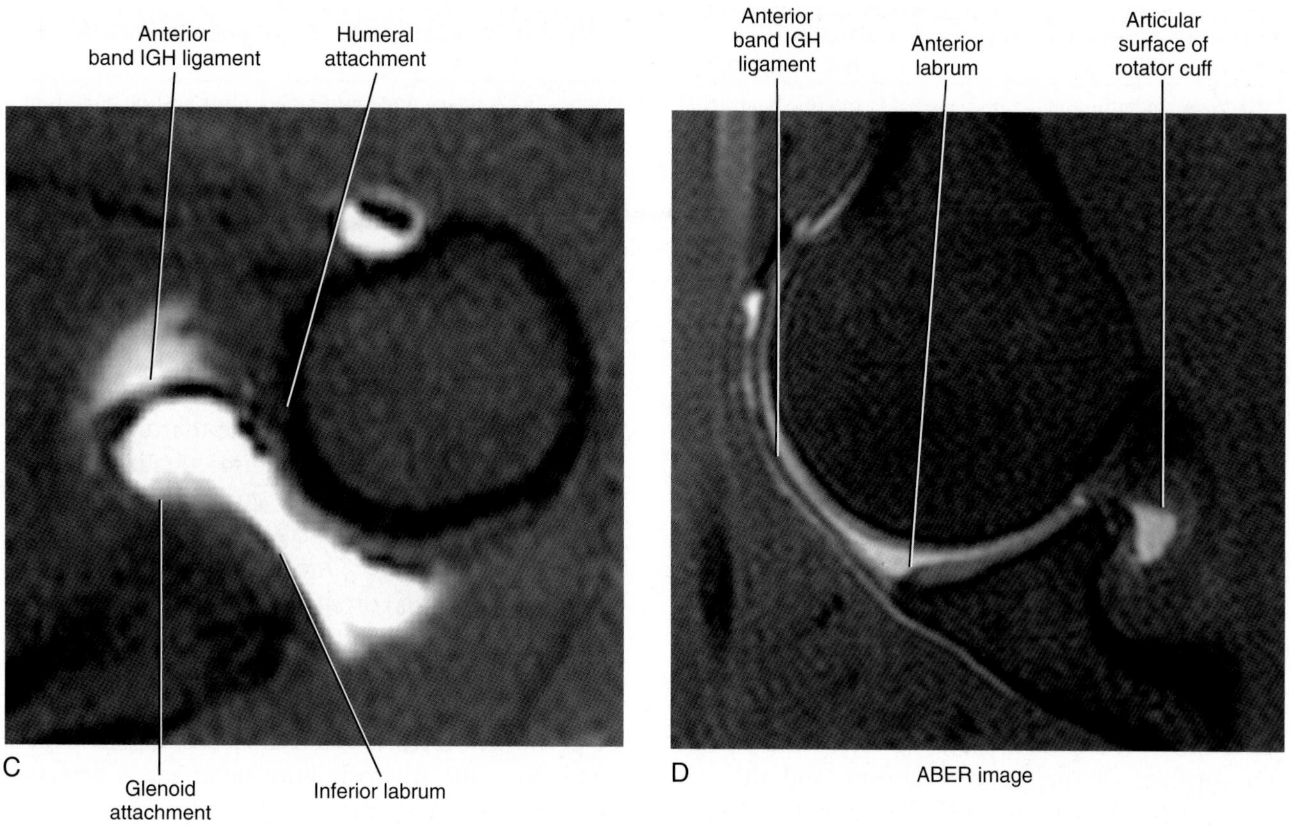
Anterior band IGH ligament
Humeral attachment
C
Glenoid attachment
Inferior labrum
Anterior band IGH ligament
Anterior labrum
Articular surface of rotator cuff
D
ABER image

Figure 7-38, cont'd **C,** Axial image shows the anterior band of the inferior glenohumeral (IGH) ligament. It originates from the inferior glenoid rim and inserts along the medial aspect of the proximal humeral shaft. With the arm imaged in neutral position, the IGH ligament is redundant and lax. Imaging of the shoulder while in abduction and external rotation (ABER) position (**D**) places tension on the anterior band of the IGH ligament resulting in a taut appearing IGH ligament.

head with the arm in 0-degree abduction (down by the side). It also serves to stabilize the long head of the biceps tendon.

The middle glenohumeral ligament (MGHL) is the most variable of the three ligaments, ranging from a thick cordlike ligament to a wispy threadlike structure. It also originates near the superior glenoid tubercle but courses more obliquely across the anterior aspect of the glenohumeral joint and eventually blends with the deep fibers of the subscapularis muscle to insert on the inferior aspect of the lesser tuberosity. As the MGHL crosses the anterior glenohumeral joint, it is located just superficial to the anterior labrum and sits just deep to the subscapularis muscle. Like the SGHL, the MGHL is also best visualized on axial MR images since it courses obliquely across the anterior joint space (see Fig. 7-38B). The MGHL serves to prevent excessive external rotation of the humeral head with the arm between 45 and 60 degrees of abduction.

The inferior glenohumeral ligament (IGHL) is the most important of the three ligaments regarding glenohumeral stability. It prevents anterior subluxation of the humeral head when the arm is fully abducted and externally rotated (late cocking phase, early acceleration phase of throwing). The IGHL is composed of three parts: the anterior band, the axillary pouch, and the posterior band. It originates along the inferior glenoid rim and extends in a cufflike fashion to attach to the humeral neck. When the arm is in a neutral position (as during standard MRI of the shoulder), the IGHL is redundant and lax (see Fig. 7-38C). By placing the arm in the fully abducted and externally rotated (ABER) position, the IGHL is stretched taut, thus improving visualization of the ligament (see Fig. 7-38D).

Table 7-8 Normal Variants of the Capsule and Labrum

Normal Variant	MR Imaging Tips
Cartilage undermining	Intermediate signal intensity hyaline cartilage undermines dark fibrocartilage of labrum; smooth, tapering
Sublabral foramen (hole)	Detached superior labrum; only in anterior superior quadrant
Sublabral recess	Smooth, tapering recess deep to superior labrum
Buford complex	Cordlike thick medial glenohumeral ligament, absent anterior superior labrum

Normal Anatomic Variants of the Labrum and Capsule

Several normal anatomic variations of the labrum and capsule can mimic labral pathology (Table 7-8). The glenoid labrum is composed of fibrocartilage and appears dark on all pulse sequences, and the articular surface of the glenoid fossa is covered with hyaline articular cartilage. The hyaline cartilage differs from the fibrocartilage in that hyaline cartilage demonstrates intermediate signal intensity on MRI. Occasionally, the hyaline cartilage undermines the fibrocartilage of the glenoid labrum, and this can mimic a labral tear on MRI. The undermining of hyaline cartilage should be easily differentiated from a tear because cartilage undermining appears smooth and tapering and does not extend completely beneath the labrum (see Fig. 7-37A and B), whereas a tear is irregular in appearance, demonstrates high fluid signal undermining the labrum, and may extend completely beneath the labrum, separating it from the adjacent osseous glenoid.

The *sublabral foramen* or *hole* is a normal anatomic variant in which the anterior superior labrum is completely detached from the underlying osseous glenoid (Fig. 7-39A). This variant occurs only in the anterior superior quadrant of the glenoid. When present, the sublabral foramen variant is often misinterpreted as either an anterior labral tear or as a superior labral (SLAP) tear. The key to distinguishing the sublabral hole from a labral tear is the location of the labral detachment. The sublabral foramen occurs only in the anterior superior quadrant of the glenoid, and the presence of a detached labrum in any other location is diagnostic of a tear. On MRI, certain landmarks make it simple to determine whether the detached labrum is isolated to the anterosuperior quadrant. First, evaluate the area using the coronal MRI plane. A detached labrum located anterior to the biceps anchor in the coronal plane represents a sublabral foramen. Extension of the labral detachment to involve the biceps anchor or posterior to the level of the biceps anchor represents a SLAP tear. Next, evaluate the axial MR images to ensure that the detached labrum is isolated to the superior quadrant. When imaging through the superior quadrant of the glenohumeral joint, the axial images contain the coracoid process on the image. Once the coracoid process is no longer visualized on the axial images, the imaging plane has moved from the superior to the inferior quadrant of the glenoid rim. Alternatively, use of cross-referencing with the other imaging planes can be performed to ensure that the labral detachment is confined to the anterosuperior quadrant. A detached labrum isolated to the anterior superior quadrant must be considered a labral foramen. Any extension of the labral detachment into the posterosuperior labrum or the inferior labrum represents a tear.

The *sublabral recess* is defined as a tapering recess that extends beneath the free edge of the superior labrum, separating it from the osseous glenoid and creating a potential space between the two structures. It differs from the sublabral foramen in that although there is a recess deep to the labrum, the labrum remains firmly attached to the glenoid. At the time of arthroscopy, a probe can be placed into the recess and the labrum pulled back away from the glenoid, but the labrum remains firmly attached at its base. The undersurface of the labrum appears smooth with no fraying or irregularity. This anatomic variant can mimic a SLAP tear; however, it is usually easy to distinguish between the two on MRI. The recess smoothly tapers toward the osseous glenoid and never results in signal extending into the substance of the superior labrum. The superior labrum should demonstrate a dark triangular appearance with smooth surfaces, and any signal extending into the substance of the triangle represents a superior labral tear and not a superior labral recess.

Finally, the *Buford complex* is an anatomic variant that is composed of a cordlike thickened middle glenohumeral ligament combined with an absent or

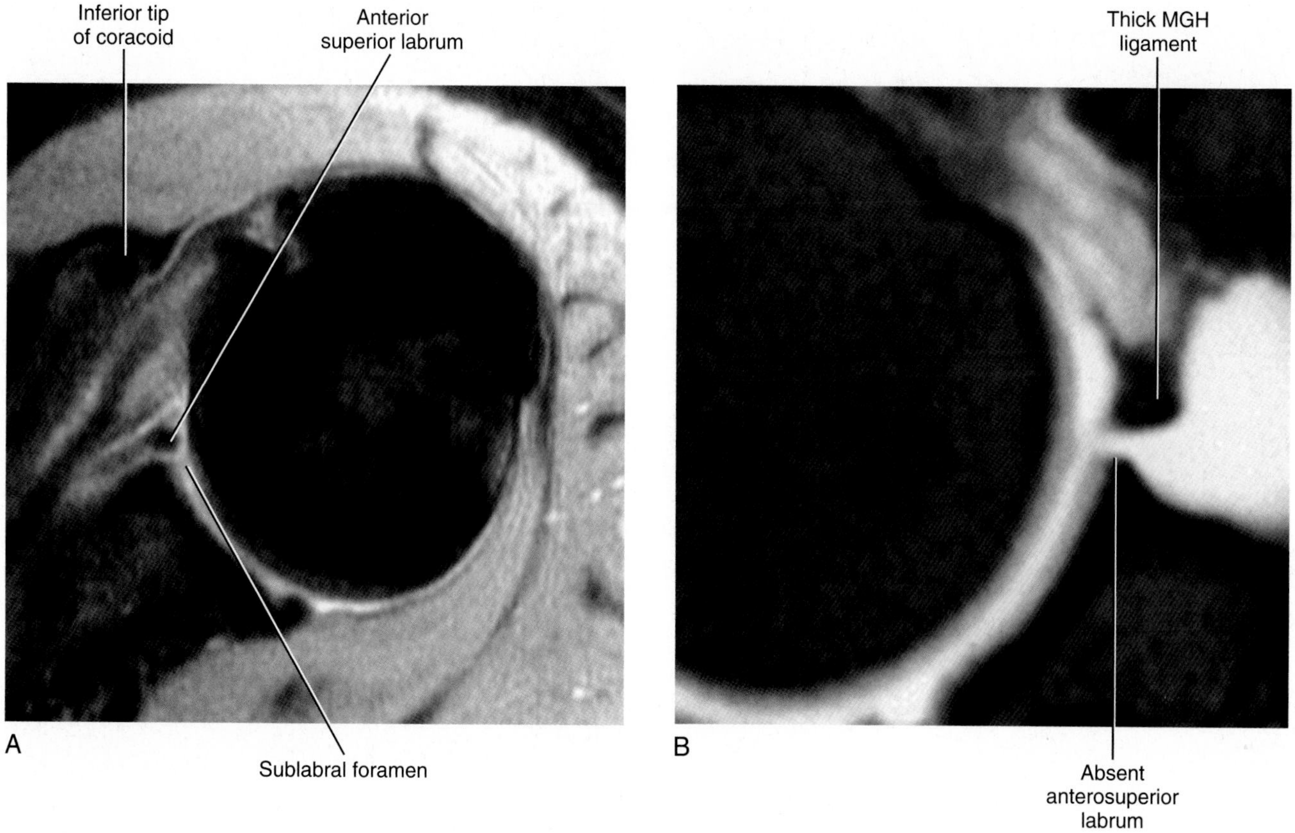
Inferior tip
of coracoid
Anterior
superior labrum
A
Sublabral foramen
Thick MGH
ligament
B
Absent
anterosuperior
labrum

Figure 7-39 **Normal variants of the labrum. A,** The anterior superior labrum is completely detached from the underlying osseous glenoid representing a sublabral foramen. **B,** Buford complex is composed of a thickened middle glenohumeral (MGH) ligament and absence of the anterosuperior labrum. This appearance can mimic an avulsion of the anterosuperior labrum.

diminutive anterior superior labrum (see Fig. 7-39B). With this anatomic variant, the thickened MGHL can be easily misinterpreted as an avulsed anterior labrum. Familiarity with the appearance and the course of the MGHL helps to avoid this pitfall. A thickened MGHL can be easily traced on multiple serial axial sections as it arises from the superior glenoid tubercle and courses obliquely across the anterior glenohumeral joint to blend with the deep fibers of the subscapularis tendon. The ligament is located just anterior to the expected position of the anterosuperior glenoid labrum. Again, absence of the anterior labrum at or above the level of the coracoid process on axial MR images is a normal anatomic variant, whereas absence of the labrum below the level of the coracoid on axial images represents a tear of the inferior glenoid labrum.

Although each of these anatomic variants can be detected on conventional MRI, the use of either intravenous or intra-articular contrast can further enhance the features that differentiate these variants from the lesions they mimic.

Lesions of Instability

Traumatic glenohumeral dislocation usually results in a lesion of one or more of the static or dynamic stabilizers of the glenohumeral joint. The specific lesion that occurs depends on many factors. The direction of the dislocation is obviously an important factor. Anterior dislocation results in disruption of the anterior stabilizers, whereas a posterior dislocation results in injury to the posterior capsule and posterior labrum. The age of the patient also plays a key role in predicting which lesion is most likely to occur. A first-time dislocation in an individual under 35 years of age usually results in a tear of the anterior labrum or capsule structures, whereas a first-time

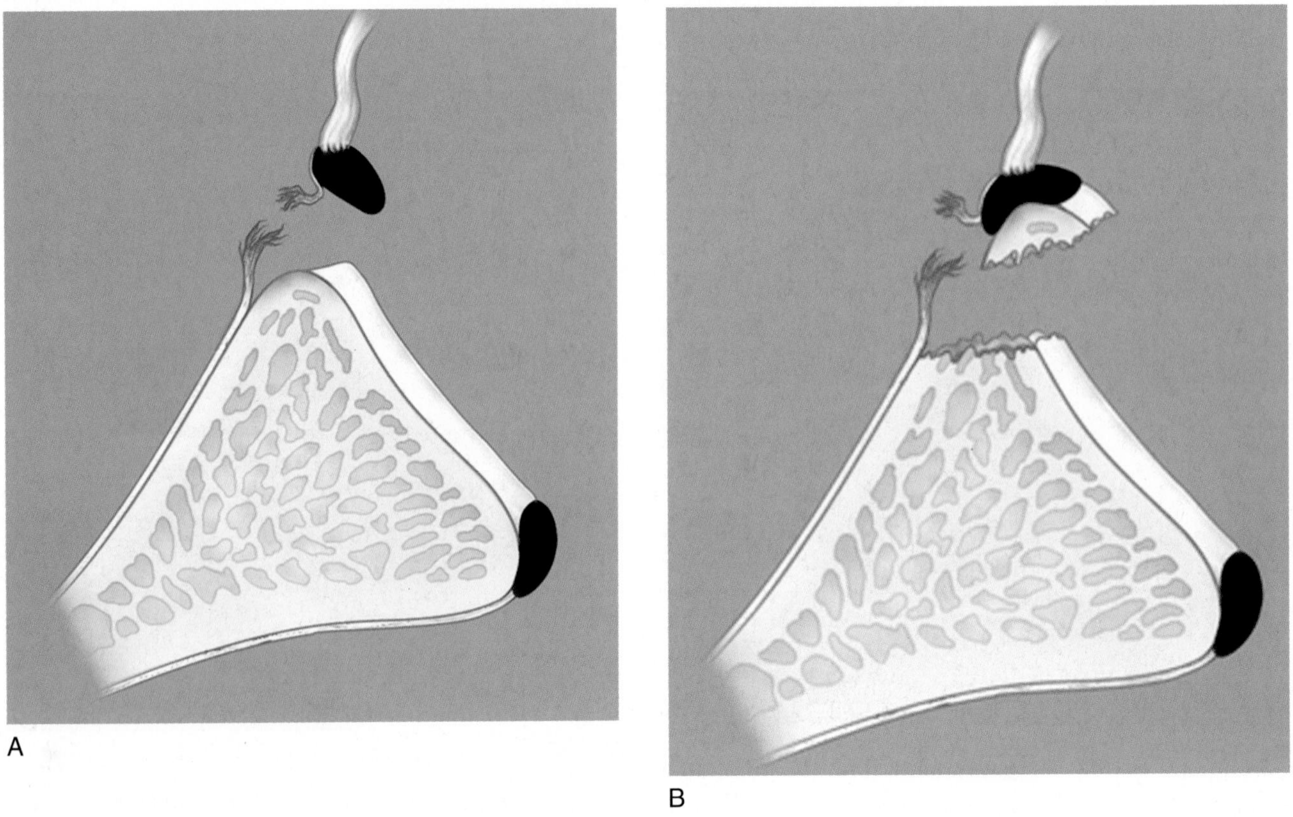

Figure 7-40 Bankart variants. A, Bankart lesion. **B,** Osseous Bankart.

dislocation in a patient over the age of 35 usually results not in a labral tear, but in a tear of the rotator cuff or in an avulsion of the greater tuberosity of the humeral head. Not all labral pathology results from a shoulder dislocation. Repetitive microtrauma, as occurs in throwers, weight-lifters, and swimmers can also result in labral pathology. Finally, trauma without dislocation, such as an impaction injury of the humeral head against the labrum and articular surface of the osseous glenoid, can lead to a tear of the labrum.

The term *Bankart lesion* was originally defined as a disruption of the anterior labroligamentous complex with disruption of the medial scapular periosteum. Over time, however, the phrase has come to be synonymous with any tear of the anteroinferior labrum, whereas the term *reverse Bankart lesion* describes a tear of the posteroinferior labrum. The term *SLAP tear* was first coined to describe a tear of the superior labrum extending from anterior to posterior, but SLAP tear is now commonly used to describe any tear involving the superior labrum and is usually associated with micro-instability of glenohumeral joint. Although the terms Bankart, reverse Bankart, and SLAP tear describe three broad categories of labral pathology, there are many subtle variations of these lesions that can have significant implications regarding proper diagnosis and treatment of glenohumeral instability. So although it is commonly accepted to use the terms "Bankart" lesion to describe any anterior labral tear, "reverse Bankart" lesion to describe a posterior labral tear, and "SLAP" tear to describe any superior labral tear, an accurate description of the subtle variations of labral pathology will improve diagnostic accuracy and provide a better roadmap for the surgeon in presurgical planning (Fig. 7-40).

The Bankart Variants

Classic Bankart Lesion The classic *Bankart lesion* is defined as a tear of the anterior labroligamentous complex with disruption of the medial scapular periosteum (Table 7-9). On MRI, the labrum may lose its normal triangular appearance or become amorphous-appearing. Abnormal signal may be detected within

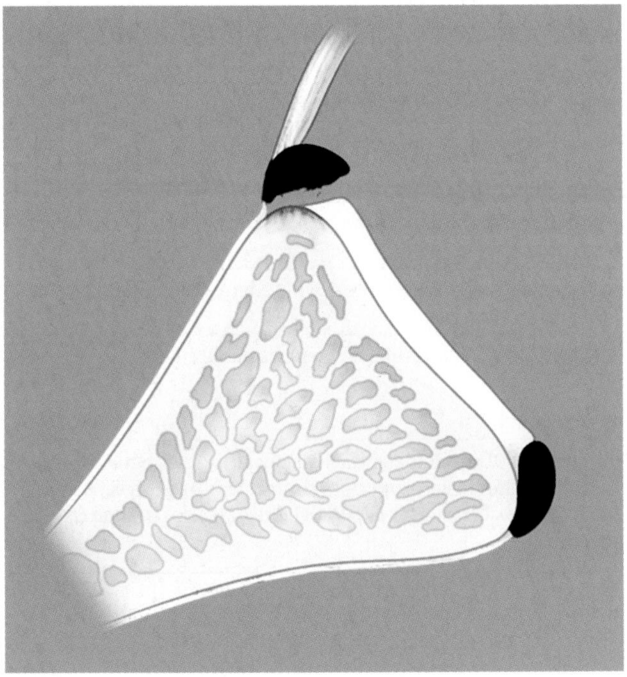

C

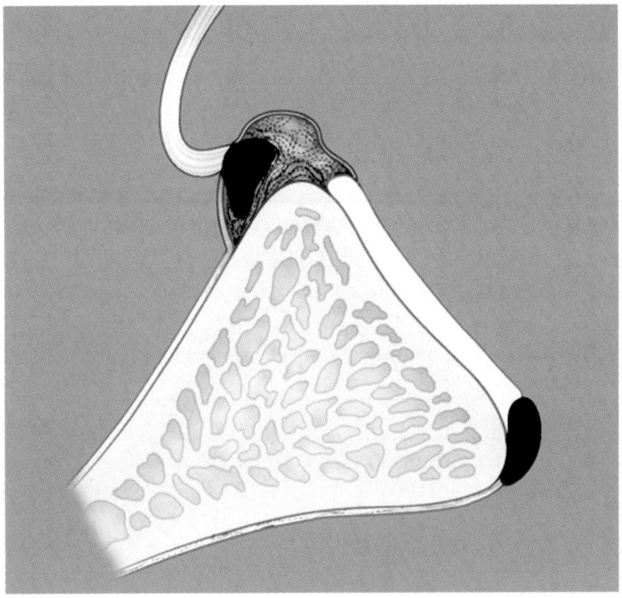

D

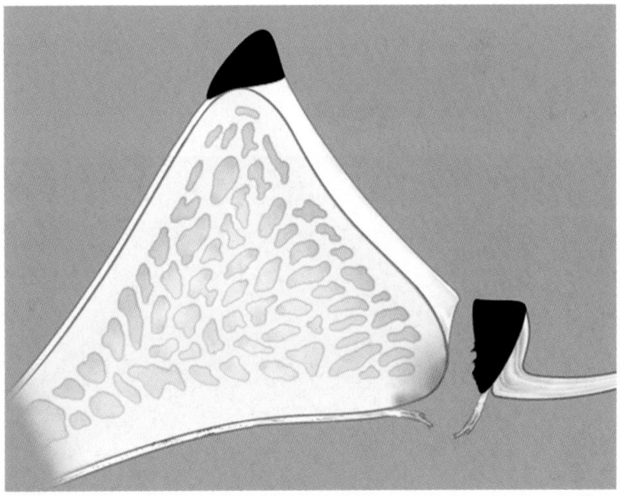

E

Figure 7-40, cont'd **C,** Perthes lesion (nondisplaced Bankart). **D,** Anterior labroligamentous sleeve avulsion (ALPSA) or medialized Bankart. **E,** Reverse Bankart.

the labrum, and the labrum may appear detached from the adjacent osseous glenoid (Fig. 7-41A). The axial plane is the primary plane for evaluating anterior and posterior labral pathology; however, the coronal imaging plane is complementary and often very helpful in detecting subtle lesions or in confirming the presence of a labral tear suspected on axial imaging. The *double axillary pouch* sign, is defined as a small collection of fluid or contrast extending deep to or into the substance of the inferior labrum as seen on coronal images and can be very helpful in detecting or confirming the presence of a suspected labral tear (Fig. 7-42). Direct Bankart repair may be performed using either an arthroscopic or open technique. Suture anchors are typically placed in the 3, 4, and 5 o'clock positions of the glenoid rim and the labrum is sutured to the osseous rim. Adjunctive capsulorrhaphy or stapling of the redundant capsule is often performed at the time of direct repair.

Osseous Bankart Osseous Bankart lesion describes a tear of the anterior inferior glenoid labrum associated with a fracture of the adjacent glenoid rim. In addition to the labral abnormality, MRI demonstrates a fracture and marrow edema involving the anterior inferior glenoid (see Fig. 7-41B). These lesions are typically repaired with screw fixation of the osseous fragment, and because the surgical repair differs from that of the classic Bankart, it is important to alert the arthroscopist to the presence of the osseous

Table 7-9 Bankart Variants

Lesion	Description
Classic Bankart	Anterior inferior labral tear; medial scapular periosteum disrupted
Osseous Bankart	Anterior inferior labral tear with adjacent glenoid fracture
Perthes (nondisplaced Bankart)	Anterior inferior labral tear; medial scapular periosteum intact
ALPSA (Anterior labroligamentous periosteal sleeve avulsion; medialized Bankart)	Anterior inferior labral tear; torn labrum displaced medially by an intact medial scapular periosteum
GLAD (glenolabral articular disruption)	Nondisplaced anterior inferior labral tear with adjacent articular cartilage injury
HAGL (humeral avulsion of the glenohumeral ligament)	Disruption of the anterior band inferior glenohumeral ligament
Reverse Bankart	Posterior inferior labral tear
PSGI (posterior superior glenoid impingement; internal impingement)	Internal impingement of the undersurface of posterior cuff between the humeral head and the posterosuperior labrum; tear of posterior cuff, degenerative fraying of posterior superior labrum, cystic change in greater tuberosity

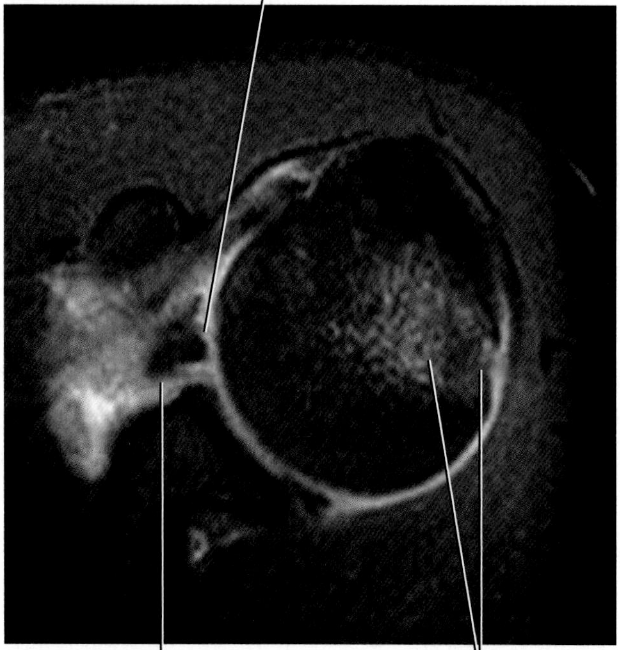
Avulsed anteroinferior labrum
A
Disrupted medial scapular periosteum
Hill-Sachs lesion with marrow edema

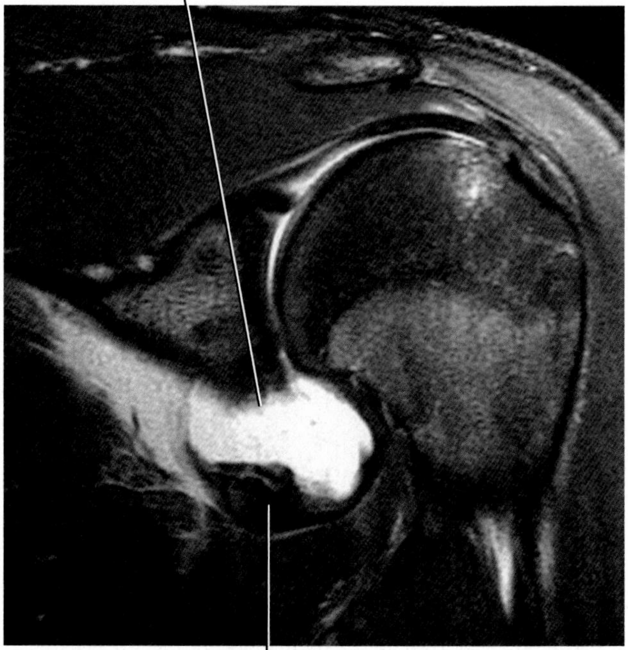
Cortical disruption inferior glenoid rim
B
Displaced osseous Bankart lesion

Figure 7-41 MR appearance of Bankart variants. A, Bankart lesion: Complete avulsion of the anterior labrum. **B,** Osseous Bankart lesion: A large osseous fragment of the inferior glenoid is avulsed along with the anterior labrum.

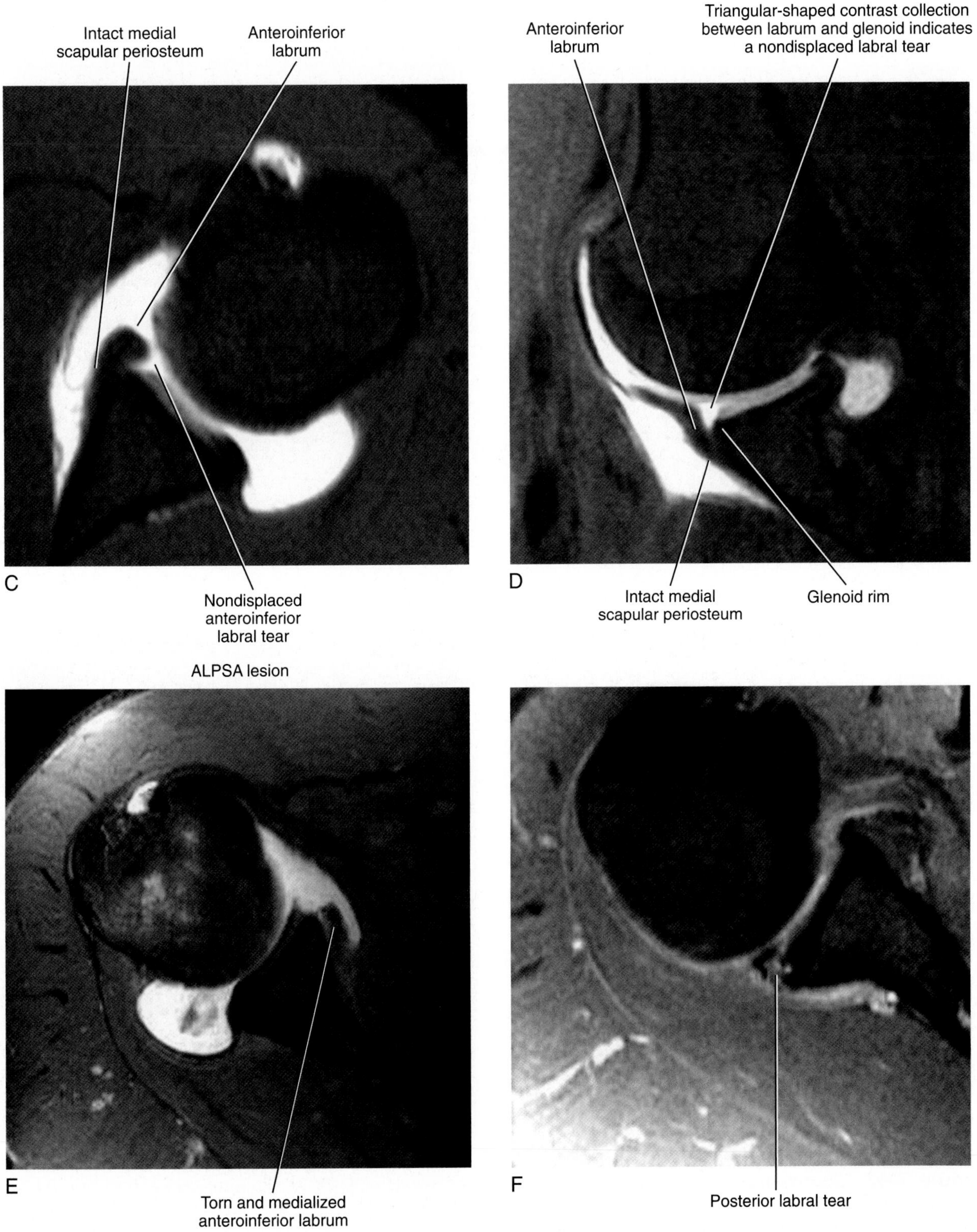
Intact medial scapular periosteum
Anteroinferior labrum
C
Nondisplaced anteroinferior labral tear
Anteroinferior labrum
Triangular-shaped contrast collection between labrum and glenoid indicates a nondisplaced labral tear
D
Intact medial scapular periosteum
Glenoid rim
ALPSA lesion
E
Torn and medialized anteroinferior labrum
F
Posterior labral tear

Figure 7-41, cont'd **C,** Perthes lesion: A small collection of contrast between the medial aspect of the inferior labrum and the glenoid rim represents a nondisplaced Bankart lesion. Note that the medial scapular periosteum remains intact. **D,** Perthes lesion on ABER imaging: A small triangular contrast collection between the anterior labrum and the osseous glenoid is diagnostic of a nondisplaced Bankart lesion. **E,** ALPSA (anterior labroligamentous periosteal sleeve) lesion: The anterior labrum is torn and displaced medially. **F,** Reverse Bankart lesion: A nondisplaced tear of the posteroinferior labrum.

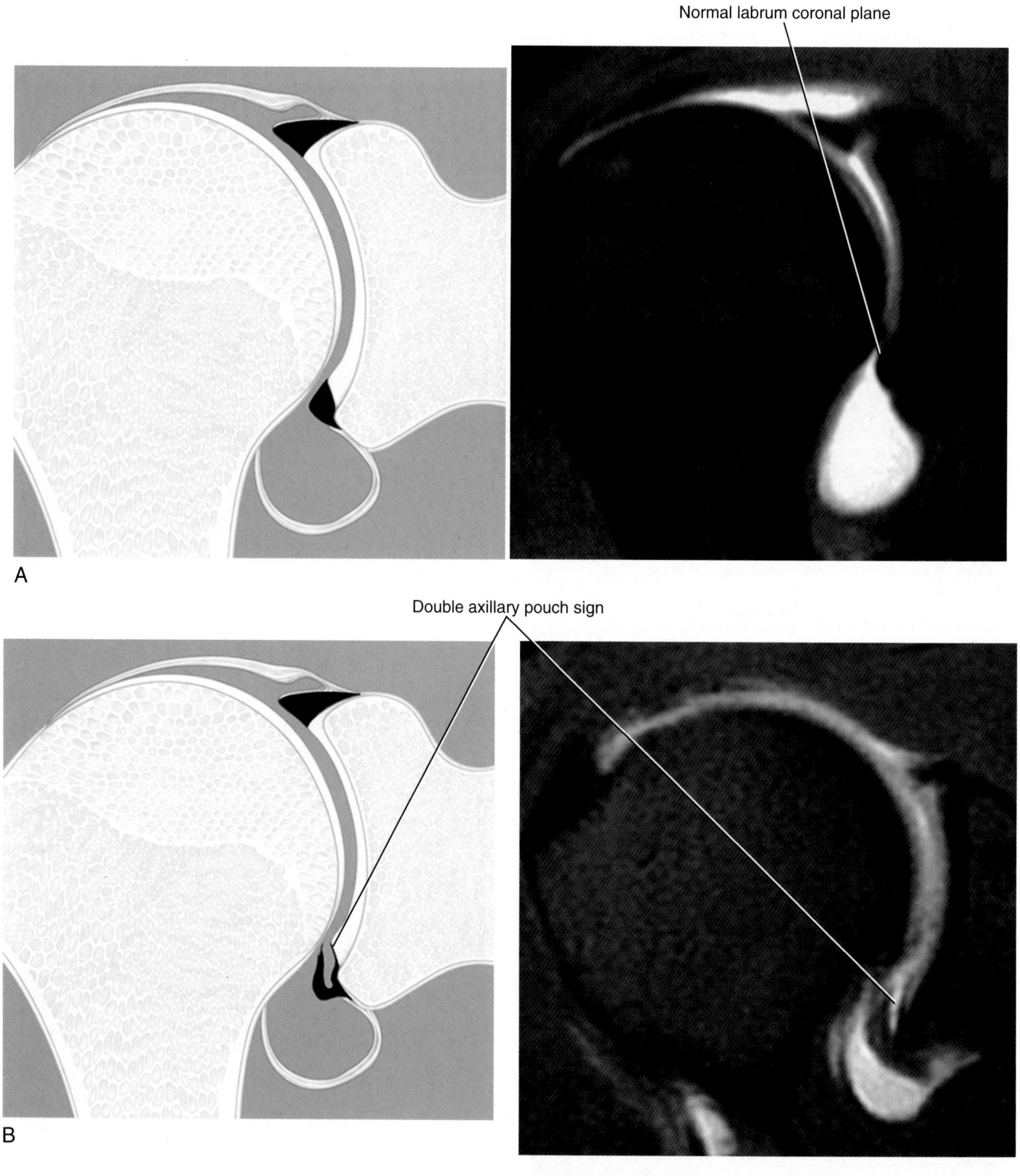
Normal labrum coronal plane
A
Double axillary pouch sign
B

Figure 7-42 **Double axillary pouch sign. A,** The surface of the anteroinferior labrum is smooth, and there is no fluid collection within the labrum or irregularity of the labrum in the coronal imaging plane. **B,** A small collection of fluid extending into the anteroinferior labrum is referred to as the "double axillary pouch" sign and is specific for a labral tear.

component. It is critical to accurately describe the amount of bone loss of the anteroinferior glenoid rim because this information helps the surgeon to determine whether bone graft material will be required at the time of Bankart repair. The extent of bone loss is usually best detected and described using the sagittal imaging plane. Although MRI is accurate in this regard, many surgeons prefer CT imaging with sagittal reconstructions to depict the extent of the osseous defect (Fig. 7-43). Glenoid bone loss in the anteroinferior quadrant can produce an appearance on the sagittal imaging plane that has been likened to an *inverted pear* appearance.

Perthes Lesion Also referred to as a "nondisplaced" Bankart lesion, the Perthes lesion demonstrates a tear of the anterior inferior glenoid labrum, but it differs from the classic Bankart lesion in that the medial scapular periosteum remains intact holding the torn labrum in near anatomic position. To further complicate things, the nondisplaced labrum may scar back down to the underlying glenoid and resynovialize in place. The significance of the Perthes lesion is that although the MR signs and arthroscopic findings are both very subtle, the labrum is unstable and the patient continues to demonstrate the clinical signs and symptoms of glenohumeral instability.

The Perthes lesion frequently goes undetected on conventional MRI, since the labrum remains in its normal anatomic position and usually demonstrates normal morphology and MR appearance. The presence of a native effusion may help in the detection of this lesion because a tiny linear fluid collection may be detected extending partially beneath the labrum, indicating the partial avulsion of the labrum from the adjacent osseous glenoid. Of all the Bankart variants, the detection of the Perthes lesion is often the most difficult; as a result, the detection of this lesion usually benefits the most from the use of direct MR arthrography and ABER stress imaging.

When a person demonstrates clinical evidence of glenohumeral instability in the face of a normal conventional MR examination, one should consider further evaluation with direct MR arthrography and ABER imaging (see Fig. 7-41C and D). Direct MR arthrography helps with the detection of a Perthes lesion in two ways. First, it results in distention of the joint, which helps to outline and accentuate the subtle MR findings of a nondisplaced labral tear. Second, with gadolinium in the joint, imaging can be performed using the higher signal-to-noise T1-weighted imaging rather than relying on T2-weighted imaging to detect fluid deep to the labrum. Next, by adding ABER imaging, the anterior band of the inferior glenohumeral ligament is stretched taut, placing tension on the anterior labrum. This results in subtle displacement of the anterior labrum and allows pooling of contrast deep to the anterior labrum. The presence of this tiny triangular fluid/contrast collection on the ABER image is diagnostic of the Perthes lesion and is often the only abnormality that can be detected on MR arthrography (see Fig. 7-41D).

The Perthes lesion can also be a challenge for the arthroscopist to detect and may require probing and tugging on the anteroinferior labrum to demonstrate its instability. Therefore, it is important to alert the arthroscopist to the presence of a nondisplaced Bankart lesion to ensure proper identification and treatment of the lesion at the time of arthroscopy. The repair technique used for the Perthes lesion is identical to the technique used for the classic Bankart lesion.

Anterior Labroligamentous Periosteal Sleeve Avulsion Lesion The anterior labroligamentous periosteal sleeve avulsion (ALPSA) lesion is also referred to as the medialized Bankart. The ALPSA lesion is similar to the Perthes lesion in that although the labrum is torn, the medial scapular periosteum remains intact. However, with the ALPSA lesion the labrum, rather than remaining in its normal position, is pulled in a medial direction by the intact scapular periosteum. The appearance of the labrum has been described as similar to that of a "sleeve" rolled up along the medial aspect of the glenoid. On MRI, the labrum may demonstrate abnormal morphology and will be medially displaced along the anterior aspect of the osseous glenoid (see Fig. 7-41E). A chronic ALPSA lesion frequently develops a mound of scar tissue adjacent to the displaced labrum, and the entire labral-scar complex may develop a thin synovial lining. This can make recognition of the lesion difficult at the time of arthroscopy. Alerting the arthroscopist to the medialized location of the torn labrum can help ensure detection and proper surgical management of the lesion. The recommended treatment is to surgically complete the Bankart lesion, debride the scar tissue, and then reattach the labrum in its normal anatomic position.

Glenolabral Articular Disruption Lesion The glenolabral articular disruption (GLAD) lesion is described

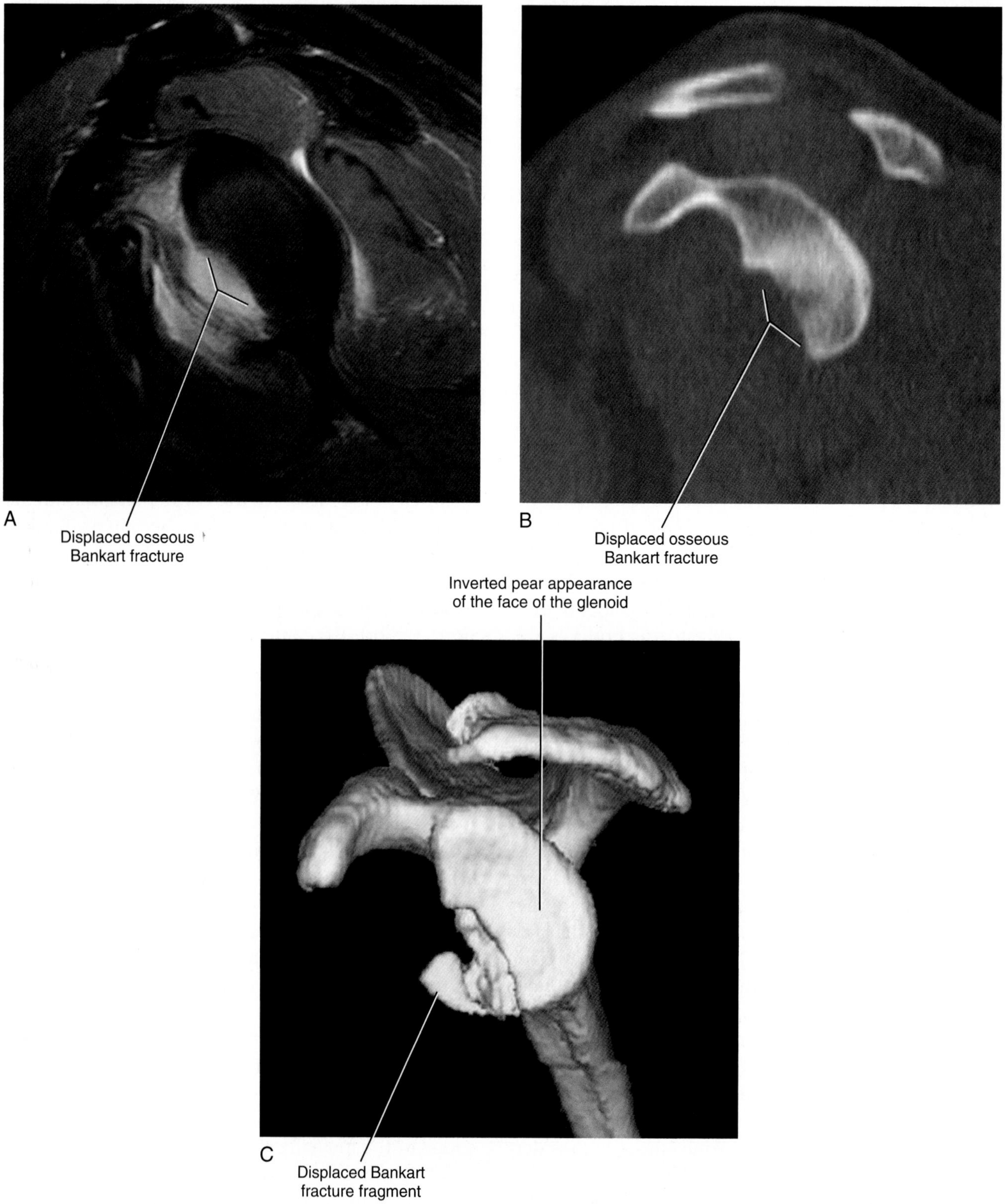
A
Displaced osseous Bankart fracture
B
Displaced osseous Bankart fracture
Inverted pear appearance of the face of the glenoid
C
Displaced Bankart fracture fragment

Figure 7-43 Osseous Bankart: inverted pear appearance. A, Oblique sagittal T2-weighted image shows a large displaced anteroinferior glenoid rim fracture. Oblique sagittal CT reconstruction (**B**) and surface rendering (**C**) images show the *inverted pear* appearance of the glenoid rim resulting from a displaced osseous Bankart fracture.

as a nondisplaced tear of the anterior inferior labrum combined with an injury of the adjacent articular cartilage. There is some controversy as to whether this lesion actually exists as a separate entity or whether it simply represents a Bankart lesion with an adjacent chondral abnormality possibly resulting from recurrent impaction of the glenoid rim that resulted from chronic instability of the humeral head. The original description of the GLAD lesion describes a lesion that results from an impaction of the humeral head against the glenoid fossa without subluxation or dislocation at the time of injury. The impaction injury of the humeral head against the glenoid occurs as the result of a fall on an outstretched hand with the arm in abduction and external rotation. The patient typically presents with the history of a fall and subsequent shoulder pain but gives no history of dislocation and demonstrates no evidence of instability on physical examination. The absence of the clinical findings of instability may delay the use of MRI in the evaluation of the patient with a GLAD lesion. It is the mechanism of injury and lack of glenohumeral instability on physical examination that differentiates this lesion from a chronic Bankart lesion with chondral abnormality. These two lesions cannot usually be differentiated on the basis of imaging alone.

The MR findings seen with the GLAD lesion are often subtle and difficult to detect using only conventional MRI. MR arthrography with stress view ABER imaging is the optimal method for visualizing the nondisplaced labral tear and the associated articular cartilage injury. On MR arthrography, the articular cartilage injury is located in the anteroinferior quadrant of the glenoid and may appear as an osteochondral defect or as an articular cartilage flap tear (Fig. 7-44). The nondisplaced labral tear is best seen on ABER imaging as a small collection of contrast material filling a triangular-shaped gap between the anterior inferior labrum and the osseous glenoid. The anterior band of the inferior glenohumeral ligament and the medial scapular periosteum remain intact. This lesion is usually treated with debridement of the osteochondral injury and direct repair of the labral tear.

Humeral Avulsion of the Glenohumeral Ligament Lesion Humeral avulsion of the glenohumeral ligament or the HAGL lesion describes a disruption of the anterior band of the inferior glenohumeral ligament at its humeral attachment site. The anterior labroligamentous complex is the most important structure with regard to anterior shoulder stability and comprises the anterior band of the inferior glenohumeral ligament and the anterior inferior labrum. The term Bankart lesion and its many variants describe injuries involving the labral portion of the anterior labroligamentous complex. However, a disruption of the anterior labroligamentous complex anywhere along its course also results in anterior instability of the glenohumeral joint similar to that from a Bankart lesion. The term HAGL lesion was originally used to describe a tear of the anterior band of the inferior glenohumeral ligament at its humeral attachment site. However a tear can occur anywhere along the course of the ligament, including the humeral attachment, mid substance, or at the labral attachment site (Fig. 7-45).

On MRI, the HAGL lesion is seen as disruption of the anterior band of the inferior glenohumeral ligament anywhere along its course, but most commonly at or near its humeral attachment site (see Fig. 7-45). In the setting of acute trauma, edema is present within the soft tissues immediately adjacent to the disrupted ligament. MR arthrography can help with the detection of the lesion since extravasation of contrast can be seen extending through the defect in the ligament. Disruption or avulsion of the adjacent subscapularis tendon often occurs in conjunction with a HAGL lesion. It is critical to alert the arthroscopist to the presence of a HAGL lesion because it can be difficult to detect through the standard arthroscopic portals. It has been suggested that many of the cases of recurrent shoulder instability following arthroscopy may actually be secondary to a missed HAGL lesion. A miniarthrotomy is typically required to identify and repair a HAGL lesion, and surgical repair is mandatory to reestablish shoulder stability.

Reverse Bankart A tear of the posterior labrum is referred to as a reverse Bankart lesion (see Fig. 7-41F). Such lesions are less common than the anterior labral lesions and can result from either a single traumatic event or, more commonly, from repetitive microtrauma to the posterior capsule and labrum as occurs in weight-lifting and swimming. The mechanism for traumatic posterior dislocation is a fall on an outstretched hand with the arm in adduction and external rotation. In this position, the posterior capsule is taut, and the posteriorly directed force of the humeral head results in a disruption of the posterior stabilizers. Many of the Bankart variants that are seen in the anterior labrum can also occur in the posterior

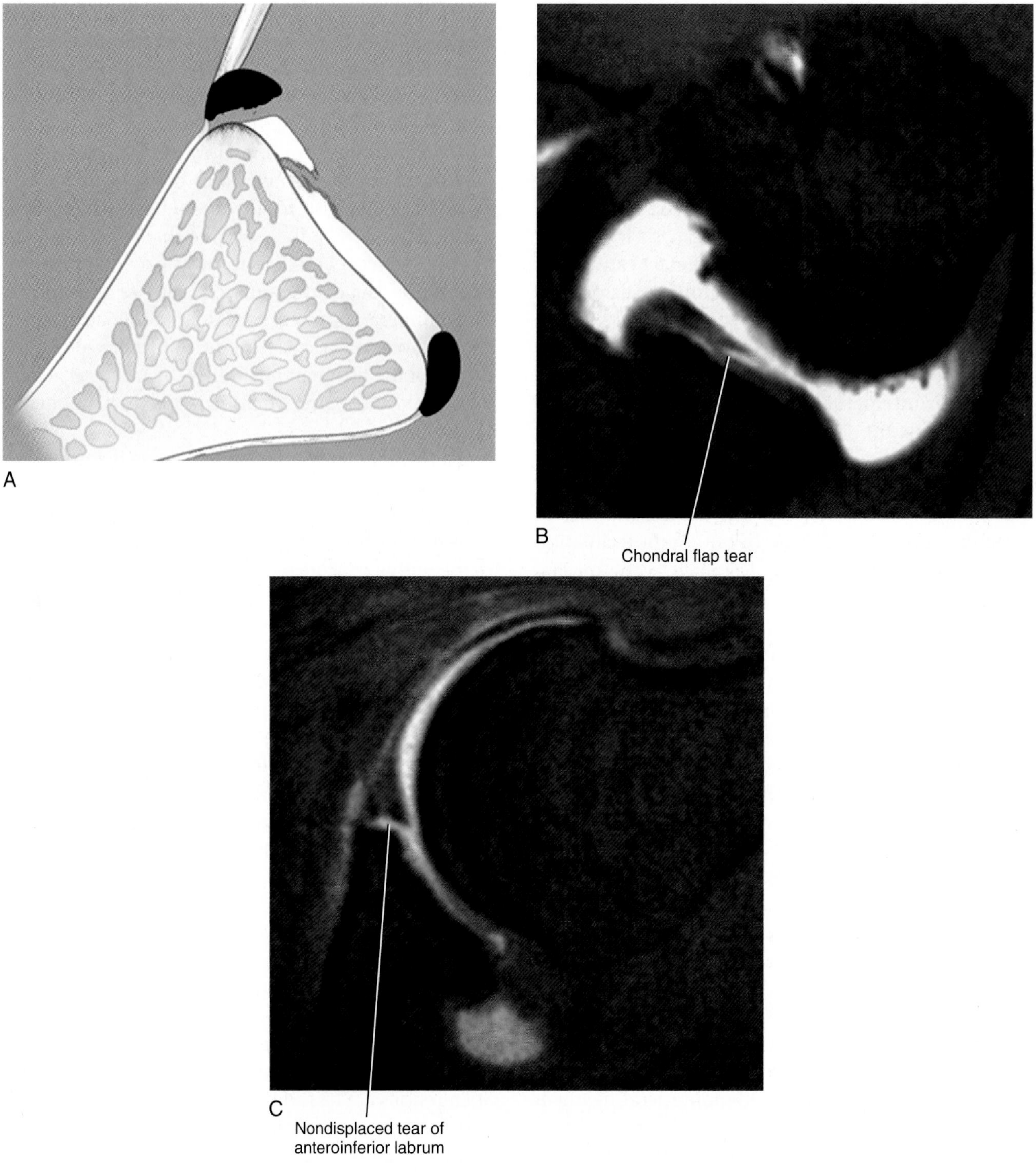
A
B
Chondral flap tear
C
Nondisplaced tear of anteroinferior labrum

Figure 7-44 GLAD (glenohumeral articular disruption) lesion. A, Artwork demonstrates the two components of a GLAD lesion; a nondisplaced tear of the anterior inferior labrum and an adjacent articular cartilage injury. **B,** Axial image demonstrates a chondral flap tear. **C,** ABER view demonstrates a nondisplaced tear of the anterior inferior labrum.

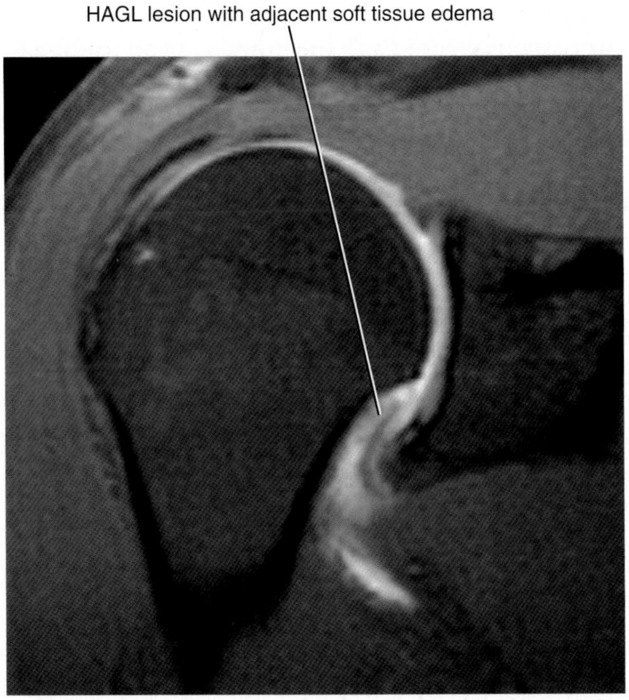
HAGL lesion with adjacent soft tissue edema

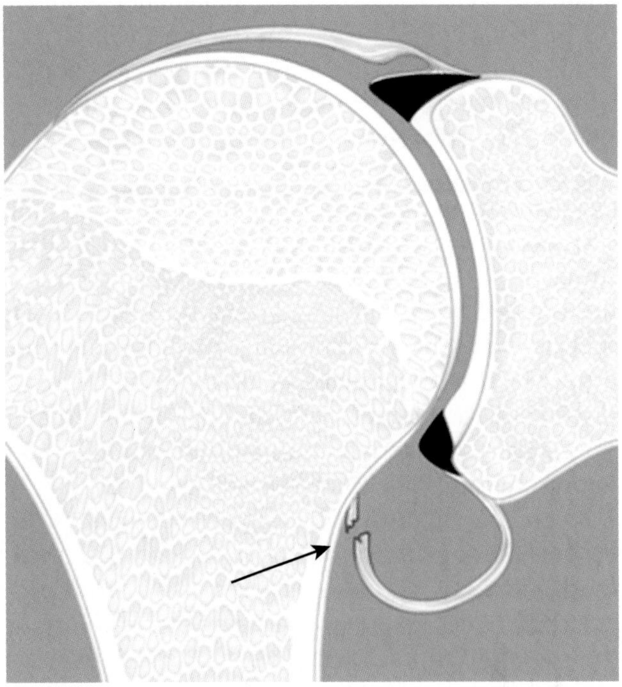

Figure 7-45 HAGL (humeral avulsion of the glenohumeral ligament). Artwork demonstrates avulsion of the anterior band of the glenohumeral ligament at the level of its humeral attachment and coronal T1-weighted image with contrast in the joint shows complete avulsion of the inferior glenohumeral ligament at its humeral attachment site with mild adjacent soft tissue edema.

labrum. The term "reverse" is typically used to describe the posterior glenoid lesions (reverse Bankart or reverse Hill-Sachs lesion). The term PHAGL has been used to describe a *posterior* HAGL lesion. Findings on MRI are similar to those seen with anterior labral/capsular injury and include abnormal morphology of the posterior labrum, a partially or completely detached posterior labrum, and an associated fracture of the posterior glenoid. Posterior labral lesions can be difficult to diagnose clinically and are more challenging to repair than the anterior labral lesions.

Superior Labral Tear Anterior to Posterior Lesion Superior labral tear anterior to posterior or SLAP lesion describes a tear that involves the superior labrum. The original classification scheme included four types of SLAP tears (Fig. 7-46). The type I lesion is defined as fraying and degeneration of the surface of the superior labrum, but the labrum remains firmly attached to the glenoid with no displaced or unstable fragment. The type II lesion is defined as an avulsion of the labrum from the osseous glenoid resulting in

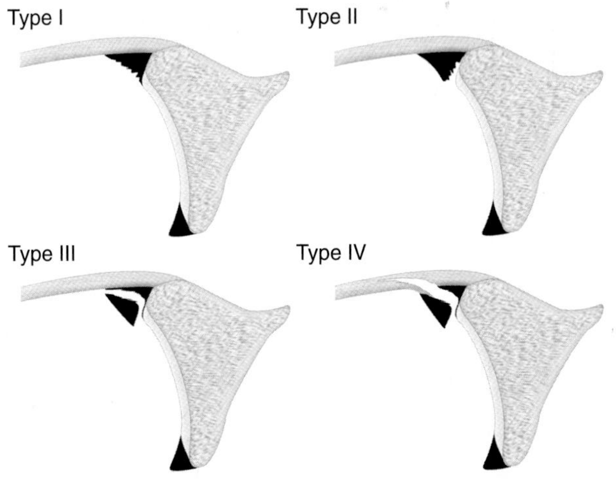
Type I
Type II
Type III
Type IV

Figure 7-46 SLAP tears. Type I—degenerative fraying of the surface of the superior labrum. Type II—avulsion of the superior labrum from the osseous glenoid, which can result in an unstable biceps anchor. Type III—displaced bucket-handle tear of the superior labrum with an intact biceps anchor. Type IV—displaced bucket-handle tear of the superior labrum that involves the biceps anchor. SLAP, superior labral tear anterior to posterior.

an unstable labral fragment and potentially an unstable biceps anchor. The type III lesion is defined as a displaced bucket-handle tear of the superior labrum with an intact biceps anchor, whereas the type IV lesion is a displaced bucket-handle tear of the superior labrum with involvement of the biceps anchor. Since the original description of the SLAP lesion, the classification scheme has been expanded to include a total of 10 types of SLAP tears. In addition, some of the original types of SLAP lesions have also been subclassified. These additional types of SLAP tears primarily describe extension of the SLAP tear to involve adjacent structures including the anteroinferior labrum, posteroinferior labrum, MGHL, and rotator interval (SGHL) complex (Table 7-10).

Several mechanisms of injury are thought to be responsible for the various SLAP lesions. The three most common mechanisms are a fall on the outstretched hand resulting in a compressive injury of the superior labrum, repetitive overhead activity as seen in throwing athletes or swimmers resulting in traction forces on the biceps anchor, and finally internal impingement of the shoulder resulting in compression of the posterior superior labrum between the osseous glenoid and the humeral head leading to injury of the posterior superior labrum. Treatment varies according to the type of lesion. A type I lesion is usually treated conservatively or with surgical debridement. A type II lesion may require debridement as well as suturing to stabilize the superior labrum and biceps anchor. Type III and IV lesions are treated with debridement of the unstable labral fragments and suturing to stabilize the biceps anchor. Extension of the SLAP tear into adjacent structures including the anterior or posterior inferior labrum may require additional repair of the involved structures.

Table 7-10 Expanded Classification of SLAP Lesions

Type	Description
I	Degenerative fraying; no unstable fragment
II	In addition to degenerative fraying: Avulsion of superior labrum from glenoid resulting in an unstable biceps anchor IIA—limited to anterosuperior labrum IIB—limited to posterosuperior labrum IIC—both anterior and posterior components
III	Bucket-handle tear
IV	Bucket-handle tear with extension into biceps anchor
V	Bankart lesion with superior extension to involve biceps anchor and superior labrum
VI	Anterior or posterior flap tear with separation of biceps tendon superiorly
VII	Biceps tendon separation, anterosuperior labral tear with extension into middle glenohumeral ligament
VIII	SLAP lesion with posteroinferior extension
IX	Complete or near-complete detachment of entire labrum; SLAP lesion with extensive anterior and posterior extension
X	SLAP lesion with extension into rotator cuff interval

SLAP, superior labral tear anterior to posterior.

MRI is an excellent noninvasive means of evaluating the superior labrum. The coronal plane is the primary plane for the evaluation of the superior labrum, but a thorough evaluation in all three imaging planes is crucial if one is to provide a thorough description of the SLAP tear and its involvement of adjacent structures. The normal superior labrum is triangular, arises from the superior glenoid, and demonstrates low signal intensity on all MR pulse sequences. The superior glenoid labrum demonstrates more variations than any other part of the labrum, and it is these anatomic variations that create the most difficulty with regard to correctly identifying and classifying the various SLAP lesions. These variations include the sublabral recess, the sublabral foramen, and the Buford complex (see Figs 7-37 through 7-39) and are described in detail in a previous section.

It is not always possible to clearly distinguish among the 10 types of SLAP tear or to accurately categorize a SLAP lesion on the basis of MR imaging. However, direct or indirect MR arthrography may help to better define the lesion and add a level of confidence when differentiating superior labral pathology from the normal variants (Fig. 7-47). A thorough evaluation and description of the SLAP lesion can provide important information for preoperative planning by the surgeon, and the description of a SLAP lesion should always include the following information (Table 7-11).

First, one must detect and accurately differentiate a SLAP tear from the normal labral variants (see previous section on normal variants of the labrum and capsule). A labral tear is diagnosed on the basis of abnormal morphology of the superior labrum or on the basis of abnormal signal within the substance of or involving the surface of the superior labrum. Next,

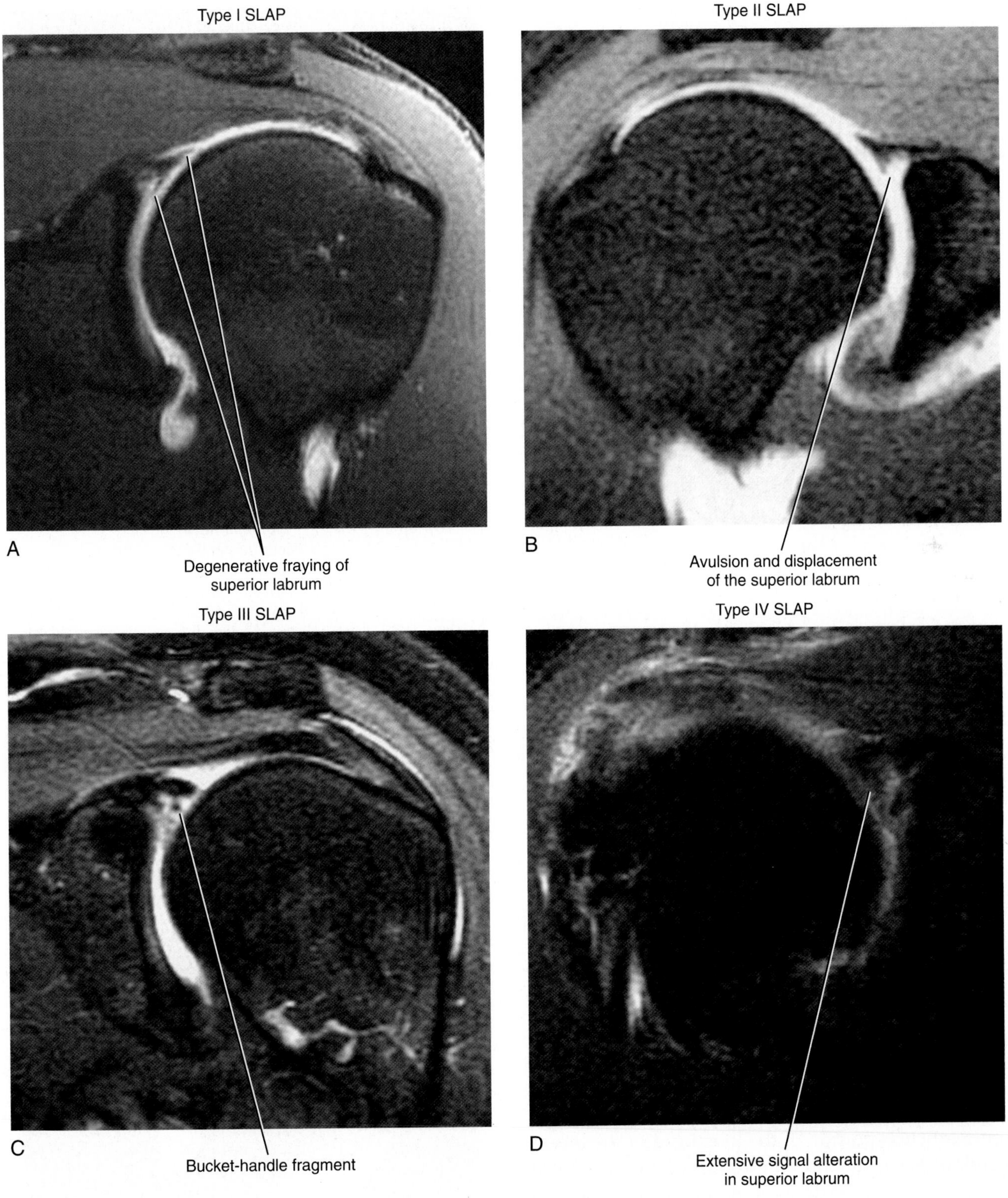
Type I SLAP
A
Degenerative fraying of superior labrum
Type II SLAP
B
Avulsion and displacement of the superior labrum
Type III SLAP
C
Bucket-handle fragment
Type IV SLAP
D
Extensive signal alteration in superior labrum

Figure 7-47 MR appearance of SLAP tears. A, Type I. There is undersurface fraying and irregularity of the superior labrum, but the labrum remains firmly attached to the osseous glenoid. **B,** Type II. The labrum is avulsed or pulled away from the adjacent osseous glenoid, but there is no bucket-handle fragment and no involvement of the biceps anchor. **C,** Type III. There is undersurface fraying and irregularity of the superior labrum and a small unstable bucket-handle fragment is present.

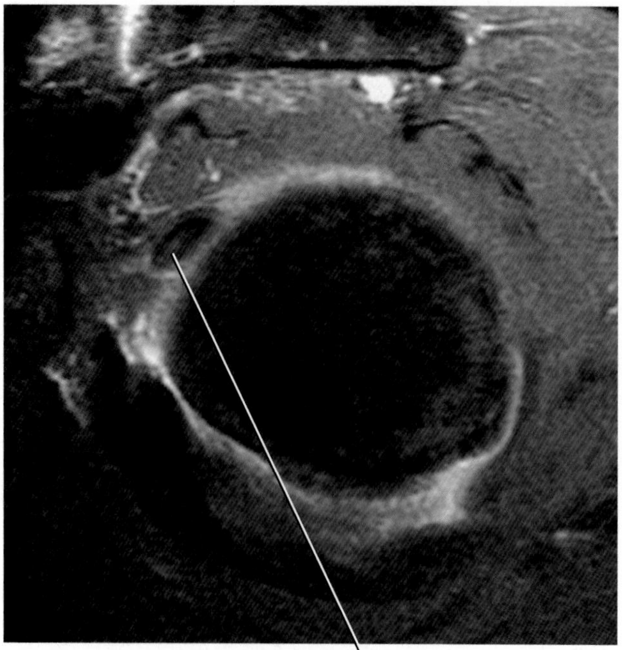
Type IV SLAP
E
Signal abnormality in biceps anchor indicating extension of SLAP tear

Figure 7-47, cont'd **D** and **E,** Type IV. The coronal image (**D**) demonstrates marked surface irregularity of the undersurface of the superior labrum, whereas the sagittal image (**E**) demonstrates abnormal signal within the substance of the biceps anchor representing extension of the tear into the intra-articular portion of the long head of the biceps tendon. SLAP, superior labral tear anterior to posterior.

Table 7-11 Description of a SLAP Tear

Detection of SLAP tear	Abnormal morphology of superior labrum Abnormal signal within labrum
Differentiate from normal variants (see Table 7-8)	Cartilage undermining Sublabral recess Sublabral foramen Buford complex
Extent of Tear from Anterior to Posterior	
Presence of a displaced fragment	Bucket handle tear Flap fragment
Involvement of biceps anchor	Tear extends into biceps anchor Detached/displaced biceps anchor Complete disruption of biceps tendon
Involvement of adjacent structures	Anterior inferior labrum (anterior extension) Posterior inferior labrum (posterior extension) MGHL, SGHL, rotator interval
Associated abnormalities	Chondral abnormalities (glenoid, humeral head) Glenohumeral osteoarthritis Glenoid fractures Marrow edema Paralabral cyst

MGHL, middle glenohumeral ligament; SGHL, superior glenohumeral ligament; SLAP, superior labral tear anterior to posterior.

describe whether the SLAP tear results in a displaced fragment, such as a bucket-handle or flap fragment. The status of the biceps anchor should then be evaluated to determine whether the tear extends into the intra-articular portion of the long head of the biceps tendon. Next, describe the extent of the SLAP tear from anterior to posterior and describe involvement of adjacent structures including the anteroinferior labrum (Fig. 7-48), posteroinferior labrum (Fig. 7-49), MGHL, SGHL (Fig. 7-50), and rotator interval. Finally, describe associated abnormalities such as chondral injuries (Fig. 7-51), glenoid fractures, marrow edema, and the presence of an adjacent paralabral cyst (Fig. 7-52).

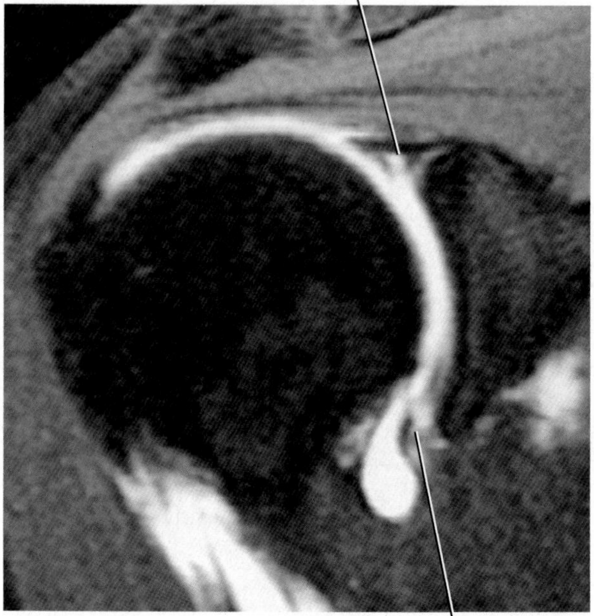
SLAP tear
Bankart lesion

Figure 7-48 SLAP tear with extension into anterior inferior labrum. Oblique coronal image shows a Bankart lesion with extension into the superior labrum.

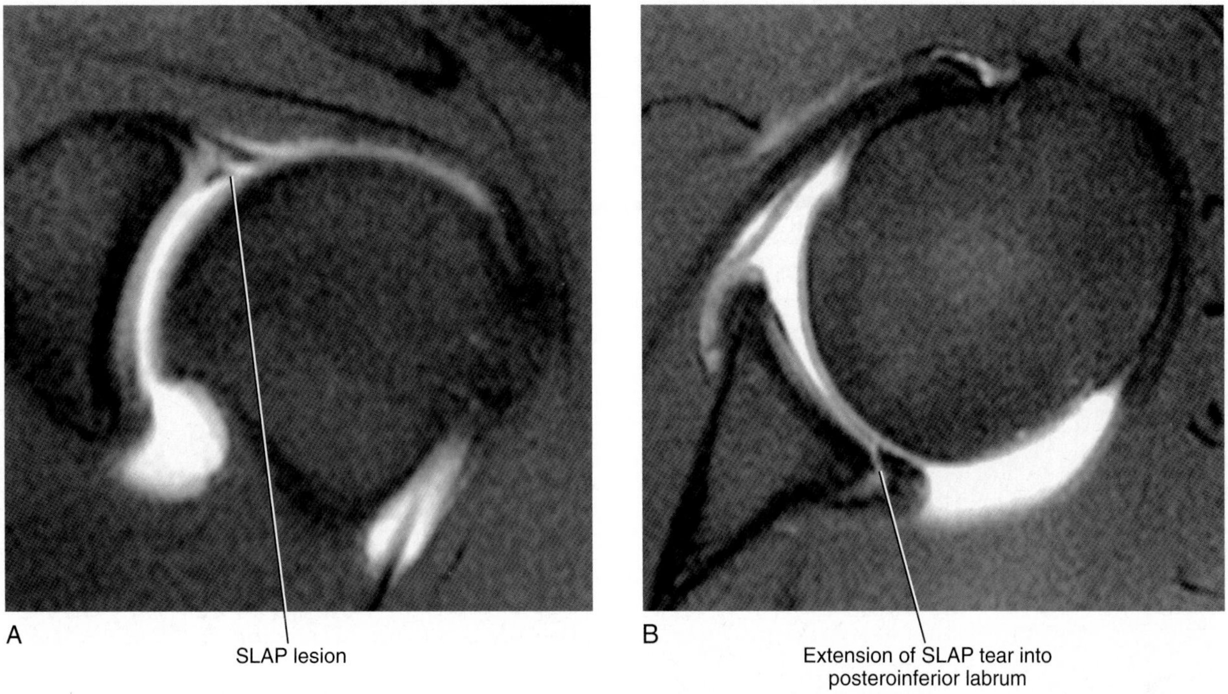
A
SLAP lesion
B
Extension of SLAP tear into posteroinferior labrum

Figure 7-49 **SLAP tear with extension into the posterior inferior labrum. A,** Coronal image demonstrates a bucket-handle tear of the superior labrum with extension of the tear into the posterior inferior labrum demonstrated on the axial image (**B**).

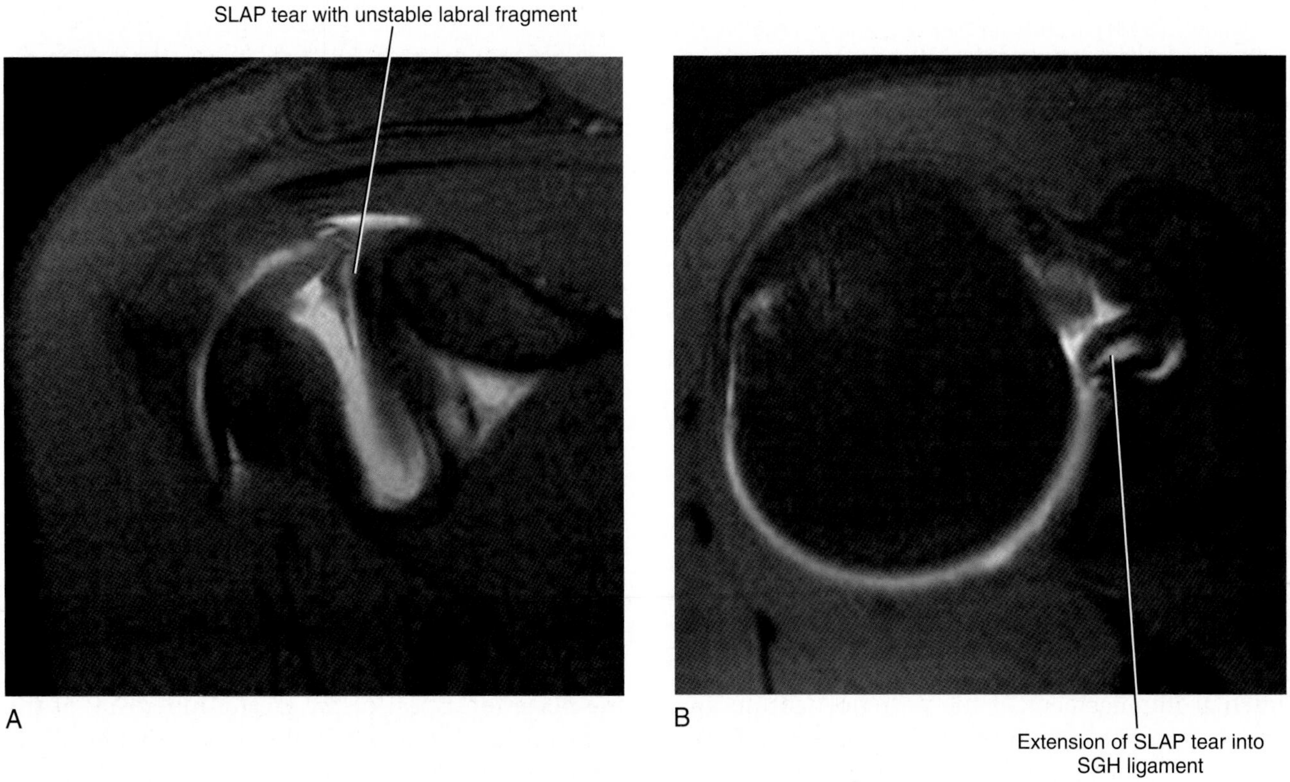
SLAP tear with unstable labral fragment
A
B
Extension of SLAP tear into SGH ligament

Figure 7-50 **SLAP tear with extension into SGHL. A,** Coronal image demonstrates undersurface fraying and an unstable fragment of the superior labrum consistent with a SLAP tear. **B,** Axial image demonstrates extension of the tear into the superior glenohumeral (SGH) ligament. SLAP, superior labral tear anterior to posterior.

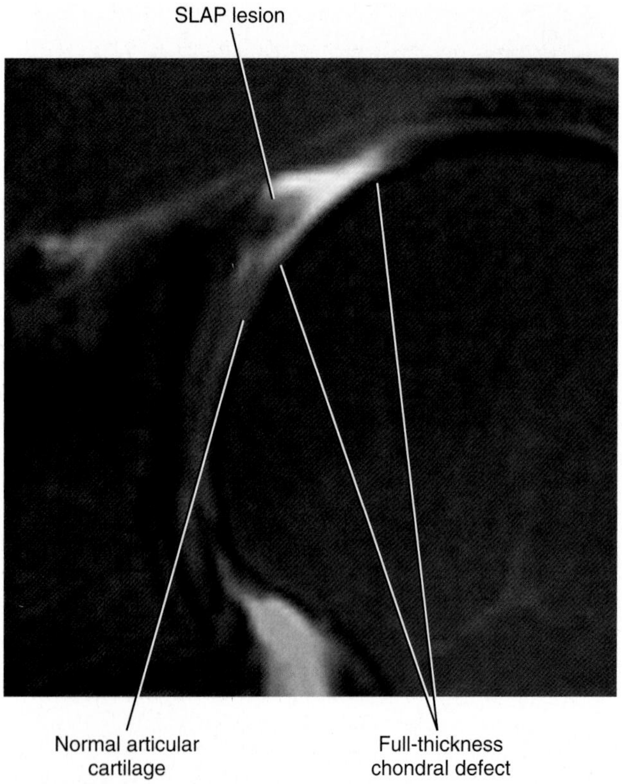
SLAP lesion
Normal articular cartilage
Full-thickness chondral defect

Figure 7-51 SLAP tear with articular cartilage defect. Oblique coronal T1-weighted image with intra-articular gadolinium shows a SLAP tear with a large adjacent full-thickness chondral defect of the humeral head.

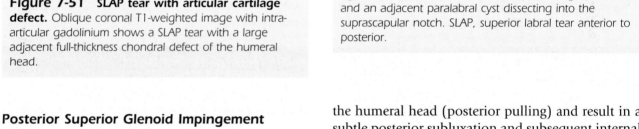

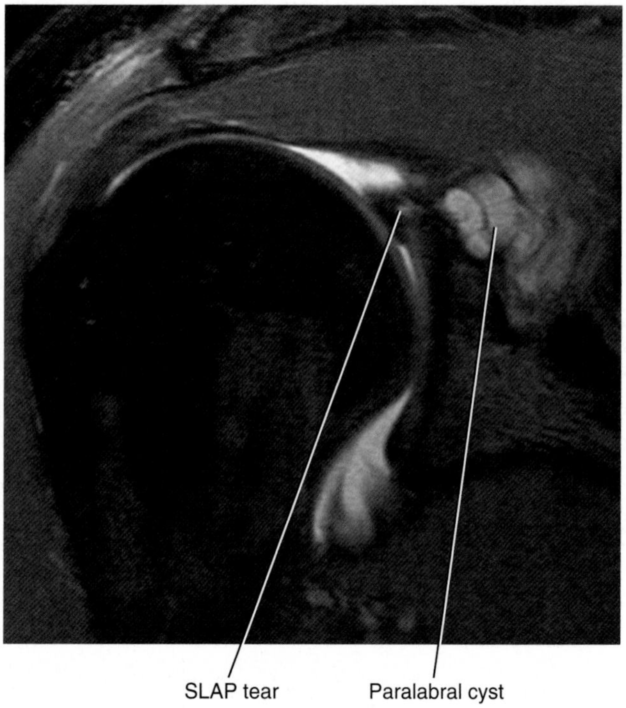
SLAP tear
Paralabral cyst

Figure 7-52 SLAP tear with adjacent paralabral cyst. Coronal T2-weighted image demonstrates abnormal signal within the superior labrum representing a SLAP tear and an adjacent paralabral cyst dissecting into the suprascapular notch. SLAP, superior labral tear anterior to posterior.

Posterior Superior Glenoid Impingement (Internal Impingement)

Internal impingement occurs primarily in athletes who participate in repetitive overhead activities such as throwing or swimming. The injury occurs during maximum abduction and external rotation of the humeral head (late cocking phase of throwing) and results from impingement of the undersurface of the posterior aspect of the rotator cuff between the posterior superior labrum and the posterior aspect of the humeral head. Two mechanisms are proposed for this type of impingement. The first suggests that anterior capsular laxity allows the humeral head to minimally sublux in a posterior direction, leading to the internal impingement of the posterior labrum and the undersurface of the posterior rotator cuff. The second proposed mechanism suggests that stresses of repetitive throwing lead to posterior capsular thickening, scarring, and contracture. These changes of the posterior capsule in turn place posterior tension on the humeral head (posterior pulling) and result in a subtle posterior subluxation and subsequent internal impingement. Internal impingement is usually treated initially with conservative means and requires surgical intervention only if the proper biomechanics cannot be restored with rest of the injured structures (Table 7-12).

The person with internal impingement demonstrates a constellation of MR findings including degenerative fraying of the posterior superior glenoid labrum and partial-thickness undersurface tearing of the posterior aspect of the rotator cuff. This may include the posterior fibers of the supraspinatus tendon or the infraspinatus tendon. Subchondral cystic change or marrow edema may be present in the posterior aspect of the greater tuberosity of the humeral head, but this is the most variable of the associated findings and is often absent. If ABER imaging is performed, entrapment of the undersurface of the posterior rotator cuff between the humeral head and the posterosuperior labrum may actually be

Table 7-12 Internal Impingement

Epidemiology	Young, throwing athletes
Mechanism of injury	Impingement of posterior cuff and superior labrum between greater tuberosity and osseous glenoid
Proposed etiologies	Anterior capsular laxity allows posterior subluxation Posterior capsular scarring pulls humeral head posteriorly
Treatment	Early: Conservative Late: Treat cause of instability
MRI findings	Fraying of posterior superior labrum Fraying/partial-thickness tear undersurface of posterior rotator cuff Cystic changes in greater tuberosity Impingement of soft tissue structures seen on ABER imaging

visualized at the time of imaging (Fig. 7-53). Other associated findings may include a lesion of the anterior labroligamentous complex leading to anterior instability and thickening and scarring of the posterior capsule. The findings of internal impingement are often very subtle, but this combination of MR findings in a young throwing athlete with shoulder pain is diagnostic of internal impingement.

BICEPS TENDON

Normal Anatomy

The long head of the biceps tendon (LHBT) demonstrates a broad triangular intra-articular origin, with fibers variably arising from the superior glenoid tubercle and the superior glenoid labrum. The short head of the biceps tendon has an extra-articular origin arising from the coracoid process along with the

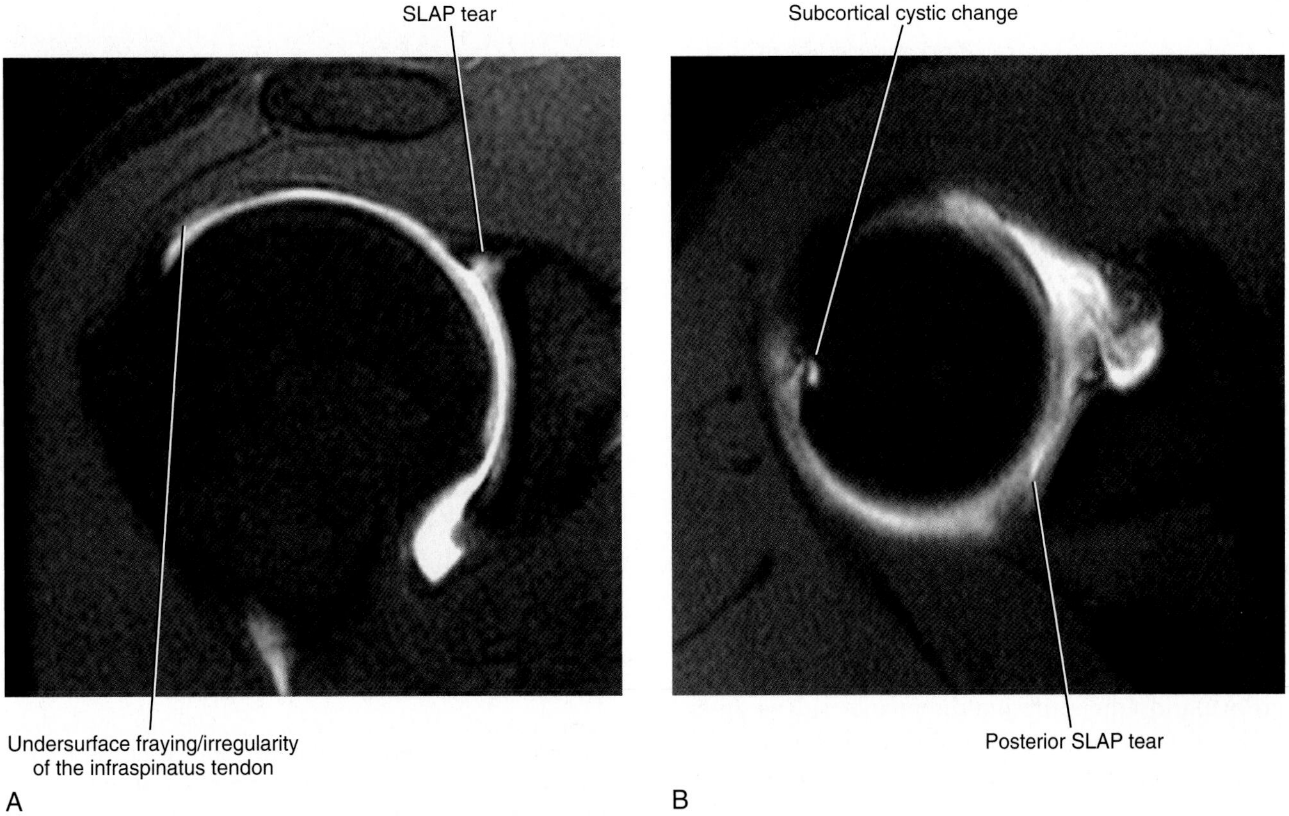
SLAP tear
Undersurface fraying/irregularity of the infraspinatus tendon
A
Subcortical cystic change
Posterior SLAP tear
B

Figure 7-53 Internal impingement. A, Coronal image in a 19-year-old pitcher with shoulder pain demonstrates subtle irregularity and fraying of the articular surface of the infraspinatus tendon. There is also fraying of the undersurface of the posterior superior labrum representing a subtle SLAP lesion. **B,** Axial image demonstrates minimal cystic change in the greater tuberosity of the humeral head and a posterior SLAP tear. *Continued*

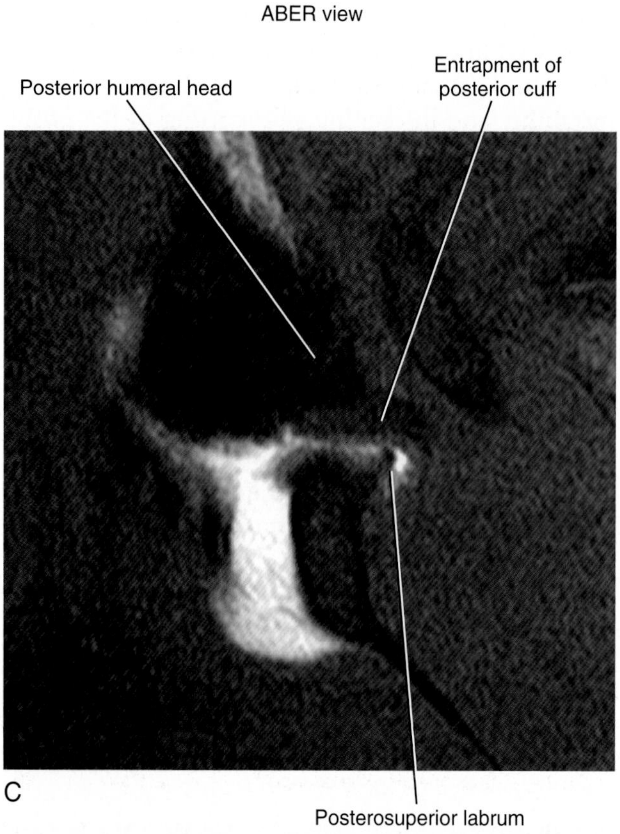
ABER view
Posterior humeral head
Entrapment of posterior cuff
C
Posterosuperior labrum

Figure 7-53, cont'd **C,** ABER image demonstrates impingement of the posterior rotator cuff between the posterior superior labrum and the greater tuberosity of the humeral head.

tendon of the coracobrachialis. The long and short heads of the biceps tendon are both accurately depicted on MRI of the shoulder, but it is the long head of the biceps tendon that is most frequently affected by injury or disease. After its origin, the long head of the biceps follows an intra-articular course traversing the anterior joint space obliquely within the rotator cuff interval (described previously under Rotator Interval), covered by the coracohumeral and the superior glenohumeral ligaments (Fig. 7-54). The LHBT exits the joint at the level of the intertubercular groove and enters the intertubercular sulcus anteriorly. At the transition level, the coracohumeral and superior glenohumeral ligaments are the main stabilizers preventing medial subluxation of the tendon. As the LHBT courses more distally, it encounters secondary stabilizers, which include the transverse humeral ligament proximally and the pectoralis major tendon distally.

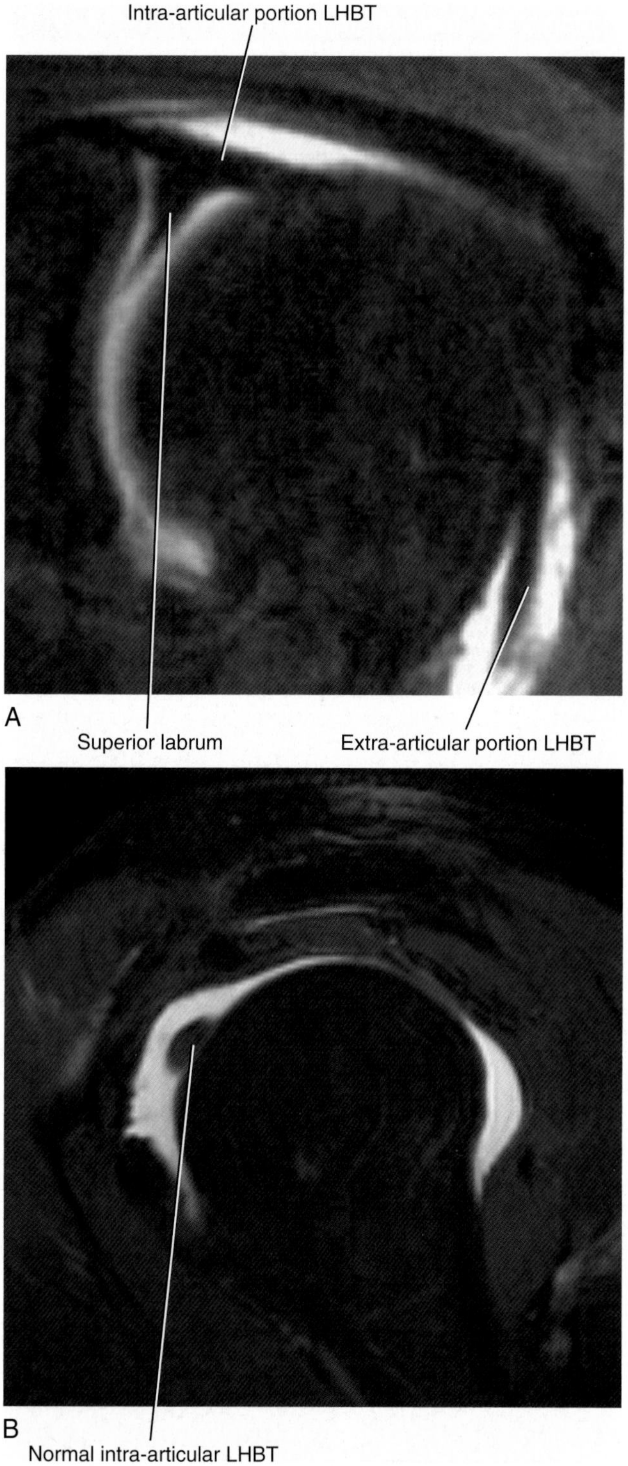
Intra-articular portion LHBT
A
Superior labrum
Extra-articular portion LHBT
B
Normal intra-articular LHBT

Figure 7-54 Normal MRI appearance of the intra-articular portion of the long head of the biceps tendon (LHBT). A, Normal intra-articular portion of the LHBT in the coronal plane arising from the superior glenoid tubercle. The extra-articular portion of the tendon is also visualized. **B,** Normal intra-articular portion of the LHBT in the sagittal imaging plane.

Pathology of the Long Head of the Biceps Tendon

Like any other tendon, the LHBT can be involved in a variety of injuries including tenosynovitis, tendinopathy, and partial- or full-thickness tear, and finally entrapment. Because of its unique anatomic configuration, it can also undergo medial subluxation or dislocation if there is injury or disruption of its stabilizers. This usually occurs in association with a large rotator cuff tear or secondary to an isolated tear of the subscapularis tendon and coracohumeral ligament. Complete MR evaluation of the LHBT should include an evaluation of both the intra-articular and extra-articular (intertubercular groove) portions of the tendon. The oblique sagittal and oblique coronal imaging planes are the primary planes for evaluating the intra-articular portion of the tendon. The oblique sagittal plane allows visualization of the intra-articular portion of the tendon in cross-section from its origin to its exiting point at the level of the intertubercular groove. The normal tendon appears oval when viewed in the sagittal plane and dark on all pulse sequences. With tendinopathy, the tendon demonstrates thickening and intrinsic signal abnormality, whereas a partial-thickness tear demonstrates thinning or attenuation of the tendon or fluid signal within the substance of the tendon (Fig. 7-55). With a complete tear, the tendon is "nonvisualized" and may demonstrate distal retraction. An "empty" intertubercular groove indicates disruption and distal retraction of the tendon extra-articular portion of the tendon.

Subluxation Patterns of the Long Head of the Biceps Tendon

The extra-articular portion of the LHBT is best evaluated using the axial imaging plane (Fig. 7-56 ; see Fig. 7-18D). The intertubercular groove portion of the LHBT should be evaluated for thickening, intrinsic signal abnormality, partial- or full-thickness tear, adjacent fluid out of proportion to the joint fluid, loose bodies, and finally medial subluxation. A tear of the coracohumeral ligament results in medial subluxation of the LHBT, and three patterns of sublux-

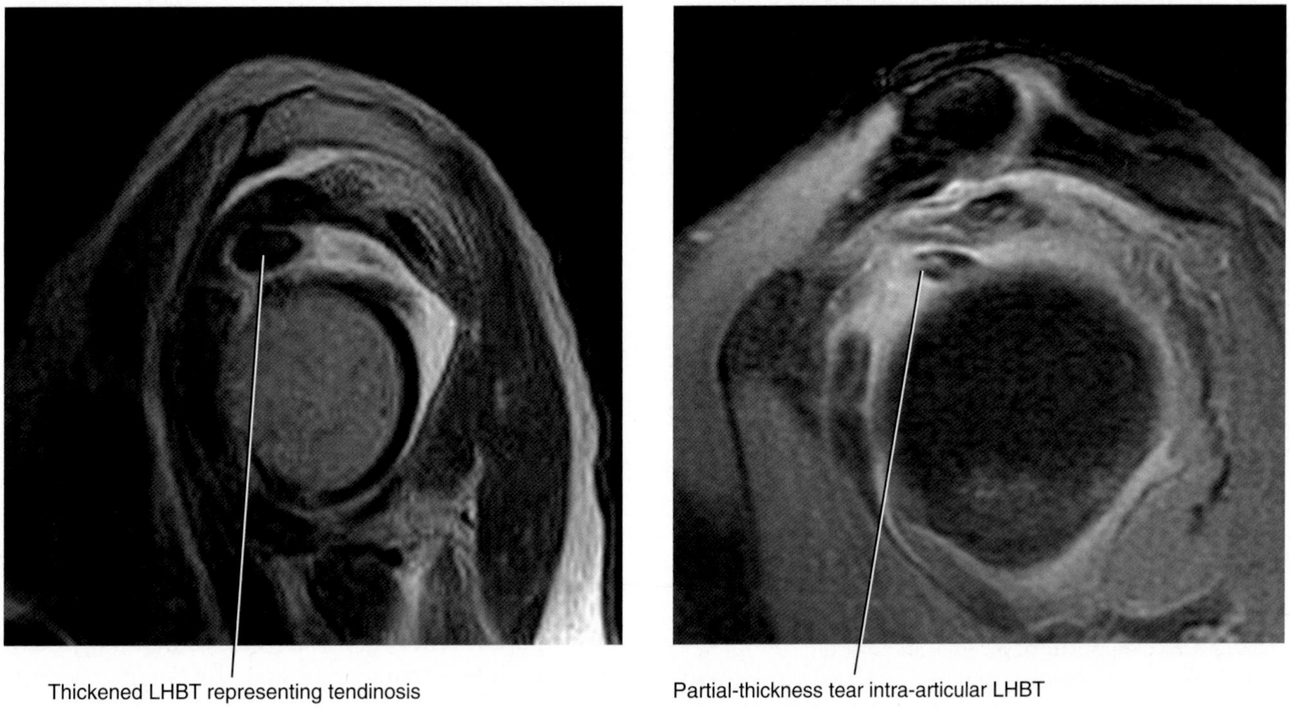
Thickened LHBT representing tendinosis
A
Partial-thickness tear intra-articular LHBT
B

Figure 7-55 Intra-articular long head biceps tendon (LHBT) pathology. A, Coronal T2-weighted image shows marked thickening and intermediate intrinsic signal abnormality within the intra-articular portion of the LHBT consistent with tendinopathy. **B,** Coronal T2-weighted image reveals a focal linear area of fluid signal within the substance of the LHBT consistent with a partial-thickness tear.

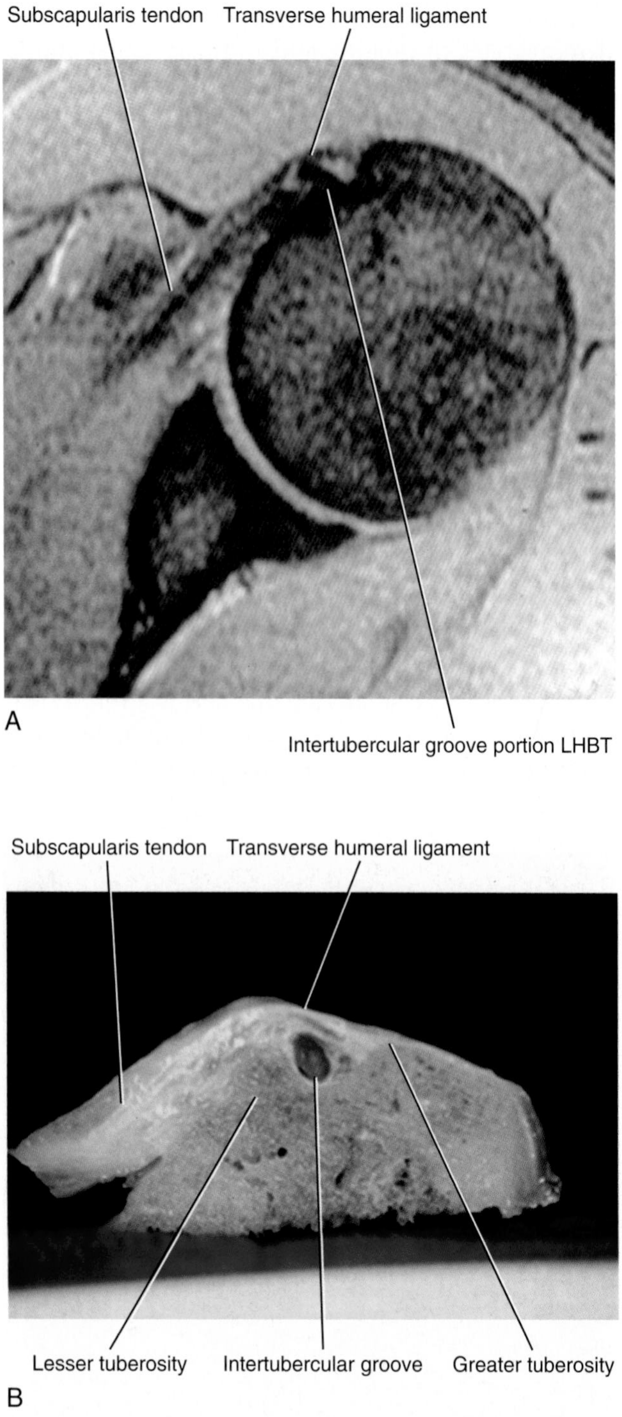
Subscapularis tendon
Transverse humeral ligament
A
Intertubercular groove portion LHBT
Subscapularis tendon
Transverse humeral ligament
Lesser tuberosity
Intertubercular groove
Greater tuberosity
B

Figure 7-56 Long head of biceps tendon (LHBT) extra-articular portion. A, Axial MR image demonstrates the normal appearance of the LHBT within the intertubercular groove covered by the transverse humeral ligament (superficial fibers of the subscapularis tendon). **B,** Gross axial section through the humeral head demonstrates the normal appearance of the fibro-osseous tunnel that contains the LHBT.

Table 7-13 Patterns of Medial Subluxation of LHBT

Structures Torn	Location of LHBT
Deep fibers of subscap and CHL	Intra-articular medial subluxation
THL and CHL	Extra-articular medial subluxation
Isolated CHL tear (subscap intact)	Medial subluxation into substance of subscapularis tendon/muscle
Isolated subscap tear (CHL intact)	No subluxation: LHBT remains within intertubercular groove

CHL, coracohumeral ligament; LHBT, long head of biceps tendon; subscap, subscapularis tendon; THL, transverse humeral ligament.

ation have been described that are related to the status of the subscapularis tendon and the coracohumeral ligament (Table 7-13).

First, disruption of the coracohumeral ligament in conjunction with a complete tear or avulsion of the subscapularis tendon off of the lesser tuberosity results in an intra-articular subluxation of the LHBT (Fig. 7-57). The LHBT is medially subluxed into the anterior joint space, medial to the intertubercular groove, and the subscapularis tendon is torn and retracted medially. Next, a tear of the coracohumeral ligament in conjunction with a tear of the subscapularis tendon isolated to the transverse humeral ligament results in extra-articular subluxation of the LHBT, and the tendon is located medial to the intertubercular groove but superficial to the intact fibers of the subscapularis tendon. Finally, an isolated tear of the coracohumeral ligament with an intact subscapularis tendon and transverse humeral ligament allows medial migration of the LHBT into the substance of the subscapularis tendon, resulting in interstitial tearing of the tendon. The LHBT is visualized medial to the intertubercular groove, but sitting within the substance of the subscapularis tendon and muscle. The combination of an isolated tear of the subscapularis tendon or transverse humeral ligament and an intact coracohumeral ligament prevents medial subluxation of the LHBT (Fig. 7-58).

Entrapment of the Long Head of the Biceps Tendon (Hourglass Biceps)

The "hourglass" biceps tendon describes a condition of marked tendinosis and hypertrophy of the

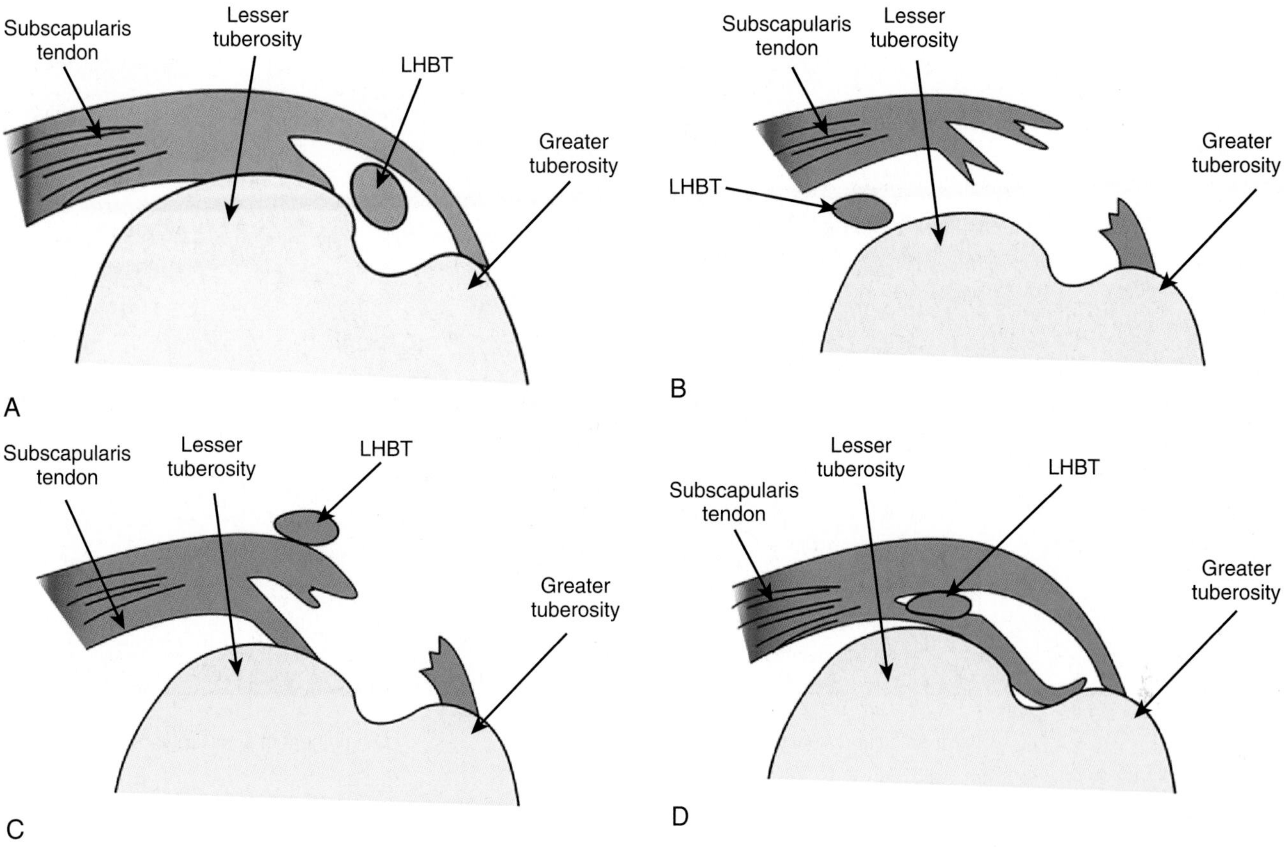
Subscapularis tendon
Lesser tuberosity
LHBT
Greater tuberosity
A
Subscapularis tendon
Lesser tuberosity
LHBT
Greater tuberosity
B
Subscapularis tendon
Lesser tuberosity
LHBT
Greater tuberosity
C
Lesser tuberosity
Subscapularis tendon
LHBT
Greater tuberosity
D

Figure 7-57 Long head of biceps tendon (LHBT), patterns of medial subluxation. A, Normal position of the LHBT in the intertubercular groove. **B,** Disruption or avulsion of the deep fibers of the subscapularis tendon off of the lesser tuberosity in conjunction with disruption of the coracohumeral ligament allows intra-articular subluxation of the LHBT. **C,** Disruption of the transverse humeral ligament along with disruption of the coracohumeral ligament allows extra-articular medial subluxation of the LHBT. **D,** Disruption of the coracohumeral ligament with an intact subscapularis tendon allows the LHBT to sublux medially into the substance of the subscapularis tendon, resulting in an interstitial tear of the subscapularis tendon and muscle.

intra-articular portion of the LHBT, which prevents the tendon from sliding into the bicipital groove during elevation of the arm. A mechanical block occurs with entrapment of the LHBT, causing entrapment and pain. This condition occurs most often in association with a full-thickness tear of the rotator cuff, although there are case reports of entrapment occurring in association with partial-thickness rotator cuff tears as well. Patients present with anterior arm pain and loss of passive elevation of the arm averaging approximately 10 to 20 degrees. Treatment is with resection of the abnormal segment and tenodesis of the biceps tendon followed by appropriate treatment of any concomitant injury of the rotator cuff after which patients experience immediate recovery of their full range of motion. MRI shows marked tendinosis and thickening limited to the intra-articular portion of the LHBT, which is usually associated with either a partial- or full-thickness rotator cuff tear (Fig. 7-59).

PECTORALIS MAJOR MUSCLE AND TENDON

Tears of the pectoralis major muscle and tendon have become more common over the past decade with most occurring in weight-lifters, especially during the bench press. Injuries of the pectoralis major have also been reported during other strenuous sporting activities such as football, rugby, and wrestling. The pectoralis major is a powerful internal rotator, flexor, and

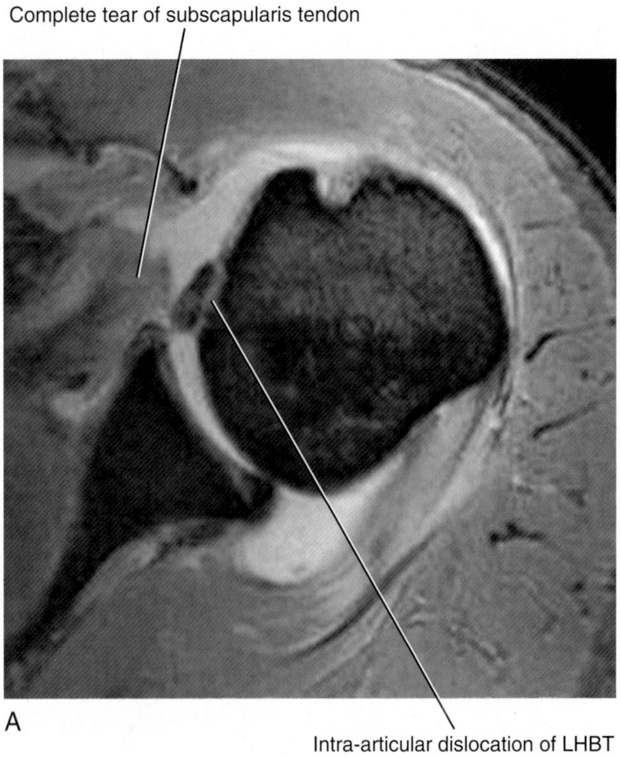
Complete tear of subscapularis tendon
A
Intra-articular dislocation of LHBT

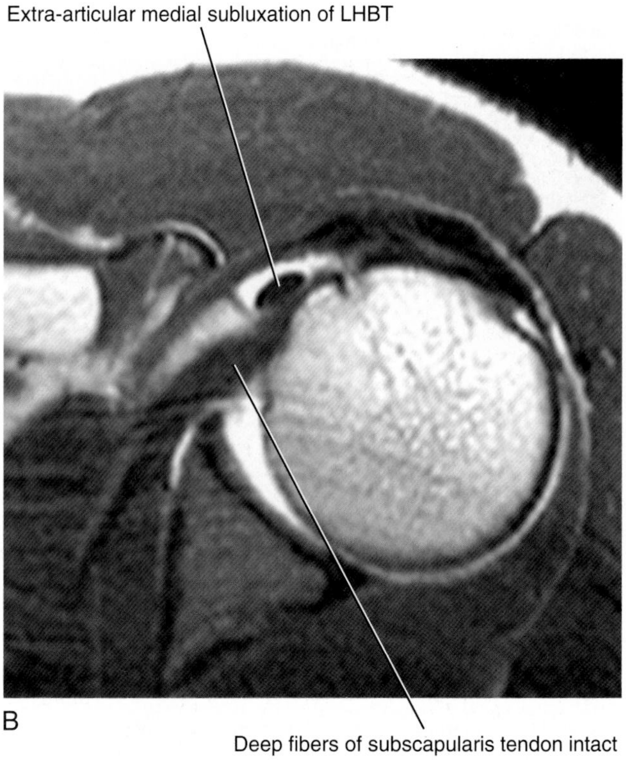
Extra-articular medial subluxation of LHBT
B
Deep fibers of subscapularis tendon intact

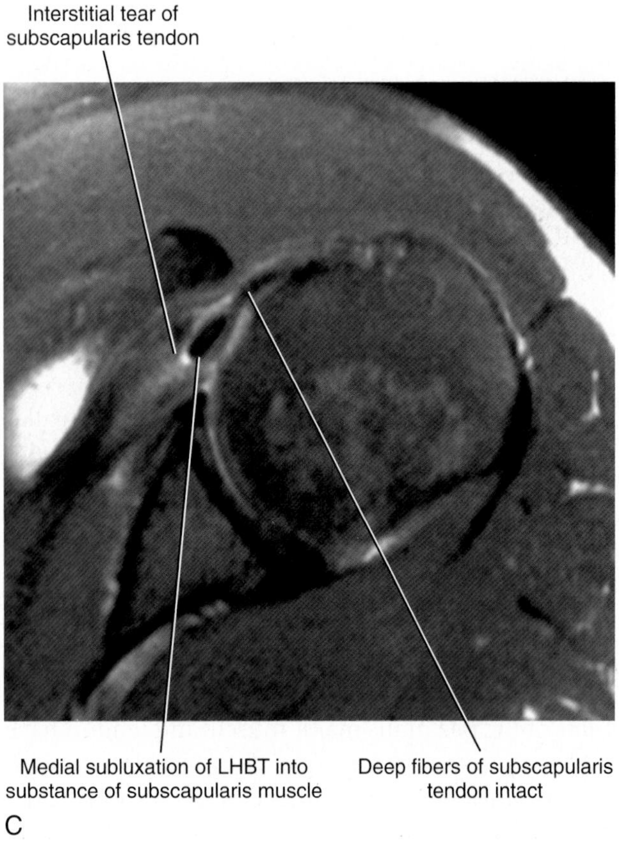
Interstitial tear of subscapularis tendon
Medial subluxation of LHBT into substance of subscapularis muscle
Deep fibers of subscapularis tendon intact
C

Figure 7-58 MR appearance of the long head of the biceps tendon (LHBT) subluxation patterns. **A,** Intra-articular medial dislocation of the LHBT indicates disruption of the deep fibers of the subscapularis as well as disruption of the coracohumeral ligament. **B,** Extra-articular medial subluxation of the LHBT indicates disruption of the transverse humeral ligament and the coracohumeral ligament. The deep fibers of the subscapularis tendon remain intact. **C,** Medial subluxation of the LHBT into the substance of the subscapularis tendon. This type of subluxation results from an isolated tear of the coracohumeral ligament. The subluxation of the LHBT is the precipitating event leading to an interstitial tear of the subscapularis tendon.

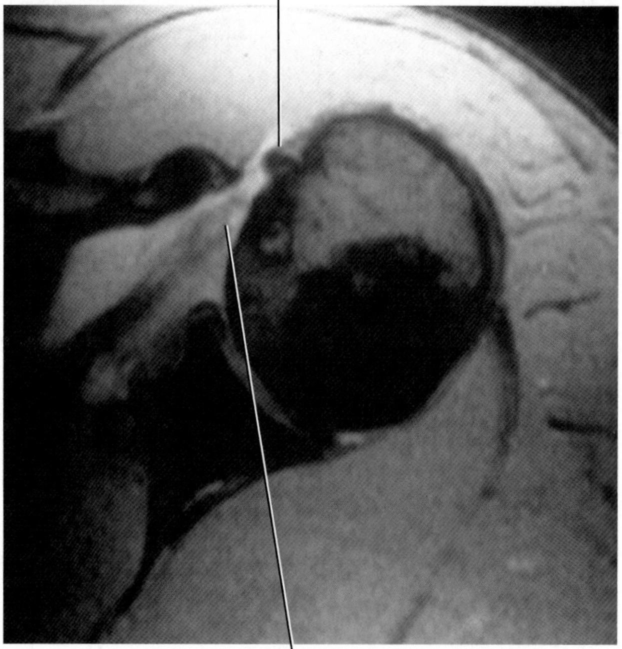
LHBT normal position in intertubercular groove
D
Complete tear and retraction of subscapularis tendon

Figure 7-58, cont'd **D,** The subscapularis tendon is completely torn and retracted; however, the LHBT remains normally positioned within the intertubercular groove. This pattern of injury indicates that the coracohumeral ligament remains intact stabilizing the LHBT and preventing medial subluxation.

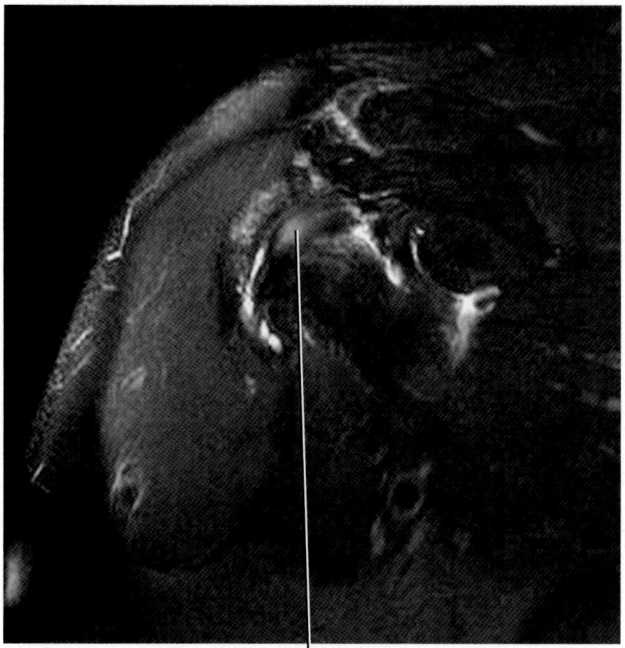
A
Tendinosis with thickening and edema of the intra-articular portion of the LHBT

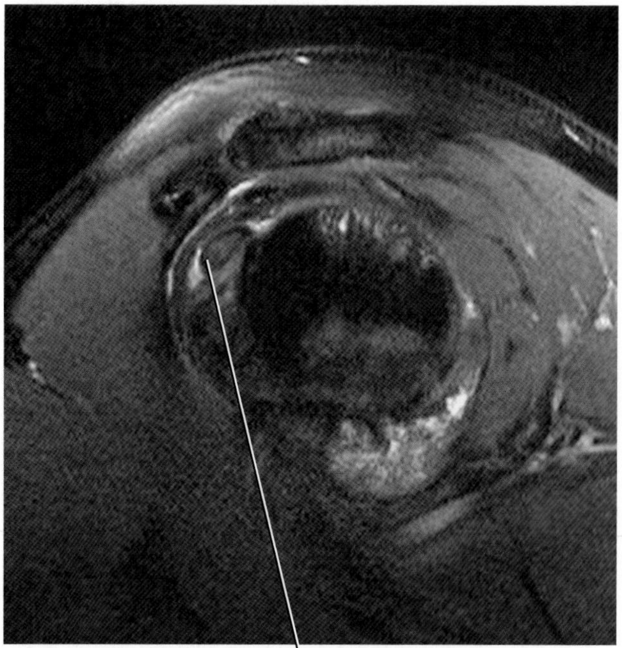
B
Tendinosis with thickening and edema of the intra-articular portion of the LHBT

Figure 7-59 **Entrapment of the long head of the biceps tendon (LHBT) "hourglass" biceps.** Coronal (**A**) and sagittal (**B**) images show marked thickening and tendinosis of the intra-articular portion of the LHBT. *Continued*

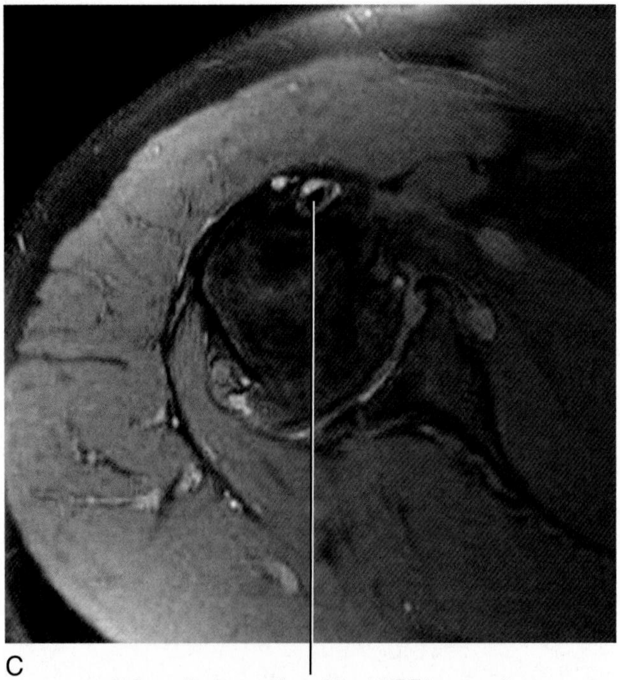
C
Extra-articular portion of the LHBT is normal

Figure 7-59, cont'd The extra-articular portion of the LHBT shows normal appearance on axial image (**C**). This patient demonstrated clinical signs of LHBT entrapment with loss of passive elevation of the arm.

adductor of the arm and is important for strenuous activity of the upper extremity. The muscle is broad, flat, and triangular and is composed of two separate heads. The smaller superior (clavicular) head originates on the medial third of the clavicle and the upper third of the sternum, whereas the larger inferior (sternal) head arises from the inferior two thirds of the sternum, the costal cartilage of the first six ribs, and the aponeurosis of the external oblique muscle (Fig. 7-60). The two heads converge laterally to form the apex of the triangle, which is a 5-cm wide bilaminate tendon that inserts onto the anterior aspect of the humeral shaft just lateral to the bicipital groove. The clavicular head forms the anterior lamina of the tendon and inserts more superficially, and its tendon measures approximately 1 cm in length. The posterior lamina is formed by the sternal head, which inserts deep to the clavicular head; this portion of the tendon is approximately 2.5 cm long.

Injuries to the pectoralis major muscle and tendon typically occur during strenuous activity, and the patient often reports the sensation of tearing and may hear a popping sound. Onset of pain is immediate. Point tenderness over the tear and extensive ecchymosis occur. Injuries are classified as muscle strains, type I; partial-thickness tears, type II; and full-thickness tears, type III. Type III injuries are further subdivided into tears of the muscular origin, belly of the muscle, musculotendinous junction, and the tendon. Although any of the full-thickness tears can be treated surgically, a full-thickness tear of the tendon appears to benefit the most from surgical repair. This scheme should be used when describing the MR appearance of pectoralis major injuries, and it should be remembered that differentiation between a partial- and full-thickness tear is usually the determining factor as to whether the individual will benefit from surgical repair of the tendon (Table 7-14).

Acute injuries of the pectoralis muscle and tendon are best evaluated on axial and coronal T2-weighted images centered over the anterior chest wall and the proximal humeral shaft just inferior to the subscapularis tendon insertion. A larger field of view is helpful to evaluate the entire pectoralis muscle, whereas additional images with a smaller field of view centered over the humeral insertion site of the pectoralis major tendon can be helpful in better defining the extent of injury to the tendon. If one uses only the larger field-of-view images to evaluate the distal tendon, it is often difficult to accurately detect the full extent of injury because of the small size of the structure.

Description of a pectoralis major injury should include the location and extent of the tear, including which head is involved and whether the injury involves the origin of the muscle, the muscle belly, the musculotendinous junction, or the tendon. The size and location of any hematoma should also be described. The overall muscle is best visualized on large field-of-view coronal images, whereas the tendon is best visualized with small field-of-view axial images at the level of the insertion. Tears of the muscle or musculotendinous junction often result in a large hematoma that can make differentiation between a full- and partial-thickness tear difficult. The coronal views can be very helpful in this regard because a full-thickness tear will result in retraction of the musculotendinous junction and loss of the anterior axillary fold (Fig. 7-61), whereas with a partial-thickness tear the axillary fold will still be present. The axillary fold is best demonstrated on the coronal images (see Fig. 7-60).

One word of caution is in order: One of the most common injury patterns is a full-thickness tear isolated to the sternal head of the pectoralis major tendon with an intact clavicular head. This injury pattern results in retraction of the musculotendinous junction of the sternal head, whereas the tendon of the clavicular head remains intact. It is best treated by surgically repairing the sternal head. This pattern is often misinterpreted on physical examination and on MRI as a partial-thickness tear of the tendon because the sternal portion of the bilaminate tendon remains intact, maintaining the anterior axillary fold and giving the appearance on MR imaging of a partial-thickness tendon tear. On the coronal images, this pattern of injury can be confirmed by identifying proximal retraction of the musculotendinous junction of the sternal head, with an intact clavicular head.

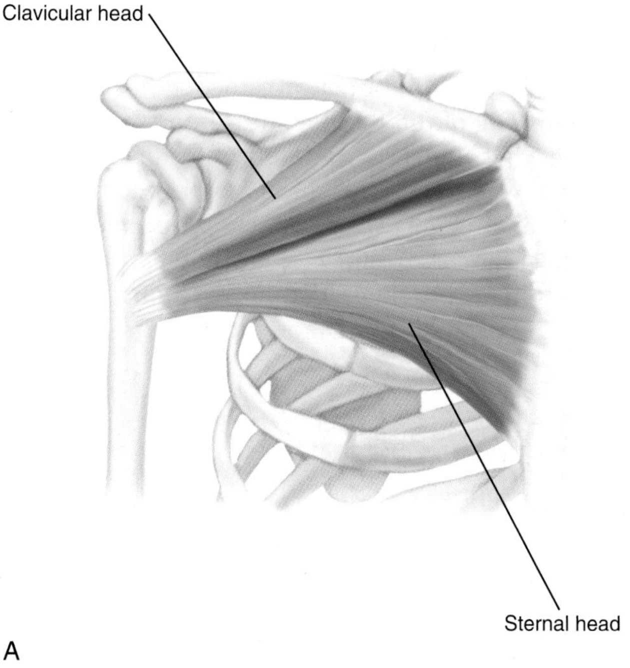
Clavicular head
Sternal head
A

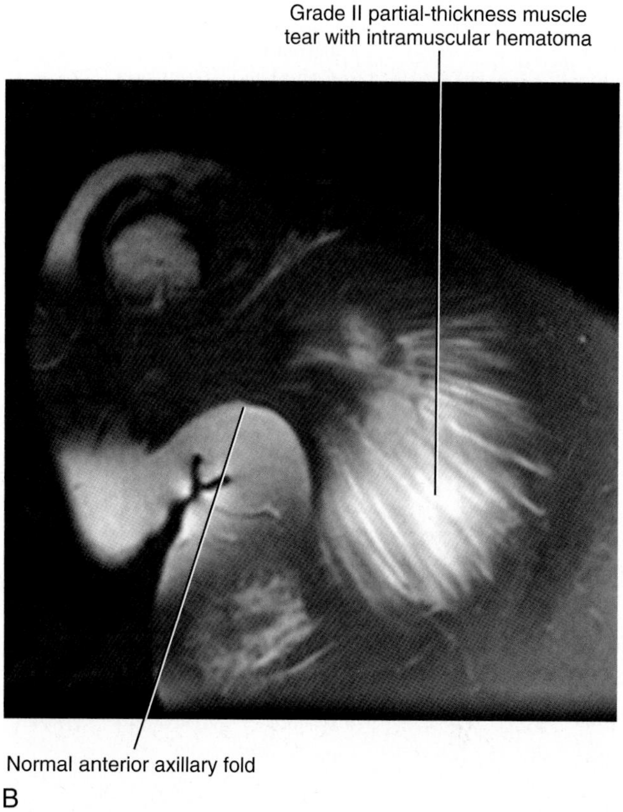
Grade II partial-thickness muscle tear with intramuscular hematoma
Normal anterior axillary fold
B

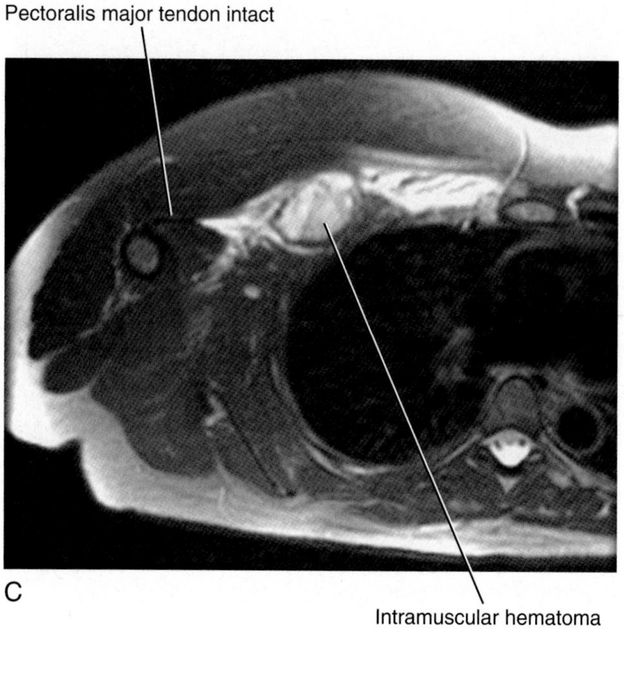
Pectoralis major tendon intact
C
Intramuscular hematoma

Figure 7-60 Grade II pectoralis muscle tear with intramuscular hematoma. A, Artwork shows normal anatomy of clavicular and sternal heads of pectoralis major. Coronal (**B**) and axial (**C**) T2-weighted images with fat saturation show a partial-thickness tear of the pectoralis major muscle with a large intramuscular hematoma. The musculotendinous junction and tendon are intact, and the anterior axillary fold is normal in appearance. An intact anterior axillary fold indicates the lack of a full-thickness tear of the bilaminate tendon.

Table 7-14 Scheme for Describing Pectoralis Major Injuries

Location of tear	Muscle Musculotendinous junction Tendon
Description of tear	Muscle Strain Partial-thickness tear Complete tear Hematoma Tendon Partial-thickness tear Complete tear/avulsion Sternal or clavicular head tendon involvement

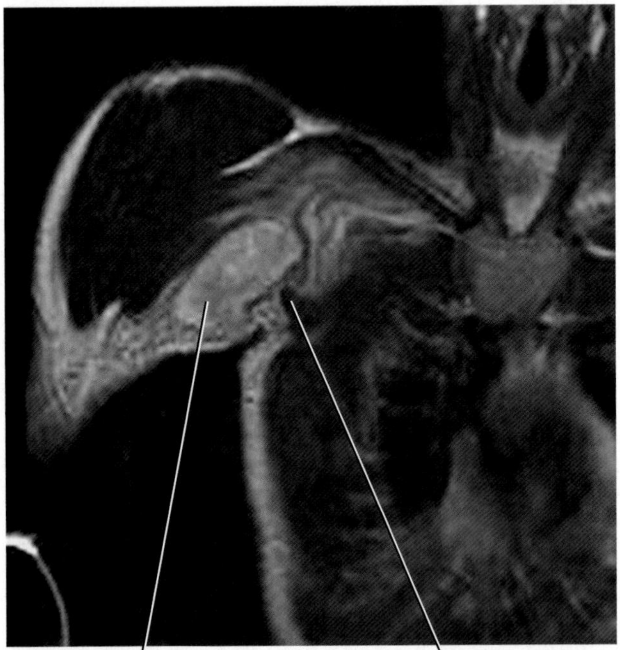
Hematoma and absence of the anterior axillary fold
Complete tear with tendon retraction

Figure 7-61 Complete tear of the pectoralis major tendon. Coronal T2-weighted image shows a complete tear of the pectoralis major tendon. There is retraction of the torn tendon end, with a large adjacent hematoma and absence of the anterior axillary fold.

THE POSTOPERATIVE SHOULDER

Interpretation of the postoperative MR examination of the shoulder can be a difficult and challenging task. Extensive postoperative artifact is frequently located in the area of interest following repair of either the rotator cuff or labrum, and the anatomy can be surgically altered. MRI signs that would indicate pathology in the nonoperative shoulder can represent normal findings in the postoperative shoulder. To maximize the information gained from postoperative imaging of the shoulder, it is important to have an imaging strategy to minimize postoperative MR artifact. One should also have a basic knowledge of the common surgical procedures performed on the shoulder and how they alter shoulder anatomy. Finally, the MRI signs of recurrent injury or postoperative complications should be understood.

MRI Strategies to Minimize Postoperative Artifact

Surgical hardware including prosthesis, screws, suture anchors, and even suture material can result in extensive susceptibility artifact in the postoperative shoulder, which can obscure the evaluation of normal anatomy as well as recurrent pathology. Minimizing these artifacts is often one of the biggest challenges facing imagers when performing MR examinations on the postoperative shoulder. Although total elimination of susceptibility artifact is rarely achieved, careful selection of the MR pulse sequences and imaging parameters can minimize this artifact (Box 7-2).

A dedicated shoulder coil should always be used when possible and standard imaging planes and pulse sequences should include T2-weighted imaging

BOX 7-2 STRATEGIES TO MINIMIZE POSTOPERATIVE MR ARTIFACT

- Avoid gradient-echo imaging (blooming artifact)
- Spin-echo or preferably fast spin-echo in place of gradient-echo imaging
- Long echo trains when performing fast spin-echo
- STIR (short tau inversion recovery) preferable to frequency-selective fat saturation
- Increase bandwidth
- Frequency encoding away from area of interest
- Use of high-matrix imaging

in the axial, oblique coronal, and oblique sagittal planes and T1-weighted images in the oblique coronal and oblique sagittal planes. Gradient-echo imaging, often performed in the axial plane to evaluate the labrum in the nonoperative shoulder, should be avoided in the postoperative patient, since it results in blooming artifact, which amplifies susceptibility artifact and often results in uninterruptible images. The one advantage of gradient-echo imaging is that it can help identify an area of prior surgery if not known from the history. Conventional spin-echo and preferably fast spin-echo imaging minimize susceptibility artifact and should be used in place of gradient-echo imaging. The use of a long echo train reduces susceptibility artifact even further. When using fat-saturation techniques, short tau inversion recovery (STIR) techniques are preferable to frequency-selective fat saturation for minimizing susceptibility artifact.

Other imaging techniques that can minimize artifact include the use of higher bandwidths, frequency-encoding axis directed away from the area of interest, and high-matrix imaging.

Finally, direct MR arthrography can be useful in the evaluation of the postoperative shoulder. It is particularly helpful when evaluating for a recurrent labral tear after a Bankart or SLAP repair and may also be of value when assessing for recurrent partial-thickness tears of the undersurface of the rotator cuff.

Common Surgical Procedures of the Shoulder

Subacromial Decompression

Extrinsic compression of the rotator cuff between the humeral head and the overlying osseous outlet is thought to be a common cause of the clinical syndrome of impingement. Subacromial decompression is a commonly performed surgical procedure aimed at correcting the anatomic abnormality or configuration that results in compression of the underlying cuff. During subacromial decompression, the surgeon removes a portion of the anterolateral acromion. The goal of the procedure is to increase the distance between the humeral head and the overriding osseous outlet, thus providing more room for the rotator cuff. This may involve shaving the undersurface of the anterior acromion or removal of a spur or anterior hook. Subacromial decompression can be accomplished via open or arthroscopic technique (Fig. 7-62). Impingement caused by AC joint hypertrophy

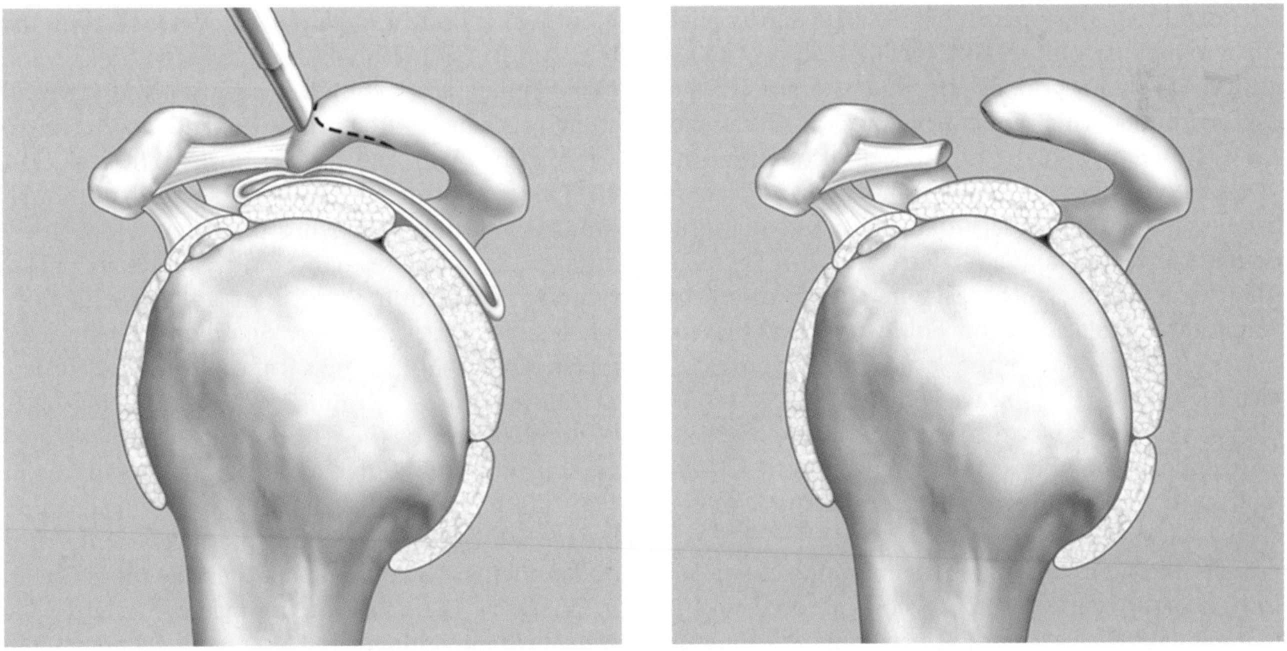

A B

Figure 7-62 Subacromial decompression. *A,* The anterior hook is removed arthroscopically and the coracoacromial ligament is either transected or debrided. ***B,*** The postoperative appearance demonstrates a flat undersurface of the acromion and absence or thinning of a portion of the coracoacromial ligament.

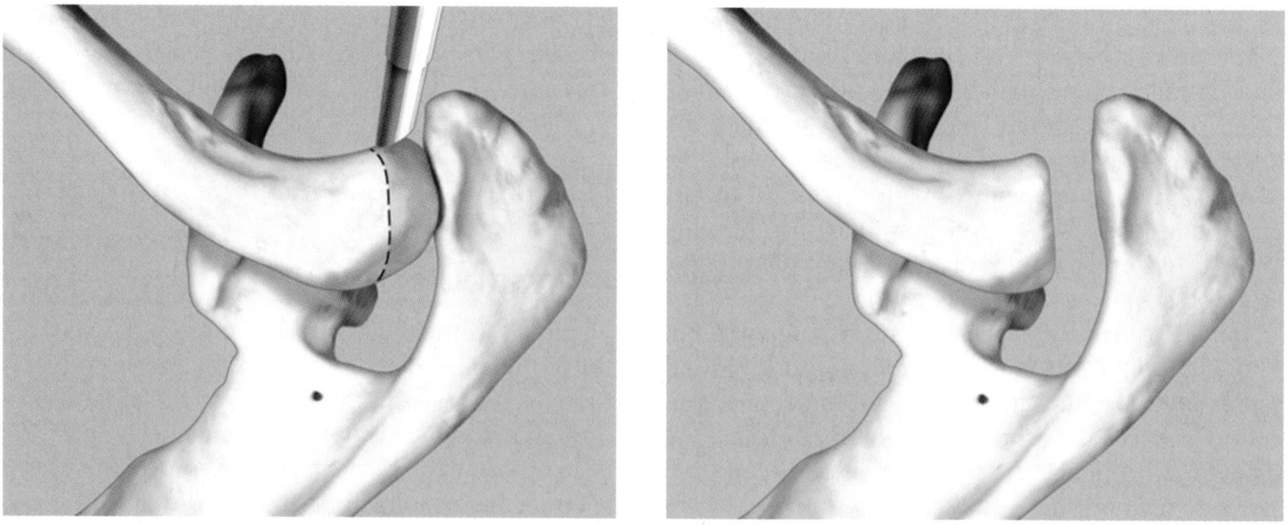

A B

Figure 7-63 Mumford procedure. The acromioclavicular joint before (**A**) and after (**B**) resection of the distal clavicle results in apparent widening of the joint.

and osteophyte formation can be corrected either by removing the distal 1 to 2 cm of the clavicle or by resecting the entire acromioclavicular joint (Fig. 7-63). Finally, thickening of the coracohumeral ligament can be addressed by debridement or resection of a portion of the ligament.

The normal postoperative MR appearance after subacromial decompression includes susceptibility artifact in the region of the undersurface of the osseous outlet. This results from surgical burrs and shavers used at the time of surgical decompression. The postoperative acromion should have a flat or mildly undulating undersurface with no inferiorly directed osteophyte (Fig. 7-64A and B). There is often scar tissue or fibrosis in the location of surgically resected acromion. Following distal clavicle or acromioclavicular joint resection, the acromioclavicular joint often appears widened (Fig. 7-64C). Finally, after section or debridement of the coracoacromial ligament, the ligament may appear irregular or disrupted near its acromial attachment (Fig. 7-64D).

Signs and symptoms of recurrent impingement following subacromial decompression can occur in up to 10% of patients. Causes of persistent or recurrent pain include inadequate resection of structures, osteoarthritis of the acromioclavicular joint, progression of rotator cuff pathology, and undiagnosed glenohumeral instability as the original source of impingement (Fig. 7-65). Another potential source of persistent impingement is the presence of an undiagnosed and untreated os acromiale.

At the time of subacromial decompression, the cuff is thoroughly evaluated and is also repaired if an abnormality is identified. Traditionally, cuff repairs were performed by means of an open surgical technique, using bone tunnels and sutures to reattach the torn cuff to the humeral head. Over the past several years, cuff repair techniques have evolved from all open procedures, to mini-open, and finally to all arthroscopic, with the use of suture anchors to reattach the torn cuff to the humeral head. Although more technically challenging, the arthroscopic procedure results in decreased morbidity, allows for a more thorough evaluation of the intra-articular structures, and enables a faster recovery. Standard guidelines for repair of a partial-thickness tear of the rotator cuff are as follows: A tear extending through more than 70% of the thickness of the tendon is usually completed and repaired similar to a complete rotator cuff repair (Fig. 7-66); 30% to 70%, debride the cuff tear, suture the tendon (tendon-to-tendon) to reinforce the area of debridement; less than 30%, debride the cuff tear. In all cases, the cause of impingement should be identified and addressed.

Rotator Cuff Repair

The normal postoperative MR appearance of the rotator cuff may include distortion of the cuff and

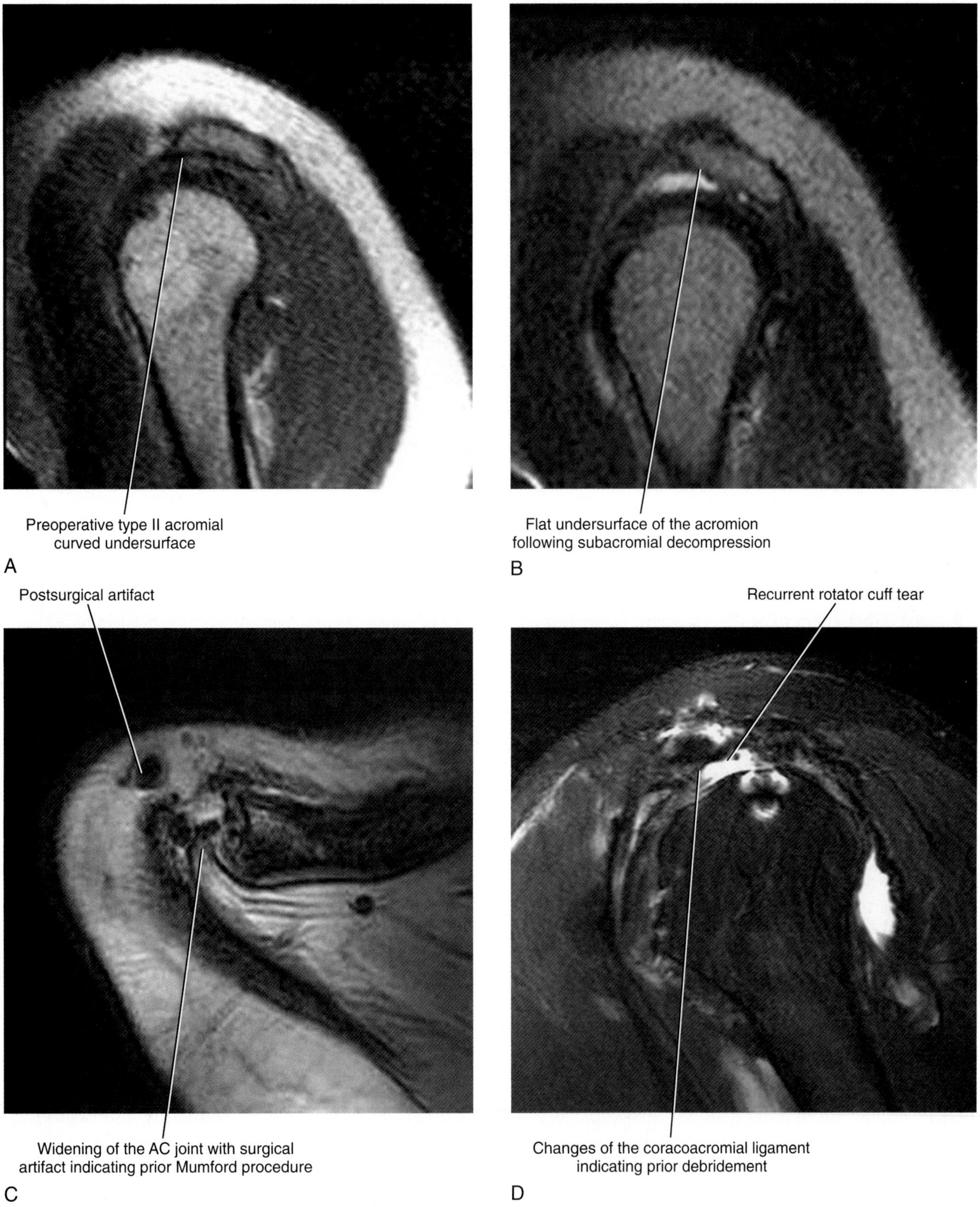
Preoperative type II acromial curved undersurface
A
Flat undersurface of the acromion following subacromial decompression
B
Postsurgical artifact
Recurrent rotator cuff tear
Widening of the AC joint with surgical artifact indicating prior Mumford procedure
C
Changes of the coracoacromial ligament indicating prior debridement
D

Figure 7-64 Normal MRI appearance following various decompression procedures. A, Sagittal image demonstrates a type II acromion with undersurface curvature resulting in the clinical syndrome of impingement. **B,** The undersurface of the acromion is flat following subacromial decompression. **C,** The acromioclavicular (AC) joint is widened and postsurgical artifact is noted following a Mumford procedure. **D,** The coracoacromial ligament has been resected at the level of its attachment to the anterior acromion.

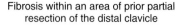

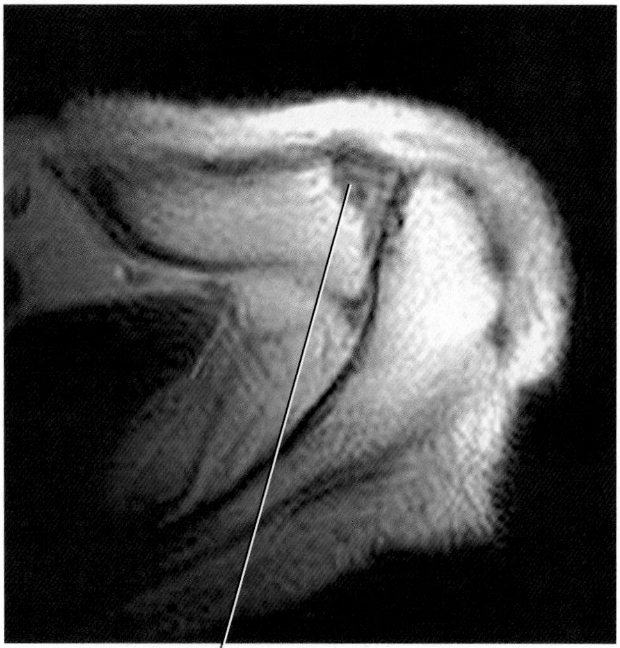
Fibrosis within an area of prior partial resection of the distal clavicle
A

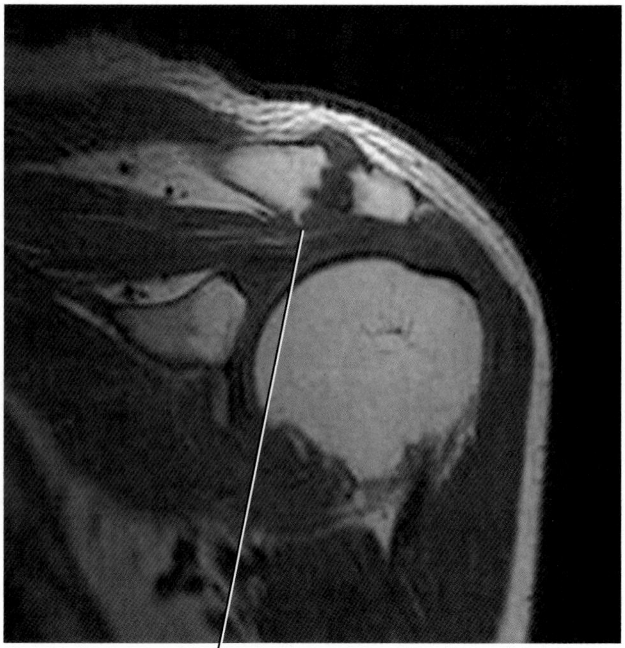
Persistent inferiorly directed osteophyte following an inadequate Mumford procedure
B

Figure 7-65 Persistent impingement following inadequate decompression. Axial (**A**) and coronal (**B**) images following an inadequately performed Mumford procedure demonstrate persistent osteophyte formation extending off of the undersurface of the acromioclavicular joint resulting in persistent symptoms of impingement.

shortening or medialization of the tendon. The tendon may demonstrate intermediate signal abnormality representing granulation tissue or thickening and fibrosis in the region of repair. If a bone tunnel was used to reattach the tendon, the humeral trough is visualized, whereas adjacent artifact usually results from suture material, screws, or suture anchors used to reattach the tendon (Fig. 7-67).

After rotator cuff repair, recurrent symptoms may indicate recurrent impingement, progression of rotator cuff disease, or a recurrent partial- or full-thickness rotator cuff tear. Although postsurgical artifact may obscure a portion of the tendon, optimization of the images as described in the previous section allows adequate visualization of the tendon in most cases. MR findings diagnostic of a full-thickness recurrent tear include fluid signal on T2-weighted images in the expected location of the tendon, nonvisualization of a portion of the tendon, or complete absence of the tendon (Fig. 7-68). Recurrent partial-thickness tears are much more difficult to diagnose because the postoperative tendon is often thinned or attenuated and often irregular in the region of previous repair. Always evaluate the postoperative muscle for the degree of muscular atrophy, and compare with preoperative images when available to determine whether the degree of atrophy has progressed. The location of the musculotendinous junction should be evaluated. However, it is often medially positioned after rotator cuff repair, and medialization does not necessarily indicate a recurrent tear. Finally, a complication of aggressive subacromial decompression may include avulsion of a portion of the deltoid tendon slip from the acromion. The deltoid muscle should be evaluated for retraction or fatty atrophy (Fig. 7-69).

Potential pitfalls when evaluating the postoperative rotator cuff include the following:

1. Artifact may obscure small focal areas of tendon mimicking a focal recurrent tear.
2. Granulation tissue in the postoperative tendon may appear bright on the T2-weighted images and mimic a tear; however, granulation tissue should not appear as bright as a fluid.

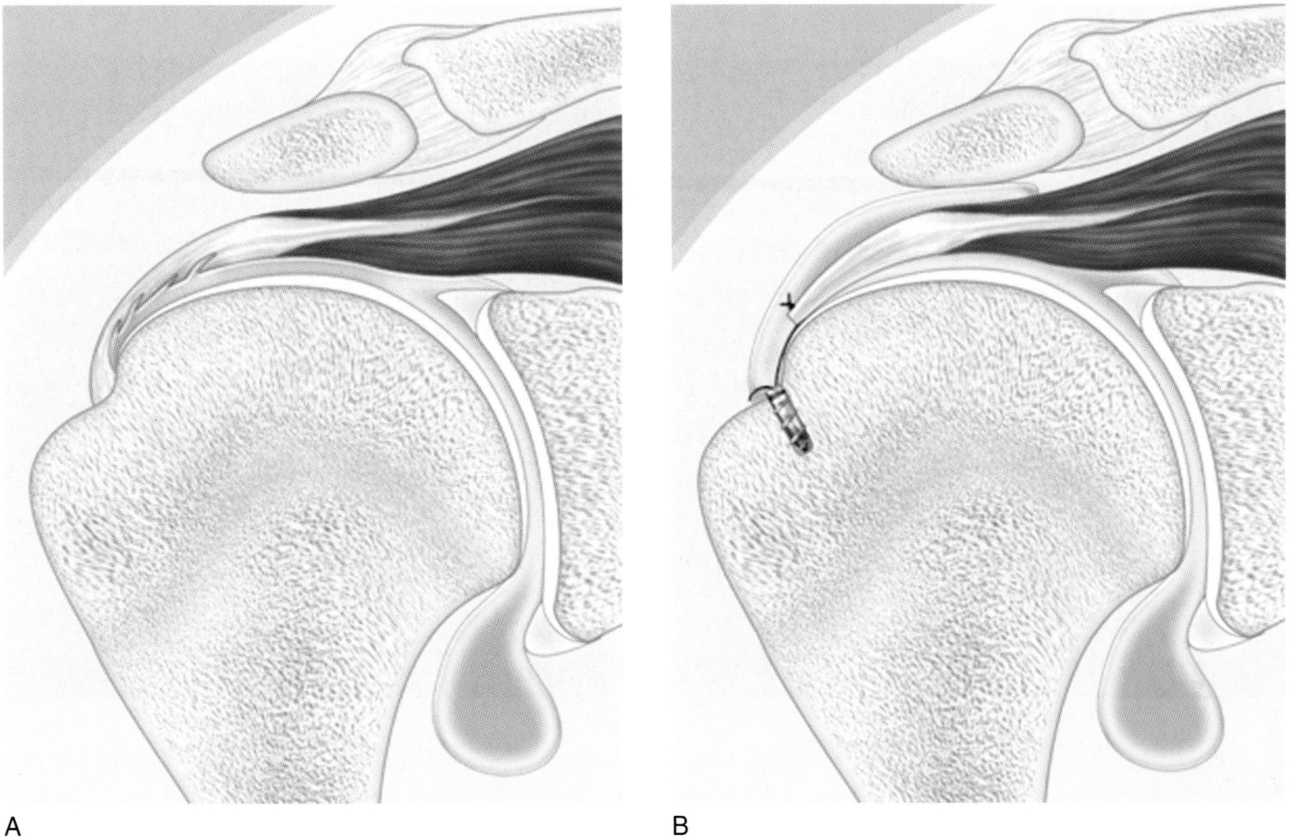
A
B

Figure 7-66 Arthroscopic rotator cuff repair technique. A, An extensive undersurface tear of the rotator cuff is demonstrated. **B,** The cuff tear is completed surgically and the tendon debrided and reattached to the humeral head via suture and suture anchor.

3. Intra-articular contrast, although occasionally helpful, can also be potentially confusing when evaluating the postoperative rotator cuff. The normal postoperative cuff may demonstrate surface irregularity and mild thinning and is not always water-tight; hence, the leakage of contrast through a small perforation in the cuff is not always a significant finding and does not necessarily indicate a recurrent tear.

Labral Repair

Although various procedures have been used in the past, most labral tears are now repaired directly using either an open or an arthroscopic technique. Suture anchors are typically placed at the 3, 4, and 5 o'clock positions of the glenoid, and suture material is used to reattach the labrum (Fig. 7-70). A staple capsulorrhaphy is often performed in conjunction with the labral repair to tighten the capsule. Thermal capsulorrhaphy has fallen out of favor and is no longer routinely used on the shoulder because of unacceptable complications. An osseous Bankart lesion is usually repaired by placing a screw through the osseous fragment. This surgical technique can result in significant postsurgical artifact, making reevaluation difficult with MRI.

MR evaluation of the postoperative labrum can be very difficult since the adjacent suture anchors or fixation screws often result in significant artifact immediately adjacent to the area of concern (Fig. 7-71). Intra-articular gadolinium can be of considerable value in evaluating the postoperative labrum. At the time of repair, the labrum is often debrided, and as a result the normal postoperative appearance may include fraying and blunting of the labrum. However, the labrum should appear firmly reattached to the glenoid after repair. The diagnosis of recurrent labral tear should therefore be made only when contrast extends completely beneath the repaired labrum or

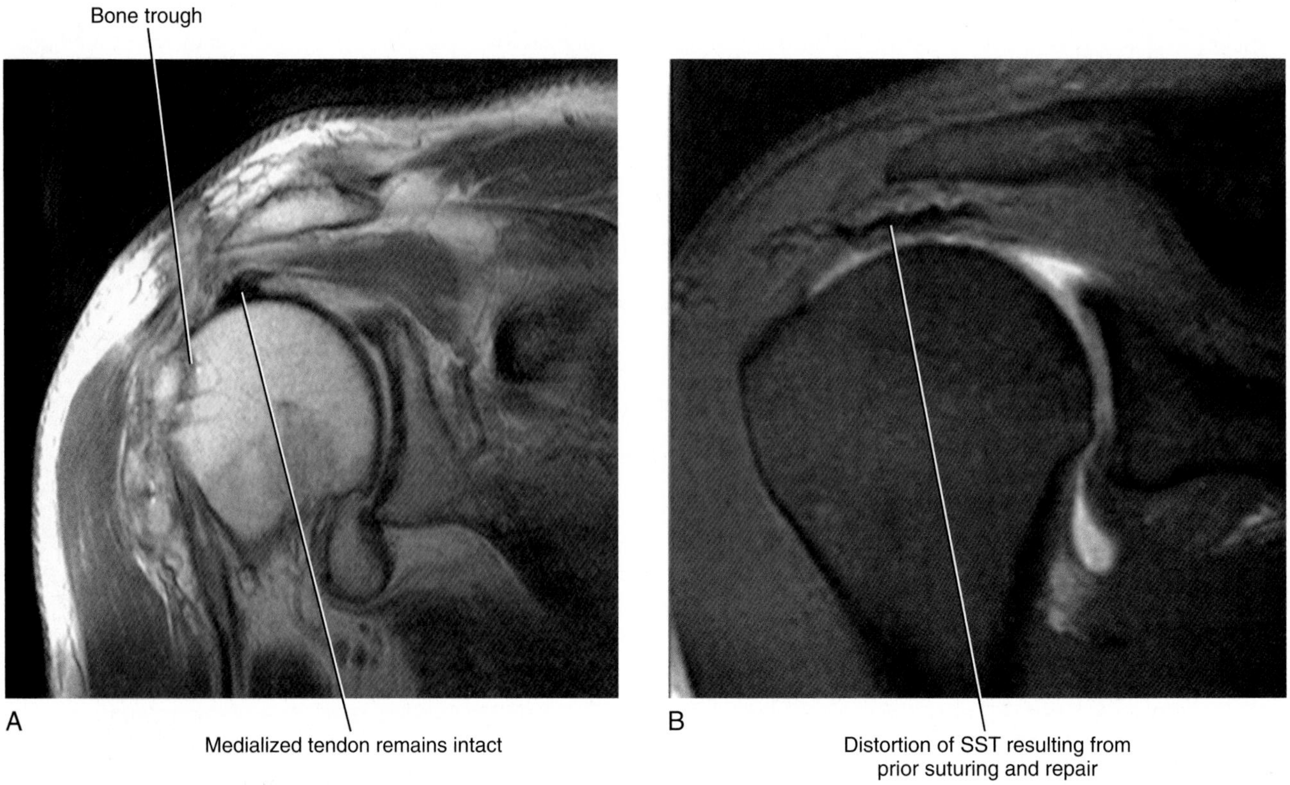
Bone trough
A
Medialized tendon remains intact
B
Distortion of SST resulting from prior suturing and repair

Figure 7-67 Normal MRI appearance of the postoperative rotator cuff. A, An intact rotator cuff following repair. The tendon is medialized and the humeral trough used to secure the suture is seen in the region of the greater tuberosity. **B,** Normal postoperative appearance of the rotator cuff tendon following rotator cuff repair. There is distortion of the tendon in the region of prior suturing but no recurrent tear. SST, supraspinatus tendon.

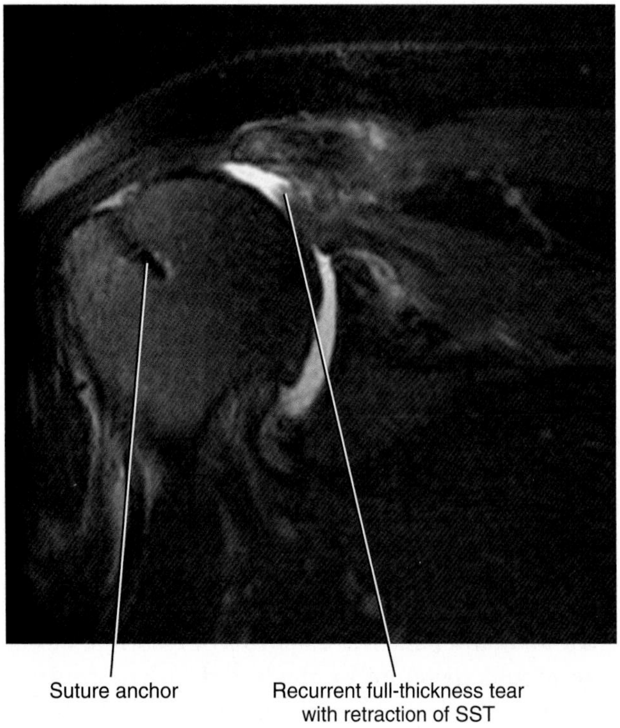
Suture anchor
Recurrent full-thickness tear with retraction of SST

Figure 7-68 Recurrent tear following rotator cuff repair. Coronal T2-weighted image demonstrates the suture anchor used to repair the cuff and a full-thickness recurrent tear. The tendon is retracted medially and there is now a fluid-filled gap in the expected location of the rotator cuff tendon. SST, supraspinatus tendon.

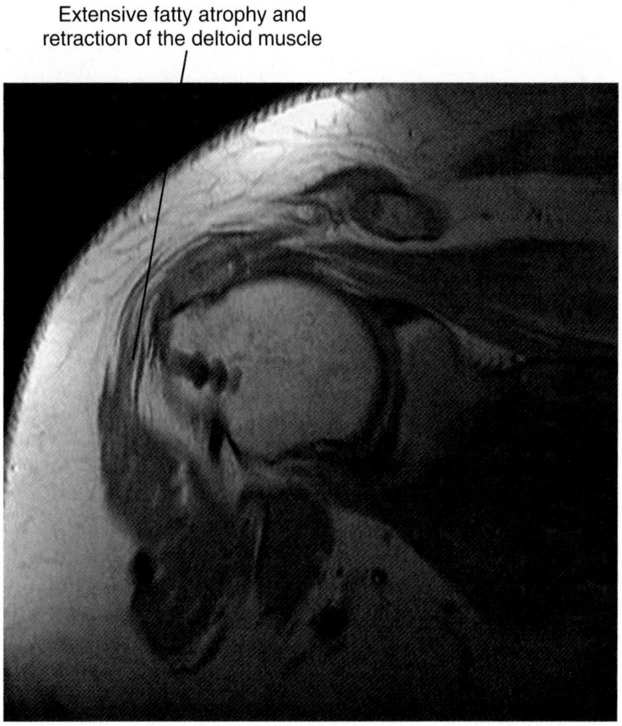
Extensive fatty atrophy and
retraction of the deltoid muscle

Figure 7-69 Deltoid muscle atrophy. Coronal T1-wieghted image demonstrates marked atrophy of the deltoid muscle after rotator cuff repair and subacromial decompression. This is a potential complication of an overly aggressive acromioplasty.

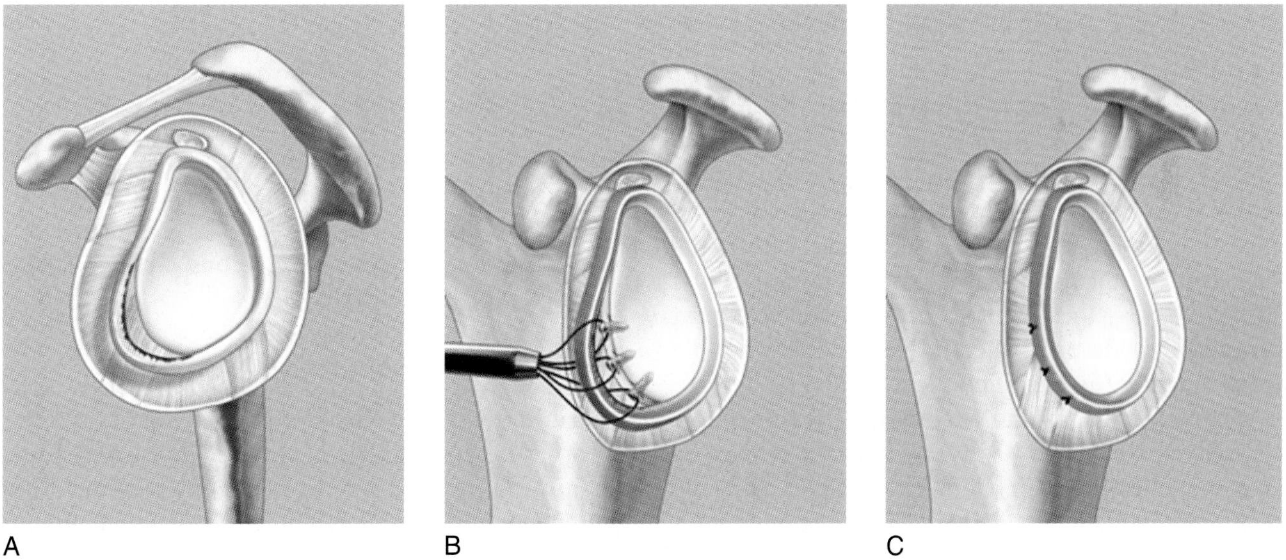
A
B
C

Figure 7-70 Standard arthroscopic technique for Bankart repair. A, Torn anterior inferior labrum. **B,** Drill holes and suture anchors are placed in the 3, 4, and 5 o'clock positions, and suture material is used to secure the labrum to the osseous glenoid **C.**

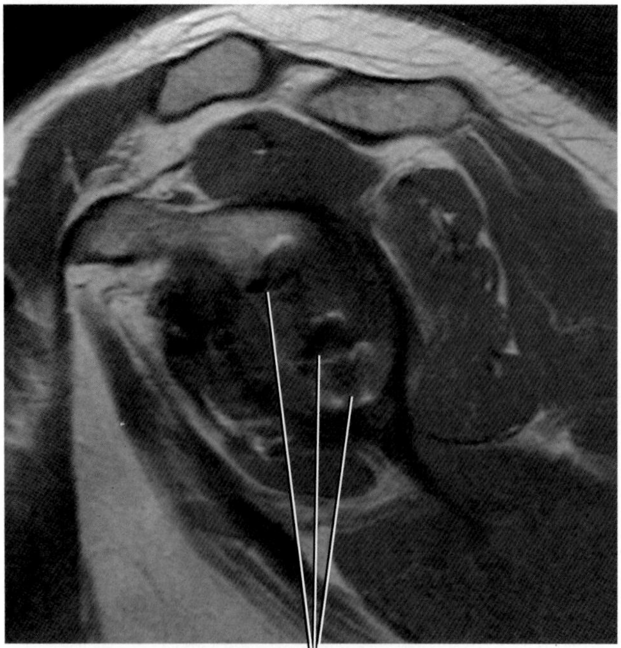
Extensive postsurgical artifact
resulting from suture anchors

Figure 7-71 Suture anchor artifact. After Bankart repair, the suture anchors can create extensive artifact that limit evaluation of the adjacent labrum.

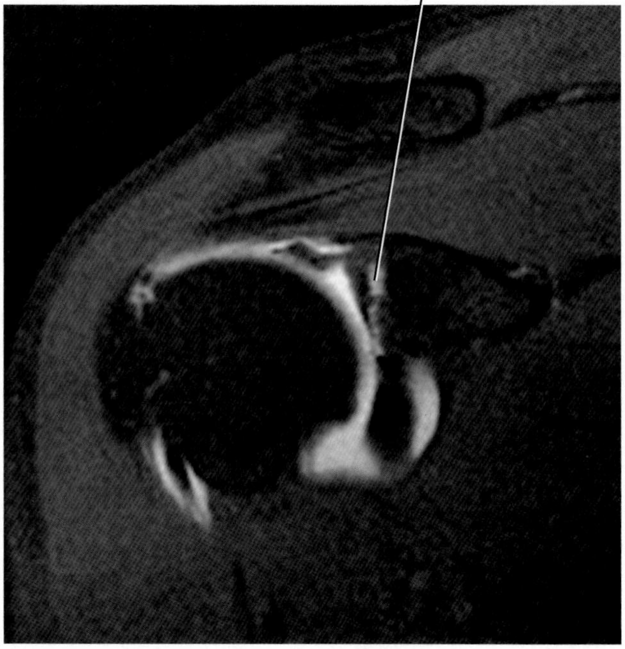
Recurrent tear following SLAP repair

Figure 7-72 Recurrent SLAP (superior labral tear anterior to posterior) tear following repair. Coronal T1-weighted image with fat saturation and intra-articular gadolinium demonstrates detachment of the superior labrum representing a recurrent SLAP tear.

when the labrum is detached or displaced. Similarly, with a SLAP repair, the surgeon usually debrides loose labral fragments and then reattaches avulsed fragments (Fig. 7-72). The normal postoperative appearance may therefore demonstrate signal within the substance of the labrum as well as fraying of the surface. Hence, the diagnosis of recurrent SLAP tear should be made only when a displaced or unstable labral fragment is identified.

When a Bankart repair is combined with a staple capsulorraphy, marked capsular thickening may be seen on follow-up MRI. Complications occasionally seen after Bankart repair include the presence of a loose or malpositioned suture anchor within the glenohumeral joint. Computed axial tomography with or without contrast can help detect hardware complications such as displaced or malpositioned screws or suture anchors (Fig. 7-73). Synovitis and postoperative infection are infrequent complications that may accompany rotator cuff or labral repair. These entities may be difficult to differentiate solely on the basis of MRI. Patients with synovitis usually present with capsular thickening and nodularity with enhancement after the administration of intravenous gadolinium. Infection may have similar findings; however, the presence of a thickened enhancing capsule, joint effusion, joint destruction, cartilage loss, subchondral cyst formation, or osseous erosions all suggest the possibility of infection (Fig. 7-74).

Glenohumeral Chondrolysis

Glenohumeral chondrolysis is a rare but devastating complication that has been reported following shoulder arthroscopy and is most frequently seen in young patients typically between the ages of 20 and 30 after shoulder reconstruction for glenohumeral instability. The exact cause is unclear, but it may be associated with the use a thermal probe at the time of capsulorrhaphy. Acute onset of chondrolysis is manifested by rapid destruction of the glenohumeral articular cartilage and leads to progressive shoulder pain and disability and rapidly developing glenohumeral osteoarthritis. MRI reveals complete loss of the glenohumeral articular cartilage on both sides of the joint, joint space narrowing, and subchondral cyst formation.

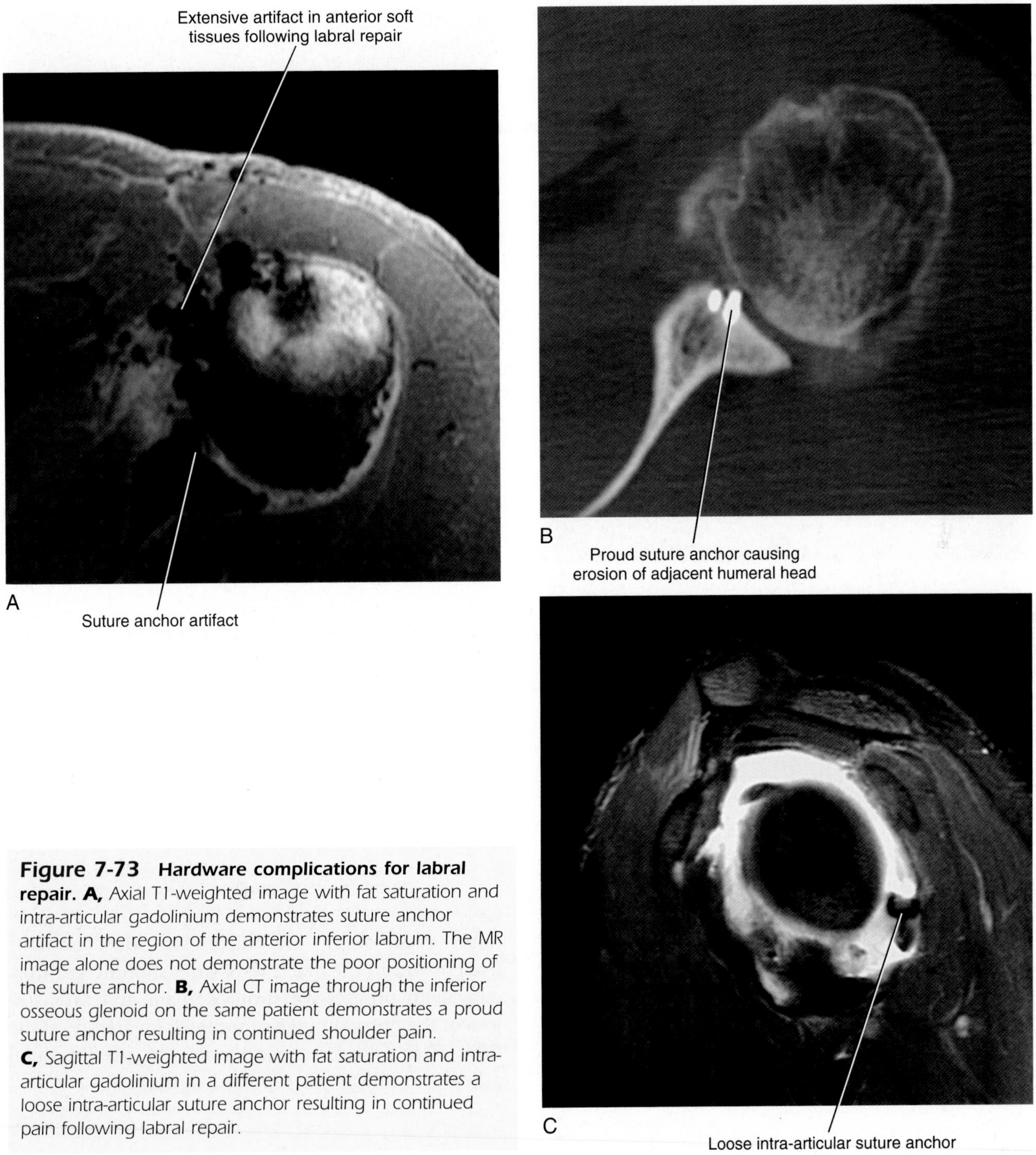
Extensive artifact in anterior soft tissues following labral repair
A
Suture anchor artifact
B
Proud suture anchor causing erosion of adjacent humeral head
C
Loose intra-articular suture anchor

Figure 7-73 Hardware complications for labral repair. A, Axial T1-weighted image with fat saturation and intra-articular gadolinium demonstrates suture anchor artifact in the region of the anterior inferior labrum. The MR image alone does not demonstrate the poor positioning of the suture anchor. **B,** Axial CT image through the inferior osseous glenoid on the same patient demonstrates a proud suture anchor resulting in continued shoulder pain. **C,** Sagittal T1-weighted image with fat saturation and intra-articular gadolinium in a different patient demonstrates a loose intra-articular suture anchor resulting in continued pain following labral repair.

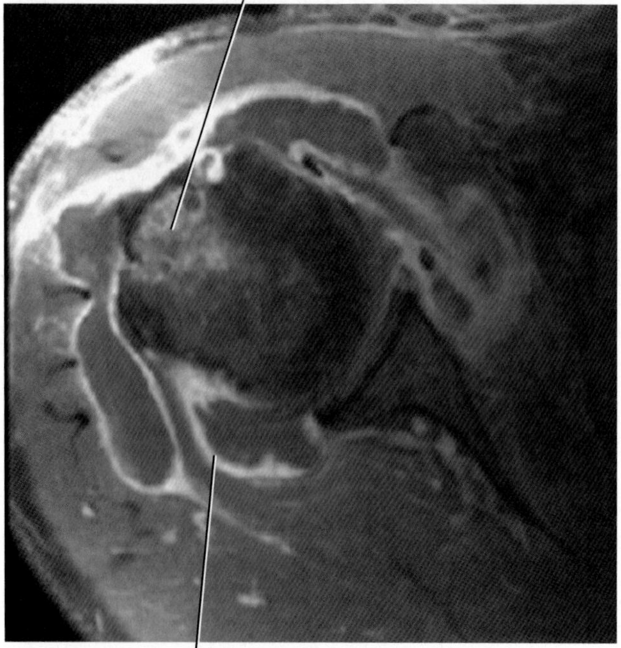
Subchondral marrow enhancement
Thickened enhancing synovium

Figure 7-74 MR appearance of postoperative infection. Axial T1-weighted image with fat saturation after administration of intravenous gadolinium demonstrates a large joint effusion with marked capsular thickening and enhancement of the capsule.

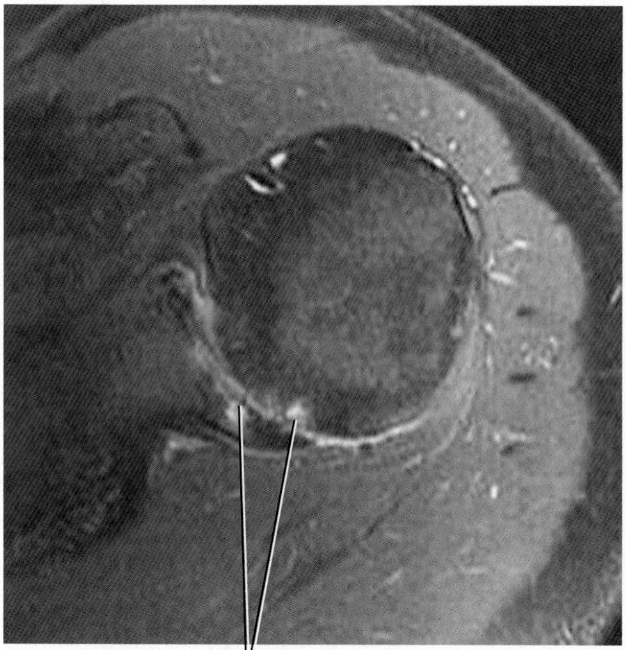
Complete articular cartilage loss with subchondral reactive marrow edema

Figure 7-75 Acute chondrolysis of the glenohumeral joint. Axial T2-weighted image shows complete loss of the normal articular cartilage on both sides of the glenohumeral joint. There is early subchondral reactive marrow edema. As is often the case in acute chondrolysis, there is a paucity of joint effusion and no significant osteophyte formation. The articular cartilage in this individual was completely normal 3 months before this MR scan at the time of shoulder arthroscopy.

The MR appearance is similar to that of advanced osteoarthritis of the glenohumeral joint. Treatment is supportive and most patients eventually require arthroplasty of the involved joint (Fig. 7-75). There is usually a paucity of joint effusion, and early MR findings indicate no significant osteophyte formation, which may be used to differentiate glenohumeral chondrolysis from other causes of osteoarthritis. Also, the surgical history is very important in accurately establishing this diagnosis. Most patients present within the first 2 years after shoulder arthroscopy with progressive shoulder pain and extensive loss of the normal range of motion. Invariably, at the time of shoulder reconstruction, the glenohumeral articular cartilage was reported as normal.

Suggested Readings

Beltran J, Kim DH. MR imaging of shoulder instability in the athlete. Magn Reson Imaging Clin N Am 2003;11:221–238.

Bencardino JT, Beltran J. MR imaging of the glenohumeral ligaments. Radiol Clin North Am 2006;44:489–502.

Carrino JA, Chandnanni VP, Mitchell DB, et al. Pectoralis major muscle and tendon tears: diagnosis and grading using magnetic resonance imaging. Skeletal Radiol 2000;29:305–313.

Gordon BH, Chew FS. Isolated acromioclavicular joint pathology in the symptomatic shoulder on magnetic resonance imaging: a pictorial essay. J Comput Assist Tomogr 2004;28:215–222.

Jung JY, Jee WH, Chun HJ, et al. Adhesive capsulitis of the shoulder: evaluation with MR arthrography. Eur Radiol 2006;16:791–796.

Kassarjian A, Bencardino JT, Palmer WE. MR imaging of the rotator cuff. Magn Reson Imaging Clin N Am 2004;12:39–60.

Kijowski R, De Smet AA. The role of ultrasound in the evaluation of sports medicine injuries of the upper extremity. 2006;Clin Sports Med 25:569–590.

Mohana-Borges AVR, Chung CB, Resnick D. MR imaging and MR arthrography of the postoperative shoulder: spectrum of normal and abnormal findings. RadioGraphics 2004;24:69–85.

Mohana-Borges AVR, Chung CB, Resnick D. Superior labral antero-posterior tear: classification and diagnosis with MRI and MR arthrography AJR 2003;181:1449–1462.
Moosikasuwan JB, Miller TT, Dines DM. Imaging of the painful shoulder in throwing athletes. Clin Sports Med 2006;25:433–443.
Morag Y, Jacobson JA, Shields G, et al. MR arthrography of rotator interval, long head of the biceps brachii, and biceps pulley of the shoulder. Radiology 2005;235:21–30.
Sanders TG, Jersey SL. Conventional radiography of the shoulder. Semin Roentgenol 2005;40:207–222.
Steinbach LS. Magnetic resonance imaging of glenohumeral joint instability. Semin Musculoskelet Radiol 2006;9:44–55.
Wu J, Covey A, Katz LD. MRI of the postoperative shoulder. Clin Sports Med 2006;25:445–464.
Zlatkin MB. MRI of the postoperative shoulder. Skeletal Radiol 2002;31:63–80.

Chapter 8

IMAGING OF THE ELBOW

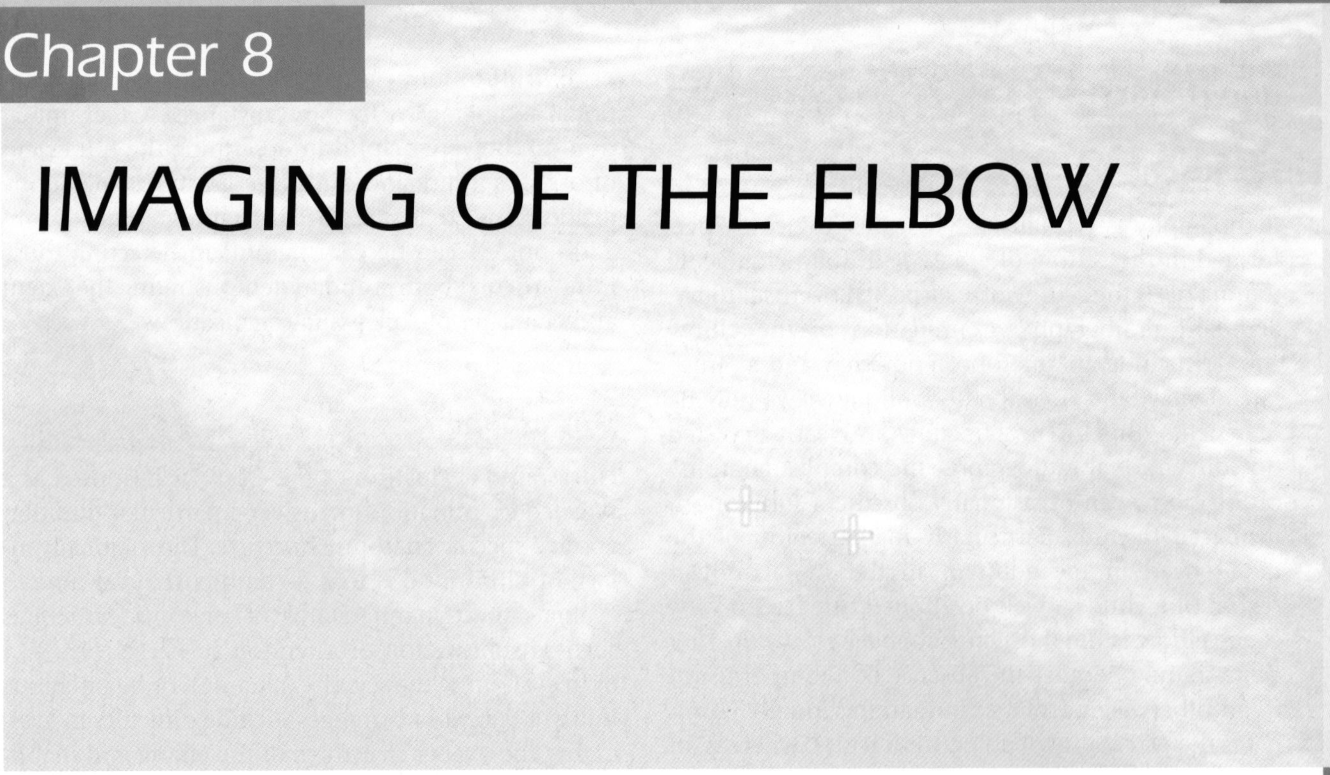

CHAPTER OUTLINE

MODALITIES

Radiology

Radiography is typically the first imaging study performed in the setting of elbow pain following acute trauma or in the setting of a suspected overuse injury. Standard radiographic examination of the elbow should include an anteroposterior view and a "true" lateral view, and occasionally oblique views may be of benefit. Athough most fractures are clearly depicted on conventional radiographs, the complex anatomy of the elbow can occasionally obscure a subtle nondisplaced fracture, particularly in the region of the radial head in the adult or in the supracondylar region of a child. A well-positioned true lateral view of the elbow is the most critical image to obtain after acute trauma because the absence of a joint effusion in an otherwise normal examination virtually eliminates the possibility of an occult fracture, whereas an effusion in the setting of trauma indicates a fracture until proven otherwise.

The "radial head" view is a special view obtained when there is suspicion of a radial head or neck fracture that is either radiographically occult on standard views or that requires better delineation. The view is obtained with the patient sitting, prone, or standing, with the humerus abducted 90 degrees and the elbow flexed 90 degrees. The x-ray beam is directed along the long axis of the humerus and tilted 45 degrees toward the shoulder. This view usually provides an improved view of the radial head and neck and better defines the degree of angulation and the amount of articular surface step-off. The search pattern should include evaluation of the soft tissues, since swelling may be an indirect sign of associated soft tissue injury.

Radiographs should also be evaluated for soft tissue calcifications, which may indicate the presence of an intra-articular body, calcific tendinitis, calcific bursitis, or myositis ossificans. Numerous ossification centers about the elbow in the child can make evaluation of the radiograph particularly difficult, and comparison with the contralateral elbow may be of occasional benefit.

Computed Tomography

The osseous anatomy of the elbow is complex, and fractures can occasionally be radiographically occult or difficult to fully delineate on the basis of conventional radiography. In these instances, CT examination can be very helpful in describing the full extent of osseous injury and can detect fractures and subtle dislocations that are occult radiographically. In addition, CT can be very helpful in detecting loose intra-articular bodies and in demonstrating the extent and character of soft tissue calcifications.

Ultrasound

Ultrasound evaluation of the elbow is best used as a targeted examination to answer a particular question about a specific anatomic structure. The major advantage of ultrasound is that it can be used real-time to evaluate the dynamic status of anatomic structures such as subluxation of a tendon or nerve (Fig. 8-1) or in evaluating the severity of tendon or ligamentous injury. Major disadvantages include difficulty in evaluating the deeper structures of the elbow and inability to adequately assess the osseous structures. Also, it can be difficult for those who did not perform the examination to determine whether the study is accurate and complete.

Ultrasound has proved useful in the evaluation of the ulnar collateral ligament and is capable of differentiating between a partial-thickness tear and a full-thickness tear and is also capable of demonstrating chronic changes related to repetitive trauma. The distal biceps and triceps tendons can also be fully evaluated with ultrasound. Differentiation among tendinosis, partial- and full-thickness tear, and the extent of retraction can all be clearly demonstrated. Ultrasound has been shown to be clinically useful in the evaluation of lateral epicondylitis and can clearly depict the extent of common extensor tendon injury.

Magnetic Resonance Imaging

Magnetic resonance imaging (MRI) is the most versatile and robust of imaging modalities available for the evaluation of the elbow and is capable of accurately depicting both soft tissue and osseous abnormalities. For instance, MRI can accurately depict the extent of soft tissue injury in a suspected biceps or triceps tendon rupture or tendinosis. It can also accurately depict the extent of tendon and ligamentous injury in a patient with signs of medial or lateral epicondylitis. MR imaging accurately depicts osseous

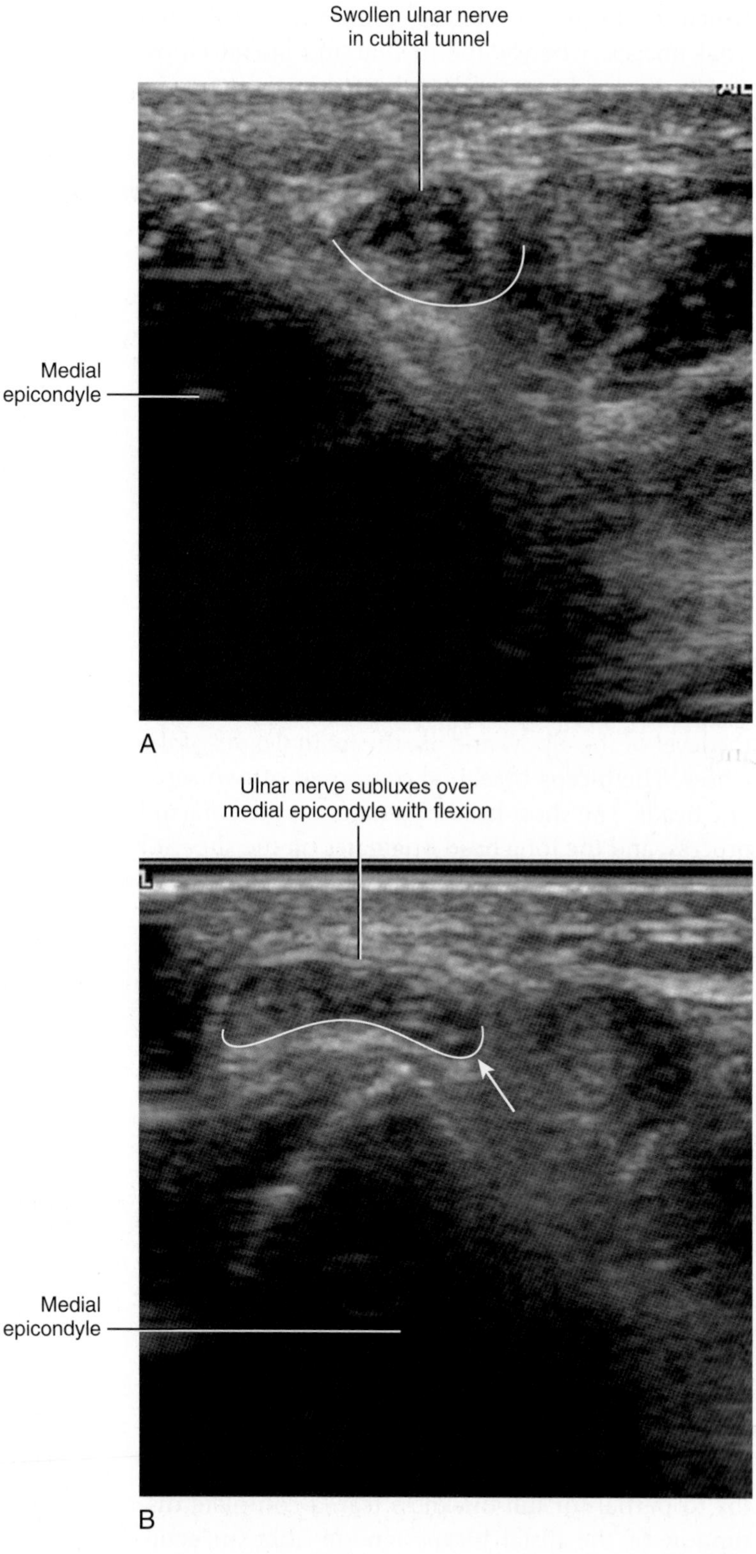
Swollen ulnar nerve in cubital tunnel
Medial epicondyle
A
Ulnar nerve subluxes over medial epicondyle with flexion
Medial epicondyle
B

Figure 8-1 Dynamic ultrasound of the elbow demonstrates ulnar nerve subluxation in a patient with painful medial snapping during elbow flexion associated with paresthesias.

abnormalities such as radiographically occult fractures and osteochondral injuries of the capitellum or the radial head. It can also accurately delineate intra-articular abnormalities, including synovial-based processes and intra-articular bodies.

Standard elbow imaging protocols typically include T2-weighted sequences with fat saturation in the axial, sagittal, and coronal imaging planes and short echo time sequences in both the sagittal and coronal planes. The anterior and posterior compartment structures are best evaluated using the sagittal and axial images, whereas the medial and lateral elbow structures are best depicted on coronal and axial images. The osseous structures should be evaluated using all available imaging planes to look for areas of marrow edema and cortical disruption. Direct or indirect MR arthrography is useful in grading osteochondral injuries and in depicting the presence of loose intra-articular bodies. MR arthrography may also be of some value in the evaluation of ligamentous structures of the elbow, particularly in depicting subtle partial-thickness articular-sided tears of the ulnar collateral ligament.

ANTERIOR COMPARTMENT ANATOMY AND INJURY PATTERNS

The biceps brachii and the brachialis are the two muscles located within the anterior compartment at the level of the elbow and are the main flexors of the elbow. The biceps brachii is composed of two separate heads. The short head originates on the coracoid process, and the long head originates on the superior glenoid tubercle. The two heads sit closely applied in the anterior compartment of the upper arm and do not merge but rather give rise to a common tendon at a level approximately 7 cm above the distal attachment on the radial tuberosity (Fig. 8-2). The *bicipitoradial bursa* separates the distal tendon from the adjacent radial tuberosity, and a broad medial expansion of the distal tendon referred to as the *bicipital aponeurosis* or *lacertus fibrosus* arises from the distal tendon and descends medially to cross the brachial artery and blend with the deep fascial layer that covers the origin of the common flexor muscle group. The brachialis muscle sits deep to the biceps brachii, originating along the distal aspect of the anterior surface of the humeral shaft. Distally, the brachialis muscle gives rise to a short thick tendon that inserts on the ulnar tuberosity.

Although injuries range from chronic tendinopathy to partial- or full-thickness tear, a complete disruption of the distal biceps tendon after an acute traumatic event is the most common injury. Less than 5% of all complete biceps brachii disruptions, however, occur distally, with most injuries involving the proximal long head of the biceps tendon at the level of the shoulder. Disruption of the distal biceps tendon typically occurs in men between the ages of 40 and 70 years and usually involves the dominant arm. Injury occurs during heavy lifting and results from sudden forceful contraction or prolonged contraction of the biceps tendon against a high-load resistance with the arm flexed at 90 degrees. Disruption is usually complete and most frequently occurs at the level of distal attachment on the radial tuberosity.

The individual usually describes a popping or tearing sensation and develops pain and ecchymosis in the region of the antecubital fossa. A complete tear leads to retraction of the musculotendinous junction of the biceps tendon, and on physical examination the distal biceps tendon is no longer palpable in the region of the antecubital fossa. The biceps muscle appears "bunched up" following retraction into the upper arm. The patient can still flex and supinate the arm because the brachialis and supinator muscles usually remain intact; however, both strength and endurance are markedly diminished. The lacertus fibrosus often remains partially or completely intact, thus preventing complete retraction of the distal biceps tendon. An intact lacertus fibrosus may help to mask the classic physical exam findings of a retracted muscle and tendon (Table 8-1).

Radiography plays little to no role in the evaluation of a suspected distal biceps tendon tear or avulsion because there is usually no associated osseous avulsion fragment. Evaluation of the distal biceps tendon is best performed on sagittal and axial T2-weighted MR images through the elbow with fat saturation. A common problem that occurs is the ordering of an MRI of the upper arm (level of the humerus) to

Table 8-1 Distal Biceps Tendon Injuries

Demographics	Dominant arm 40- to 70-year-old male
Mechanism of injury	Axial loading with elbow flexed 90°
Tendon's distal attachment site	Radial tuberosity
Injury pattern	Complete tear most common
MR evaluation	
T2 axial images	Complete versus incomplete tear
T2 sagittal images	Measure extent of tendon retraction
Pitfalls	
Lacertus fibrosus	May prevent retraction of torn tendon mimicking an incomplete tear
Bicipitoradial bursitis	Mimic of tendon pathology

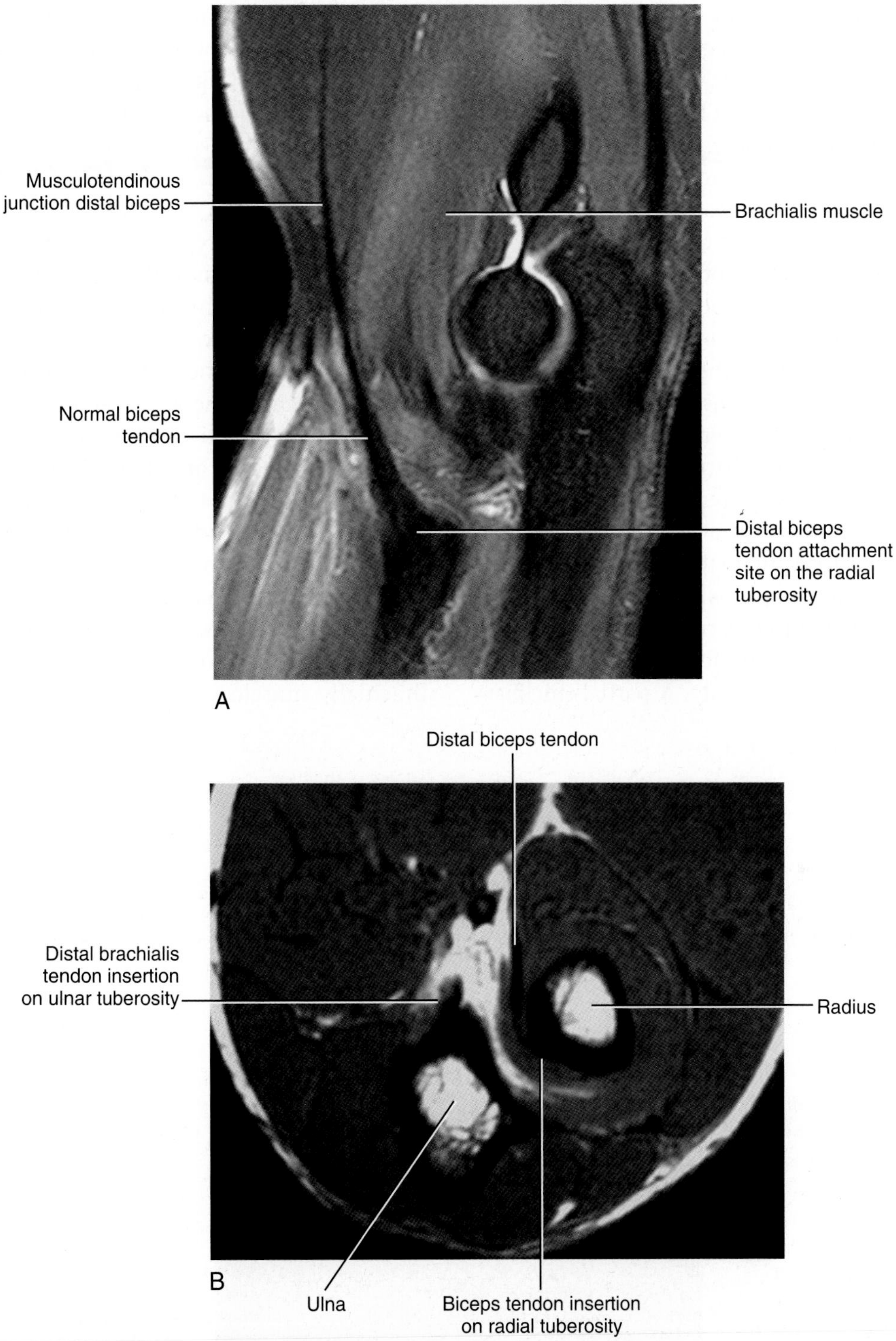
Musculotendinous junction distal biceps
Brachialis muscle
Normal biceps tendon
Distal biceps tendon attachment site on the radial tuberosity
A
Distal biceps tendon
Distal brachialis tendon insertion on ulnar tuberosity
Radius
B
Ulna
Biceps tendon insertion on radial tuberosity

Figure 8-2 Normal biceps and brachialis muscles and tendons. Sagittal T2-weighted (**A**) and axial T1-weighted (**B**) images demonstrate the normal appearance of the distal biceps tendon and the underlying brachialis muscle and tendon. The normal attachments of the biceps tendon on the radial tuberosity and the brachialis tendon on the ulna are both shown.

evaluate for a biceps tear, rather than correctly ordering an MRI of the elbow. Imaging through the level of the upper arm may not include the distal attachment site of the biceps tendon below the level of the elbow on the radial tuberosity.

The role of MR imaging is to confirm the clinical suspicion of biceps tendon tear and to differentiate partial from complete disruption as well as to determine the extent of retraction of the torn tendon (see Table 8-1). Axial images are best suited for demonstrating complete disruption or avulsion at the level of the distal attachment, whereas sagittal images demonstrates the extent of musculotendinous retraction (Fig. 8-3). An intact lacertus fibrosus prevents proximal retraction of the disrupted biceps tendon, potentially masking a biceps tendon tear on physical examination and mimicking a partial-thickness tear on MRI. The key is to evaluate the distal insertion site of the biceps tendon using axial images to determine whether the distal tendon is completely avulsed or whether a portion of the distal tendon remains attached to the radial tuberosity. A partial-thickness tear is usually manifested on MR images as thickening or attenuation of the distal tendon with intrinsic signal alteration (Fig. 8-4), whereas a complete disruption with an intact lacertus fibrosus demonstrates a complete tear/avulsion distally with minimal or no significant retraction of the torn tendon. Bicipitoradial bursitis is often seen in association with pathology of the distal biceps tendon, and on MR imaging is manifested as an oval and somewhat lobulated fluid collection within the bursa immediately adjacent to the distal biceps tendon attachment site (Fig. 8-5). Fluid within the bursa should not be misinterpreted as a tear of the distal biceps tendon. However, bicipitoradial bursitis *is* often associated with a tear of the distal tendon, and fluid within the bursa should prompt a thorough evaluation of the distal tendon.

The brachialis tendon usually remains intact when the distal biceps tendon is torn; however, the distal brachialis muscle may occasionally demonstrate evidence of a mild (grade 1) muscle strain associated with a biceps tendon injury. Isolated injury of the brachialis muscle or tendon is uncommon; when

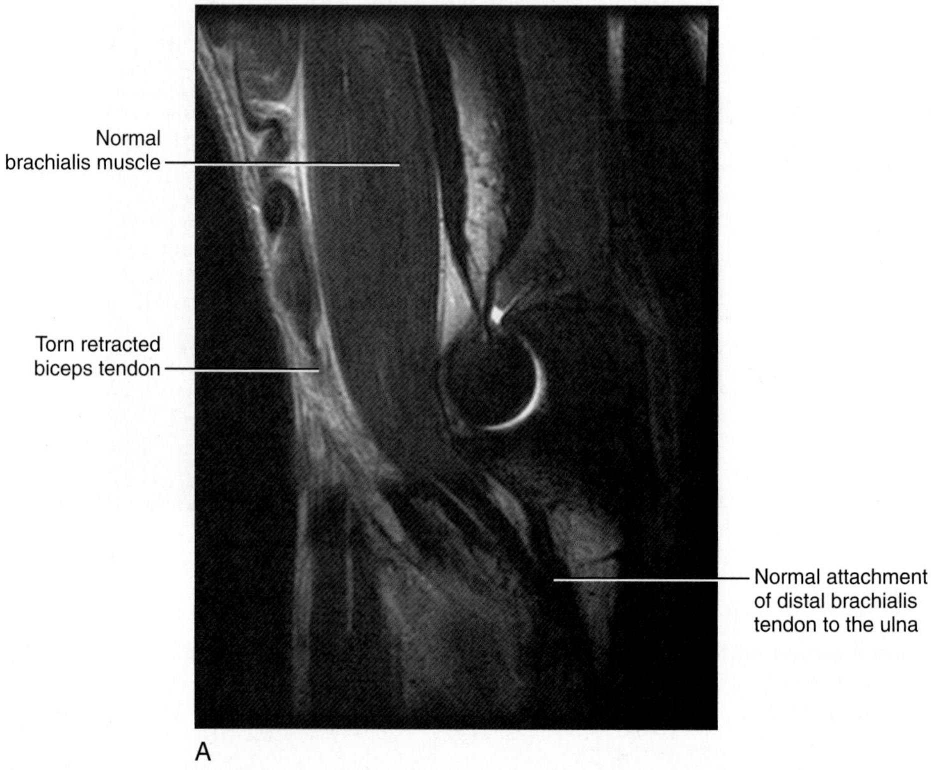
Normal brachialis muscle
Torn retracted biceps tendon
Normal attachment of distal brachialis tendon to the ulna
A

Figure 8-3 Complete disruption of the biceps tendon. Sagittal (**A**) and axial (**B**) T2-weighted images demonstrate complete disruption and marked retraction of the biceps tendon. The axial images clearly show edema and absence of the biceps tendon at the level of radial tuberosity.

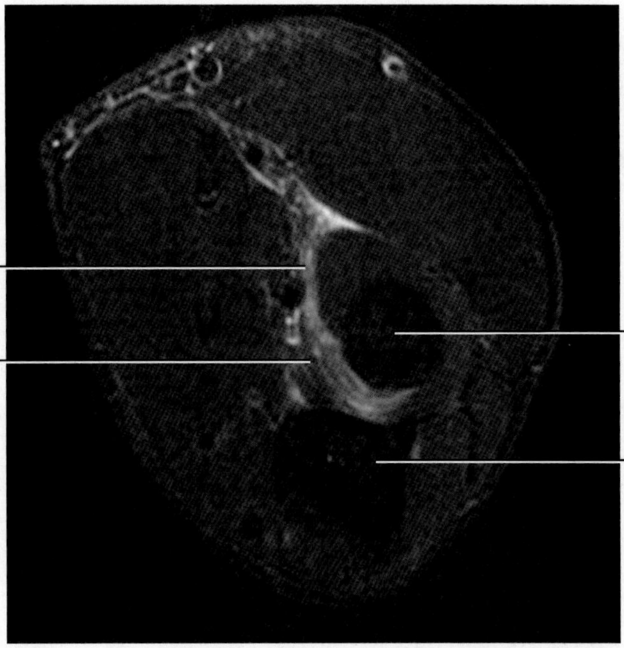
Edema in expected
biceps tendon track
Biceps tendon
absent at distal
attachment site
Radius
Ulna

B

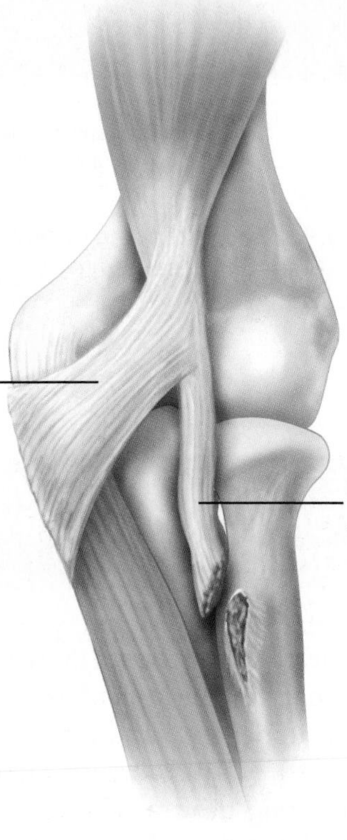
Intact
lacertus
fibrosus
Torn biceps
tendon

C

Figure 8-3, cont'd **C,** A completely torn biceps tendon at the distal attachment site; an intact lacertus fibrosus, however, will prevent proximal retractions of the torn tendon end and can mimic an incomplete tear of the tendon. Axial images at the level of distal attachment will show a complete absence of the distal tendon and fluid in the expected location of the distal attachment if a complete tear has occurred.

injury or disruption of the brachialis muscle or tendon does occur, it is usually associated with a posterior or posterolateral dislocation of the elbow. After a posterior dislocation of the elbow, brachialis tendon injury may be seen in conjunction with the other soft tissue injuries including disruption of the posterior capsule, tear of the lateral ulnar collateral ligament, and injuries of both the common flexor and extensor tendons and muscle groups.

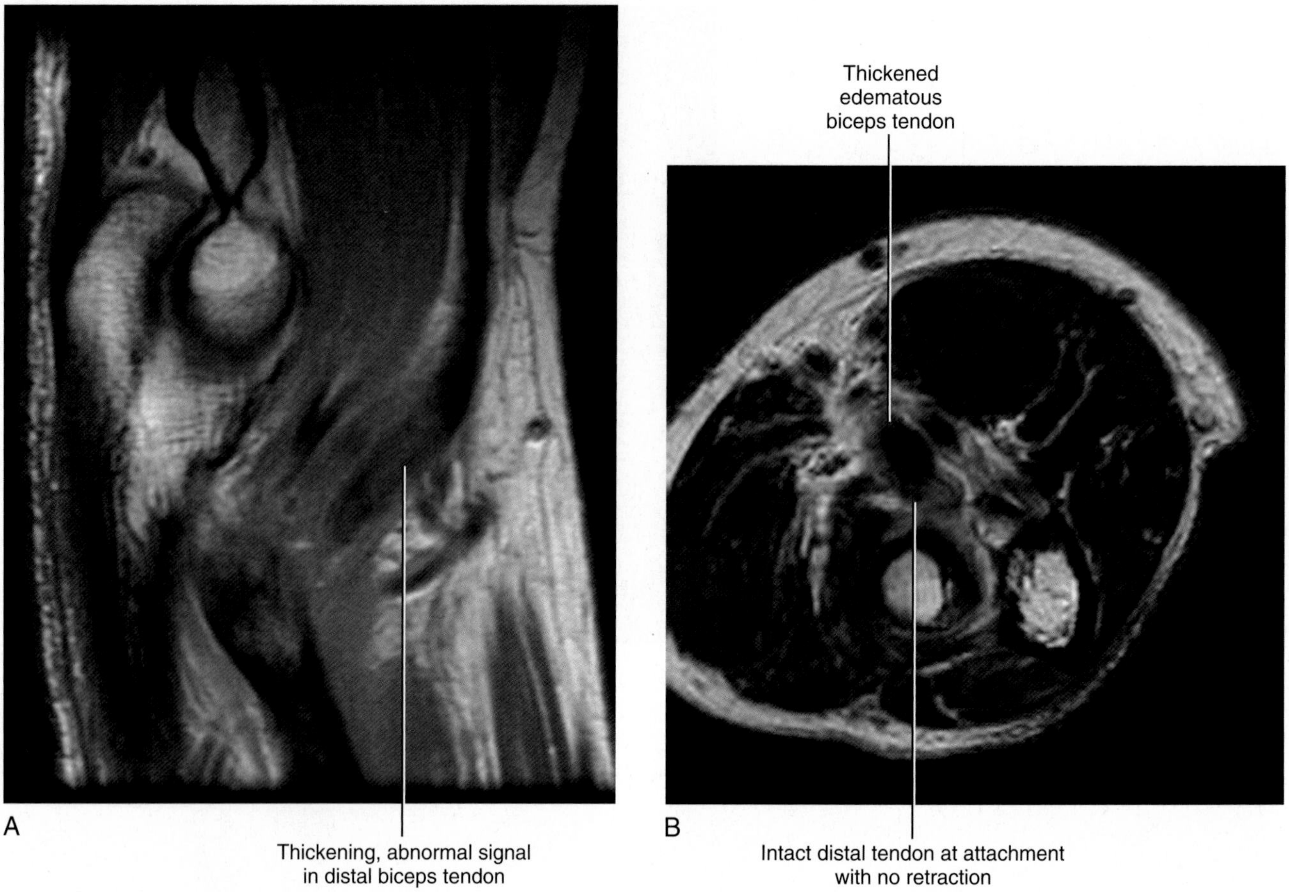

Thickened edematous biceps tendon
A
Thickening, abnormal signal in distal biceps tendon
B
Intact distal tendon at attachment with no retraction

Figure 8-4 Biceps tendinosis without evidence of a complete tear. Sagittal T1-weighted (**A**) and axial T2-weighted (**B**) images demonstrate marked thickening and intrinsic signal alteration within the substance of the distal biceps tendon, but no full-thickness tear or retraction.

POSTERIOR COMPARTMENT ANATOMY AND INJURY PATTERNS

The three heads of the triceps muscle (medial, lateral, and long) make up the bulk of the posterior compartment of the upper arm, and the triceps muscle is the major extensor of the forearm at the level of the elbow. The long head arises from the infraglenoid tubercle of the scapula. The lateral head arises along a ridge located on the posterior aspect of the proximal humeral shaft, whereas the medial head has an extensive origin along the posterior margin at the level of the middle and distal thirds of the humeral shaft. The distal triceps tendon originates as two separate slips within the mid triceps muscle, which then fuse to form a single tendon before inserting onto the proximal aspect of the dorsal olecranon. In addition, a lateral band is present that covers the anconeus muscle and inserts onto the dorsal fascia of the forearm.

Tendinosis of the triceps tendon can occur as an isolated entity or in association with lateral epicondylitis or chronic olecranon bursitis. Isolated tendinitis usually occurs as the result of repeated forced extension of the elbow and is occasionally seen in weight-lifters. Full-thickness tears are very uncommon and usually result from eccentric overload during a fall on an outstretched hand. Direct trauma to the tendon or laceration is another potential source of disruption. Minimal trauma can lead to a tear when there is underlying weakening of the tendon from exogenous steroid use or in association with a collagen vascular disease. Tendinosis is usually treated with conservative measures and does not require

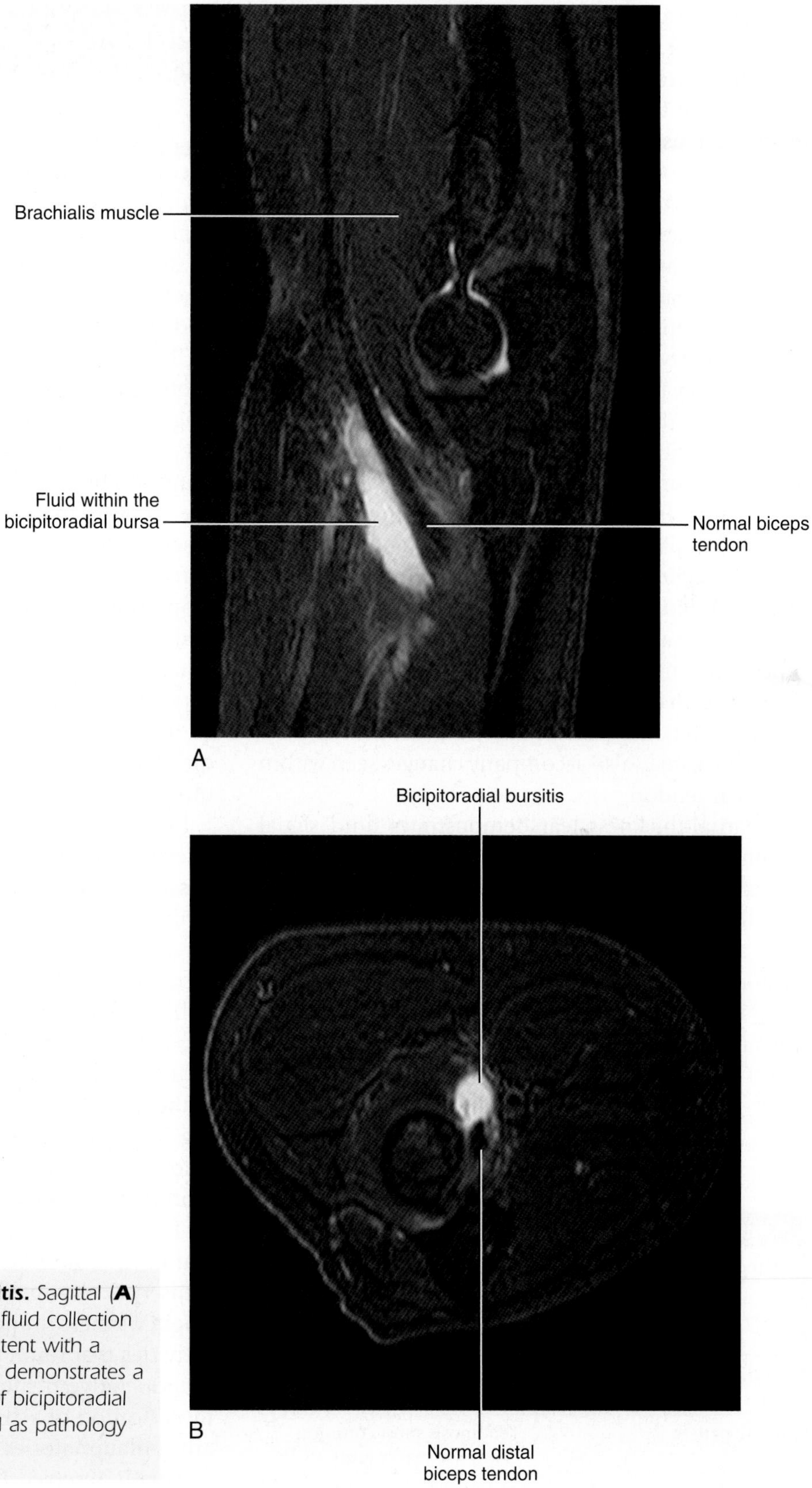
Brachialis muscle
Fluid within the bicipitoradial bursa
Normal biceps tendon
A
Bicipitoradial bursitis
B
Normal distal biceps tendon

Figure 8-5 Bicipitoradial bursitis. Sagittal (**A**) and axial (**B**) images demonstrate a fluid collection within the bicipitoradial bursa consistent with a bursitis. The adjacent biceps tendon demonstrates a normal appearance. The presence of bicipitoradial bursitis should not be misinterpreted as pathology of the biceps tendon.

surgery unless there is an associated extensive partial-thickness tear. Full-thickness disruption or avulsion of the triceps tendon is typically treated with a primary repair of the tendon and may require an allograft if there is extensive retraction or damage to the tendon (Table 8-2).

The triceps tendon is best evaluated on T2-weighted sagittal images, whereas T2-weighted axial images are complementary. The normal tendon demonstrates a striated appearance with longitudinal streaks of fibro-fatty tissue interposed between the various tendon slips at the level of attachment to the posterior olecranon. MR evaluation of the elbow is typically accomplished with the elbow in full extension, and this may result in laxity or redundancy of the distal triceps tendon in turn resulting in a wavy appearance on sagittal images. These changes should not be misinterpreted as pathology of the distal tendon (Fig. 8-6). On MR imaging, tendinitis appears as thickening and increased signal within the distal triceps tendon, and there may be associated enthesiophyte formation and subcortical marrow edema at the distal attachment site on the olecranon (Fig. 8-7). Adjacent reactive soft tissue edema and occasionally fluid within the olecranon bursa may also accompany changes seen within the distal tendon.

A partial-thickness tear demonstrates fluid signal within the expected location of the tendon, partial retraction, and thinning or attenuation of the tendon. A full-thickness tear shows complete disruption with a fluid-filled gap and retraction of the torn tendon end (Fig. 8-8). For purposes of surgical planning, it is important to describe the extent of retraction and the appearance or quality of the torn tendon end.

Table 8-2 Triceps Tendon Injury

Demographics	Steroid use Collagen vascular disease Lateral epicondylitis Chronic olecranon bursitis
Mechanism of injury	Repeated forced extension Weight-lifters
Injury pattern	Tendinosis most common Complete tear is rare
MR evaluation	T2 Sagittal and axial images
Pitfalls	Normal striations Redundancy/laxity of tendon

MEDIAL ELBOW ANATOMY AND INJURY PATTERNS

The flexor-pronator muscle group of the forearm has a common attachment on the medial epicondyle, which is typically referred to as the *common flexor tendon.* The ulnar collateral ligament (UCL) sits deep to the common flexor muscle group and consists of three separate components: the anterior, posterior, and transverse bundles. The anterior bundle of the UCL is the most important with regard to stability, protecting the elbow against excessive valgus load (Fig. 8-9). As it turns out, the anterior bundle is also the most easily evaluated using MRI. The anterior bundle is broad, thick, and very strong, arising along the inferior margin of the medial epicondyle and inserting onto the sublime tubercle along the medial coronoid margin. The posterior bundle also arises along the inferior margin of the medial epicondyle and inserts onto the medial aspect of the olecranon. Finally, the transverse bundle appears to contribute very little to medial elbow stability since it sits in a transverse orientation extending between the olecranon and the coronoid process of the proximal ulna.

Injuries of the common flexor tendon are generally referred to as *medial epicondylitis,* a term that encompasses a wide spectrum of injuries. These injuries typically result from repetitive valgus and flexor forearm stress and can be seen in those active in racquet sports, such as tennis, squash, and racquetball. Golfers develop medial epicondylitis in the trailing arm, and the injury in golfers can be attributed to the repetitive stress of the club striking the ground at the same time as the flexor muscles contract, resulting in a repetitive jolt to the medial soft tissue restraints. Medial elbow injuries are also very common among throwing athletes. The range of pathology includes tendinosis and partial- and full-thickness tear of the common flexor tendon (Fig. 8-10). Symptoms typically include pain and dull aching at the origin of the common flexor tendon, exacerbated by activities that result in valgus stress across the elbow. Nonoperative treatment is standard, which includes modification of activity combined with nonsteroidal anti-inflammatories and ice. Operative management is usually reserved for chronic recalcitrant cases and is typically accomplished with excision of the abnormal scarred portion of the tendon with repair or reattachment of the normal tendon (Table 8-3).

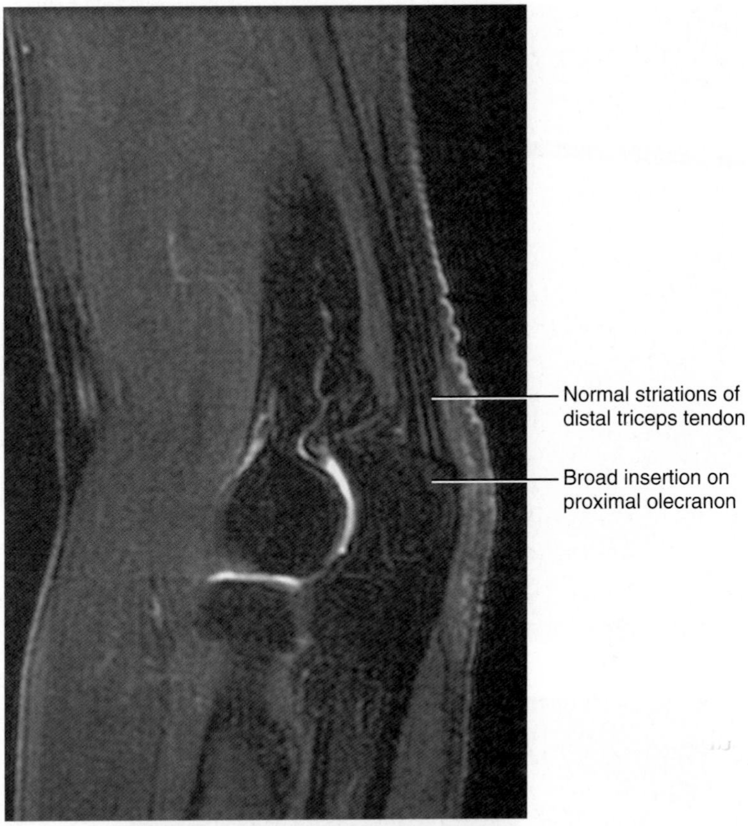
Normal striations of distal triceps tendon
Broad insertion on proximal olecranon

A

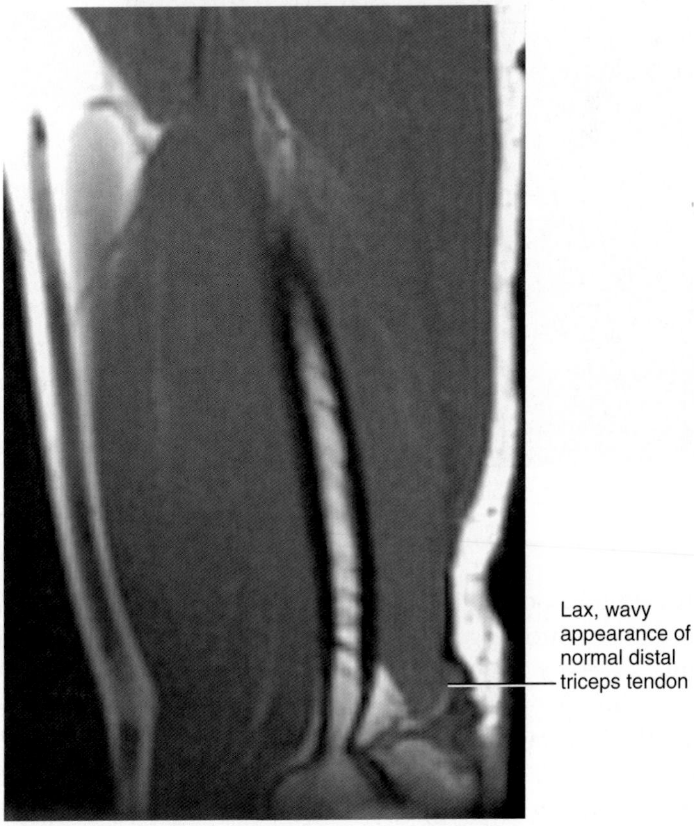
Lax, wavy appearance of normal distal triceps tendon

B

Figure 8-6 Normal MRI appearance of the triceps tendon. A, Sagittal T2-weighted image demonstrates the normal striations of the triceps tendon. **B,** Sagittal T1-weighted image shows redundancy and laxity of the triceps tendon. This appearance of the triceps tendon is often seen with the arm imaged in full extension.

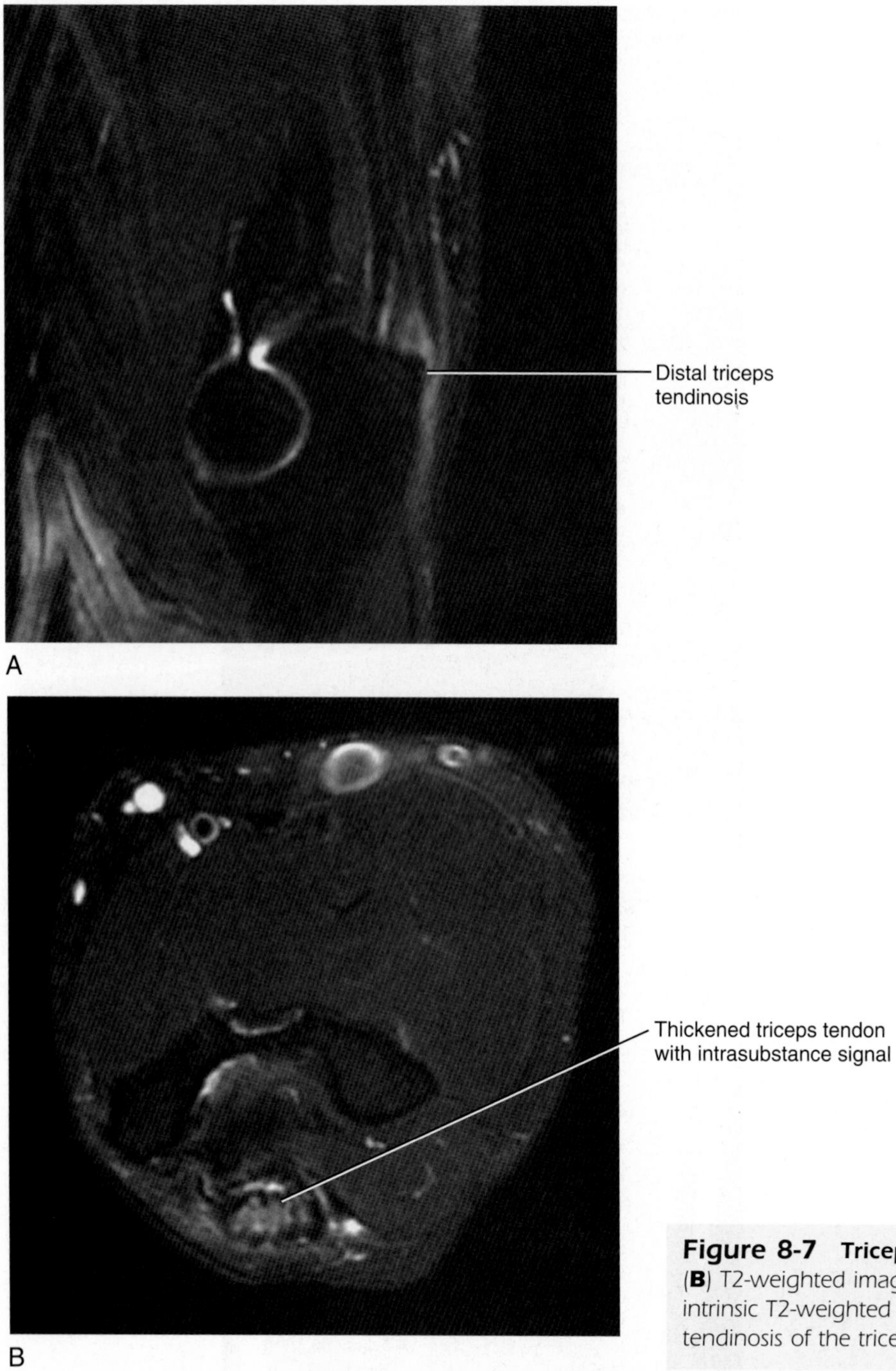
Distal triceps tendinosis
A
Thickened triceps tendon with intrasubstance signal
B

Figure 8-7 **Triceps tendinosis.** Sagittal (**A**) and axial (**B**) T2-weighted images demonstrate thickening and intrinsic T2-weighted signal abnormality representing tendinosis of the triceps tendon.

UCL injury occurs most commonly in high-performance throwing athletes and results from chronic excessive valgus stress. The tendons and muscles are the primary stabilizers of the elbow during the mid ranges of motion, whereas the UCL is the primary stabilizer at the extremes of motion (maximum valgus loading), which occurs during the late cocking phase and early acceleration phase of throwing. Injuries to the UCL are most likely to occur when the common flexor muscle group is fatigued, as occurs when a pitcher has been throwing for several consecutive innings. Less support from fatigued muscles results in increased valgus stress applied across the elbow and places the UCL at greater risk for injury. Injuries range from minimal fraying of the ligament to partial- or full-thickness tear. High-performance throwers may develop chronic thickening of the UCL as a result of repetitive valgus stress.

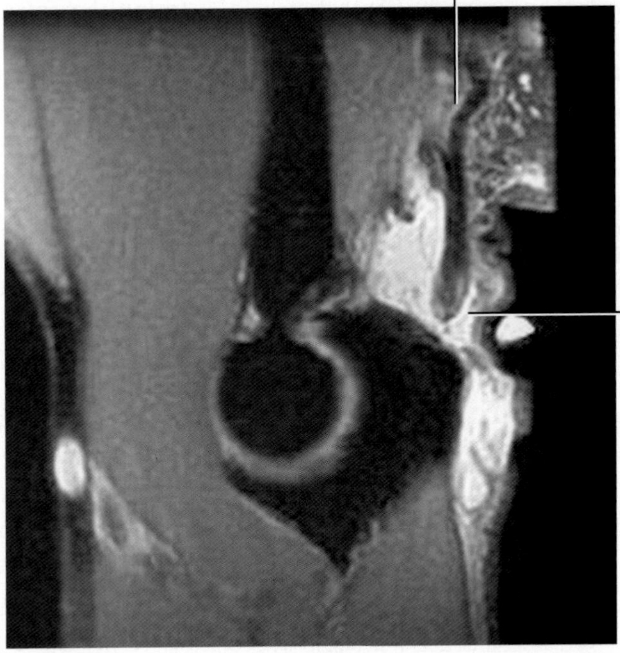
Retraction and laxity of triceps tendon
Complete avulsion of triceps tendon

Figure 8-8 Full-thickness triceps tendon tear. Sagittal T2-weighted image shows a full-thickness avulsion of the distal triceps tendon with retraction of the tendon and adjacent reactive soft tissue edema. This patient had a history of exogenous steroid use.

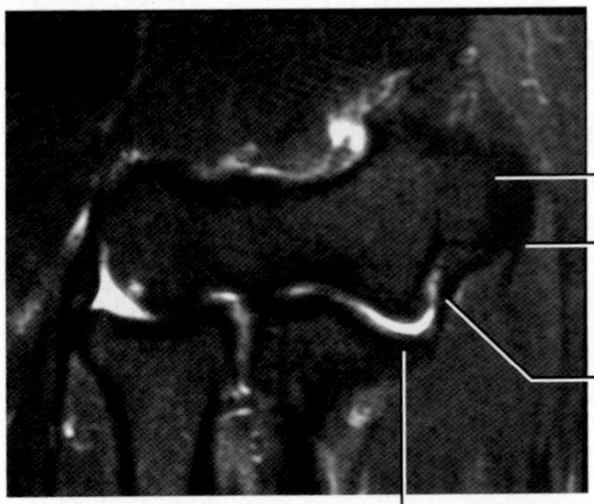
Medial epicondyle
Common flexor tendon
Anterior bundle ulnar collateral ligament
Sublime tubercle of ulna

Figure 8-9 Normal soft tissue anatomy of the medial elbow. The common flexor tendon is a short tendon that attaches directly to the medial epicondyle. It is dark on all MR pulse sequences. The common flexor muscle group directly overlies the ulnar collateral ligament (UCL). The normal UCL forms a tight attachment to the sublime tubercle of the ulna with no fluid extending deep to the distal fibers of the UCL.

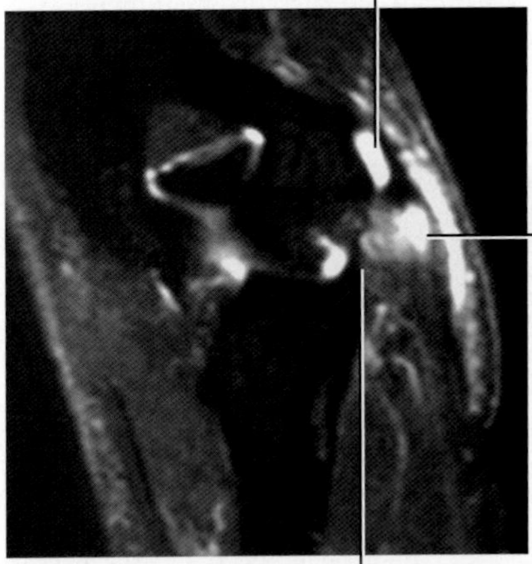
Fluid signal within substance of common flexor tendon; high-grade partial-thickness tear
Small hematoma within common flexor muscle group
Intact UCL

Figure 8-10 Medial epicondylitis with partial-thickness tear of the common flexor tendon. Coronal T2-weighted image with fat saturation demonstrates fluid signal within the substance of the common flexor tendon at the level of proximal attachment consistent with a high-grade partial-thickness tear. A moderate strain and intramuscular hematoma involving the proximal fibers of the common flexor muscle group are also found. UCL, ulnar collateral ligament.

SECTION IV

Partial-thickness tears in most cases respond to noninvasive treatment including rest, ice, and nonsteroidal anti-inflammatory medications, whereas a complete tear nearly always requires surgical management if the athlete hopes to return to a level of function close to that of pre-injury status.

Table 8-3 Medial Epicondylitis

Demographics	Racquet sports Golf Throwing or pitching
Mechanism of injury	Repetitive valgus stress across the elbow
Anatomy	Common flexor tendon Anterior bundle ulnar collateral ligament
Injury patterns	
Common flexor tendon	Tendinosis Partial- or full-thickness tear
Ulnar collateral ligament	Thickening—chronic stress Partial-thickness tear T-sign Complete tear—midsubstance
Pitfalls	Proximal attachment of ulnar collateral ligament can have an indistinct appearance on coronal MR
Associated injuries	Ulnar nerve neuritis Osteochondral impaction injuries of the lateral compartment

The primary role of MRI is to confirm the clinical suspicion of medial soft tissue injury and to determine the extent of injury. The medial elbow structures are best evaluated using coronal and axial T2-weighted MR images with fat saturation. Use of fat saturation improves conspicuity of the lesion and is very helpful in identifying subtle pathology. On MR imaging, the normal common flexor tendon should appear dark on all pulse sequences (see Fig. 8-9). Tendinosis is manifested as thickening of the tendon with intermediate intrinsic signal alteration and is often associated with mild adjacent or overlying soft tissue edema. Partial-thickness tears demonstrate fluid signal within the substance of the tendon or thinning and attenuation of the tendon. Often, partial-thickness tears are interstitial and appear on MR imaging as a linear area of fluid signal within the substance of the tendon; alternatively, a partial-thickness tear at the level of attachment may result in partial avulsion and retraction of the common flexor tendon (see Fig. 8-10). A strain of the proximal musculotendinous junction can also occur and appears as feathery edema within the substance of the common flexor muscle group at the level of the musculotendinous junction (Fig. 8-11A). A common flexor muscle strain may occur in conjunction with tendinosis or as an isolated injury. Finally, a full-thickness tear appears as complete disruption of the flexor tendon with fluid in the expected location

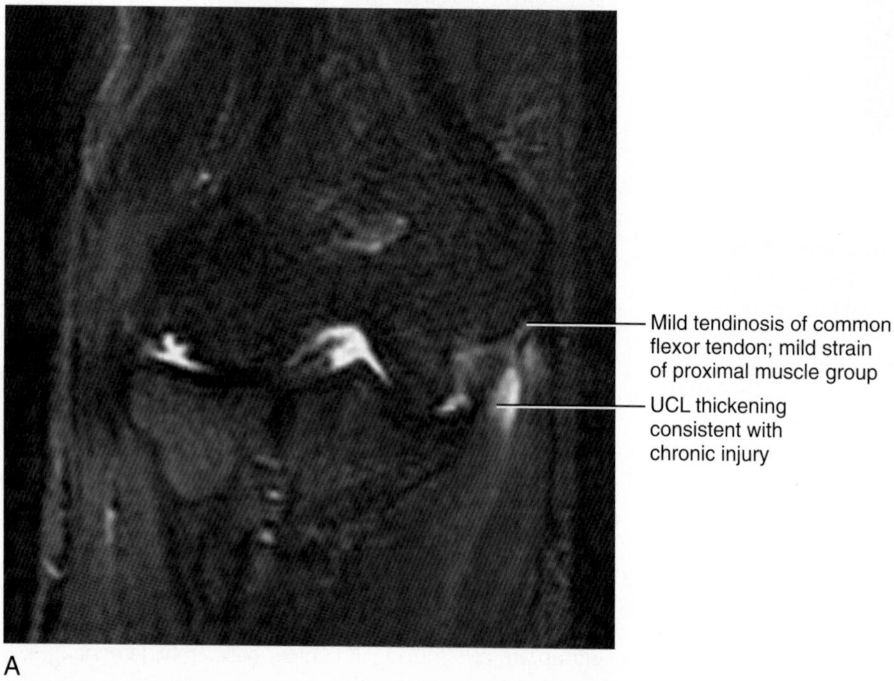
Mild tendinosis of common flexor tendon; mild strain of proximal muscle group
UCL thickening consistent with chronic injury
A

Figure 8-11 Injury patterns of the ulnar collateral ligament (UCL). **A,** Marked thickening of the UCL representing chronic changes from repetitive valgus stress across the elbow in a semiprofessional baseball pitcher.

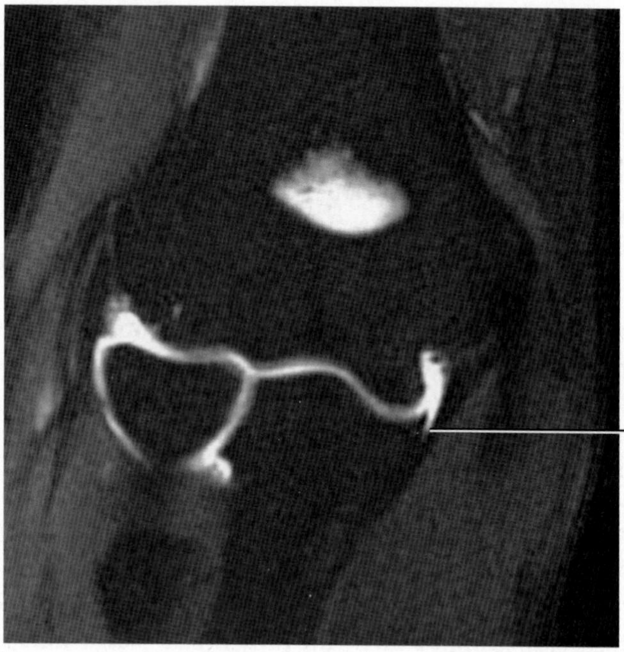
T sign
Partial-thickness
tear UCL
B

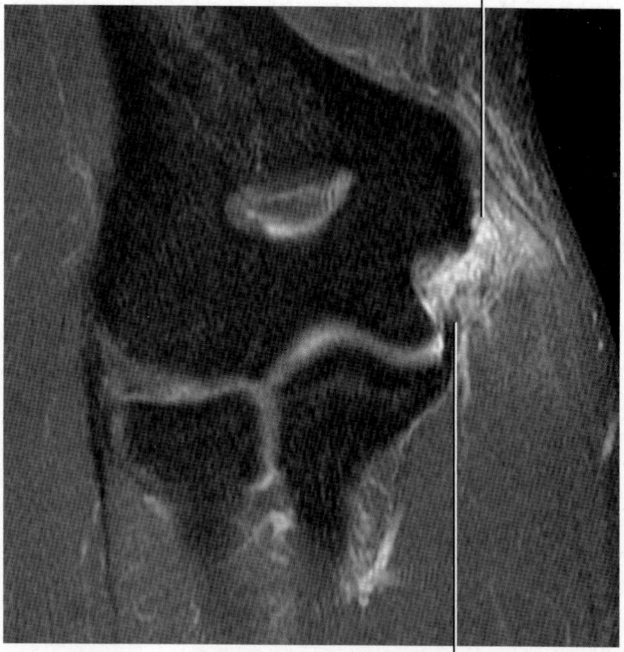
Common flexor
tendinosis
C
Complete disruption
midsubstance UCL

Figure 8-11, cont'd **B,** A partial-thickness tear with fluid extending deep to the distal attachment of the UCL known as the T sign. **C,** A complete tear of the UCL. The most common location for a complete tear of the UCL is within the midsubstance.

of the tendon, often associated with mild retraction of the torn tendon end and adjacent soft tissue edema.

Injury to the UCL is usually best depicted on T2-weighted coronal images with fat saturation (see Fig. 8-11). The normal UCL appears as a bandlike structure on coronal MR images, extending from the inferior medial epicondyle to insert on the sublime tubercle along the lateral margin of the olecranon (see Fig. 8-9). The proximal attachment site sometimes appears slightly indistinct on coronal images with interposed fibrofatty tissue, whereas the distal attachment site demonstrates a very tight-appearing osseous attachment. Marked thickening of the UCL may be seen as a result of chronic valgus stress applied to the elbow as occurs in high-performance throwing athletes and may be associated with adjacent overlying soft tissue edema (see Fig. 8-11A).

Acute injuries can range from minimal fraying and irregularity to a partial- or full-thickness tear. A partial-thickness tear most frequently occurs at the distal attachment site as a partial-thickness avulsion of the deep fibers at the level of the attachment on the sublime tubercle. On MRI, a partial-thickness avulsion of the deep fibers of the ligament is seen as a small collection of fluid extending between the distal fibers of the UCL and the coronoid tubercle. The conspicuity of this lesion is improved by the presence of a joint effusion or by the administration of either intravenous or intra-articular gadolinium. Normally, no fluid extends deep to the distal attachment of the UCL. Any fluid located between the deep fibers of the ulnar collateral ligament and its attachment to the adjacent bone is specific for a partial-thickness tear at the distal attachment site and has been referred to as the T sign (see Fig. 8-11B). A full-thickness tear typically occurs in the region of the midsubstance of the UCL and on MRI is seen as a complete disruption of the fibers with overlying soft tissue edema (see Fig. 8-11C).

Ultrasound can also be used to evaluate the status of the UCL. The normal UCL appears as an echogenic fibrillar bandlike structure that courses deep to the common flexor tendon from the medial epicondyle to insert on the coronoid process of the proximal ulna. An acute partial-thickness tear of the UCL appears as a diffusely hypoechoic and thickened ligament, with more pronounced hypoechogenicity in focal areas. An acute full-thickness tear demonstrates an anechoic fluid-filled gap within the ligament with retraction of the torn fibers, or on occasion they may be complete nonvisualization of the ligament. Chronic injury of the UCL can occur as a result of repetitive valgus stress across the elbow, as occurs in pitchers; these chronic changes are seen as a thickened UCL. One of the main benefits of ultrasonic examination is the use of dynamic imaging, which can be used to demonstrate laxity of the UCL and widening of the elbow during valgus stress (Fig. 8-12).

Medial epicondylitis may be associated with ulnar neuropathy because of the proximity of the ulnar

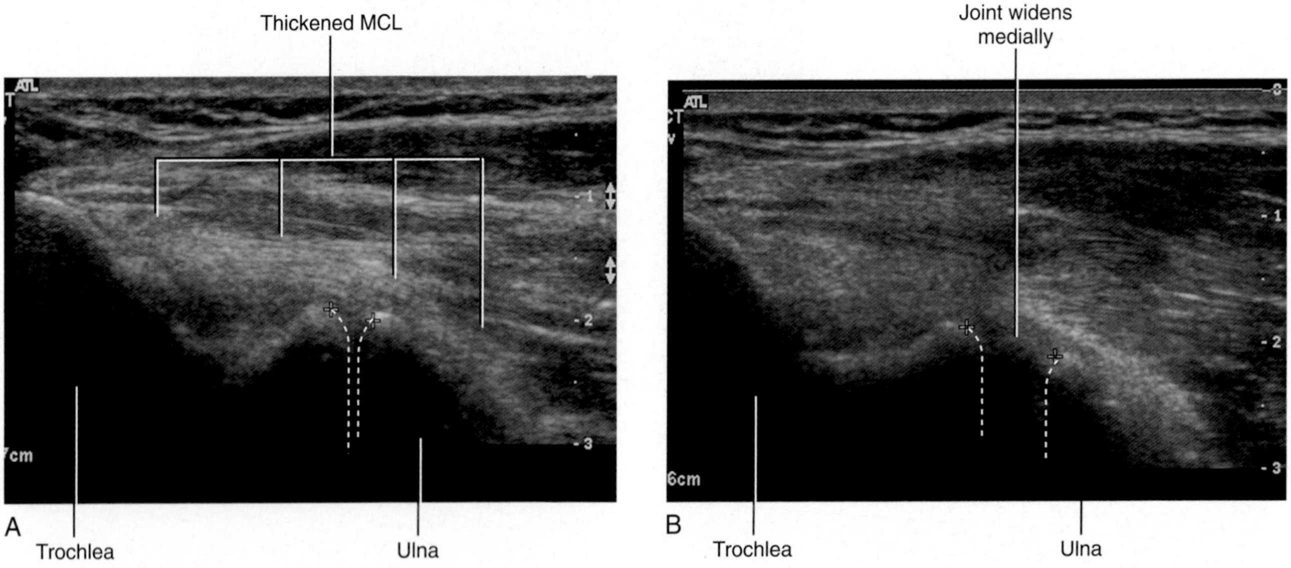
Thickened MCL
Joint widens medially
A
Trochlea
Ulna
B
Trochlea
Ulna

Figure 8-12 Dynamic ultrasound examination of the medial elbow. In addition to demonstrating the status of the ulnar collateral ligament (UCL) dynamic ultrasound imaging can also be used to demonstrate associated elbow instability. Rest (**A**) versus valgus stress (**B**) imaging shows a 4-mm opening of the medial joint (MCL) in this patient with UCL instability.

nerve to the medial epicondyle. The ulnar nerve is normally positioned within the cubital tunnel, located just posterior to the medial epicondyle, and is usually surrounded by a rim of fat. Inflammatory changes within the adjacent fat or edema and high T2-weighted signal within the substance of the ulnar nerve in combination with an enlarged diameter and fasciculation of the nerve is indicative of ulnar neuritis (Fig. 8-13). Other injuries that are sometimes associated with medial epicondylitis include osteochondral injuries of the lateral compartment of the elbow. As previously described, during the late cocking phase of throwing, injuries of the UCL and flexor tendon result from *distraction* forces applied across the medial soft tissues of the elbow. The same mechanism results in *compressive* or shearing forces applied across the lateral aspect of the elbow, which is responsible for osteochondral injuries of the capitellum and radial head. The osseous structures of the lateral elbow should be closely evaluated in any patient with MR evidence of medial epicondylitis. These injuries are further described later in chapter in the section Osseous Structures and Articular Surfaces. Tendinosis of the triceps tendon is also occasionally seen in association with medial epicondylitis.

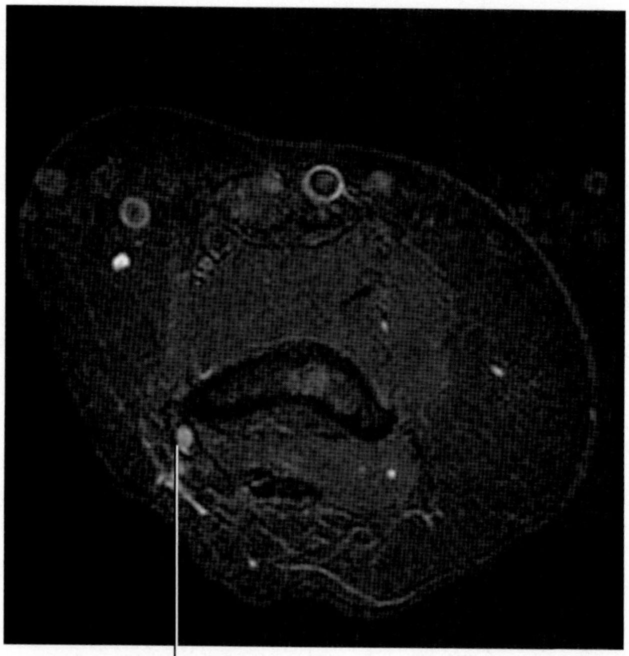
Ulnar nerve neuritis;
bright signal within nerve

Figure 8-13 Ulnar nerve neuritis associated with medial epicondylitis. This patient with medial epicondylitis demonstrated signs of ulnar neuritis on physical examination. Axial T2-weighted MR image shows bright T2 signal within the ulnar nerve representing swelling and edema of the nerve consistent with ulnar neuritis.

LATERAL ELBOW ANATOMY AND INJURY PATTERNS

Similar to the anatomy of the medial elbow, the extensor muscles of the forearm attach to the lateral epicondyle of the distal humerus via a common extensor tendon. Deep to this tendon sits the lateral collateral ligament complex, which is composed of three primary components, the radial collateral ligament, the lateral UCL, and the annular ligament. The radial collateral ligament originates along the anterior aspect of the lateral epicondyle and inserts distally onto the annular ligament. The annular ligament is a strong band that encircles the radial head and holds it tightly against the proximal ulna and is the main stabilizer of the proximal radioulnar joint. The lateral UCL arises along the posterior aspect of the lateral epicondyle slightly distal to the origin of the radial collateral ligament and courses in an oblique fashion along the posterior margin of the radial head to insert onto the posterior aspect of the proximal ulna. The lateral UCL forms a sling along the posterior margin of the radial head and is primarily responsible for preventing posterolateral rotatory instability of the radial head, thus preventing posterior subluxation or dislocation of the radial head (Fig. 8-14).

The term lateral epicondylitis describes a broad range of injuries that involve the common extensor tendon and may also involve the underlying lateral collateral ligament complex. Lateral epicondylitis is commonly referred to as "tennis elbow." Although at least 50% of all tennis players develop lateral epicondylitis sometime during their career, the majority of cases of lateral epicondylitis actually occur in nontennis players. Lateral epicondylitis is much more common in the general population than is medial epicondylitis. It is associated with repetitive flexion-extension or pronation-supination activities of the forearm or recurrent varus stress applied to the elbow, but most patients cannot identify a specific precipitating event. In tennis players, the backhand swing is responsible for lateral epicondylitis. As in medial epicondylitis, the injuries range from mild tendinosis to partial- or full-thickness tear of the tendon. Although

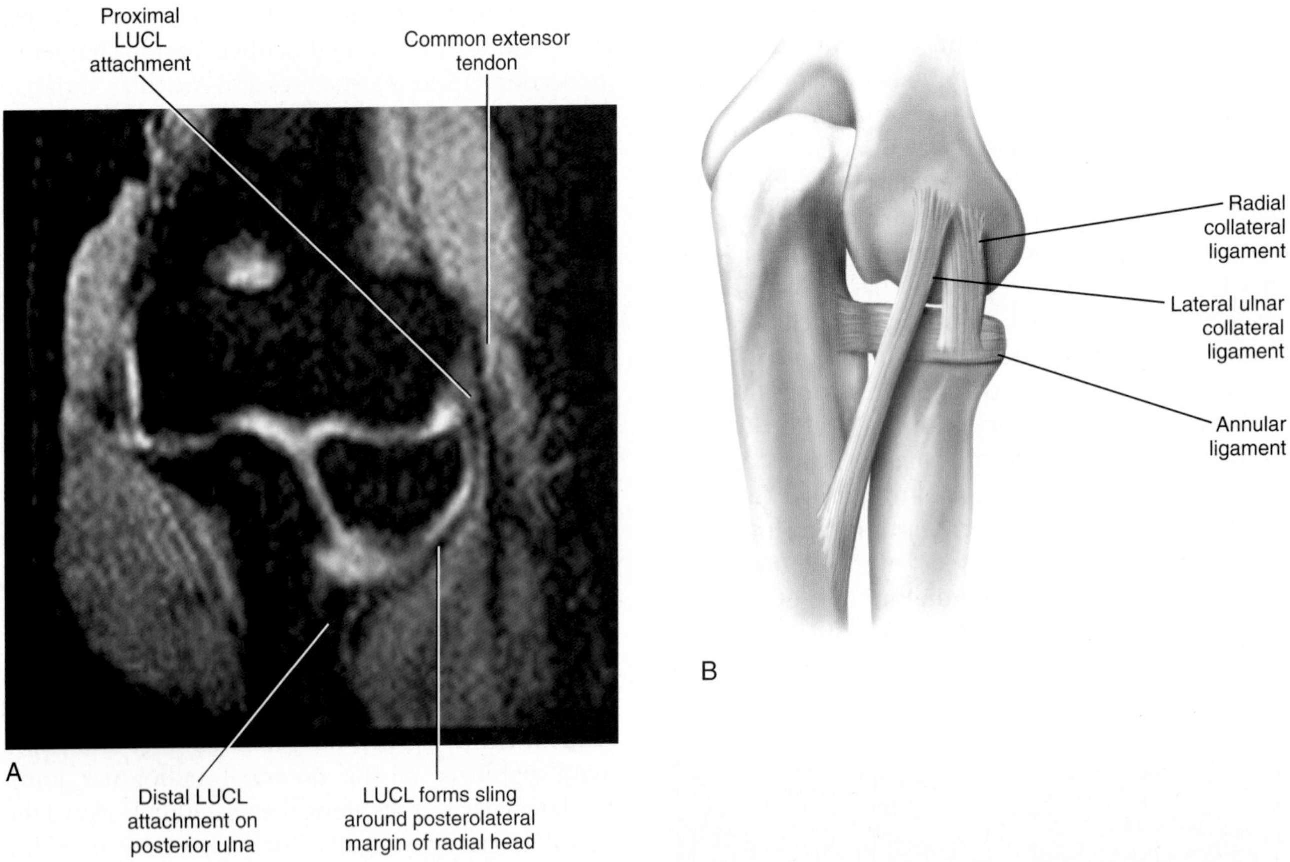
Proximal
LUCL
attachment
Common extensor
tendon
A
Distal LUCL
attachment on
posterior ulna
LUCL forms sling
around posterolateral
margin of radial head
Radial
collateral
ligament
Lateral ulnar
collateral
ligament
Annular
ligament
B

Figure 8-14 Normal soft tissue anatomy of the lateral aspect of the elbow. A, Coronal T2-weighted image shows the common extensor tendon originating on the lateral epicondyle and should demonstrate low signal on all pulse sequences. The lateral ulnar collateral ligament (LUCL) originates from the lateral epicondyle, posterior to the radial collateral ligament and then extends in a slinglike fashion around the posterolateral aspect of the radial head to attach on the proximal ulna. The LUCL is responsible for preventing posterolateral rotatory instability of the radial head. **B,** The lateral ulnar collateral ligament originates on the lateral epicondyle slightly posterior to the radial collateral ligament and forms a sling around the posterior aspect of the radial head.

the injury involves the common extensor tendon, it is the extensor carpi radialis brevis tendon that is most significantly affected. Initial treatment is usually conservative, with surgical release and repair of the tendon reserved for the chronic cases with symptoms persisting for more than a year despite conservative therapy. Injury of the underlying radial collateral ligament complex can also occur and usually results from chronic repetitive varus stress. Acute disruption can occur at the time of posterior dislocation of the elbow (Table 8-4).

MR imaging is usually reserved for patients who do not respond adequately to initial conservative treatment measures. The common extensor tendon is best evaluated on coronal and axial T2-weighted images. Fat saturation techniques improve the conspicuity of

Table 8-4 Lateral Epicondylitis

Demographics	Tennis elbow Common in general population
Mechanism of injury	Flexion-extension or pronation-supination activities of the forearm Often no known precipitating trauma
Injury patterns	
Common extensor tendon	Tendinosis Partial- or full-thickness tear
Lateral collateral ligament complex	Thickening Partial-/full-thickness tear
Associated injuries	Triceps tendinosis

lesions of the common extensor tendon. The normal tendon is dark on pulse sequences, whereas tendinosis appears as a thickened tendon with increased signal noted on both T1- and T2-weighted imaging sequences. A partial-thickness tear demonstrates fluid signal within the substance of the tendon, thinning and attenuation of the tendon, and occasionally partial retraction of the torn tendon end. Full-thickness disruption usually demonstrates abnormal morphology and thickening of the tendon, retraction of the torn tendon end, and extensive surrounding soft tissue edema (Fig. 8-15). Chronic lateral epicondylitis, resulting from repetitive varus stress is often associated with changes of the lateral collateral ligament complex, including thickening of the radial collateral ligament with increased signal within the substance of the ligament. After an acute posterior dislocation of the radial head, extensive soft tissue edema is often noted along the posterior lateral aspect of the elbow with partial to complete tear or avulsion of the common extensor tendon. In addition, there is usually extensive partial-thickness tearing or complete disruption of the lateral UCL. Lateral ulnar collateral injuries typically occur at or near the proximal attachment site along the inferior margin of the lateral epicondyle.

Ultrasound can accurately detect and depict abnormalities of the common extensor tendon in patients with suspected lateral epicondylitis. The normal common extensor tendon appears as an echogenic fibrillar structure arising from the lateral epicondyle and extending distally to give rise to the common extensor muscle group. In cases of lateral epicondylitis, the tendon appears thickened with loss of the normal fibrillar pattern and a heterogeneous appearance. There may be superimposed areas of focal decreased echogenicity. Doppler examination shows areas of hyperemia (Fig. 8-16). A partial-thickness tear appears as a focal anechoic area within the substance of the tendon, whereas a full-thickness tear demonstrates discontinuity and retraction of the tendon.

POSTERIOR DISLOCATION

Posterior dislocation of the elbow is an uncommon injury that is not related to any specific sport but typically results from a fall on an outstretched hand. Most elbow dislocations are posterior or posterolateral with only 1% to 2% occurring in the anterior direction. For the purposes of treatment, it is important to differentiate partial subluxation or a "perched" ulna and radius from a complete posterior dislocation. MRI can play a role in determining the extent of both osseous and soft tissue injury.

Posterior dislocation of the elbow results in a predictable pattern of osseous injury resulting from impaction of the bones at the time of dislocation. Areas of involvement may demonstrate contusion or fracture. In the adult, a fracture of the radial head is the most common fracture and occurs in approximately 10% of patients after a posterior dislocation. Other associated fractures that occur less frequently are the tip of the coronoid, the olecranon, and the medial or lateral epicondyle. The most common pattern of osseous injury seen on MRI after posterior elbow dislocation is that of either bone contusion and/or fracture involving the anterior margin of the radial head in conjunction with contusion or fracture of the tip of the coronoid process (Fig. 8-17). In the child, if the medial epicondyle growth plate remains unfused at the time of posterior dislocation, then an avulsion of the medial epicondyle is the most common osseous injury. Minimal displacement of the medial epicondyle is treated conservatively, but if displacement is more than 1 cm, open surgical reduction is the preferred method of treatment. Bone contusions or fractures involving the anterior radial head, posterior capitellum, and tip of the coronoid constitute an osseous injury pattern that is highly specific for posterior elbow dislocation. This pattern of osseous injury is a marker for posterior dislocation and should prompt a thorough evaluation of the specific soft tissue structures commonly injured during posterior elbow dislocation (Table 8-5).

After posterior dislocation of the elbow, the extent of soft tissue injury and the number of structures involved can be extensive. At first glance, evaluation of the MR images can be overwhelming, but understanding the sequential pattern of soft tissue injury can help ensure an adequate description of all of the important anatomic structures. The most important soft tissue structure with regard to lateral elbow stability is the lateral ulnar collateral ligament (LUCL), and evaluation of the soft tissue structures following posterior elbow dislocation should begin here. In nearly all cases of complete posterior elbow dislocation, the LUCL is injured and is usually completely disrupted. The LUCL originates on the posterior aspect of the lateral epicondyle, extends distally to form a sling around the posterior aspect of the radial

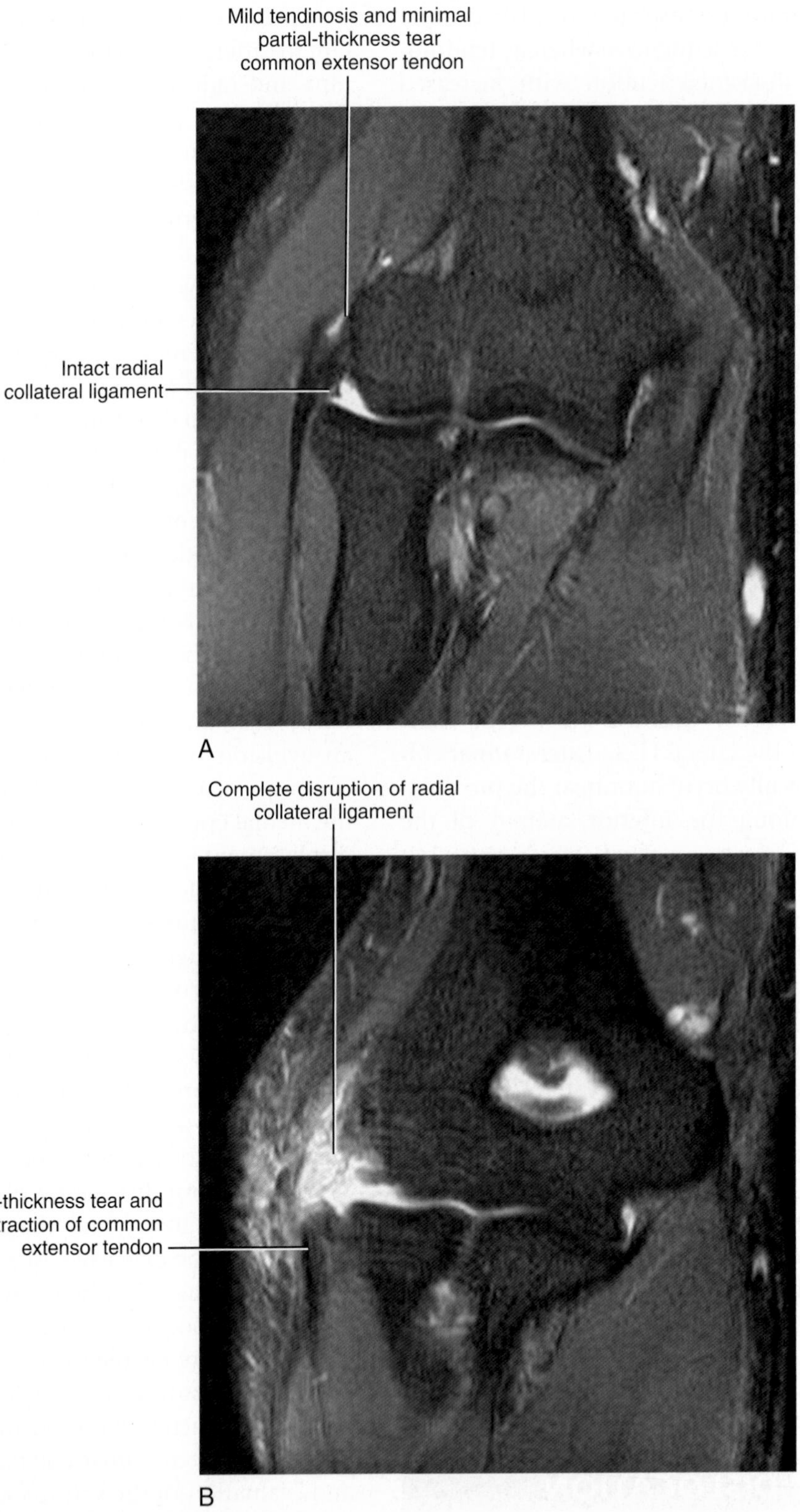

Mild tendinosis and minimal partial-thickness tear common extensor tendon
Intact radial collateral ligament
A
Complete disruption of radial collateral ligament
Full-thickness tear and retraction of common extensor tendon
B

Figure 8-15 Range of MR appearance of lateral epicondylitis. A, Minimal thickening of the common extensor tendon consistent with a mild tendinosis. In addition, there is a small focus of fluid signal within the substance of the tendon representing a small partial-thickness interstitial tear. **B,** Evidence of marked lateral epicondylitis with a complete avulsion of the common extensor tendon and approximately 2 cm of musculotendinous retraction. Seen are extensive adjacent soft tissue edema and swelling, and complete disruption of the underlying radial collateral ligament.

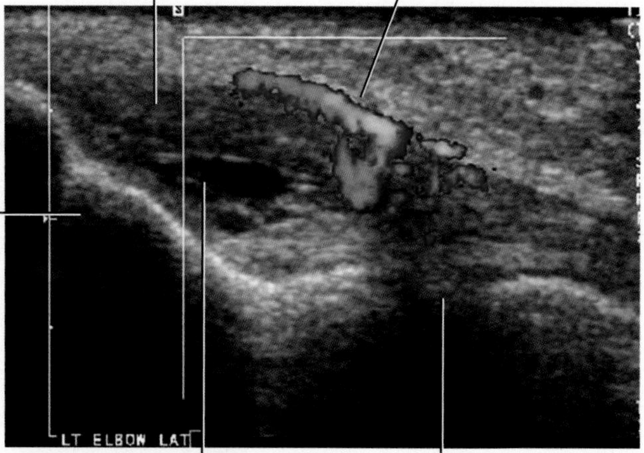
Common extensor
tendon origin
Hyperemia
Lateral epicondyle
LT ELBOW LAT
Focus of low echogenicity
representing a partial tear
Elbow joint

Figure 8-16 Ultrasound examination demonstrates lateral epicondylitis with a partial tear of the common extensor tendon. Adjacent hyperemia is also noted.

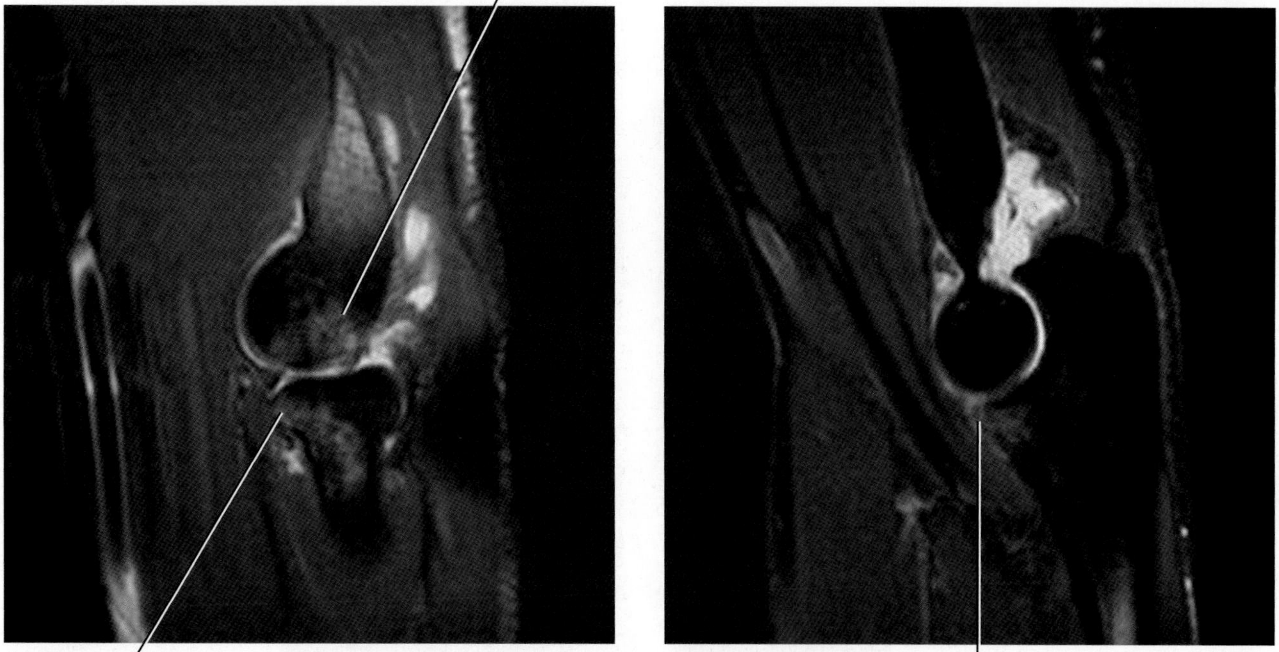
Bone contusion in
posterior capitellum
A
Bone contusion in
anterior margin
radial head
B
Bone contusion
and fracture tip of
coronoid process

Figure 8-17 **Osseous injury patterns associated with posterior elbow dislocation.** The marrow edema pattern involving the posterior aspect of the capitellum and anterior aspect of the radial head (**A**) combined with marrow edema of the tip of the coronoid process (**B**) is the classic bone contusion pattern seen after posterior dislocation of the elbow.

Continued

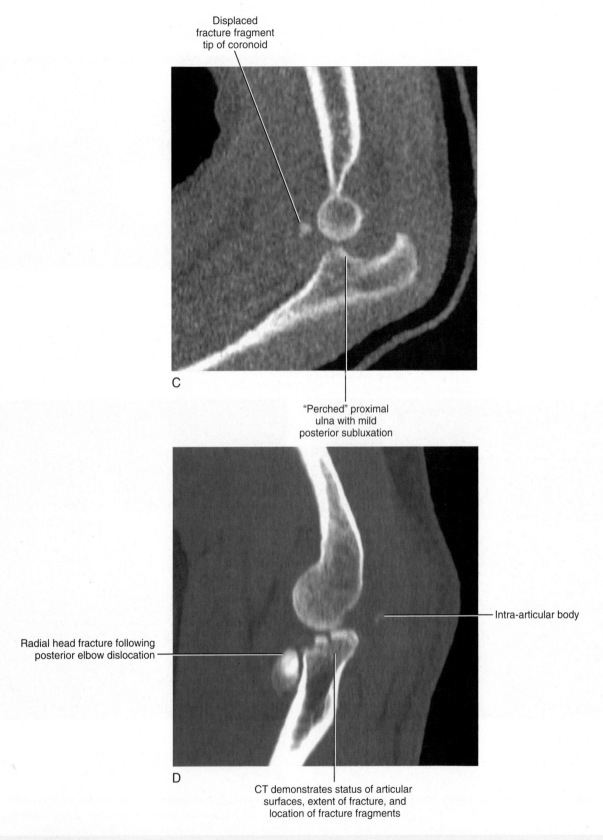

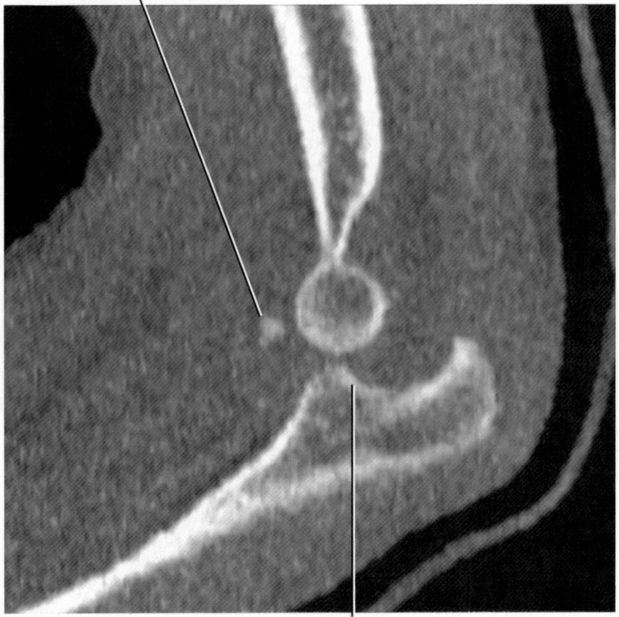
Displaced
fracture fragment
tip of coronoid
C
"Perched" proximal
ulna with mild
posterior subluxation

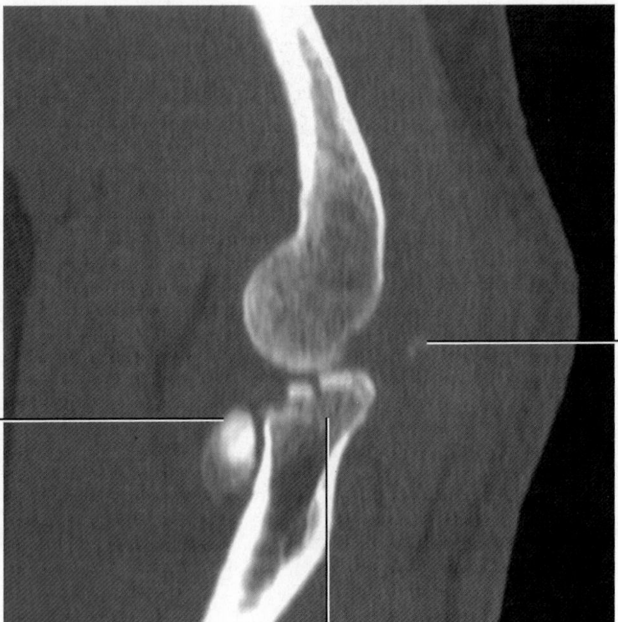
Intra-articular body
Radial head fracture following
posterior elbow dislocation
D
CT demonstrates status of articular
surfaces, extent of fracture, and
location of fracture fragments

Figure 8-17, cont'd Fractures can also occur in these locations, and CT examination can be helpful in demonstrating the extent and location of these fractures (**C** and **D**).

head, and finally inserts onto the posterior aspect of the ulna. It is the primary stabilizer of the lateral elbow with regard to posterolateral rotatory stability, and complete disruption of this structure can lead to recurrent elbow instability. Moreover, its disruption may require lateral elbow reconstruction. The LUCL is best evaluated on fat-saturated T2-weighted coronal MR images (Box 8-1). The majority of injuries occur near the proximal attachment site adjacent to the posterior lateral epicondyle, but disruption also occasionally occurs in the midsubstance (Fig. 8-18A).

With increasing severity of distraction forces at the time of dislocation, a very predictable and sequential pattern of soft tissue injury occurs (Table 8-6). The pattern of injury begins with the proximal attachment of the LUCL and then travels around the elbow circumferentially in both the anterior and posterior directions. As the disruptive forces move anteriorly, the radial collateral ligament is the next structure to be injured, and it is often completely disrupted at its proximal site or in its midsubstance. Varying degrees

Table 8-5 Posterior Elbow Dislocation

Demographics	No specific associated sport
Mechanism of injury	Fall on an outstretched arm
Injury patterns	
Osseous structures (contusion or fracture)	Anterior radial head Posterior capitellum Tip of the coronoid Child—avulsion medial epicondyle
Anterior/posterior soft tissues	Brachialis muscle Anterior and posterior capsule
Medial soft tissue structures	Common flexor tendon Anterior band UCL
Lateral soft tissue structures	Common extensor tendon RCL Proximal LUCL
Associated injuries/ complications	Myositis ossificans Persistent pain/instability Decreased range of motion

LUCL, lateral ulnar collateral ligament; RCL, radial collateral ligament; UCL, ulnar collateral ligament.

BOX 8-1 LATERAL ULNAR COLLATERAL LIGAMENT

- Stabilizes elbow against posterolateral rotatory instability
- Acts as a posterior sling for radial head
- Proximal attachment—posterior aspect of lateral epicondyle
- Distal attachment—posterior aspect of proximal ulna
- Injured during posterior elbow dislocation
- Tear—usually proximal, less often mid substance
- Best seen on coronal T2-weighted MR images

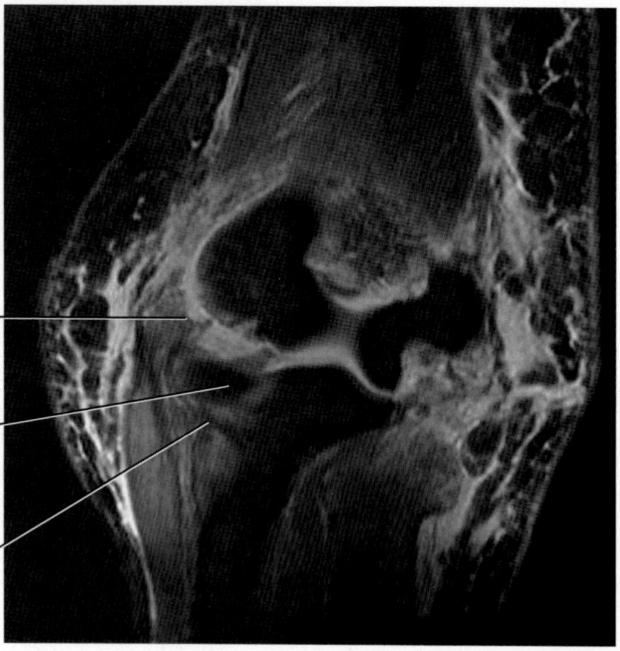
Proximal LUCL tear with minimal retraction
Radial head
LUCL intact distally
A

Figure 8-18 Soft tissue injury patterns associated with posterior elbow dislocation. A, Coronal T2-weighted image shows a complete disruption of the proximal fibers of the lateral ulnar collateral ligament (LUCL), which normally acts as a sling to prevent rotatory instability of the elbow. Disruption most often occurs proximally, but may also occur in the midsubstance. *Continued*

SECTION IV

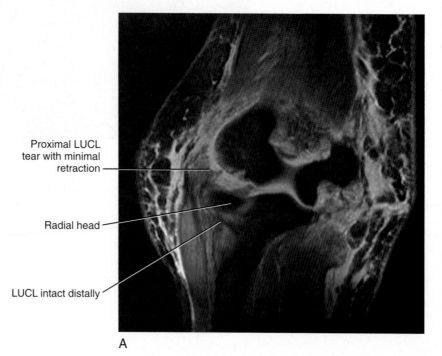

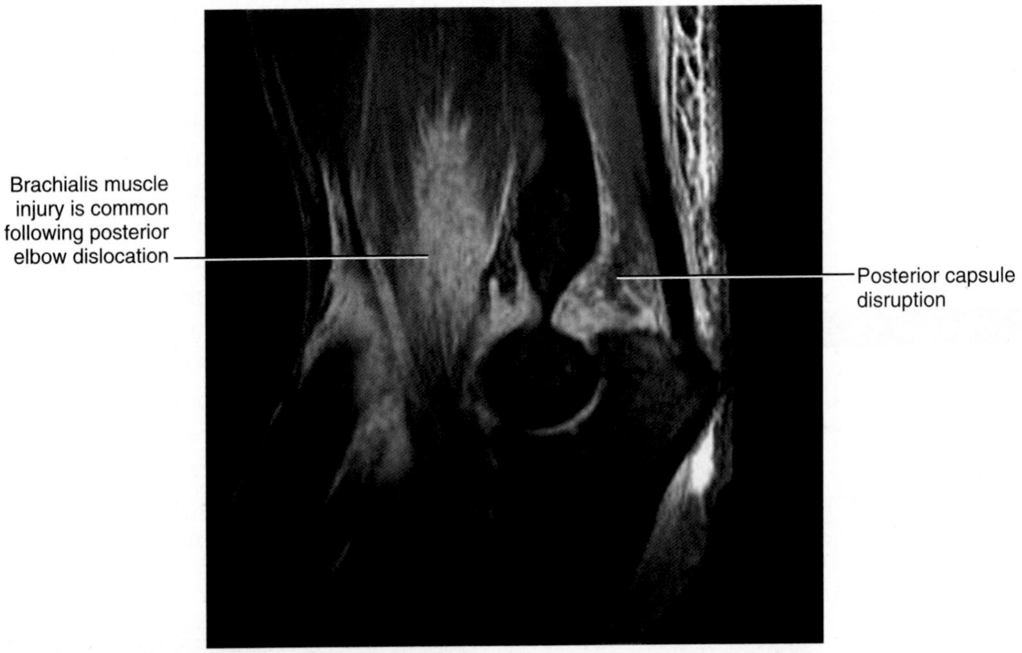
Brachialis muscle injury is common following posterior elbow dislocation
Posterior capsule disruption

B

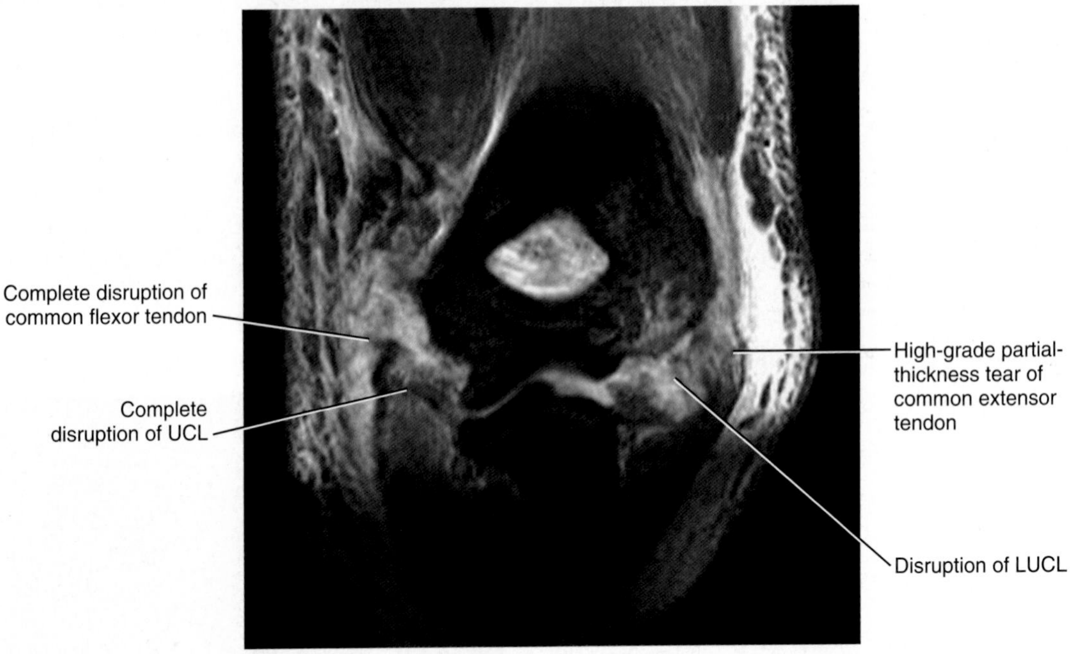
Complete disruption of common flexor tendon
Complete disruption of UCL
High-grade partial-thickness tear of common extensor tendon
Disruption of LUCL

C

Figure 8-18, cont'd **B,** Sagittal image demonstrates injury of the brachialis muscle, which can range from a mild strain to an extensive partial-thickness tear with associated intramuscular hematoma. Stretching injury or disruption of the anterior and posterior capsule is often noted along with a large joint effusion. **C,** Coronal image shows injury to the medial and lateral soft tissue structures. Injury typically ranges from a strain to a complete disruption of the common flexor and extensor tendons as well as the ulnar collateral ligament (UCL) and radial collateral ligament.

Table 8-6 Progression of Soft Tissue Injury With Posterior Elbow Dislocation

Stage	Soft Tissue Injury
1	Disruption of proximal fibers LUCL Common extensor tendon injury (strain/partial-thickness/full-thickness tear)
2	Radial collateral ligament Anterior capsule Posterior capsule
3A	Posterior bundle of UCL Common flexor tendon injury (strain/partial-thickness/full-thickness tear)
3B	Anterior bundle of UCL

LUCL, lateral ulnar collateral ligament; UCL, ulnar collateral ligament.

of injury also involve the overlying common extensor tendon ranging from a mild strain to a complete avulsion or disruption (Fig. 8-18C). Next, as the forces of injury continue in an anterior direction, the anterior capsule is stretched or disrupted, and there is nearly always a strain or partial-thickness tear of the overlying brachialis muscle (Fig. 8-18B). Injury to the brachialis muscle with a normal overlying biceps muscle and tendon is a marker that is quite specific for posterior elbow dislocation.

As the forces of injury move in the posterior direction from the LUCL, the first structure to be injured is the posterior capsule, which may be stretched or disrupted. As the forces continue along the posterior elbow, the posterior bundle of the UCL is the next structure in line and is often disrupted. With increasing severity of the distraction forces, the injury moves more anteriorly to involve the anterior bundle of the UCL and this structure is considered the primary stabilizer of the medial elbow. Finally, the overlying common flexor muscle and tendon may be injured with a strain or partial- or full-thickness disruption (see Fig. 8-18C).

In summation, the most specific markers indicating prior posterior elbow dislocation include bone contusions or fractures involving the anterior radial head, posterior capitellum, and the tip of the coronoid process. Injury to the brachialis muscle with an intact overlying biceps musculotendinous complex is also a marker that is specific for posterior elbow dislocation. The presence of these markers on MRI or the history of an elbow dislocation should prompt a thorough evaluation of the LUCL, which is the primary stabilizer of the lateral elbow with regard to rotatory instability, and the anterior band of the UCL, which is the primary stabilizer of the medial elbow with regard to excessive valgus stress.

Complications of elbow dislocation include long-term pain associated with persistent instability. Decreased range of motion is another common complication following elbow dislocation, especially among adults. Small ectopic calcifications are frequently seen within the capsule or within torn ligaments following elbow dislocation and have little clinical relevance. Myositis ossificans, on the other hand, is a rather uncommon complication that has been shown to occur most often after delayed reduction or multiple unsuccessful attempts at reduction. Myositis ossificans usually leads to a significant decrease in the normal range of motion of the elbow. It is important to differentiate between linear calcification and true myositis ossificans within the soft tissues of the elbow following dislocation, because myositis ossificans portends a much poorer prognosis. Radiographs can easily differentiate myositis ossificans from linear ectopic calcification; however, with MRI, linear calcifications may be easily overlooked (Fig. 8-19).

OSSEOUS STRUCTURES AND ARTICULAR SURFACES

Most fractures and osseous injuries about the elbow are adequately evaluated with conventional radiographs. A subset of injuries, however, are either occult radiographically or are more completely evaluated with cross-sectional imaging using either MRI or CT to identify and fully delineate the extent of injury.

Radiographically Occult Fractures

Identification of a joint effusion on conventional radiographs after elbow trauma indicates the likelihood of a radiographically occult fracture. A true lateral radiograph is essential for the detection of an elbow effusion. Fluid within the joint results in displacement of the posterior elbow fat pad beyond the borders of the posterior humeral cortex and is referred to as the *posterior fat pad sign,* whereas the anterior fat pad, which is normally visible as a thin lucent line on the lateral view, is displaced anteriorly and superiorly by a joint effusion and is referred to as the *anterior sail sign.* A radial head fracture is the most common radiographically occult fracture to occur in

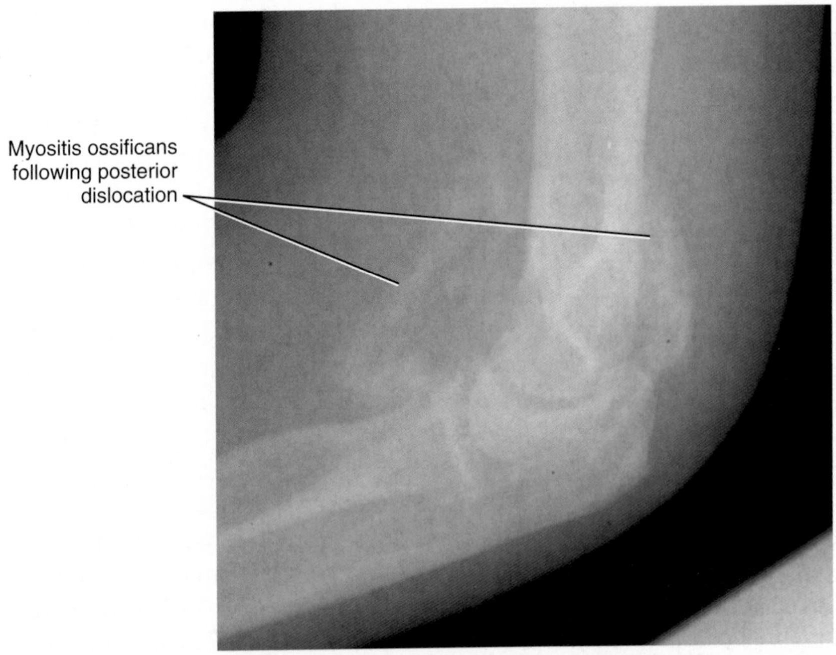
Myositis ossificans
following posterior
dislocation

A

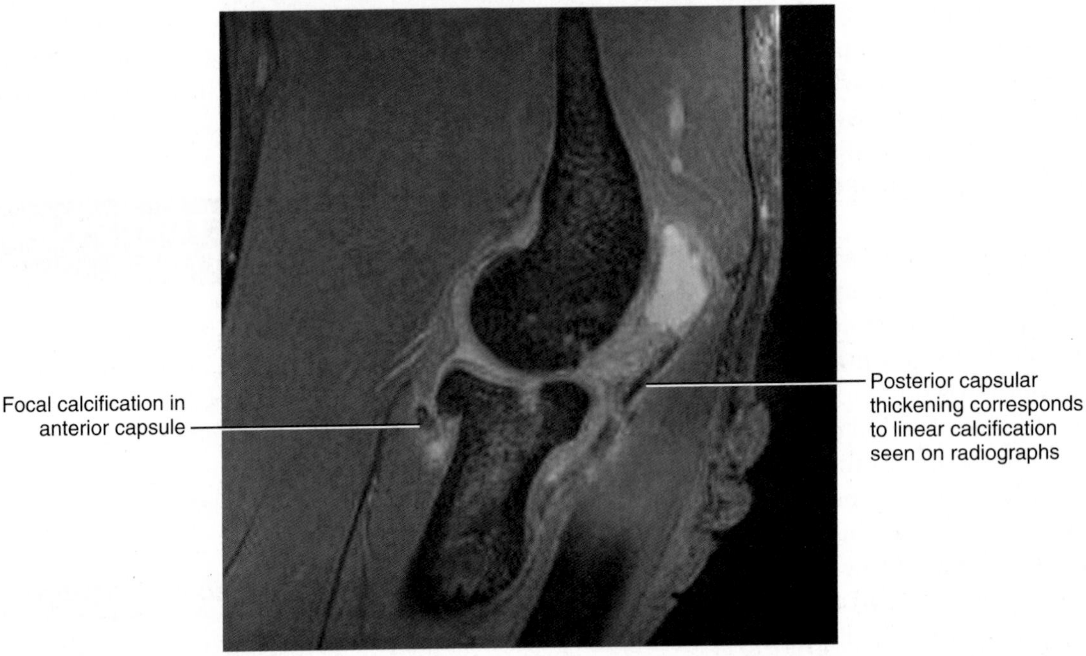
Focal calcification in
anterior capsule
Posterior capsular
thickening corresponds
to linear calcification
seen on radiographs

B

Figure 8-19 Soft tissue calcification surrounding the elbow following posterior dislocation. A, Lateral radiograph of the elbow shows extensive myositis ossificans surrounding the elbow as a complication of prior posterior dislocation. **B,** Sagittal T2-weighted MR image in a different patient shows linear calcification in the anterior and posterior capsule after posterior dislocation.

the adult, whereas in the child, it is the supracondylar fracture. Either MRI or CT examination can accurately detect these fractures.

Osteochondroses of the Elbow

Osteochondrosis is defined as a group of disorders affecting an ossification center in a child or adolescent resulting in alteration of endochondral ossification. Histologic studies have shown that the affected ossification center undergoes degeneration or avascular necrosis followed by resorption and changes of repair with recalcification. The osteochondroses of the elbow most frequently occur in adolescent athletes, with involvement of the capitellum and radial head resulting from compressive or shearing forces whereas lesions of the olecranon and medial epicondyle result from traction forces.

Osteochondral lesions of the capitellum or radial head most frequently occur in adolescent pitchers or gymnasts and almost always involve the dominant arm. Repeated valgus stress across the lateral compartment of the elbow in pitchers results in excessive compressive or shearing forces leading to these osteochondral injuries. In gymnasts, the lateral compartment of the elbow acts as a weight-bearing joint and is subjected to excessive compressive forces. These osteochondral injuries range from minimal subchondral marrow edema and microtrabecular injury to a partially or completely detached osteochondral fragment in situ or, in the most severe cases, to a displaced osteochondral fragment. The stable injuries are usually treated with conservative measures by placing the arm at rest and by eliminating the aggravating activity. Unstable or displaced osteochondral fragments require surgical reattachment or debridement.

In most cases, MRI can accurately differentiate between the various stages of injury, and the most critical decision point is to differentiate between a stable and an unstable fragment in situ because the unstable lesions require surgical intervention. On occasion, it may prove difficult using conventional MRI to differentiate between a stable and an unstable in situ lesion (Fig. 8-20). Fluid, seen on a T2-weighted image, extending completely beneath the osteochondral fragment, indicates a loose but in situ lesion. However, loose granulation tissue that holds a stable

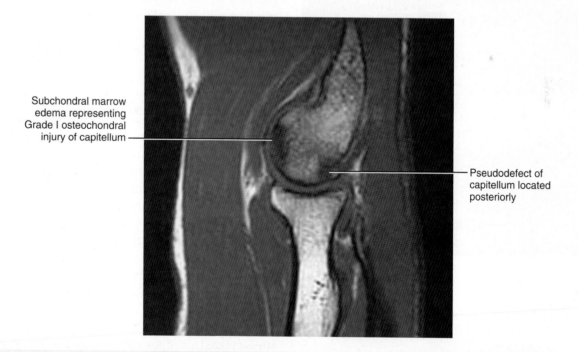

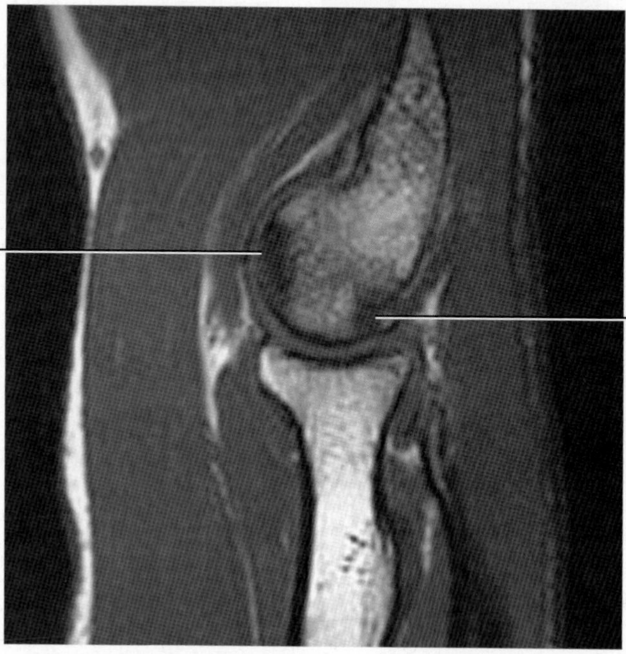
Subchondral marrow edema representing Grade I osteochondral injury of capitellum
Pseudodefect of capitellum located posteriorly

Figure 8-20 Differentiating an osteochondral injury from the pseudodefect of the capitellum. Osteochondral injuries of the capitellum typically involve the anterior margin of the capitellum because the compressive forces that occur during the mechanism of throwing are greatest when the elbow is in the flexed position, thus transmitting the greatest force to the capitellum along its anterior margin. The cortical step-off seen along the mid to posterior aspect of the capitellum represents the normal MR appearance of the posterior margin of the articular surface of the capitellum and is referred to as the pseudodefect of the capitellum.

fragment in place may appear very bright on T2-weighted MR images and mimic fluid surrounding an unstable fragment. Direct MR arthrography can increase the specificity in these cases. Gadolinium completely surrounding a fragment is indicative of an unstable fragment. Occasionally, in adolescent pitchers a purely chondral shearing injury results in a full-thickness chondral defect and resultant loose body. This injury is occult on radiographs, although a joint effusion may be present. MR imaging demonstrates a full-thickness chondral defect and resultant loose body (Fig. 8-21).

The major pitfall with regard to the diagnosis of an osteochondral injury of the capitellum is the presence of the pseudodefect of the capitellum. This is a normal anatomic finding that can mimic an osteochondral lesion of the capitellum on MR imaging. Along the posterolateral margin of the articular surface of the capitellum, the articular cartilage ends abruptly, and on sagittal and coronal images this gives the appearance of an abrupt step-off of the chondral surface, which can mimic an osteochondral lesion but actually represents the normal appearance of the interface between the articular cartilage and the nonarticular surface of the posterior capitellum. The key to differentiating this from a true osteochondral lesion is to recognize that the osteochondral lesions occur in the anterior aspect of the capitellum as seen on sagittal images, whereas the pseudodefect of the capitellum is located posteriorly and usually demonstrate little to no subchondral signal abnormality (see Fig. 8-20).

The medial epicondyle is another location of common injury in adolescent pitchers, and osteochondrosis of the medial epicondyle usually results from excessive traction forces that are applied across the elbow during the motion of throwing. The incidence of this injury has decreased significantly over the past decade in the little league age group as a result of education of parents and coaches. The lesion is now more commonly seen in the slightly older age group and in athletes of early high school age (Fig. 8-22).

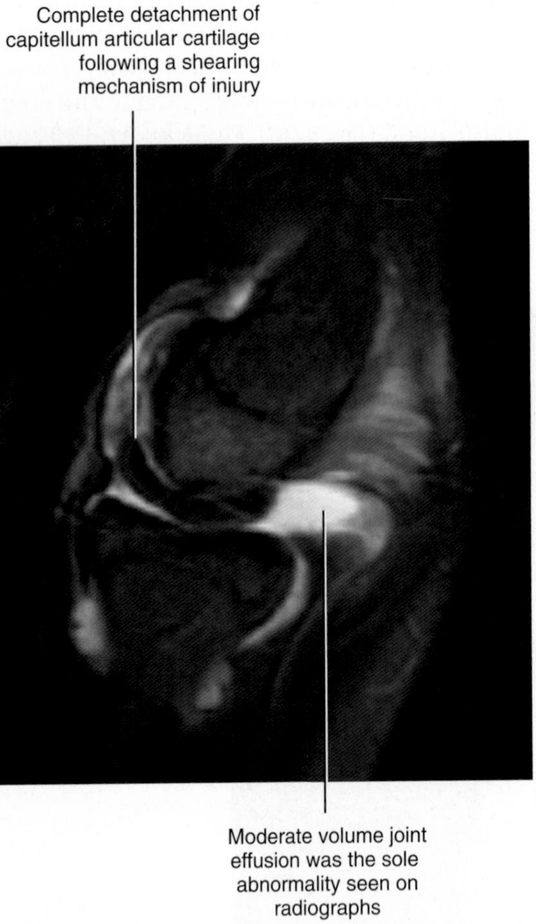
Complete detachment of capitellum articular cartilage following a shearing mechanism of injury
Moderate volume joint effusion was the sole abnormality seen on radiographs

Figure 8-21 Sagittal T2-weighted image shows the elbow of a 12-year-old pitcher who suffered an elbow injury during throwing. Shearing forces have resulted in a complete avulsion of the articular cartilage of the capitellum. The underlying bone demonstrates only mild marrow edema but is otherwise normal. Radiographs (not shown) demonstrate only a small joint effusion but are otherwise normal.

Olecranon Stress Fractures

Stress fractures of the olecranon occur as a result of tension overload of the triceps tendon during the acceleration phase of throwing and usually occur in high-performance throwers. Although stress-related injuries of the olecranon are more common in the adolescent thrower, they are not uncommon in adult throwers. Patients usually present with pain to palpation over the olecranon, and posterior elbow pain during the acceleration phase of throwing. Radiographs may demonstrate an incomplete fracture line that is oriented transverse to the long axis of the proximal ulna with adjacent sclerosis. MRI depicts stress-related changes earlier than radiographs, and findings may include marrow edema isolated to the olecranon, often with accompanying overlying soft tissue edema and enthesiophyte formation at the distal triceps attachment site. An incomplete nondisplaced fracture may be seen as a dark line on T1- and T2-weighted images (Fig. 8-23). In advanced cases, a complete fracture with a displaced fragment,

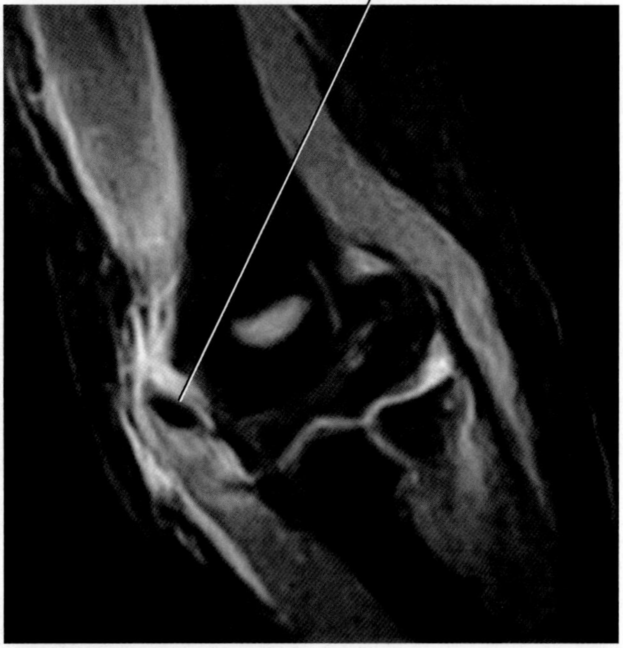
Minimally displaced medial epicondyle avulsion with adjacent soft tissue edema

Figure 8-22 Medial epicondyle avulsion. In the adolescent, the apophyseal growth plate is the "weak link," and excessive repetitive traction forces applied across the medial aspect of the elbow during the motion of throwing more commonly results in an avulsion of the medial epicondyle rather than in disruption of the common flexor tendon.

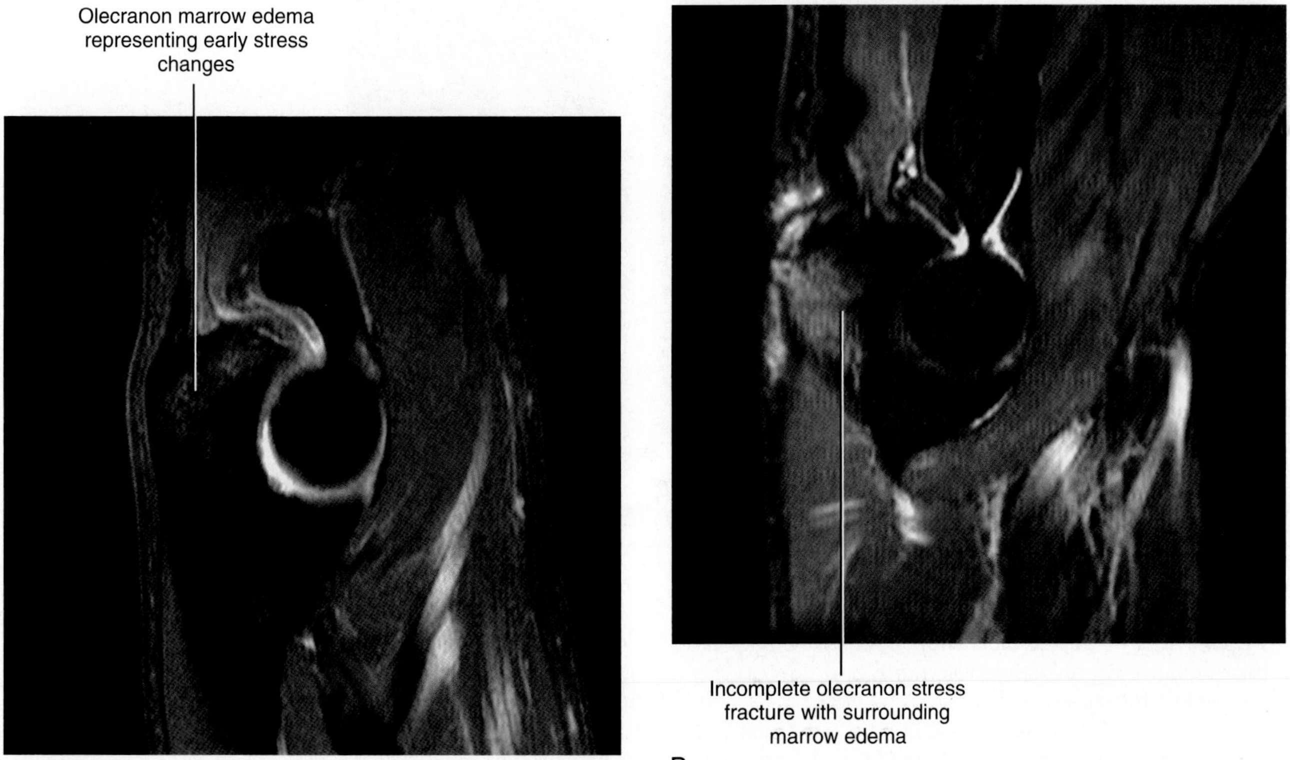
Olecranon marrow edema representing early stress changes
A
Incomplete olecranon stress fracture with surrounding marrow edema
B

Figure 8-23 Olecranon stress injuries. A, Sagittal T2-weighted image with fat saturation shows marrow edema within the olecranon of a 16-year-old pitcher with posterior elbow pain. This represents stress-related marrow changes resulting from excessive traction applied at the level of the distal triceps attachment. **B,** Sagittal T2-weighted image with fat saturation shows a chronic incomplete, nondisplaced stress fracture of the olecranon in a 17-year-old pitcher with posterior elbow pain aggravated by throwing.

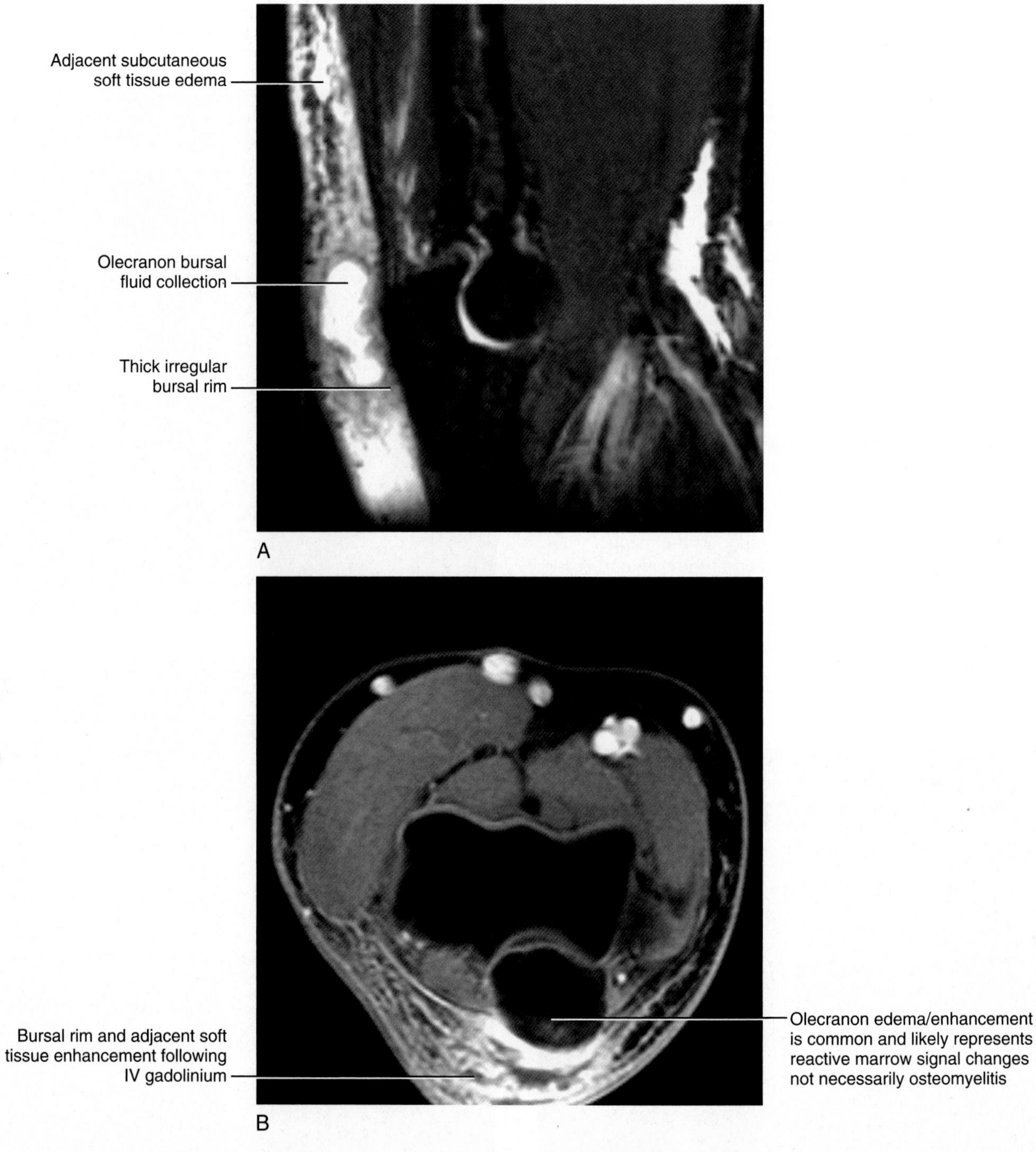
Adjacent subcutaneous soft tissue edema
Olecranon bursal fluid collection
Thick irregular bursal rim
A
Bursal rim and adjacent soft tissue enhancement following IV gadolinium
Olecranon edema/enhancement is common and likely represents reactive marrow signal changes not necessarily osteomyelitis
B

Figure 8-24 Septic olecranon bursitis. A, Sagittal T2-weighted image shows fluid within the olecranon bursa with a thick irregular rim of intermediate signal and surrounding soft tissue edema. **B,** Axial T1-weighted image with intravenous gadolinium reveals enhancement of the thick bursal wall, adjacent subcutaneous soft tissues, and olecranon. Enhancement can be seen with septic or aseptic bursitis, but the absence of enhancement excludes the presence of infection. Reactive marrow edema or enhancement is a common finding and is not indicative of osteomyelitis.

fragmentation of the fracture fragment, or intra-articular bodies may occur.

COMPRESSION SYNDROMES AROUND THE ELBOW

Olecranon Bursitis

Inflammation of the olecranon bursa may be acute, chronic, or infectious and most often results from repetitive trauma to the posterior aspect of the elbow. Olecranon bursitis is seen more often in occupations that result in repetitive trauma to the posterior aspect of the elbow and has been referred to as *miner's elbow* and *student's elbow*. It has also been commonly reported in football and hockey players, and in this population it is thought to result from repetitively falling on the flexed elbow. Chronic cases can be associated with inflammatory processes such as hydroxyapatite deposition disease (HADD) or gout. Imaging typically plays little role in the diagnosis and evaluation of olecranon bursitis, but has been shown to be useful in the differentiation of septic from aseptic bursitis and in the evaluation of associated soft tissue abnormalities.

There is considerable overlap on MRI between the appearance of septic and of aseptic bursitis. Both can present with complex-appearing fluid within the distended bursa and a thick irregular bursal lining with surrounding soft tissue edema. Edema can be seen in the distal triceps tendon as well as within the marrow of the overlying olecranon. These osseous changes are nearly always reactive in origin and do not necessarily indicate the presence of osteomyelitis. Intravenous gadolinium can be helpful in differentiating septic from aseptic olecranon bursitis. Enhancement of the rim of the bursa and the adjacent subcutaneous soft tissues is commonly seen in both septic and aseptic bursitis (Fig. 8-24). However, the absence of rim and adjacent soft tissue enhancement excludes the possibility of an infectious etiology.

Suggested Readings

Anderson MA. Imaging of upper extremity stress fractures in the athlete. Clin Sports Med 2006;25:489–504.

Bencardino JT, Rosenberg ZS. Entrapment neuropathies of the shoulder and elbow in the athlete. Clin Sports Med 2006;25: 465–487.

Cain EL Jr, Dugas JR, Wolf RS, Andrews JR. Elbow injuries in throwing athletes: a current concepts review. Am J Sports Med 2003;31:621–635.

Chung CB, Stanley AJ, Gentili A. Magnetic resonance imaging of elbow instability. Semin Musculoskelet Radiol 2005;9: 67–76.

Floemer F, Morrison WB, Bongartz G, Ledermann HP. MRI characteristics of olecranon bursitis. AJR Am J Roentgenol 2004;183: 29–34.

Fowler KA, Chung CB. Normal MR imaging anatomy of the elbow. Magn Reson Imaging Clin N Am 2004;12:191–206.

Fritz RC. MR imaging of osteochondral and articular lesions. Magn Reson Imaging Clin N Am 1997;5:579–602.

Kaplan LJ, Potter HG. MR imaging of ligament injuries to the elbow. Magn Reson Imaging Clin N Am 2004;12:221–232.

Kijowski R, De Smet AA. The role of ultrasound in the evaluation of sports medicine injuries of the upper extremity. Clin Sports Med 2006;25:569–590.

Kijowski R, Tuite M, Sanford M. Magnetic resonance imaging of the elbow. Part I: normal anatomy, imaging techniques, and osseous abnormalities. Skelet Radiol 2004;33:685–697.

Kijowski R, Tuite M, Sanford M. Magnetic resonance imaging of the elbow. Part II: abnormalities of the ligaments, tendons, and nerves. Skelet Radiol 2005;34:1–18.

O'Driscoll SW. Classification and evaluation of recurrent instability of the elbow. Clin Orthop Relat Res 2000;370:34–43.

Ouellette H, Kassarjian A, Tretreault P, Palmer W. Imaging of the overhead throwing athlete. Semin Musculoskeletal Radiol 2005;9:316–333.

Pudas T, Hurme T, Mattila K, Svedstrom E. Magnetic resonance imaging in pediatric elbow fractures. Acta Radiol 2005;46: 636–644.

Tuite MJ, Kijowski R. Sports-related injuries of the elbow: an approach to MRI interpretation. Clin Sports Med 2006;25: 387–408.

Chapter 9

IMAGING OF THE WRIST

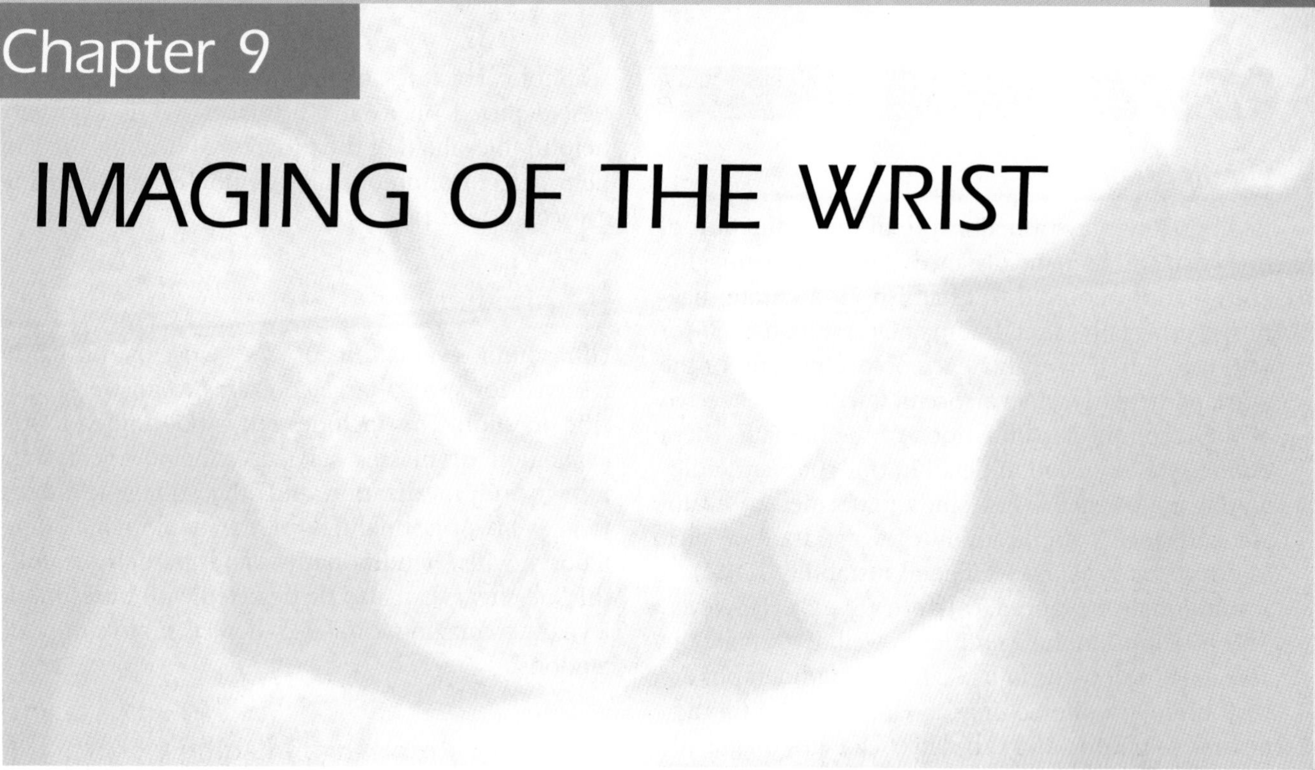

CHAPTER OUTLINE

MODALITIES

Radiography

Radiography plays a major role in the evaluation of the wrist, and in many instances it is the only imaging examination required to establish an accurate diagnosis, especially after trauma. Occasionally, CT or MRI is required to evaluate for occult fractures of the wrist, particularly when an occult fracture is suspected of the scaphoid or of the hook of the hamate. These entities are discussed in detail in this chapter. Radiographs are often the first study performed to evaluate end-stage complications of wrist trauma such as dorsal intercalated segmental instability (DISI) or scapholunate advanced collapse (SLAC). However, MRI is helpful in these entities as well to evaluate the associated soft tissue injuries. Finally, radiographs are very useful in the setting of wrist pain without a history of trauma and can detect changes diagnostic of entities such as inflammatory or degenerative arthropathies, impingement syndromes, and avascular necrosis. In most instances, radiographs are helpful in the early evaluation of wrist pain and can help guide or direct more advanced imaging.

The standard radiographic views of the wrist include the posteroanterior, oblique, and lateral views. Numerous specialized views have been developed to help in the evaluation of the wrist, especially with regard to instability of the wrist. These include the views of the wrist in radial or ulnar deviation, in flexion and extension, and in the "clenched fist" view. The scaphoid view is a specialized view that can aid in the detection of subtle fractures of the scaphoid, whereas the carpal tunnel view is helpful in evaluating the hook of the hamate.

Computed Tomography

Computed tomography (CT) is most commonly used to assess the extent of complex fractures of the wrist or to evaluate for the presence of an occult fracture. Multidetector CT allows high-resolution submillimeter imaging in any plane. CT accurately depicts the extent of articular surface incongruity when fractures involve the distal radial articular surface and also accurately depicts complex fractures of each of the carpal bones. The scaphoid is best evaluated with images obtained or reformatted in an oblique sagittal or coronal plane paralleling the long axis of the scaphoid. Fractures of the hook of the hamate are best depicted on axial CT images. CT is also very helpful in evaluating the progress of healing and can help detect nonunion, fibrous union, and evolving avascular necrosis.

Ultrasound

Ultrasound evaluation of the wrist is primarily reserved for special targeted exams to answer a specific question. This includes but is not limited to the evaluation of masses such as ganglia, aneurysms, foreign body localization, and other soft tissue masses (Fig. 9-1). Abnormalities of the tendon including tenosynovitis, tendinopathy, and partial- or full-thickness tears can also be depicted with ultrasound. Dynamic imaging can also depict subluxation of tendons.

Magnetic Resonance Imaging

MRI is especially well suited for evaluation of the small soft tissue structures of the wrist, including the tendons, the intrinsic ligaments, and the neurovascular structures. The intrinsic ligaments are best evaluated with high-resolution 1-mm thick images using three-dimensional gradient-echo images. Occasionally, intra-articular gadolinium is of help in evaluating the integrity of the intrinsic ligaments. MRI also accurately depicts abnormalities of the osseous structures including fracture, avascular necrosis, and impingement syndromes.

TENDONS

At the level of the wrist, the tendons are broadly classified as either flexor or extensor tendons. The extensor tendons are located along the dorsal aspect of the wrist and are arranged in six separate compartments (numbered one through six) with the first compartment located along the radial aspect of the wrist and the sixth compartment located along the ulnar side of the wrist (Fig. 9-2A). The number of tendons varies within the six compartments, but each compartment contains only a single common tendon sheath, which is shared by all tendons within that compartment (Table 9-1). The flexor tendons are divided into two separate groups based on whether they are located within or outside of the carpal tunnel (Fig. 9-2B and Table 9-2).

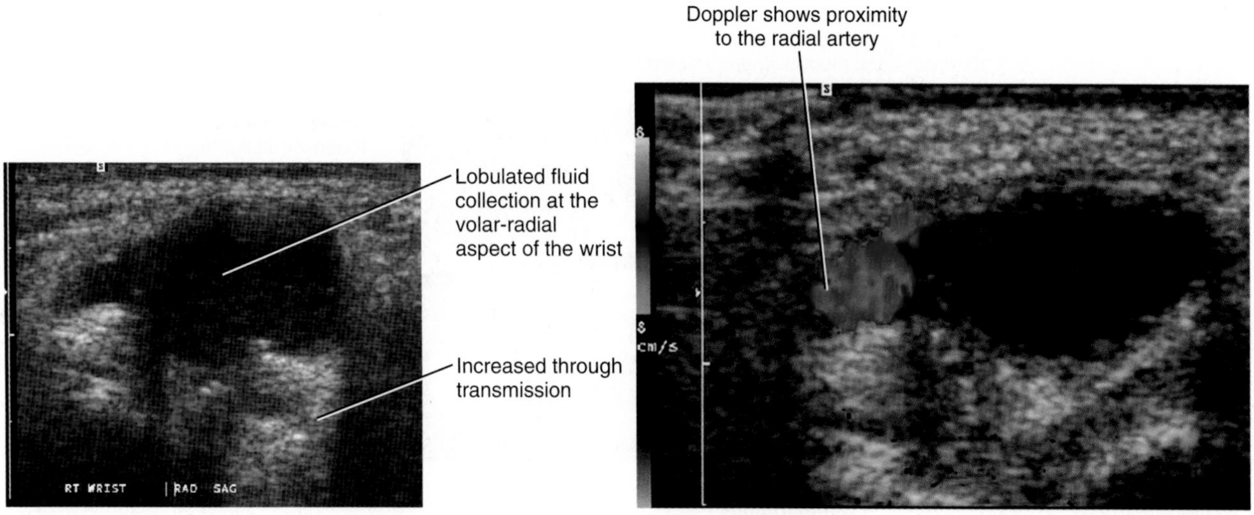
Doppler shows proximity
to the radial artery
Lobulated fluid
collection at the
volar-radial
aspect of the wrist
Increased through
transmission
RT WRIST
RAD SAG
cm/s

Figure 9-1 Ultrasound examination of the wrist with power Doppler shows a focal anechoic structure representing a ganglion. Doppler clearly shows flow within the adjacent radial artery with lack of flow in the ganglion, confirming the presence of a ganglion rather than a vascular lesion.

Table 9-1 Extensor Compartment Anatomy

Compartment	Tendons
1	Abductor pollicis longus Extensor pollicis brevis
2	Extensor carpi radialis brevis Extensor carpi radialis longus Extensor pollicis longus (distal to the radioulnar joint)
3	Extensor pollicis longus (proximal to the radioulnar joint)
4	Extensor digitorum tendons Extensor indicis tendons
5	Extensor digiti minimi tendon
6	Extensor carpi ulnaris tendon

Table 9-2 Flexor Compartment Anatomy

Compartment	Anatomic Structures
Inside carpal tunnel	Flexor digitorum superficialis tendons Flexor digitorum profundus tendons Flexor pollicis longus tendon Median nerve
Outside carpal tunnel	Flexor carpi radialis Flexor carpi ulnaris Palmaris longus (variable) Radial neurovascular bundle
Inside Guyon's canal	Ulnar artery and nerve

The range of tendon pathology in the wrist is similar to the range of pathology found in tendons elsewhere in the body. Inflammation isolated to the tendon sheath is referred to as tenosynovitis and may be sterile or infectious (Fig. 9-3). Noninfectious tenosynovitis is most common and typically results from repetitive trauma or mechanical irritation of the tendon sheath but may also occur in association with an inflammatory arthropathy. Tenosynovitis usually leads to the accumulation of fluid and/or synovial proliferation within the tendon sheath and may occasionally be associated with scarring within the tendon sheath. Scarring or fibrosis within the tendon sheath is referred to as *stenosing tenosynovitis* and may lead to entrapment and loss of function of the tendon. When this occurs at the level of the distal hand or fingers, it may lead to trigger finger.

Infectious tenosynovitis is usually bacterial in origin but may result from mycobacterium. Tendinosis typically occurs in association with repetitive trauma or overuse and results in tendon degeneration leading to an initial thickening of the tendon. Over time, repetitive trauma may lead to attenuation or thinning of the tendon. Finally, a partial- or full-thickness tear of the tendon may occur. Disruption most often occurs in a previously diseased tendon after chronic attritional change in association with repetitive trauma, but it may also result from an acute injury such as a laceration.

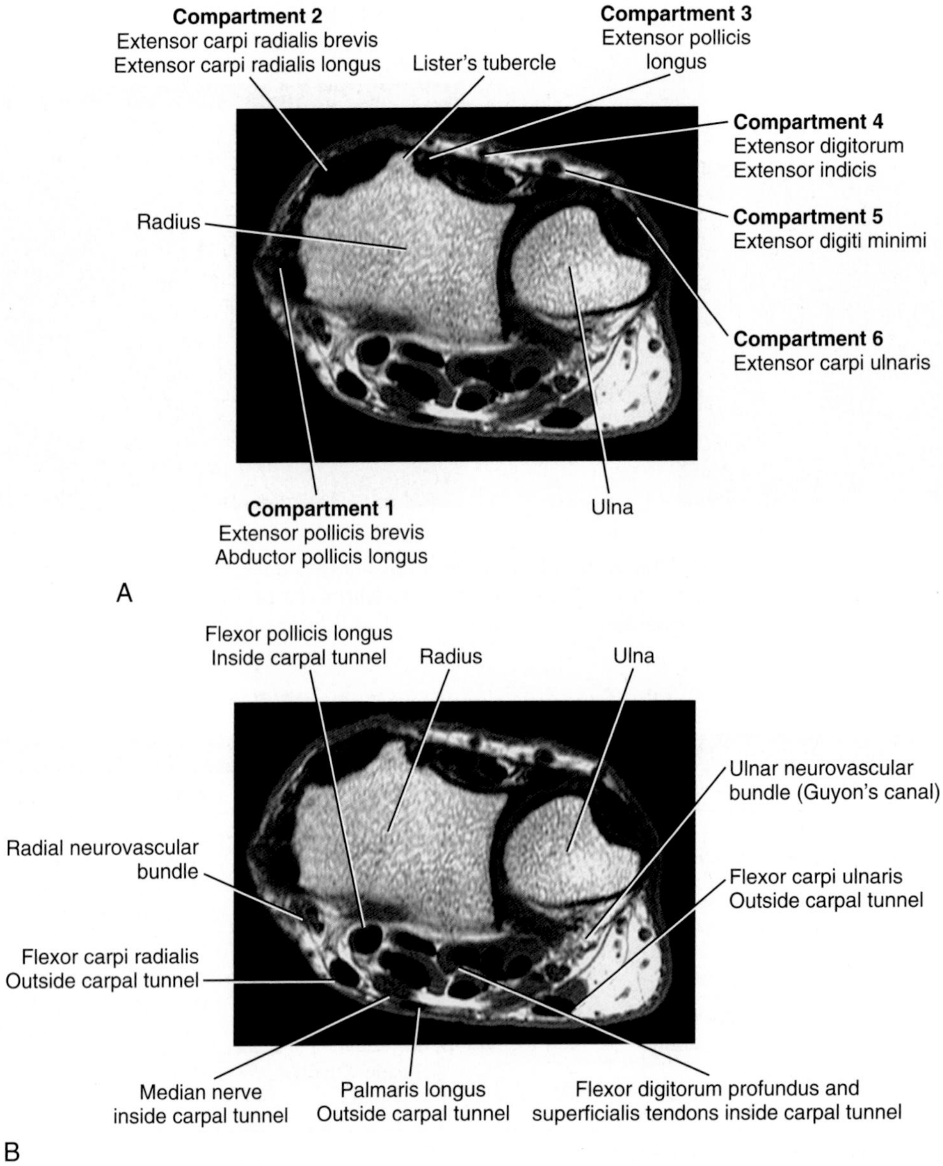
Compartment 2
Extensor carpi radialis brevis
Extensor carpi radialis longus
Lister's tubercle
Compartment 3
Extensor pollicis longus
Compartment 4
Extensor digitorum
Extensor indicis
Radius
Compartment 5
Extensor digiti minimi
Compartment 6
Extensor carpi ulnaris
Compartment 1
Extensor pollicis brevis
Abductor pollicis longus
Ulna
A
Flexor pollicis longus
Inside carpal tunnel
Radius
Ulna
Ulnar neurovascular
bundle (Guyon's canal)
Radial neurovascular
bundle
Flexor carpi ulnaris
Outside carpal tunnel
Flexor carpi radialis
Outside carpal tunnel
Median nerve
inside carpal tunnel
Palmaris longus
Outside carpal tunnel
Flexor digitorum profundus and
superficialis tendons inside carpal tunnel
B

Figure 9-2 Normal extensor (**A**) and flexor (**B**) tendon anatomy.

The compartmental anatomy of the tendons of the wrist makes the axial image at the level of Lister's tubercle best suited for identifying a specific tendon. As a result, tendon anatomy and pathology are usually best depicted on axial MR images, whereas coronal and sagittal images are complementary. The use of fat saturation increases the conspicuity of abnormalities such as minimal fluid within a tendon sheath and subtle surrounding soft tissue edema. Although frequency-selective fat saturation is the preferred method on a high field strength system, STIR (short tau inversion recovery) imaging can be substituted when frequency-selective fat-saturation techniques produce inhomogeneous fat saturation or when using a low field strength magnet. On MRI, the normal tendon typically demonstrates homogeneous low signal. Each tendon, however, is composed of multiple bundles, and on occasion this anatomic configuration can result in intermediate striations within the substance of the tendon, which can mimic tendinosis or an interstitial tear of the tendon. The normal tendon, however, lacks other signs of inflammation such as tenosynovitis and adjacent reactive soft tissue edema.

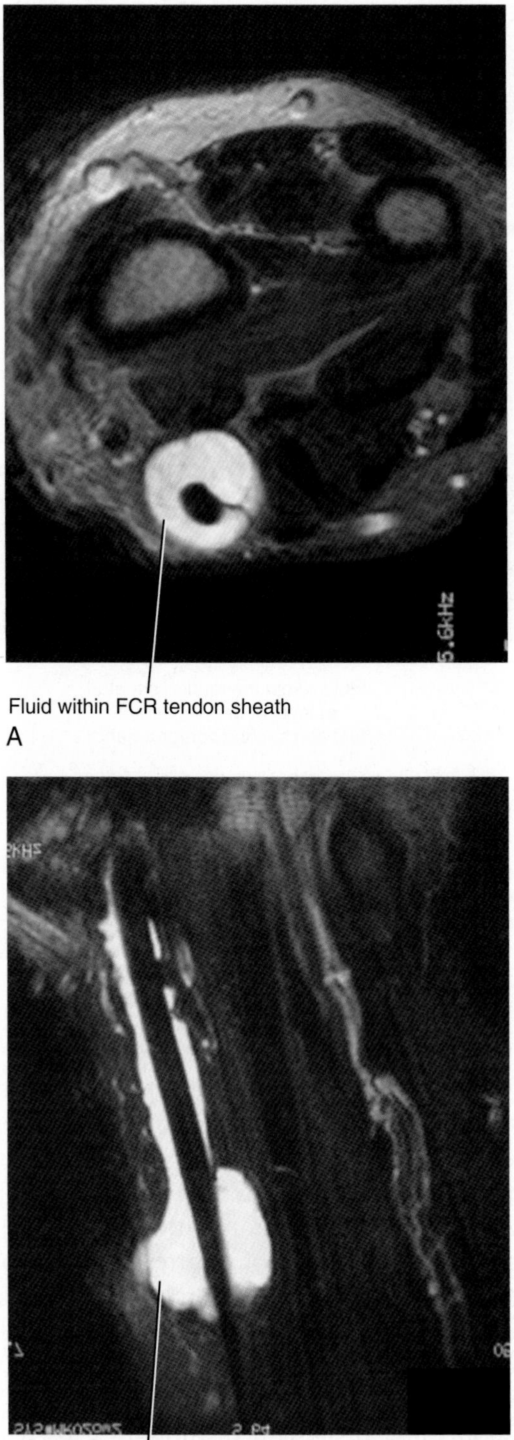
Fluid within FCR tendon sheath
A
Fluid within FCR tendon sheath
B

Figure 9-3 Tenosynovitis of the flexor carpi radialis (FCR) tendon sheath. Axial (**A**) and coronal (**B**) T2-weighted images with fat saturation show a large quantity of fluid within the FCR tendon sheath consistent with marked tenosynovitis. The tendon is normal without tendinopathy or tear.

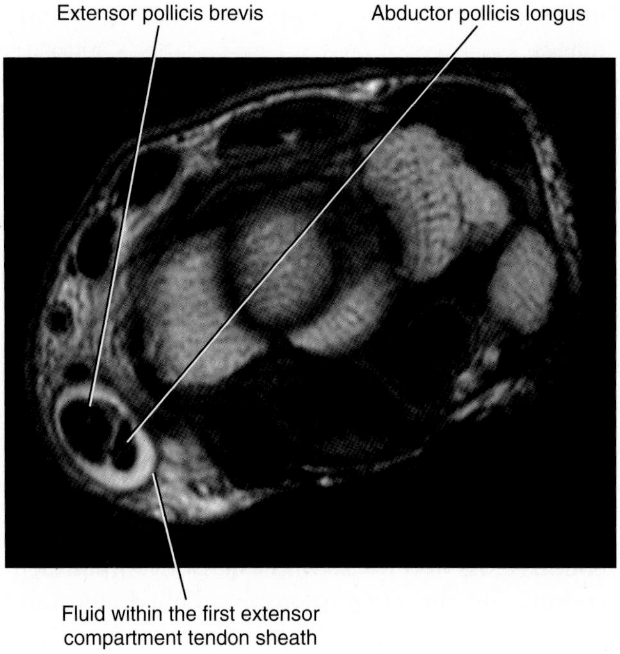
Extensor pollicis brevis
Abductor pollicis longus
Fluid within the first extensor compartment tendon sheath

Figure 9-4 De Quervain disease. Axial T2-weighted image of the wrist shows thickening and intrinsic signal abnormality within the extensor pollicis brevis and abductor pollicis longus tendons as well as moderate fluid within the tendon sheath.

Tenosynovitis involving the first extensor compartment at the level of the wrist is referred to as *de Quervain disease* (Fig. 9-4). The first extensor compartment contains the extensor pollicis brevis and the abductor pollicis longus tendons, and inflammatory changes of this compartment typically result from chronic microtrauma associated with repetitive ulnar and radial deviation of the wrist. There appears to be an increased incidence of de Quervain disease in young women during the third trimester of pregnancy and in the early postpartum period. Postpartum de Quervain disease may be associated with breast-feeding, and speculation has been made that the increased incidence in these young women results from the position of the wrist while feeding or possibly carrying the young infant. Patients with de Quervain's disease usually present with pain and swelling over the radial aspect of the wrist at the level of the radial styloid, and there is usually little confusion regarding the diagnosis on the basis of clinical examination. On MRI, changes within the tendon sheath may include tenosynovitis, stenosing tenosynovitis, and tendinopathy. Reactive marrow edema within the underlying radial styloid is a common finding seen best on fat-suppressed T2-weighted MR images.

Intersection syndrome refers to a tenosynovitis that occurs in the distal forearm at the crossing levels of the first and second extensor compartments. This condition most often results from chronic overuse and has been associated with rowing and racquet sports. Intersection syndrome is common in helicopter skiing and in aggressive downhill alpine skiing (in up to 11% of participants); in this setting intersection syndrome has also been referred to as bugaboo forearm. The mechanism of injury in this subset of patients is likely repetitive dorsiflexion and radial deviation of the wrist against the resistance of deep snow on withdrawal of the planted ski pole. The extensor pollicis brevis and abductor pollicis longus tendons cross over the second extensor compartment tendons and the extensor carpi radialis longus and brevis tendons at a level approximately 4 to 5 cm proximal to the radiocarpal joint. At the point of crossover, repetitive friction can lead to tenosynovitis, stenosing tenosynovitis, and occasionally adventitial bursa formation. On MRI, intersection syndrome is manifested as fluid within and surrounding the two tendon sheaths at the point of crossover (Fig. 9-5). The primary differential diagnosis is that of de Quervain disease. Decussation syndrome refers to a friction tenosynovitis caused by the third compartment tendons crossing superficial to the second compartment tendons.

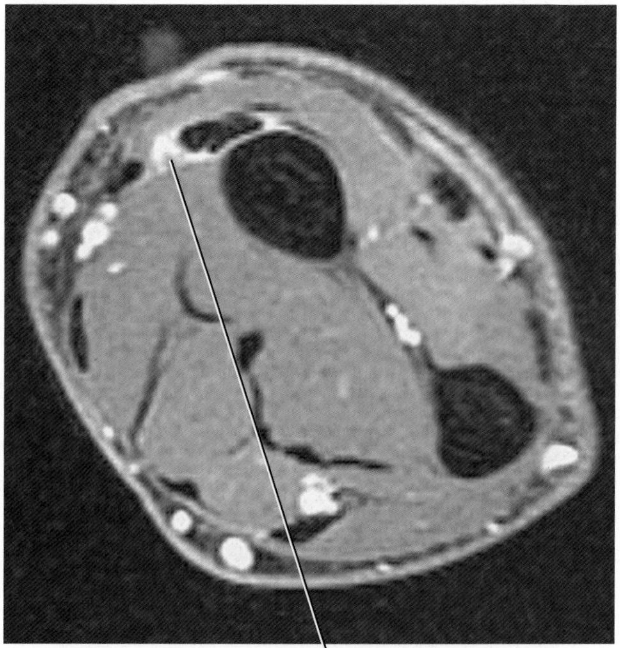
Fluid within the tendon sheaths
at level of intersection of
first and second compartments

Figure 9-5 Intersection syndrome (bugaboo forearm). Axial T2-weighted image with fat saturation approximately 4 to 5 cm proximal to the radiocarpal joint shows fluid within the two tendon sheaths at the level of crossover of the first and second extensor compartments.

Extensor carpi ulnaris tenosynovitis is also common and often results from excessive repetitive ulnar deviation as occurs in racquet sports. The extensor carpi ulnaris tendon sheath is considered to be a part of the triangular fibrocartilage complex (TFC; see Fig. 9-16), and injuries of the TFC are often accompanied by abnormalities of the extensor carpi ulnaris tendon. As a result, MRI evidence of extensor carpi ulnaris tenosynovitis/tendinosis should prompt a thorough evaluation of the TFC and especially its peripheral attachment for evidence of injury or tear. Extensor carpi ulnaris tendinopathy and tenosynovitis can mimic other ulnar-sided wrist abnormalities such as injury of the triangular fibrocartilage, lunotriquetral ligament tear, or one of the ulnar-sided abutment syndromes. MRI can be useful in differentiating these various entities. Traumatic injury of the extensor carpi ulnaris tendon sheath at the level of the distal ulna can result in tendon instability and recurrent dislocation (Fig. 9-6). Dislocation of the extensor carpi ulnaris tendon often accompanies tenosynovitis and may require dynamic MRI of the wrist or axial MRI of the wrist in the pronated and supinated positions to correctly establish this diagnosis. Subluxation of the extensor carpi ulnaris tendon can result in ulnar wrist pain accompanied by reproducible snapping sensation during wrist motion. Ultrasound is uniquely suited for the evaluation of recurrent subluxation of the extensor carpi ulnaris tendon because a dynamic exam can demonstrate the change in position of the tendon during motion of the wrist (Fig. 9-7).

Laceration or penetrating trauma to the wrist is a common cause of tendon disruption. Closed tears can also occur and are often attritional in etiology, occurring in association with inflammatory processes such as rheumatoid arthritis or occurring secondary to changes in the underlying osseous anatomy, as occurs after carpal fracture or dislocation. A complete description of a tendon tear should include the extent of tear as partial or complete. The location of the torn tendon end is usually described as it relates to the adjacent osseous anatomy. When a full-thickness

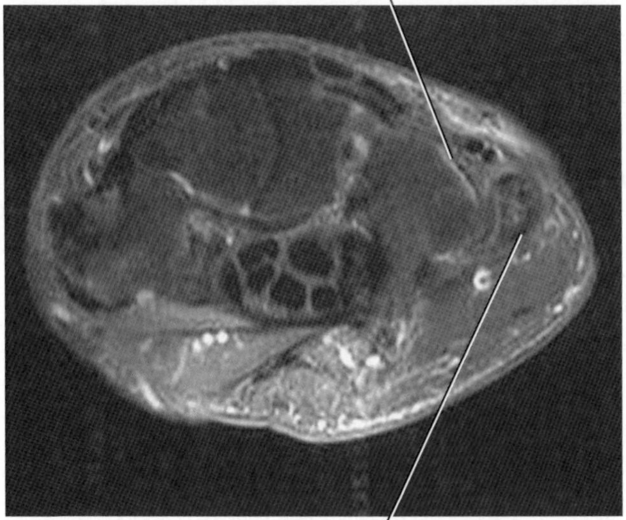
Expected location of ECU tendon
ECU tendon demonstrating marked tendinosis and subluxation

Figure 9-6 Extensor carpi ulnaris (ECU) tendinosis and subluxation. Axial T2-weighted image with fat saturation shows marked thickening of the ECU tendon with intrinsic signal alteration consistent with a marked tendinosis. There is also ulnar subluxation of the ECU tendon indicating instability.

tear is identified, it is important to accurately describe the length of the gap between the tendon ends. A gap of more than 3 cm often requires a tendon graft for adequate repair. Finally, the integrity of adjacent tendons should be described, since injuries often involve neighboring tendons.

Pitfalls of Tendon Pathology

Several known MRI pitfalls can obscure or mimic tendon pathology at the level of the wrist. Inhomogeneous or failed fat saturation is a common problem that may decrease the conspicuity of fluid located within or surrounding a tendon sheath. Inadequate fat saturation is more likely to occur when the wrist is imaged by the patient's side, which places the wrist out of the isocenter of the magnet. Recognition of failed fat saturation should be remedied by repositioning the wrist or by adding an axial STIR sequence. Motion artifact is another common pitfall that can result either from patient motion or from pulsating blood within adjacent vessels. Motion artifact can either obscure abnormalities of the tendon or result in spurious intrasubstance signal mimicking pathology. Patient motion can be minimized by ensuring patient comfort and by minimizing the length of the

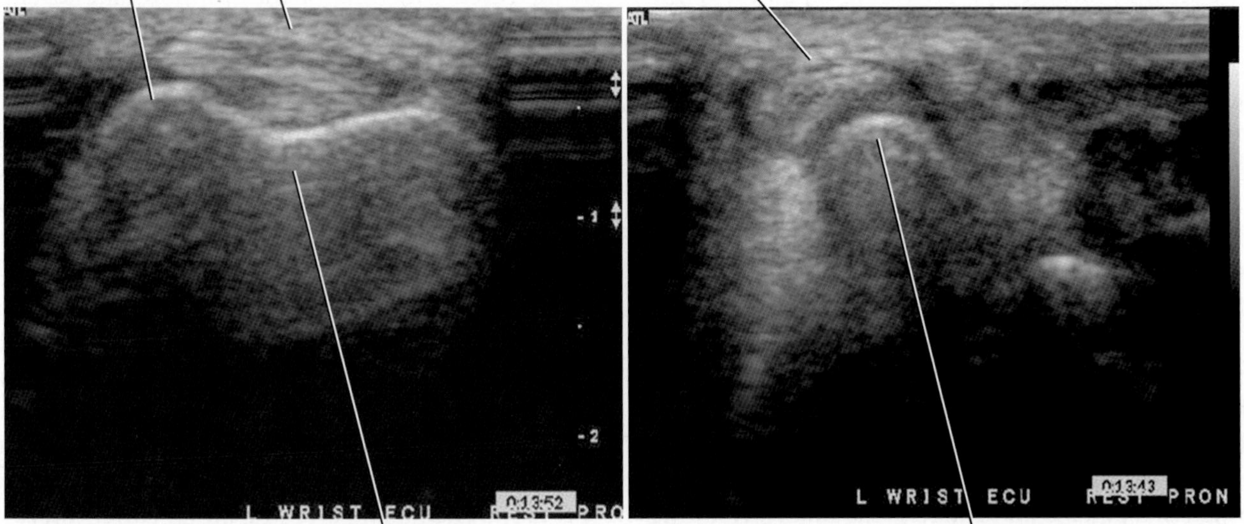
Ulnar styloid
ECU
ECU subluxed
L WRIST ECU
0:13:52
L WRIST ECU
0:13:43
PRON
Groove
Ulnar styloid

Figure 9-7 Dynamic ultrasound examination of the wrist shows subluxation of the extensor carpi ulnaris (ECU) tendon during active motion; the patient described a recurrent, reproducible snapping sensation during wrist motion.

exam time. Phase encoding should be directed in the vertical plane on axial images of the wrist to minimize artifact from pulsating blood over the region of the tendons. Magic angle effect, seen on short echo time sequences, is another potential pitfall that may result in spurious intrasubstance signal and mimic tendinosis. This phenomenon is most likely to occur in the flexor pollicis longus tendon as it courses from the distal aspect of the carpal tunnel toward the base of the thumb, but it has also been described in the extensor carpi ulnaris and extensor pollicis longus tendons. Intrasubstance signal resulting from magic angle can be differentiated from tendon pathology by recognizing that the signal diminishes or resolves on the T2-weighted sequences. The tendon morphology will be normal and there will be a lack of adjacent inflammatory changes when intrinsic signal alteration is the result of magic angle.

Table 9-3 Common Carpal Instability Patterns

Pattern	Radiographic Findings
Scapholunate (SL) dissociation (rotatory subluxation)	Posteroanterior (PA) view Widened SL distance (>3 mm) Cortical "ring sign" distal pole scaphoid PA "Clenched fist" view Accentuates SL distance widening
DISI (dorsal intercalated segmental instability)	PA view Widening SL distance (>3 mm) Lateral view Lunate: dorsal tilt Distal pole scaphoid: volar tilt SL angle > 60 degrees
VISI (volar intercalated segmental instability)	PA view Widened SL distance (>3 mm) Lateral view Lunate: volar tilt SL angle < 30 degrees

LIGAMENTS

Carpal stability is primarily provided by the synergistic effects of the intrinsic and extrinsic ligaments of the wrist. The intrinsic ligaments include the scapholunate and lunotriquetral ligaments, which help to link and stabilize the proximal carpal row, and the TFC complex, which is the primary stabilizer of the distal radioulnar joint. The extrinsic ligaments are classified by their location as either volar or dorsal and are responsible for providing stability to the carpus in both the transverse and longitudinal planes. It is the extrinsic ligaments that provide linkage between the radius and the proximal carpal row as well as between the proximal and distal carpal rows. The volar extrinsic ligaments are thicker and stronger than the dorsal ligaments and are more important with regard to stability. Specifically, the volar radioscapholunate ligament is the primary stabilizer of the proximal pole of the scaphoid.

A fall on an outstretched hand is the most common mechanism of injury leading to ligamentous injury and carpal instability. Injury typically begins with disruption of the scapholunate ligament, however, with increasing severity of injury. The forces are transmitted in a pattern that encircles the lunate, resulting in disruption of both the volar and dorsal capsular attachments with the most severe injuries resulting in complete disruption of the ligamentous support for the lunate (Table 9-3). Four stages of injury have been described, ranging from isolated scapholunate ligament disruption to complete perilunate dislocation. Disruption of the scapholunate ligament is associated with an injury pattern referred to as dorsal intercalated segmental instability (DISI), which results in the loss of linkage of the scaphoid, lunate, and capitate. Radiographic and MRI findings indicative of a DISI injury pattern include widening of the scapholunate intercarpal distance, dorsal tilt of the lunate, and volar rotation of the distal pole of the scaphoid (Fig. 9-8). Over time, proximal carpal row instability leads to increased widening of the scapholunate distance and radioscaphoid articular cartilage loss and osteoarthritis referred to as stage I scapholunate advanced collapse (SLAC wrist). Proximal migration of the capitate is a late sequela of instability and results in an end-stage degenerative collapse of the midcarpus with loss of the midcarpal congruity, referred to as stage II scapholunate advanced collapse (SLAC) wrist (Figs. 9-9 and 9-10).

Although the extrinsic ligaments of the wrist are vital for maintaining proper carpal alignment, MR imaging lacks sensitivity and specificity with regard to the evaluation of the integrity of these ligaments, and for the most part MRI plays only a minor role in the evaluation of these structures. The presence of soft tissue edema and swelling along either the volar or dorsal aspect of the capsule of the wrist in the setting of trauma is an indicator of extrinsic ligament injury and is usually best identified on axial images, whereas the abnormality may also be identified on sagittal and coronal T2-weighted images with fat

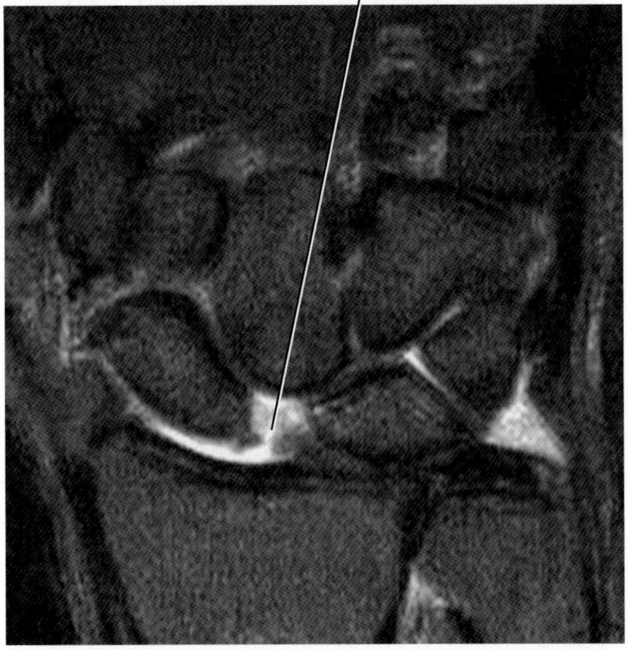
Disruption of SL ligament with
widening of intercarpal distance
A

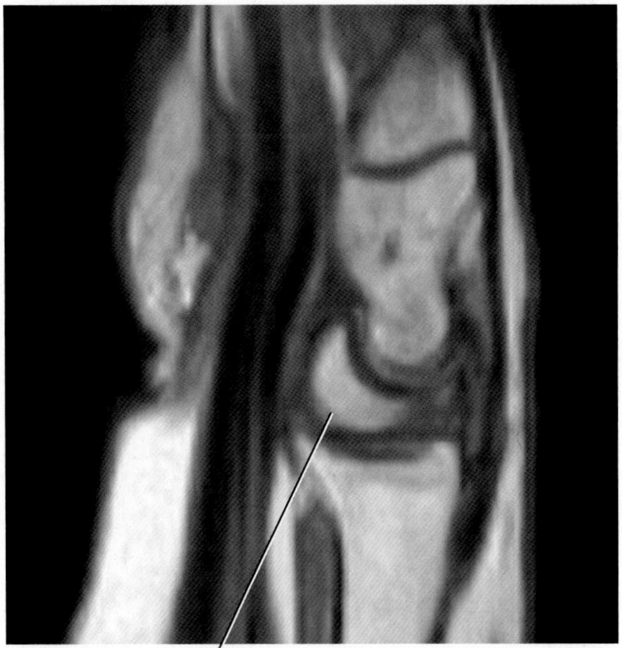
B
Dorsal tilt of the lunate

Figure 9-8 Dorsal intercalated segmental instability (DISI). A, Coronal T2-weighted image with fat saturation shows disruption of the scapholunate (SL) ligament with widening of the intercarpal distance. **B,** Sagittal T1-weighted image shows a dorsal tilt of the lunate. This combination of findings indicates a loss of the linkage between the scaphoid and the lunate and represents a DISI deformity of the wrist.

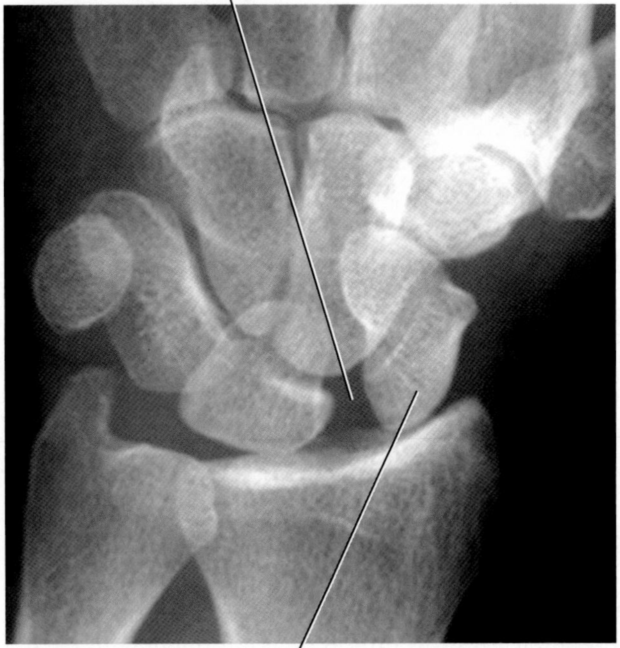
Widening of the scapholunate interval
A
Distal pole of scaphoid rotates in volar direction
losing its normal relationship to the radius

Figure 9-9 Radiographic progression of scapholunate advanced collapse (SLAC) wrist. A, The precursor findings of a SLAC wrist. There is widening of the scapholunate distance and radioscaphoid incongruity. The distal pole of the scaphoid rotates in a volar direction and migrates out of its normal position within the scaphoid fossa of the distal radius. *Continued*

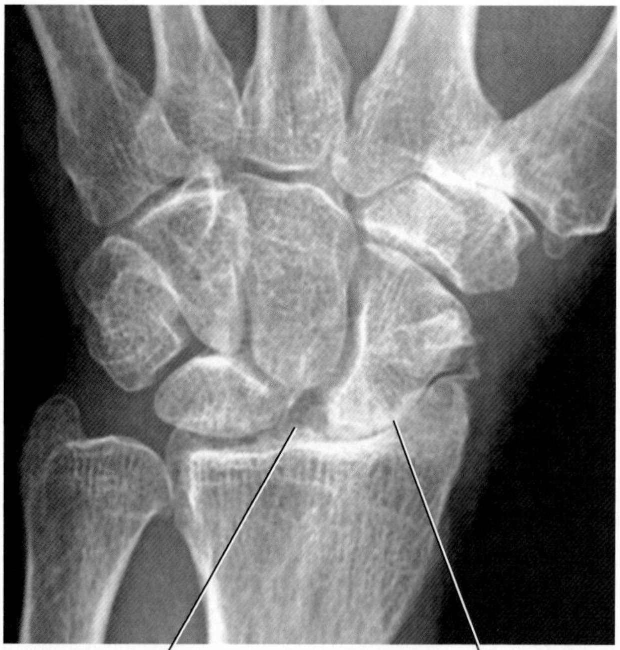
Stage I SLAC wrist
Widening of intercarpal distance
Radioscaphoid osteoarthritis
B

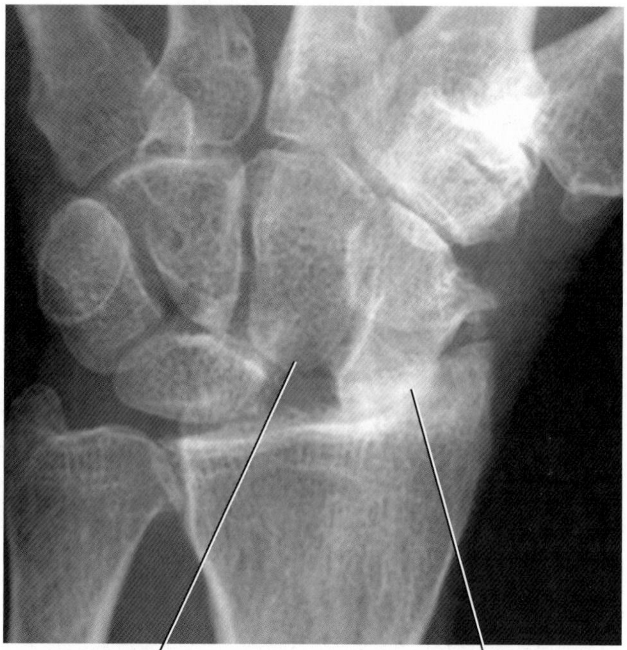
Stage II SLAC wrist
Proximal migration of capitate and loss of midcarpal congruity
Radioscaphoid osteoarthritis
C

Figure 9-9, cont'd **B,** Stage I scapholunate advanced collapse with loss of the radioscaphoid articular cartilage. **C,** Stage II SLAC with extensive radioscaphoid arthritis and proximal migration of the capitate and loss of midcarpal congruity.

suppression (Fig. 9-11). The possibility of injury should be suggested on the basis of these findings, but it is difficult to accurately determine the status of the individual extrinsic ligaments. The presence of capsular edema should also prompt a thorough search for small cortical avulsion fractures of the carpal bones, such as a dorsal triquetral avulsion fracture, and radiographic correlation or CT examination may be necessary to accurately depict such avulsion injuries.

Scapholunate Ligament

The scapholunate (SL) ligament is composed of a thin central membranous portion, and thicker and stronger dorsal and volar components. The dorsal and volar components differ histologically from the central membranous portion, being composed of strong transverse collagen bundles. The dorsal component is the most important component with regard to SL stability. Nontraumatic age-related perforations or fenestrations of the central membranous portion of the SL ligament are common in older persons, but are rarely seen in persons younger than the mid to late 20s. Traumatic injury of the SL ligament usually results from a fall on an outstretched hand with excessive force applied across the hyperextended hand.

The spectrum of abnormalities of the SL ligament includes degeneration, sprain, partial-thickness tear and full-thickness tear and can involve any combination of the three components of the SL ligament (Table 9-4). The SL ligament is best evaluated using a combination of high-resolution thin-section 3D-gradient-echo and fluid-sensitive T2-weighted coronal images. Minor injury may result in a partial-thickness tear of the SL ligament, which is seen as a focal area of thinning, attenuation, or fluid extending partially through the thickness of the ligament (Fig. 9-12). A partial-thickness tear of the central component is often associated with a sprain or stretching injury of either the dorsal or volar component. A stretching injury appears as a focal area of thickening with increased intrinsic T2-weighted signal and abnormal

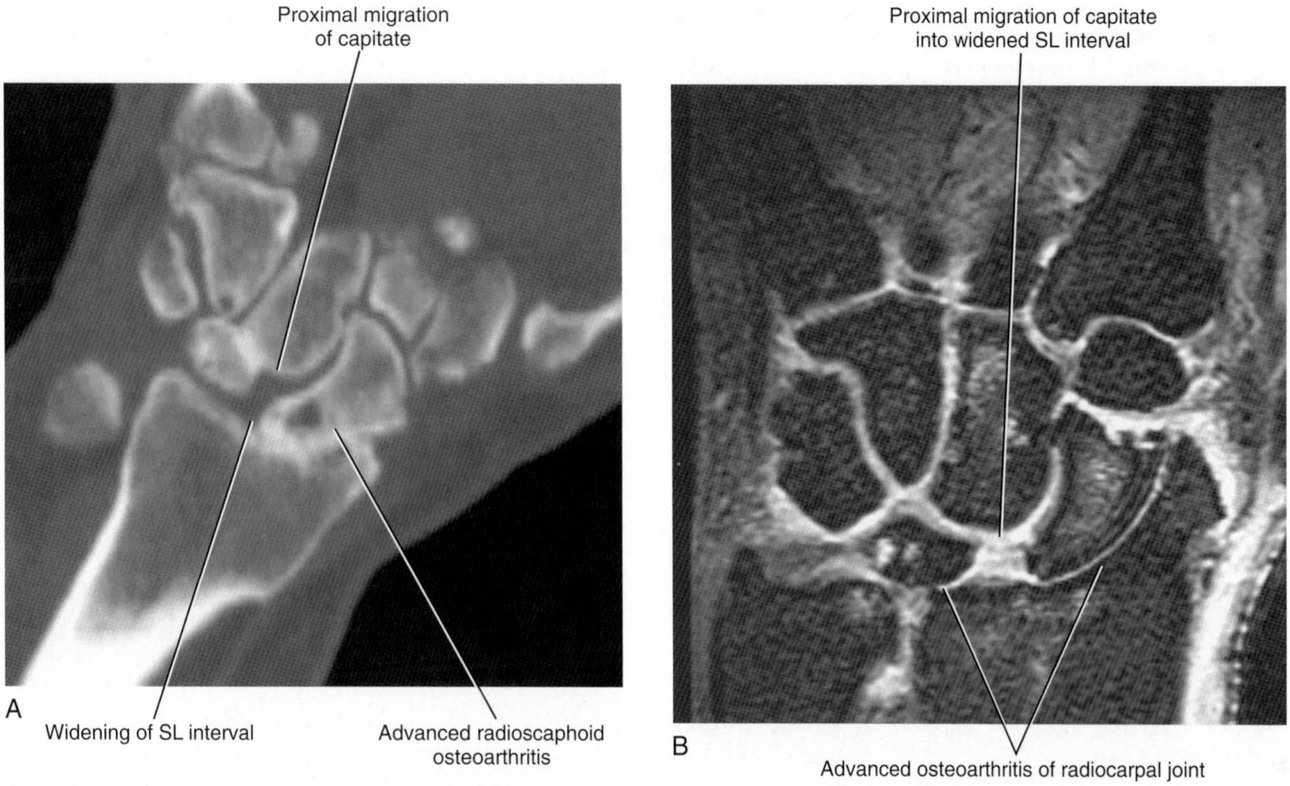

Proximal migration of capitate
A
Widening of SL interval
Advanced radioscaphoid osteoarthritis
Proximal migration of capitate into widened SL interval
B
Advanced osteoarthritis of radiocarpal joint

Figure 9-10 CT and MRI of scapholunate advanced collapse (SLAC) wrist. A, Coronal CT image shows widening of the scapholunate (SL) interval, proximal migration of the capitate and extensive osteoarthritis of the radioscaphoid articulation indicating a SLAC wrist. **B,** Coronal T2-weighted image from a different patient demonstrates similar MR findings with widening of the SL interval, proximal migration of the capitate, and extensive end-stage osteoarthritis of the radiocarpal joint.

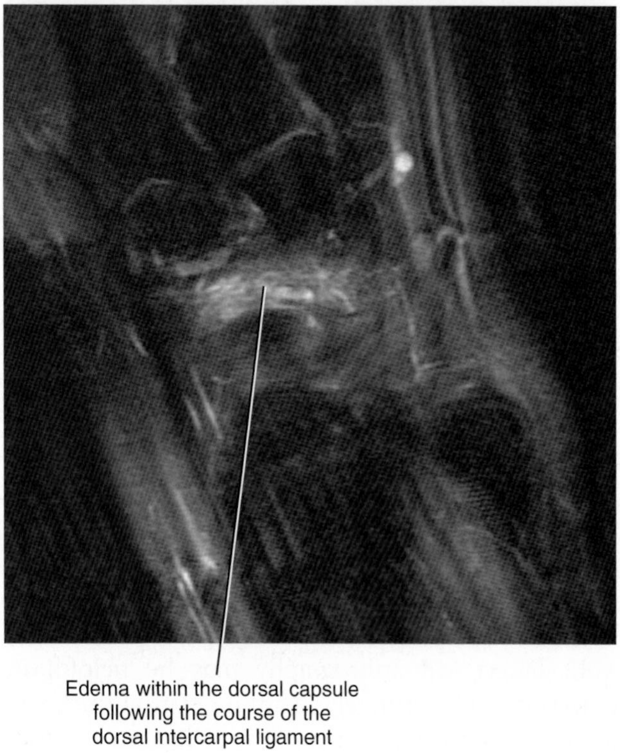

Edema within the dorsal capsule following the course of the dorsal intercarpal ligament

Figure 9-11 Dorsal extrinsic ligament injury. Coronal T2-weighted image with fat saturation shows edema within the dorsal capsule isolated to the course of the dorsal intercarpal ligament, which takes its origin from the triquetrum and inserts with three separate slips onto the scaphoid, trapezium, and trapezoid. This finding should prompt a thorough search for an avulsion fracture of the dorsal aspect of the triquetrum.

Table 9-4 Scapholunate (SL) Ligament Injury Patterns Seen on MRI

SL Ligament MR Appearance	Injury
Normal morphology	None
Fibrillation/fraying of surface	Degeneration Partial-thickness tear
Perforation central component	Normal aging (incidence increases with age; typically lacks mechanism of injury) Tear (young athletic person with mechanism of injury and pain)
Dorsal or volar component thickening	Old partial-thickness tear with scarring/fibrosis
Dorsal or volar component disruption (often associated with intercarpal distance widening)	Traumatic disruption

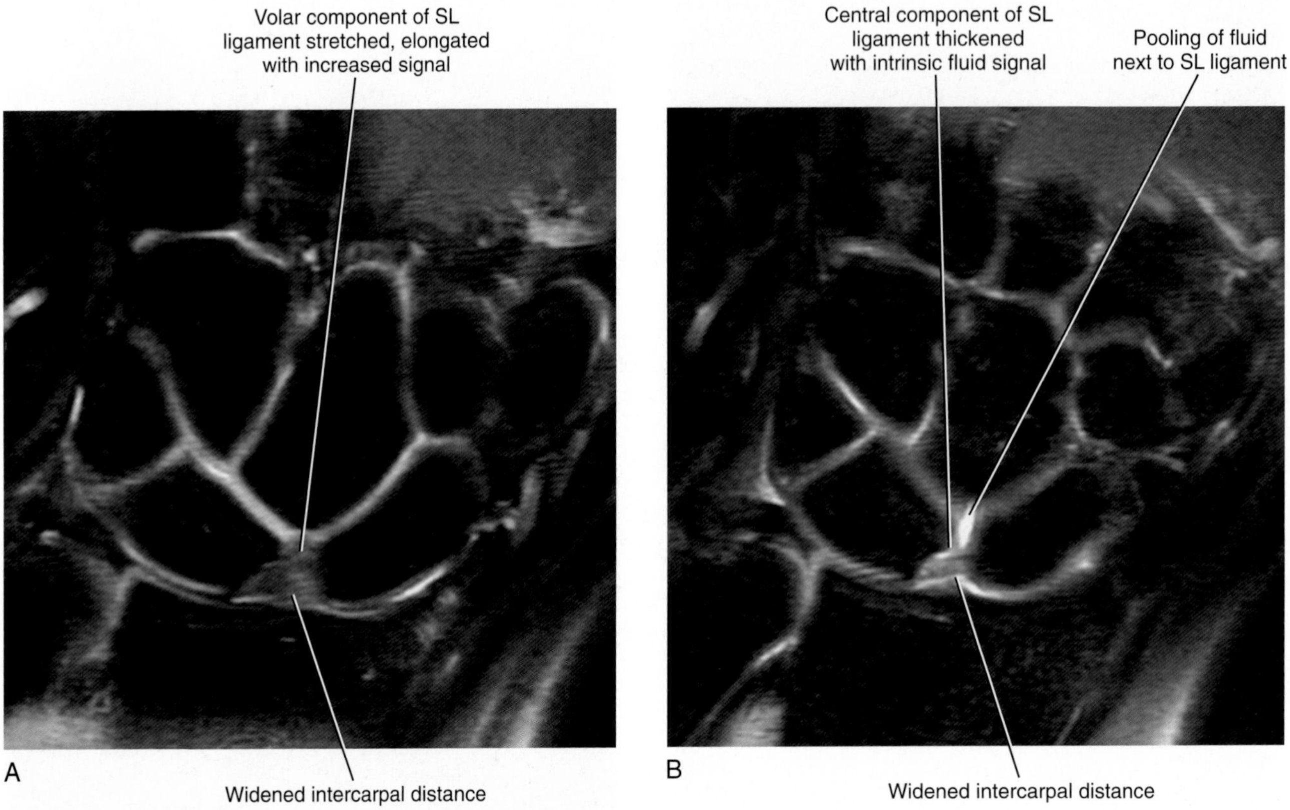
Volar component of SL ligament stretched, elongated with increased signal
Widened intercarpal distance
A
Central component of SL ligament thickened with intrinsic fluid signal
Pooling of fluid next to SL ligament
Widened intercarpal distance
B

Figure 9-12 Partial-thickness scapholunate (SL) ligament tear. Consecutive coronal T2-weighted images with fat suppression show marked thickening of the volar component of the SL ligament (**A**) with increased intrinsic signal abnormality but no full-thickness perforation. The central component (**B**) is also mildly thickened with fluid signal noted within the substance of the ligament. Again, there is no full-thickness perforation. Mild widening of the intercarpal distance is noted, indicating dysfunction of the SL ligament in spite of the lack of a complete tear or a fluid-filled defect. Pooling of fluid adjacent to the SL ligament is a secondary sign of injury.

morphology of the involved portion of the ligament, but no full-thickness perforation can be noted on MRI. Direct MR arthrography may be helpful in detecting and accurately defining partial-thickness tears and stretching injuries of the SL ligament. A full-thickness tear is present when fluid is seen unequivocally extending through the entire thickness of the ligament (Fig. 9-13). It is important to note which of the three components are involved, since this may have surgical implications. The precise location of SL

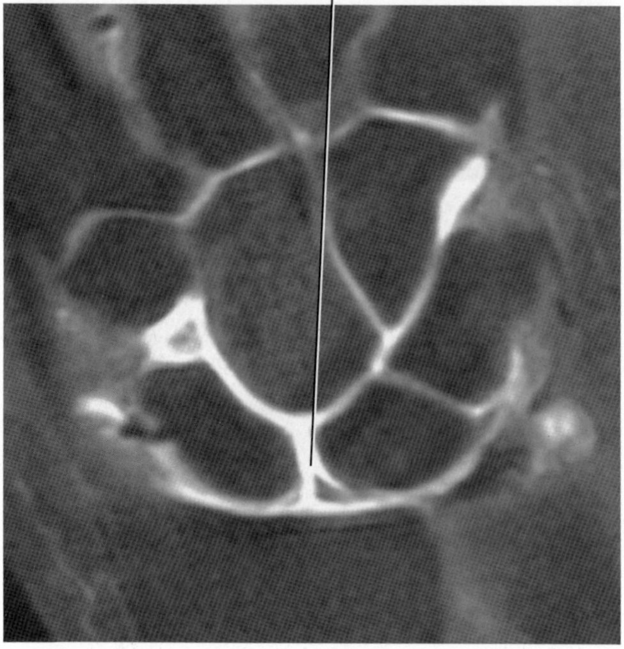
Full-thickness tear of central component of SL ligament

Figure 9-13 Full-thickness scapholunate (SL) ligament tear. Coronal T1-weighted image with fat suppression and intra-articular gadolinium shows a fluid-filled defect completely traversing the central component of the SL ligament, indicating a full-thickness tear. There is also minimal widening of the SL intercarpal distance.

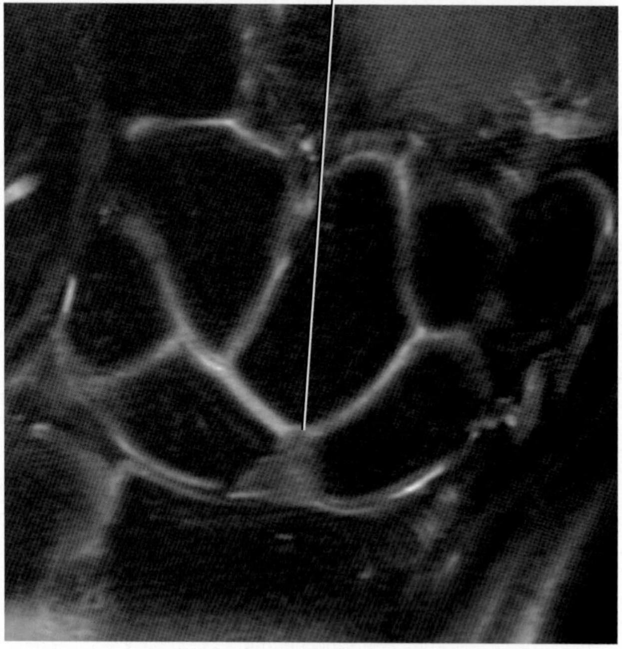
Thickened SL ligament with increased T2 signal and widening of SL interval
A

Figure 9-14 Secondary signs of SL injury. **A,** Coronal T2-weighted image with fat saturation shows thickening and stretching of the SL ligament indicating a partial-thickness tear of the ligament with adjacent scarring and fibrosis. Widening of the SL interval indicates underlying instability. *Continued*

ligament injury (dorsal or volar component) can be determined by cross-referencing the area of abnormality seen on coronal images with either the sagittal or axial images. Widening of the scapholunate distance may occur following disruption of any two components of the SL ligament (see Fig. 9-8A).

Secondary signs that have been described in associated with SL ligament injury include the presence of ganglia originating in the vicinity of the SL ligament, adjacent marrow edema, loss of scapholunate articular cartilage, and pooling of fluid adjacent to the SL ligament (Fig. 9-14). Thickening of the SL ligament with or without widening of the SL intercarpal distance or fibrillation and fraying of the surface of the SL ligaments are both signs of chronic injury. An MRI finding that argues against a full-thickness perforation of the SL ligament is the presence of an isolated joint effusion in one carpal compartment and not the other.

Lunotriquetral Ligament

The lunotriquetral (LT) ligament is usually a delta-shaped structure that is smaller than the scapholunate ligament and, as a result,is usually more difficult to accurately assess on MRI. As with the SL ligament, the LT ligament is often injured as the result of a fall on the outstretched hand (see Table 9-3). The LT ligament is also composed of a thin central membranous portion and thicker dorsal and volar components. Disruption is diagnosed using MR imaging when fluid is seen unequivocally extending completely through the thickness of the ligament. Direct MR arthrography is often very helpful in the evaluation of the LT ligament (Fig. 9-15). Injury to this ligament may also be seen in association with ulnar-sided abutment syndromes, which are discussed in more detail in the text that follows.

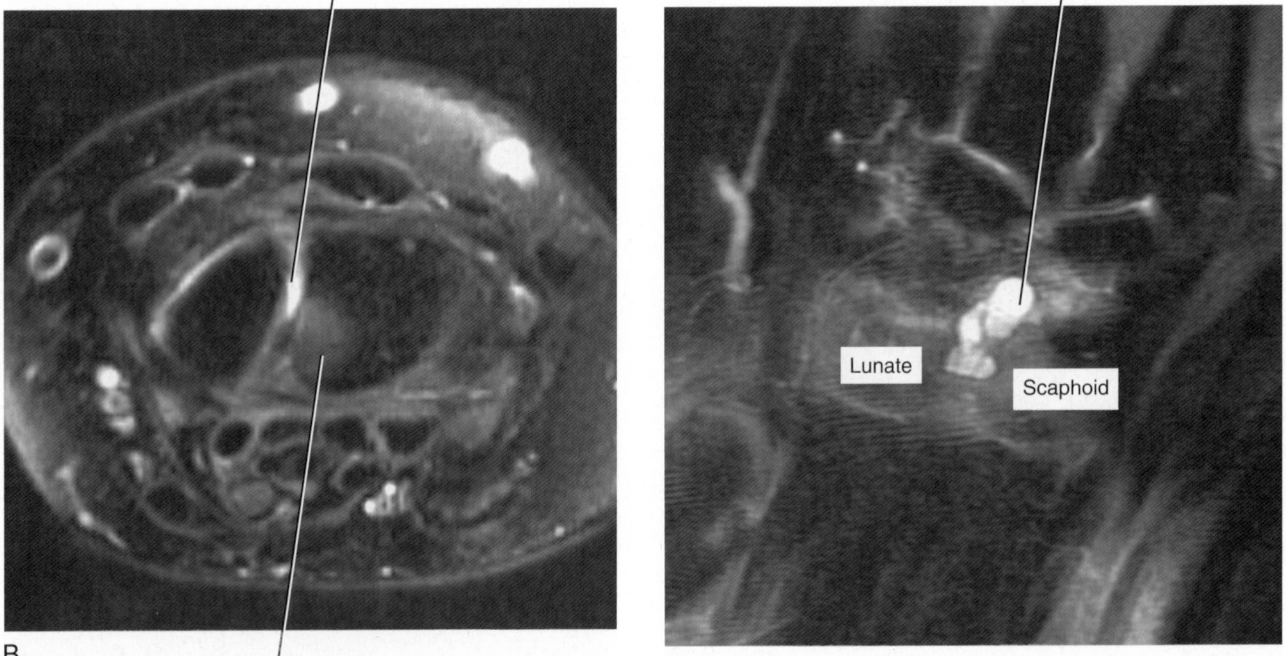

Pooling of fluid near the SL ligament
B
Lunate marrow edema
Ganglia arising dorsal to the SL ligament
Lunate
Scaphoid
C

Figure 9-14, cont'd **B,** Axial T2-weighted image with fat saturation shows pooling of fluid next to the SL ligament and a contusion of the lunate, both of which are secondary signs of SL ligament injury. **C,** Coronal T2-weighted image with fat saturation shows a ganglion located along the dorsal aspect of the wrist adjacent to the SL ligament, another secondary sign associated with SL ligament injury.

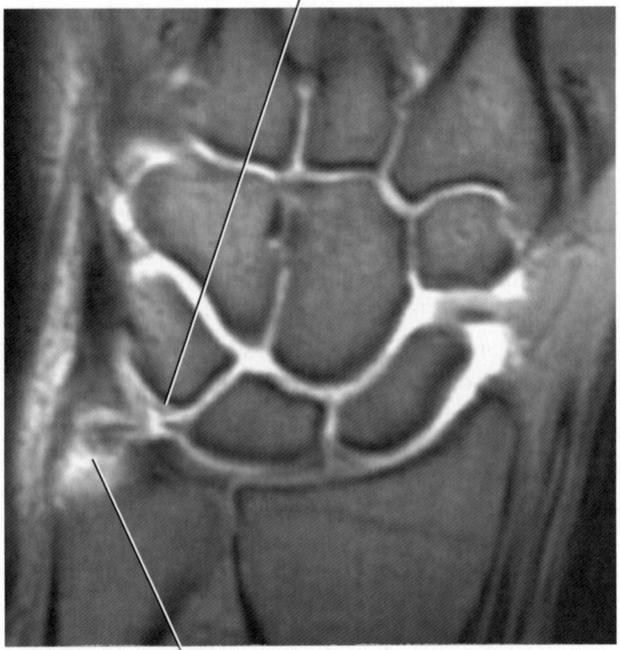

LT ligament tear
Tear of ulnar attachment of TFC

Figure 9-15 **Lunotriquetral (LT) ligament tear.** Coronal T1-weighted image with fat saturation and intra-articular gadolinium shows a full-thickness tear of the LT ligament with gadolinium extending completely through the thickness of the ligament. Note the adjacent injury of the ulnar attachment of the triangular fibrocartilage. LT ligament tears are often seen in conjunction with other injuries to the ulnar side of the wrist.

Triangular Fibrocartilage Complex

The TFC is primarily responsible for stability of the distal radioulnar joint. Abnormalities of the TFC are the most common cause of ulnar-sided wrist pain and may be post-traumatic or degenerative in origin. Palmer proposed a classification system for TFC tears distinguishing traumatic (class I) from degenerative (class II) lesions. He further subclassified traumatic lesions to accurately describe the location of tear and the degenerative lesions to describe the extent of degeneration. The Palmer classification can be very helpful in providing an accurate MR description of TFC abnormalities and in guiding proper clinical/surgical management (Table 9-5). Variant anatomy of the ulnar aspect of the wrist (i.e., ulnar-positive variance) can predispose to abnormalities of the TFC and altered wrist function.

The TFC is a complex anatomic structure with several interrelated components, each of which is vital to the ensuring of proper motion and function of the wrist. The TFC forms a water-tight seal between the distal radioulnar joint and the adjacent radiocarpal joint, and an intact TFC allows the proper articulation of the distal ulna and radius with the adjacent lunate and triquetrum. The TFC is composed of a central articular disk, dorsal and volar radioulnar ligaments, lunotriquetral ligament, meniscal homologue, and the tendon sheath of the extensor carpi ulnaris tendon.

The central articular disk of the TFC is an avascular triangular-shaped structure that is composed of fibrocartilage and therefore appears dark on all MRI pulse sequences, similar to the meniscus of the knee (Fig. 9-16). The central disk attaches to the articular cartilage of the distal radius at the level of the sigmoid notch. The articular cartilage of the distal radius undermines the TFC radial attachment and on MR imaging can be a potential pitfall, mimicking a radial-sided TFC avulsion. A tear and cartilage undermining can be easily differentiated, however, because the distal radial articular cartilage is intermediate in signal intensity and is smooth and tapering in appearance, whereas an avulsion of the TFC from the distal radius results in an irregular margin of the TFC with fluid signal extending between the articular disk and

Table 9-5 Palmer Classification for Triangular Fibrocartilage Complex (TFC) Tears with MR Findings

Class of Injury	MR Findings	Clinical Significance
Traumatic (Class I)		
Central perforation—IA	Slit-like perforation of central articular disk	Avascular portion of TFC treated with surgical debridement
Traumatic avulsion of TFC from ulnar fovea—IB	Fluid signal at ulnar attachment; associated with injury of palmar and dorsal distal radioulnar ligaments	Associated with radioulnar instability; vascular portion of TFC repaired by suturing
Traumatic avulsion of peripheral TFC attachment—IC	Avulsion of TFC from its osseous attachment to ulna and triquetrum; increased signal and thickened peripheral portion of TFC	Associated with ulnocarpal instability; surgical repair attempted in acute injury
Traumatic avulsion of radial TFC attachment—ID	Avulsion of TFC from radial attachment at sigmoid notch	Associated with distal radial fractures; avascular portion of TFC; treated with debridement
Degenerative (Class II)		
Degenerative thinning/wear central articular disk—IIA	Fraying of proximal or distal aspect of TFC central articular disk without perforation; best depicted on MRA	Associated with ulnar variance and axial loading of the wrist; conservative treatment
TFC articular disk wear and chondromalacia—IIB	Progressive articular disk fraying; chondromalacia of ulna, lunate, triquetrum	Conservative treatment or debridement; ulnar shortening when ulnar variance is present
Further TFC degeneration with perforation—IIC	Progressive degeneration with central disk perforation (oval) and chondromalacia	TFC debridement and ulnar decompression/shortening
TFC perforation, chondromalacia, and lunotriquetral (LT) perforation—IID	Class IIC findings plus LT ligament disruption	Associated with LT instability; TFC debridement and ulnar decompression/shortening
Large TFC perforation, chondromalacia, LT tear, ulnocarpal/radioulnar arthritis—IIE	End-stage TFC degeneration with ulnocarpal/radioulnar arthritis/impaction	Treat with TFC debridement and ulnar decompression/shortening

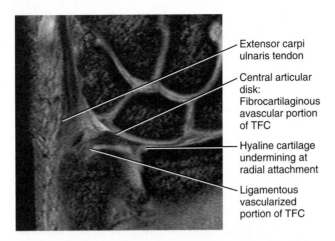

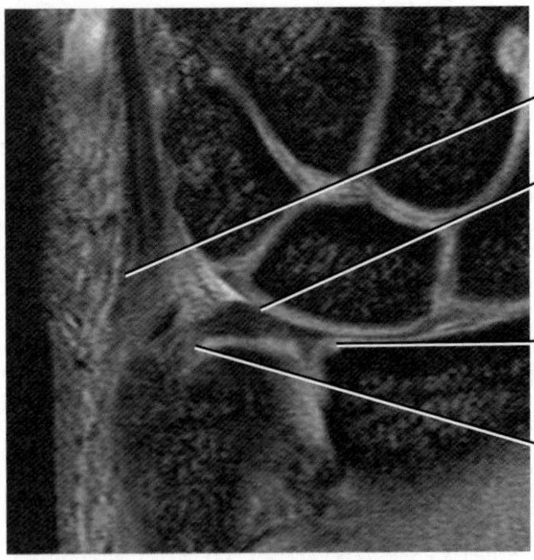
Extensor carpi ulnaris tendon
Central articular disk: Fibrocartilaginous avascular portion of TFC
Hyaline cartilage undermining at radial attachment
Ligamentous vascularized portion of TFC

Figure 9-16 Normal MR imaging appearance of the triangular fibrocartilage (TFC). Coronal three-dimensional gradient-echo image shows a thick low-signal intensity fibrocartilaginous central articular disk. There is intermediate signal intensity hyaline cartilage undermining the radial attachment. Histologically, the TFC transitions to ligamentous-type structure near its ulnar attachment, demonstrating intermediate signal internal striations on MRI in this region. Note the close proximity of the extensor carpi ulnaris tendon to the peripheral aspect of the TFC complex.

the radius. The central disk is often thicker in the presence of negative ulnar variance.

As the TFC extends peripherally, the avascular fibrocartilage of the central disk undergoes a transition to a vascularized structure whose histologic composition more closely resembles that of a ligament. The TFC fans out, becoming broader and thicker, and attaches to the distal ulna at the level of the fovea and ulnar styloid. This histologic transition from an avascular fibrocartilage to a vascularized ligamentous-like structure is responsible for the changing MR appearance of the TFC as it approaches its site of ulnar attachment. On MRI, the ulnar attachment of the TFC has an appearance that more closely resembles that of the anterior cruciate ligament rather than that of the meniscus, as seen in the region of the central articular disk (see Fig. 9-16). As a result, traumatic tears near the ulnar or peripheral attachments of the TFC are more difficult to detect and accurately classify on the basis of MR imaging.

Traumatic tears of the TFC occur most frequently in young active individuals and are classified on the basis of the location of the tear (see Table 9-5). Tears of the central articular disk are usually 2 to 3 mm in diameter and are described as slitlike in appearance. On MRI, traumatic tears of the central disk (class IA) or at the level of radial attachment (class ID) are best detected on coronal images and appear as fluid signal completely traversing the TFC. High-resolution imaging with a small field of view is essential for the accurate detection of these lesions, since they are often only 2 to 3 mm in diameter. MR arthrography improves the conspicuity and accuracy of detection of these lesions, which is attributed to joint distention and high-contrast gadolinium within the tear (Fig. 9-17). Since the central articular disk portion of the TFC is avascular, tears of the disk or radial attachment are usually treated with debridement because this area does not heal following suturing.

On MRI, a traumatic tear of the peripheral aspect of the TFC may appear as a complete avulsion of the peripheral attachment. The attachment of the TFC should be evaluated at the level of the fovea and at the level of the ulnar styloid. Disruption or fluid signal at the level of either the fovea or the ulnar styloid is evidence of a peripheral tear. Traumatic peripheral TFC tears (class IB and class IC tears) can appear on MRI as altered morphology and excessive fluid within or adjacent to the peripheral portion of the TFC (see Fig. 9-17). The presence of marrow edema within the ulnar styloid or adjacent synovitis has also been shown to correlate with peripheral TFC tears after acute trauma to the wrist. In the setting of trauma, tendinosis/tenosynovitis of the extensor carpi ulnaris tendon is also associated with an increased incidence of peripheral TFC tears. The peripheral aspect of the TFC is vascularized, and, as a result, ulnar-sided or peripheral tears or avulsions of the TFC can be repaired surgically by suturing the torn TFC to the adjacent capsule.

As individuals age, the central articular disk often undergoes degeneration with progressive thinning or wear of the proximal or distal aspect, resulting in fibrillation and fraying of the surface of the central articular disk. Positive ulnar variance increases the risk of TFC degeneration. Degenerative tears of the TFC (class II) are further categorized on the basis of the extent of degeneration (see Table 9-5). Early degeneration results in only minimal fraying and irregularity of the central articular disk. With increasing wear and tear, a central perforation of the articular disk will occur. These degenerative tears are typically larger than the slitlike tears that occur in the setting

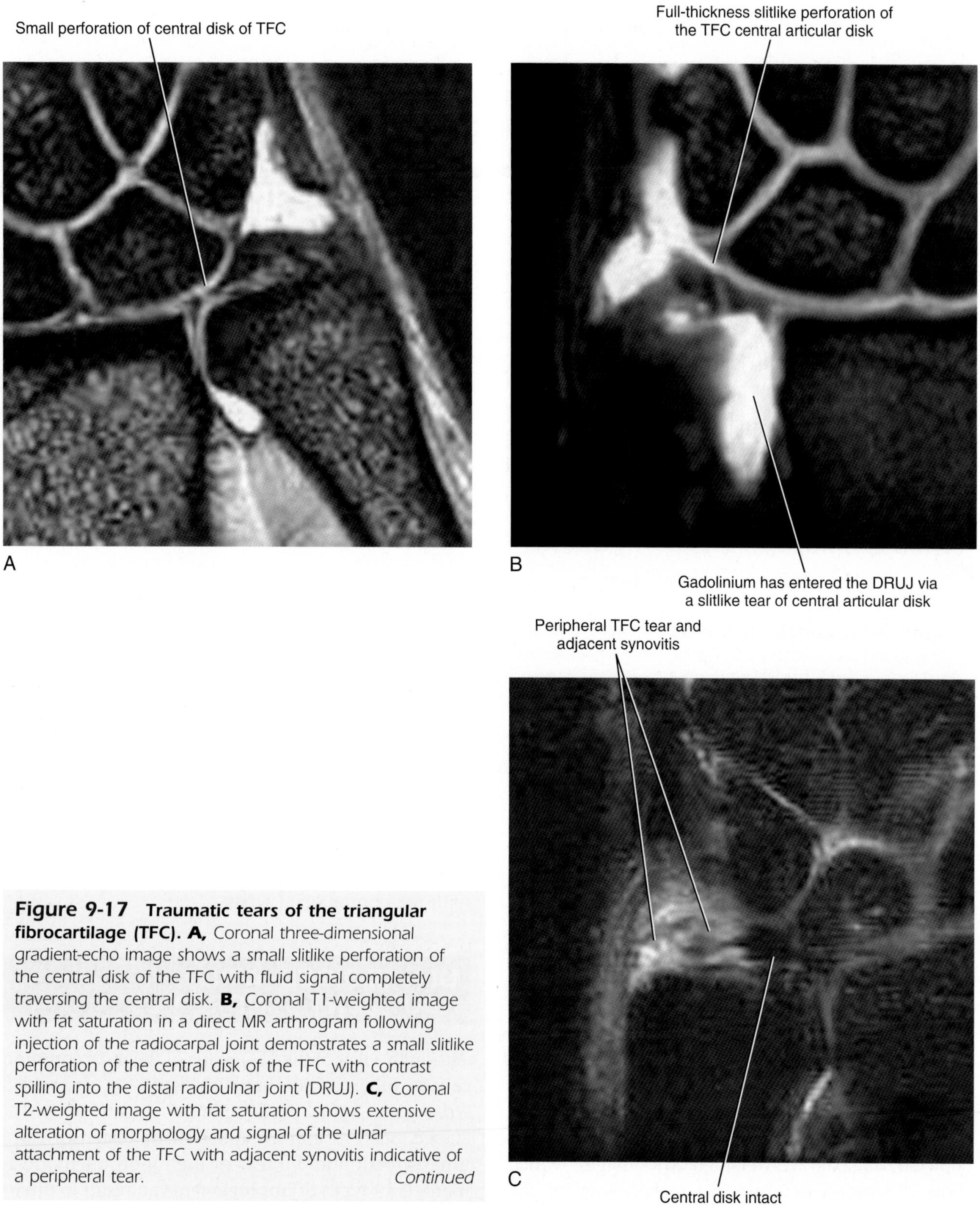

Small perforation of central disk of TFC
A
Full-thickness slitlike perforation of the TFC central articular disk
B
Gadolinium has entered the DRUJ via a slitlike tear of central articular disk
Peripheral TFC tear and adjacent synovitis
C
Central disk intact

Figure 9-17 Traumatic tears of the triangular fibrocartilage (TFC). A, Coronal three-dimensional gradient-echo image shows a small slitlike perforation of the central disk of the TFC with fluid signal completely traversing the central disk. **B,** Coronal T1-weighted image with fat saturation in a direct MR arthrogram following injection of the radiocarpal joint demonstrates a small slitlike perforation of the central disk of the TFC with contrast spilling into the distal radioulnar joint (DRUJ). **C,** Coronal T2-weighted image with fat saturation shows extensive alteration of morphology and signal of the ulnar attachment of the TFC with adjacent synovitis indicative of a peripheral tear. *Continued*

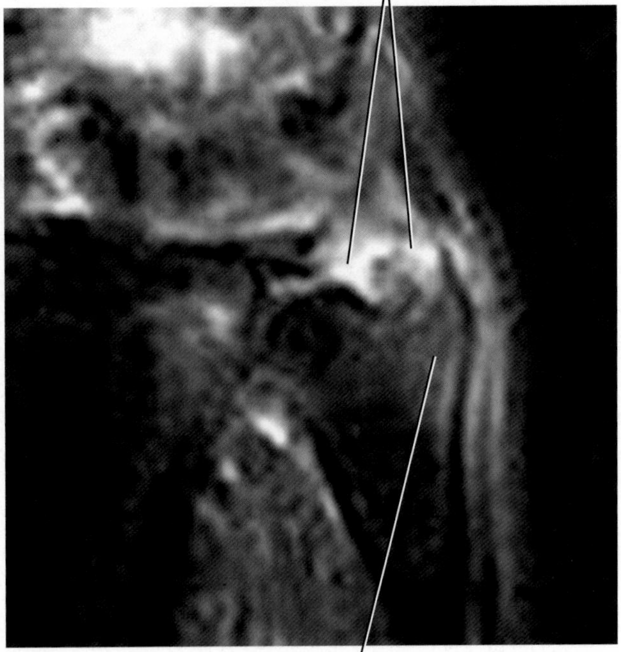
Tear of peripheral TFC with adjacent synovitis and fluid
Marrow edema at ulnar styloid
D

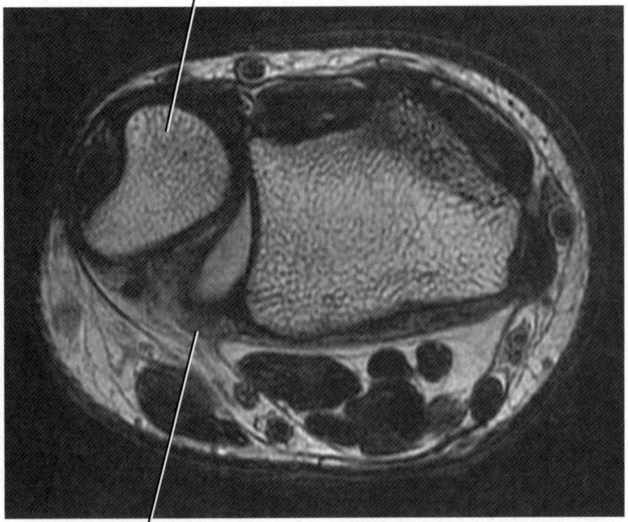
Dorsal subluxation of distal ulna
Thickened edematous volar distal radioulnar ligament
E

Figure 9-17, cont'd **D,** Coronal STIR image demonstrates a complete avulsion of the peripheral attachment of the TFC with marrow edema involving the ulnar styloid. **E,** Axial T2-weighted image shows thickening and edema of the volar distal radioulnar ligament with dorsal subluxation of the distal ulna. This represents an injury of the volar component of the distal radioulnar ligament and often accompanies ulnar-sided injuries of the TFC and indicates instability of the distal radioulnar joint.

of trauma and are usually oval in appearance. Progressive changes lead to chondromalacia of the ulna, lunate, and triquetrum. End-stage changes usually include a tear of the lunotriquetral ligament along with ulnocarpal and radioulnar arthritis (Fig. 9-18).

The volar and dorsal distal radioulnar ligaments are important contributors to the stability of the distal radioulnar joint, and disruption can lead to subluxation of the distal ulna. Tears most commonly involve the volar ligament and result in dorsal subluxation of the ulna. These tears are usually best depicted on axial T2-weighted MR images, which show disruption or abnormal morphology of the ligament in association with dorsal subluxation of the distal ulna (see Fig. 9-17E). Axial imaging of the wrist using either MR or CT can be performed to evaluate for distal radioulnar subluxation. The wrist is imaged in both the supinated and pronated positions, and it is often helpful to compare these images with the contralateral wrist.

ULNAR-SIDED WRIST ABUTMENT SYNDROMES

Although a tear of the TFC is one of the most common causes, other causes can also result in ulnar-sided wrist pain. Some of these have already been discussed, such as abnormalities of the extensor carpi ulnaris tendon and a tear of the lunotriquetral ligament. Four types of impingement can result in ulnar-sided wrist pain, and MRI accurately depicts each of these types of ulnar-sided impingement (Table 9-6): (1) ulnar-lunate abutment, (2) ulnar-styloid abutment, (3) distal radioulnar impingement, and (4) hamatolunate impingement.

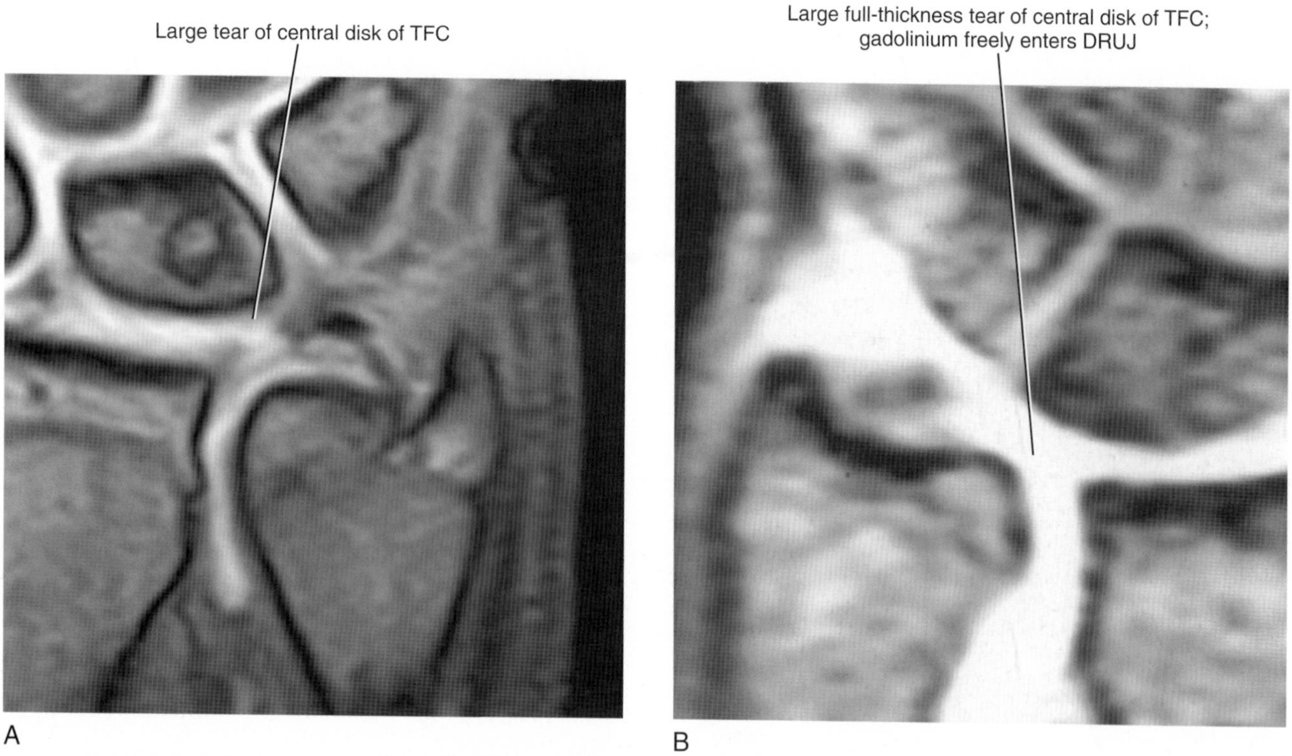
Large tear of central disk of TFC
A
Large full-thickness tear of central disk of TFC; gadolinium freely enters DRUJ
B

Figure 9-18 Degenerative tears of the TFC. A, Coronal gradient-echo image shows a large oval-appearing tear of the central aspect of the TFC representing a degenerative tear. **B,** Coronal gradient-echo image following administration of intra-articular gadolinium shows a large degenerative tear of the central articular disk with extensive chondral thinning and arthrosis of the distal ulna and adjacent lunate. DRUJ, distal radioulnar joint.

Table 9-6 Ulnar-Sided Impaction Syndromes

Syndrome	Symptoms
Ulnar-lunate abutment	Positive ulnar variance Tear of central disk TFC Marrow edema arthrosis, ulnar head and adjacent lunate
Ulnar-triquetral abutment (ulnar-styloid abutment)	Elongated ulnar styloid Marrow edema ulnar styloid and triquetrum Intact TFC with adjacent synovitis
Ulnar impingement (distal radioulnar impingement)	Short ulna Osteoarthritis of distal radioulnar joint Remodeling of distal radius
Hamatolunate impingement	Type II hamatolunate articulation Marrow edema and arthrosis of lunate and adjacent hamate

Ulnar-Lunate Abutment

Positive ulnar variance or a prominent ulnar head can lead to abutment of the TFC between the distal ulna and the adjacent lunate. Over time, the impaction results in attritional and degenerative changes of the TFC, eventually leading to a perforation of the central articular disk. Arthrosis of the distal ulnar articular surface and the adjacent lunate is the hallmark of this type of abutment and eventually leads to subchondral marrow changes, including edema and subchondral cyst formation (Fig. 9-19). Ulnar-lunate abutment is a potential source of ulnar-sided wrist pain and is often treated by an ulnar shortening procedure and, if necessary, by debridement of the central articular disk of the TFC. Differential diagnosis includes avascular necrosis of the lunate (Kienböck disease). This is differentiated on the basis of MRI when marrow signal alterations are limited to the lunate with no involvement of the adjacent TFC or distal ulna.

SECTION IV

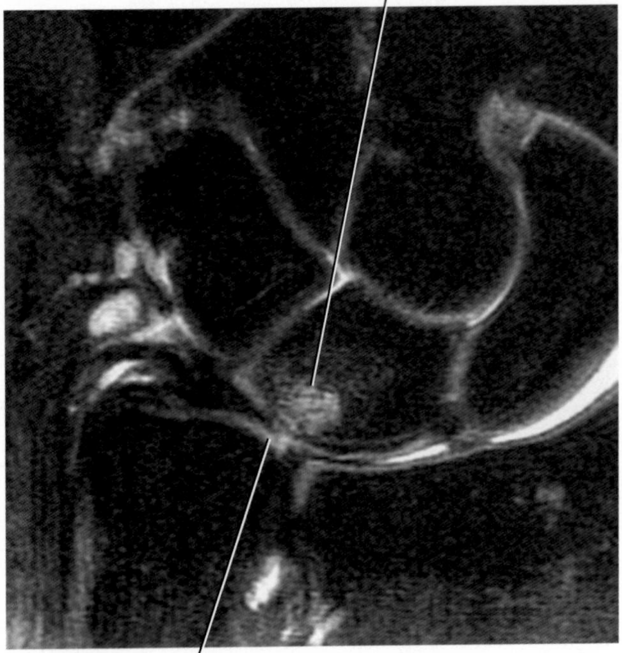
Subchondral marrow edema
and arthrosis lunate
Slight positive ulnar variance
with disruption of TFC

Figure 9-19 Ulnar-lunate abutment. Coronal T2-weighted image with fat saturation shows a positive ulnar variance with a small perforation of the central articular disk of the triangular fibrocartilage (TFC). Subchondral marrow edema and thinning of the articular cartilage of the adjacent lunate are found.

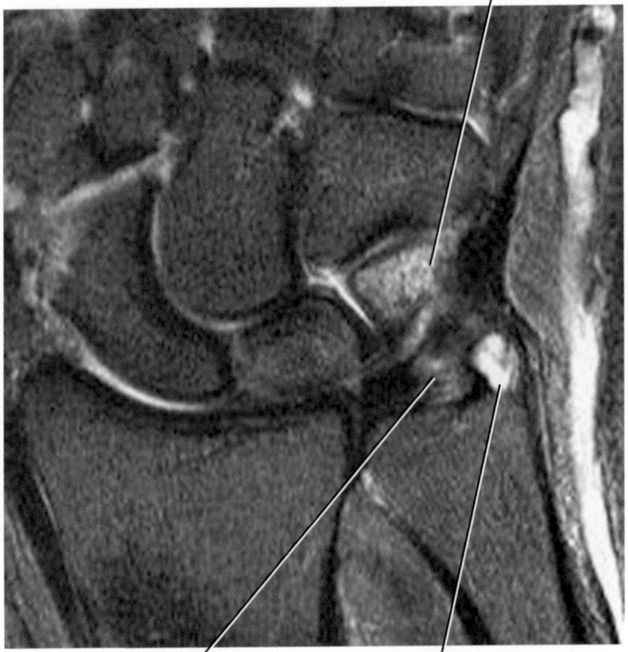
Marrow edema
within triquetrum
Intact TFC with
adjacent synovitis
Elongated ulnar styloid
with marrow edema

Figure 9-20 Ulnar-triquetral abutment. Coronal T2-weighted image with fat saturation shows an elongated ulnar styloid with marrow edema within both the ulnar styloid and the adjacent triquetrum indicating abutment. Typically, in this type of ulnar-sided impaction, the triangular fibrocartilage complex (TFC) remains intact but reveals mild adjacent synovitis.

Ulnar-Triquetral Abutment (Ulnar-Styloid Abutment)

Ulnar-triquetral abutment refers to an impaction of the triquetrum resulting from an elongated ulnar styloid. On MRI, subcortical marrow edema is noted within the elongated ulnar styloid. In addition, focal articular cartilage loss is often noted involving the proximal articular surface of the triquetrum with subchondral marrow edema and subchondral cystic change (Fig. 9-20). The TFC usually remains intact, but there may be increased T2 signal adjacent to the ulnar attachment of the TFC representing synovitis.

Ulnar Impingement (Distal Radioulnar Impingement)

This type of impingement is associated with a short ulna resulting in an abnormal articulation of the distal radioulnar joint (DRUJ), which occurs proximal to the level of the sigmoid notch and in turn leads to an impingement of distal ulna against the distal radius. This abnormal articulation leads to premature osteoarthritis of the distal radioulnar joint with subchondral marrow edema, subchondral cyst formation, joint effusion, and osteophyte formation. Longstanding distal radioulnar impingement may lead to remodeling of the distal radius (Fig. 9-21).

Hamatolunate Impingement

The normal lunate has a single distal articular facet (type I lunate) that articulates with the capitate (described as a C-shaped midcarpal joint). An anatomic variation of the lunate exists in which a second distal articular facet (type II lunate) articulates with a broad facet located on the proximal aspect of the

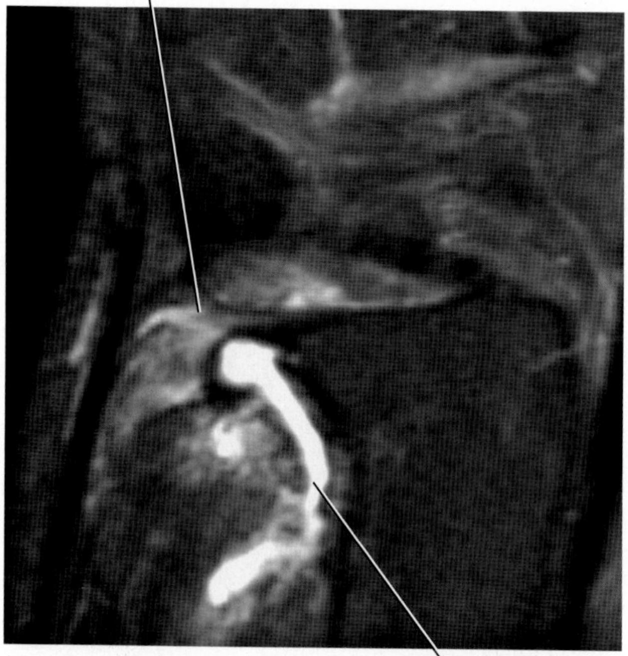
Intact TFC
Short ulna with DRUJ osteoarthritis

Figure 9-21 Ulnar impingement. Coronal T2-weighted image with fat saturation shows a short ulna resulting in distal radioulnar impingement and secondary osteoarthritis of the distal radioulnar joint (DRUJ). There is remodeling of the radius, subchondral reactive marrow edema on both sides of the joint and early subchondral cyst formation. The triangular fibrocartilage complex (TFC) is abnormally thickened and edematous but remains intact.

hamate (described as a W-shaped midcarpal joint). The type II lunate configuration results in altered load bearing across the carpus during ulnar deviation, which in turn leads to repeated abrasion of the adjacent articular surface of the hamate. Eventually, the impingement results in arthrosis of the adjacent articular facet of the hamate, cartilage loss, and osteoarthritis (Fig. 9-22). This type of impingement results in ulnar-sided wrist pain that is exacerbated when the wrist is placed in full ulnar deviation.

OSSEOUS STRUCTURES

Occult Fractures

An occult fracture is defined as a fracture that is not visible on radiographs. The complex anatomy of the wrist makes this area particularly difficult to evaluate with radiographs, and occult fractures of the carpal bones are common. When an occult fracture is suspected clinically, several additional imaging options are available. These include additional or special radiographic views, or, in some instances, cross-sectional imaging such as CT, MRI, or nuclear medicine bone scan may be indicated.

Occult Scaphoid Fractures

The prototypical occult fracture of the wrist is that of the scaphoid. Scaphoid fractures usually occur after a fall on an outstretched hand. The patient presents clinically with snuff-box tenderness. It is important to make a timely diagnosis of a scaphoid fracture because delay in diagnosis and immobilization is one of the major risk factors for developing avascular necrosis of the proximal pole of the scaphoid, a devastating complication that often leads to significant secondary osteoarthritis and chronic wrist pain.

The scaphoid is the largest bone of the proximal carpal row and forms a link between the proximal and distal carpal rows. It is tilted in a slightly volar direction distally. This tilt is in large part responsible for the increased incidence of radiographically occult fractures of the scaphoid. The x-ray beam in a standard anteroposterior view of the wrist is directed partially down the long axis of the scaphoid rather than aligned perpendicular to the long axis, whereas fracture detection is usually optimized if the beam is aligned perpendicular to the long axis of a bone. Simply by obtaining an oblique projection, the beam of the x-ray becomes more perpendicular to the long axis of the scaphoid and can improve the detection rate of transverse fractures. The scaphoid view is a special radiographic view that is obtained by positioning the wrist in maximum ulnar deviation while directing the beam in the straight anteroposterior projection with 15 degrees of craniocaudal angulation. Ulnar deviation of the wrist results in the dorsal elevation of the distal pole of the scaphoid and aids in detection of fractures because the beam once again is more perpendicular to the long axis of the bone. If these techniques fail to demonstrate a suspected fracture, then two options remain; one can immediately proceed to a cross-sectional imaging modality if available, or, if unavailable, the wrist can be immobilized and treated as if it is fractured. Repeat radiographs can then be obtained in

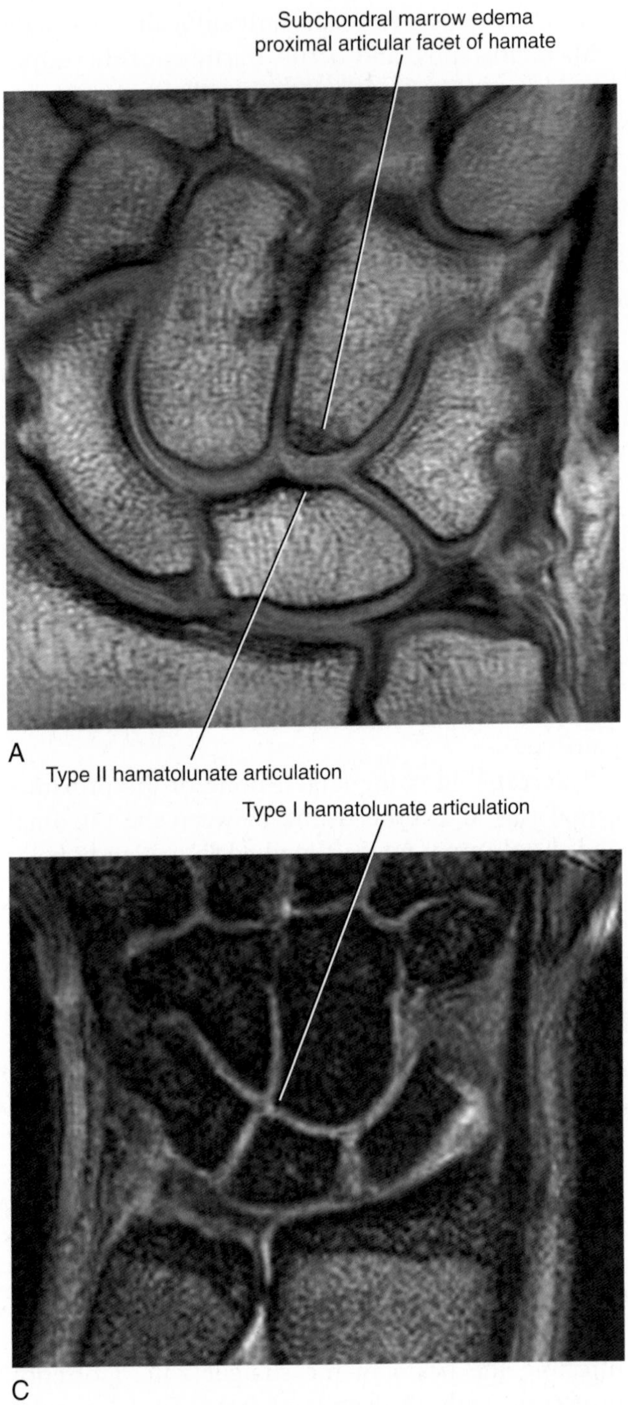
Subchondral marrow edema
proximal articular facet of hamate
A
Type II hamatolunate articulation
Chondral loss and subchondral
reactive marrow edema
B
Minimal adjacent synovitis
Type I hamatolunate articulation
C

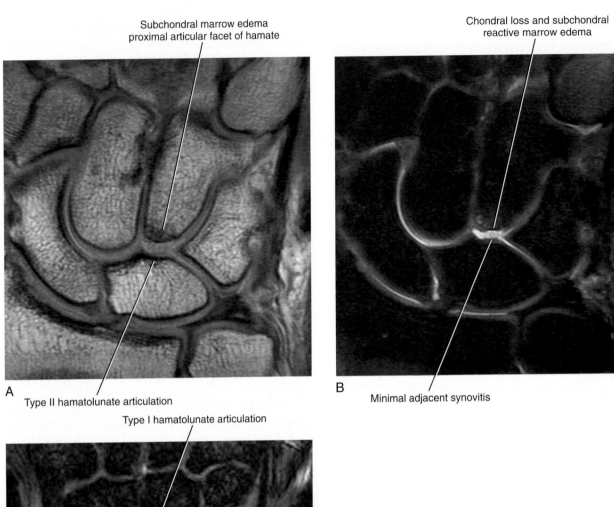

Figure 9-22 Hamatolunate impingement. Coronal T1-weighted image (**A**) and coronal T2-weighted image (**B**) with fat saturation shows a type II lunate with an additional articular facet that articulates with the hamate (W-shaped midcarpal joint). There is arthrosis with chondral loss, subchondral reactive marrow edema, and mild adjacent reactive synovitis. **C,** Coronal T2-weighted image with fat saturation shows the appearance of a type I lunate (C-shaped midcarpal joint). Note the absence of a separate hamatolunate articular facet.

7 to 10 days, at which time the repair process often results in a fracture that is more readily detected on radiographs.

Multidetector CT examination through the wrist with sagittal and coronal reformations can be very helpful in detecting occult fractures of the wrist. This technique is especially helpful in defining the extent of fracture, determining the location of fracture fragments, and detecting small cortical avulsion fractures, which can be challenging to detect on radiographs or MRI.

MRI is the modality of choice in most instances to evaluate the wrist for suspected radiographically occult fractures. The value of MRI is that it can

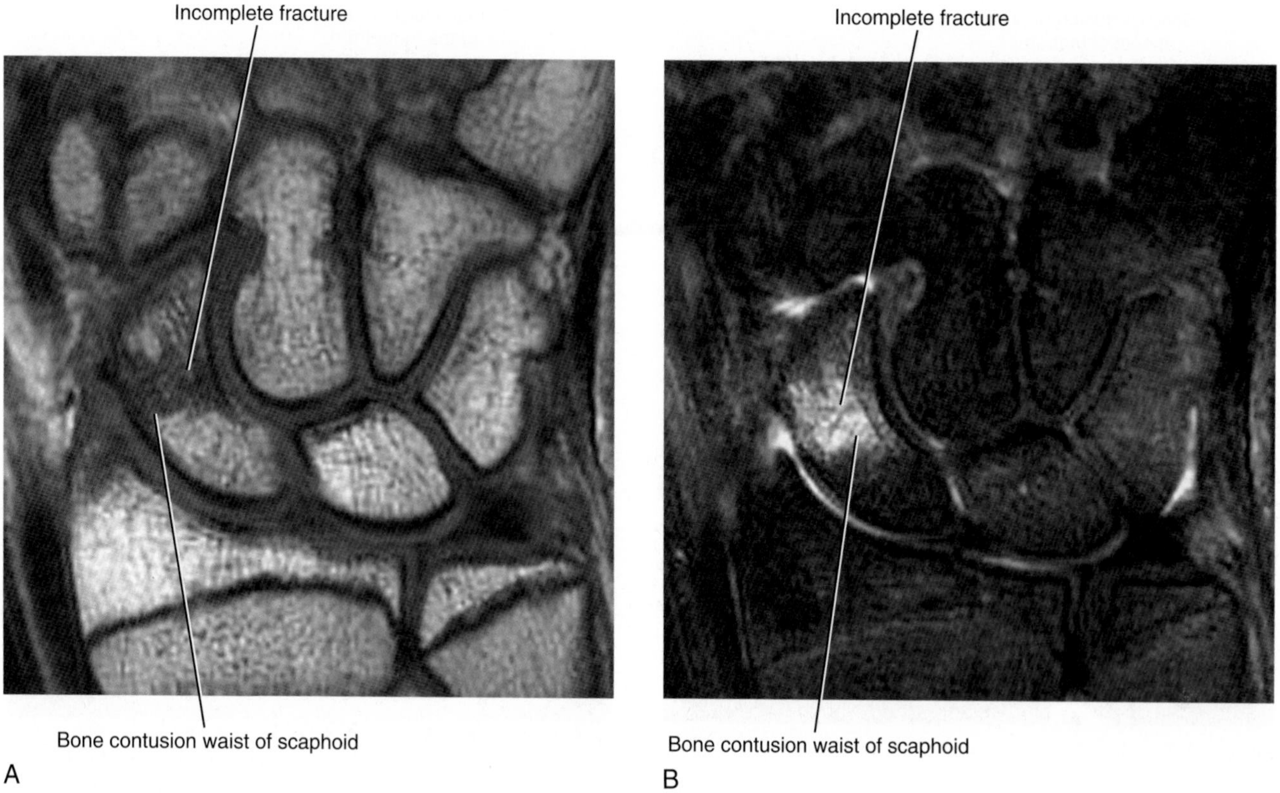
Incomplete fracture
Bone contusion waist of scaphoid
A
Incomplete fracture
Bone contusion waist of scaphoid
B

Figure 9-23 **Radiographically occult scaphoid fracture seen on MR imaging.** Coronal T1 (**A**) and T2-weighted (**B**) images show a focal area of bone contusion with an incomplete nondisplaced dark line seen on both T1- and T2-weighted images, representing an incomplete nondisplaced fracture.

accurately detect the presence of a fracture and can also depict associated soft tissue injures such as disruption of the intrinsic ligaments of the wrist. The use of T2-weighted imaging with fat suppression or a STIR sequence is the most accurate for detecting the area of edema surrounding the fracture, which appears bright on the T2-weighted images. The use of T1-weighted images without fat suppression can then accurately differentiate between fracture and bone contusion because the fracture can be seen as a dark line on the T1-weighted images (Fig. 9-23).

Cortical avulsion fractures, which occur along the dorsal aspect of the triquetrum can be very difficult to detect on MRI and are often overlooked. This is because the small cortical fragment is black on MR images and blends imperceptibly with the adjacent capsular structures of the wrist. Minimal bone marrow edema is usually present in association with an avulsion fracture, and overlying capsular edema is often noted. If a cortical avulsion fracture is suspected on MRI, then comparison with radiographs or follow-up CT examination is often helpful in depicting the avulsion fracture fragment (Fig. 9-24).

Hook of the Hamate Fracture

A fracture of the hook of a hamate may result from direct trauma during a fall on an outstretched hand; however, in athletes these fractures most often involve the nondominant hand and result from the transmission of shear forces through ligaments that insert on the hook of the hamate during forced hyperextension of the wrist while gripping a racquet, golf club, or baseball bat. The individual presents with point tenderness along the volar aspect of the hook of the hamate and usually has difficulty continuing to participate in the sport because of significant pain while holding the racquet, club, or bat. Fractures of the hook of the hamate are usually occult on standard radiographic views of the wrist, which may lead to a delay in diagnosis. When the diagnosis is suspected

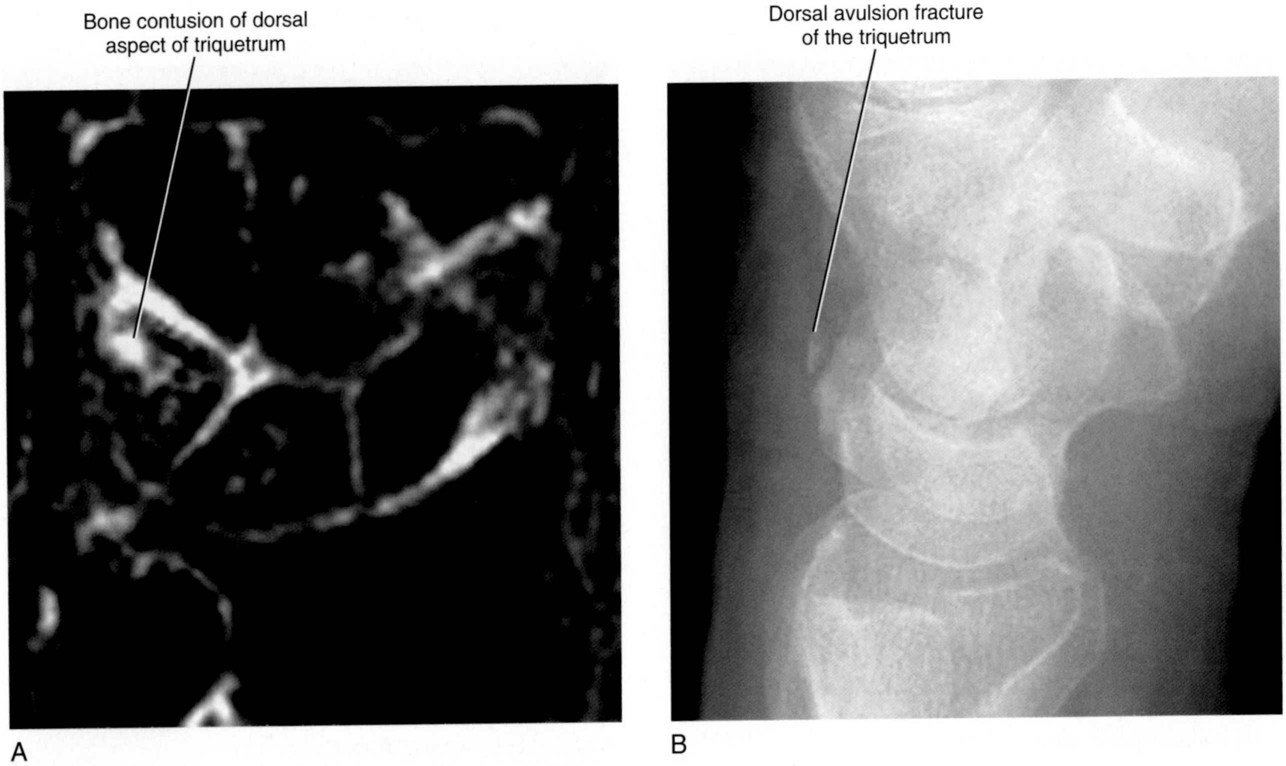
Bone contusion of dorsal aspect of triquetrum
Dorsal avulsion fracture of the triquetrum
A
B

Figure 9-24 Dorsal avulsion fracture of the triquetrum. A, Coronal STIR image of the wrist shows an area of marrow edema involving the triquetrum, but no fracture or cortical disruption was identified on the MR images. **B,** Lateral radiograph shows a small cortical avulsion fracture of the dorsal aspect of the triquetrum.

clinically, the carpal tunnel view can improve detection rate on radiographs, which demonstrates the hook in profile. The fracture is best depicted on cross-sectional imaging in the axial plane, using either CT or MRI. Pain relief is obtained after resection of the fracture fragment (Fig. 9-25).

Gymnast Wrist

Gymnast wrist describes a stress-related epiphysiolysis of the distal radial growth plate and is so named because it has been described almost exclusively in gymnasts. The injury occurs as a result of excessive compressive and rotation forces that occur when the upper extremity becomes weight-bearing; the injury is often bilateral. Radiographs demonstrate distal radial epiphyseal widening and irregularity. MRI is more sensitive than radiographs in depicting early epiphysiolysis, and shows increased T2 signal and widening and irregularity of the distal radial epiphysis (Fig. 9-26).

Avascular Necrosis

Avascular necrosis (AVN) is defined as death of the osteocytes in a region of bone resulting from interruption of the blood supply. The list of potential etiologies for osseous AVN is usually quite extensive. In the wrist, however, the two most common locations for AVN include the proximal pole of the scaphoid, where AVN is a complication of fracture, and the lunate, where AVN usually results from repetitive trauma and a tenuous blood supply.

Lunate (Kienböck Disease)

Avascular necrosis of the lunate may have several potential causes, but in most cases, it is thought to result from chronic repetitive trauma and is often seen in manual laborers. AVN of the lunate is frequently associated with negative ulnar variance because this anatomic variation may expose the ulna to increased axial loading across the lunate, which increases the significance of repetitive trauma. The vascular supply of the lunate is also a consideration

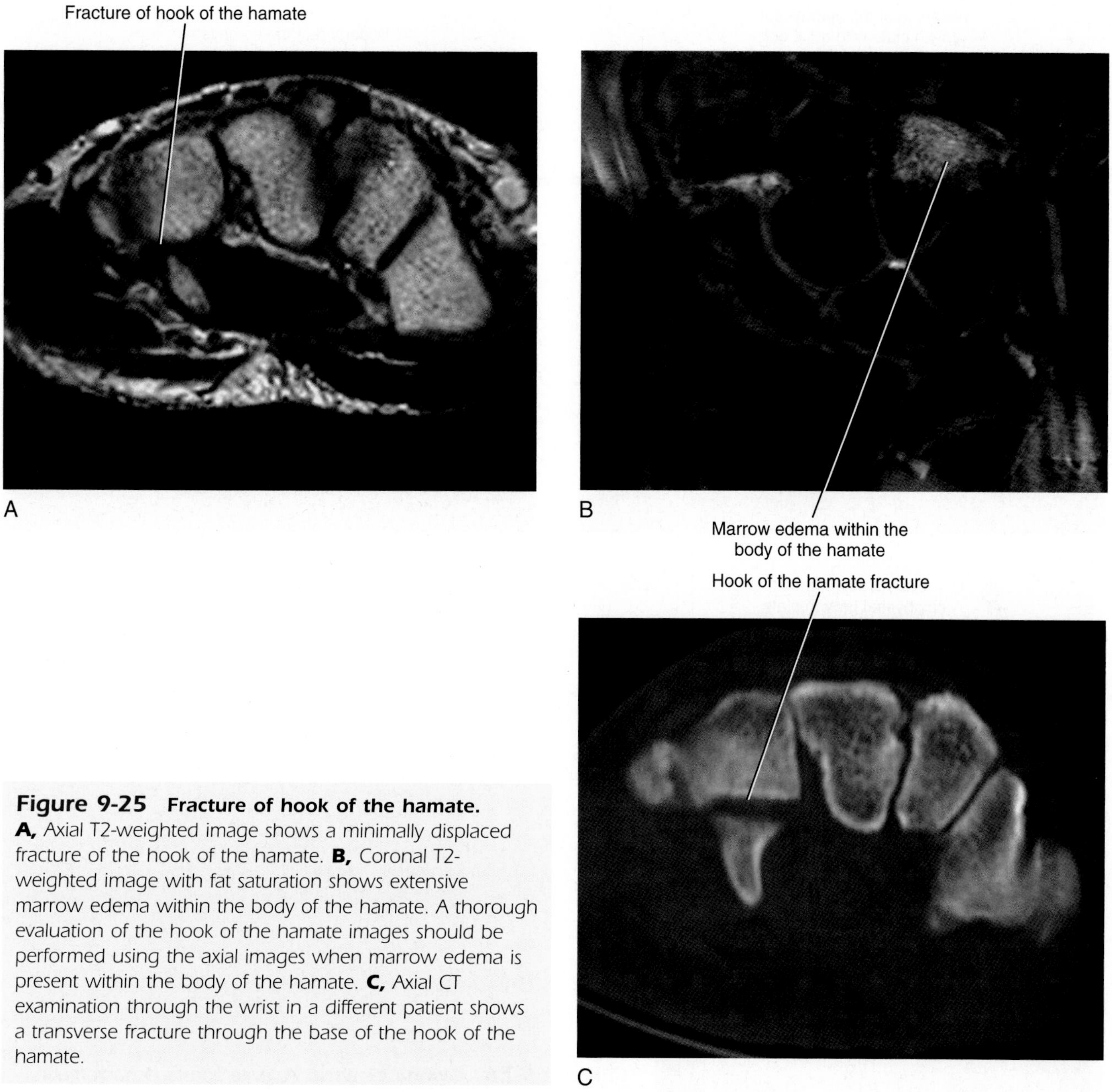
Fracture of hook of the hamate
A
B
Marrow edema within the body of the hamate
Hook of the hamate fracture
C

Figure 9-25 Fracture of hook of the hamate. **A,** Axial T2-weighted image shows a minimally displaced fracture of the hook of the hamate. **B,** Coronal T2-weighted image with fat saturation shows extensive marrow edema within the body of the hamate. A thorough evaluation of the hook of the hamate images should be performed using the axial images when marrow edema is present within the body of the hamate. **C,** Axial CT examination through the wrist in a different patient shows a transverse fracture through the base of the hook of the hamate.

in the pattern and distribution of AVN of the lunate, since vessels enter from both the dorsal and volar aspects of the lunate and only terminal arteries supply the proximal pole of the lunate, where AVN is most likely to originate.

Several classification systems have been devised to describe the stages of AVN of the lunate. However, a system suggested by Lichtman and Ross is one of the most commonly used systems and combines the use of radiography, MRI, and CT (Table 9-7). In stage I, the radiographs are normal; homogeneous marrow edema is present on MRI within the area of AVN, with homogeneous enhancement of the areas of involvement after administration of intravenous gadolinium. In stage II, there is early sclerosis and cystic formation noted on radiographs without cortical collapse. These changes are most frequently noted involving the proximal pole of the lunate, and CT may show these changes slightly earlier than radiographs. MRI shows heterogeneous signal abnormality with mixed high and low T2 signal and heterogeneous enhancement (Fig. 9-27). Stage IIIA shows progressive fracture and collapse of the lunate without carpal instability. Radiographs and CT demonstrate increased areas of sclerosis with cortical collapse and fragmentation. MRI demonstrates mixed areas of high and low signal

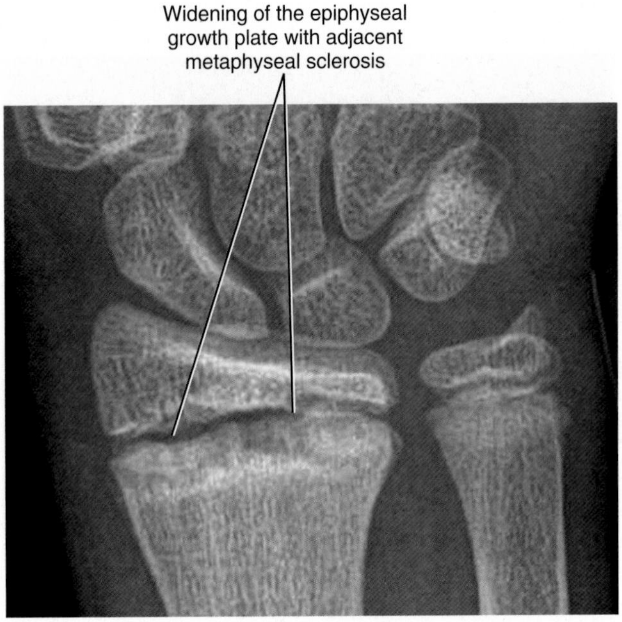
Widening of the epiphyseal growth plate with adjacent metaphyseal sclerosis
A

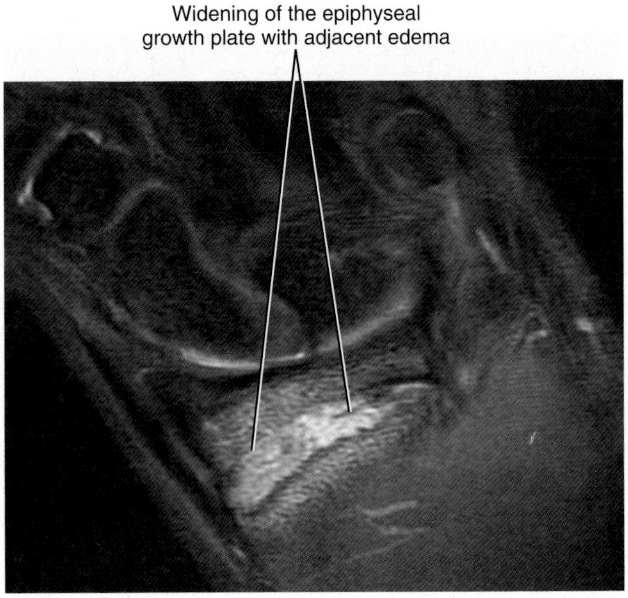
Widening of the epiphyseal growth plate with adjacent edema
B

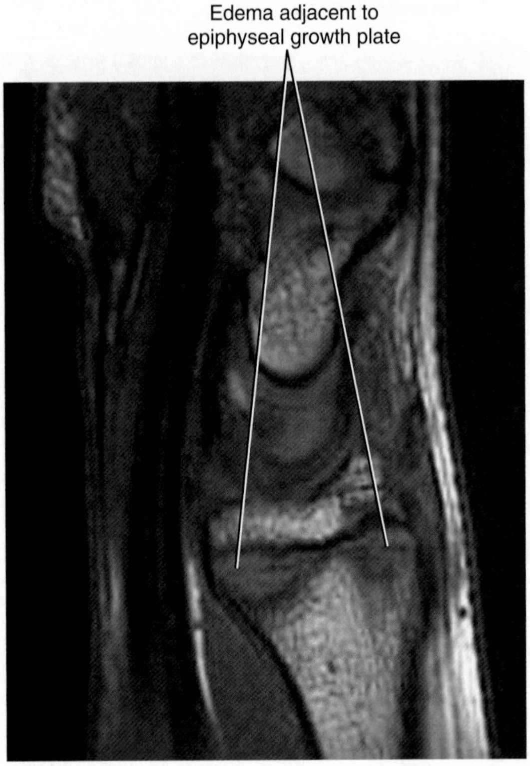
Edema adjacent to epiphyseal growth plate
C

Figure 9-26 Gymnast's wrist. A, Anteroposterior radiograph of the wrist shows widening of the distal radial epiphyseal growth plate and adjacent metaphyseal mixed sclerosis and lucency. This represents advanced epiphysiolysis. Coronal T2-weighted image (**B**) with fat saturation and sagittal T1-weighted image (**C**) shows widening of the growth plate and extensive adjacent marrow edema.

with the low signal corresponding to areas of sclerosis. Stage IIIB, shows progressive fracture and fragmentation of the lunate with the onset of rotatory instability of the scaphoid and carpal collapse. Stage IV shows progressive carpal collapse and development of end-stage osteoarthritis of the wrist, or scapholunate advanced collapse (SLAC) wrist.

The use of dynamic intravenous gadolinium in the evaluation of AVN of the lunate has been advocated by some to assess for blood flow indicating potential viability of the bone. Intense homogeneous enhancement is seen in stage I, whereas in stage II the enhancement is less intense and heterogeneous since the areas of sclerosis lack enhancement. Finally, there is

Table 9-7 Staging of Avascular Necrosis of the Lunate

Stage	Radiographic Findings	MR Findings
I	Normal	Homogeneous marrow edema
II	Subchondral cysts/sclerosis No cortical collapse	Heterogeneous mixed high and low T2-weighted signal
IIIA	Progressive fracture/collapse	Mixed high and low T2 signal Progressive fracture/collapse
IIIB	Same as IIIA with onset of carpal instability	Same as IIIA with onset of carpal instability
IV	Same as IIIA with scapholunate advanced collapse (SLAC)	Same as IIIA with SLAC

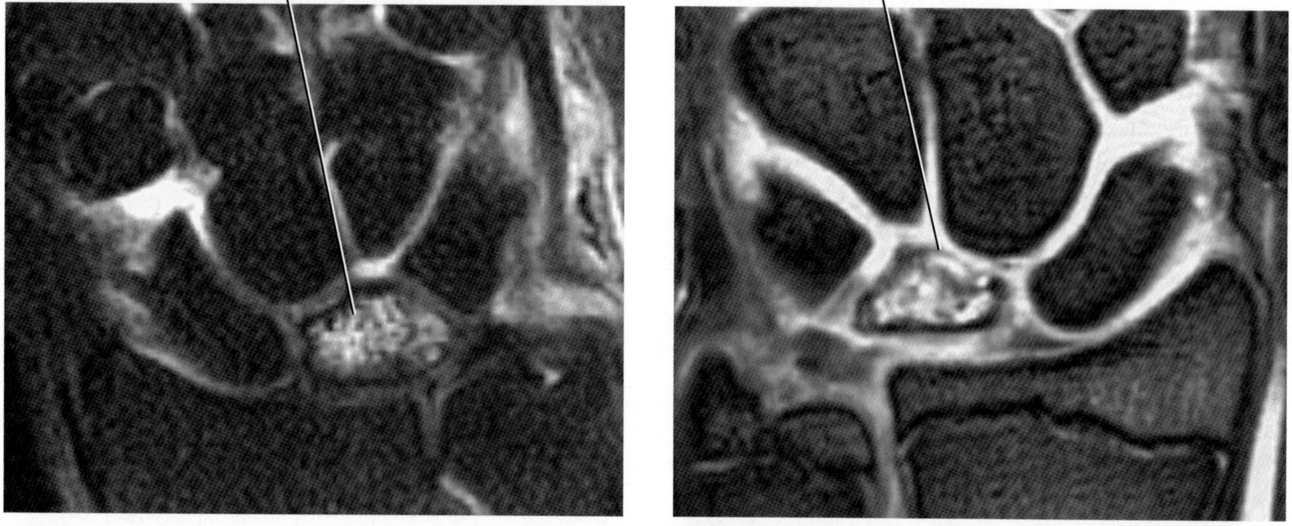
Heterogeneous T2 signal with no cortical collapse or fracture
Heterogeneous mixed T2 signal with early collapse
Grade II
A
Grade IIIA
B

Figure 9-27 Kienböck disease (avascular necrosis of the lunate). A, Coronal T2-weighted image with fat saturation shows extensive edema and heterogeneous mixed T2 signal within the lunate, but no cortical collapse or fragmentation (grade II). **B,** Coronal T2-weighted image with fat saturation shows heterogeneous T2 signal and early cortical collapse of the distal articular surface (grade IIIA).

a total lack of enhancement in stages III and IV, indicating nonviable bone.

Scaphoid Fracture: Nonunion and Avascular Necrosis

Nonunion of a scaphoid fracture is a serious complication that leads to osteoarthritis of the radiocarpal joint and chronic wrist pain. Risk factors for nonunion include a delay in diagnosis and immobilization, significant displacement or fragmentation of fracture fragments at the time of initial injury, and a fracture that is located proximally in the scaphoid. Imaging plays an important role in the evaluation of the healing process of a scaphoid fracture and in the assessment of potential nonunion.

A classification system for staging nonunion of scaphoid fractures was developed by Trojan and Jahna and is a useful scheme for understanding and describing the radiographic sequence that accompanies the development of nonunion. The scheme was originally developed to describe radiographic changes that occur, but CT also demonstrates each of the stages nicely and depicts many of the changes more completely and earlier than radiographs (Table 9-8).

Table 9-8 Staging System for Nonunion of Scaphoid Fractures

Stage	Radiographic/CT Findings
I	Bandlike resorption zones on both sides of fracture Nonunion considered reversible at this stage
II	Small resorptional cysts and marginal sclerosis on both sides of fracture Nonunion irreversible without surgical intervention
IIIA	Smooth sclerotic edges on both sides of fracture No carpal instability
IIIB	Smooth sclerotic edges on both sides of fracture Carpal instability
IV	Osteoarthritis and carpal collapse

Stage I demonstrates bandlike resorption zones along the fracture line; at this stage, the nonunion remains reversible. During stage II, tiny resorptional cysts and marginal sclerosis begin to develop along both fracture margins, and at this point the nonunion is considered irreversible without some sort of surgical intervention (Fig. 9-28). Stage IIIA and IIIB demonstrate smooth sclerotic edges at the level of fracture with and without carpal instability. Finally, stage IV demonstrates osteoarthritis and carpal collapse, which has been termed scaphoid nonunion-advanced collapse or SNAC wrist (Fig. 9-29). Humpback deformity at the level of scaphoid fracture describes a deformity of the scaphoid in which there is palmar flexion of the distal pole and dorsiflexion of the proximal pole and lunate. This leads to an incongruent radioscaphoid joint, which in turn leads to osteoarthritis and eventually to a SNAC wrist.

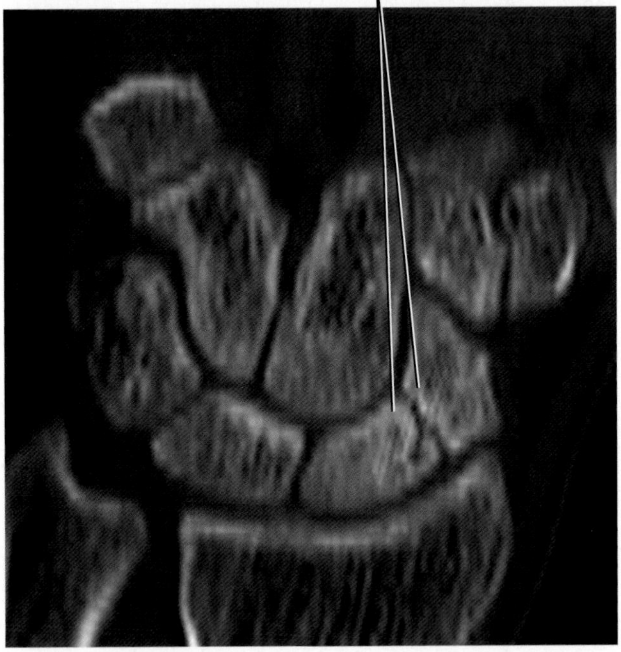
Small resorptional cysts and marginal sclerosis on both sides of fracture

Figure 9-28 Nonunion of a scaphoid fracture. Coronal reconstruction CT image of the wrist shows a transverse fracture across the waist of the navicular bone. Small resorptional cysts and marginal sclerosis are on both sides of the fracture indicating a stage II nonunion of the scaphoid. At this stage, the nonunion is nonreversible without surgical intervention.

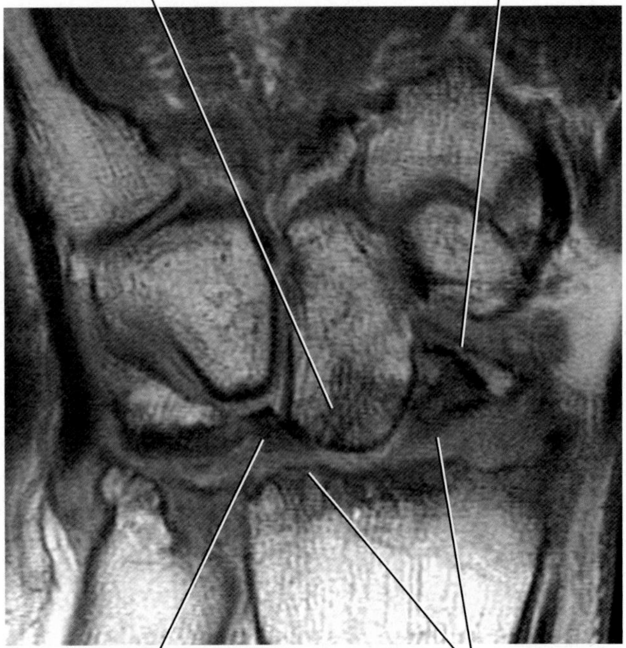
Proximal migration capitate
Proximal pole scaphoid
Distal pole scaphoid
Advanced OA radiocarpal joint proximal carpal row collapse

Figure 9-29 Scaphoid nonunion advanced collapse (SNAC) wrist. Coronal T1-weighted image shows nonunion of a scaphoid fracture with advanced collapse of the midcarpus. The capitate has migrated proximally and is interposed between the proximal and distal pole fracture fragments of the scaphoid with complete collapse of the proximal carpal row and advanced osteoarthritis (OA) of the radiocarpal joint.

In addition to these changes, MRI can also demonstrate a fibrous union depicted as low-signal material filling the fracture gap on both T1- and T2-weighted images consistent with fibrosis rather than new bone formation (Fig. 9-30). On MRI, stage IV nonunion

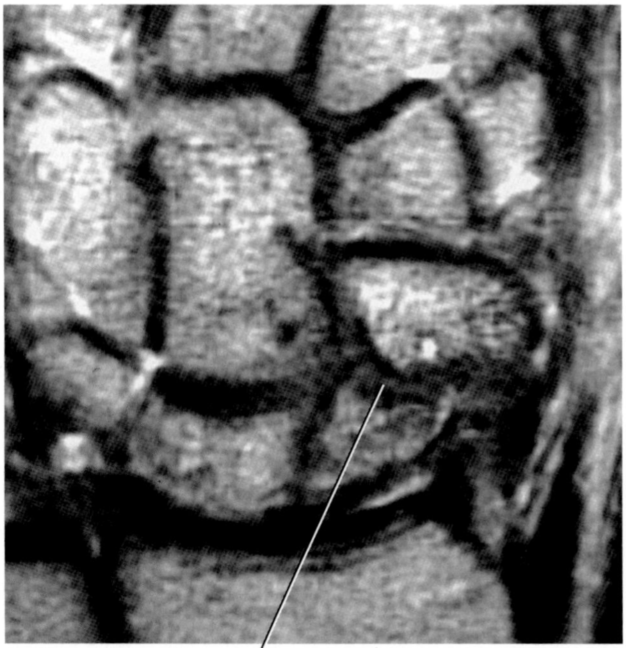
A
Low-signal material fills the fracture site

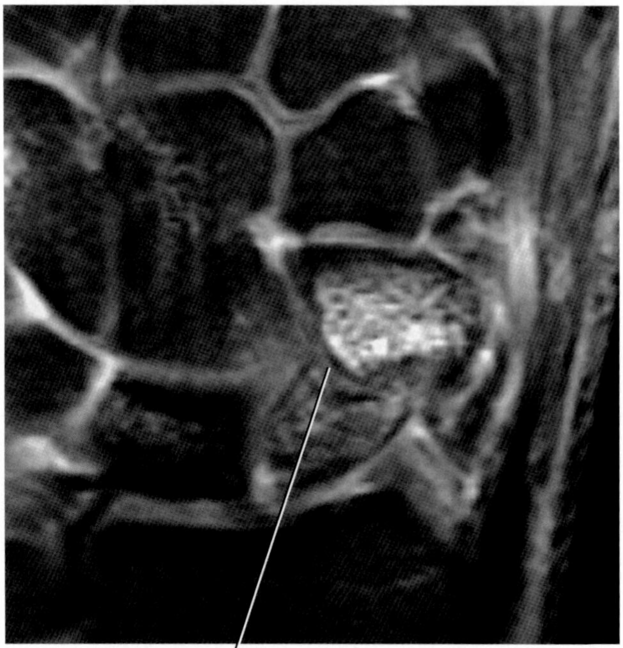
B
Low-signal material fills the fracture site

Figure 9-30 Fibrous union of a scaphoid fracture. Coronal T1-weighted (**A**) and T2-weighted (**B**) images show low-signal material bridging the fracture site on both T1- and T2-weighted images. This represents a fibrous union rather than new bone formation across the fracture site.

demonstrates sclerotic fracture margins with a fluid-filled gap between the fracture fragments. The gap demonstrates intermediate signal on T1- and bright fluid signal on T2-weighted images (Fig. 9-31).

Osteoarthritis is inevitable following scaphoid nonunion and is first seen at the level of articulation between the distal scaphoid fracture fragment and the radial styloid while sparing the articulation between the proximal scaphoid fracture fragment and the radius. Next, osteoarthritis develops between the lunate and the capitate. End-stage changes include proximal migration of the capitate combined with a dorsal tilt of the lunate (DISI configuration) accompanied by osteoarthritis at the level of articulation between the proximal scaphoid fracture fragment and the adjacent radius—SNAC wrist (Fig. 9-32).

AVN can accompany nonunion of the scaphoid, and because the blood supply to the scaphoid is recurrent, a fracture traversing the waist or proximal pole of the scaphoid has the potential to disrupt the blood supply to the proximal pole. Nonunion of the scaphoid is typically treated with open fixation and bone grafting across the fracture site, but this procedure will fail if the proximal fragment lacks an adequate blood supply. At the time of the operation, the surgeon scrapes the proximal pole of the scaphoid with a scalpel. Bleeding is an indication of adequate blood supply to the proximal pole of the scaphoid, whereas the lack of bleeding indicates AVN of the proximal pole of the scaphoid. The presence of proximal pole AVN demands that a vascular pedicle be brought to the proximal pole, which is a more complicated and lengthy surgical procedure. MRI can accurately determine the vascular status of the proximal pole of the scaphoid and can thus play an important role in preoperative planning.

AVN of the scaphoid manifests radiographic changes similar to those previously described in the section Lunate (Kienböck Disease).

Early AVN of the proximal pole manifests a normal radiographic appearance, but as the AVN progresses, subtle sclerosis and cystic formation can be noted without cortical collapse, followed by a progressive increase in sclerosis, cortical collapse, and fragmentation (Fig. 9-33). The advanced stages of AVN are easily depicted on radiographs and CT, whereas MRI

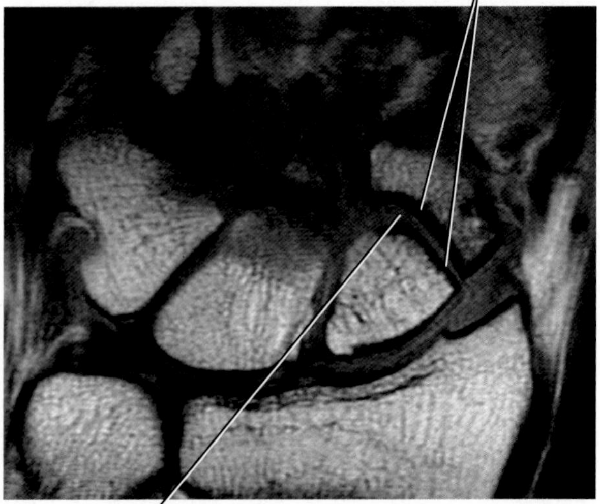
Smooth sclerotic margins
A
Fluid-filled gap

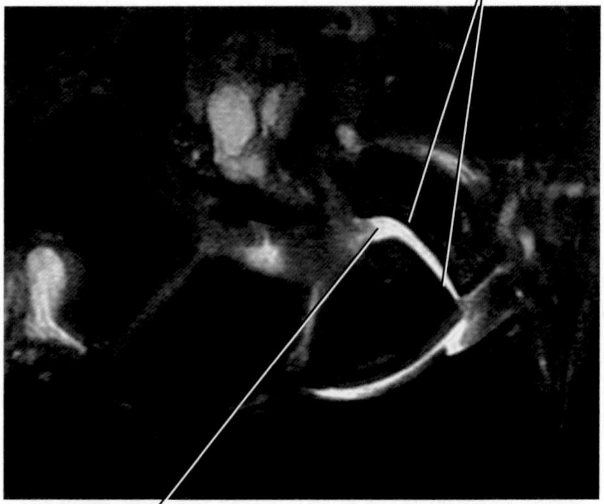
Smooth sclerotic margins
B
Fluid-filled gap

Figure 9-31 Nonunion of a scaphoid fracture. Coronal T1-weighted (**A**) and T2-weighted (**B**) images show smooth sclerotic margins on both sides of the fracture with a fluid-filled gap representing a nonunion fracture of the scaphoid.

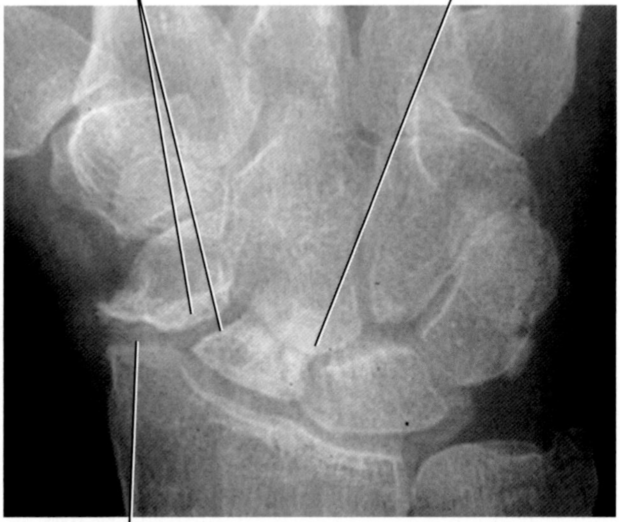
Sclerotic fracture margins
Proximal capitate migration
Radiocarpal osteoarthritis

Figure 9-32 Stage IV nonunion of a scaphoid fracture. Anteroposterior radiograph of the wrist demonstrates end-stage nonunion of a scaphoid fracture. Smooth sclerotic margins are on both sides of the fracture indicating a irreversible nonunion. Also seen are extensive osteoarthritis of the radiocarpal joint, proximal capitate migration, and early carpal collapse.

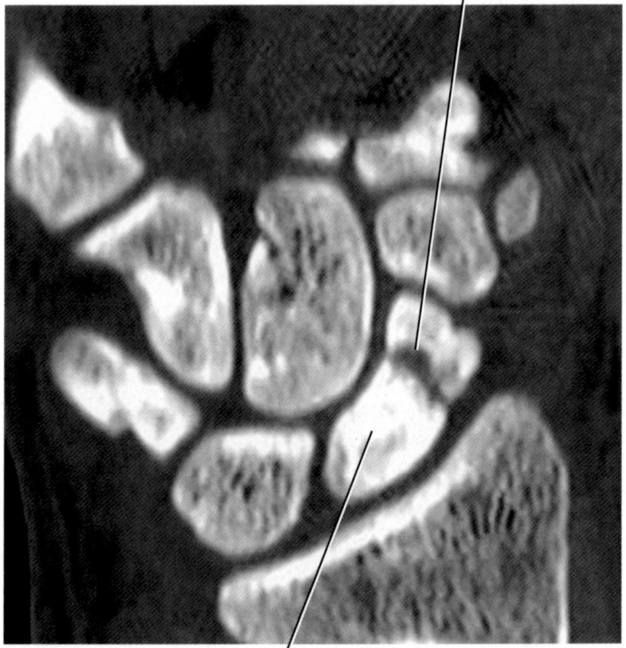
Fracture waist of the scaphoid
Sclerosis of proximal pole

Figure 9-33 Avascular necrosis of proximal pole of the scaphoid. Coronal reconstructed CT image of the wrist demonstrates a transverse fracture across the waist of the scaphoid with marked sclerosis of the proximal pole indicating advanced avascular necrosis.

with intravenous gadolinium is helpful in evaluating for early changes of AVN. The presence of low T1 and bright T2 signal within the proximal pole of the scaphoid combined with bright homogeneous enhancement of the marrow after administration of intravenous gadolinium indicates revascularization of the proximal pole and an intact blood supply. There is no need for a vascular graft at the time of fracture fixation and bone graft. During early stages of AVN, conventional MRI demonstrates low T1 signal and heterogeneous T2 signal with mixed areas of increased and decreased signal intensity, with the areas of low signal corresponding to the areas of sclerosis seen on radiographs. In the later stages of AVN, homogeneous low signal on both T1- and T2-weighted images and a complete lack of enhancement are seen. This indicates a complete lack of blood supply to the proximal pole and requires a vascular graft at the time of fracture fixation to allow adequate healing (Fig. 9-34).

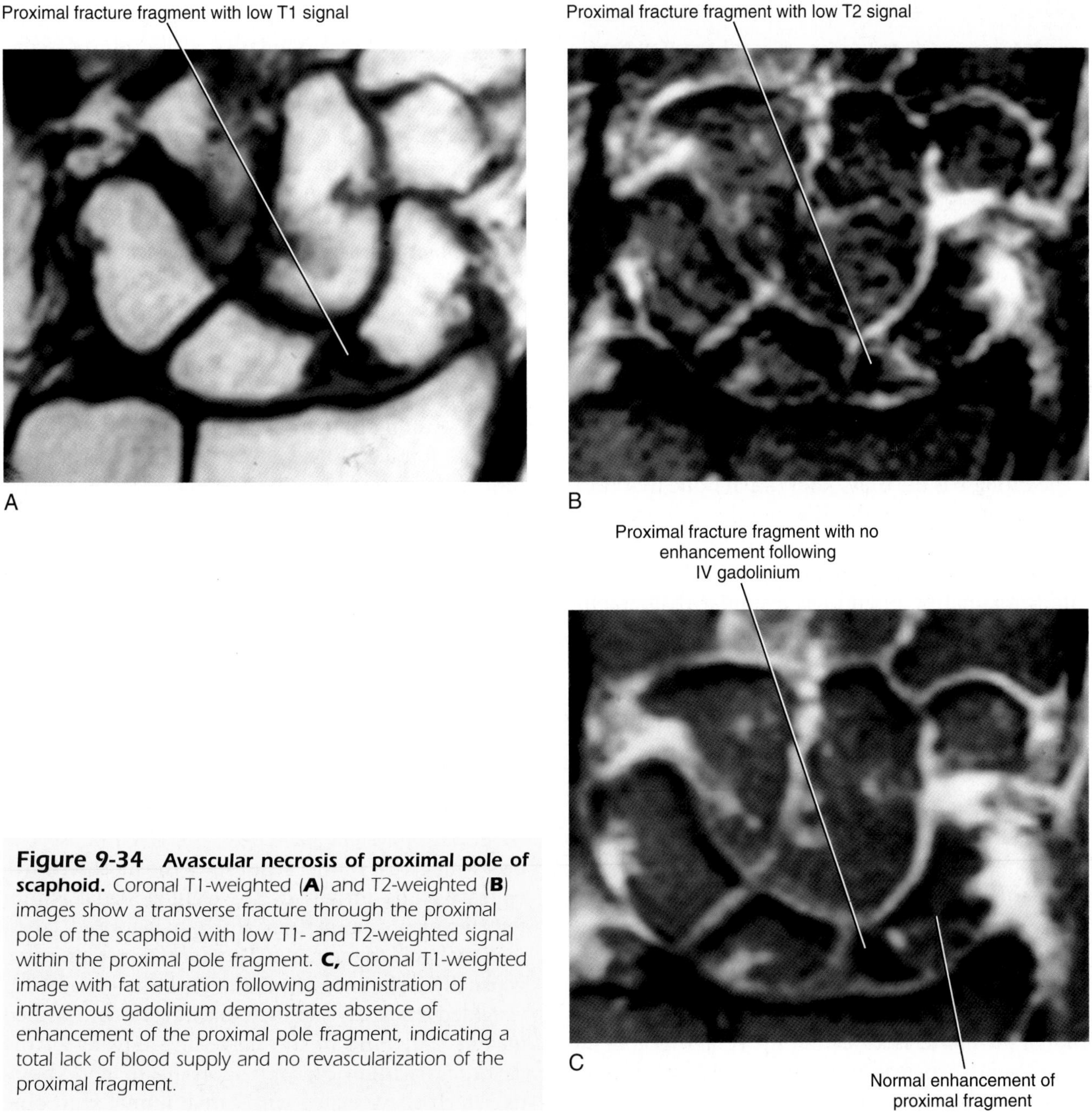
Proximal fracture fragment with low T1 signal
A
Proximal fracture fragment with low T2 signal
B
Proximal fracture fragment with no enhancement following IV gadolinium
C
Normal enhancement of proximal fragment

Figure 9-34 Avascular necrosis of proximal pole of scaphoid. Coronal T1-weighted (**A**) and T2-weighted (**B**) images show a transverse fracture through the proximal pole of the scaphoid with low T1- and T2-weighted signal within the proximal pole fragment. **C,** Coronal T1-weighted image with fat saturation following administration of intravenous gadolinium demonstrates absence of enhancement of the proximal pole fragment, indicating a total lack of blood supply and no revascularization of the proximal fragment.

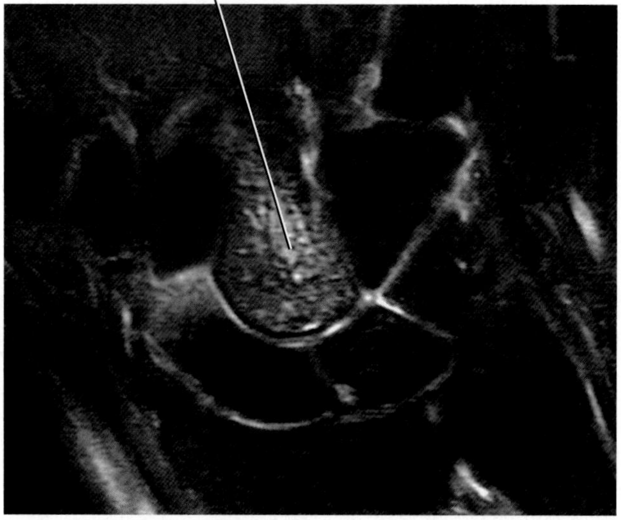
Heterogeneous bright T2 signal within the capitate

Figure 9-35 Avascular necrosis (AVN) of the capitate. Coronal T2-weighted image shows heterogeneous T2-signal in the capitate in this patient with early AVN of the capitate. There is no fracture or cortical collapse at this time.

Avascular Necrosis of Other Carpal Bones

The capitate is the only other carpal bone that occasionally undergoes AVN. The blood supply is recurrent, similar to that of the scaphoid. Therefore, when AVN occurs, it typically involves the head of the capitate (proximal pole) and has a similar radiographic and MRI appearance as seen in AVN of the proximal pole of the scaphoid (Fig. 9-35). There is a rich anastomotic blood supply to the other carpal bones, and therefore AVN rarely if ever occurs in the remainder of the carpal bones.

CARPAL TUNNEL

The carpal tunnel is a fibro-osseous tunnel located along the volar aspect of the wrist. The radial boundary of the tunnel includes the tubercles of the scaphoid and the trapezium, and the hook of the hamate and pisiform form the ulnar boundary. The dorsal roof of the tunnel is formed by the volar aspect of the carpal bones, whereas the palmar boundary is formed by a thick flexor retinaculum that extends from the hook of the hamate to the tubercles of the scaphoid and trapezium.

The contents of the canal include the flexor pollicis longus tendon, the flexor digitorum profundus, the superficialis tendons to each of the second through fifth digits, and finally the median nerve. Sometimes a persistent vessel lies next to the median nerve. The median nerve is normally located superficially within the radial aspect of the tunnel and sits just deep to the flexor retinaculum (see Fig. 9-2B), but variant anatomy can occasionally result in the nerve sitting deep to the tendons.

Carpal tunnel syndrome describes an entrapment neuropathy of the median nerve as it traverses the carpal tunnel. The boundaries of the fibro-osseous tunnel are quite rigid; therefore, any process that increases the volume of the contents of the canal results in compression of the median nerve, leading to symptoms of pain and paresthesias located within the first three and one-half digits of the hand. The most common cause of carpal tunnel syndrome is tenosynovitis of the flexor tendon sheaths resulting from repetitive motion. An entire laundry list of causes has been described, including inflammatory conditions, masses, variant anatomy, and deposition arthropathies, but the common pathway remains an increased volume contained within a limited space, resulting in increased pressure on the median nerve as it traverses the tunnel. In most cases, carpal tunnel syndrome can be accurately diagnosed on the basis of history, physical examination, and electromyography.

Controversy exists regarding the exact role of MRI in the diagnosis of carpal tunnel syndrome. Most of the MRI signs described in association with carpal tunnel syndrome lack either sensitivity or specificity. As a result, MRI is usually reserved for atypical cases in which the diagnosis is not clearly established on the basis of clinical findings, in which a mass is suspected, or in which surgical release has failed (Fig. 9-36).

Several MRI signs have been described in association with carpal tunnel syndrome. The most sensitive appears to be increased T2-weighted signal within the nerve in conjunction with an increased cross-sectional area of the nerve. The normal median nerve is usually isointense to muscle on both T1- and T2-weighted images. Other signs that have been described include flattening of the nerve and bowing of the flexor retinaculum. Flexor tendon sheath tenosynovitis, which is associated with carpal tunnel syndrome

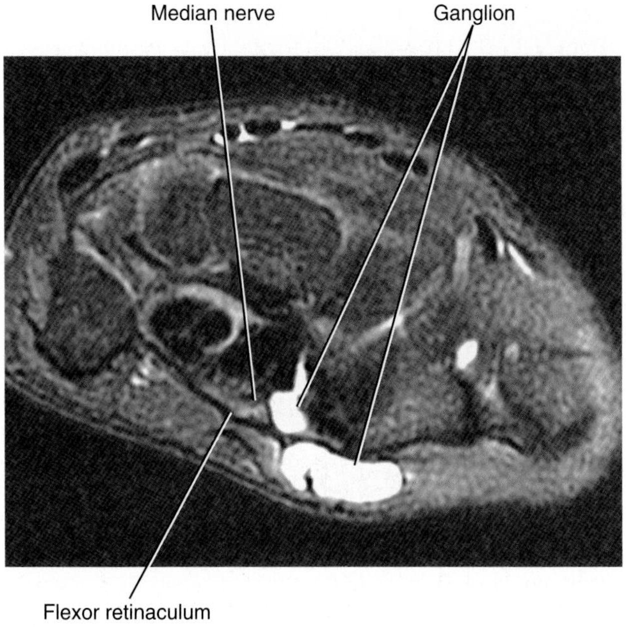
Median nerve
Ganglion
Flexor retinaculum

Figure 9-36 Ganglion in carpal tunnel. Axial T2-weighted image shows a ganglion within and superficial to the carpal tunnel resulting in mass effect on the median nerve in this patient with symptoms of carpal tunnel syndrome.

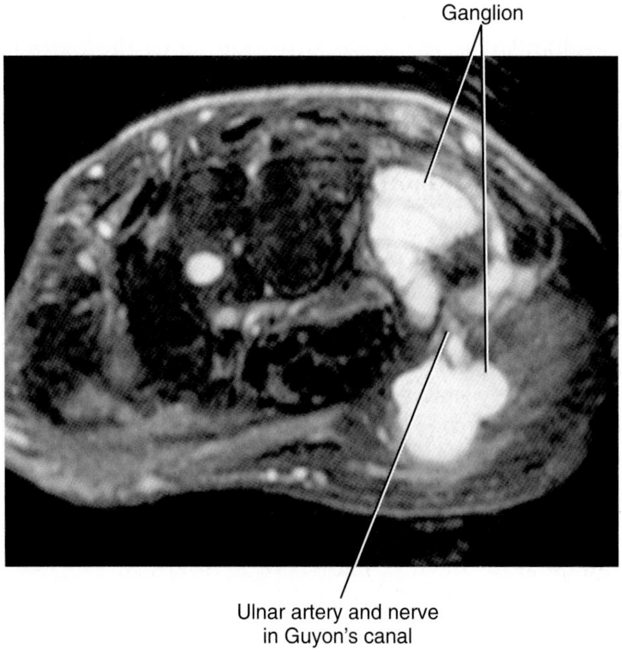
Ganglion
Ulnar artery and nerve
in Guyon's canal

Figure 9-37 Ganglion resulting in mass effect on the ulnar nerve at the level of Guyon's canal. Axial T2-weighted image shows a large ganglion arising along the ulnar aspect of the wrist, resulting in mass effect on the ulnar neurovascular bundle in this patient with symptoms of ulnar nerve entrapment.

can be diagnosed on MRI by intermediate signal separating the tendons, and occasionally fluid may be seen surrounding the tendons proximal to the carpal tunnel. MRI is very accurate in the evaluation of a mass within the carpal tunnel (see Fig. 9-36). A ganglion is the most common mass lesion to occur within the carpal tunnel, but other masses that are easily depicted are lesions such as a lipoma, displaced fracture fragment, aneurysm, gouty tophous, and pannus formation associated with rheumatoid arthritis.

GUYON'S CANAL

The ulnar artery and nerve traverse the wrist through a fibro-osseous tunnel referred to as Guyon's canal or the ulnar tunnel, which is located along the ulnar aspect of the wrist just superficial to the flexor retinaculum (see Fig. 9-2B). The lateral boundary is formed by the hook of the hamate and the pisiform, whereas the volar carpal ligament forms the superficial margin. The ulnar artery and nerve are easily visualized on MRI within the ulnar tunnel since they are surrounded by abundant fat. Compressive neuropathy of the ulnar nerve at the level of Guyon's canal is usually the result of a space-occupying lesion such as a ganglion, variant anatomy, or pseudoaneurysm of the ulnar artery (Fig. 9-37). As a result, unlike with carpal tunnel syndrome, MRI is usually very helpful in the evaluation of a compressive neuropathy of the ulnar nerve. It usually demonstrates a space-occupying lesion and distal muscle atrophy.

HYPOTHENAR HAMMER SYNDROME

Overuse or repetitive trauma to the palmar aspect of the hand can result in thrombosis or vasospasm of the digital arteries of the hand. This syndrome most frequently affects the ulnar artery at the level of the hook of the hamate. In the past, hypothenar hammer syndrome was most commonly reported as a result of occupational trauma as seen in jackhammer operators, mechanics, and those who use power tools. Hyponthenar hammer syndrome has also been reported in pianists and keyboard operators and more recently has been described in several types of athletes including practitioners of martial arts, baseball catchers, tennis players, and golfers. The common mechanism is repeated blunt trauma to the palmar aspect of the hand or wrist. The affected person presents with pain and "numbness" in the fourth and fifth digits.

MR angiography is a noninvasive method of evaluation and demonstrates occlusion of the ulnar artery, typically at the level of the hook of the hamate (Fig. 9-38). The ulnar artery is the primary source of blood supply to the common palmar digital artery of the fourth and fifth digits, but collateral flow from the radial artery may supply these vessels after occlusion of the ulnar artery. The severity of symptoms is related to the degree of collateral flow, with individuals who demonstrate good collateral flow complaining of only minor symptoms and those with a lack of collateral flow having significant symptoms. Doppler ultrasound and conventional angiography may also be of benefit in establishing the correct diagnosis and in defining the extent of vascular occlusion and collateral blood supply following occlusion of the ulnar artery.

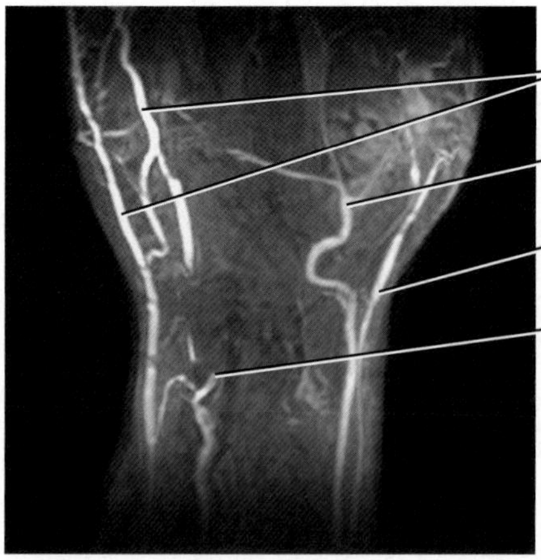
Venous structures
Radial artery
Venous structure
Complete occlusion of ulnar artery

Figure 9-38 Hypothenar hammer syndrome with occlusion of the ulnar artery. MR angiogram demonstrates thrombosis and complete occlusion of the ulnar artery at the level of the wrist. This patient was a manual laborer working on an oil rig and had been experiencing numbness in the fourth and fifth digits for 2 years.

Suggested Readings

Anderson MW. Imaging of upper extremity stress fractures in the athlete. Clin Sports Med 2006;25:489–504.

Andreisek G, Crook DW, Burg D, et al. Peripheral neuropathies of the median, radial, and ulnar nerves: MR imaging features. RadioGraphics 2006;26:1267–1287.

Bencardino JT, Rosenberg ZS. Sports-related injuries of the wrist: an approach to MRI interpretation. Clin Sports Med 2006;25: 409–432.

Brown RR, Fliszar E, Cotton A, et al. Extrinsic and intrinsic ligaments of the wrist: normal and pathologic anatomy at MR arthrography with three-compartment enhancement. RadioGraphics 1988;18: 667–674.

Cerezal L, Pinal F, Abascal F, et al. Imaging findings in ulnar-sided wrist impaction syndromes. RadioGraphics 2002;22:105–121.

Coggins CA. Imaging of ulnar-sided wrist pain. Clin Sports Med 2006;25:505–526.

Lima JE, Kim HJ, Albertotti F, Resnick D. Intersection syndrome: MR imaging with anatomic comparison of the distal forearm. Skeletal Radiol 2004;33:627–631.

Loredo RA, Sorge DG, Garcia G. Radiographic evaluation of the wrist: a vanishing art. Semin Roentgenol 2005;40:248–289.

Memarsadeghi M, Breitenseher MJ, Schaefer-Prokop C, et al. Occult scaphoid fractures: comparison of multidetector CT and MR-imaging-initial experience. Radiology 2006;240:169–176.

Oneson SR, Scales LM, Timins ME, et al. MR imaging interpretation of the palmer classification of triangular fibrocartilage complex lesions. RadioGraphics 1996;16:97–106.

Rosner JL, Zlatkin MB, Clifford P, et al. Imaging of athletic wrist and hand injuries. Semin Musculoskelet Radiol 2004;8:57–79.

Schmitt R, Heinze A, Fellner F, et al. Imaging and staging of avascular osteonecrosis at the wrist and hand. Eur J Radiol 1997; 25:92–103.

Smith DK. Dorsal carpal ligaments of the wrist: normal appearance on multiplanar reconstructions of three-dimensional fourier transform MR imaging. AJR 1993;161:119–125.

Sofka CM, Potter HG. Magnetic resonance imaging of the wrist. Semin Musculoskelet Radiol 2001;5:217–226.

Zlatkin MB, Rosner JL. MR imaging of ligaments and triangular fibrocartilage complex of the wrist. Radiol Clin North Am 2006;44:595–623.

Chapter 10

IMAGING OF THE HAND AND FINGERS

CHAPTER OUTLINE

MODALITIES

Radiography

Imaging evaluation of the hand and fingers often begins with conventional radiographs, especially in the setting of acute trauma for suspected fracture or dislocation. Radiographs are usually adequate to delineate the specific osseous abnormality following trauma. Evaluation in other clinical settings such as suspected arthritis, infection, or mass usually begins with radiographs as well but often proceeds to more advanced imaging. Anteroposterior, lateral, and oblique radiographs of the hand are usually adequate in the setting of trauma to visualize fractures or malalignment. The reverse anteroposterior oblique view, sometimes referred to as the ball-catcher's view, is helpful in demonstrating the early erosive disease seen in inflammatory arthritis. Anterolateral, lateral, and oblique views of the fingers and thumb are also usually adequate to demonstrate osseous abnormalities. If the suspected abnormality is isolated to a single digit, radiographs can be coned down to that particular digit. A good-quality lateral view of the finger is mandatory when evaluating for fracture. If multiple fingers are included in the same view, care must be taken to avoid overlap of the digits on the lateral view.

Computed Tomography

Computed tomography (CT) is rarely required in the evaluation of the hand and fingers, although it may occasionally be helpful in delineating the exact nature of complex fractures or in demonstrating the matrix of a lesion.

Ultrasound

Ultrasound may be particularly useful in the dynamic evaluation of tendon and pulley injuries of the hand and fingers and can be very useful in the localization of suspected foreign bodies within the soft tissues of the hand and fingers. Moreover, ultrasound can be useful in the evaluation of soft tissue masses such as ganglion and giant cell tumor of the tendon sheath. A thorough evaluation requires either an ultrasound technologist who is highly skilled in musculoskeletal imaging or a physician to direct or perform the imaging. A small parts transducer is mandatory for the evaluation of the small soft tissue structures of the digits, and comparison with the adjacent normal fingers can be very helpful.

Magnetic Resonance Imaging

Recent advances in MR technology such as improvement in coil technology and improved pulse sequences resulting in enhanced signal-to-noise ratios have made high-quality magnetic resonance imaging (MRI) of the small anatomic structures of the hand and fingers a reality. It is becoming common for the clinician to request MRI of the hand or even of an individual finger to evaluate for a specific soft tissue injury following acute trauma or to evaluate a palpable mass or a suspected infection. With improved treatment options for early arthritis, MRI is being used increasingly more frequently for the evaluation of early inflammatory arthropathies to detect subtle osseous changes such as marrow edema and tiny erosions that are not yet visible on conventional radiographs.

In the past, conventional radiography was the primary means available for imaging the hand and fingers in the setting of acute trauma, and evaluation was limited to the osseous structures or to indirect signs that would indicate a specific soft tissue injury. Now, however, MRI can accurately depict even the smallest of soft tissue structures of the hand and fingers. It has therefore become increasingly important for the radiologist to have a detailed understanding of the anatomy of the soft tissue structures and to have knowledge of the specific injury patterns that occur in the hand and fingers. When a soft tissue injury of a specific finger is suspected, inclusion of the two adjacent digits on MRI is helpful to allow comparison with the normal anatomy.

SOFT TISSUE ANATOMY AND INJURY PATTERNS

Metacarpophalangeal Joint

The metacarpophalangeal joints each have a strong fibrous capsule that is composed of two cord-like collateral ligaments and a thickened volar component referred to as the volar plate (Fig. 10-1A). The second through fifth metacarpal heads are also stabilized in the coronal plane by deep transverse metacarpal ligaments. These ligaments extend along the

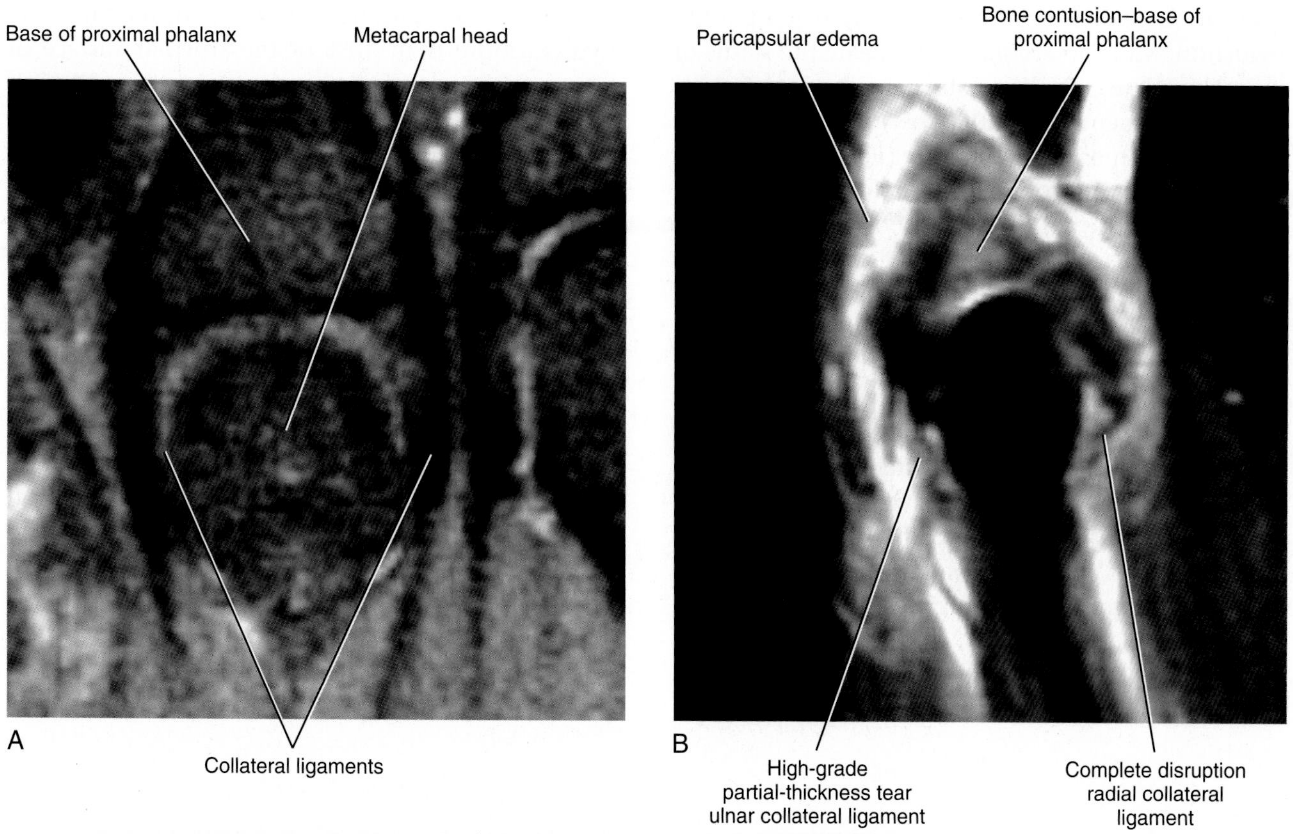
Base of proximal phalanx
Metacarpal head
A
Collateral ligaments
Pericapsular edema
Bone contusion–base of proximal phalanx
B
High-grade partial-thickness tear ulnar collateral ligament
Complete disruption radial collateral ligament

Figure 10-1 Metacarpophalangeal joint capsule. A, The normal capsule is composed of two cordlike collateral ligaments that are best demonstrated on T2-weighted coronal images. **B,** Coronal T2-weighted image of the fifth metacarpophalangeal joint demonstrates complete disruption of the proximal aspect of the radial collateral ligament and a high-grade partial-thickness tear of the ulnar collateral ligament. There is marked thickening of more distal fibers of the radial collateral ligament, and there is extensive adjacent soft tissue edema and a bone contusion involving the base of the proximal phalanx.

volar aspect of the metacarpophalangeal joints connecting the volar plates of adjacent metacarpophalangeal joints and have also been referred to as the "intervolar plate ligaments." The dorsal aspect of the joint is stabilized primarily by the extensor "hood" and the extensor tendon. This complex capsular anatomy provides tremendous stability at the level of the second through fifth metacarpophalangeal joints, and, as a result, complete dislocation at this level is uncommon.

Although full-blown medial or lateral dislocation of the metacarpophalangeal joint only rarely occurs, valgus or varus stress injuries can result in a sprain or disruption of the collateral ligaments. Injuries to the collateral ligaments are described either as a sprain (thickening of the collateral ligament with adjacent soft tissue edema) or as a partial- or full-thickness disruption (Fig. 10-1B). Acute injuries show extensive pericapsular soft tissue edema, whereas chronic injuries demonstrate thickening but lack the associated soft tissue edema. Bone contusions are often seen accompanying capsular injuries and usually result from the impaction of two bones at the time of injury. They may indicate subluxation or dislocation at the time of injury. Contusions may be accompanied by small cortical avulsion fractures, which occur at the level of attachment of the collateral ligament. Bone contusions are best depicted on fat-suppressed T2-weighted images, whereas avulsion fractures are best seen on T1-weighted images without fat saturation or gradient-echo images and may require evaluation with radiographs for detection.

Volar plate injury can result from a significant hyperextension injury or from either a dorsal or volar dislocation of the metacarpophalangeal joint. After reduction, MRI can accurately delineate the status of the volar plate, which usually remains intact at its distal attachment site, with most injuries occurring near the proximal attachment site (Fig. 10-2). Injuries range from a mild sprain to complete disruption or avulsion, and the volar plate may become entrapped within the metacarpophalangeal joint, resulting in an incomplete reduction or preventing full range of motion after reduction. Volar plate injuries are described as either a partial or complete disruption. Intra-articular entrapment of a portion of the volar plate should also be noted. Volar plate injuries of the metacarpophalangeal joint are often accompanied by a fracture of the volar aspect involving the articular surface at the base of the proximal phalanx, which typically occurs at the time of dorsal dislocation. The size of the fragment and the congruence of the articular surface should be described. A fracture that involves more than 50% of the articular surface or demonstrates significant articular surface step-off usually requires open reduction and fixation.

MR evaluation of the collateral ligaments is best performed in the coronal and axial imaging planes, whereas volar plate injuries are best detected on sagittal and axial images. A T2-weighted sequence with fat saturation or an STIR (short tau inversion recovery) sequence can aid in the detection of soft tissue edema, which often accompanies an acute injury. Use of a three-dimensional gradient-echo sequence allows visualization of these very small soft tissue structures, whereas T1-weighted images are very helpful in the evaluation of associated osseous abnormalities and in particular small avulsion fractures that often accompany volar plate and collateral ligament injuries.

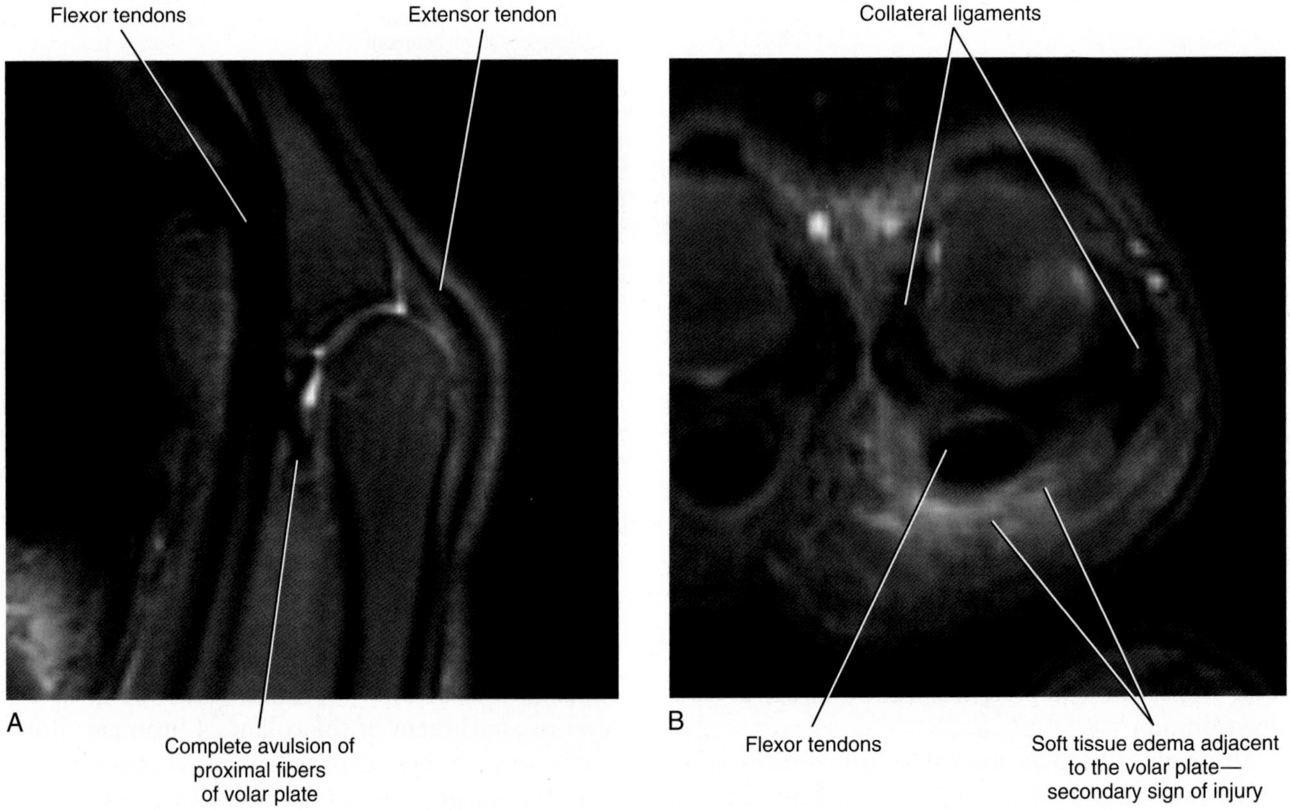
Flexor tendons
Extensor tendon
A
Complete avulsion of proximal fibers of volar plate
Collateral ligaments
B
Flexor tendons
Soft tissue edema adjacent to the volar plate—secondary sign of injury

Figure 10-2 Volar plate injury of metacarpophalangeal joint. A, Sagittal T2-weighted image shows complete avulsion of the proximal fibers of the volar plate from its normal attachment site on the metacarpal neck. **B,** Axial T2-weighted images are often helpful because they demonstrate soft tissue edema located along the volar aspect of the involved joint.

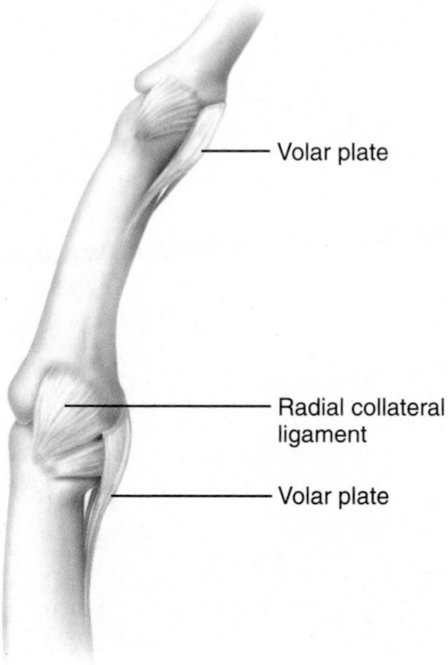
Volar plate
Radial collateral ligament
Volar plate

Figure 10-3 Normal anatomy of the volar plate shown in the lateral projection. The distal aspect of the volar plate is thick and attaches tightly to the base of the more distal phalanx while thin periscoping ligamentous-like attachments extend approximately 1 cm proximal to the interphalangeal joint.

Interphalangeal Joint

The capsular anatomy of the interphalangeal joint is very similar to that of the metacarpophalangeal joint. There is a strong fibrous capsule that is composed of medial and lateral collateral ligaments and a strong thickened volar component referred to as the volar plate (Figs. 10-3 and 10-4). The extensor apparatus including the extensor tendon and its numerous attachments provides the major support along the dorsal aspect of the interphalangeal joint.

Collateral ligament injuries result from excessive valgus or varus force and are described as a sprain, seen as capsular thickening and adjacent edema, or as a partial- or full-thickness tear or avulsion. Small avulsion fractures can occur at either the proximal or the distal attachment site (Fig. 10-5).

Dorsal dislocation of an interphalangeal joint is such a common injury across the entire array of athletic pursuits that it has been referred to as "coach's finger." Dorsal dislocations occur most commonly at the level of the proximal interphalangeal joint but also occur at the distal interphalangeal joint (Fig. 10-6). Dorsal dislocation can result in an injury to the volar plate and is often associated with a fracture of the volar aspect of the base of the dislocated

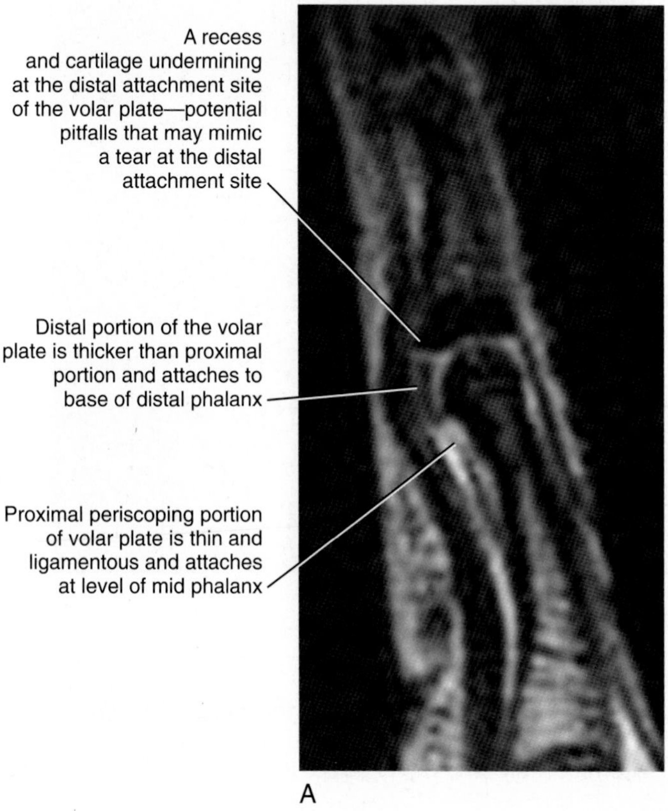
A recess and cartilage undermining at the distal attachment site of the volar plate—potential pitfalls that may mimic a tear at the distal attachment site
Distal portion of the volar plate is thicker than proximal portion and attaches to base of distal phalanx
Proximal periscoping portion of volar plate is thin and ligamentous and attaches at level of mid phalanx
A

Figure 10-4 Normal capsular anatomy of the interphalangeal joints. A, Sagittal T2-weighted image shows the volar plate, a thickening of the capsule along the volar aspect of the joint that sits deep to the flexor tendon. The distal aspect of the volar plate is thick and attaches tightly to the base of the distal phalanx. The volar plate has thin periscoping ligamentous-like attachments approximately 1 cm proximal to the joint. A distal recess is present, which compresses in flexion. This recess combined with cartilage undermining is a potential pitfall that may mimic a tear of the distal attachment of the volar plate. *Continued*

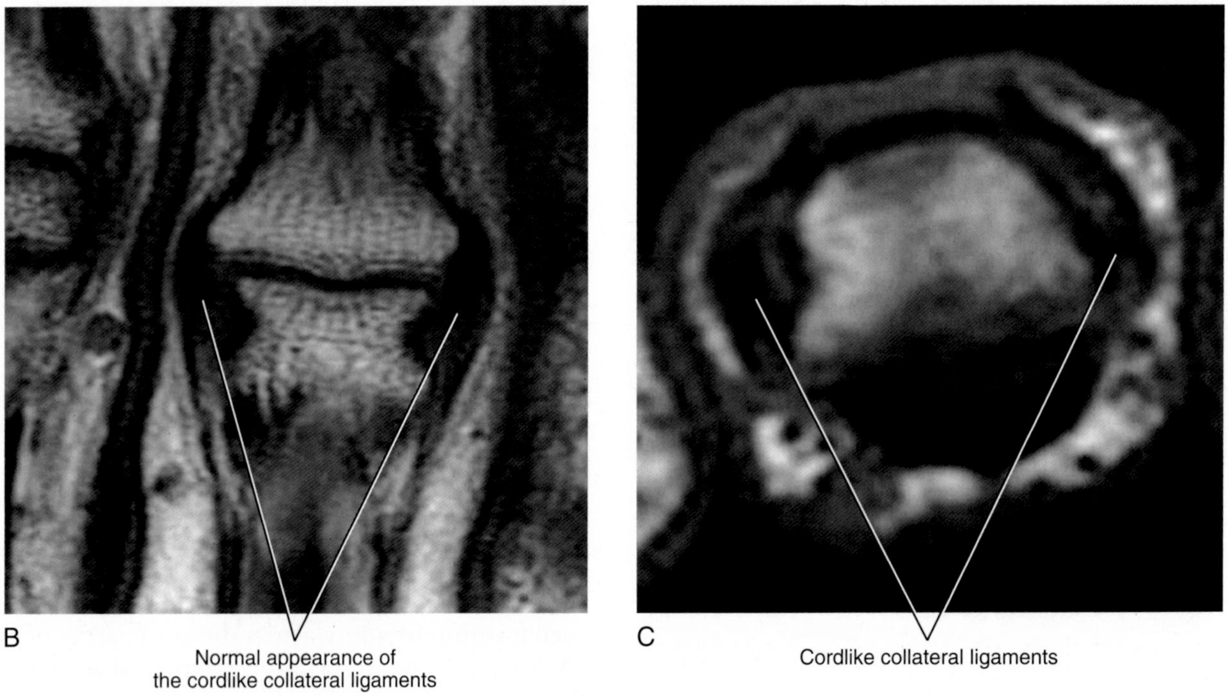
B
Normal appearance of
the cordlike collateral ligaments
C
Cordlike collateral ligaments

Figure 10-4, cont'd Coronal (**B**) and axial (**C**) T2-weighted images demonstrate the normal appearance of the cordlike collateral ligaments.

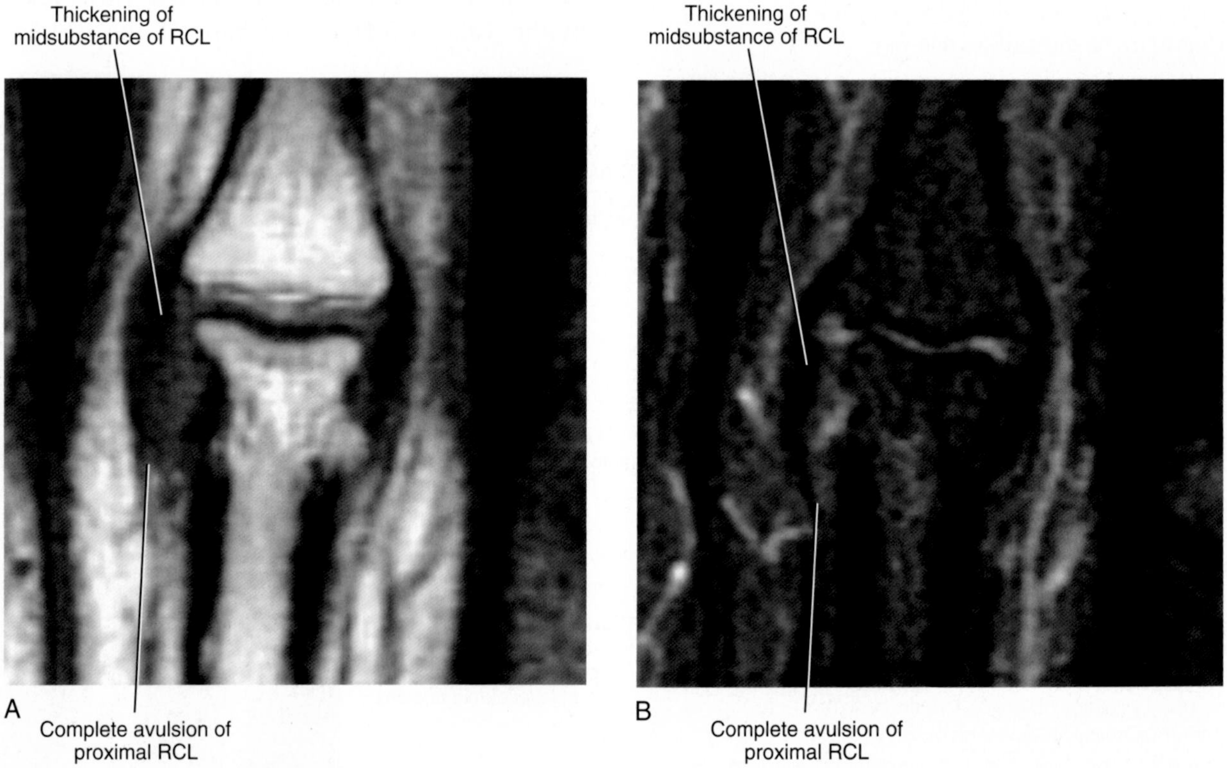
Thickening of
midsubstance of RCL
A
Complete avulsion of
proximal RCL
Thickening of
midsubstance of RCL
B
Complete avulsion of
proximal RCL

Figure 10-5 **Interphalangeal joint capsular injury.** Coronal T1-weighted (**A**) and T2-weighted (**B**) images show mild thickening of the midsubstance of the radial collateral ligament (RCL) with a complete avulsion at its proximal attachment site. The lack of adjacent soft tissue edema indicates that this injury is either subacute or chronic.

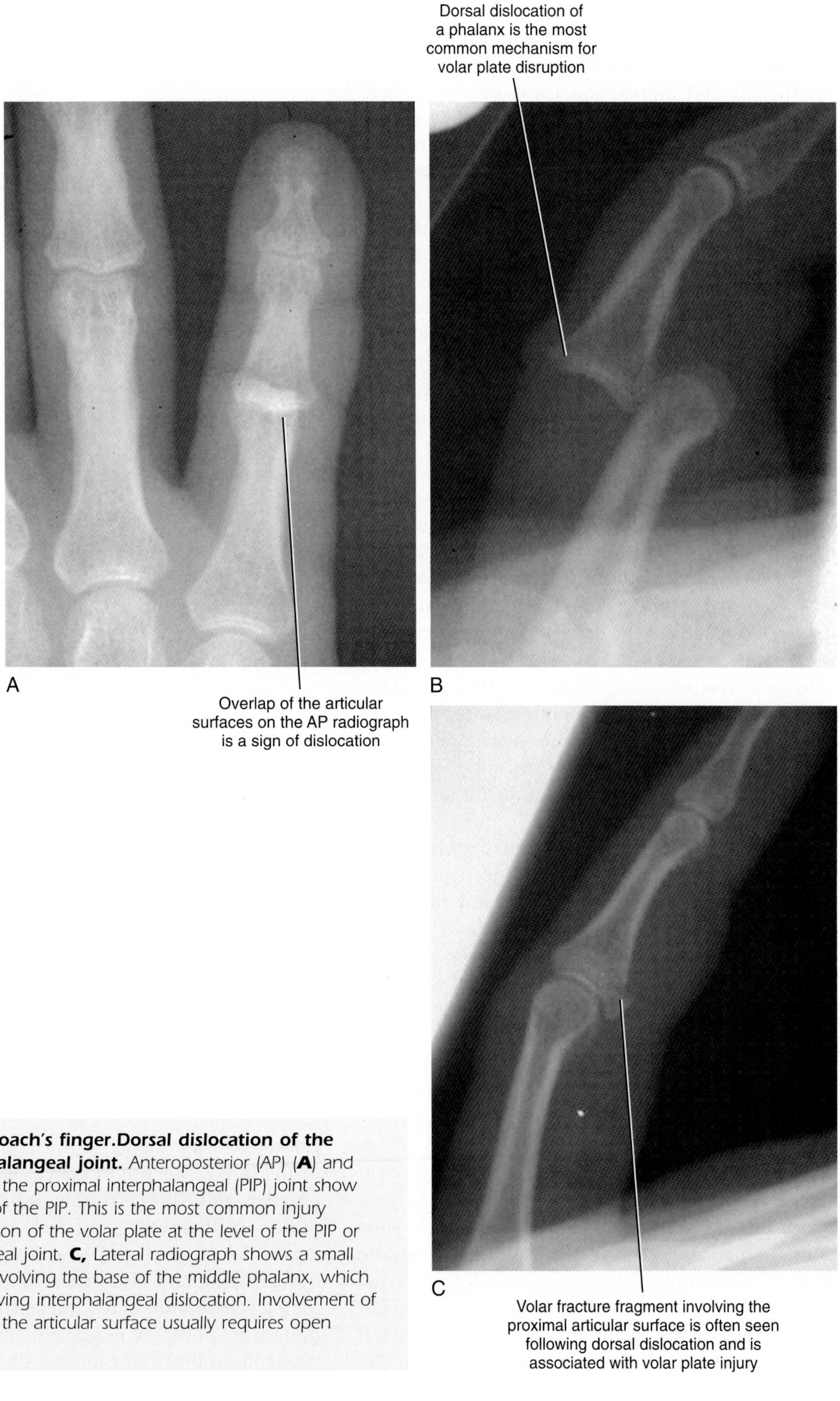
Dorsal dislocation of a phalanx is the most common mechanism for volar plate disruption
A
B
Overlap of the articular surfaces on the AP radiograph is a sign of dislocation
C
Volar fracture fragment involving the proximal articular surface is often seen following dorsal dislocation and is associated with volar plate injury

Figure 10-6 Coach's finger.Dorsal dislocation of the proximal interphalangeal joint. Anteroposterior (AP) (**A**) and lateral (**B**) views of the proximal interphalangeal (PIP) joint show dorsal dislocation of the PIP. This is the most common injury resulting in disruption of the volar plate at the level of the PIP or distal interphalangeal joint. **C,** Lateral radiograph shows a small avulsion fracture involving the base of the middle phalanx, which may be seen following interphalangeal dislocation. Involvement of more than 50% of the articular surface usually requires open fixation.

phalanx (Fig. 10-6C). Fractures/dislocations are usually treated with dorsal splinting, with the interphalangeal joint in mild flexion to allow healing of the fracture and injured soft tissue structures. Fractures that involve more than 50% of the articular surface of the base of the dislocated phalanx are considered unstable and require open fixation.

MRI of the interphalangeal joints is performed in a similar manner as previously described for the metacarpophalangeal joints, with coronal and axial imaging planes best suited for the evaluation of the collateral ligaments and sagittal and axial imaging planes best suited for evaluation of the volar plate injuries. In addition to a description of the extent of soft tissue injury, it is important to search for adjacent osseous injuries and to describe avulsion fractures or involvement of the adjacent articular surface.

Flexor Tendons and Pulley System

Flexion of the digits is accomplished by a complex system of muscles, tendons, pulleys, and vincula. A basic knowledge of this complex anatomy is crucial if one is to adequately describe injuries involving these structures. The flexor pollicis longus tendon exits the carpal tunnel at the level of the base of the first metacarpal and passes obliquely between the opponens pollicis and the oblique head of the adductor pollicis, enters a synovial sheath, and then inserts on the volar aspect of the base of the distal phalanx of the thumb.

Flexion of the second through fifth digits is accomplished by the combined action of two tendons, the flexor digitorum superficialis (FDS) and the flexor digitorum profundus (FDP). The two flexor tendons travel together with the FDP tendon located just deep to the FDS tendon as they exit the carpal tunnel at the level of the wrist and enter the hand. The tendons then enter a common digital flexor tendon sheath at the level of the metacarpophalangeal joint. Prior to the level of the proximal interphalangeal joint, the flexor superficialis tendon splits into two slips and allows passage of the flexor profundus tendon, which becomes superficial at this level. The separate tendon slips of the superficialis tendon then reunite deep to the profundus and insert as radial and ulnar slips onto the palmar aspect of the base of the middle phalanx. This normal splitting and reuniting or decussation of the FDS tendon to allow passage of the FDP tendon has been referred to as the *camper's chiasm* (Fig. 10-7). After passing through the decussation, the FDP tendon continues distally to attach on the base of the distal phalanx. This anatomic configuration allows the FDS tendon to control flexion of the proximal interphalangeal joint, while the FDP tendon controls flexion at the level of the distal interphalangeal joint (Fig. 10-8).

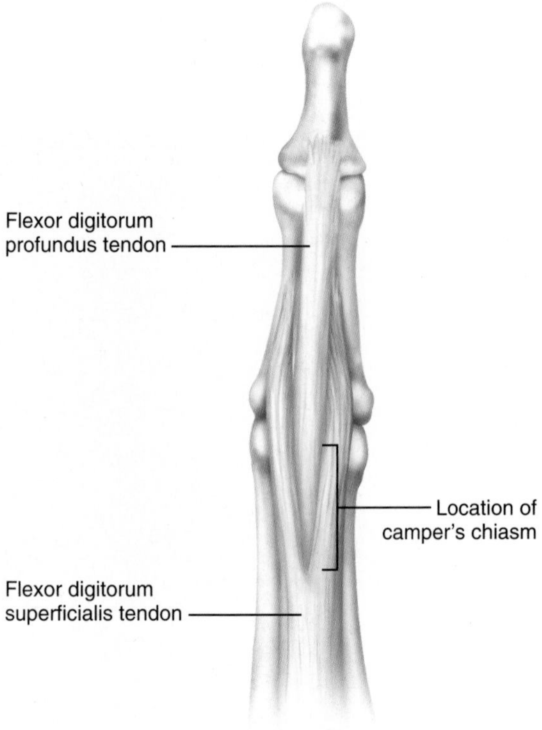
Flexor digitorum profundus tendon
Location of camper's chiasm
Flexor digitorum superficialis tendon

Figure 10-7 Flexor tendon anatomy. Decussation or splitting of the flexor digitorum superficialis tendon (camper's chiasm) at the level of the proximal interphalangeal joint allows passage of the flexor digitorum profundus tendon, which continues on to attach on the base of the distal phalanx.

A complex system of fibrous bands or retinacular sheaths, referred to as "pulleys" is responsible for maintaining the proper position of the flexor tendons firmly against the volar aspect of the phalanges and prevents "bowstringing" of the tendons during flexion of the finger. The pulley system is composed of five annular and three cruciate pulleys. The annular pulleys (primarily A2 and A4) are vital for normal digital function (Fig. 10-9). They prevent tendon bowstringing and also ensure optimal joint flexion for a given amount of tendon excursion. The cruciate pulleys are primarily responsible for maintaining the proper flexibility of the tendon sheath, thus allowing

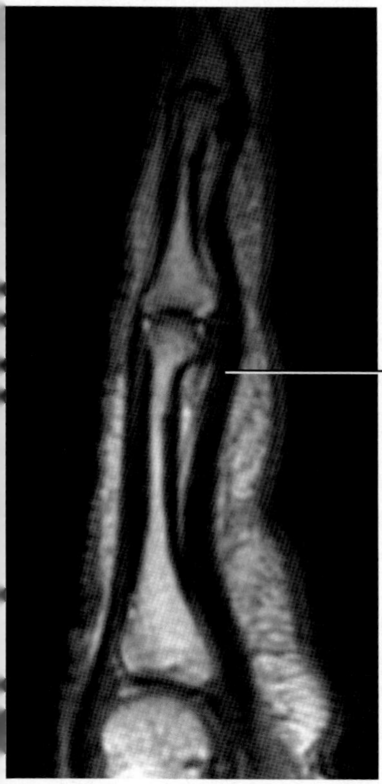
The FDP and FDS tendons share a common tendon sheath beyond the level of the MCP joint and are indistinguishable from one another at this level in the sagittal imaging plane
A

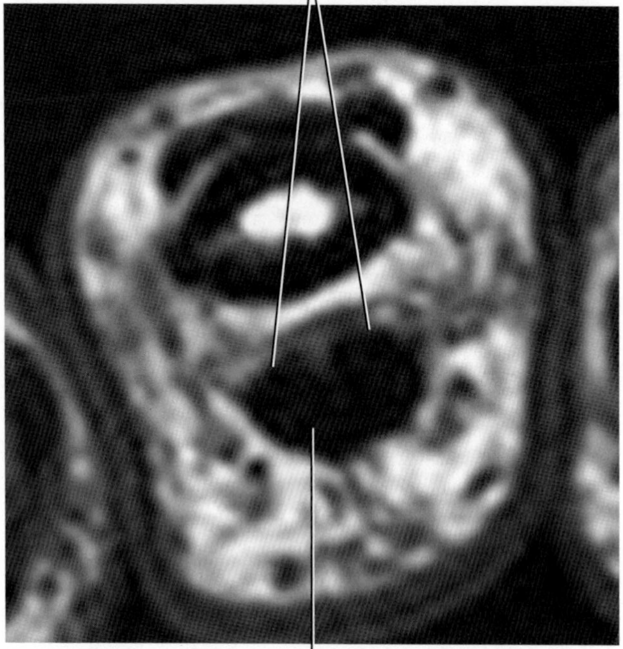
Just beyond the level of the PIP joint, this axial image clearly demonstrates the separate slips of the FDS tendon allowing passage of the FDP tendon
B
At this level, the FDP tendon has passed between the separate slips of the split FDS tendon and the FDP is located superficial to the split FDS tendon

Figure 10-8 Flexor tendon anatomy at the level of the proximal interphalangeal (PIP) joint. The normal anatomy of the flexor tendons. The flexor digitorum superficialis (FDS) and the flexor digitorum profundus (FDP) tendons are indistinguishable from one another in the sagittal imaging plane (**A**) whereas the axial imaging plane (**B**) nicely demonstrates the separate FDS tendon slips, allowing passage of the FDP tendon at the level of the PIP joint. MCP, metacarpophalangeal.

the sheath to conform to the various shapes required for normal digital flexion. The cruciate pulleys also allow access of the digital arteries, which provide the tendon blood supply (Fig. 10-10).

The vinculum system is an arrangement of triangular fibrous bands that extend from the dorsal surface of the flexor tendons of the digit to the nearby capsule of the interphalangeal joint and the adjacent phalanx. These fibrous bands are located just proximal to the insertion of the tendon to the underlying bone and are responsible for conveying small vessels to the tendons. The vinculum breve superficialis provides the blood supply for the FDS at the level of the proximal interphalangeal joint, whereas the vinculum breve profundus provides the blood supply for the FDP at the level of the distal interphalangeal joint.

The range of abnormalities involving the flexor tendons includes tenosynovitis of the tendon sheath, which may be sterile or infectious. Sterile tenosynovitis often results from repetitive trauma or can be associated with inflammatory arthropathies such as rheumatoid arthritis. Infectious tenosynovitis is most commonly bacterial in origin but may result from an atypical infectious agent such as mycobacterium. Infectious tenosynovitis is most often associated with a history of penetrating trauma, usually a punch to the mouth. Tendinopathy represents a degenerative process of the tendon that may be age-related or may result from repetitive trauma. Finally, a partial- or full-thickness tear of the tendon may occur. Flexor tendon tears most commonly result from a laceration. Closed tears, though less common, have been shown to be associated with rheumatoid arthritis,

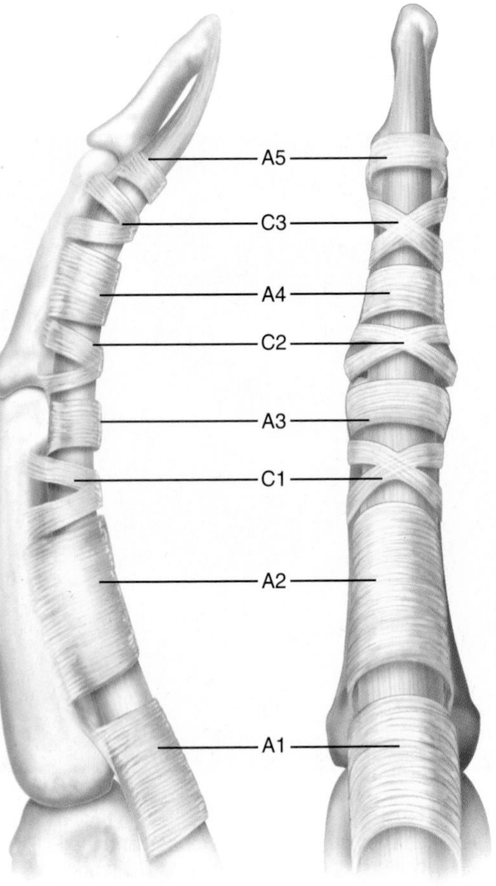
A5
C3
A4
C2
A3
C1
A2
A1

Figure 10-9 Normal anatomy of the flexor tendon pulley system.

osteoarthritis, scaphoid nonunion, Kienböck disease, hook-of-the-hamate fracture, and carpal dislocation. Closed flexor tendon injuries can also result from sudden extension of a flexed joint, and these injuries are commonly seen in rugby and football participants.

Flexor tendon tear or avulsion has been referred to as "jersey finger" because the closed injury often occurs when a player catches his or her finger on an opponent's jersey resulting in forced hyperextension of an actively flexed finger. The most common pattern of injury is an isolated tear of the FDP, followed by a combined tear of the FDP and FDS; the least common injury is an isolated tear of the FDS tendon. Avulsion injuries of the tendon may be associated with an avulsion fracture, and contraction of the flexor muscle can result in proximal displacement of the osseous fragment. Occasionally, an avulsed osseous fragment arising from the base of the distal phalanx is significantly displaced, sometimes to the level of the proximal interphalangeal joint. As a result, this displacement may mimic an avulsion fracture arising from the base of the middle phalanx.

On MRI, tenosynovitis manifests as fluid contained within the tendon sheath and a peritendinous edema of the involved tendon, and it is best demonstrated on axial T2-weighted images (Fig. 10-11). The tendon maintains normal morphology and intrinsic signal. Tenosynovitis may involve a single or multiple adjacent tendon sheaths and is typically graded as mild, moderate, or severe based on the quantity of fluid within the sheath. Ultrasound also demonstrates thickening of the sheath and fluid within the sheath, and power Doppler demonstrates increased flow and hyperemia of the surrounding soft tissues (Fig. 10-12) Tendinopathy appears as thickening and increased intrinsic signal within the tendon on both T1- and T2-weighted images and is usually best demonstrated on axial and sagittal images.

Trigger finger describes a specific subgroup of tendinopathy in which the tendon develops a focal area of thickening (tendinopathy) that catches on the surrounding sheath during flexion and extension of the digit, thus preventing full range of motion. MRI shows a focal area of tendon thickening, which is often palpable on physical examination. Complex fluid is often noted within the adjacent tendon sheath. Initial treatment may involve injection of the sheath with steroids. If this fails, a surgical release of the sheath can be performed to try to allow the tendon to once again glide smoothly within the tendon sheath. A partial-thickness tear appears as a focal area of thinning or attenuation, or a partial-thickness defect of the tendon and MRI may demonstrate fluid signal on the T2-weighted images extending partially through the thickness of the tendon. A full-thickness tear is seen as a complete disruption with retraction of the ends of the torn tendon (Fig. 10-13).

A complete description of tendon tears on MR imaging should include the following information (Table 10-1): the location of the tear, the length of the gap or retraction of the tendon ends (describe the exact location of the proximal and distal ends of the tendon), and a description of the integrity of the adjacent tendons (Fig. 10-14). The location of the tear is described in relation to the adjacent osseous structures (at the level of the metacarpal phalangeal joint, at the level of the mid-shaft of the proximal phalanx, and so on). The exact location of both ends of the

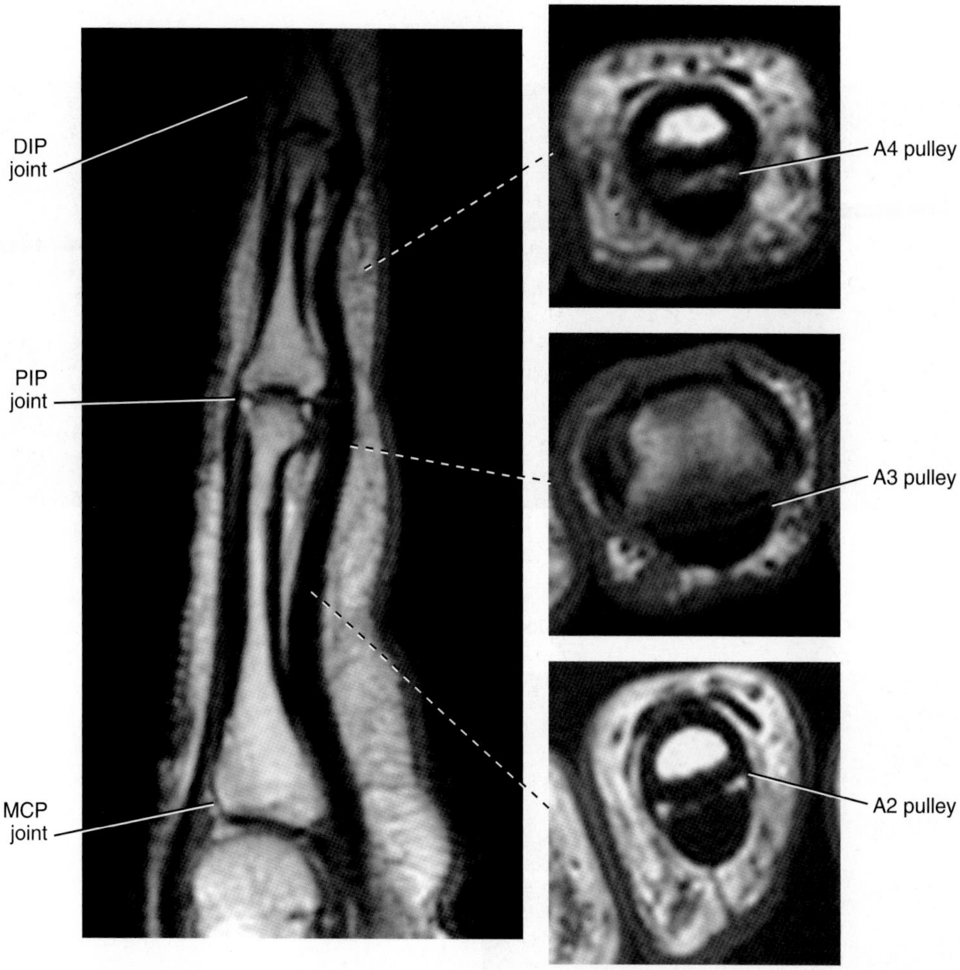
DIP
joint
PIP
joint
MCP
joint
A4 pulley
A3 pulley
A2 pulley

Figure 10-10 MR appearance of the flexor tendon pulley system. Sagittal and axial images show the normal MR appearance of the flexor tendons, their supporting pulley mechanism, and the relation of one to the other at the various levels. DIP, distal interphalangeal; MCP, metacarpophalangeal; PIP, proximal interphalangeal.

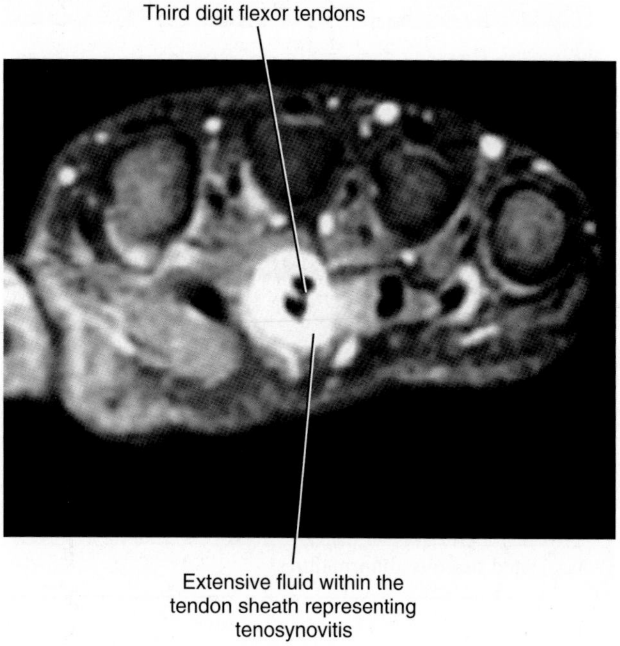
Third digit flexor tendons
Extensive fluid within the tendon sheath representing tenosynovitis

Figure 10-11 Tenosynovitis of the flexor tendon sheath. Axial T2-weighted image of the hand demonstrates extensive fluid within the flexor tendon sheath of the third digit with mild surrounding soft tissue edema consistent with tenosynovitis of the flexor tendon sheath.

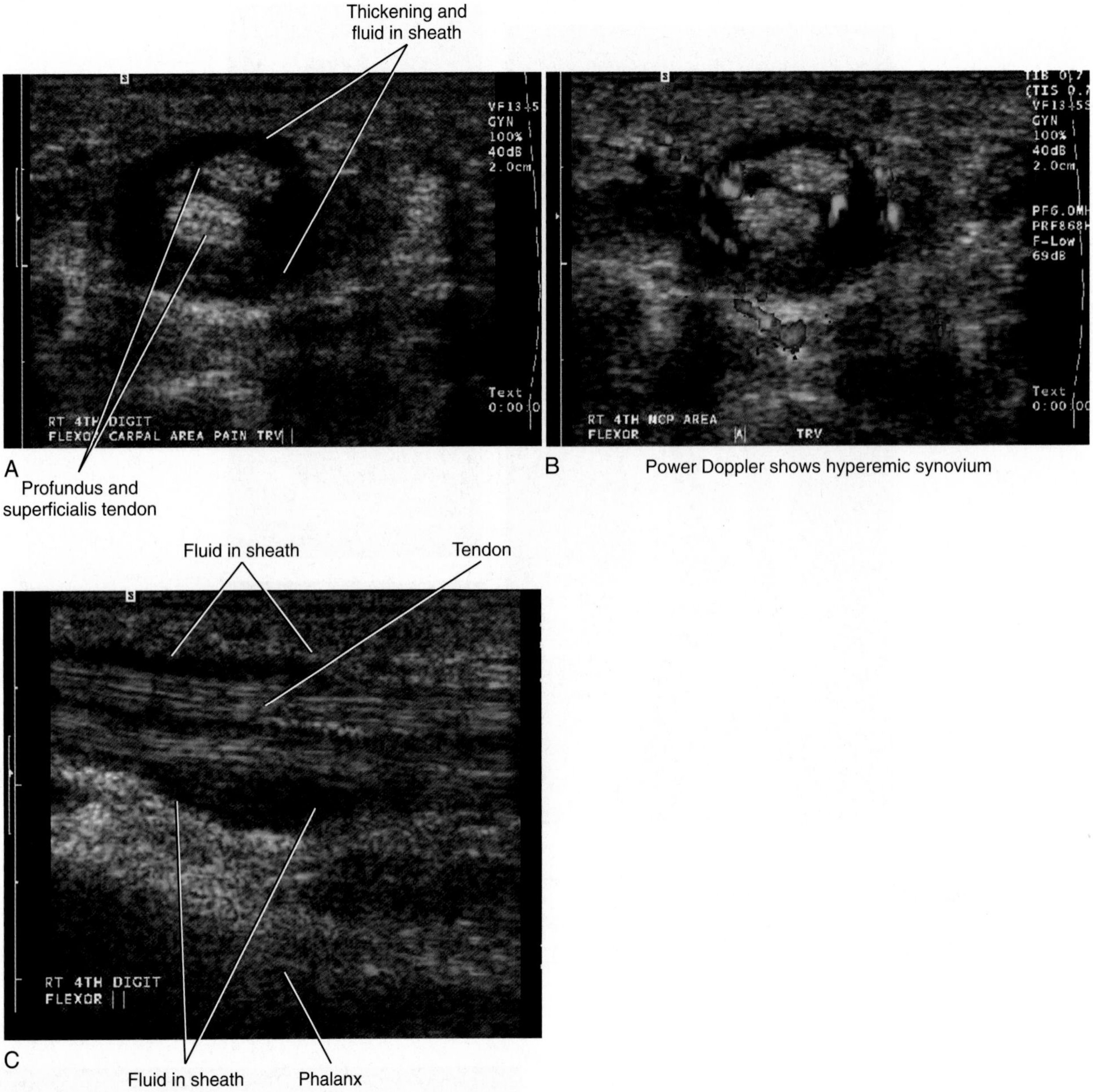
Thickening and fluid in sheath
RT 4TH DIGIT
FLEXOR CARPAL AREA PAIN TRV
A
Profundus and superficialis tendon
RT 4TH MCP AREA
FLEXOR
TRV
B
Power Doppler shows hyperemic synovium
Fluid in sheath
Tendon
RT 4TH DIGIT
FLEXOR
C
Fluid in sheath
Phalanx

Figure 10-12 Ultrasound findings of tenosynovitis of the flexor tendon sheath in the transverse (**A** and **B**) and sagittal (**C**) planes.

Table 10-1 Description of Tendon Tears on MRI

Extent of tear	Complete versus incomplete tear
Location of tear (exact location of both ends of the torn tendon)	Based on adjacent anatomy (at the level of the metacarpophalangeal joint; proximal interphalangeal joint, etc)
Length of gap	Describe in centimeters
Description of tendon ends	Smooth, frayed, irregular, etc
Integrity of adjacent tendons	Multiple tendon tears
Associated soft tissue injuries	Volar plate, capsular ligaments
Associated osseous abnormalities	Avulsion fracture: Size, location, articular surface involvement

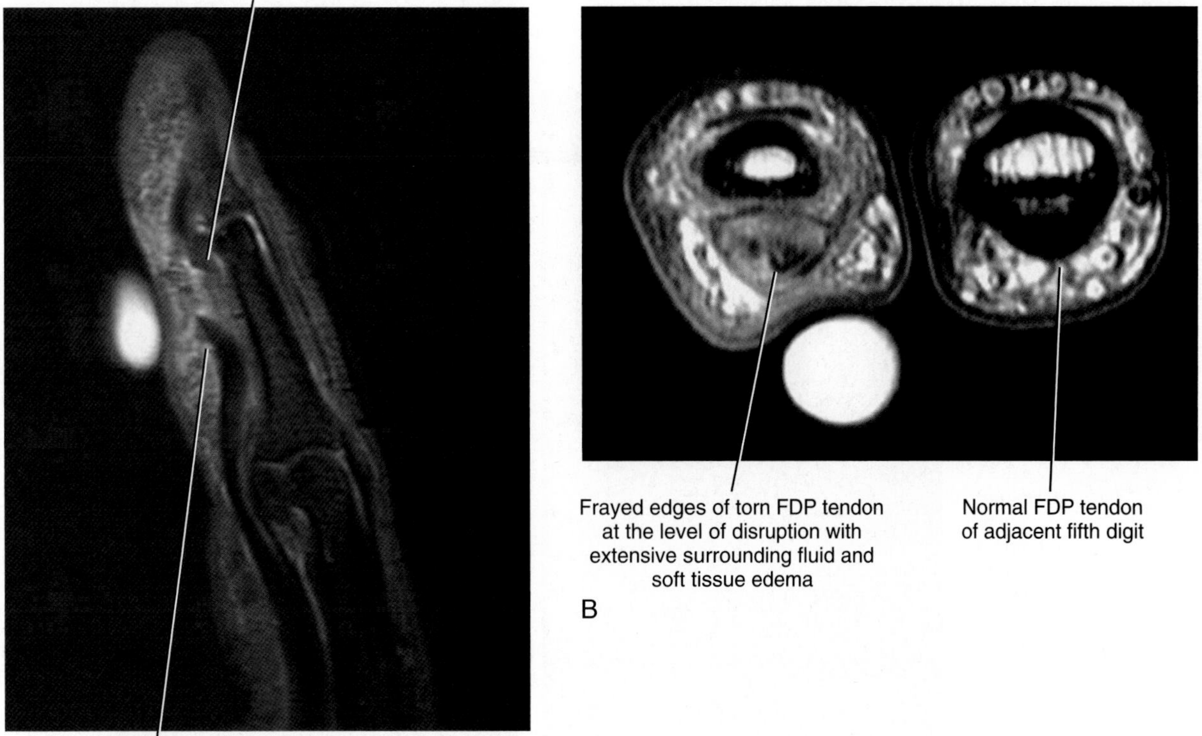
Distal end of torn FDS tendon
Retracted proximal end of torn FDP tendon with a 1-cm gap between torn tendon ends
A
Frayed edges of torn FDP tendon at the level of disruption with extensive surrounding fluid and soft tissue edema
Normal FDP tendon of adjacent fifth digit
B

Figure 10-13 Flexor digitorum profundis (FDP) tendon disruption at the level of the distal interphalangeal (DIP) joint. A, Sagittal T2-weighted image demonstrates complete disruption of the FDP tendon of the fourth digit at the level of the DIP joint with 1 cm of retraction of the proximal tendon end. **B,** Axial T1-weighted image shows edema and the torn tendon ends within the flexor tendon sheath.

torn tendon provides an important road map for the surgeon to minimize the extent of incision at the time of repair. The length of the gap between torn tendon ends is important to describe because a gap of more than 30 mm usually requires a tendon graft rather than a direct repair. Finally, associated fractures and other soft tissue injuries (volar plate and capsule) should be described.

Injuries isolated to the flexor tendon pulley mechanism are referred to as *rock climber's injury* and are often seen in rock climbers as a result of forced extension of the flexed finger. The tendon remains intact, but the supporting retinacular bands disrupt, resulting in bowstringing of the flexor tendons. The injury most commonly occurs at the A2 level, and progression occurs in a predictable pattern involving, in sequence, the A2-A3-A4, and rarely, the A1 pulley (Fig. 10-15). The A2 and A4 pulleys are the most crucial with regard to normal digital function and are responsible for preventing bowstringing of the tendons as well as for providing optimal joint flexion for a given amount of tendon excursion. The A3 and A5 pulleys are relatively insignificant with regard to tendon function, and the A3 pulley is often lysed at the time of surgery. Dynamic ultrasound imaging can nicely depict bowstringing of the flexor tendon during flexion of the involved digit following disruption of the pulley mechanism (Fig. 10-16).

Extensor Tendons

Each digit is typically supplied by a single extensor digitorum tendon unlike the flexor compartment of the second through fifth digits, which has two flexor

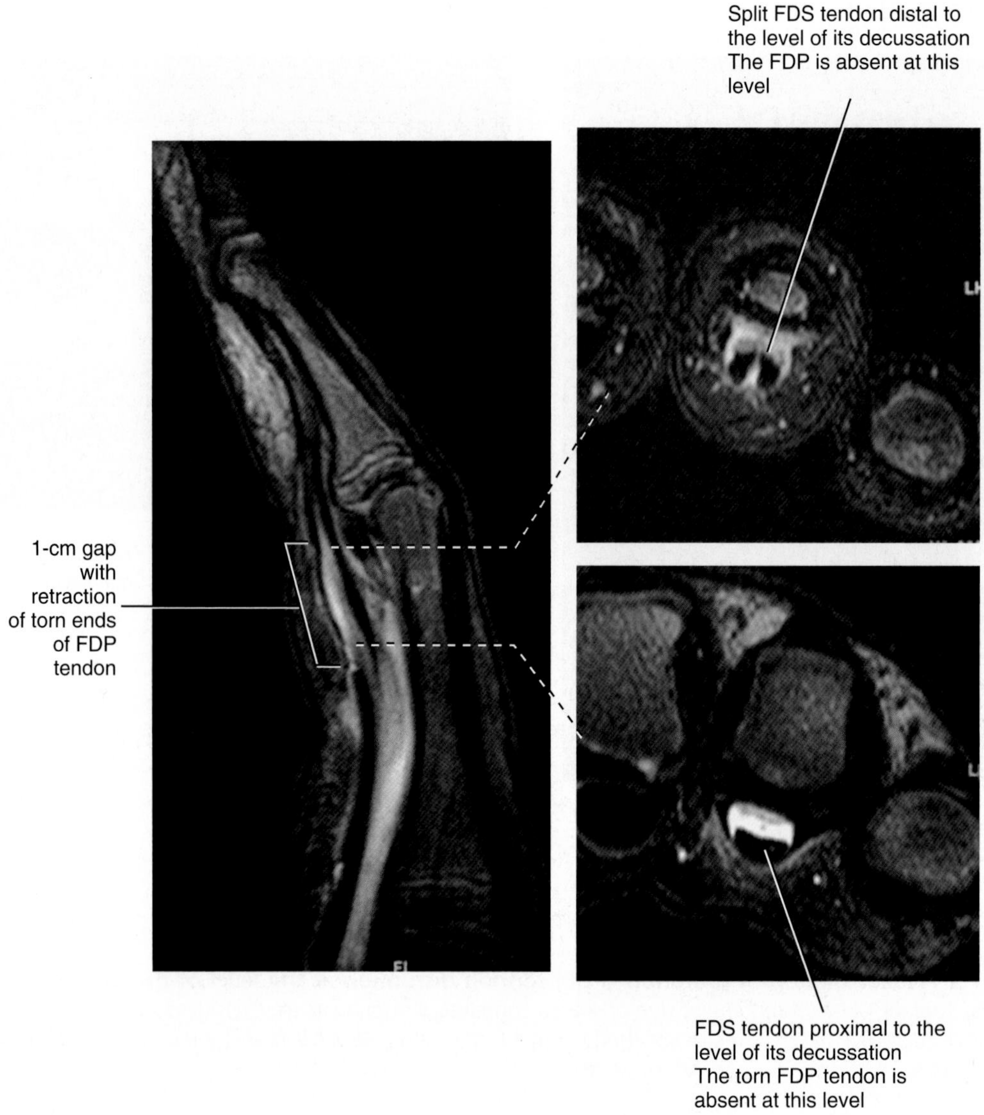
Split FDS tendon distal to the level of its decussation The FDP is absent at this level
1-cm gap with retraction of torn ends of FDP tendon
FDS tendon proximal to the level of its decussation The torn FDP tendon is absent at this level

Figure 10-14 Flexor digitorum profundus (FDP) tendon disruption. Sagittal T2-weighted image shows complete disruption of the FDP tendon at the level of the proximal interphalangeal joint with approximately a 1-cm gap between the torn tendon ends. The axial images show the FDS tendon to be intact with fluid present in the expected location of the FDP. The more distal axial T2-weighted image shows the normal splitting of the FDS. Normally, the FDP would pass through this split, but in this patient it is torn and retracted and not present at this level.

tendons. Anatomic variations of the extensor digitorum tendon anatomy may occur, such as a congenital absence of the tendon or more commonly two or even three separate extensor tendon slips to a single digit. The distal attachments of the extensor digitorum tendon are variable but typically include insertions along the dorsal aspect of the digit at the level of the metacarpophalangeal, distal interphalangeal, and proximal interphalangeal joints via slips that attach to the adjacent joint capsule and collateral ligaments (Fig. 10-17). The extensor hood is a fibrous expansion at the level of the metacarpophalangeal joint responsible for maintaining proper position of the extensor tendon in the coronal plane.

Injury patterns of extensor tendons are similar to the flexor tendons, with tenosynovitis, tendinopathy, and partial- and full-thickness tears all occurring. Tears of the extensor tendon usually result from a laceration or penetrating injury. A complete tear of the extensor digitorum tendon at the level of the distal interphalangeal joint leads to a *mallet finger deformity,* resulting from unopposed flexion at the

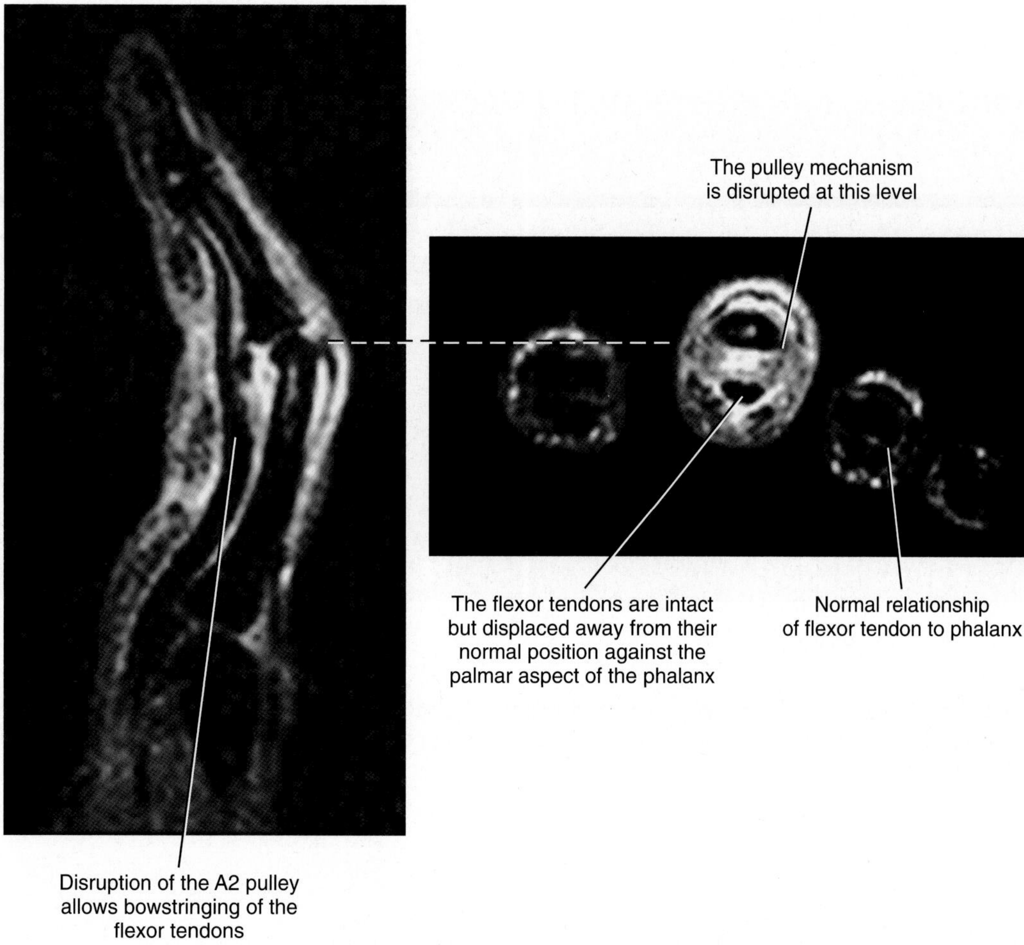
The pulley mechanism
is disrupted at this level
The flexor tendons are intact
but displaced away from their
normal position against the
palmar aspect of the phalanx
Normal relationship
of flexor tendon to phalanx
Disruption of the A2 pulley
allows bowstringing of the
flexor tendons

Figure 10-15 Isolated pulley injury. Sagittal and axial T2-weighted images demonstrate bowstringing of the flexor tendons at the level of the mid proximal phalanx and at the level of the proximal interphalangeal joint with surrounding soft tissue edema. This indicates isolated disruption of the A2 and A3 pulleys. The axial T2-weighted image shows the flexor tendon to be displaced away from the underlying phalanx with surrounding edema. Normally, the flexor tendon sits immediately adjacent to the flexor tendon as seen in the adjacent fingers. This finding on the axial image indicates disruption of the pulley mechanism.

level of the distal interphalangeal joint. A tear at the level of the proximal interphalangeal joint results in unopposed flexion at the level of the proximal interphalangeal joint and leads to the *swan neck deformity*. Avulsion injuries of the tendon may be associated with small avulsion fractures. Partial-thickness tears are usually treated with splinting of the digit, whereas complete tears are repaired surgically.

The extensor tendon is smaller in caliber than the flexor tendon, and high-quality well-positioned sagittal MR images are crucial for adequate visualization on MRI. As in flexor tendon tears, it is important to describe the injury as a partial- or full-thickness disruption of the tendon. For example, when a full-thickness tear is present, an exact description of the location of the proximal and distal ends of the torn extensor tendon, the length of the gap, and complete evaluation of the adjacent extensor tendons are mandatory for adequate surgical planning (Fig. 10-18). The presence of an avulsion fracture fragment should also be described.

Extensor hood disruption may occur as a complication of rheumatoid arthritis or in the setting of trauma usually as a result of punching an object with a closed fist. Tears most often involve the radial band of the extensor hood resulting in ulnar subluxation of the tendon, which is accentuated with flexion of the metacarpophalangeal joint. MR imaging demonstrates edema overlying the dorsal aspect of the metacarpophalangeal joint and subluxation of the extensor

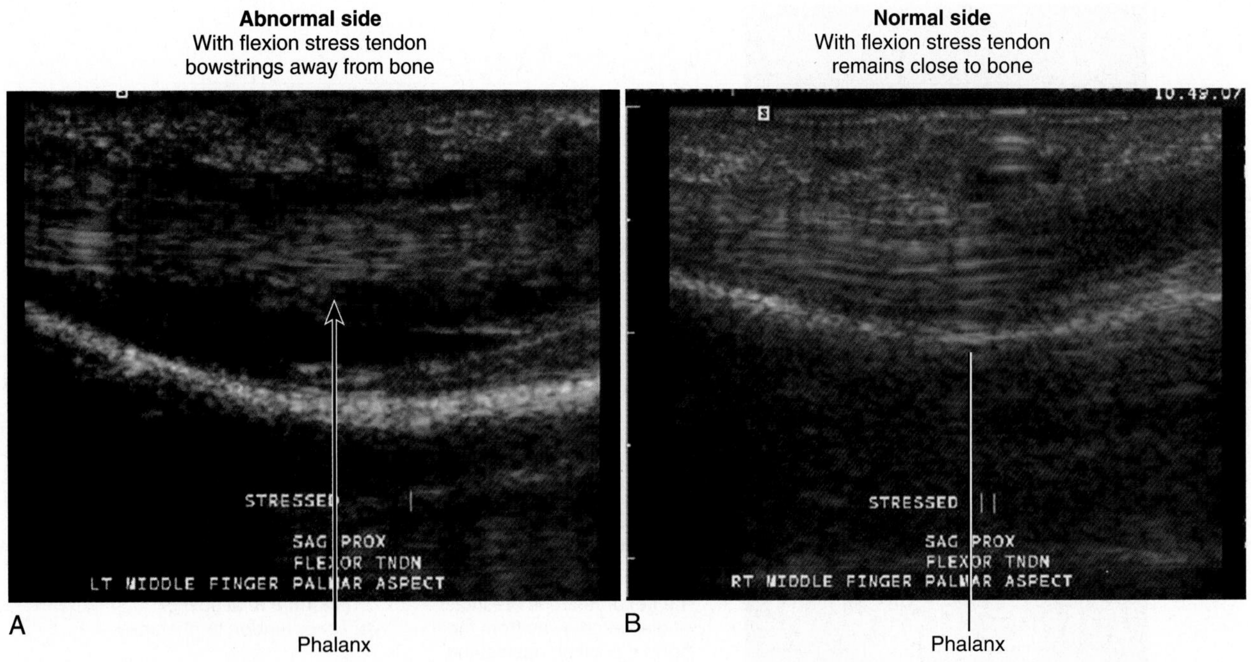
Abnormal side
With flexion stress tendon bowstrings away from bone
Normal side
With flexion stress tendon remains close to bone
STRESSED
SAG PROX
FLEXOR TNDN
LT MIDDLE FINGER PALMAR ASPECT
RT MIDDLE FINGER PALMAR ASPECT
A
B
Phalanx
Phalanx

Figure 10-16 **A,** Dynamic ultrasound with flexion stress imaging demonstrates bowstringing of the flexor tendon indicating disruption of the third finger A2 pulley rupture. **B,** Imaging of the normal side demonstrates normal positioning of the flexor tendon during stress imaging.

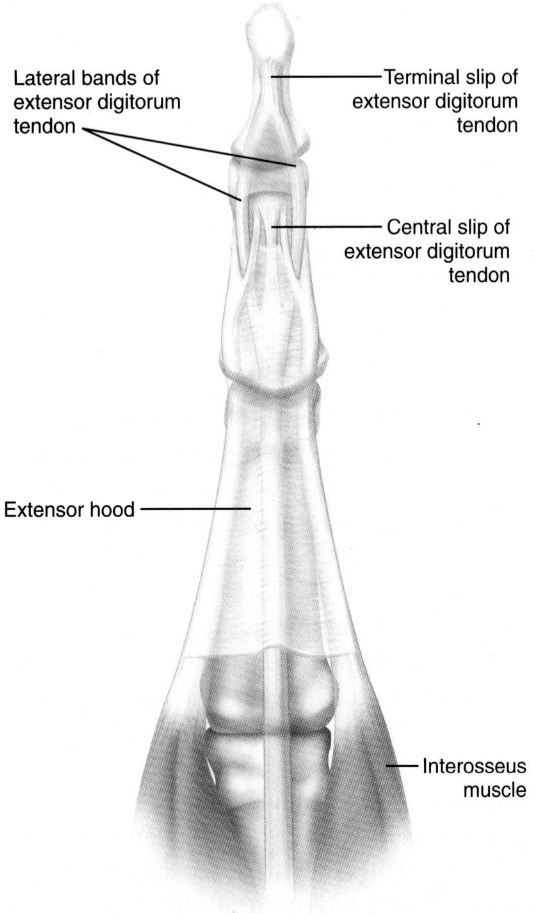
Lateral bands of extensor digitorum tendon
Terminal slip of extensor digitorum tendon
Central slip of extensor digitorum tendon
Extensor hood
Interosseus muscle

Figure 10-17 **Anatomy of the extensor tendon attachment.** Complex attachments are responsible for stabilizing the extensor tendon at the level of the proximal interphalangeal and distal interphalangeal joints.

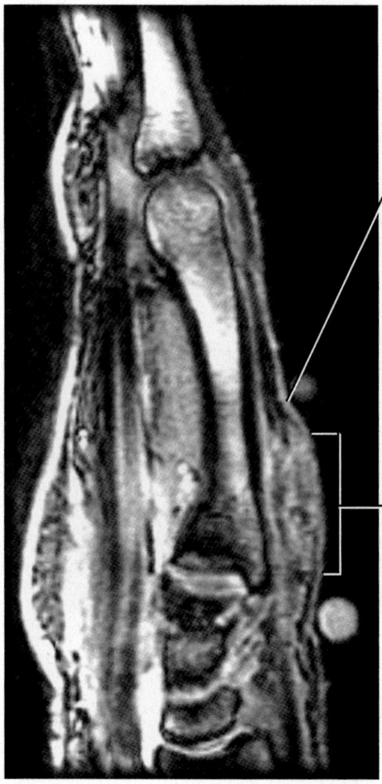
Distal end of torn extensor tendon demonstrates fraying and irregularity
2-cm gap between torn tendon ends

Figure 10-18 Extensor tendon disruption. Sagittal T2-weighted image shows complete disruption of the extensor tendon of the long finger at the level of the mid metacarpal shaft.

tendon. Subluxation of the extensor tendon results in the tendon moving out of the plane on the sagittal images and may mimic a tear or disruption of the tendon. Axial images demonstrate an intact extensor tendon that is subluxed most often in the ulnar direction (Fig. 10-19).

SOFT TISSUE ANATOMY AND INJURY PATTERNS OF THE THUMB

Although the anatomy and injury patterns are similar when comparing the thumb with the other digits, enough variation exists to warrant a separate discussion. The unprotected position of the thumb puts the first metacarpophalangeal joint at much greater risk for injury than the second through fifth metacarpophalangeal joints. Stability against valgus and varus stress at this level is provided primarily by the proper radial and ulnar collateral ligaments. Like the other metacarpophalangeal joints, the volar portion of the first metacarpophalangeal joint capsule is stabilized by a thickened volar plate. Stabilization along the extensor surface is provided by the extensor pollicis longus tendon and its capsular attachments. The interphalangeal joint is also stabilized by radial and ulnar collateral ligaments and a strong volar plate. The flexor pollicis longus tendon inserts onto the volar aspect of the base of the distal phalanx, and the extensor pollicis longus inserts dorsally at this same level. The flexor tendon pulley system is similar to that of the other digits; however, the thumb has only three annular pulleys responsible for stabilizing the position of the flexor tendon.

Ulnar Collateral Ligament Injury (Gamekeeper's Thumb)

Disruption of the ulnar collateral ligament (UCL) at the level of the first metacarpophalangeal joint has historically been referred to as *gamekeeper's thumb*. More recently, its high incidence among skiers has led to use of the term *skier's thumb;* the injury, however, is actually quite common among a variety of athletes. Suspected injury of the UCL at the level of the metacarpophalangeal joint is the most common indication for obtaining an MRI of the thumb.

Injuries of the UCL result from excessive valgus force (hyperextension) applied to the metacarpophalangeal joint and are graded as a sprain, partial-thickness tear, or full-thickness tear. Avulsion fractures at the distal attachment site may also occur, and fracture fragments may range from a tiny fleck of cortical bone to a large fragment that involves the articular surface. At the level of the first metacarpophalangeal joint, the adductor pollicis muscle crosses the joint at an angle that is oblique or almost transverse to the long axis of the thumb. This unique anatomic configuration allows for the thumb to oppose the fingers during gripping, but it is also responsible for occasional entrapment of the UCL superficial to the adductor aponeurosis after complete disruption and retraction of the UCL (Fig. 10-20).

Entrapment of the UCL is referred to as the *Stener lesion* and requires open surgical reapproximation of the ligament to its normal attachment site if proper healing is to occur. Although in the past, nondisplaced complete disruptions of the UCL were usually treated with closed reduction, more recently most orthopedic surgeons advocate open repair for all complete disruptions of the UCL or high-grade

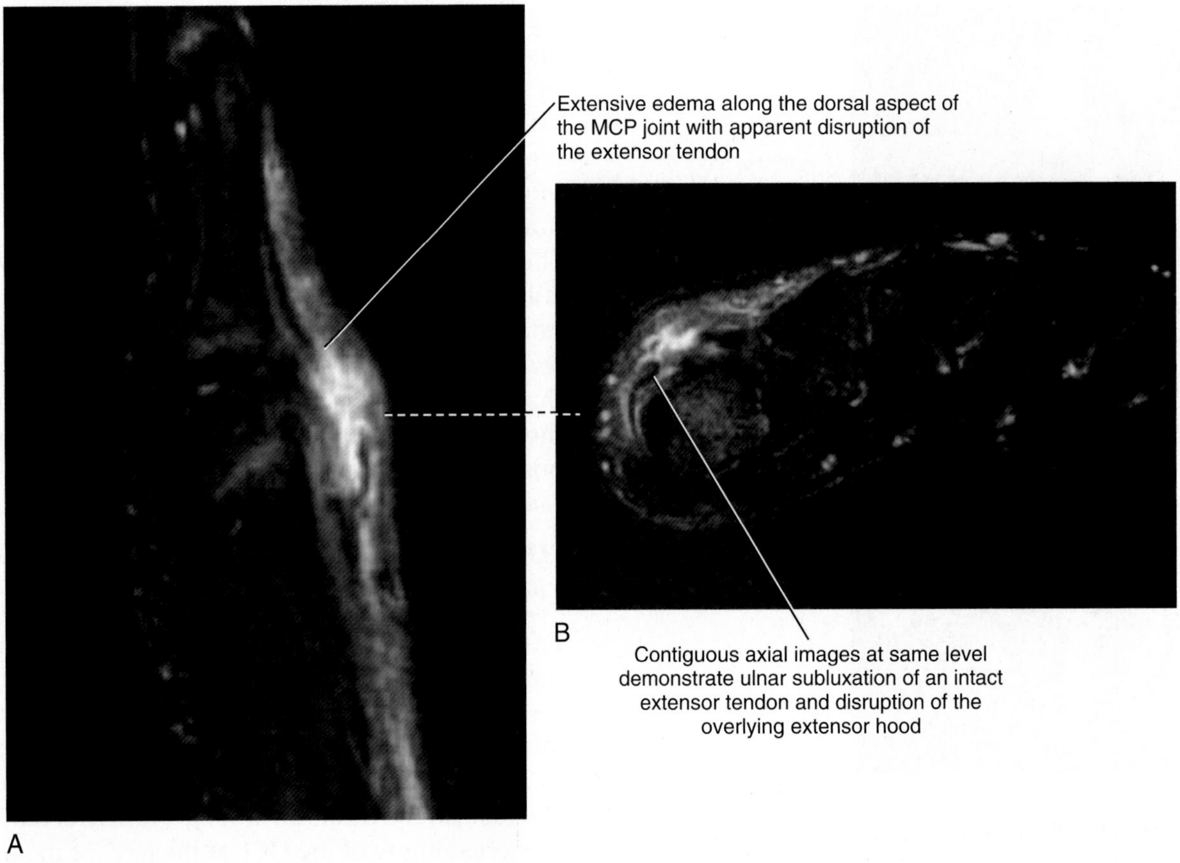
Extensive edema along the dorsal aspect of the MCP joint with apparent disruption of the extensor tendon
B
Contiguous axial images at same level demonstrate ulnar subluxation of an intact extensor tendon and disruption of the overlying extensor hood
A

Figure 10-19 Extensor hood injury. Sagittal (**A**) and axial (**B**) images at the level of the MCP joint demonstrate dorsal soft tissue edema. There is apparent disruption of the extensor tendon as the tendon moves out of plane on the midsagittal image. Axial image at this level reveals that the tendon has simply subluxed in an ulnar direction but remains intact, indicating an extensor hood tear rather than an extensor tendon injury.

partial-thickness tears that do not demonstrate a good end point on physical examination. Some surgeons are concerned that physical examination of the thumb in the setting of a possible UCL disruption can actually create a Stener lesion and would prefer MRI when disruption of the UCL is suspected clinically. In addition, extensive swelling, ecchymosis, and pain can prevent adequate physical examination in the setting of acute trauma. MRI is a powerful tool that provides noninvasive evaluation of the UCL, thus eliminating some of the difficulties encountered with the physical examination, and it has been shown to be very accurate in the grading of these injuries and in guiding proper surgical management. In experienced hands, ultrasound has also been shown to accurately depict injuries of the UCL. A large avulsion fracture involving the base of the proximal phalanx is usually treated with open reduction and pinning of the osseous fragment, whereas a partial-thickness tear of the UCL with a good end point of the ligament on physical examination requires only splinting.

Good MR technique and patient positioning are mandatory to ensure proper evaluation of the UCL. A small field of view should be used with imaging limited to the thumb rather than the entire hand. To optimize visualization of the UCL, the imaging planes must be performed coronal and sagittal to the thumb rather than the hand. Setting up the imaging plane coronal to the hand rather than the thumb is a common mistake made by technicians, and this alteration in positioning can make adequate visualization and evaluation of the UCL very problematic. Properly aligned T2-weighted images with fat saturation in the coronal and axial imaging planes as well as a coronal three-dimensional gradient-echo sequence usually provides for good visualization and assessment.

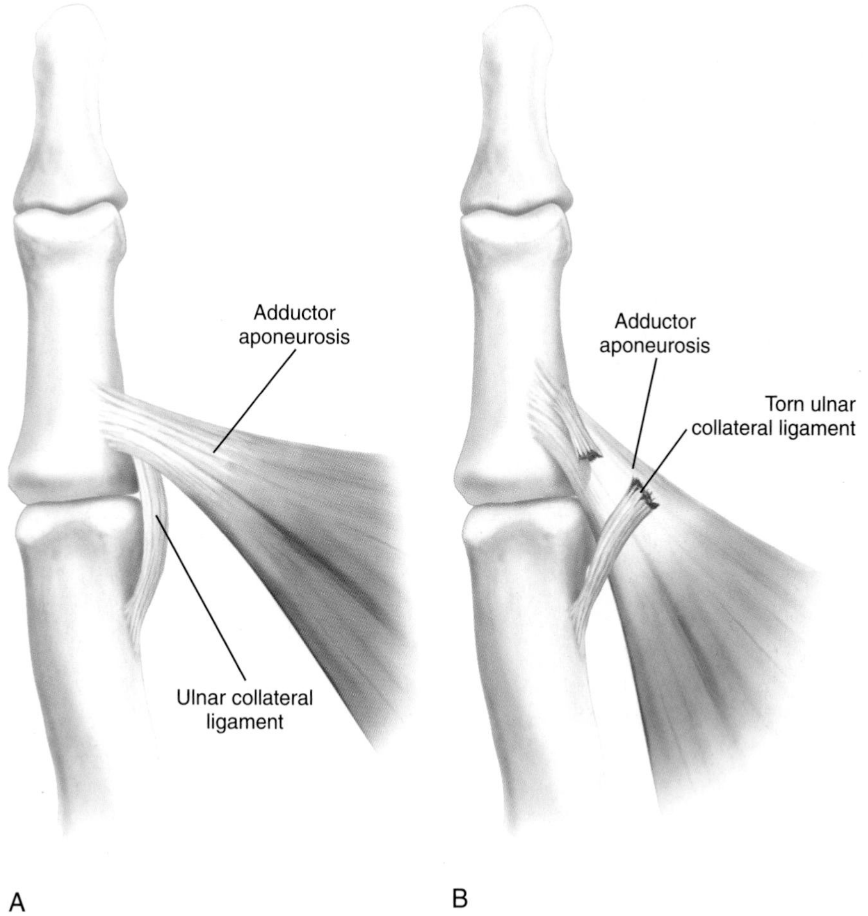
Adductor aponeurosis
Ulnar collateral ligament
Adductor aponeurosis
Torn ulnar collateral ligament
A
B

Figure 10-20 Ulnar collateral ligament (UCL) anatomy. A, Normal anatomy of the UCL and its relation to the overlying adductor aponeurosis. **B,** Stener lesion with retraction of the torn UCL proximal to the adductor aponeurosis.

A sprain of the UCL appears as soft tissue swelling and edema superficial to the UCL. There may also be thickening and intermediate signal within the substance of the ligament, but the ligament appears intact. A partial-thickness tear shows thinning or attenuation of the ligament or fluid, partially traversing the ligament with some fibers remaining intact. A thorough description of a completely disrupted UCL should include the location of the tear (proximal, midsubstance, or distal) as well as whether the tear is dorsal or volar in location (Fig. 10-21). Mention should also be made of the presence of an avulsion fracture fragment. It is important to describe retraction and entrapment of the UCL superficial or proximal to the adductor aponeurosis because this configuration is always considered a surgical lesion (Fig. 10-22).

Radial Collateral Ligament Injury

Radial collateral ligament (RCL) injuries reportedly make up as much as 40% of all ligamentous injuries of the first metacarpophalangeal joint. Injury results from a varus-type mechanism or hyperextension of the first metacarpophalangeal joint and is most often seen in ball-handling athletes. In the past, it was recommended that all RCL injuries be treated conservatively with splinting, but it is now recommended that complete disruption resulting in an incompetent RCL be treated with open repair to prevent the development of premature osteoarthritis of the metacarpophalangeal joint. Osseous avulsion injuries occur less commonly with RCL than with UCL, and although a complete tear can occur anywhere along the course of the ligament, they are most often seen at the proximal attachment site. The overlying soft tissue anatomy differs from that seen on the ulnar side of the thumb. The abductor pollicis muscle is oriented parallel rather than perpendicular to the long axis of the thumb, as seen on the ulnar side (Fig. 10-23). As a result, the disrupted and retracted RCL continues to lie deep to the overlying musculature, and no Stener-type lesion counterpart occurs on the radial side of the metacarpophalangeal joint of the thumb.

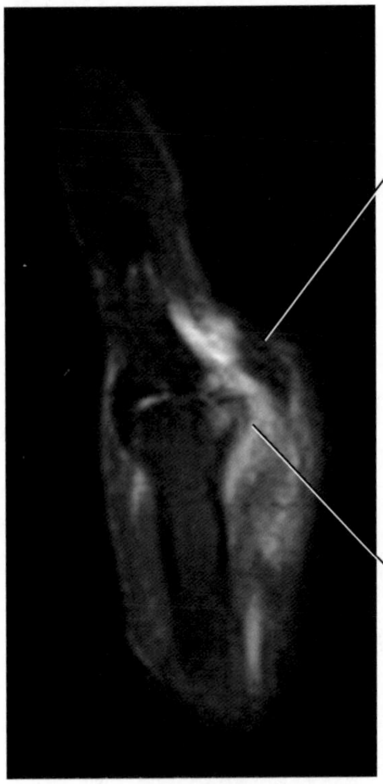
Adductor
aponeurosis
Ulnar collateral
ligament

Figure 10-21 Disruption of the ulnar collateral ligament (UCL) of the thumb. T2-weighted coronal image shows complete disruption of the UCL at the distal attachment site with thickening of the UCL more proximally and adjacent soft tissue edema. The UCL is not retracted, but remains normally positioned deep to the adductor aponeurosis.

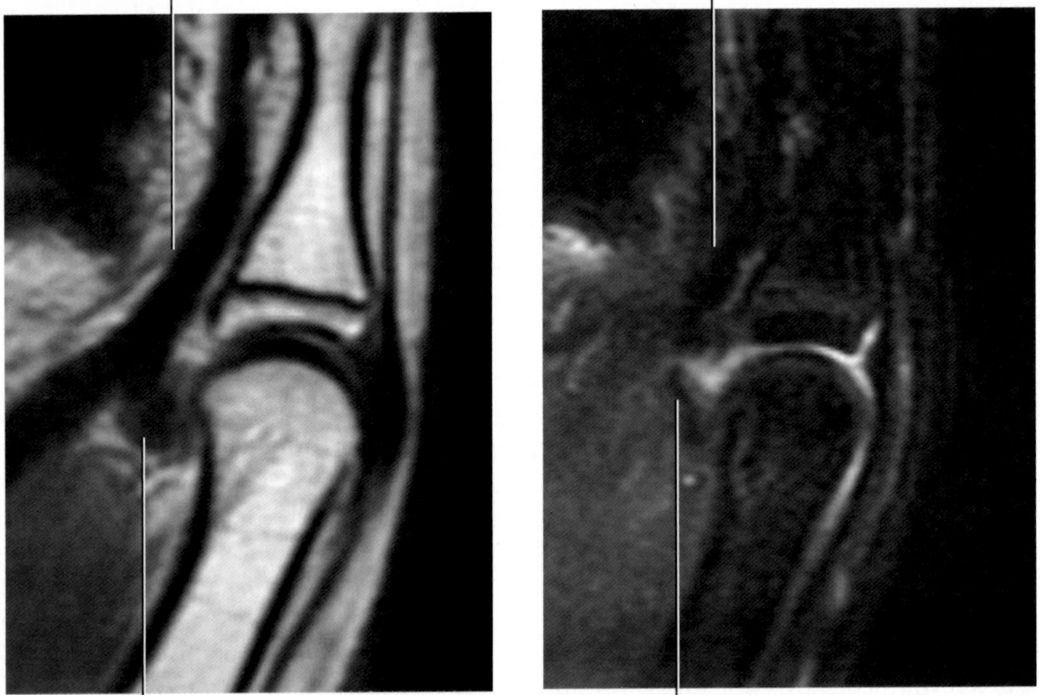
Flexor pollicis
longus tendon
A
Torn and retracted
UCL demonstrates "balled-up"
appearance
Flexor pollicis
longus tendon
B
Torn and retracted UCL

Figure 10-22 Stener lesion. Coronal T1-weighted (**A**) and T2-weighted (**B**) images show complete disruption of the ulnar collateral ligament (UCL) with retraction of the fibers proximal to the adductor aponeurosis.

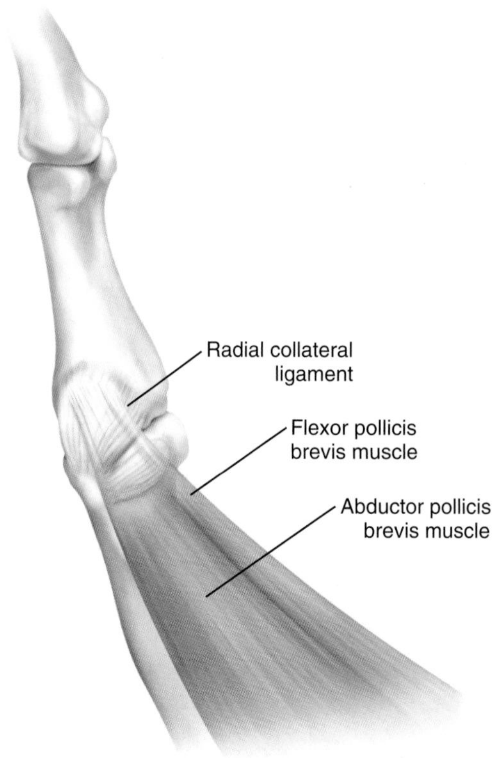
Radial collateral ligament
Flexor pollicis brevis muscle
Abductor pollicis brevis muscle

Figure 10-23 Radial collateral ligament (RCL) anatomy. Note that the abductor pollicis muscle is oriented parallel with the long axis of the thumb rather than perpendicular to the long axis as occurs with the adductor aponeurosis as on the ulnar side. This prevents a Stener-type lesion from occurring on the radial side of the thumb.

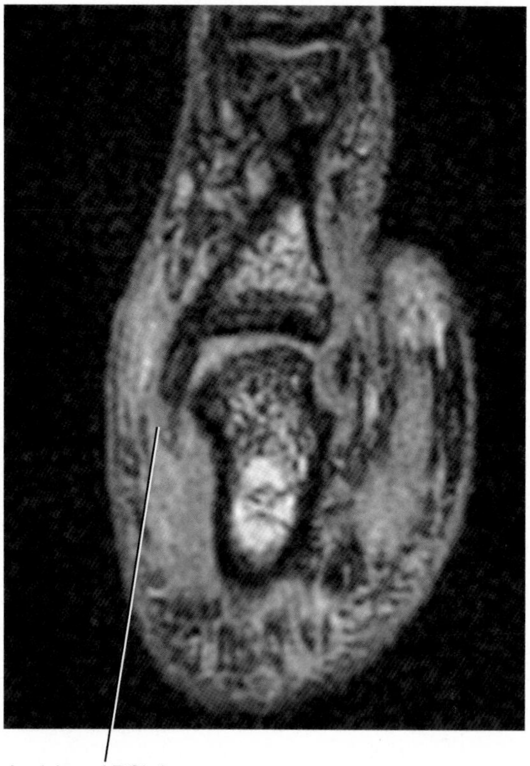
Avulsion of RCL from proximal attachment

Figure 10-24 Radial collateral ligament (RCL) disruption. Coronal three-dimensional gradient-echo image shows complete avulsion of the proximal fibers of the RCL at the proximal attachment site on the neck of the first metacarpal. Mild adjacent soft tissue edema is present. The RCL is most often injured at the proximal attachment site.

Evaluation of the RCL with MRI follows the same recommendations as those provided previously for UCL injuries. Well-positioned coronal images are the key to proper evaluation. Injuries are graded as a sprain, partial-thickness tear, or complete disruption. The location of injury should be reported as a proximal attachment site, mid substance or distal attachment site, and the presence of an avulsion fracture or a fracture involving the articular surface of the metacarpophalangeal joint should be described (Fig. 10-24).

First Carpometacarpal Joint Injury

The first carpometacarpal joint has a strong and multipart ligamentous complex that provides stability while allowing for full range of motion. There are four primary ligamentous components that provide the majority of the stability of the joint: anterior oblique ligament, dorsal radial ligament, posterior oblique ligament, and intermetacarpal ligament (Fig. 10-25). The most important stabilizer against valgus stress is the anterior oblique ligament (AOL), which is a short thick ligament that arises from the palmar tubercle of the trapezium and extends obliquely to insertion along the volar aspect of the base of the first metacarpal. Injury to the first metacarpophalangeal joint may result in disruption of the AOL, leading to instability; complete tears are often repaired surgically to prevent the inevitable progression to osteoarthritis.

Injury to the first carpometacarpal joint is usually initially evaluated with radiographs, which may demonstrate a Bennett-type or Rolando-type fracture of

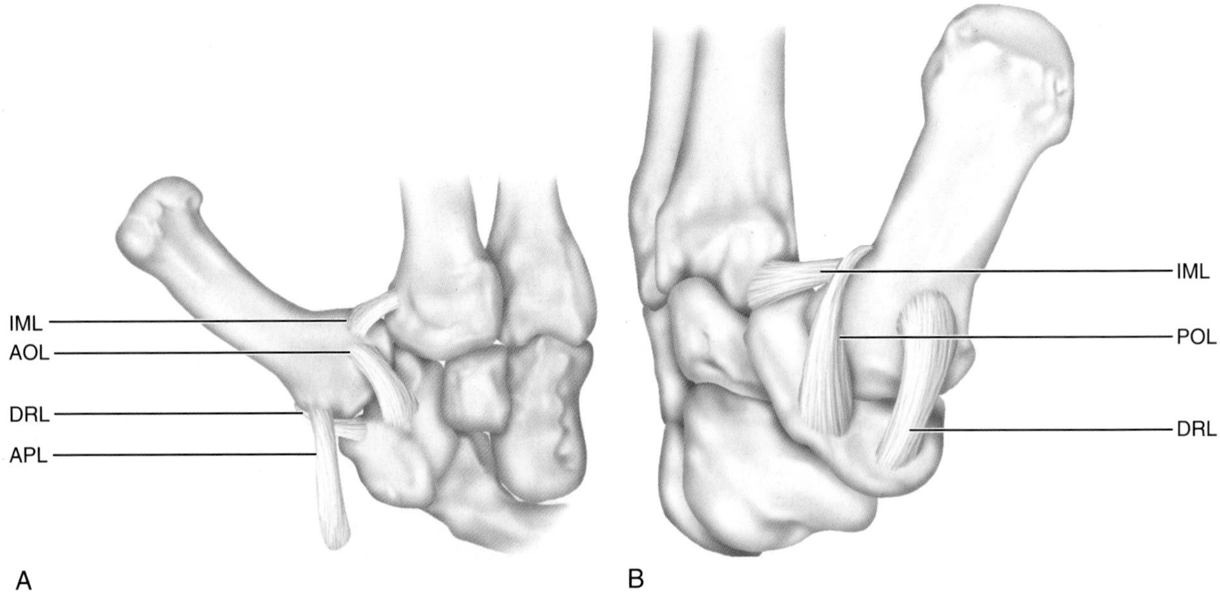
IML
AOL
DRL
APL
A
IML
POL
DRL
B

Figure 10-25 Ligamentous anatomy of the first carpometacarpal joint. A, Palma view. **B,** Dorsal view. AOL, anterior oblique ligament; APL, abductor pollicis longus tendon; DRL, dorsal radial ligament; IML, intermetacarpal ligament; POL, posterior oblique ligament.

the base of the first metacarpal. A Bennett fracture is a noncomminuted fracture involving the articular surface of the base of the first metacarpal, whereas a Rolando fracture represents a comminuted fracture involving the proximal articular surface of the first metacarpal. Significant soft tissue swelling and tenderness in the absence of a fracture may indicate AOL injury, and although stress views may indicate disruption, MRI can provide direct visualization of the AOL and show partial- or full-thickness disruption (Fig. 10-26). Disruption of the AOL can lead to long-term complications of first carpometacarpal osteoarthritis and tear/tenosynovitis of the flexor carpi radialis tendon.

SOFT TISSUE MASSES OF THE HAND AND FINGERS

The most common soft tissue mass found in the hand and fingers is a ganglion, which is a synovial–lined, fluid-filled mass that typically arises adjacent to a joint or tendon sheath. The giant cell tumor of the tendon sheath (GCTTS) is the second most common soft tissue mass found in the hand, and this lesion represents a localized extra-articular form of pigmented villonodular synovitis and is composed of variable components of villous, fibrous, pigmented (hemosiderin), and inflammatory tissue. Occasionally, it can be a challenge to differentiate between a ganglion and a GCCTS on the basis of MR imaging; however, both lesions have characteristic MRI features, which, when present, allow one to confidently differentiate between the two lesions (Table 10-2).

Ganglion

A ganglion typically follows water signal intensity on all MR pulse sequences and usually arises in close proximity to an adjacent joint or tendon sheath. Occasionally, however, a ganglion may contain fluid that is highly proteinaceous or complicated by hemorrhage, resulting in atypical MR signal characteristics. Ganglia vary in size from a few millimeters to several centimeters and may be unilocular or multiseptated. A small neck is often identified, which extends toward the adjacent joint or tendon sheath; this is nearly diagnostic of a ganglion and can be a very useful sign when trying to differentiate a ganglion from other soft tissue masses (Fig. 10-27). Rarely, a ganglion can arise within the substance of a tendon and remain completely within the tendon sheath. After the administration of intravenous gadolinium, peripheral rim enhancement is characteristic, and internal septations may also enhance. Occasion-

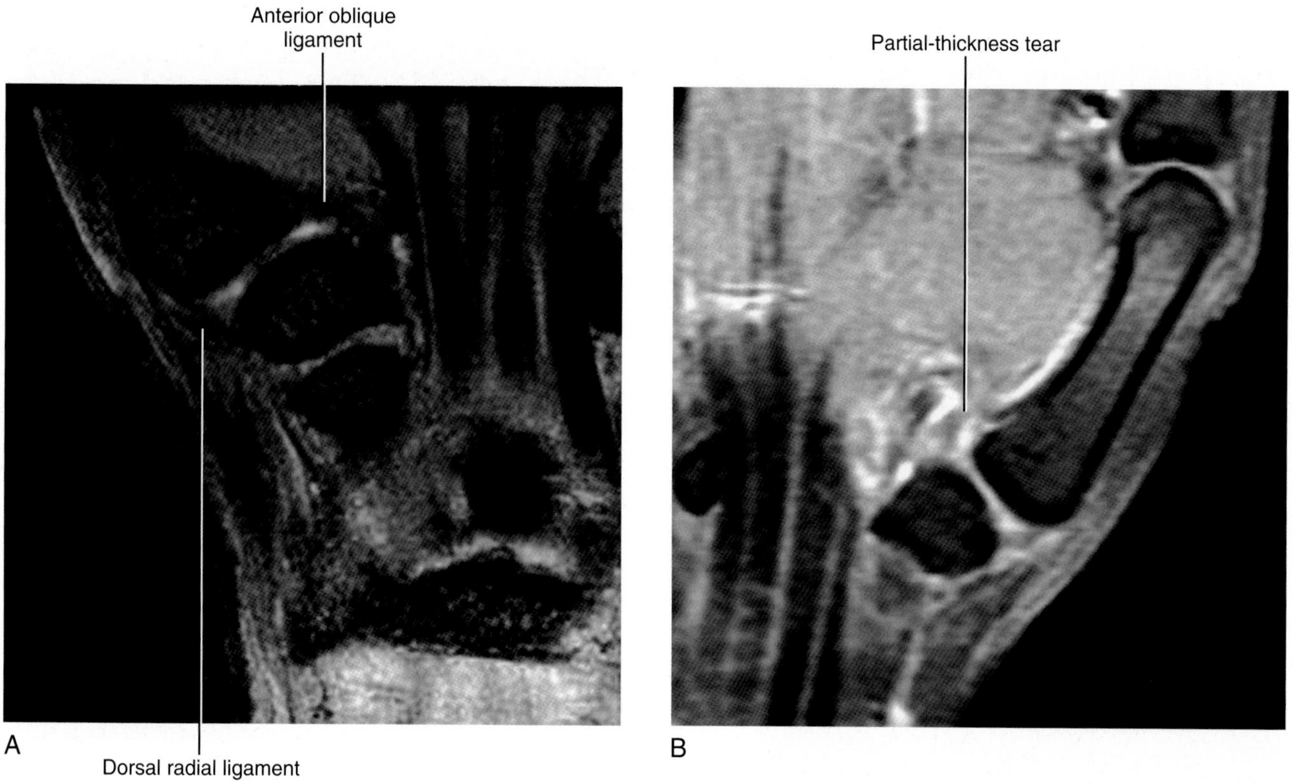
Anterior oblique ligament
Dorsal radial ligament
A
Partial-thickness tear
B

Figure 10-26 Anterior oblique ligament of the first carpometacarpal joint. A, Normal anatomy of the anterior oblique ligament and coronal image of the base of the thumb shows a short thick ligament that arises from the palmar tubercle of the trapezium and extends obliquely to insertion along the volar aspect of the base of the first metacarpal. **B,** Thickening and edema of the anterior oblique ligament with a partial-thickness tear near the distal attachment.

Table 10-2 Differentiating Ganglion from Giant Cell Tumor of the Tendon Sheath (GCTTS)

	Ganglion	GCTTS
Histology	Synovial-lined, fluid-filled	Villous, fibrous, hemosiderin, inflammatory components
T1 signal	Intermediate (water)	Low (fibrous)
T2 signal	Bright (water)	Low (fibrous/hemosiderin)
Location	Proximity to joint	Volar, proximity to tendon
Unique features	Neck leading to adjacent joint	
Enhancement	Peripheral, rim	Diffuse
Adjacent osseous structures	Normal	+/− Pressure erosions

ally, it is difficult to distinguish between a normal joint recess filled with fluid and a ganglion. Internal septations, a neck, or mass effect on the adjacent structures all are imaging characteristics that are specific for a ganglion rather than a joint recess. A complete description of the location of the ganglion is important for presurgical planning, especially in relation to adjacent anatomic structures such as neurovascular bundles.

Giant Cell Tumor of the Tendon Sheath

Giant cell tumor of the tendon sheath (GCTTS) is a benign tumor that typically presents as a nodular

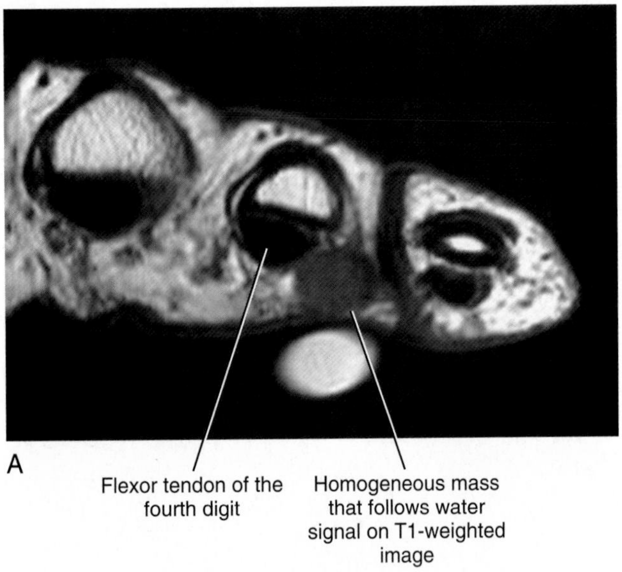
A
Flexor tendon of the fourth digit
Homogeneous mass that follows water signal on T1-weighted image

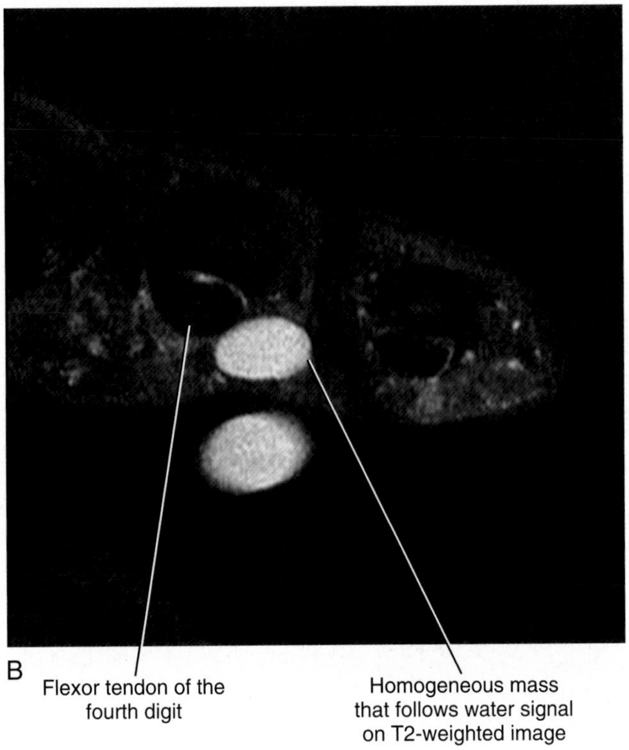
B
Flexor tendon of the fourth digit
Homogeneous mass that follows water signal on T2-weighted image

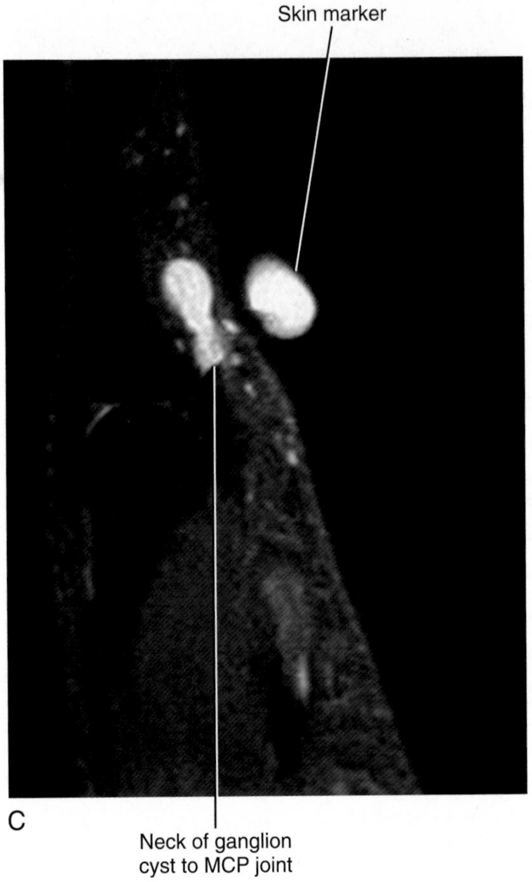
Skin marker
C
Neck of ganglion cyst to MCP joint

Figure 10-27 Ganglion arising from the fourth metacarpophalangeal (MCP) joint. Axial T1-weighted (**A**) and T2-weighted (**B**) images demonstrate a homogeneous mass located along the volar aspect of the proximal phalanx of the fourth digit, which follows water signal intensity on both pulse sequences. **C,** Sagittal T2-weighted image shows the presence of a thin neck extending toward the joint or tendon sheath (in this case the fourth MCP joint), which is highly specific for a ganglion.

mass arising along the volar aspect of a flexor tendon of the hand or fingers. These tumors are usually less than 2 cm in diameter at the time of presentation. Hemosiderin and fibrous material within these lesions are responsible for the typical MR signal characteristics of low signal intensity on both T1- and T2-weighted images (Fig. 10-28). These lesions usually demonstrate some degree of heterogeneity on MRI as a result of variable histologic components. The T2-weighted imaging appearance of a GTCCS, however, can range from homogeneous low signal to a mixed pattern of high and low signal to an occasional appearance of intermediate to high signal throughout the lesion. In most instances, however, low T2-weighted signal predominates. The presence of a long-standing lesion can result in scalloping of the adjacent bone. After the administration of intravenous contrast, these lesions demonstrate intense diffuse enhancement (Fig. 10-29).

Glomus Tumor

Glomus tumors (neuromyoarterial glomus) are benign lesions containing neural, muscle, and arterial components. Although these lesions can be found anywhere in the body, they typically arise along the dorsal aspect of the terminal phalanx of the finger. They are often subungual and most commonly occur in patients between 20 and 40 years of age. On physical examination, a glomus tumor is seen as a red-blue superficial nodule with paroxysms of radiating pain, often exacerbated by changes in temperature. On

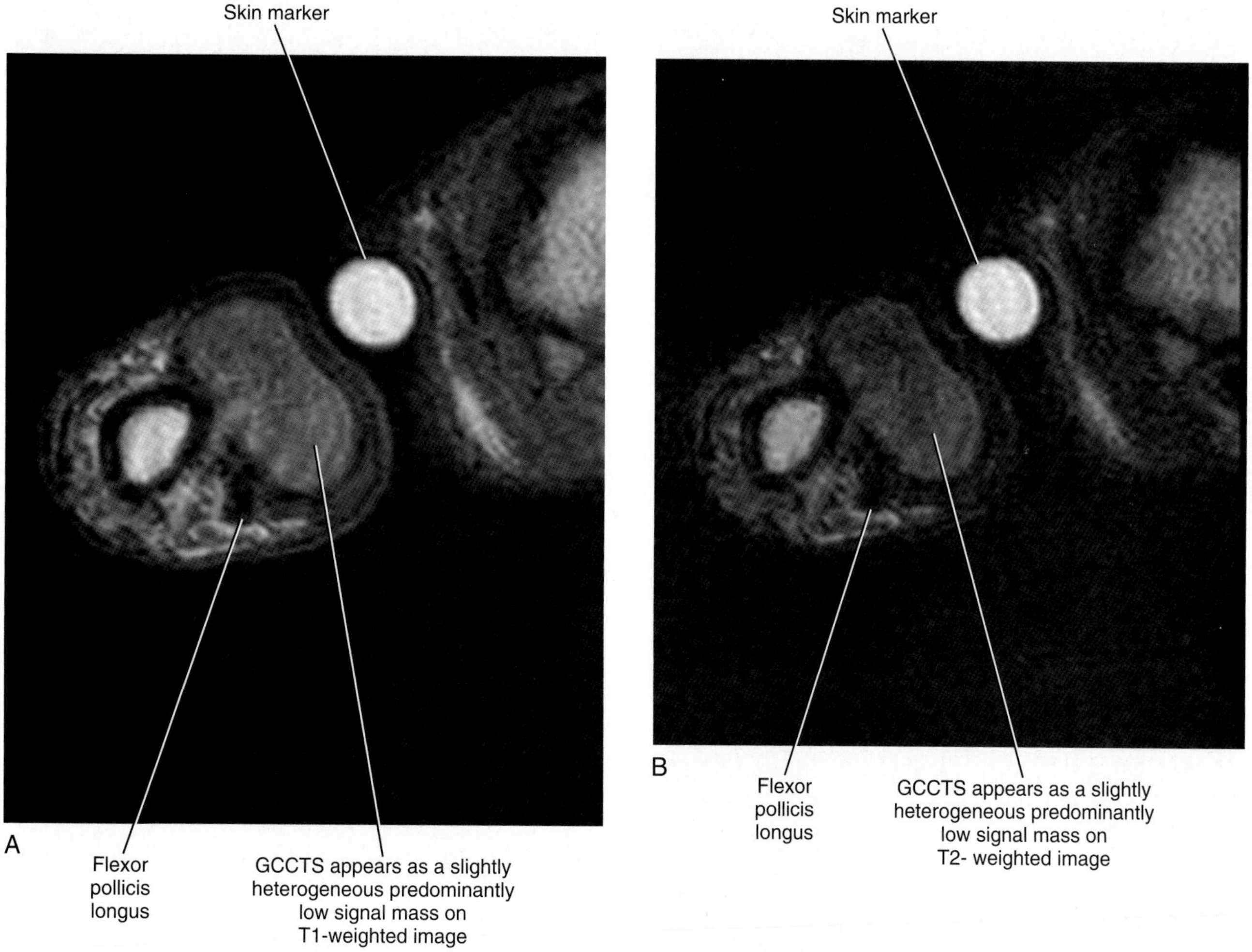
Skin marker
A
Flexor pollicis longus
GCCTS appears as a slightly heterogeneous predominantly low signal mass on T1-weighted image
Skin marker
B
Flexor pollicis longus
GCCTS appears as a slightly heterogeneous predominantly low signal mass on T2- weighted image

Figure 10-28 Giant cell tumor of the tendon sheath (GSTTS) arising adjacent to the flexor tendon of the thumb. Axial T1-weighted (**A**) and T2-weighted (**B**) images through the base of the proximal phalanx of the thumb show a slightly heterogeneous mass demonstrating predominantly low signal on both T1- and T2-weighted images. The mass is slightly lobular in appearance and eccentric in location and sits in direct contact with the adjacent flexor tendon of the thumb. GCTTS is the most common soft tissue mass in the digits. Because of hemosiderin, it is generally intermediate to low signal on T1- and T2-weighted sequences and may have areas of blooming (low signal) artifact on gradient-echo image. These characteristics as well as close association with a tendon are specific for GCTTS.

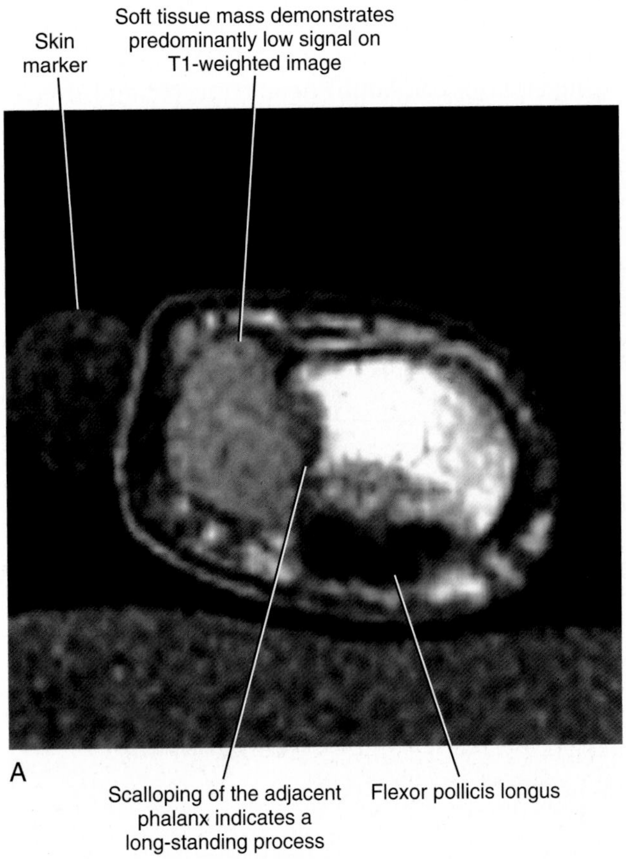
Skin marker
Soft tissue mass demonstrates predominantly low signal on T1-weighted image
Scalloping of the adjacent phalanx indicates a long-standing process
Flexor pollicis longus

A

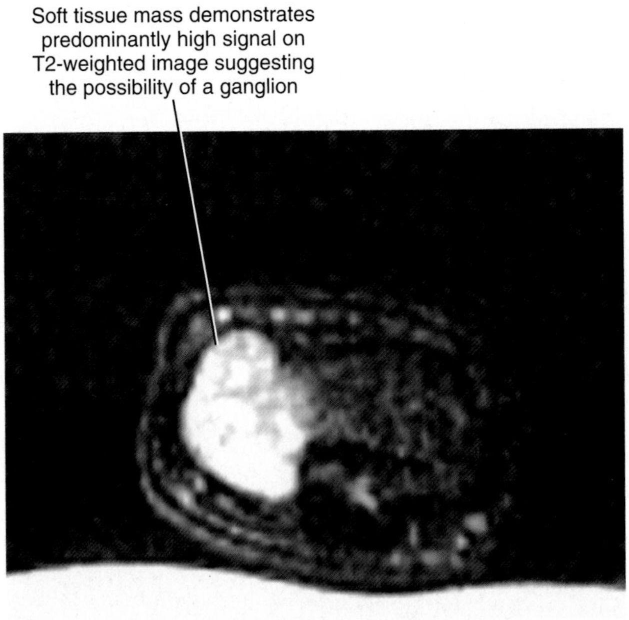
Soft tissue mass demonstrates predominantly high signal on T2-weighted image suggesting the possibility of a ganglion

B

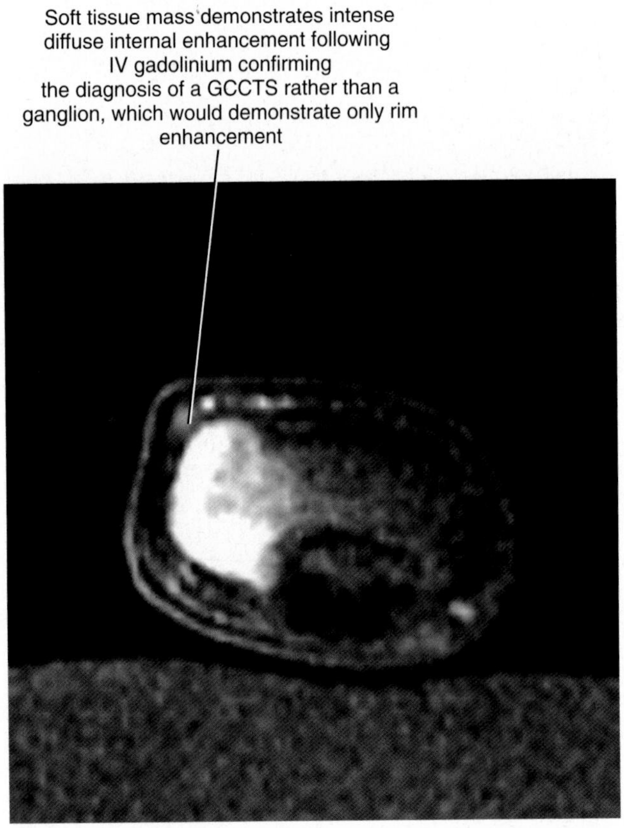
Soft tissue mass demonstrates intense diffuse internal enhancement following IV gadolinium confirming the diagnosis of a GCCTS rather than a ganglion, which would demonstrate only rim enhancement

C

Figure 10-29 Enhancement pattern of a giant cell tumor of the tendon sheath (GCCTS). A, Axial T1-weighted image shows a slightly lobulated homogeneous-appearing mass with low to intermediate T1-weighted signal intensity. **B,** Axial T2-weighted image shows a predominantly high signal mass, which is slightly atypical for a GCTTS. However, there are areas of low signal within the lesion. **C,** Axial T1-weighted image with fat saturation following administration of intravenous gadolinium shows diffuse enhancement throughout the lesion. This is typical of a GCTTS and differentiates this lesion from a ganglion, which would show only rim enhancement.

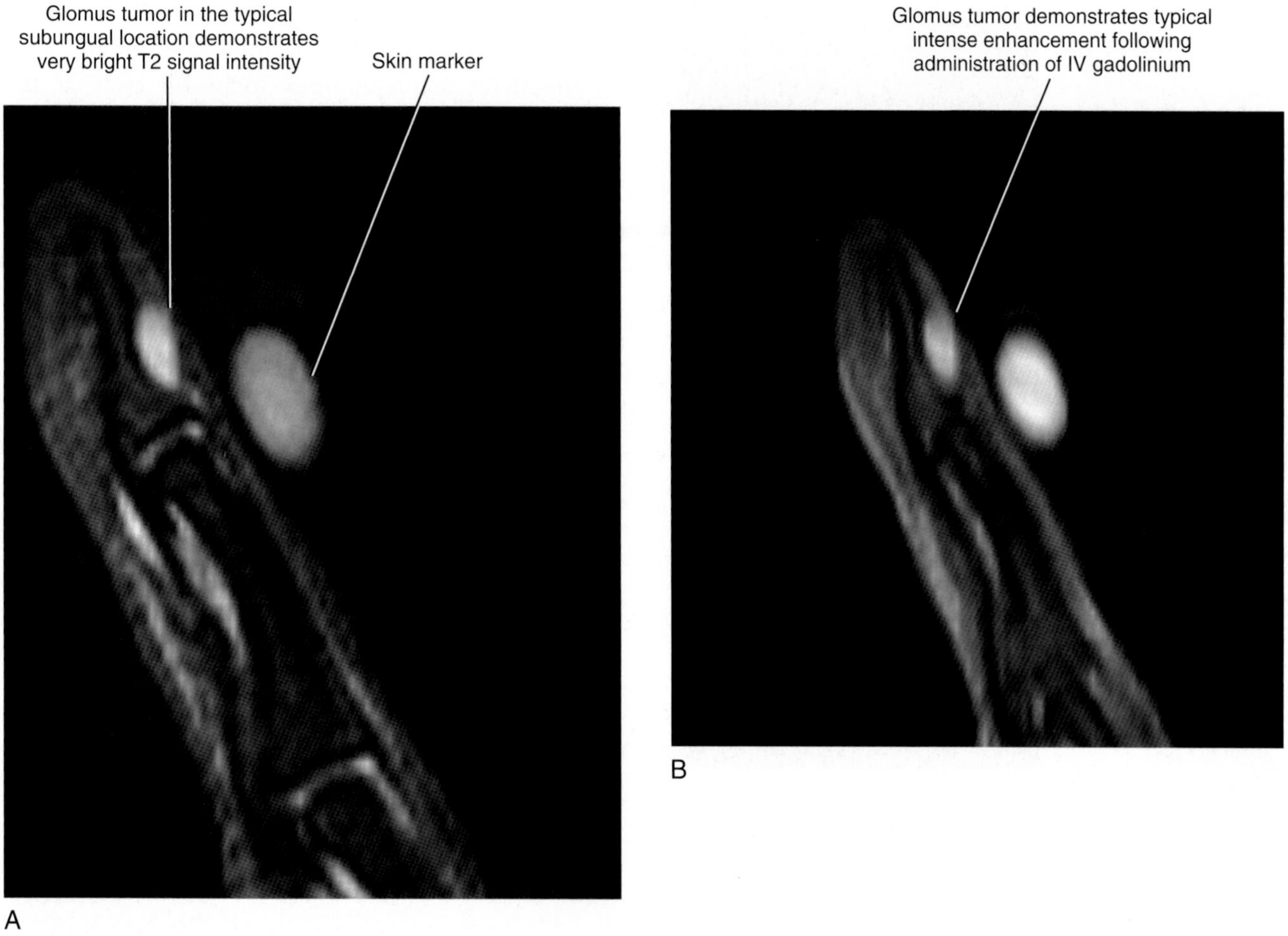
Glomus tumor in the typical subungual location demonstrates very bright T2 signal intensity
Skin marker
A
Glomus tumor demonstrates typical intense enhancement following administration of IV gadolinium
B

Figure 10-30 Glomus tumor. *A,* *T2-weighted sagittal image demonstrates homogeneous high signal throughout the lesion.* ***B,*** *T1-weighted sagittal image with fat saturation after administration of intravenous gadolinium demonstrates intense enhancement of a small oval lesion, subungual in location. Glomus tumor is intensely painful and tender. Characteristic history as well as location (distal digit) and intense enhancement are specific for the diagnosis.*

MRI, these tumors appear as a small mass, typically less than 1 cm in diameter, and they are very bright on T2-weighted images. They demonstrate intense homogeneous enhancement with intravenous contrast (Fig. 10-30). Treatment is surgical resection, and incomplete excision leads to a recurrence of the lesion. The main role of MRI is to detect and accurately localize these lesions and on follow-up postsurgical imaging to ensure complete resection and to monitor for recurrence.

Foreign Body Granuloma

Like the foot, the hand is susceptible to penetrating trauma and foreign body granuloma. Although the history of penetrating trauma is often available, on occasion no such history is provided. MR imaging demonstrates an ill-defined nonspecific soft tissue mass with high T2 and low T1 signal intensity. Intravenous gadolinium can help identify a small adjacent abscess, which appears as a fluid collection with low T1 signal surrounded by enhancing reactive inflammatory tissue. The MR images should be evaluated for signs of adjacent cellulitis, infectious tenosynovitis, and osteomyelitis. Occasionally, the foreign body is identified on MRI within the area of soft tissue abnormality. When present, it can help establish the correct diagnosis (Fig. 10-31). Gradient-echo imaging can help identify the foreign body, which often contains material that results in magnetic susceptibility artifact (blooming artifact). Suspicion of a foreign body on the basis of clinical history and/or MRI can

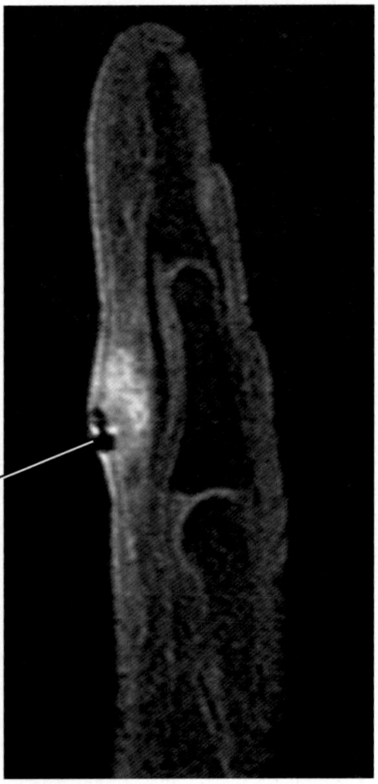
Foreign body with
surrounding granuloma

Figure 10-31 Foreign body granuloma. Sagittal T2-weighted image shows a nonspecific soft tissue mass of the finger with high T2-weighted signal intensity within the mass. A foreign body is identified within the mass, which is specific for a foreign body granuloma in this patient with a history of penetrating trauma to the index finger.

be further evaluated with radiography or ultrasonography or both, which may help confirm the presence of and localize the foreign body.

Miscellaneous Soft Tissue Masses

Other benign and malignant soft tissue lesions are occasionally seen in the hand and fingers. In the adult, some of the most common malignant soft tissue neoplasms seen in the hand are synovial cell sarcoma, malignant fibrous histiocytoma, and fibrosarcoma. These all manifest as nonspecific soft tissue masses on MRI, and usually only a differential diagnosis can be provided when a nonspecific MR appearance is noted.

Certain benign lesions can be confidently diagnosed on the basis of MR appearance. Aside from those previously mentioned, these lesions include hemangioma and lipoma. The typical MR appearances of these lesions are discussed in detail in Chapter 6. Other benign lesions occasionally seen in the hand are squamous inclusion cysts at the nail bed, nerve sheath tumors, and macrodystrophia lipomatosa.

OSSEOUS LESIONS OF THE HAND

Enchondroma is the most common benign tumor to involve the small bones of the hand and fingers. These lesions are often found incidentally on radiographs but may also present as a mass or with a pathologic fracture. Radiographs typically demonstrate a small lucent lesion with endosteal scalloping (Fig. 10-32A). Only 30% of enchondromas demonstrate a visible chondroid matrix on conventional radiographs. MRI reveals a lobulated intramedullary mass often with endosteal scalloping and expansion of the adjacent cortex. On MRI, signal characteristics of enchondromas usually demonstrate intermediate T1 signal and high T2 signal intensity (Fig. 10-32). A pathologic fracture may result in periostitis as well as edema within the adjacent bone and soft tissues (Fig. 10-33).

ARTHROPATHIES OF THE HAND

Aggressive treatment with new and improved drugs during the early stages of rheumatoid arthritis has been shown to minimize deformity and limit the progression of disease. As a result, early diagnosis and treatment of rheumatoid arthritis have become more important than ever and can have a significant impact of the long-term outcome and associated morbidity. MRI has been shown to be more effective than radiography in identifying the early changes of rheumatoid arthritis. The earliest changes on MRI are subchondral marrow edema and tiny erosions (Fig. 10-34). These changes are usually seen first in the region of the second and third metacarpal heads of the hand and in the lunate when there is involvement of the wrist. Subchondral marrow edema indicates that the disease is active and that the patient will likely benefit from drug therapy. Small effusions of the involved joints, though nonspecific, can indicate the presence of synovitis, and joint capsule thickening may also be present. Mild tenosynovitis often accompanies early bone changes and most often

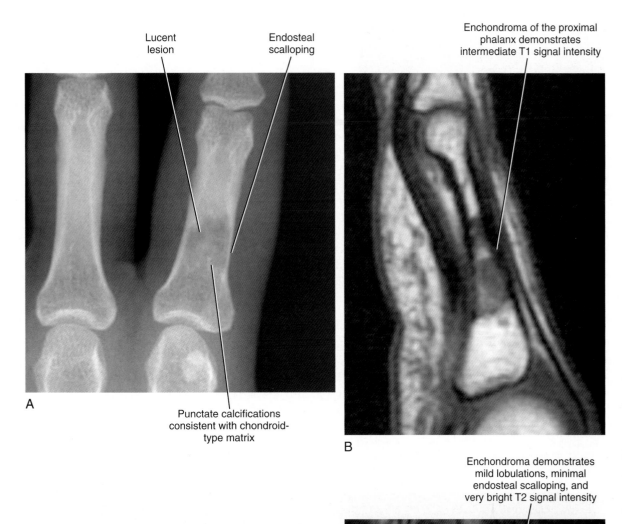

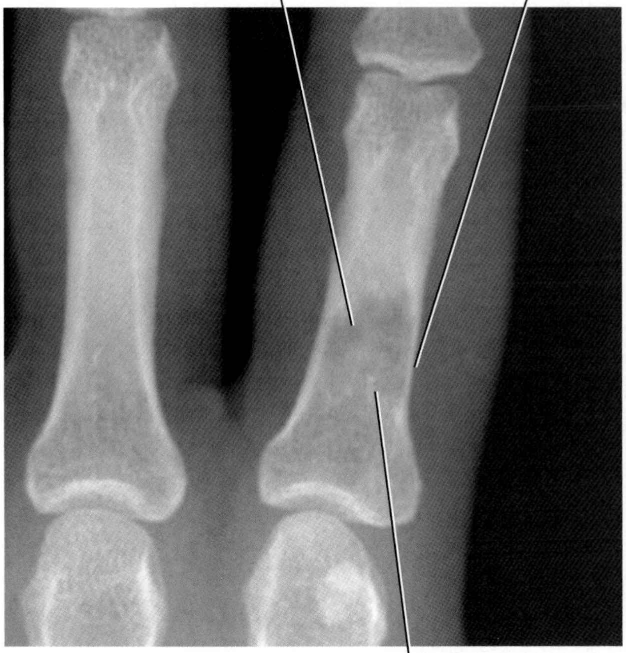
Lucent
lesion
Endosteal
scalloping
A
Punctate calcifications
consistent with chondroid-
type matrix

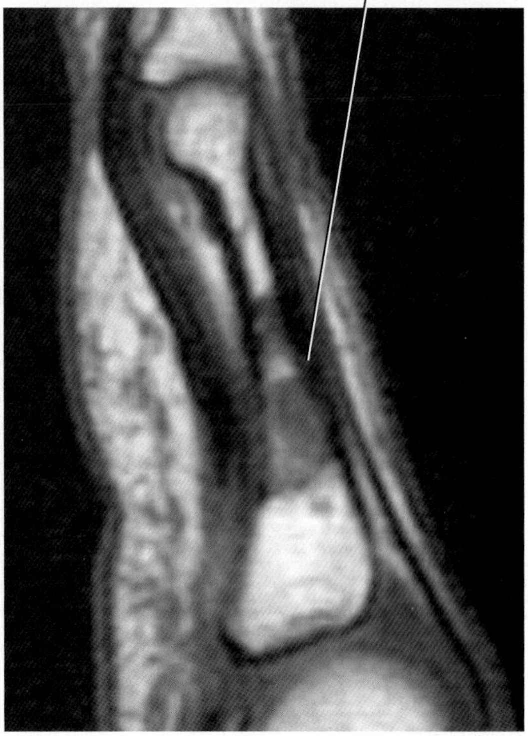
Enchondroma of the proximal
phalanx demonstrates
intermediate T1 signal intensity
B

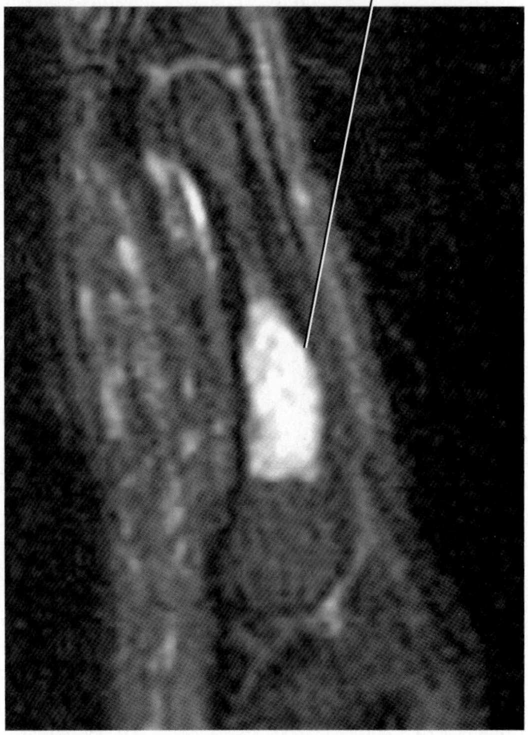
Enchondroma demonstrates
mild lobulations, minimal
endosteal scalloping, and
very bright T2 signal intensity
C

Figure 10-32 Enchondroma of the fifth metacarpal. **A,** Anteroposterior radiograph of the hand shows a well-defined lucent intramedullary lesion of the fifth metacarpal containing chondroid matrix and demonstrating mild endosteal scalloping. Sagittal T1-weighed (**B**) and T2-weighted (**C**) images shows a mildly lobulated intramedullary mass that contains chondroid matrix. Chondroid tissue is intermediate on T1 and classically is "bright as a light bulb" on T2. Rim and septal enhancement helps to differentiate from a cyst.

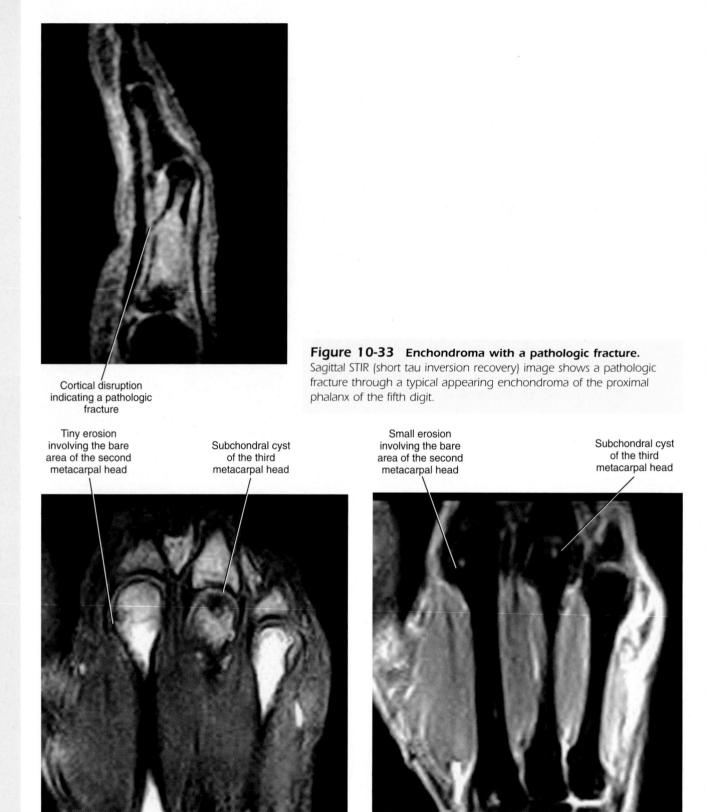

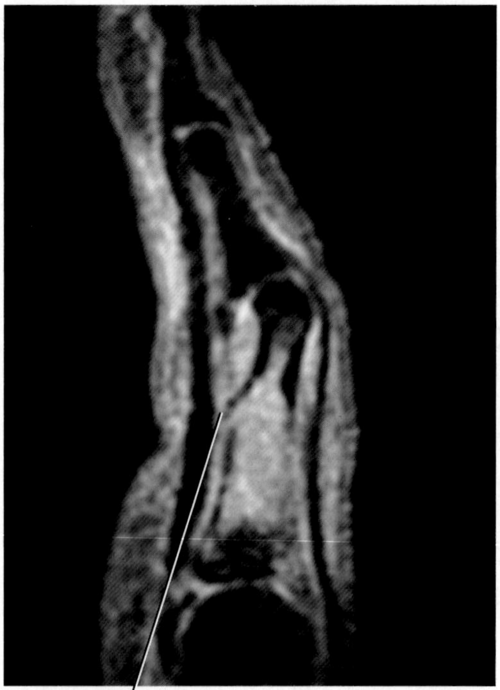
Cortical disruption
indicating a pathologic
fracture

Figure 10-33 Enchondroma with a pathologic fracture. Sagittal STIR (short tau inversion recovery) image shows a pathologic fracture through a typical appearing enchondroma of the proximal phalanx of the fifth digit.

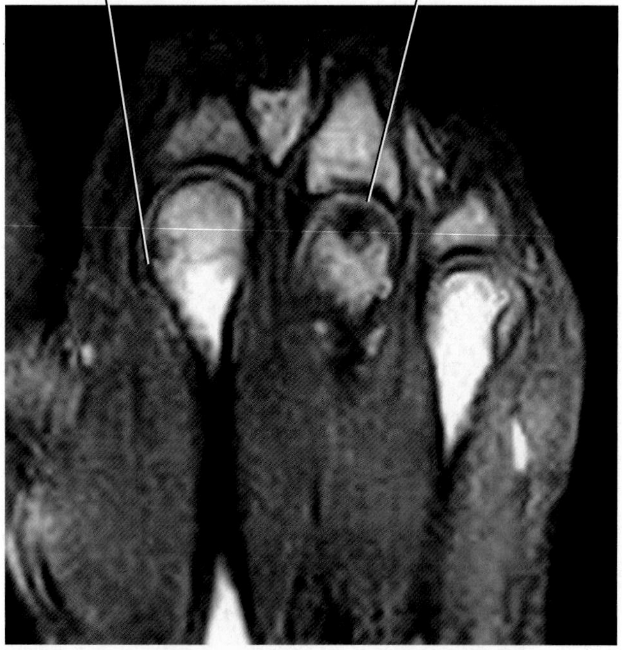
Tiny erosion
involving the bare
area of the second
metacarpal head
Subchondral cyst
of the third
metacarpal head
A

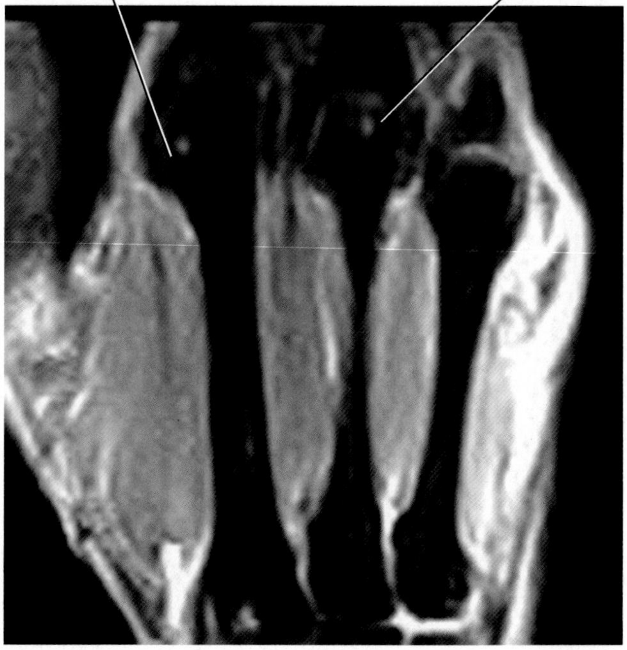
Small erosion
involving the bare
area of the second
metacarpal head
Subchondral cyst
of the third
metacarpal head
B

Figure 10-34 Rheumatoid arthritis. Coronal T1-weighted (**A**) and T2-weighted (**B**) images through the level of the metacarpophalangeal joints shows an erosion involving the second metacarpal head, subchondral cyst of the third metacarpal head and minimal adjacent marrow edema. These findings are indicative of an ongoing active inflammatory process.

involves the extensor tendon sheaths. More advanced disease may demonstrate subluxation of the tendons, tendinopathy, and even tendon disruption. Ulnar deviation at the level of the metacarpophalangeal joints is a late finding and is often accompanied by extensive erosive disease. Rice bodies represent excessive fibrinous exudate and are occasionally found within the joint or tendon sheath. On MRI, these appear as low signal intensity round or oval bodies within the involved joint or tendon sheath (Fig. 10-35).

When evaluating for early changes of rheumatoid arthritis, MRI of the hand should be centered over the metacarpophalangeal joints. The wrist can also be included within the field of view if symptoms are in this area. Coronal three-dimensional spoiled-gradient (SPGR) images are best suited for identifying early erosions of the metacarpal heads. Coronal T2-weighted images with fat saturation demonstrate subchondral marrow edema. Axial T2-weighted images reveal small fluid collections within the flexor and extensor tendon sheaths. This topic is covered in more detail in Chapter 4.

INFECTION

Infection involves the hands less often than the feet, but can occur as a result of penetrating trauma, prior surgery, or hematogenous spread. Soft tissue infections of the hand can be superficial or deep and can be accompanied by abscess formation. Most soft tissue infections are bacterial in origin, but fungal and tuberculosis soft tissue infections also occur and are usually associated with a more indolent clinical course (Fig. 10-36). MRI shows soft tissue swelling and edema with intermediate to high T2-weighted signal alterations within the soft tissues. Abscess formation appears on MRI as a focal fluid collection within the soft tissues, often with a thick irregular border that enhances after administration of intravenous contrast. A soft tissue infection of the pulp of

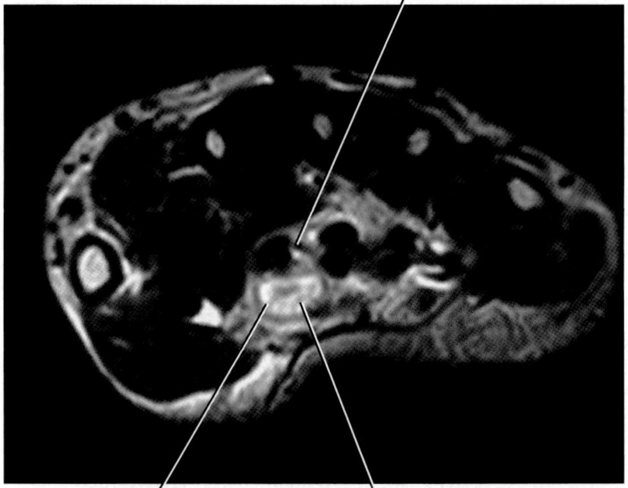
Flexor tendons of the second digit
Fluid within the tendon sheath representing tenosynovitis
Multiple small low-signal foci within the tendon sheath representing rice bodies

Figure 10-35 Tenosynovitis and rice bodies of the tendon sheath associated with rheumatoid arthritis. Axial T2-weighted image shows fluid within the flexor tendon sheath of the index finger consistent with tenosynovitis. Multiple focal loose bodies within the tendon sheath result from excessive fibrinous exudation and represent rice bodies occasionally seen in rheumatoid arthritis.

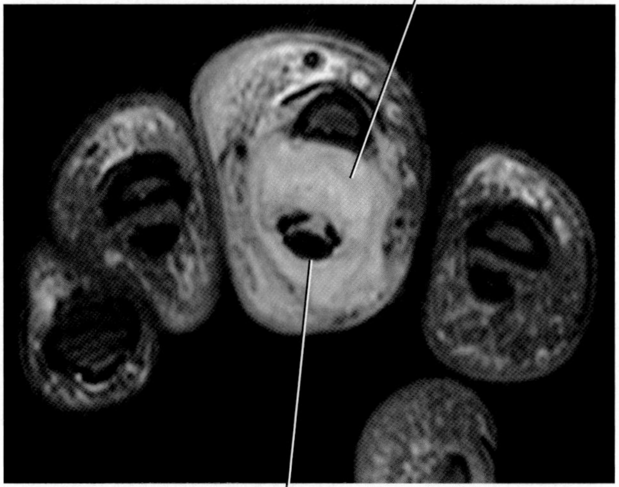
Extensive enhancing inflammatory tissue within and surrounding flexor tendon sheath
Flexor tendons of third digit

Figure 10-36 *Mycobacterium marinum* infectious tenosynovitis. Axial T1-weighted images with fat saturation after administration of intravenous gadolinium show marked enhancement of inflammatory tissue surrounding the flexor tendon consistent with tenosynovitis.

SECTION IV

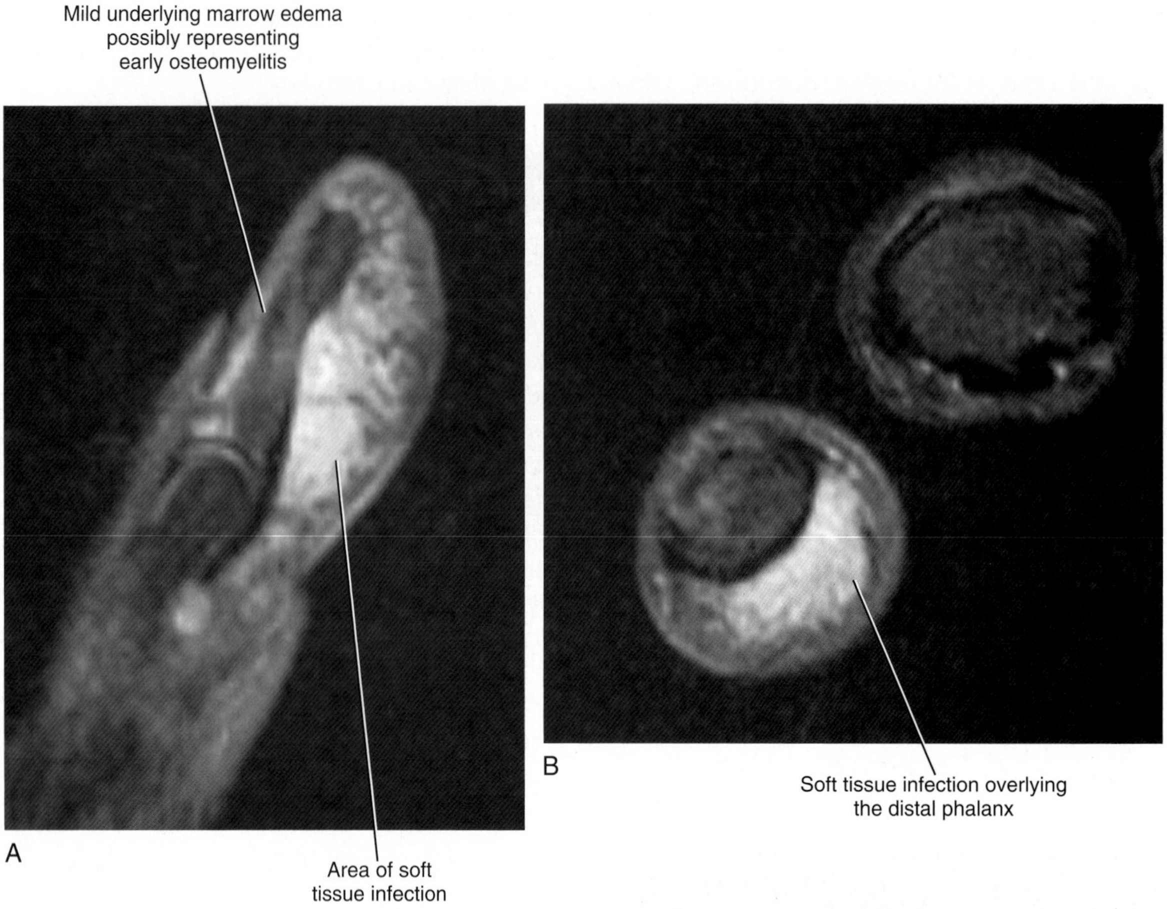
Mild underlying marrow edema possibly representing early osteomyelitis
A
Area of soft tissue infection
B
Soft tissue infection overlying the distal phalanx

Figure 10-37 Soft tissue infection (felon) of the distal finger tip. Sagittal (**A**) and axial (**B**) T2-weighted images with fat saturation show a focal area of soft tissue edema within the pulp of the finger. This represents a soft tissue infection and is referred to as a felon. The underlying phalanx shows minimal marrow edema and may represent early osteomyelitis.

the finger tip is referred to as a felon and is often associated with osteomyelitis of the adjacent distal phalanx (Fig. 10-37).

Infectious tenosynovitis can be bacterial in origin following penetrating trauma, but the tendon sheath is the most common location for atypical mycobacterial infections to involve the hand. MRI reveals fluid within the tendon sheath, which is often complex and filled with debris. The tendon sheaths are a common path of spread for infection within the hands and fingers. Infectious arthritis should be considered any time a single joint is involved. MRI signs of infectious arthritis include joint effusion, adjacent soft tissue swelling, and edema. Articular cartilage destruction, osseous erosions, and subchondral or subcortical marrow edema are often present but may be of little help in differentiating from an inflammatory arthropathy. Monarticular disease is probably the single most important imaging feature that suggests the possibility of an infectious arthritis.

Osteomyelitis of the small bones of the hands and fingers is uncommon but can result from either penetrating trauma or secondary to hematogenous spread. Fracture of the distal phalanx is occasionally associated with disruption of the overlying nail bed, especially when a fracture results from a crushing injury as when a finger is caught in a slamming door. In this situation, the fracture should be considered an open fracture, and the patient should be monitored for the possibility of secondary osteomyelitis. MRI is sensitive for the detection of osteomyelitis, particularly if there has been no prior trauma or

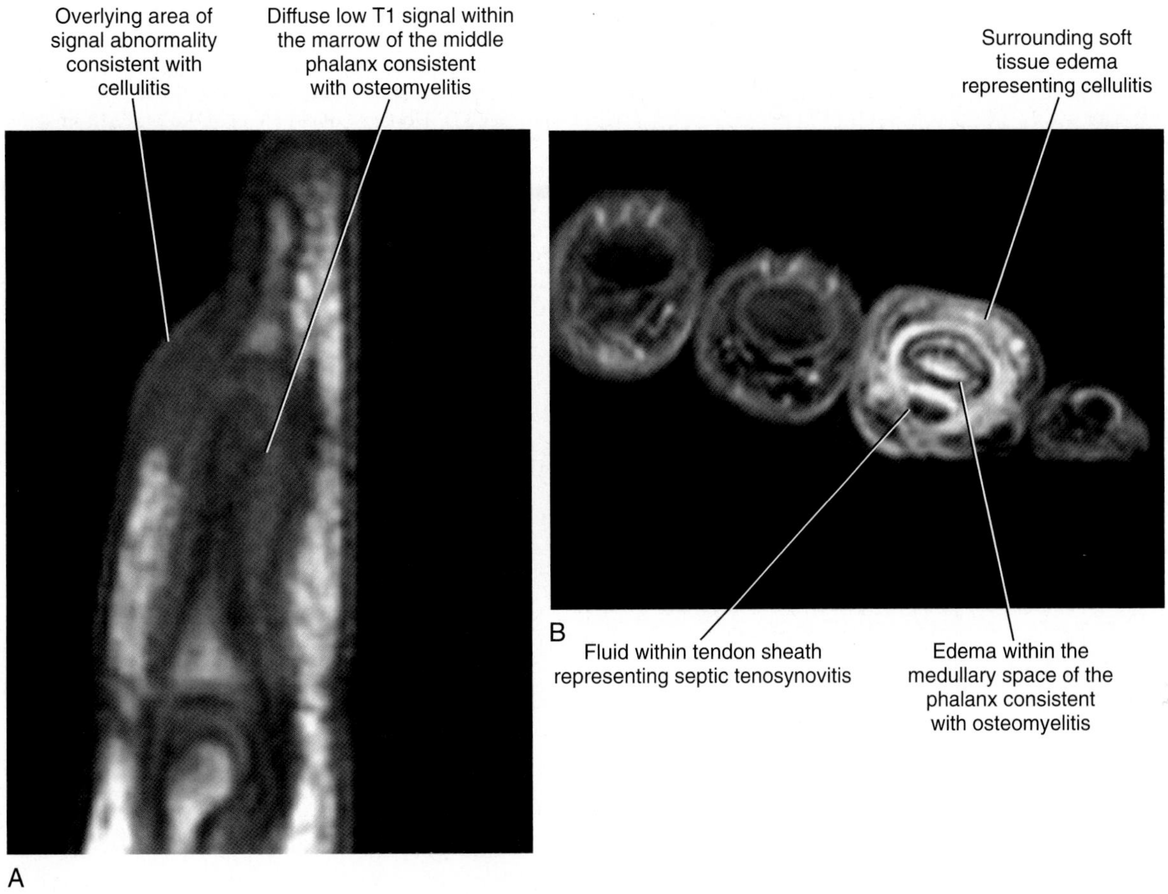
Overlying area of signal abnormality consistent with cellulitis
Diffuse low T1 signal within the marrow of the middle phalanx consistent with osteomyelitis
Surrounding soft tissue edema representing cellulitis
A
B
Fluid within tendon sheath representing septic tenosynovitis
Edema within the medullary space of the phalanx consistent with osteomyelitis

Figure 10-38 Osteomyelitis of the middle phalanx. A, Sagittal T1-weighted image of the index finger demonstrates abnormal marrow signal within the middle phalanx representing osteomyelitis after penetrating trauma by a palm branch. **B,** Axial T2-weighted image shows abnormal increased T2 signal within the medullary space as well as surrounding soft tissue edema consistent with cellulitis and fluid surrounding the middle phalanx representing periostitis.

surgery. MR imaging demonstrates decreased T1- and increased T2-weighted signal within the medullary space of the involved bone, and there may be associated cortical destruction (Fig. 10-38). Inhomogeneous fat suppression can be a problem when imaging the fingers for evidence of osteomyelitis. When this problem arises, a STIR sequence can be added to the MRI protocol to ensure adequate fat saturation. T1-weighted images are also very helpful in confirming the presence of edema in areas of concern on fat-saturated T2-weighted images. The presence of osteomyelitis results in marrow edema and replacement of the normal bright T1 intramedullary fat signal with low signal. To avoid the pitfall of misinterpreting failure of fat saturation as marrow edema, all areas of signal alteration on T2-weighted fat-saturated images should be confirmed on either a T1-weighted non–fat-saturated sequence or on a STIR sequence.

Suggested Readings

Bencardino JT. MR imaging of tendons of the hand and wrist. Magn Reson Imaging North Am 2004;12:333–347.

Clavero JA, Alomar X, Monill JM, et al. MR imaging of ligament and tendon injuries of the fingers. RadioGraphics 2002;22:237–256.

Connell DA, Pike J, Koulouris G, et al. MR imaging of thumb and carpometacarpal joint ligament injuries. J Hand Surg [Br] 2004;29:46–54.

Haramati N, Hiller N, Dowdle J, et al. MRI of the Stener lesion. Skeletal Radiol 1995;24:515–518.

Hauger O, Chung CB, Lektrakul N, et al. Pulley system in the fingers: normal anatomy and simulated lesions in cadavers at MR imaging, CT, and US with and without contrast material distention of the tendon sheath. Radiology 2000; 21:201–212.

Hergan K, Mittler C, Oser W. Ulnar collateral ligament: differentiation of displaced and nondisplaced tears with US and MR imaging. Radiology 1995;194:65–71.

Hoving JL, Buchbinder R, Hall S, et al. A comparison of magnetic resonance imaging, sonography, and radiology of the hand in patients with early rheumatoid arthritis. J Rheumatol 2004;31: 663–675.

Jbara M, Patnana M, Kazmi F, Beltran J. MR imaging: arthropathies and infectious conditions of the elbow, wrist, and hand. Magn Reson Imaging North Am 2004;12:361–379.

Lopez-Ben R, Lee DH, Nicolodi DJ. Boxer Knuckle (injury of the extensor hood with extensor tendon subluxation): diagnosis with dynamic US—report of three cases. Radiology 2003;228: 642–646.

Martinoli C, Bianchi S, Cotton A. Imaging of rock climbing injuries. Semin Musculoskelet Radiol 2005;9:334–345.

Peterson JJ, Bancroft LW. Injuries of the fingers and thumb in the athlete. Clin Sports Med 2006;25:527–542.

Plancher KD, Ho CP, Cofield SS, et al. Role of MR imaging in the management of "skier's thumb" injuries. Magn Reson Imaging North Am 1999;7:73–84.

Schoellnast H, Deutschmann HA, Hermann J, et al. Psoriatic arthritis and rheumatoid arthritis: findings in contrast-enhanced MRI. AJR Am J Roentgenol 2006;187:351–357.

Theumann NH, Goettmann S, Le Viet D, et al. Recurrent glomus tumors of fingertips: MR imaging evaluation. Radiology 2002; 223:143–151.

Theumann NH, Pfirrmann CW, Chung CB, et al. Ligamentous and tendinous anatomy of the intermetacarpal and common carpometacarpal joints: evaluation with MR imaging and MR arthrography. J Comput Assist Tomogr 2002;26:145–152.

Yu JS, Habib PA. Normal MR imaging anatomy of the wrist and hand. Magn Reson Imaging North Am 2004;12:207–219.

Chapter 11

IMAGING OF THE HIP AND PELVIS

CHAPTER OUTLINE

Imaging of the hip is a rapidly growing area of interest to orthopedic surgeons, especially with regard to dysplasia, impingement, labral tear, and groin injuries. This chapter focuses on newly emerging areas, issues in which controversy exists, and management conundrums that commonly affect the practicing radiologist.

MODALITIES

Radiography

Radiography remains the initial tool for evaluation of the majority of musculoskeletal conditions involving the hip and pelvis. These include acute and chronic injury, infection, avascular necrosis, arthritis, metabolic disease, tumor, and dysplasia/impingement. Radiography is the mainstay for diagnosis of fractures, both acute and stress-related. In the acute trauma setting, views such as oblique Judet views and inlet/outlet views (with craniocaudal angulation) can be helpful. Anteroposterior (AP; actually AP with internal rotation) and "frog lateral" (AP with external rotation) views are excellent for detection of femoral neck fracture; the surgical lateral view is used to detect AP fracture angulation. The frog lateral view is especially useful for detection of avascular necrosis of the femoral head, as well as slipped capital femoral epiphysis. Evaluation of sacroiliitis is best performed with a modified Ferguson view (cranially angulated AP), which elongates the joint. Some radiologists prefer oblique views to image along the joint. The AP pelvis is useful as a screening examination for a variety of pathologic conditions, but care should be taken to align the pubic symphysis with the coccyx to ensure that the image is directly anteroposterior. On a properly positioned AP pelvis, the hips can be evaluated for symmetry as well as for dysplasia and femoral-acetabular impingement. A specialized view, the faux profile, has been described for evaluation of hip pathology, especially arthritis, dysplasia, and impingement. When evaluating a hip prosthesis, radiographs are especially useful for detection of loosening; using fluoroscopy, the joint can be aspirated for fluid analysis and culture. Confirmation of loosening can be obtained by injecting iodinated contrast and visualizing its extension around the bone/cement interface. The surgical lateral view is especially useful for evaluation of retroversion of the acetabular cup, which can lead to dislocation. The flamingo view (AP view acquired while standing on one foot, then the other) can be used to evaluate pelvic instability in patients with chronic pain and osteitis pubis.

Computed Tomography

In the setting of acute trauma, CT is essential for diagnosis of subtle fractures and for planning surgical intervention. It offers advantages over radiography in some situations, as when evaluating cortices, avulsions, matrix mineralization, and soft tissue calcifications. With multidetector CT offering high-quality reformatted images, CT has also become more valuable for evaluation of hip prostheses and other hardware. In addition, use of multidetector CT has resulted in a resurgence of CT arthrography.

Ultrasound

Ultrasound is very useful for evaluation of the hip joint for effusion, and aspiration can be performed at the same setting. Fluid collections (bursitis, ganglia, paralabral cyst, abscess, hematoma) can similarly be evaluated and aspirated if necessary. As elsewhere in the body, ultrasound is excellent for detection of tendon pathology and can dynamically evaluate tendon motion (useful for evaluating a "snapping hip" for iliopsoas tendon deflection over the anterior acetabulum or iliotibial band friction over the greater trochanter).

Nuclear Medicine

Bone scan can be useful for screening for avascular necrosis (AVN), evaluation of suspected stress fracture, prosthesis loosening, osteomyelitis (in conjunction with labeled-WBC scan), and tumor (to differentiate benign from malignant sclerotic lesions or to look for multiplicity of lesions). Bladder uptake may obscure the sacrum and pubic symphysis, which can be overcome when lateral/sitting views or single photon emission computed tomography (SPECT) are used.

Magnetic Resonance Imaging

For patients with acute trauma, nondisplaced fractures may not be visible radiographically or even on CT. This is especially true in elderly patients with osteoporosis; the combination of low bone density, thin cortices, volume averaging, and osteoarthritis/enthesopathy can make detection of fracture lines and cortical step-off very difficult. In this situation, MRI is the best test for detection of fracture as well as for the associated soft tissue injury. MRI is also excellent for diagnosis of stress-related injuries, which may not be apparent radiographically. In its early stages, AVN of the femoral head is also not visualized on radiographs. MRI is highly sensitive and can guide rapid intervention such as core decompression. It is also the test of choice for infection because it can give an overall picture of soft tissue disease and spread as well as underlying osseous involvement. MR arthrography is the test of choice for detection of acetabular labral tear; an additional advantage of this invasive procedure is that although the needle is in the joint, anesthetic can be injected to give additional information regarding the site of pain generation.

The approach to hip pain requires a flexible approach to imaging protocols. For example, hip MRI should not be approached from the perspective that one protocol can answer all questions. Most musculoskeletal radiologists have a number of protocols aimed at diagnosing different conditions at the hip and pelvis. (See also the protocols in the accompanying CD.)

AVASCULAR NECROSIS OF THE HIP (Figs. 11-1 through 11-6)

A number of predisposing conditions can result in AVN (the most common are listed in Box 11-1). Often, however, no cause is found (idiopathic is common). Patients present with groin pain, which becomes worse with weight-bearing.

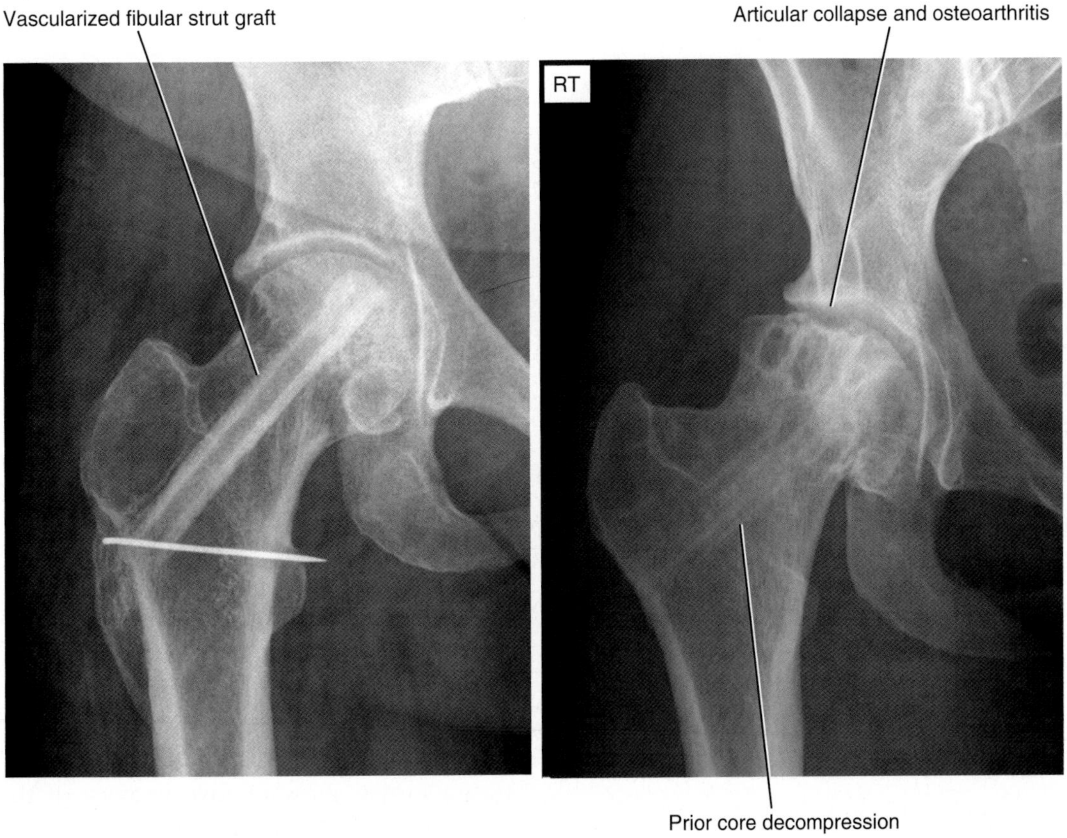
Vascularized fibular strut graft
RT
Articular collapse and osteoarthritis
Prior core decompression

Figure 11-1 Radiographic signs of treatment for avascular necrosis. Core decompression (drilling through the femoral neck into the head) is commonly performed in early stage (i.e., stage 1 or 2) avascular necrosis. Some surgeons prefer to insert a vascularized fibular strut graft; the nutrient vessels of the autograft are connected to the circumflex femoral artery and vein, and blood supply is theoretically restored to the subchondral bone in addition to providing added structural support against collapse. It remains controversial whether treatments affect the ultimate course.

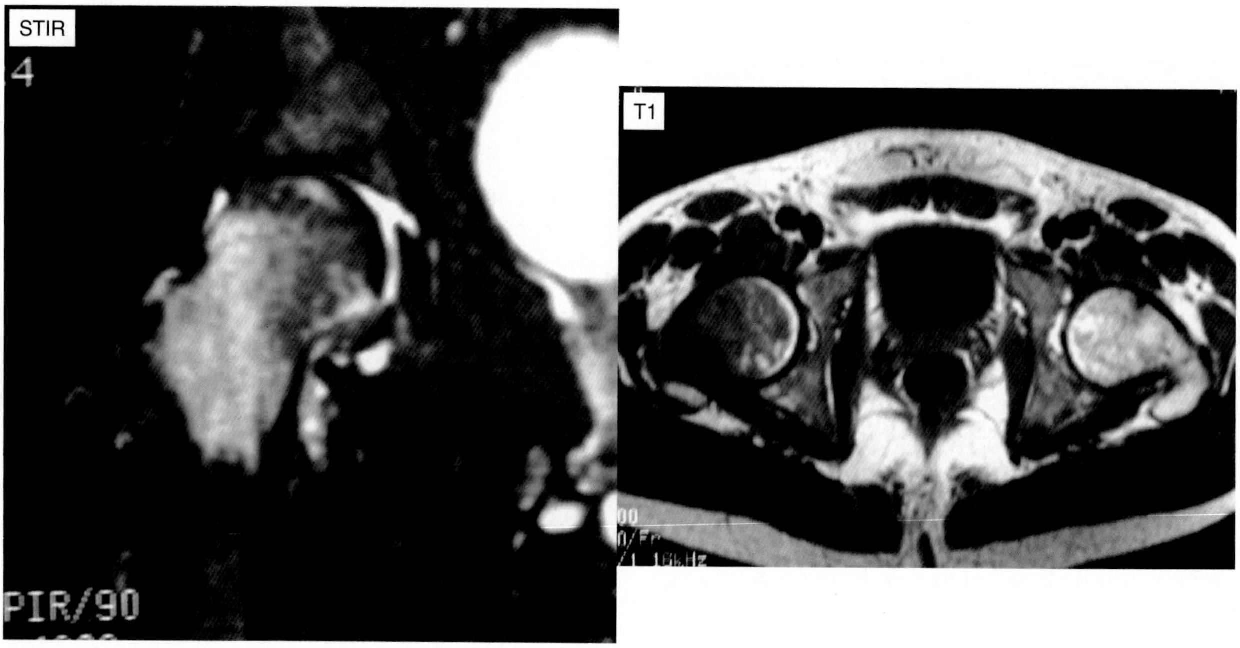
STIR
4
PIR/90
T1

Figure 11-2 Early avascular necrosis on MRI shows diffuse marrow edema.

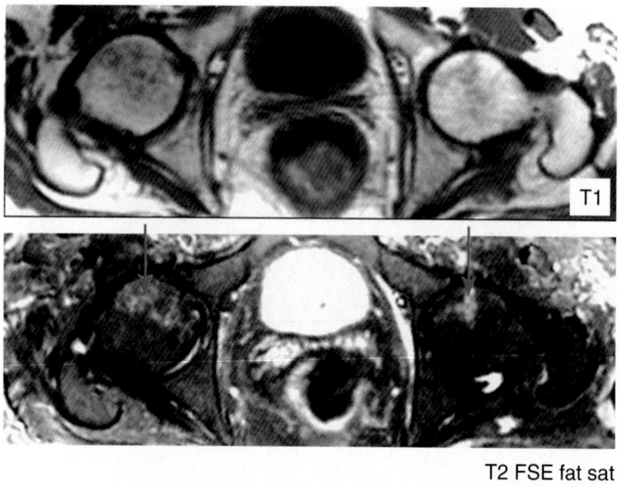
T1
T2 FSE fat sat

Figure 11-3 Subacute avascular necrosis on MRI. FSE fat sat, fast spin-echo fat saturation. Consolidation of marrow edema in subchondral bone. Note anterosuperior location, typical of avascular necrosis of the hip.

BOX 11-1 CAUSES OF AVASCULAR NECROSIS OF THE HIP

- Trauma (subcapital fracture or dislocation)
- Steroids
- Sickle cell disease
- Alcoholism
- Radiation therapy
- Chemotherapy
- Systemic lupus erythematosus/vasculitis
- Infection
- Miscellaneous (chronic pancreatitis, Gaucher disease, Cushing disease, Caisson disease)

In the early stages of AVN, radiographs are negative. MRI will show diffuse marrow edema of the femoral head, possibly with some subchondral crescentic signal. At this stage, the differential diagnosis includes subchondral stress fracture or transient osteoporosis of the hip (TOPH). AVN does not show bone resorption because there is no blood flow. Therefore, to differentiate these entities the radiologist can perform a dynamic contrast-enhanced MRI looking for lack of enhancement (AVN) versus hyperemia (stress fracture, TOPH). Alternatively, noncontrast CT may show relative lucency of the femoral head in TOPH but not in the other conditions. However, care should be taken when comparing with the opposite side in patients who may have AVN bilaterally.

The Ficat staging system is a radiographic staging system, but it is still the most widely used. It has since been modified by the Subcommittee of

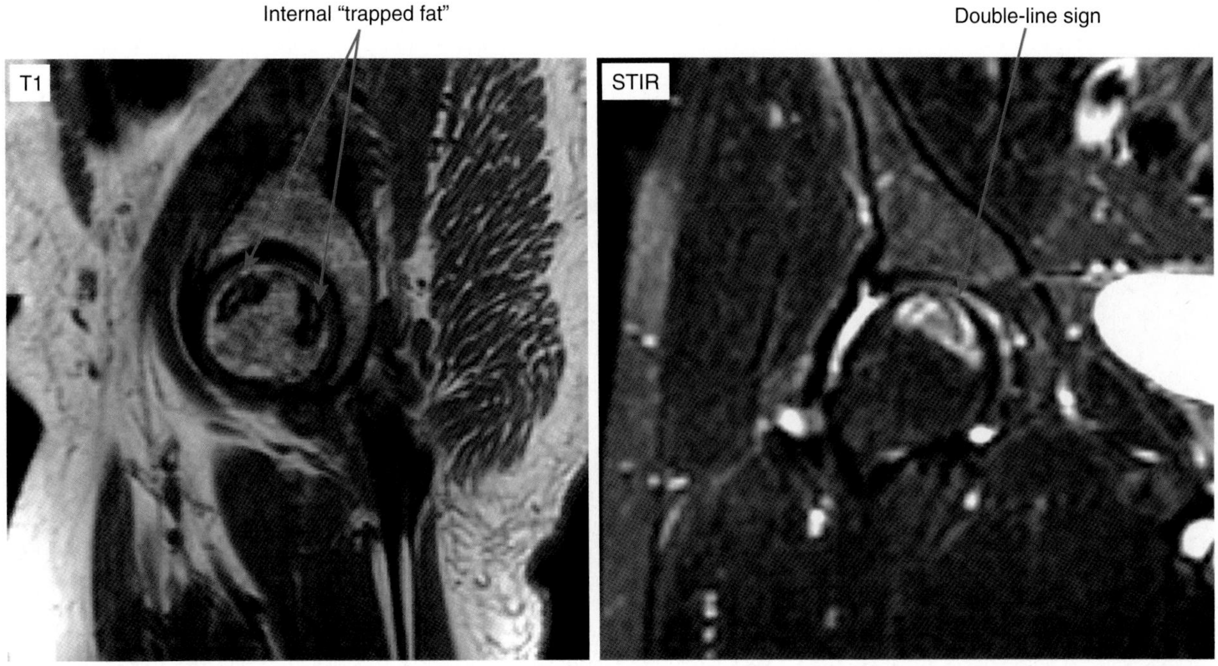
Internal "trapped fat"
Double-line sign
T1
STIR

Figure 11-4 Avascular necrosis: double-line sign on MRI. Zone of hyperintense signal represents granulation tissue at the margin of dead and living bone.

Table 11-1 Modified Ficat Staging System for Avascular Necrosis of the Hip

Stage	X-ray	MRI	Clinical Symptoms	Treatment
Stage 0	Neg.	—	No symptoms; + risk factors	—
Stage 1	Neg.	Neg.	+ Pain	Core decompression
Stage 2	Increased density	Well defined Double line	+/– Pain	Core decompression
Stage 3	Subchondral lucency*	Diffuse edema Subchondral fluid	+ Acute pain	Hemiarthroplasty
Stage 4	Femoral head collapse	Diffuse edema Flat head	+ Acute-on-chronic pain	Hemiarthroplasty
Stage 5	OA	OA	+ Chronic pain	THA
Stage 6	Extensive destruction of joint	Extensive destruction of joint	+ Chronic pain	THA

*Subchondral crescentic lucency represents subchondral fracture. Subcategories have been proposed: 3a: crescent <15% of articular surface; 3b: 15% to 30%; 3c: >30%.
OA, osteoarthritis; THA, total hip arthroplasty.

Nomenclature of the International Association on Bone Circulation and Bone Necrosis; Table 11-1 summarizes the stages. The key is that appearance and progression are similar no matter what bone is affected. In other words, the disease progresses from radiographically occult to an increase in density, to collapse and fragmentation, to osteoarthritis. Treatment is based on the modified Ficat stage. However, in radiologic reports it always better to be descriptive rather than to list the stage because some surgeons

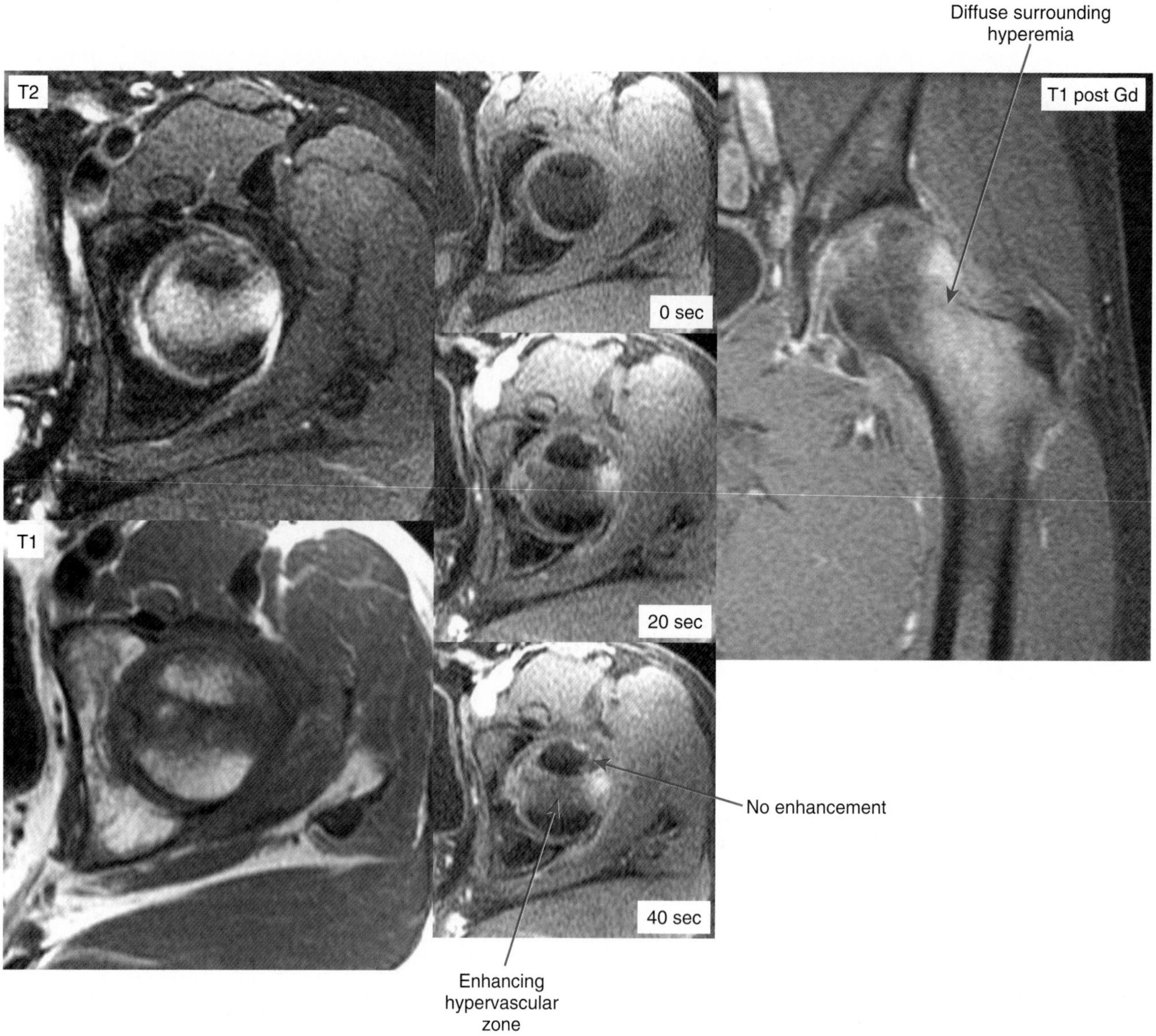
Diffuse surrounding hyperemia
T2
T1 post Gd
0 sec
T1
20 sec
No enhancement
40 sec
Enhancing hypervascular zone

Figure 11-5 Dynamic contrast-enhanced MRI (DCEMRI). Diagnosis of acute avascular necrosis.

may refer to the original Ficat staging, which is numbered differently.

In later stages, it is easier to document the finding as AVN. In stage 2 in which increased radiographic density is seen, MRI demonstrates a focal subchondral geographic signal abnormality, usually centered anterosuperiorly. The central signal is variable, often high on T1 (trapped/mummified fat) but occasionally bright on T2 or dark on all sequences (fibrotic). The margins demonstrate the classic "double line sign" of Mitchell, representing the interface between living and dead bone with a rim of granulation tissue. Typically, the surrounding marrow edema has resolved. At this point, patients may be asymptomatic.

Patients may go on for many years at the prior stage. When a patient with established AVN presents with acute pain, the suspicion and imaging should be directed toward finding articular collapse, which is often very subtle. On radiographs, a subchondral lucent line may be seen, representing a fracture. Flattening of the normally spherical femoral head indicates collapse. If no radiographic signs of collapse are seen, CT with sagittal and coronal reformats is very useful, especially when using multidetector CT

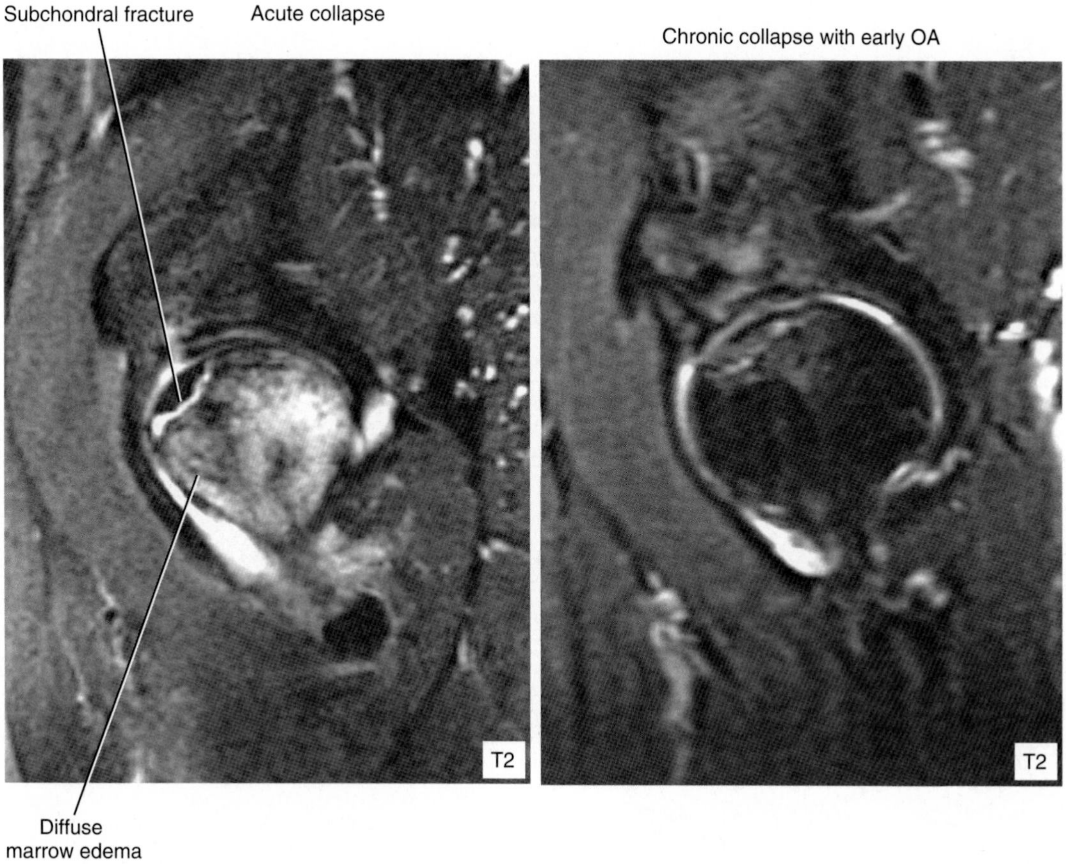
Subchondral fracture
Acute collapse
Chronic collapse with early OA
T2
T2
Diffuse marrow edema

Figure 11-6 Avascular necrosis: collapse. When the articular surface collapses, the patient becomes acutely symptomatic. On MRI, the articular surface is flattened. Often a linear hyperintensity represents the fracture line. Marked surrounding edema and moderate joint effusion are present and can suggest a differential diagnosis of early avascular necrosis or transient osteoporosis. OA, osteoarthritis.

with thin cuts. MRI can also be used, although CT has higher resolution. The advantage of MRI is visualization of the diffuse marrow edema that results from collapse, edema that extends to the intertrochanteric region simulating early AVN. If established AVN is seen in addition to this finding, certainly acute-on-chronic AVN is a possibility, but subtle articular surface collapse should be sought. Like AVN, the collapse is usually anterosuperior. TOPH is in the differential for diffuse femoral head edema, but underlying established AVN (or AVN on the other side) helps exclude this possibility.

Osteoarthritis is the last stage of AVN, but distinction should be made between patients with AVN, collapse and subsequent osteoarthritis and those with incidental AVN, no collapse, and osteoarthritis from some other cause. These patients may be treated differently.

Description of Findings

The MR imaging (or radiographic) report should not only diagnose AVN but also discuss features that will help the orthopedist decide on appropriate treatment such as the following:

Location of AVN (e.g., anterosuperior)
Percent articular surface area involved (can be estimated based on coronal and sagittal images)
Articular surface collapse
Osteoarthritis

TRANSIENT OSTEOPOROSIS OF THE HIP

Transient osteoporosis of the hip is a painful condition that was first described in patients in the third

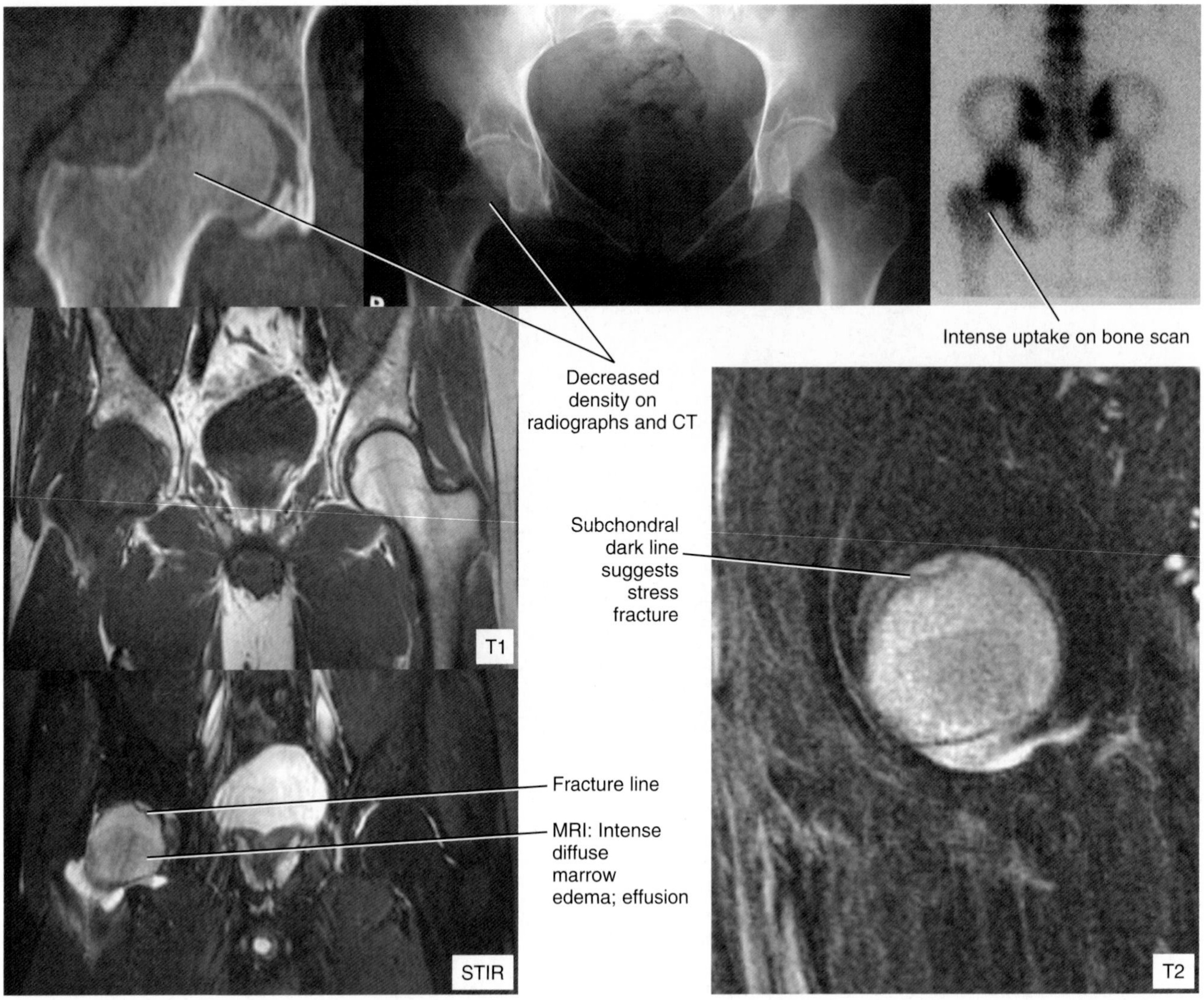

Intense uptake on bone scan
Decreased density on radiographs and CT
Subchondral dark line suggests stress fracture
T1
Fracture line
MRI: Intense diffuse marrow edema; effusion
STIR
T2

Figure 11-7 Transient osteoporosis of the hip. Osteopenia of the femoral head is seen on radiographs and CT. This suggests lack of avascular necrosis, since blood flow is necessary to resorb bone. Intense marrow edema is seen on MRI, often with a subchondral line. Proposed etiology is that this actually represents a subchondral stress fracture, like spontaneous osteonecrosis of the knee. If the diagnosis remains unclear, MRI can be performed with dynamic contrast enhancement to differentiate marrow edema related to hyperemia (transient osteoporosis) from ischemia (avascular necrosis).

trimester of pregnancy (Figs. 11-7 through 11-9). Radiographs and CT show asymmetric osteopenia of the femoral head. MRI shows diffuse edema of the femoral head extending to the intertrochanteric region, an appearance that mimics early AVN. However, unlike AVN, TOPH resolves spontaneously. One theory is that TOPH is ischemia that does not go on to frank necrosis; another theory is that TOPH represents a subchondral stress fracture, much like spontaneous osteonecrosis of the knee. Appearance in late pregnancy supports a stress-related etiology. Also supporting a stress origin is the presence of a subchondral crescentic low-signal region in many cases. CT (showing osteopenia) or dynamic contrast-enhanced MRI (showing early contrast enhancement) should be able to differentiate TOPH from AVN.

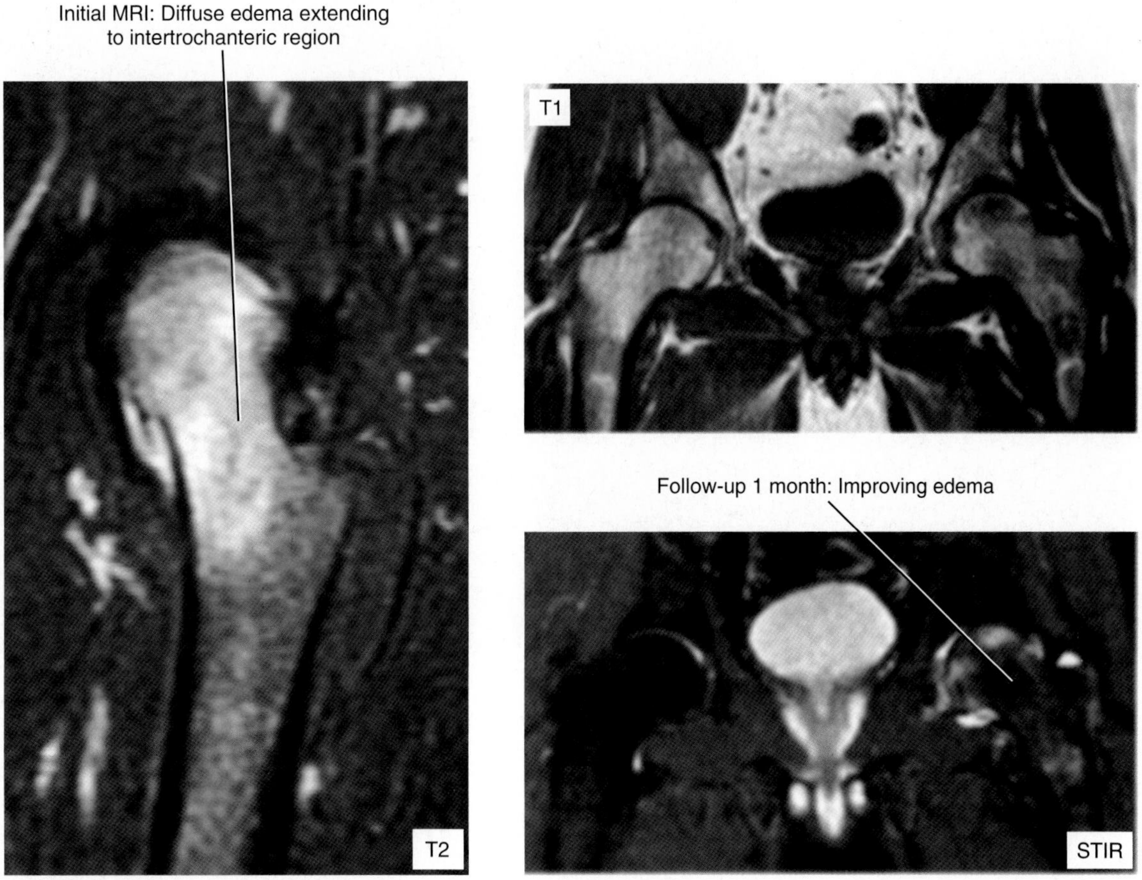
Initial MRI: Diffuse edema extending to intertrochanteric region
T1
Follow-up 1 month: Improving edema
T2
STIR

Figure 11-8 Transient osteoporosis. Follow-up shows improvement.

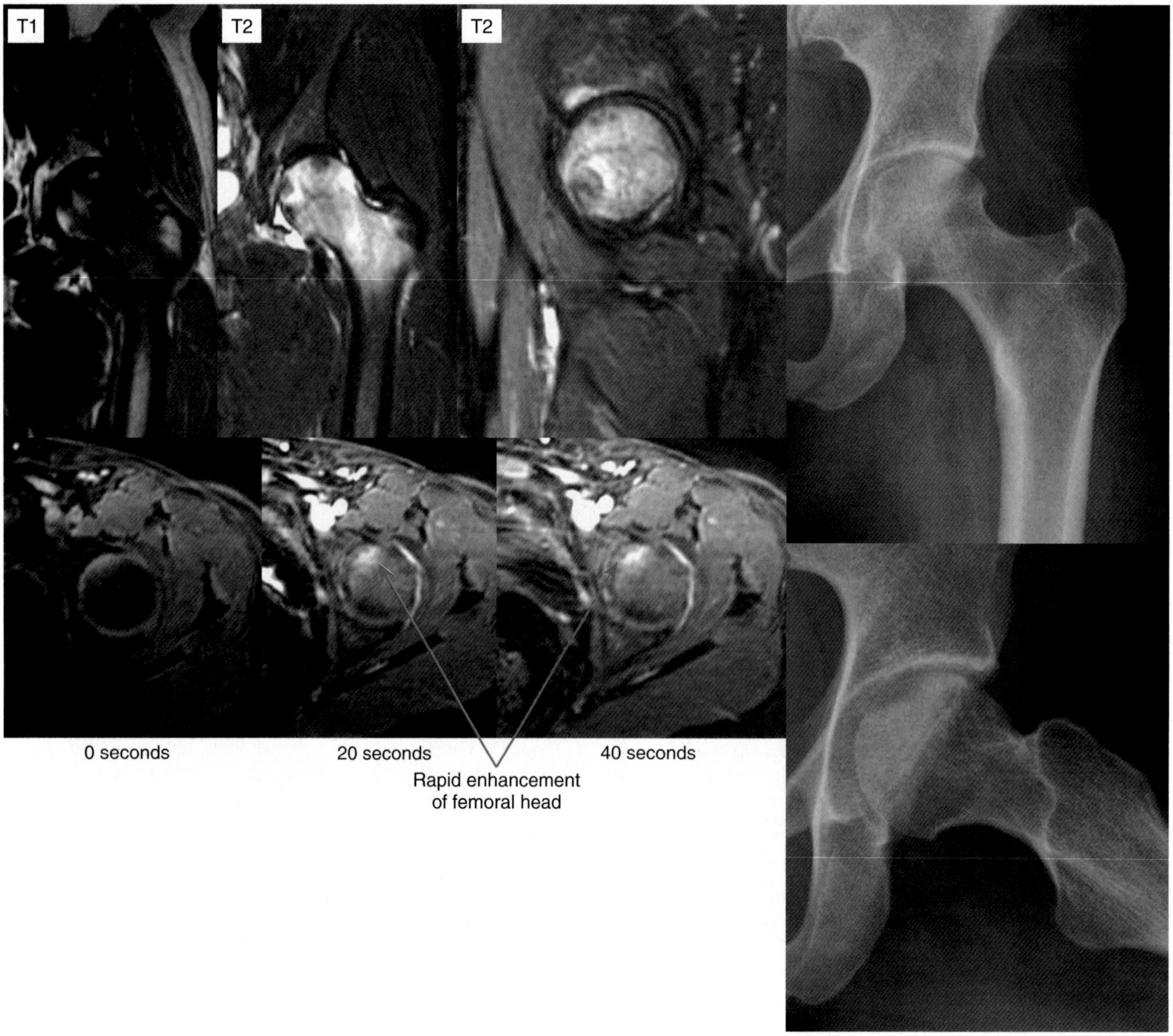
T1
T2
T2
0 seconds
20 seconds
40 seconds
Rapid enhancement
of femoral head

Figure 11-9 Dynamic contrast-enhanced MRI (DCEMRI) is useful for distinguishing transient osteoporosis of the hip (most likely a stress fracture and should result in hyperemia) from avascular necrosis (which shows a region of nonenhancement).

STRESS FRACTURE (Figs. 11-10 through 11-13)

Stress fracture is divided into two categories: fatigue (normal bone undergoing abnormal stress) and insufficiency (abnormal bone undergoing normal stresses). Stress fracture is a relatively common source of hip pain in certain populations, such as teens or young adults undergoing new physical activity (fatigue) and older patients with radiation therapy to the pelvis or with underlying osteoporosis and alteration of activity (e.g., recent total knee arthroplasty with shifting of weight-bearing to the other side) (insufficiency).

If MRI is ordered for a stress fracture, which is suspected either based on the clinical history or hip pain in a susceptible population, it is recommended to use a large field of view because these injuries often are multiple and bilateral in expected locations around the pelvic ring.

In young patients, common sites for stress fracture around the pelvis include the superior and inferior pubic ramus and the femoral neck. In older patients, the sacral alae and supra-acetabular region are more common.

Stress fractures at the femoral neck tend to be solitary and unilateral. They tend to occur most frequently by far at the base of the medial femoral neck (the compressive aspect, where each step pushes the fracture sides together). Since bony apposition is essential for healing, stress fractures in this location have a good prognosis for healing. If the fracture occurs laterally, it is more unstable (this is the tensile

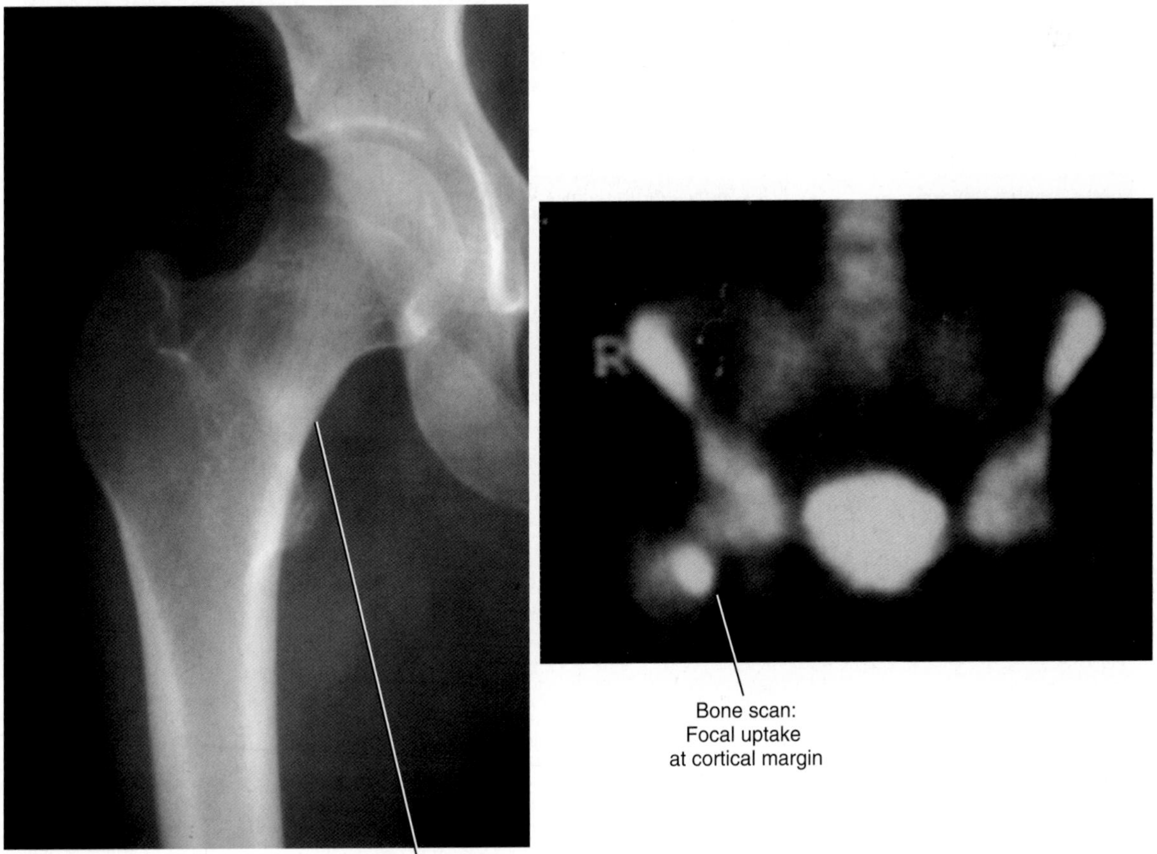
R
Bone scan:
Focal uptake
at cortical margin
Radiographs:
Late finding—subcortical
linear density

Figure 11-10 Classic stress fracture of the hip in a young patient at the medial aspect of the base of the femoral neck. Fractures at the medial aspect (compressive side) are usually treated conservatively, whereas fractures at the lateral aspect (distractive side) are often treated aggressively with pinning.

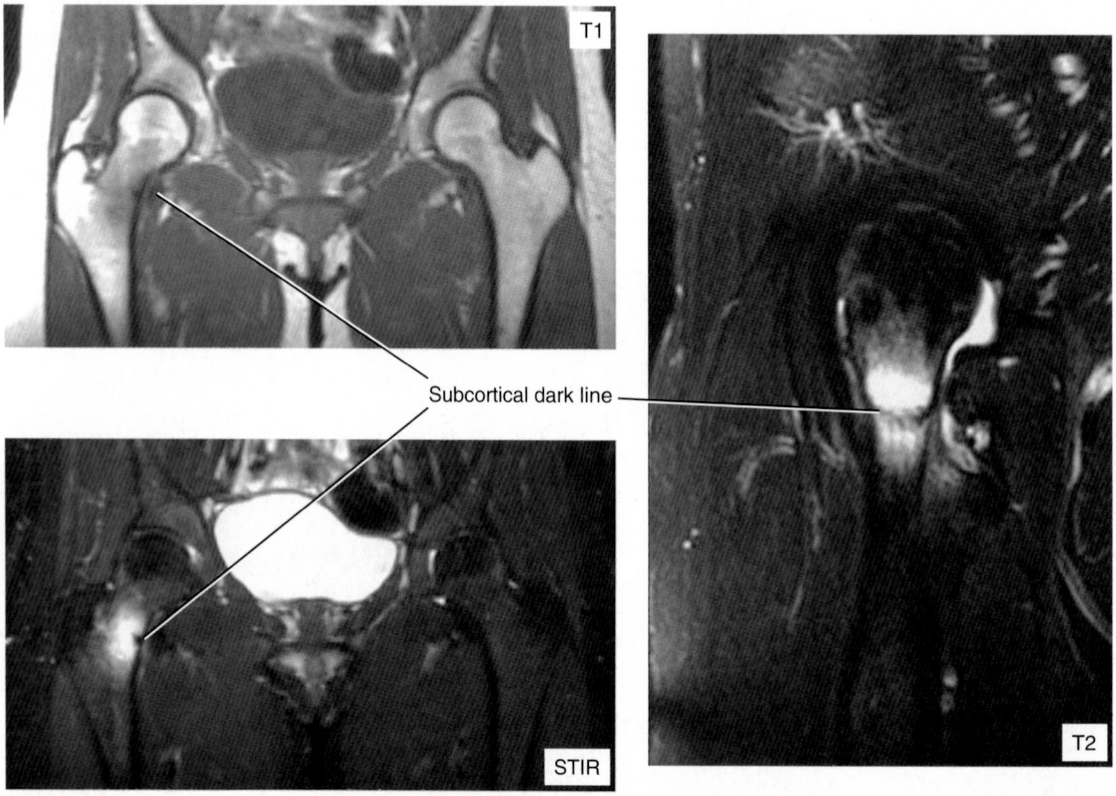
T1
Subcortical dark line
STIR
T2

Figure 11-11 Stress fracture on MRI. The subchondral density on radiographs corresponds to a low-signal subcortical line on T1 and fluid-sensitive sequences. This represents trabecular callus and is surrounded by marrow edema. This line is very specific for stress fracture, and MRI is the test of choice to exclude other etiologies such as tumor. Follow-up MRI can be useful for tracking therapeutic response, but radiologic findings lag behind clinical improvement.

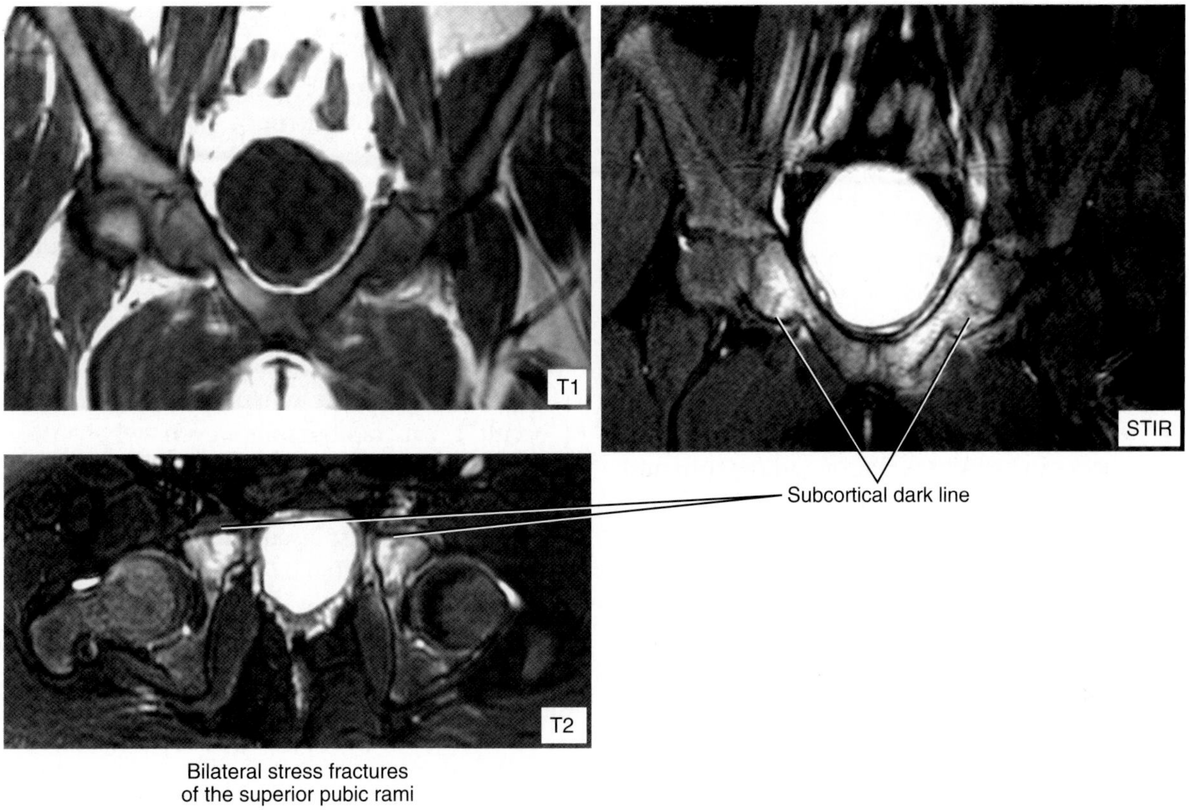
T1
STIR
T2
Subcortical dark line
Bilateral stress fractures of the superior pubic rami

Figure 11-12 Stress fractures around the hip in young patients often occur at the pubic rami. Whenever a fracture is seen at the pelvic ring, other fractures of the ring should be sought, whether the cause is acute trauma or stress. In older patients, they are seen more frequently at the sacrum and supra-acetabular region; in this older population, they may be mistaken for tumor. The finding of a dark line with surrounding edema is highly specific.

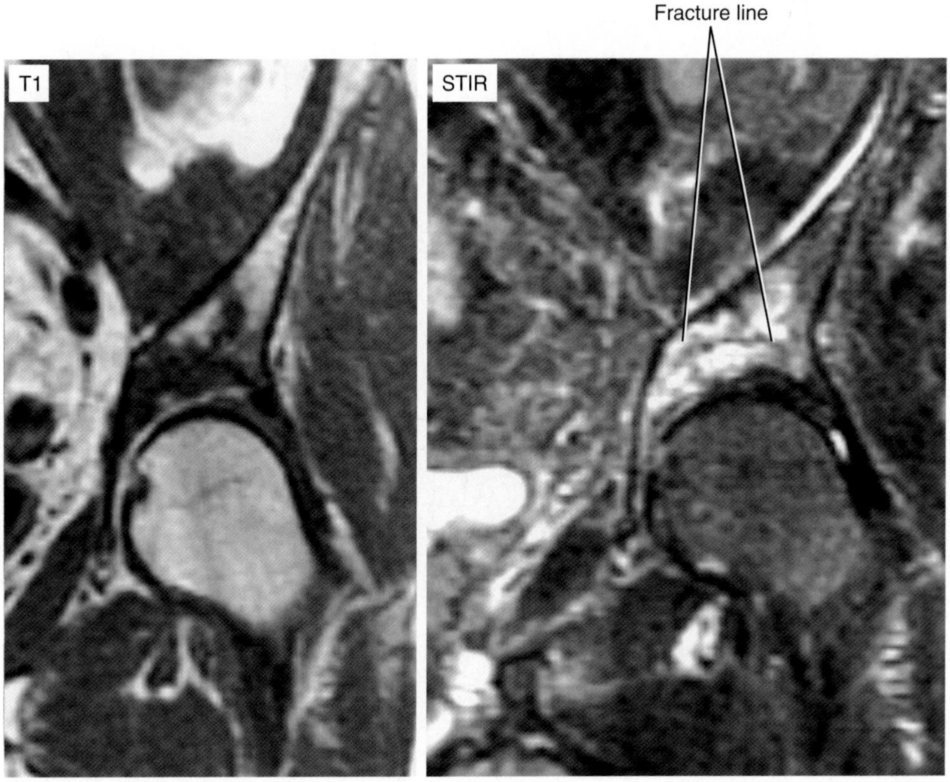
Fracture line
T1
STIR

Figure 11-13 Acetabular insufficiency fracture. On T1-weighted images, the fracture and surrounding edema can resemble a malignancy. However, on fluid-sensitive images the low-signal fracture line is seen, set apart by surrounding edema. MRI with in-phase and out-of-phase imaging can be used to document residual marrow fat if the diagnosis remains unclear on routine sequences.

aspect; weight-bearing tends to pull the fracture apart). The latter may be prophylactically treated with pin fixation.

Stress fracture has a characteristic appearance on most modalities and should not be confused with tumor or another pathology. Despite this, sacral stress fracture is often referred for biopsy or more imaging, based on concern over the patient's age and the presence of a sclerotic lesion.

Radiographs show a sclerotic region, which is linear and extends from the cortex. Sacral fractures are vertically oriented at the ala and often cross the midline, leading to the classic H sign on bone scan. Sacral stress fractures can be nonspecific on radiographs and present with ill-defined sclerosis. CT or MRI is the next test to confirm the diagnosis. Bone scan is useful if the injury is bilateral or if unilateral uptake in one sacral ala is nonspecific. CT shows sclerosis, which, if inspected closely or with reformatted images, shows a linear pattern. In the sacrum, inspection of the foraminal cortices often shows very subtle cortical step-off that can help confirm the diagnosis. MRI shows a subcortical low signal line on T1- and T2-weighted images, representing microcallus, surrounded by marrow edema.

TRAUMA

Occult Fracture (Figs. 11-14 through 11-17)

Hip and/or pelvic fractures may be undetectable ("occult") on radiographs, even when they are reviewed after learning of the precise location. This situation is especially common in elderly patients who suffer a nondisplaced fracture through osteoporotic bone during a fall. Usually, a more severe injury is suspected clinically because the patient often cannot bear weight on the affected side, and additional imaging is requested. The best modality for definitive diagnosis of occult fracture is MRI. In fact,

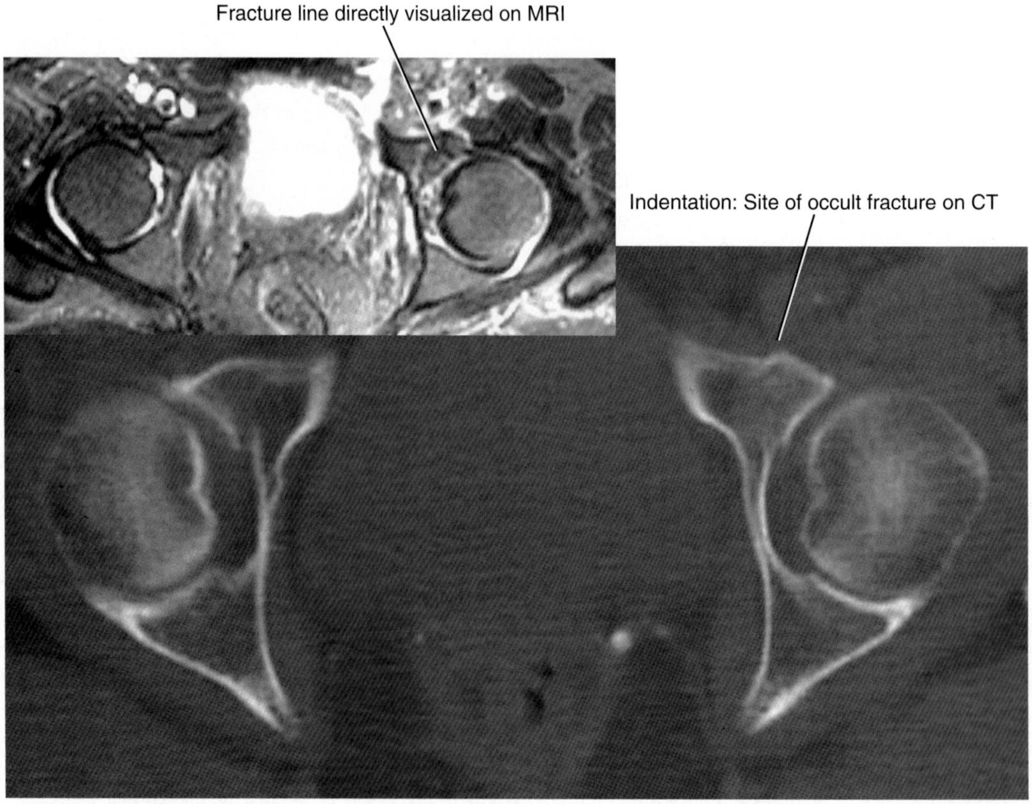
Fracture line directly visualized on MRI
Indentation: Site of occult fracture on CT

Figure 11-14 Occult fracture. CT (especially multidetector CT) can be very useful for diagnosis of clinically suspected fracture. However, nondisplaced fractures (presenting on CT as a small asymmetric dent or cortical step-off) can still be difficult to detect.

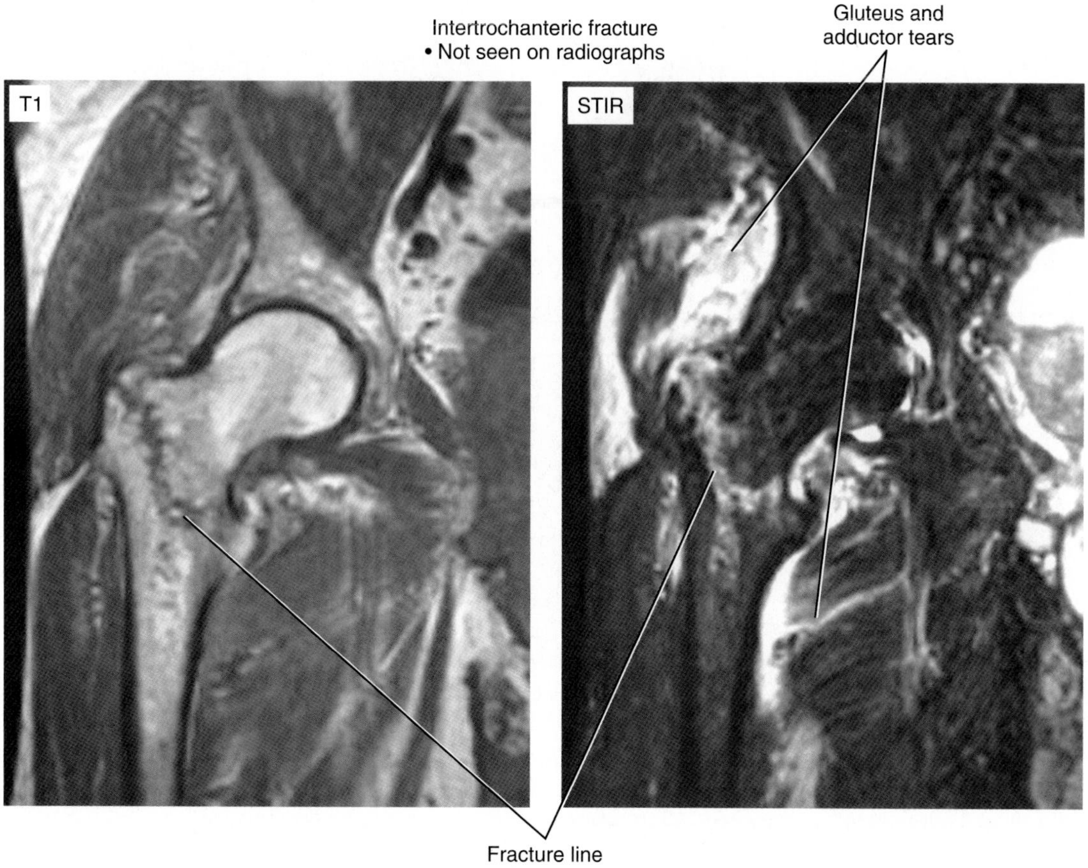
Intertrochanteric fracture
• Not seen on radiographs
Gluteus and
adductor tears
T1
STIR
Fracture line

Figure 11-15 Occult fracture of the hip. MRI is generally preferred over CT and can be performed as an abbreviated, rapid protocol. There is a high association of muscle strain and fracture. When edema of the hip adductors, obturators, and/or gluteus muscles is seen in the setting of trauma, careful inspection should be made for underlying fracture.

this exam is considered one of the few "musculoskeletal emergencies" (outside of spine imaging) that would prompt calling in the night technologist. During the day, an abbreviated hip survey exam (refer to protocols) can be performed in approximately 10 minutes, sandwiched between routine exams.

The survey exam is acquired using a large field of view to detect associated soft tissue injury and contralateral injury to the rigid pelvic ring. A coronal STIR sequence is used to provide maximal fluid conspicuity while limiting artifact from field heterogeneity. Bone marrow edema is easily seen, as are muscle tears and traumatic bursitis. Muscles that commonly tear include the adductors, glutei, and obturator externus and internus. In the acute stage, wherever they occur, fractures can be hard to distinguish from bone bruises on fluid-sensitive sequences (STIR or fat-suppressed T2-weighted imaging) because the fracture line is bright and so is the surrounding marrow. Although this is less of an issue in the pelvis after acute trauma, acquisition of a coronal T1-weighted sequence facilitates visualization of the fracture line itself. Location, whether complete or partial, and associated soft tissue injury should be reported. Just as on trauma radiographs, when one fracture is found, others should be sought.

CT can be used as an alternate modality, but this is less sensitive than MRI, especially for nondisplaced fractures that may have only slight cortical indentation or step-off or impacted femoral neck fractures that can be confused for a healed fracture or ring of osteophytes. Comparison from side to side is useful, as is close inspection of commonly fractured sites (femoral neck, acetabulum, superior/inferior pubic rami, sacral alae) and close inspection of bone adjacent to traumatic soft tissue infiltration.

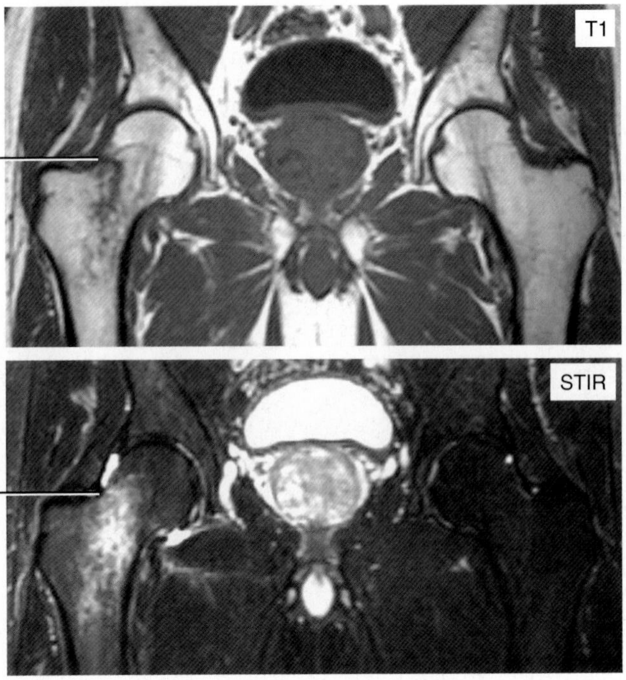
T1
Fracture line
STIR
Fracture line can be obscured by surrounding edema on T2/STIR
Acute incomplete femoral neck fracture

Figure 11-16 Occult fracture on MRI. The fracture line may be obscured on fluid-sensitive images, since the fracture line and surrounding marrow are both bright. T1-weighted images are essential for visualizing the fracture line (this is the opposite of a stress fracture in which the dark fracture line is best seen on fluid-sensitive images).

Nuclear medicine bone scan is too insensitive in the acute phase of occult fracture. A traditional low-cost alternative to advanced imaging, that being conservative therapy with follow-up radiographs, is not an option in this setting because the fracture can displace and become more complicated in addition to pulmonary embolism and other dreaded complications resulting from prolonged immobilization of the elderly.

Avulsion Fracture (Figs. 11-18 through 11-21)

Avulsion fractures are seen with sudden, forceful muscle contraction; adolescents are susceptible to avulsion of the sartorius from the anterior superior iliac spine (ASIS), and the rectus femoris from the anterior inferior iliac spine (AIIS). Hip pain in a young patient should always draw attention to these attachment sites, regardless of the modality. MRI of the hip with a small field of view can miss the ASIS, and if included, near field brightening or artifact can simulate pathology. Again, a large field-of-view STIR sequence is very useful as a survey for this and other pathology. In high-performance adolescent athletes, hamstring avulsion can be seen. Avulsions acquired during youth may heal back to the underlying bone leaving a bony prominence that can be mistaken for an osteochondroma. Often the avulsion remains separate from the native bone, becoming rounded and proliferative over time.

In the elderly, the greater trochanter is especially susceptible to avulsion, usually from the gluteus medius (fragment heads superiorly) or the obturator internus (fragment heads medially). Often there is associated greater trochanteric bursitis and, when visualized, care must be taken not to miss underlying avulsion or muscle/tendon tear. Lesser trochanter avulsions are very uncommon but should prompt evaluation for an underlying lesion (pathologic fracture).

CALCIFIC TENDINOSIS

The differential diagnosis of hip pain includes hydroxyapatite deposition disease (HADD), which can manifest as calcific tendinosis, calcific bursitis, or

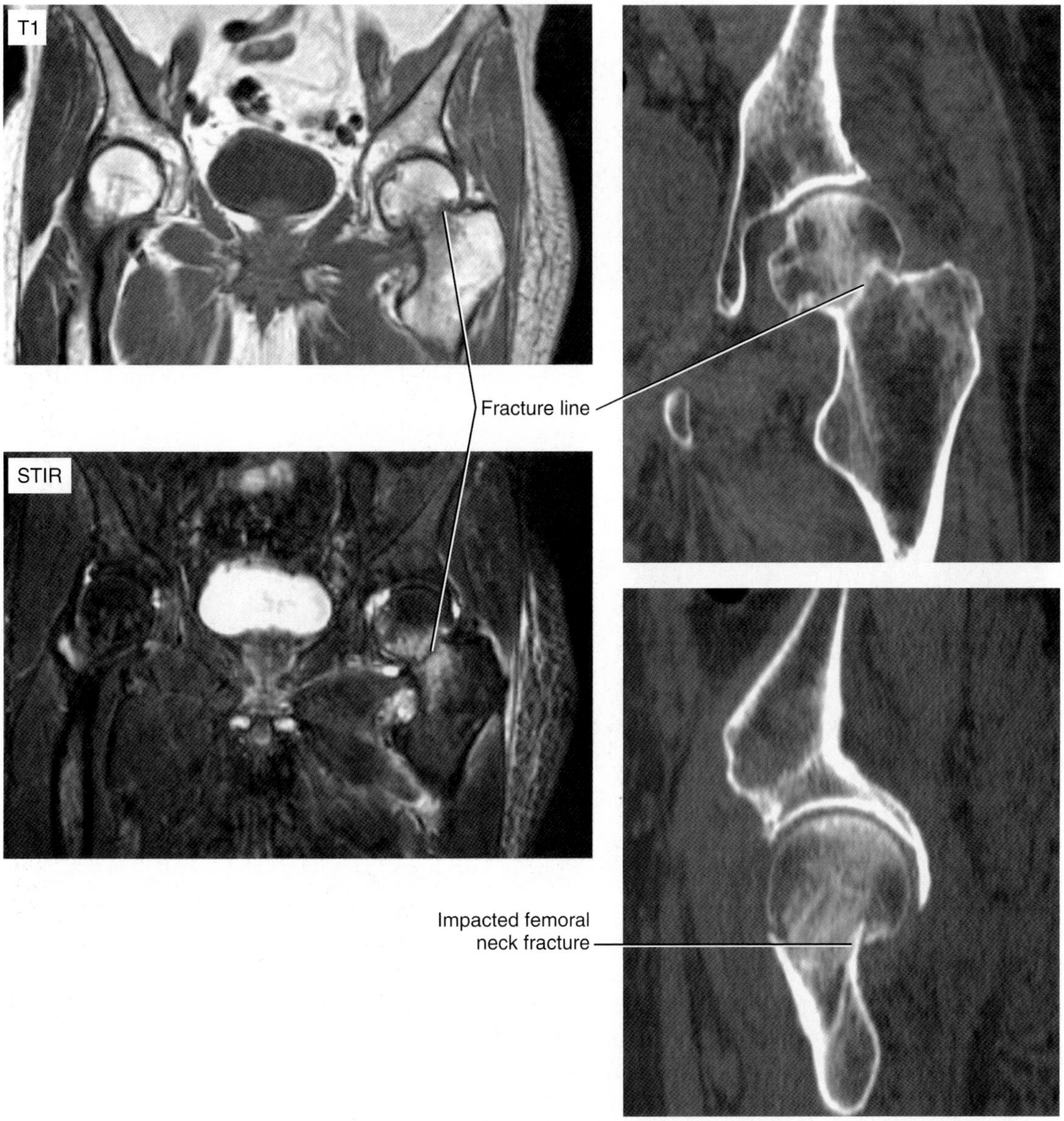
T1
STIR
Fracture line
Impacted femoral neck fracture

Figure 11-17 Occult femoral neck fracture with impaction. Trabecular compression can also result in a low signal line similar to stress or subacute fracture. History and other findings (e.g., adjacent soft tissue edema) point to acute injury.

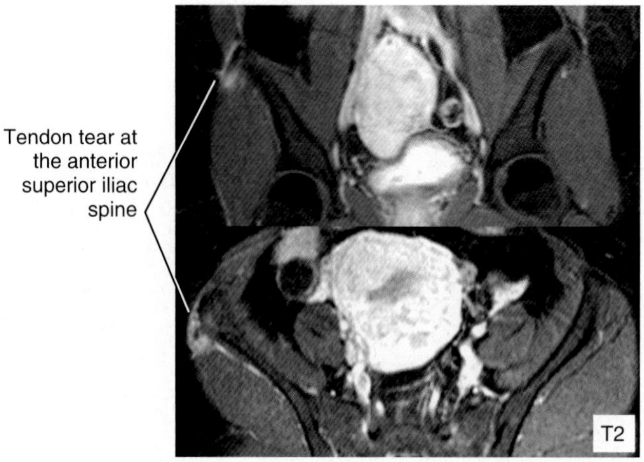
Tendon tear at the anterior superior iliac spine
T2

Figure 11-18 Avulsion fracture. Avulsions at the hip are common in adolescent athletes, especially at the anterior superior iliac spine (ASIS; from the sartorius or tensor fascia lata origin, referred to clinically as a "hip pointer") or the anterior inferior iliac spine (AIIS; rectus femoris origin).

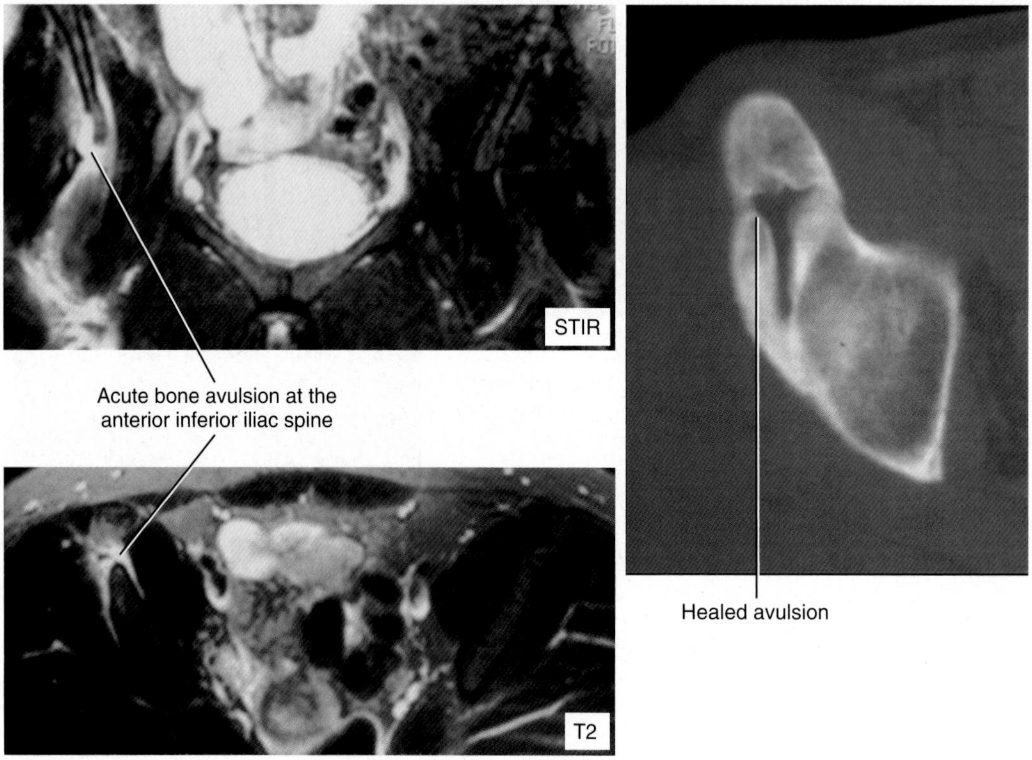
STIR
Acute bone avulsion at the anterior inferior iliac spine
T2
Healed avulsion

Figure 11-19 Avulsion of the anterior inferior iliac spine—acute and chronic appearance.

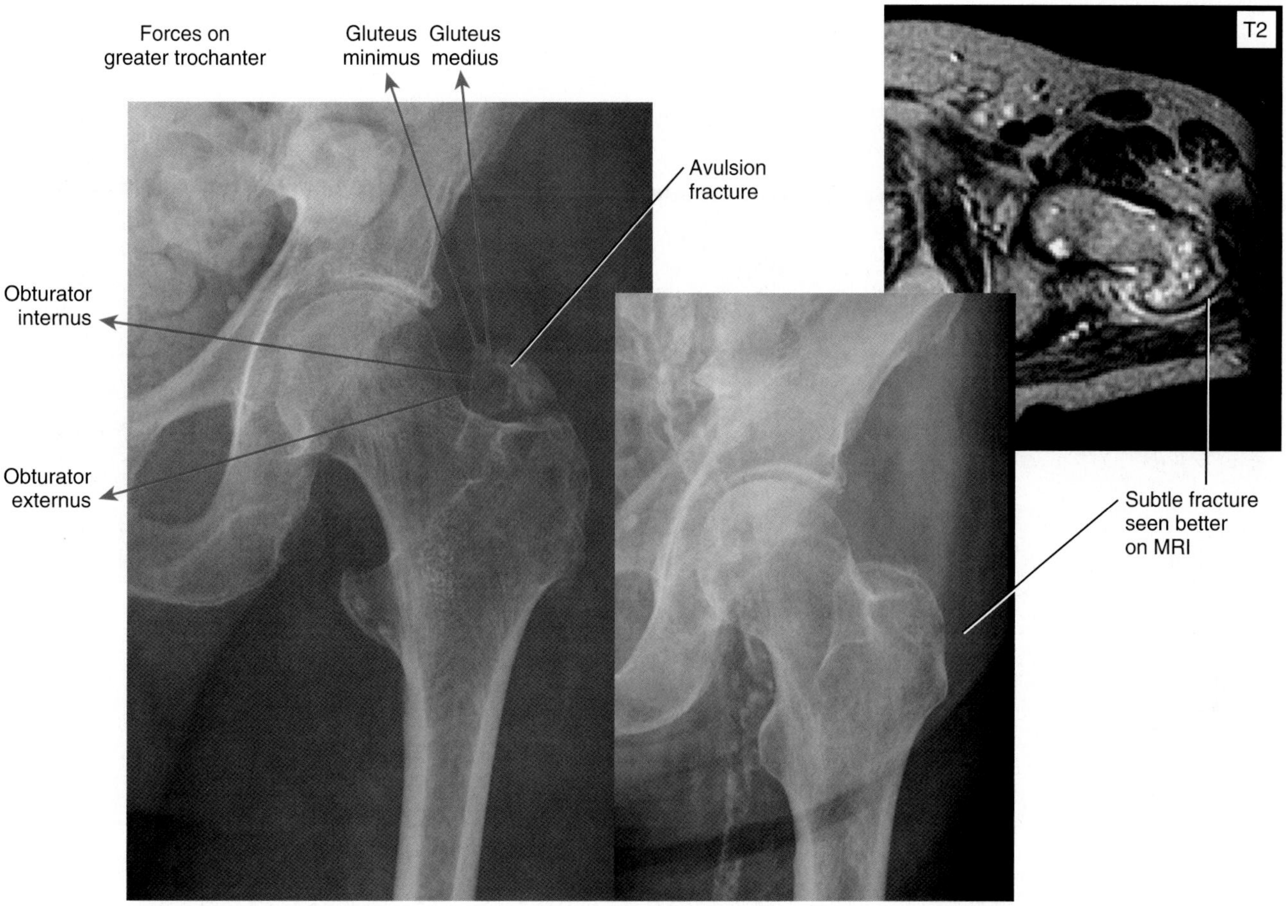
Forces on
greater trochanter
Gluteus minimus
Gluteus medius
Avulsion
fracture
Obturator
internus
Obturator
externus
T2
Subtle fracture
seen better
on MRI

Figure 11-20 Avulsion fractures are fairly common in the older population, but tend to occur at the greater trochanter, from the attachment of the obturator internus and externus as well as the gluteus medius and minimus. Note traction forces depicted in red.

calcific periarthritis. All forms look similar, with a glob of homogeneous calcification corresponding to a tendon or bursa. As in the shoulder, calcific tendinosis is common around the hip, especially at the greater trochanter or gluteus maximus insertion. This finding is often overlooked on radiographs, but with pain and a typical calcification, the diagnosis should be considered as a potential source of pain. HADD can be associated with severe pain, tenderness, and low-grade fever. This is discussed in more detail in Chapter 4.

METASTATIC DISEASE AND MYELOMA

The pelvis and hips are a common location for metastatic disease and myeloma, corresponding to areas of red marrow. Distribution of hematopoietic marrow, as well as diagnosis of malignancy, is discussed in Chapter 6.

OSTEOMYELITIS

At the hip and pelvis, contiguous spread of infection is most common (similar to that in foot); this is because most infection in this location is seen in paralyzed patients with decubitus ulcers. Infection in paralyzed patients corresponds to locations that are subject to pressure and friction, which then break down into an ulcer. Infection then enters the subcutaneous tissues and progresses to involve the underlying bone. The most common sites are the ischium, the sacrum, and the greater trochanter. Specific imaging characteristics are discussed in Chapter 5.

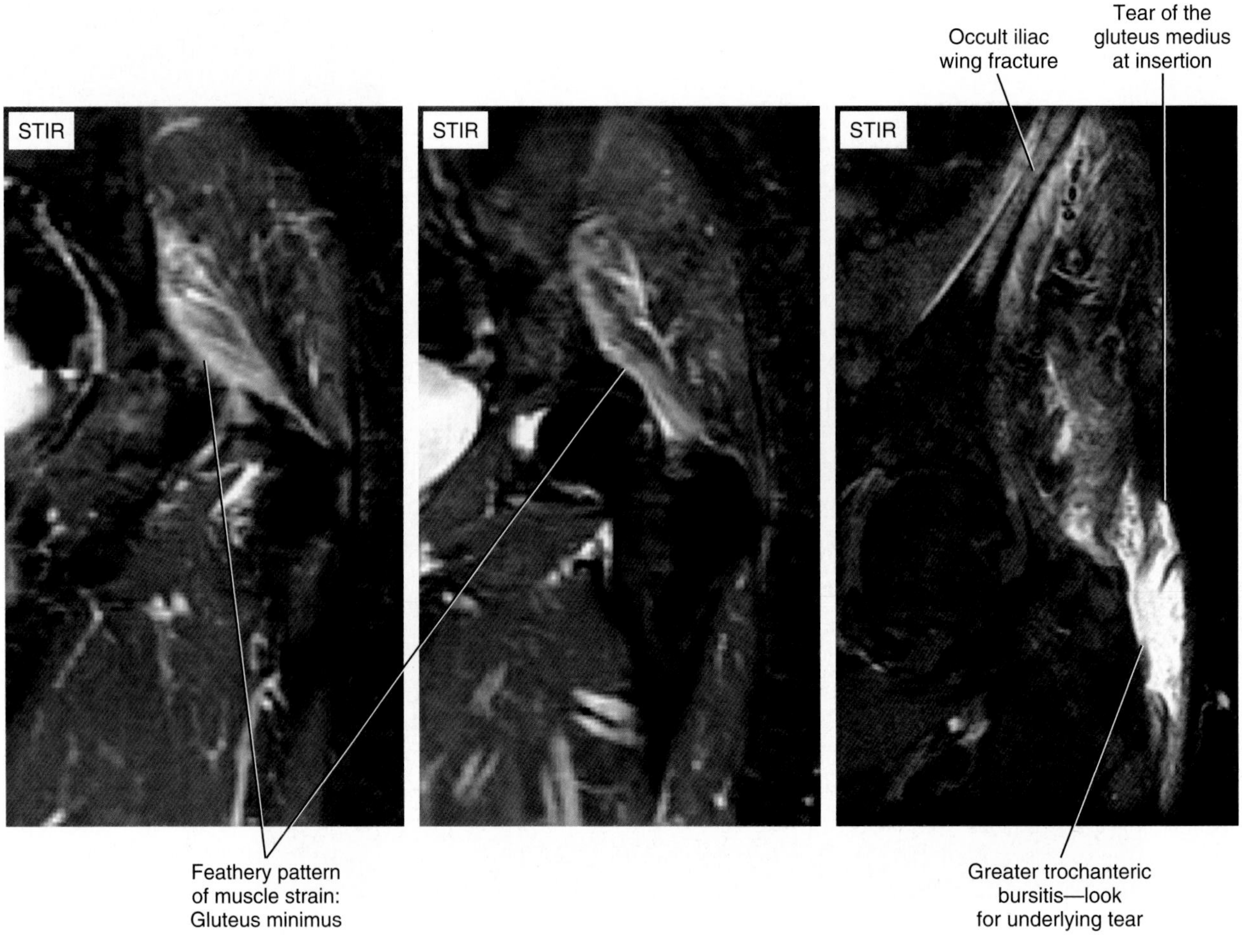
Occult iliac wing fracture
Tear of the gluteus medius at insertion
STIR
STIR
STIR
Feathery pattern of muscle strain: Gluteus minimus
Greater trochanteric bursitis—look for underlying tear

Figure 11-21 Muscle tear of gluteus medius and minimus. The feathery pattern of muscle edema is characteristic of strain. Greater trochanteric bursal fluid is very common, but when asymmetric or on the side of pain, look closely at the insertion sites of the gluteus medius and minimus on the greater trochanter for tear.

However, it is helpful to understand the patterns of spread of infection along fascial planes to predict the extent of involvement.

PROSTHESIS IMAGING

Imaging hip prostheses for complications is a common request. Patients present with pain; severity, acuity, and presence of fever help form the clinical differential (Figs. 11-22 through 11-30). Fever obviously raises concern for infection, in which case the most useful test is aspiration. (The technique is described in more detail in Chapter 2.) The patient with infection typically has severe pain and often cannot bear weight. An 18-g needle must be used since the secretions are thick. In cases of infection, the fluid in the joint is under pressure, and rapidly decompresses through the needle, yielding thick, yellowish purulent material. If no fluid is aspirated, the needle can be walked around the neck since the fluid can be compartmentalized. If no fluid is acquired after this, sterile saline can be injected (not water, which is bacteriocidal owing to hypotonicity) and re-aspirated to send for culture. However, it can be difficult to re-aspirate injected fluid.

After aspiration, injection of iodinated contrast can be performed to ensure that the fluid was acquired from the joint and not an adjacent bursa (although feeling metal on metal is also a good sign) and to look for loosening (contrast extending around the prosthetic femoral stem or acetabulum). Often, an infected total hip arthroplasty communicates with an

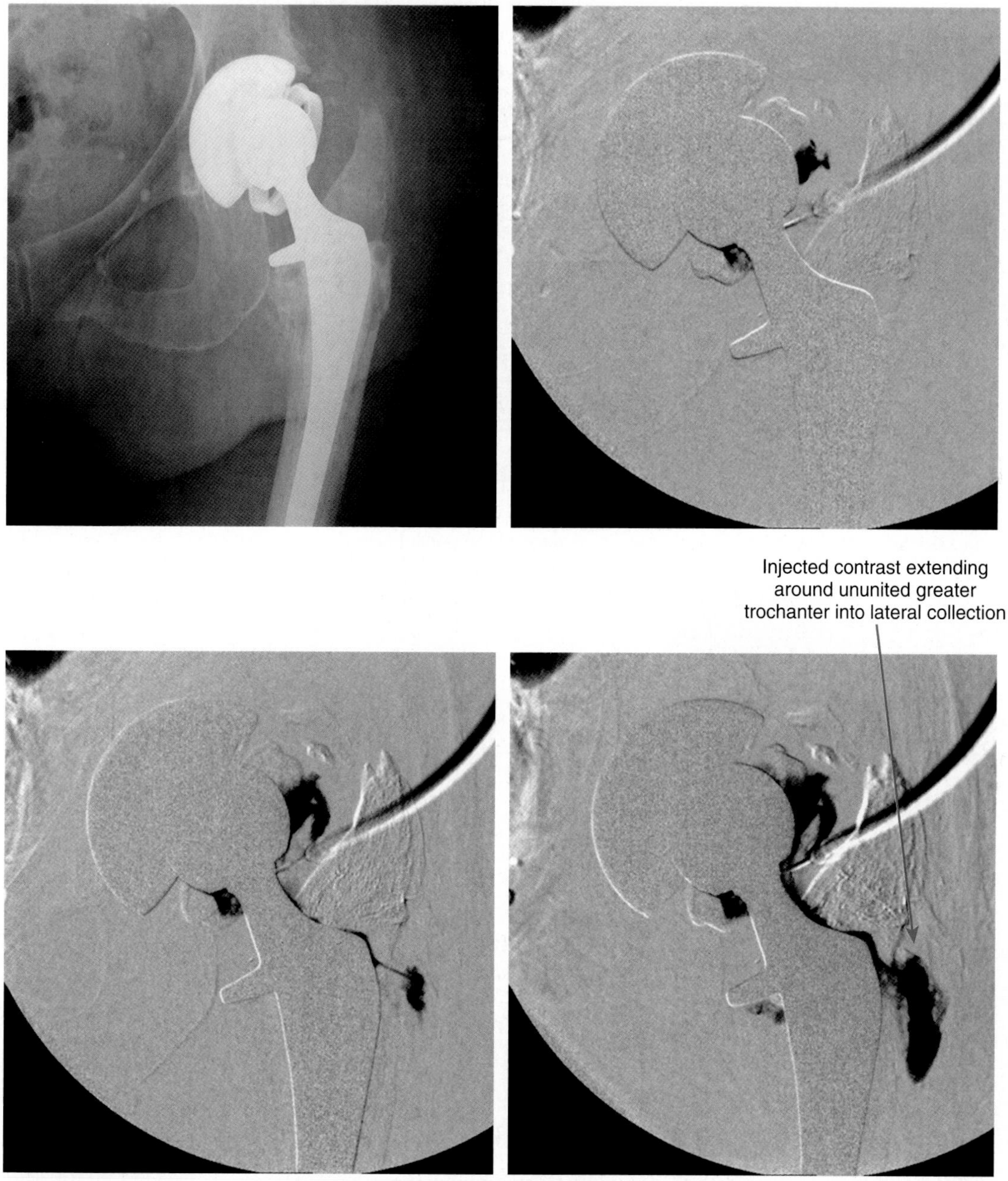
Injected contrast extending around ununited greater trochanter into lateral collection

Figure 11-22 **Total hip arthroplasty.** Digital subtraction technique is useful for distinguishing injected contrast from metal and cortex.

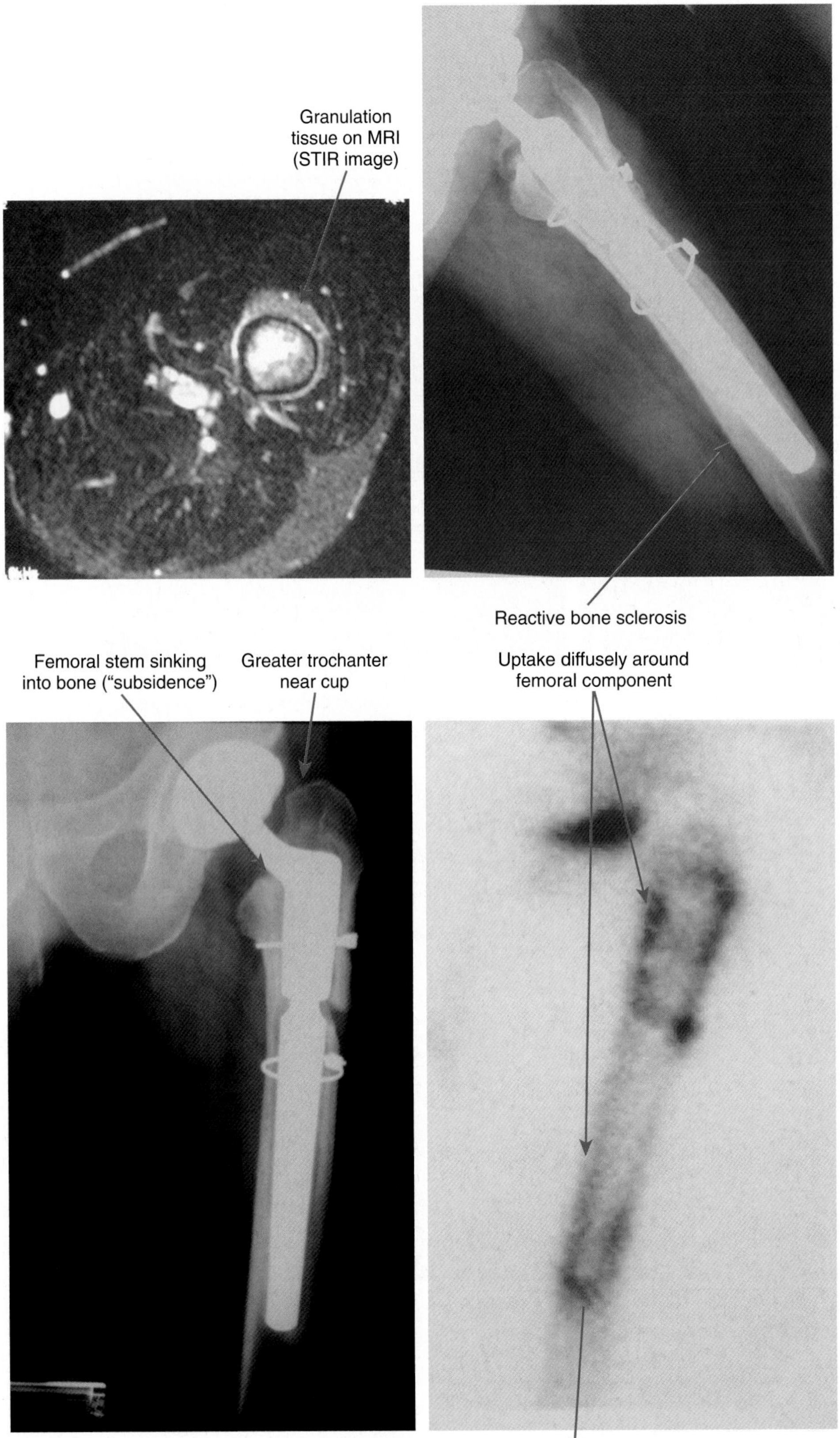
Granulation tissue on MRI (STIR image)
Reactive bone sclerosis
Femoral stem sinking into bone ("subsidence")
Greater trochanter near cup
Uptake diffusely around femoral component
Often a loosened femoral stem shows focal uptake on bone scan at the tip due to a windshield wiper effect

Figure 11-23
Noncemented total hip arthroplasty with loosening in a patient presenting with pain. On radiographs, subsidence (component progressively "sinking" into bone) is suspected based on low position of the stem relative to the greater trochanter; however, postoperative radiographs were not available. Bone scan confirms high uptake surrounding the femoral component. MRI shows granulation tissue around the femoral shaft and marrow edema.

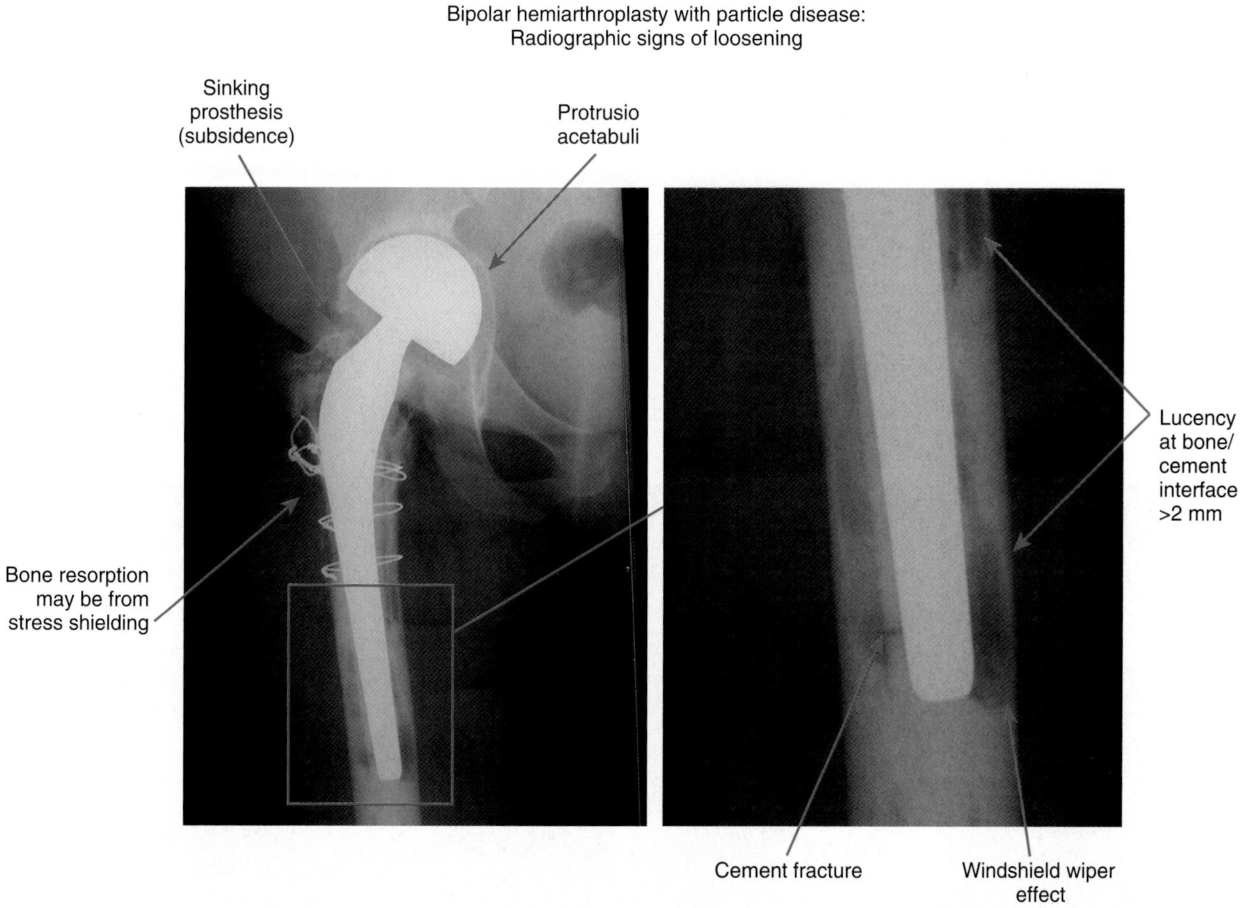
Bipolar hemiarthroplasty with particle disease:
Radiographic signs of loosening
Sinking
prosthesis
(subsidence)
Protrusio
acetabuli
Lucency
at bone/
cement
interface
>2 mm
Bone resorption
may be from
stress shielding
Cement fracture
Windshield wiper
effect

Figure 11-24 As with any prosthesis, component loosening is a major cause of failure of hip arthroplasties. Loosening can result from infection, wear, or particle disease. Particle disease results from shedding of the polyethylene spacer, the cement, or even the metal components.

abscess cavity adjacent to the joint, often near the greater trochanter.

Acute symptoms without fever may be related to mechanical failure of the prosthesis, which can range from periprosthetic fracture to dislocation of the prosthetic femoral head to catastrophic failure of the components (e.g., fracture of a ceramic femoral head). In particular, ceramic prostheses, despite having a lower risk of particle disease, have a higher risk of component fracture. These findings should be apparent on radiographs. In a patient with total hip arthroplasty dislocation, evaluation should be performed for retroversion or steep angle of the acetabular cup which can predispose. Angle (inclination) of the cup is easily measured on a centered AP view of the pelvis and should be approximately 40 to 50 degrees. Above this range (steep cup), there is increased risk of dislocation; below this, range of motion is suboptimal. The cup should also be anteverted approximately 25 degrees; if retroverted, risk of dislocation is increased when the patient bends over. Cup retroversion can be diagnosed on surgical lateral radiograph or CT (see Fig. 11-27).

Loosening/Particle Disease

Patients without fever and/or with chronic symptoms may have chronic wear of the components, or particle disease. A number of radiographic signs are listed in Box 11-2. As with other prostheses, it is very helpful to compare with the preoperative and immediate postoperative exams; for example, if acetabular lucency is present, was it there preoperatively (i.e., was it a subchondral cyst)? Also, regarding lucency around the components: Was it there postoperatively (i.e., incomplete cement filling around component)?

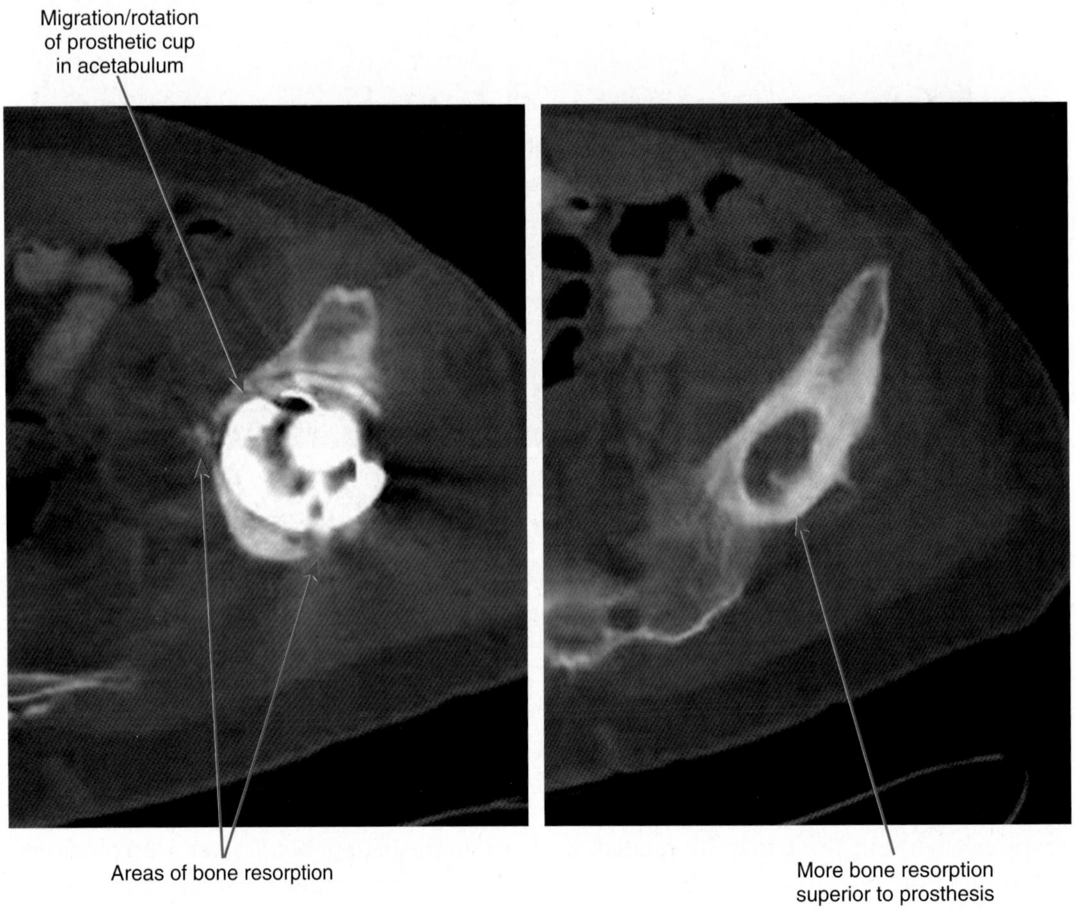
Migration/rotation
of prosthetic cup
in acetabulum
Areas of bone resorption
More bone resorption
superior to prosthesis

Figure 11-25 **Particle disease on CT.**

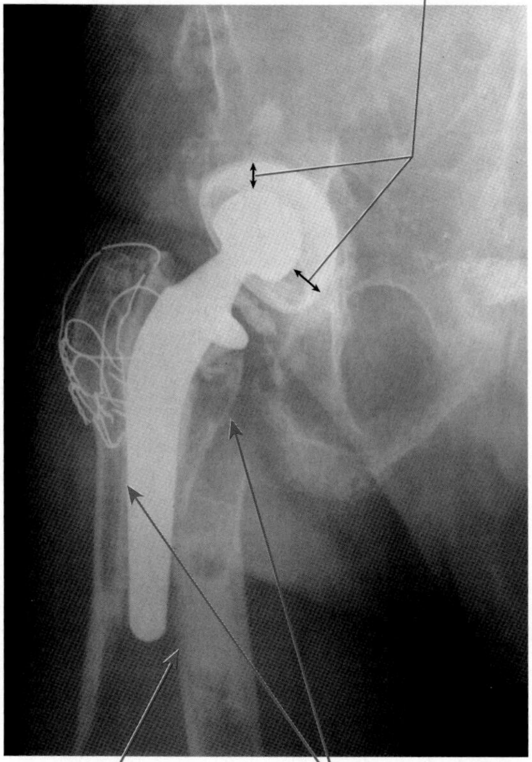
Nonuniformity of radiolucent spacer indicates wear
Fracture
Lucent zones related to particle disease

Figure 11-26 Periprosthetic fracture. Note wear of the spacer and lucency surrounding the components suggesting particle disease, which most likely contributed to the fracture.

BOX 11-2 RADIOGRAPHIC SIGNS OF LOOSENING OF TOTAL HIP ARTHROPLASTY

Spacer wear (thinning of a portion of the radiolucent spacer, usually at the superior aspect)
Shedding of metal fragments
Lucency at the bone/cement interface (especially around the distal femoral component or the central acetabular component, ≥2 mm)
Contrast extending around bone/cement interface on arthrogram
Subsidence (the prosthesis progressively "sinks" into the underlying bone)
Progressive protrusio acetabuli
Cement fracture
Periprosthetic fracture

Particle disease occurs when small particles shed off various components of the implant. Particles of a particular size range are engulfed by macrophages that die and lyse, releasing factors that stimulate osteoclastic activity. Osteoclasts resorb bone around the prosthesis, leading to loosening and making it difficult to perform a revision because of loss of bone stock. In particle disease, the osteolysis can be focal or diffuse; however, focal areas of osteolysis are classic. Osteolysis can also be seen with infection, so the clinical context must be considered. On arthrography, a loose total hip arthroplasty exhibits contrast extending around the prosthesis or the bone-cement interface. In some cases of particle disease, aspiration yields a dark-colored liquid related to the high concentration of metallic particles. The fluid should be sent for microbiology evaluation as well.

The advent of multidetector CT has made it possible to evaluate prostheses and the immediately adjacent bone in multiple planes at high resolution. The protocol should be geared toward reducing metal artifact. Similar to what occurs in MRI, titanium components result in less artifact than other metals. Lucency around the prosthetic components can be detected with high precision, and at the same time cup position/orientation can be evaluated. Bone scan can be used, with uptake around the prosthesis indicating pathology, though somewhat nonspecifically. In conjunction with labeled WBCs, specificity increases, but aspiration is faster and eventually necessary in many cases, rendering additional imaging unnecessary. MRI is useful to delineate periprosthetic fluid collections (with appropriate metal reduction protocol) and can also detect areas of osteomyelitis as well as foci of granulation tissue associated with osteolysis and particle disease. MRI is also useful in the postoperative patient with a complication, such as numbness or paralysis; MRI can detect hematoma around the sciatic or femoral nerve that may require drainage. Ultrasound is also useful for detection of hematomas and fluid collections associated with infection.

ARTICULAR PATHOLOGY

Arthrography Indications

There are two approaches for the diagnosis of labral pathology: spatial resolution and contrast resolution. A high spatial resolution noncontrast proton density

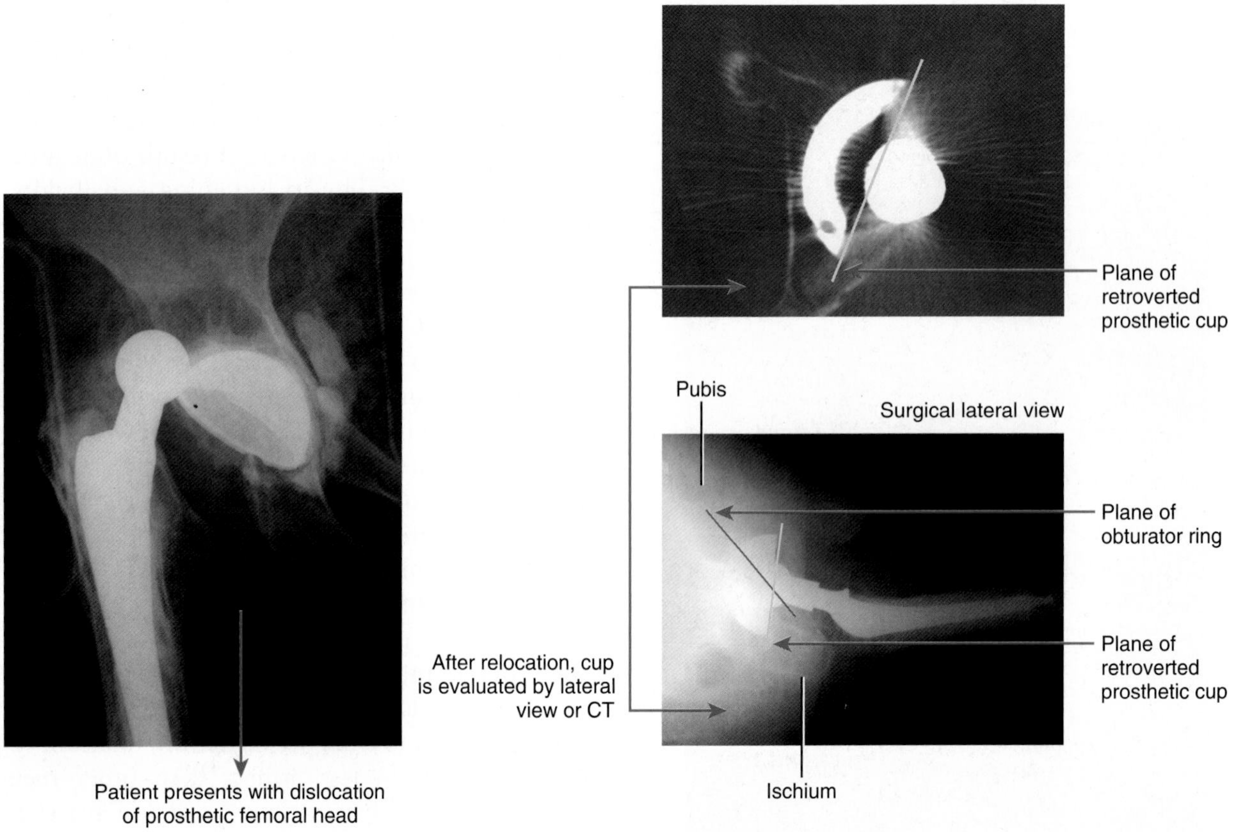
Plane of
retroverted
prosthetic cup
Pubis
Surgical lateral view
Plane of
obturator ring
Plane of
retroverted
prosthetic cup
After relocation, cup
is evaluated by lateral
view or CT
Patient presents with dislocation
of prosthetic femoral head
Ischium

Figure 11-27 Retroversion of the acetabular cup is a common cause for failure, especially dislocation. CT or a surgical lateral view is excellent for determining position of the cup. The prosthetic cup should be tilted anteriorly, similar to the plane of the native acetabulum. Retroversion can be from placement or component migration due to loosening.

sequence have been popularized recently. This sequence is excellent when optimized on a high field strength magnet, but factors can conspire to reduce the quality and consistency of resultant images: First, if the magnet or coils are not optimized for imaging of the hip, the desired resolution and signal-to-noise ratio (SNR) will be difficult to achieve. This effect is magnified by motion artifact and by obese patients, in whom the surface coil may be far from the hip, resulting in disadvantageous SNR. Injecting contrast into the joint increases overall signal regardless of physical and technical limitations, yielding a more consistently high-quality exam. Also, there is a mechanical advantage in that distention of the joint can force fluid through pathologic communications. At the same time, anesthetic can be injected, which can provide information regarding symptom relief. Therefore, most musculoskeletal radiologists prefer direct MR arthrography for evaluation of hip internal derangement (see Chapter 2 for technique). Indirect MR arthrography of the hip is generally less consistent in quality than direct MR arthrography.

DYSPLASIA, FEMORAL-ACETABULAR IMPINGEMENT, LABRAL TEAR, AND OSTEOARTHRITIS

Recent work has provided strong evidence that hip dysplasia and impingement are significant sources of chronic hip pain in young adults, and both processes may lead to labral tear, focal cartilage loss, and eventually osteoarthritis. The high rate of total hip arthroplasty in the United States is an indication of the common nature of this disease, which has only recently been recognized in its early stages.

It is increasingly becoming the job of community radiologists to detect the early signs of this spectrum of disease, since there are treatments geared toward

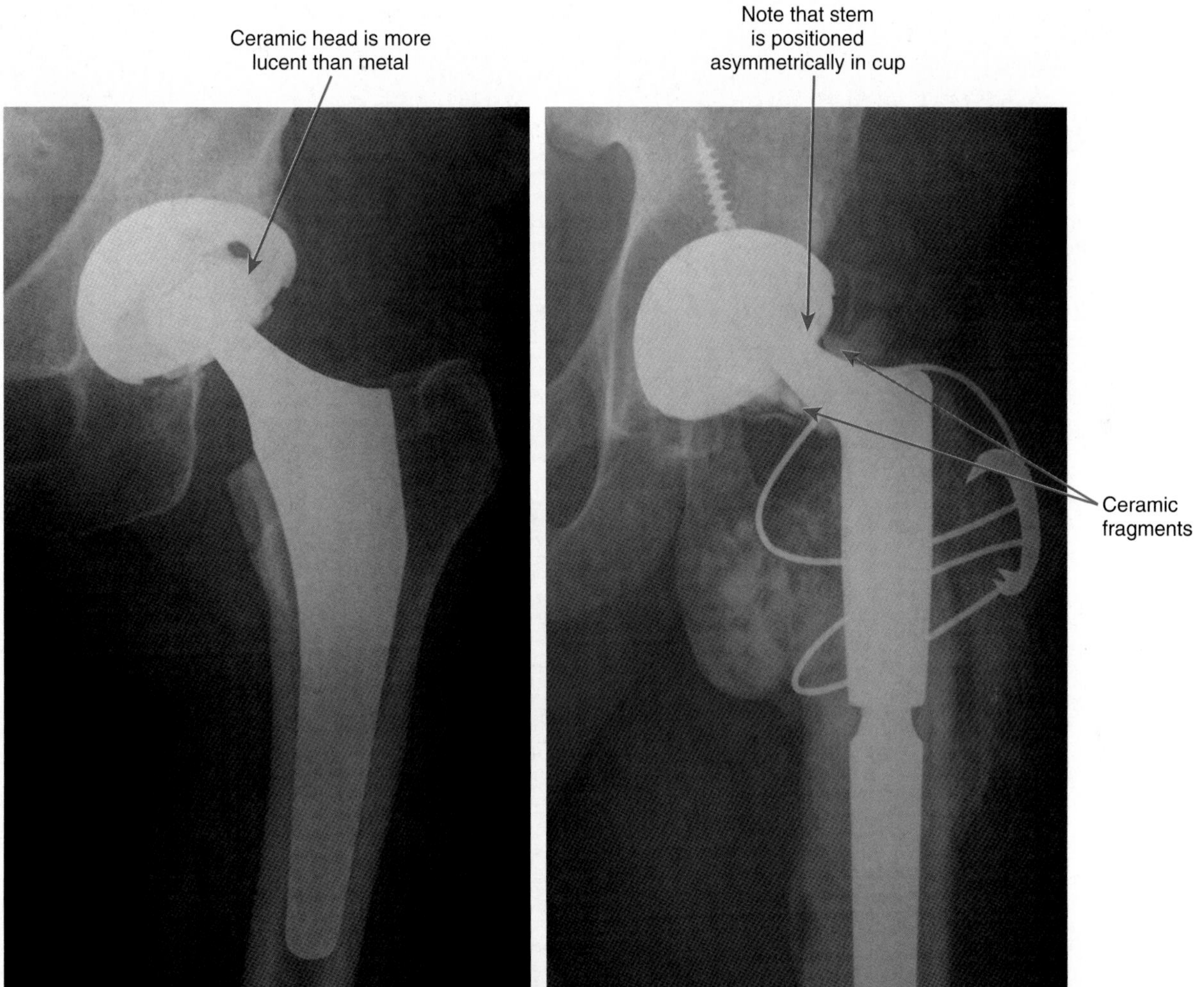
Ceramic head is more lucent than metal
Note that stem is positioned asymmetrically in cup
Ceramic fragments
Normal
Ceramic fracture

Figure 11-28 Introduction of ceramic components reduced the effect of component shedding and particle disease, but ceramic components occasionally present with catastrophic failure.

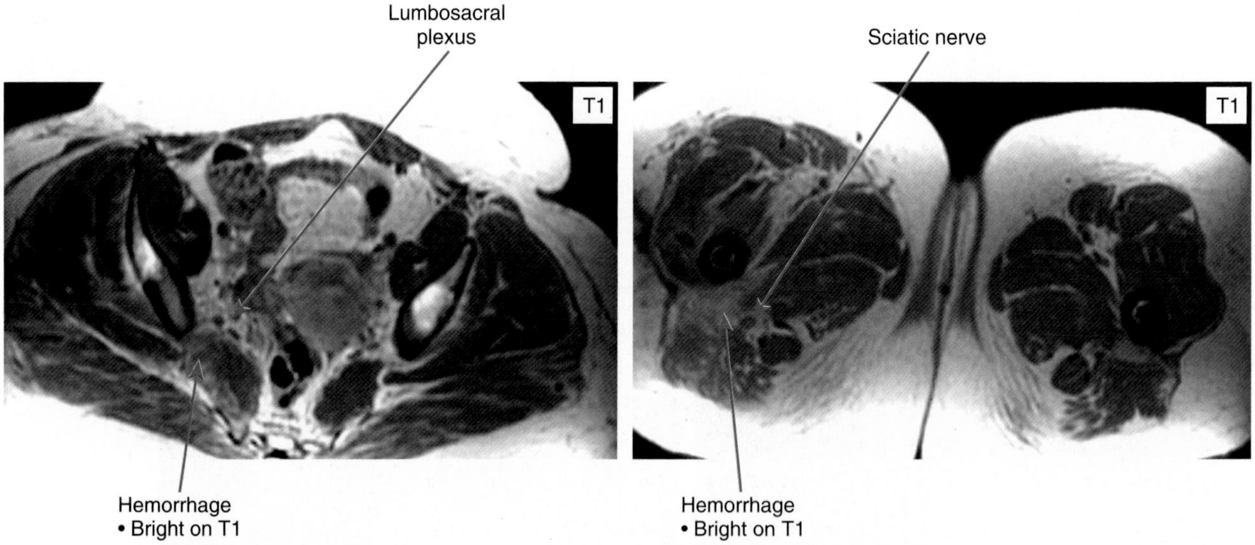
Lumbosacral plexus
Sciatic nerve
T1
T1
Hemorrhage
• Bright on T1
Hemorrhage
• Bright on T1

Figure 11-29 MRI can be useful for problem solving in the recent postoperative patient with symptoms. Occasionally, after hip surgery patients experience numbness or weakness in the extremity. This can be temporary owing to retraction during surgery, but if a hematoma is pressing on the nerve, it may need to be drained. In this case after total hip arthroplasty, MRI shows a small hematoma surrounding the right lumbosacral plexus and sciatic nerve, explaining the patient's symptoms. Because of the small size of the hematoma, the patient was treated conservatively.

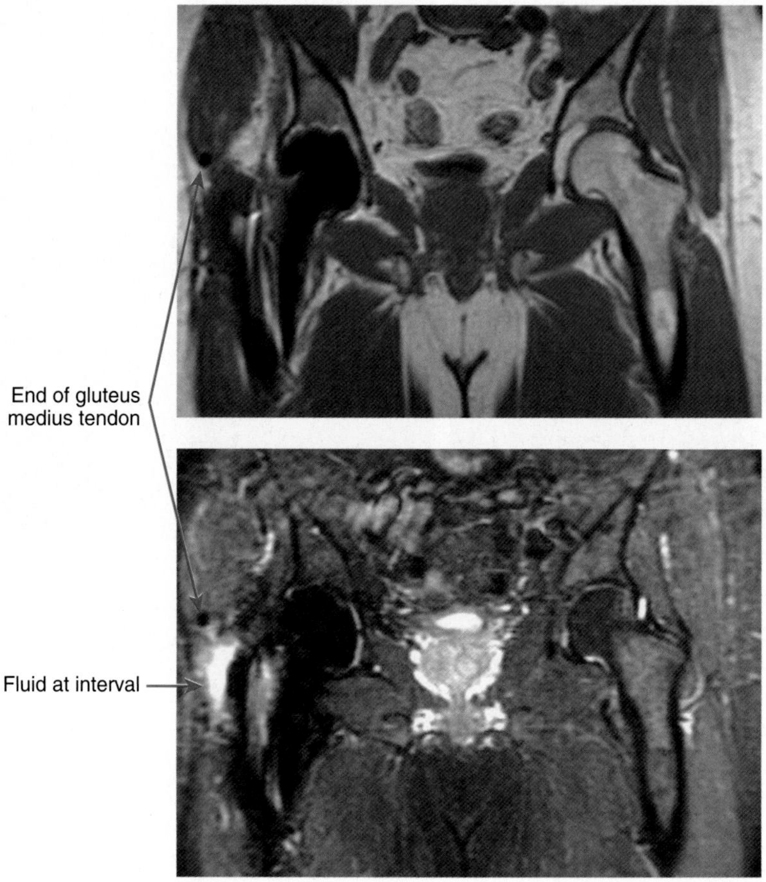
End of gluteus medius tendon
Fluid at interval

Figure 11-30 **Postoperative total hip arthroplasty.** Patient presents with pain and abductor weakness. MRI shows avulsion of the gluteus medius tendon from the greater tuberosity.

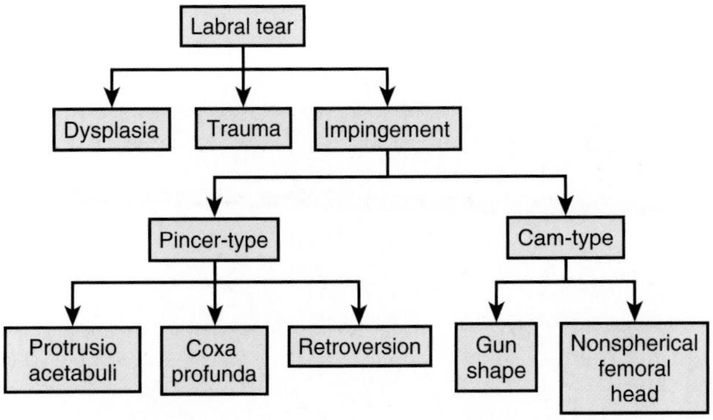
Labral tear
Dysplasia
Trauma
Impingement
Pincer-type
Cam-type
Protrusio acetabuli
Coxa profunda
Retroversion
Gun shape
Nonspherical femoral head

Figure 11-31 Schema classifying causes of acetabular labral tear. (Courtesy of Suzanne Anderson, MD, Bern, Switzerland.)

relieving the patient's pain and preventing or slowing progression to osteoarthritis.

Dysplasia and impingement are at opposite ends of a spectrum (Fig. 11-31). Both diseases result from a mechanically disadvantageous shape of the acetabulum and/or femoral head. In the case of dysplasia, acetabular coverage is inadequate, leading to instability, labral hypertrophy, and eventually labral tear and cartilage wear. In impingement, the acetabulum may be too deep, or the femoral head/neck may be misshapen, leading to abutment of articular surfaces during extremes of range of motion, which is often reduced compared with normal individuals. It is important to note that if a radiologist sees radiographs of the pelvis or hips of a young patient (20s to 40s) with chronic hip pain, signs of impingement or dysplasia should be reported.

Standardized radiographic technique is essential for diagnosis of these conditions. A straight AP view of the pelvis must be acquired. Slight angulation alters the appearance of the acetabular margins, rendering diagnosis difficult or impossible; the pubic symphysis should exactly overlap the coccyx. An AP and frog lateral view of the symptomatic hip is also part of the evaluation. Surgeons may also request a "faux profile" view (Fig. 11-32), which offers a better view of the acetabular rim.

Hip Dysplasia (Figs. 11-33 through 11-36)

Developmental hip dysplasia that presents in infancy is well described, characterized by an abnormally steep acetabular angle and lateral subluxation of the femoral head with interruption of Shenton's line. Dynamic displacement of the femoral head can be demonstrated by ultrasound. Extreme cases are easily detected on clinical exam or radiographically, and these patients are treated with bracing. However, the process that creates this condition exists relatively commonly in a more subtle form that presents with hip pain in young adulthood. Basic radiographic signs are similar; these include upturn of the lateral acetabular margin, increase in the acetabular angle, and uncovering of the lateral femoral head. However, it should be recognized that different forms of dysplasia exist based on deficiency of a portion of the acetabular rim. Therefore, the anterior and posterior acetabular margins should be evaluated on each radiograph in addition to the lateral margin.

On MRI, the acetabular deformity may not be as apparent, but the soft tissue pathology will be seen. The labrum degenerates in dysplastic hips, at first hypertrophying and later tearing.

Posterior-superior acetabular deficiency actually creates a condition of retroversion, which can cause anterior impingement. This is discussed in more detail under the category of impingement (Box 11-3).

Femoral-Acetabular Impingement

Two basic types of acetabular impingement have been described: cam and pincer. Each has subcategories.

Cam Impingement (Fig. 11-37)

Imagine a camshaft of a car: Attached to the shaft are lobes, or cams, that are eccentrically shaped, like a circle with a bump on one side. What does this have to do with the hip? To allow the widest range of motion, the femoral head and neck should be circular on transverse sections, and the femoral head should be spherical in three dimensions. If there is a bump on the side of the femoral neck, or if the head

BOX 11-3 SUMMARY OF FINDINGS IN HIP DYSPLASIA

Increased acetabular angle
Upturn of lateral acetabular margin
Lateral subluxation
  Widening of medial joint
  Uncovering of lateral femoral head

SECTION IV

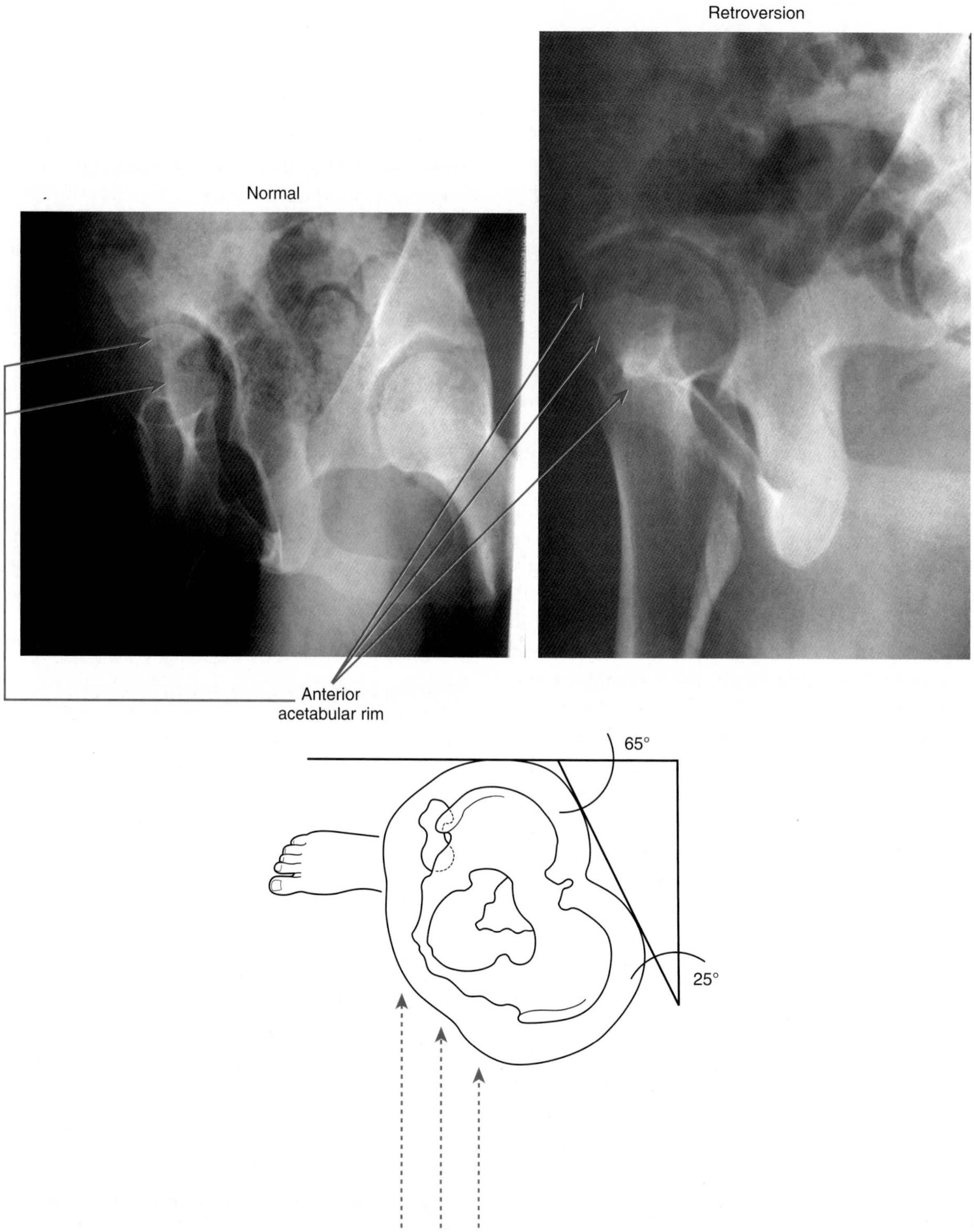
Retroversion
Normal
Anterior
acetabular rim
65°
25°

Figure 11-32 Faux profile view. Red arrows show anterior acetabular rim. (From Lequesne MG, Laredo JD: The faux profil (oblique view) of the standing position. Contribution to the evaluation of osteoarthritis of the adult hip. Ann Rheum Dis 1998;57[11]:676–681. Reproduced with permission from BMJ Publishing Group.)

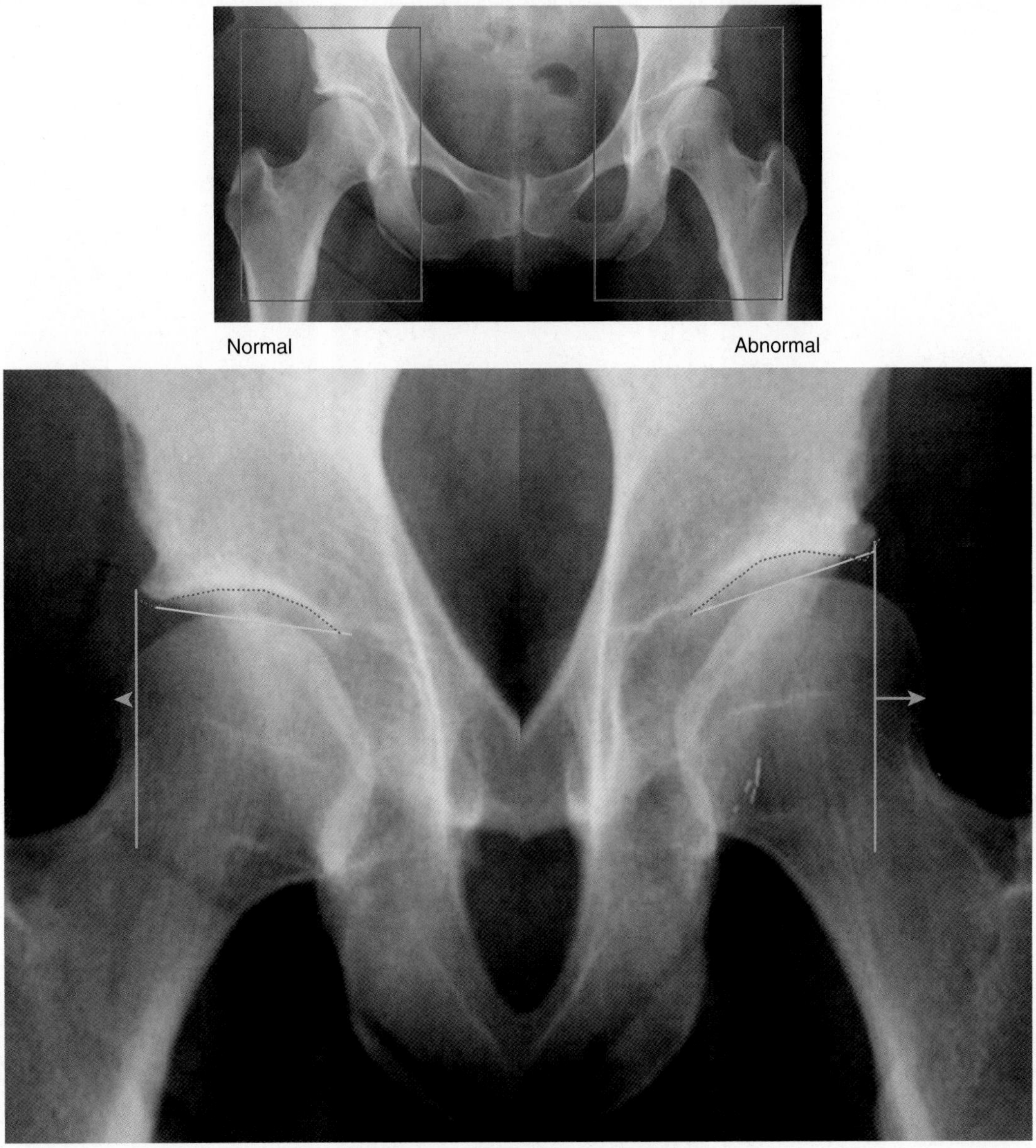
Normal
Abnormal
• Increased acetabular angle (yellow line)
• Upturn of lateral acetabular rim (red dotted line)
• Uncovering of lateral femoral head (blue line)
• Widening of medial joint

Figure 11-33 Findings of hip dysplasia.

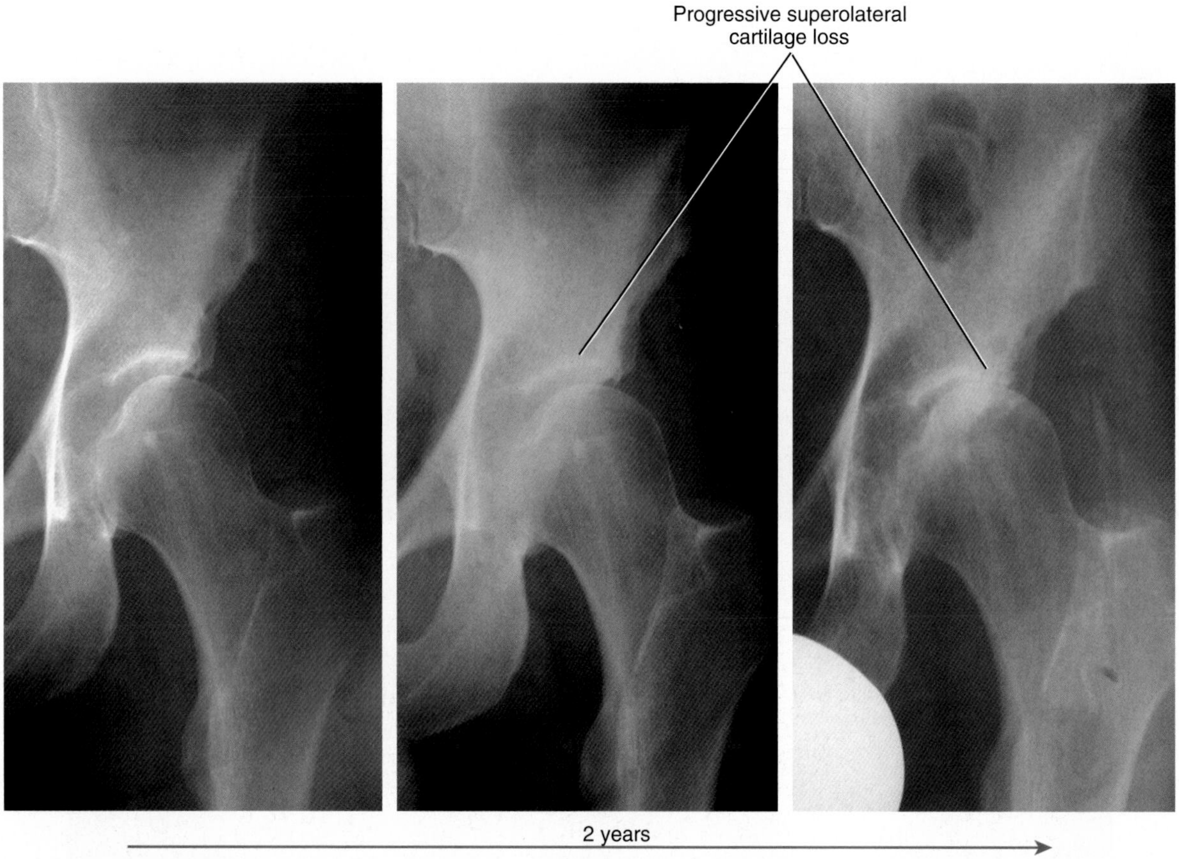
Progressive superolateral cartilage loss
2 years

Figure 11-34 Hip dysplasia in a young adult at 2-year follow-up with development of osteoarthritis. (Courtesy of Javad Parvizi, MD, Philadelphia.)

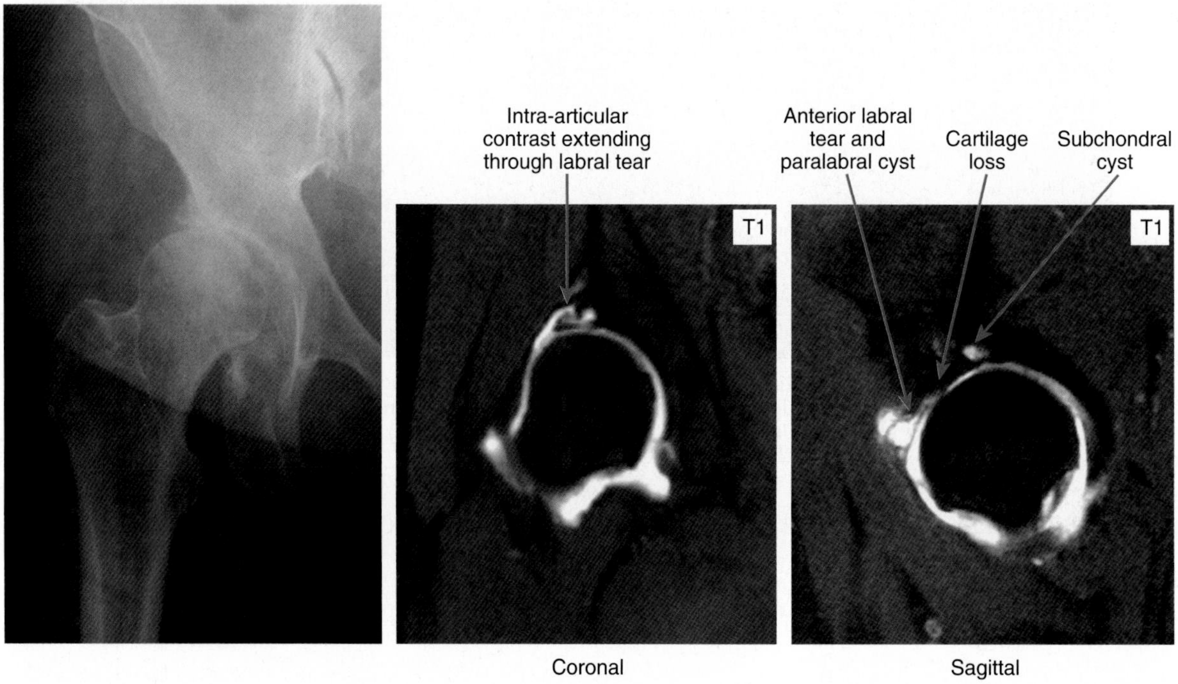
Intra-articular contrast extending through labral tear
Anterior labral tear and paralabral cyst
Cartilage loss
Subchondral cyst
T1
T1
Coronal
Sagittal

Figure 11-35 Labral tear and osteoarthritis in a dysplastic hip.

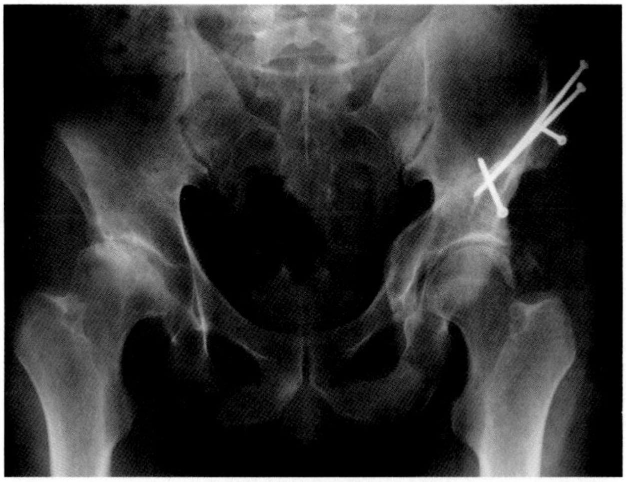

Figure 11-36 Prior treatment of hip dysplasia with acetabuloplasty on the left side. Progression of osteoarthritis on the untreated right side.

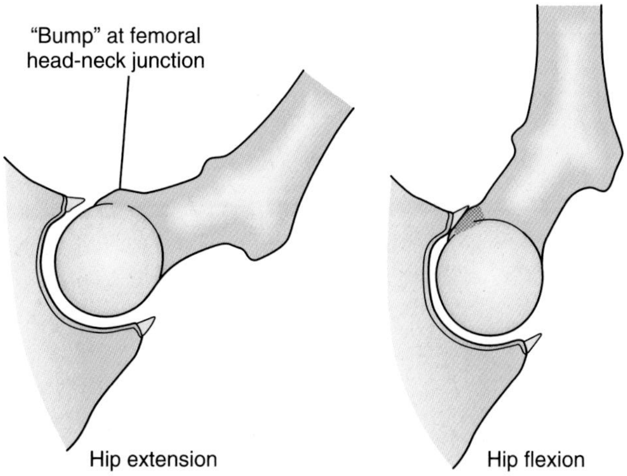

"Bump" at femoral head-neck junction
Hip extension
Hip flexion

Figure 11-38 Mechanics of cam impingement related to a nonspherical femoral head.

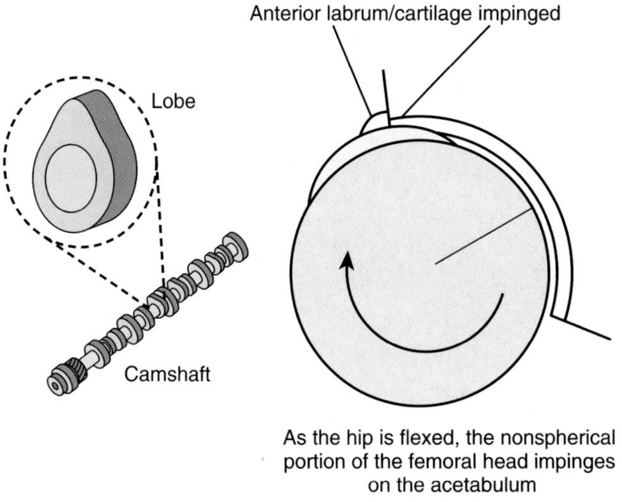

Anterior labrum/cartilage impinged
Lobe
Camshaft
As the hip is flexed, the nonspherical portion of the femoral head impinges on the acetabulum

Figure 11-37 Cam impingement.

is not spherical, it can resemble a cam on axial images and serve as a focus of impingement (Fig. 11-38; see also Fig. 11-37).

This cam configuration can be caused by two basic deformities: a nonspherical femoral head and a gun-type shape.

Nonspherical Femoral Head Deformity A nonspherical femoral head is observed radiographically as a bump at the anterolateral femoral head-neck junction (Figs. 11-39 and 11-40; see also Fig. 11-38). This may be interpreted as a spur initially, but if the patient is relatively young and there is no joint narrowing *and* there is hip pain, the diagnosis of femoral-acetabular impingement should be suggested. This bump may be best seen radiographically on a frog lateral view. On cross-sectional imaging (CT or MRI), the finding is more apparent. Other causes of femoral head deformity such as prior Perthes disease can also lead to impingement.

Gun-Type Deformity (Figs. 11-41 through 11-43) The gun-type deformity is best described as a lateral or anterolateral femoral neck deficiency. Seen on an AP view of the hip, the lateral femoral neck normally dips in symmetrically with the medial aspect; in this deformity there is little or no dip laterally. This creates an appearance similar to the handle of an old-fashioned pistol. This shape has also been described in patients with prior slipped capital femoral epiphysis, and although these patients are susceptible to future impingement, it is unclear whether patients with this type of impingement have their deformity on the basis of developmental variation or subclinical slipped capital femoral epiphysis. Once recognized, gun-type deformity is easy to spot on radiographs, but there is a method for measuring the effect called the femoral head offset, which is acquired from a surgical lateral view of the hip. The depth of

SECTION IV

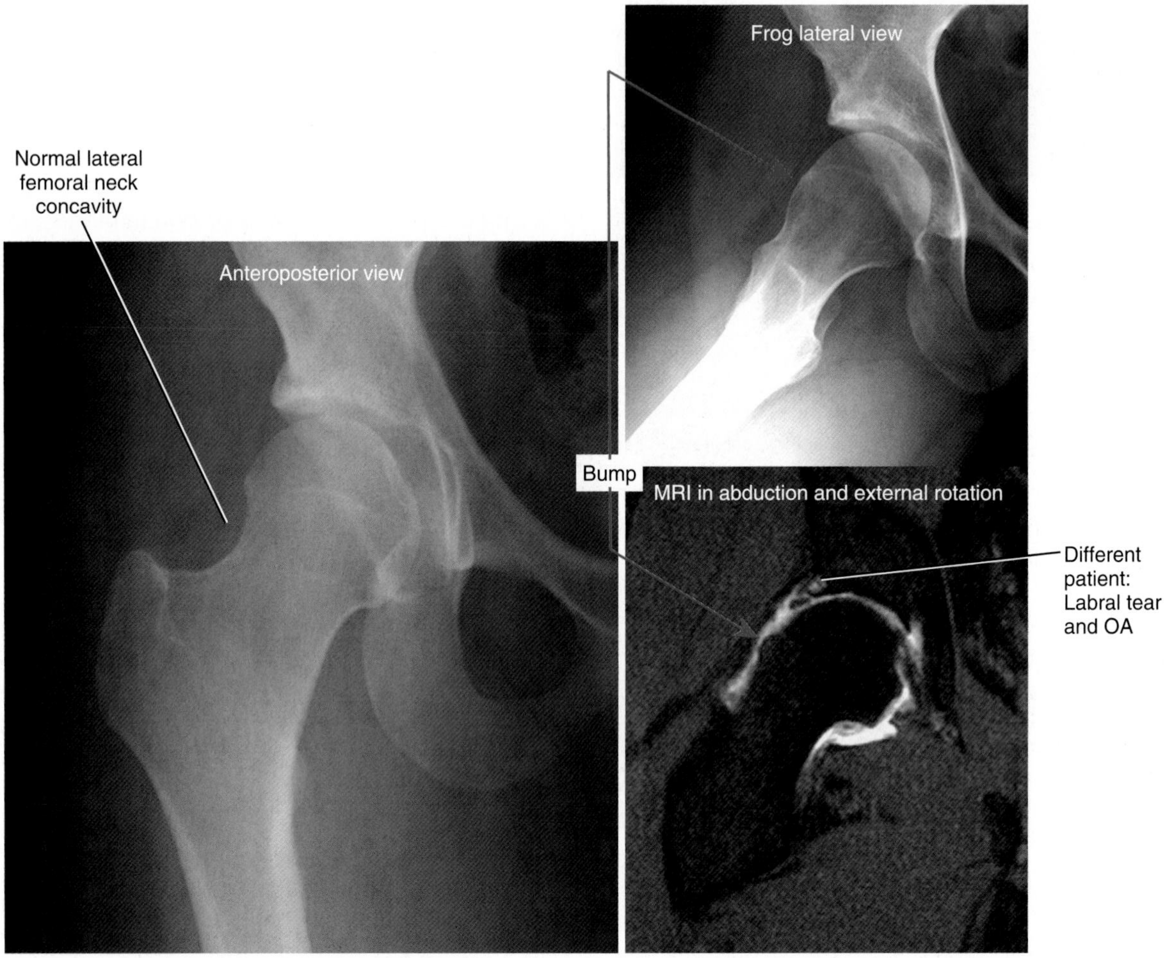
Frog lateral view
Normal lateral femoral neck concavity
Anteroposterior view
Bump
MRI in abduction and external rotation
Different patient: Labral tear and OA

Figure 11-39 Cam-type femoral-acetabular impingement. Nonspherical femoral head. Bump associated with lack of femoral head sphericity may be subtle. Located at the anterolateral femoral head/neck junction, better seen on the frog lateral radiographic view or anterior coronal slices or axial cross-sectional images. Note lack of joint narrowing and circumferential spurs on radiographs above, indicating that the finding does not represent a manifestation of osteoarthritis in this young patient. OA, osteoarthritis.

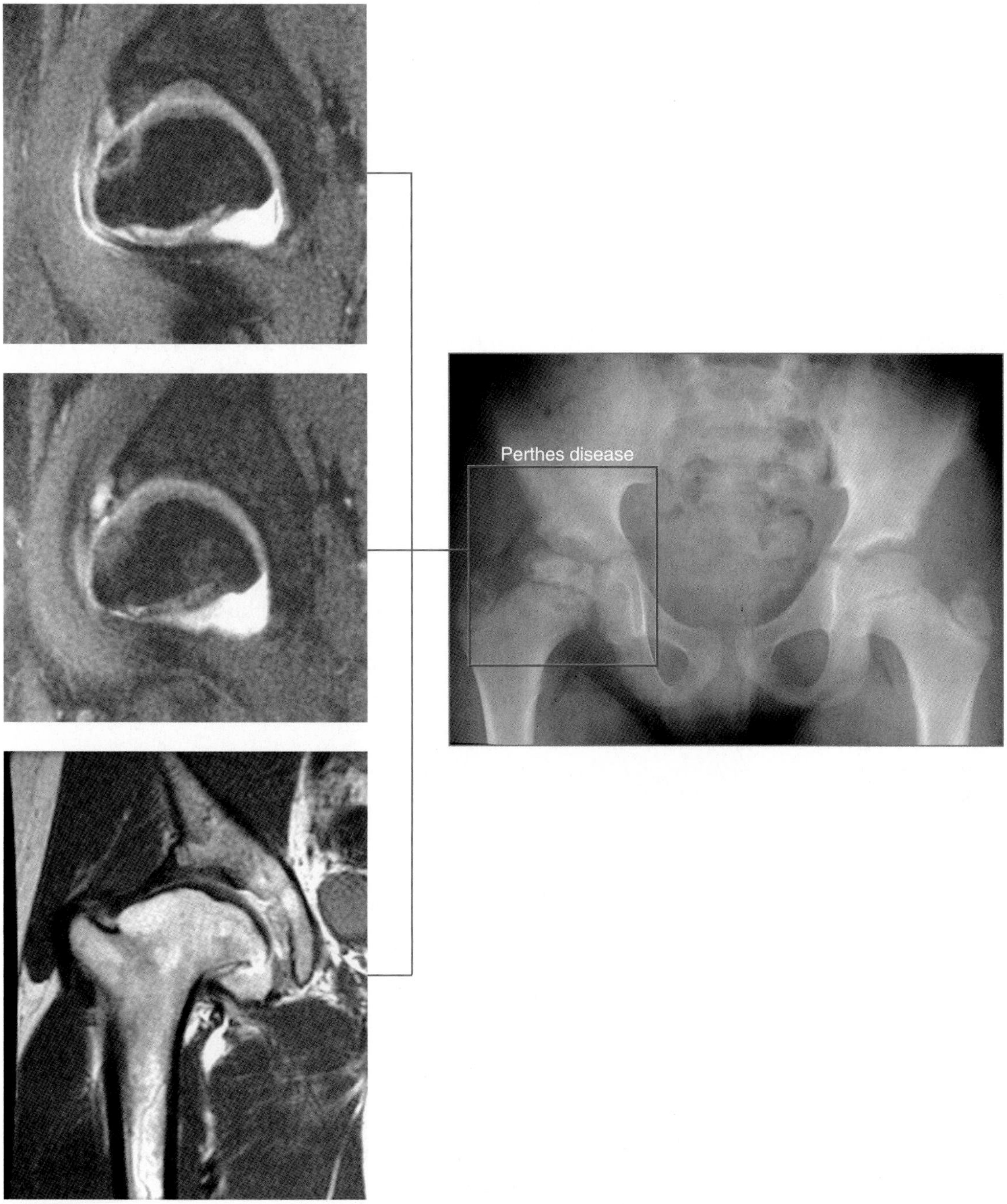
Perthes disease

Figure 11-40 **Perthes disease.** Development of femoral-acetabular deformity and secondary impingement. Resultant labral tear and osteoarthritis.

the neck anteriorly is measured; less than 7 mm is considered abnormal.

On MRI, detection of the deformity resulting from the bump or the femoral neck deficiency can be evaluated using an oblique axial plane, prescribed along the neck of the femur. On this plane, the alpha angle can be measured; although this measurement has become popular, it is usually obvious that there is a deformity (Fig. 11-44). Surgical management is directed toward reshaping the femoral head-neck junction (Fig. 11-45).

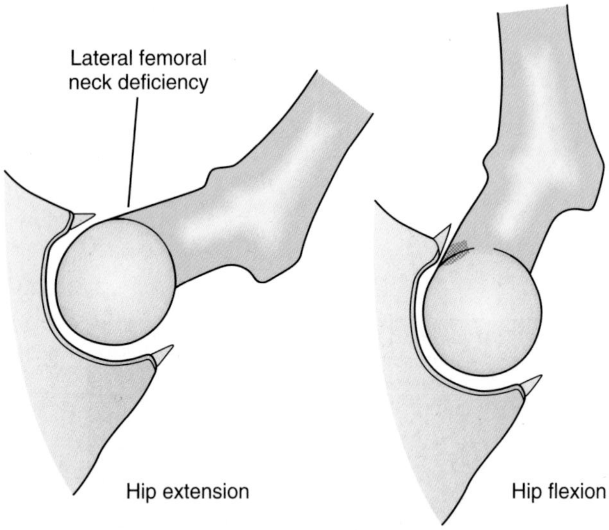
Lateral femoral
neck deficiency
Hip extension
Hip flexion

Figure 11-41 Gun-shaped cam impingement. Deficiency of the lateral femoral neck.

Labral/Acetabular Lesions in Cam Impingement

The prominence of bone at the femoral head/neck junction abuts the anterolateral acetabular margin during flexion; the labrum lifts, and the bone wears the adjacent cartilage, eventually delaminating it and rolling it back like a carpet. The labrum becomes detached or torn secondarily, or it may be torn along with the cartilage. Search should be performed for these cartilage flap lesions, which are very subtle.

Pincer-Type Impingement

(Figs. 11-46 through 11-50)

Pincer impingement occurs when the acetabulum is too deep or overhangs too much, again leading to abutment on the femoral neck. The most extreme of this class of deformity is protrusio acetabuli, in which the iliopectineal line bows inward toward the center of the pelvis. This condition can be developmental

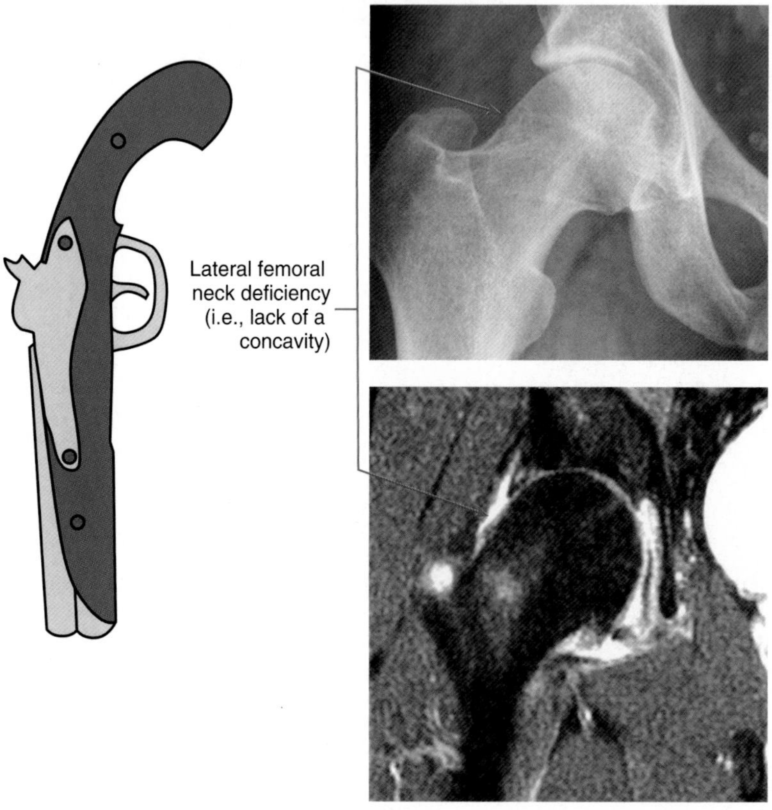
Lateral femoral
neck deficiency
(i.e., lack of a
concavity)

Figure 11-42 Lateral femoral neck deficiency results in a shape resembling an antique gun. The shape can predispose to femoral-acetabular impingement.

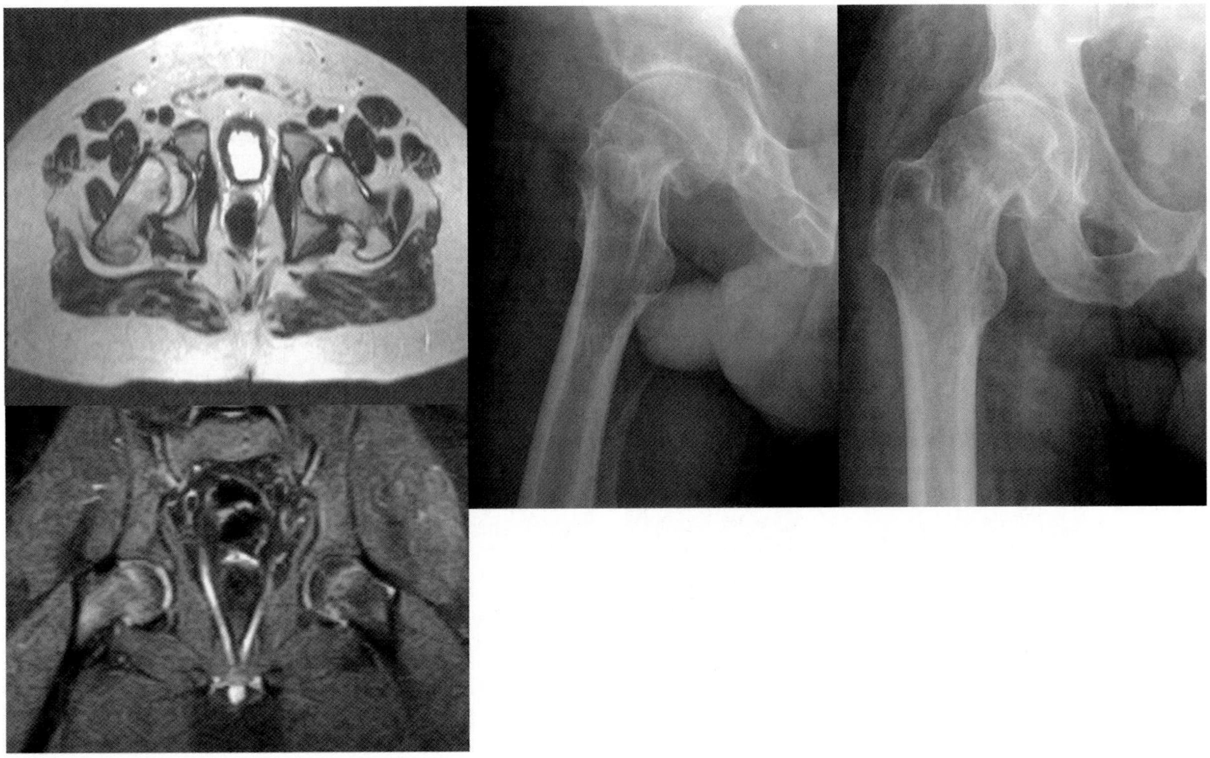

Figure 11-43 Slipped capital femoral epiphysis also results in lateral femoral neck deficiency and can lead to impingement later in life.

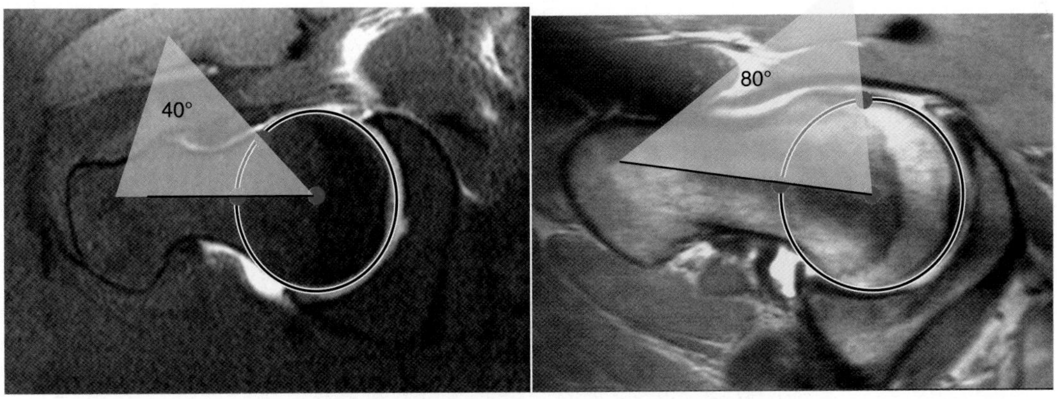
40°
80°

Normal and abnormal values	
Control group (no FAI):	avg 42 ± 2.2 degrees
FAI group:	avg 74 ± 5.4 degrees

Figure 11-44 Alpha angle: Examples of normal and abnormal measurement. Usually the bump is easily seen, but surgeons may request reporting of the angle itself. The angle is measured off an oblique axial image oriented along the femoral neck. A circle is drawn around the femoral head and a point is marked where the cortex leaves the circle anteriorly. The angle between this point and the center of the femoral neck is the alpha angle. FAI, femoral-acetabular impingement. (From Nötzli HP, Wyss TF, Stoecklin CH, et al: The contour of the femoral head-neck junction as a predictor for the risk of anterior impingement. J Bone Joint Surg Br 2002;84:556–560.)

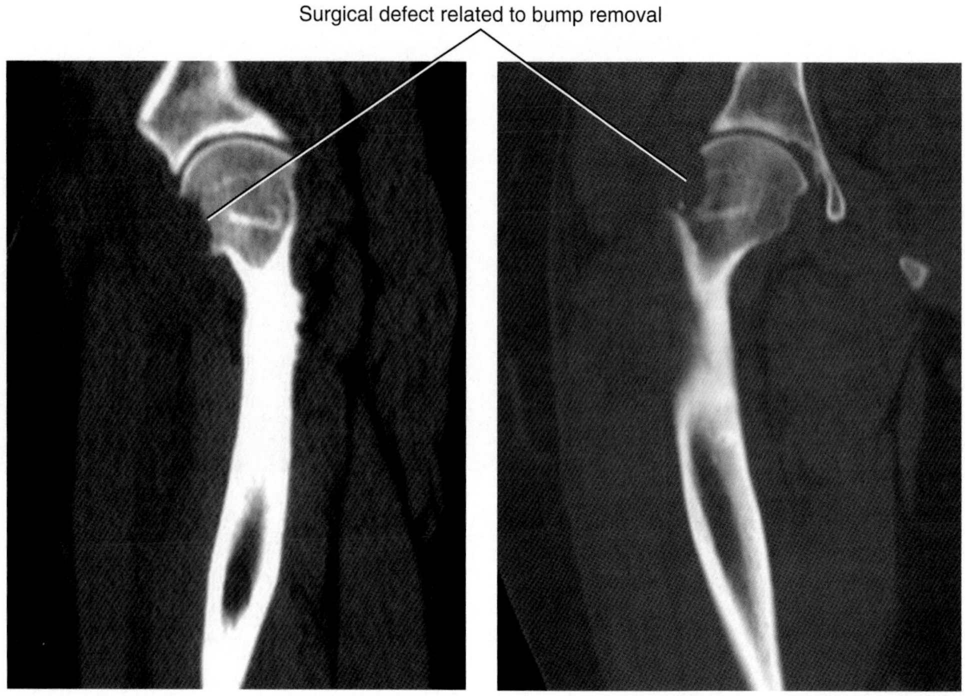
Surgical defect related to bump removal

Figure 11-45 **Postoperative appearance after hip spur removal.**

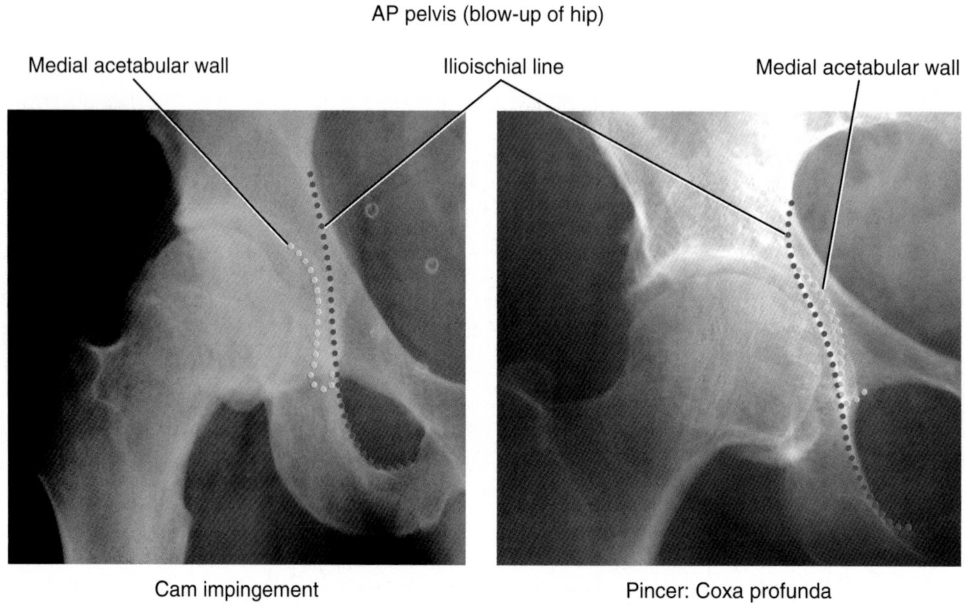
AP pelvis (blow-up of hip)
Medial acetabular wall
Ilioischial line
Medial acetabular wall
Cam impingement
Pincer: Coxa profunda

Figure 11-46 **Coxa profunda (deep acetabulum).** On a well-positioned anteroposterior (AP) view of the pelvis, the medial wall of the acetabular cup crosses medial to the ilioischial line (*right*). In more severe cases, protrusio acetabuli (inward bowing of the iliopectineal line) is seen.

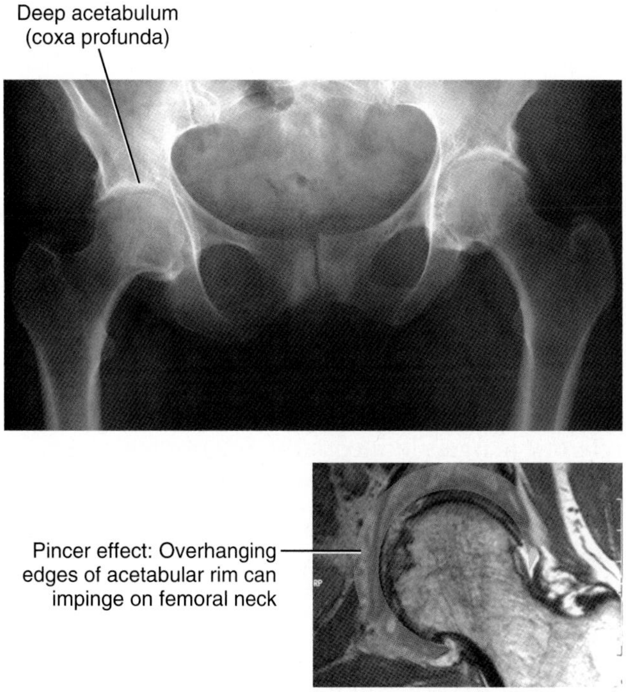
Deep acetabulum
(coxa profunda)
Pincer effect: Overhanging edges of acetabular rim can impinge on femoral neck

Figure 11-47 **Coxa profunda resulting in pincer-type femoral-acetabular impingement.**

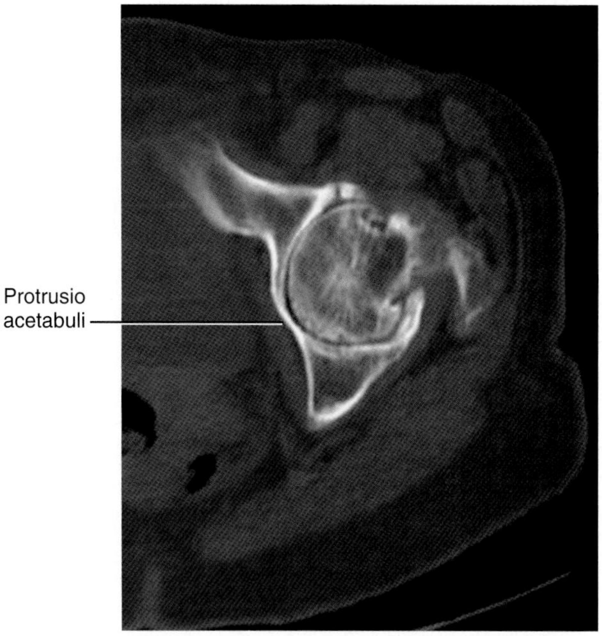
Protrusio acetabuli

Figure 11-48 **Deep acetabulum (coxa profunda) with protrusio acetabuli and pincer impingement.** This can be developmental but can also result from disorders associated with bone softening (e.g., renal osteodystrophy/osteomalacia, Paget disease) or inflammatory arthropathies (e.g., rheumatoid arthritis). Secondary osteoarthritis is present with diffuse joint narrowing and overhanging marginal osteophytes.

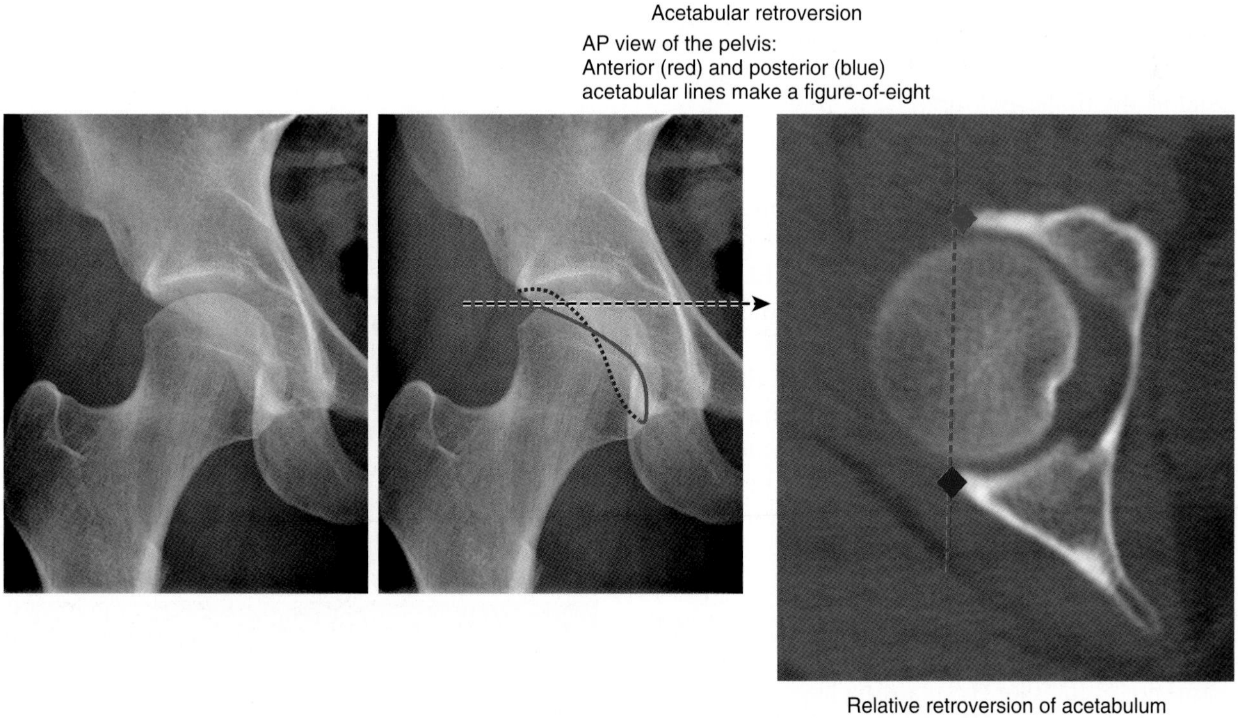
Acetabular retroversion
AP view of the pelvis:
Anterior (red) and posterior (blue) acetabular lines make a figure-of-eight
Relative retroversion of acetabulum

Figure 11-49 **Acetabular retroversion on anteroposterior (AP) pelvis radiograph and CT.**

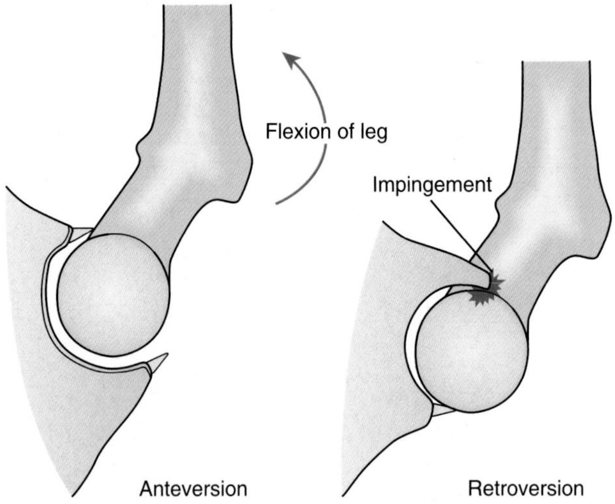
Flexion of leg
Impingement
Anteversion
Retroversion

Figure 11-50 Why is retroversion associated with impingement? An overhanging edge anteriorly or bone deficiency posteriorly results in relative posterior tilt of the acetabular cup (retroversion). This prominence anteriorly can impinge on the femoral neck during flexion of the hip.

but is commonly associated with inflammatory arthropathies (e.g., rheumatoid arthritis) and bone softening disorders (e.g., Paget's disease, osteomalacia) that lead to axial migration. A less obvious deformity is referred to as coxa profunda (deep hip); this is subtle but can be diagnosed on a straight AP pelvis when the medial wall of the acetabulum passes medial to the ilioischial line.

Finally, retroversion can also lead to pincer-type impingement. This is not as obvious, since as previously explained, retroversion is really a form of posterosuperior acetabular deficiency. This deficiency is seen on a straight AP pelvis radiograph if the anterior and posterior acetabular rim lines are traced. On an AP pelvis, these lines should not cross; the posterior rim remains lateral to the anterior rim. If the posterior rim crosses medial to the anterior rim, creating a figure-of-eight pattern, this represents retroversion (see Fig. 11-49). With this configuration, the anterior acetabular rim overhangs and abuts the femoral neck on flexion, creating pincer impingement.

Labral/Cartilaginous Lesions in Pincer Impingement In pincer impingement, the femoral neck abuts the anterior acetabular rim, causing large labral tears and detachments. Secondarily, the articular cartilage is damaged, usually without the flaps and delaminations seen in cam impingement. When the femoral neck hits the rim anteriorly, the head levers back posteriorly and can abut the inner margin of the posterior acetabulum, creating a "contrecoup" posterior cartilage defect. With chronic impingement, labral ossification and osseous hypertrophy of the acetabular rim can occur.

Other Signs That May Be Associated With Femoral-Acetabular Impingement

Synovial Herniation Pits (Fig. 11-51) A synovial herniation pit, also known as a "Pitt's pit," is seen on radiographs as a focal ovoid lucency with thin sclerotic margins located at the anterior femoral neck. For many years, this has been attributed to a normal variation, merely a "pitfall." However, recent work suggests that at least some of these lesions are associated with femoral-acetabular impingement. They occur at the locking point of impaction in femoral-acetabular impingement and show inflammation during surgery for femoral-acetabular impingement. It appears that some pits do represent normal variation, since there are penetrating vessels that also occur in this location. Cystic foci tend to occur where vessels penetrate bone at or near joints, with similar synovial herniations occurring at the waist of the capitate, at the posterior greater tuberosity of the shoulder, and at the angle of Gessane of the calcaneus. Nevertheless, if a synovial herniation pit is seen on any modality in the femoral neck in a young patient with chronic hip pain, other signs of impingement should be sought.

Os Acetabulare (Fig. 11-52) Similar to Pitt's pit, the os acetabulare (ossification at the anterolateral acetabular rim) has been attributed to normal variation for many years. However, this finding also occurs at the impaction point of femoral-acetabular impingement and has recently been implicated as a finding in the impingement spectrum. It may represent a type of pseudarthrosis, or ossification of a degenerated labrum. Again, the pathoetiology is unclear, but if this ossification is seen, the radiologist should look for other signs of impingement (Boxes 11-4 through 11-9).

DETECTION OF LABRAL TEARS

Labral Anatomy (Fig. 11-53)

The labrum is a fibrocartilaginous structure, triangular in cross-section like the glenoid labrum of the

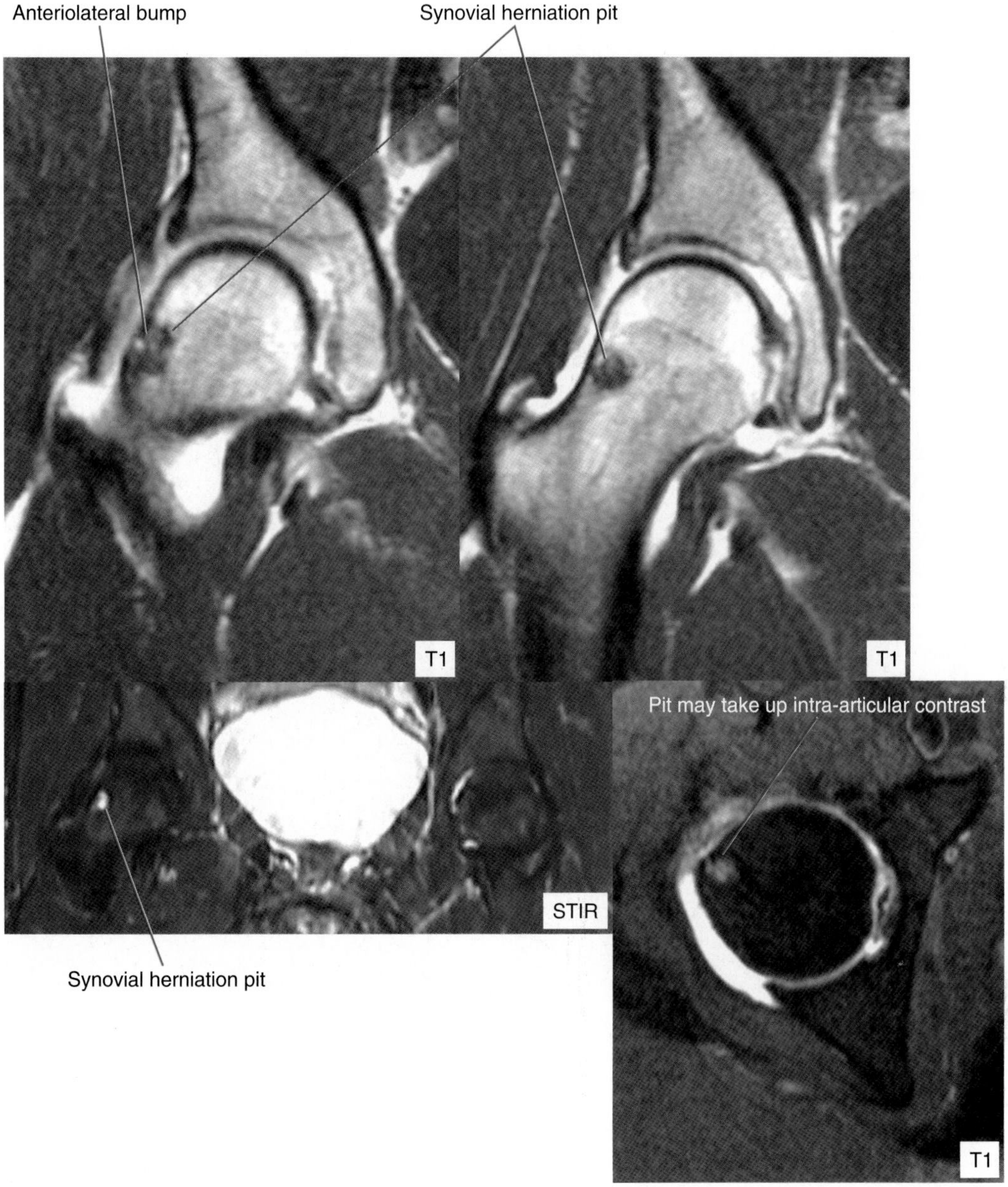
Anteriolateral bump
Synovial herniation pit
T1
T1
STIR
Synovial herniation pit
Pit may take up intra-articular contrast
T1

Figure 11-51 **MR arthrogram of a patient with clinical impingement.** Synovial herniation pits occur at the site of impingement and although frequently incidental, their presence should initiate a search for other signs of femoral-acetabular impingement in a young adult with hip pain.

BOX 11-4 FEMORAL-ACETABULAR IMPINGEMENT: CLINICAL PRESENTATION

Groin pain
Worse after prolonged sitting
Reduced range of motion
Positive impingement sign—pain in:
- 90-degree flexion and internal rotation
- Extreme extension and external rotation

BOX 11-5 POTENTIAL CAUSES OF DEFORMITY LEADING TO IMPINGEMENT

Slipped capital femoral epiphysis
Retroversion
Perthes disease
Avascular necrosis
Post-traumatic
Prior surgery (e.g., intertrochanteric osteotomy)

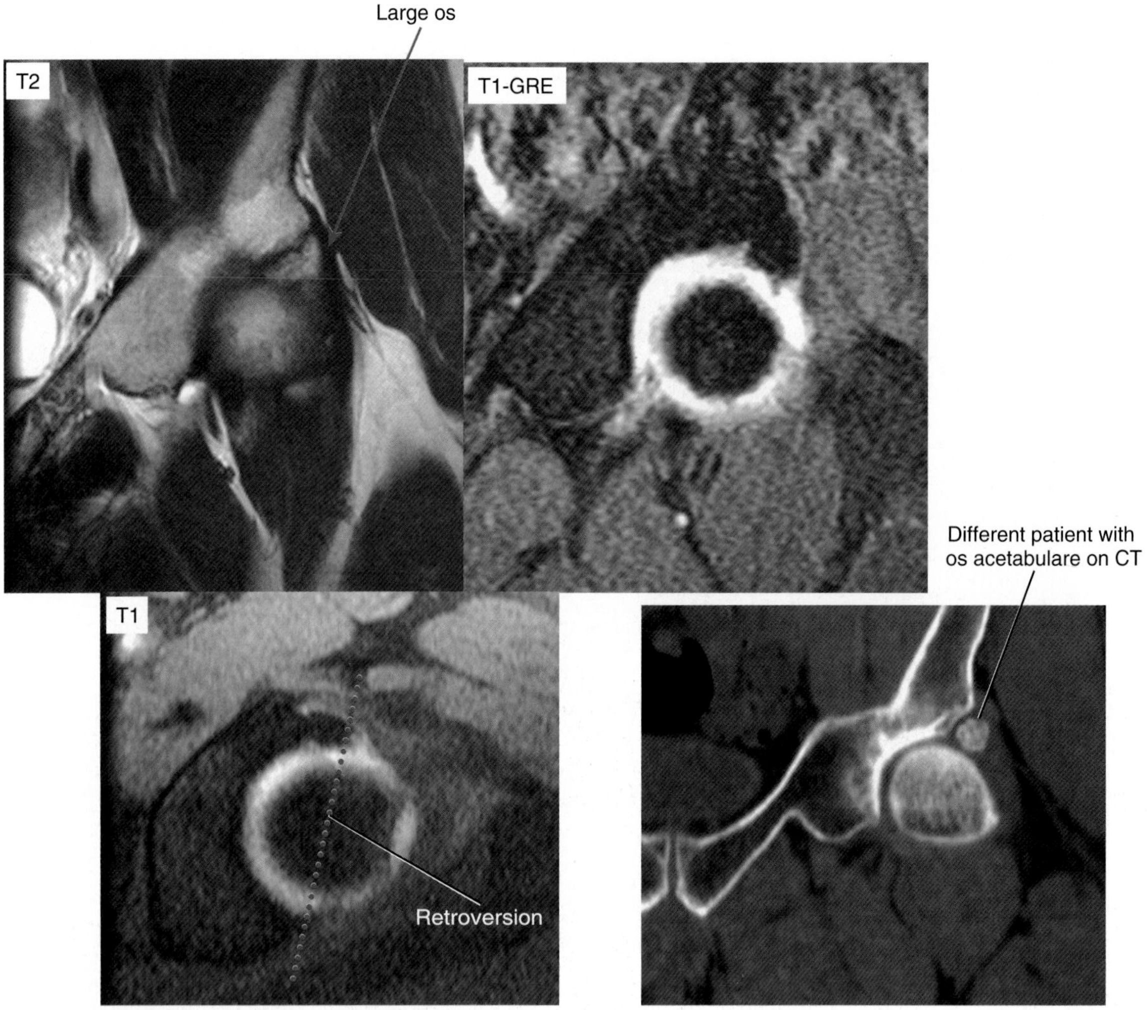
Large os
T2
T1-GRE
Different patient with os acetabulare on CT
T1
Retroversion

Figure 11-52 Os acetabulare. Ossification at the margin of the acetabular rim has been postulated to be associated with femoral-acetabular impingement in a subset of individuals. In this patient, a large os at the anterolateral rim has a fibrous connection to the underlying bone and results in an overhanging edge and potentially impingement in a similar way that retroversion can result in impingement.

BOX 11-6 SLIPPED CAPITAL FEMORAL EPIPHYSIS

More common in overweight male adolescents
Often bilateral
Result: Gun-shaped femur
- Lack of lateral femoral neck concavity
- Susceptible to cam-type impingement

BOX 11-7 LEGG-CALVÉ-PERTHES DISEASE

Avascular necrosis
Peak age, 4–7
Irregular growth; articular collapse results in deformity; aspherical head
Decreased longitudinal growth at physis with periosteal apposition leading to short, fat neck (coxa magna, coxa brevis)

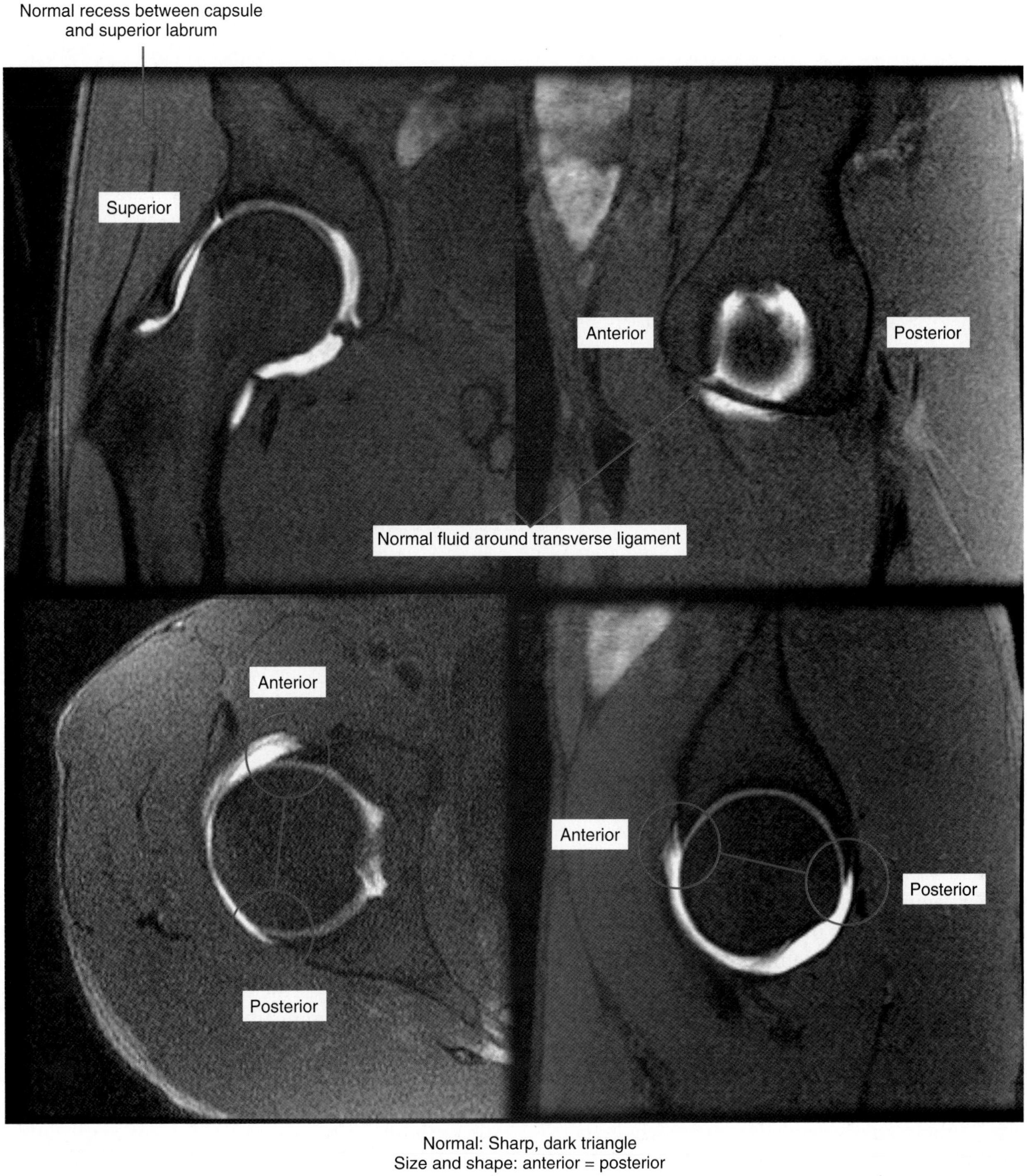
Normal recess between capsule and superior labrum
Superior
Anterior
Posterior
Normal fluid around transverse ligament
Anterior
Posterior
Anterior
Posterior
Normal: Sharp, dark triangle
Size and shape: anterior = posterior

Figure 11-53 Normal labral anatomy on an MR arthrogram. Unlike the glenoid labrum, the acetabular labrum is not a complete ring, but extends across the inferior acetabulum as a transverse ligament. Also unlike the glenoid labrum, the hip labrum is fairly uniform in size and shape in different regions. There is a recess around the transverse ligament and between the labrum and capsule. Like the glenoid labrum, the dark signal of fibrocartilaginous labrum blends with the intermediate signal hyaline cartilage.

BOX 11-8 COMPARISON OF CAM- AND PINCER-TYPE LESION

Cam
M:F = 13:1
Average age = 32
Large anterosuperior lesion
No contrecoup lesion posteriorly

Pincer
M:F = 1:3
Average age = 40
Small anterosuperior lesion
Contrecoup lesion posteriorly

BOX 11-9 SUMMARY OF FINDINGS

Femoral Acetabular Impingement
Retroversion (figure-of-8 sign)
Deep acetabular socket
Spur or bump at anterolateral femoral head-neck junction (esp without joint narrowing)
Lack of lateral femoral neck concavity
Synovial herniation pit
Os acetabulare
Anterior labral tear/cartilage loss

Spectrum of Dysplasia to Impingement
Dysplasia
- Acetabulum too small, deficient, or deformed

Impingement
- Acetabulum too big or retroverted or femoral head malformed

shoulder, which blends with the hyaline cartilage. The labrum surrounds the acetabular rim, increasing joint surface area and stability. Unlike the glenoid labrum, the acetabular labrum extends only 270 to 300 degrees around the hip, being incomplete inferiorly. At the inferior joint, the transverse ligament completes the ring, extending with a taut appearance from the anteroinferior to the posteroinferior acetabulum. At these attachment sites, there may be small sulci. Otherwise, the anterior and posterior labrum is somewhat monotonous, without recesses or foramina that characterize the range of findings in the shoulder; only blunting has been established and appears to be associated with age, likely a degenerative phenomenon. It has been speculated that there may be a normal sulcus anterosuperiorly, but this is still being debated. This also happens to be where tears are most common. Proponents suggest that a sulcus in this location is small and smooth and does not extend into the labral substance.

Between the labrum and the capsule anteriorly, superiorly, and posteriorly, there is a small recess, visualized when there is excess fluid in the joint. Inferomedially, there are larger recesses, and when there is an effusion this may resemble a ganglion cyst. The joint is surrounded by a very thick capsule composed of the iliofemoral, ischiofemoral, and pubofemoral ligaments, which wrap around the neck, with the different components becoming taut in various positions. The capsule inserts at the base of the femoral neck resulting in rounded recesses just above the intertrochanteric ridge. The distended joint has a region of constriction, or a waist, created by the zona orbicularis ligament, which is part of the capsule and surrounds the femoral neck. These ligaments and recesses have implications regarding selection of a site for joint injection (see Chapter 2).

Clinically, patients with labral tear present with pain and snapping or clicking during range of motion. Although acute injury (i.e., twisting) can result in labral tear, the current thinking is that most labral tears are caused by impingement or dysplasia. If a labral tear is found, the cause should be sought.

Diagnosis of Labral Tear (Figs. 11-54 through 11-58)

Arthrography using multidetector CT can obtain high-resolution images of labral tear; however, MRI remains the most widely used imaging exam. Low-field MRI is at a significant disadvantage because the resolution and SNR required for visualization are difficult to achieve. Noncontrast high-field MRI must incorporate small field-of-view, high-resolution sequences in at least the coronal and sagittal planes. Most experts recommend MR arthrography.

Labral tears can occasionally be seen on images from low-field scanners; in this scenario it is especially helpful to acquire a coronal STIR image including both hips. Comparing sides, asymmetric fluid, or morphologic abnormality at the acetabular rim can aid diagnosis. MR arthrography can also improve visualization if some form of fat suppression is available (e.g., Dixon fat-water separation).

Indirect MR arthrography (see Chapter 2) generally yields suboptimal SNR for the hip and does not provide the distention effect. Direct MR arthrography is preferred. Knowing the location of sublabral recesses helps distinguish tears. Apart from this, there

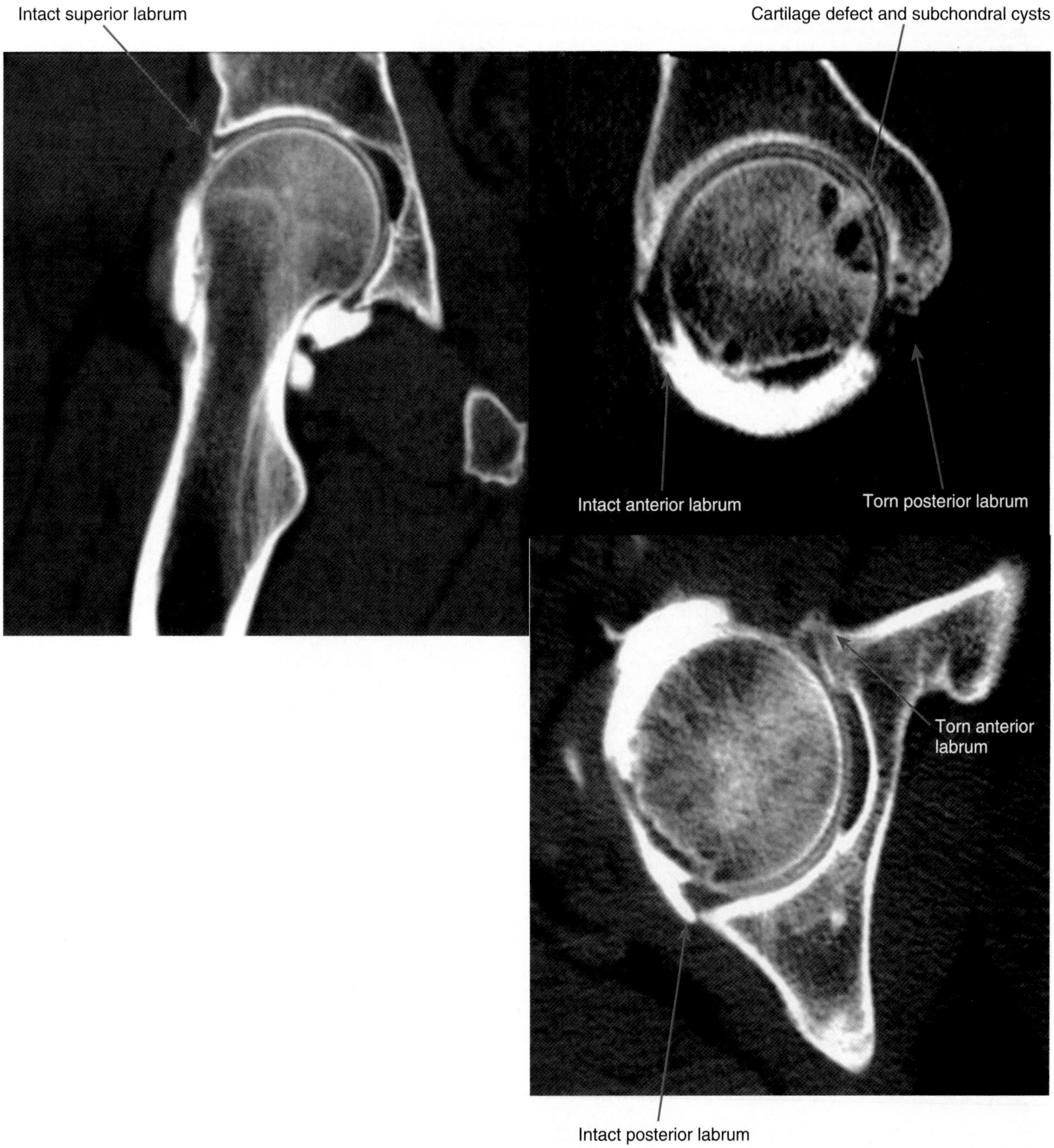
Intact superior labrum
Cartilage defect and subchondral cysts
Intact anterior labrum
Torn posterior labrum
Torn anterior labrum
Intact posterior labrum

Figure 11-54 *Arthrography using multidetector CT is excellent for diagnosis of hip pathology.*

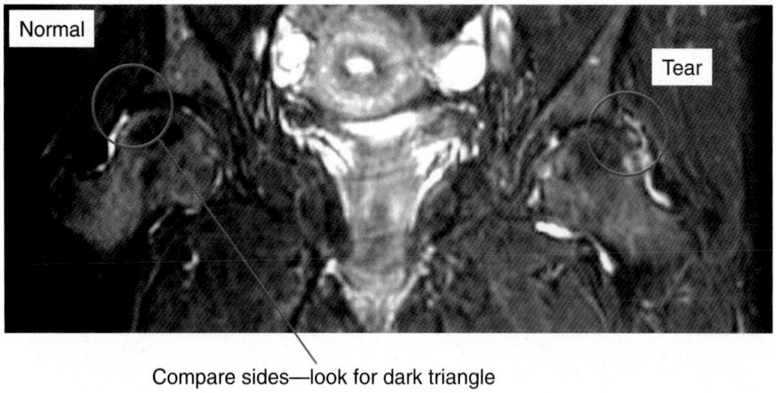
Normal
Tear
Compare sides—look for dark triangle

Figure 11-55 Labral tear can be detected on noncontrast MRI using fluid-sensitive sequences; however, MR arthrography is more sensitive.

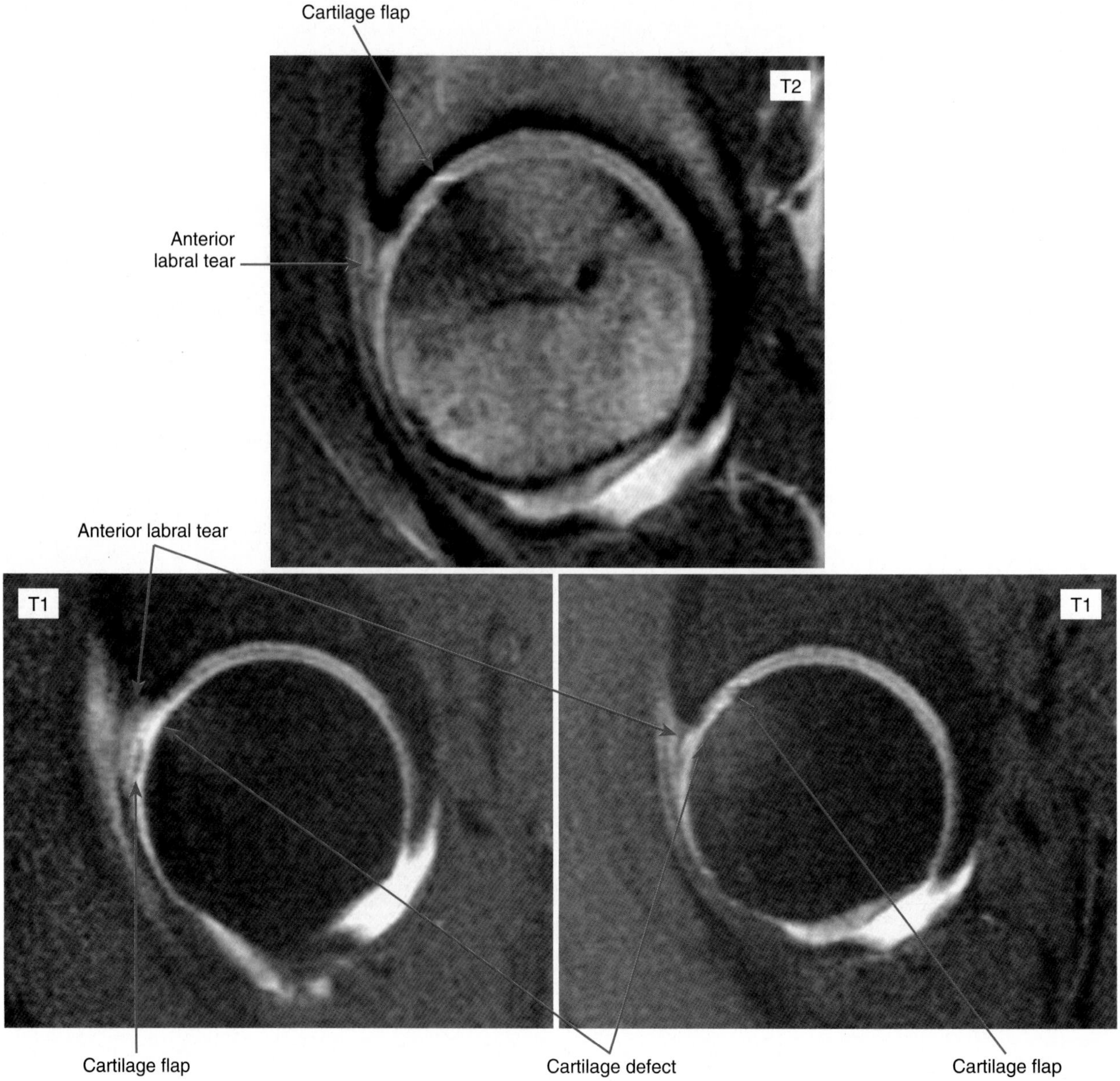
Cartilage flap
T2
Anterior labral tear
Anterior labral tear
T1
T1
Cartilage flap
Cartilage defect
Cartilage flap

Figure 11-56 Hip MR arthrogram of anterior labral tear and cartilage flap. Intermediate signal of hyaline cartilage should be evaluated for defects; anterior chondrosis and labral pathology is best seen on sagittal images.

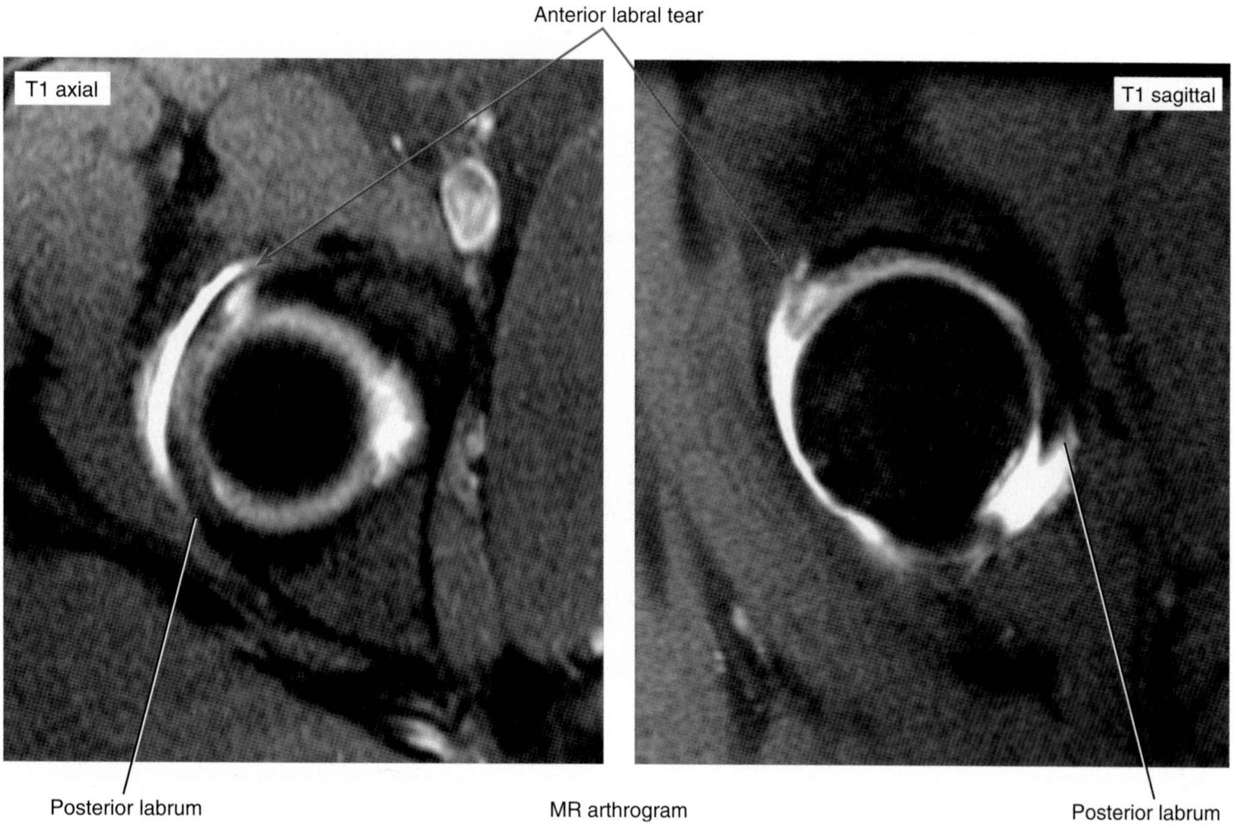
Anterior labral tear
T1 axial
T1 sagittal
Posterior labrum
MR arthrogram
Posterior labrum

Figure 11-57 Anterior labral tear on direct MR arthrogram. The anterior labrum should appear similar to the posterior labrum. This serves as a useful internal control. Axial and sagittal images are excellent for detection of anterior and posterior tears.

is little variation of the acetabular labrum, unlike its glenoid counterpart. Although the margin may be blunted or diminutive, there should not be intrasubstance (i.e., within the "dark triangle") fluid or contrast. Irregular signal is especially indicative of tear, as is separation of the triangle from the rim. It is also helpful to note that the anterior labrum and posterior labrum are usually very similar in size and signal. Therefore, comparison from side to side and from front to back is very useful.

Paralabral Cysts (Figs. 11-59 and 11-60)

As in the shoulder, the presence of a paralabral cyst is highly suggestive of underlying tear; often these are visible on large field-of-view images of the pelvis. Paralabral cysts are usually anterior or anterosuperior, are typically lobulated, disproportionate to joint fluid, and either are directly adjacent to the labrum or have a neck pointing to the acetabular rim. Cysts can erode into bone, simulating tumor, and can extend far from the joint. Care must be taken to differentiate from distended recesses (non- or minimally lobulated, proportionate to joint fluid) or iliopsoas bursitis (separate from joint, oriented along iliopsoas).

Labral tears are often associated with cartilage loss. No matter what the cause of the labral tear is, cartilage loss originates near the labral tear (the exception being in pincer impingement, with the contrecoup cartilage lesion at the posterior rim). If fluid or contrast extends under the cartilage, a flap should be diagnosed. Flaps can cause snapping like labral tears and imply a worse prognosis for repair, since they generally require debridement. Location and extent of cartilage loss, partial versus full thickness, and presence of subchondral cysts should be described. This gives the surgeon an idea of the degree of damage and facilitates surgical planning. Similarly, location and extent of tear should be discussed in the report;

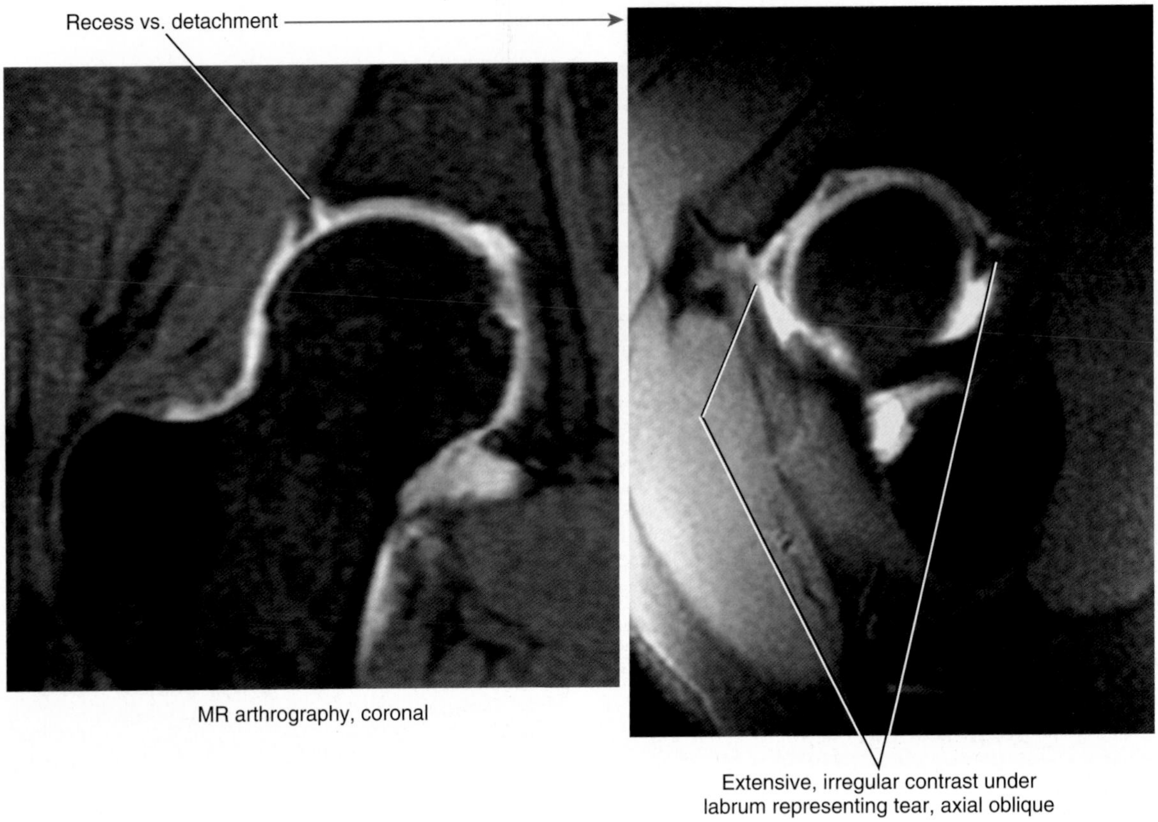
Recess vs. detachment
MR arthrography, coronal
Extensive, irregular contrast under labrum representing tear, axial oblique

Figure 11-58 It is controversial whether sublabral recesses other than those around the transverse ligament exist and, if so, whether they are observed on routine MR imaging or MR arthrogram sequences. Fluid that is prominent, extensive, and/or irregular is more likely to represent pathology. Labral findings associated with a paralabral cyst, arthritis, or impingement anatomy are likely to be pathologic. Extent of tear should be described.

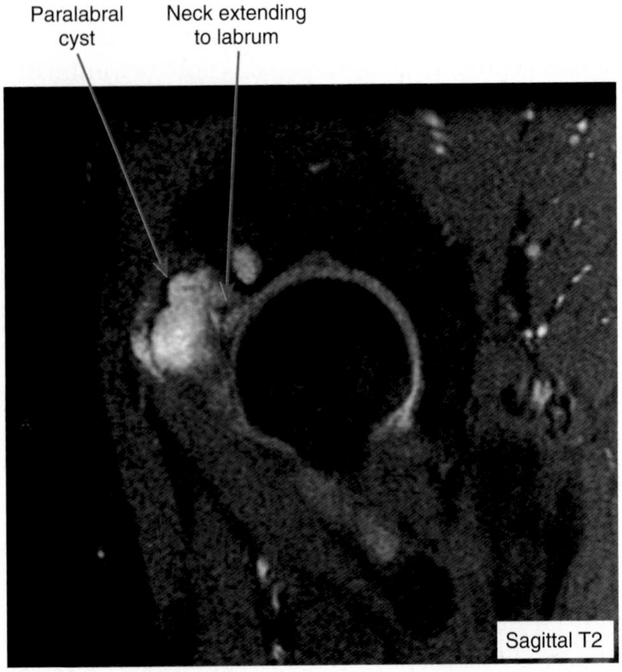
Paralabral cyst
Neck extending to labrum
Sagittal T2

Figure 11-59 Paralabral cysts are invariably associated with labral tear. Paralabral cysts are generally lobulated if large. To differentiate paralabral cysts from other pathology (i.e., iliopsoas bursitis), look for a thin neck extending to the acetabular rim.

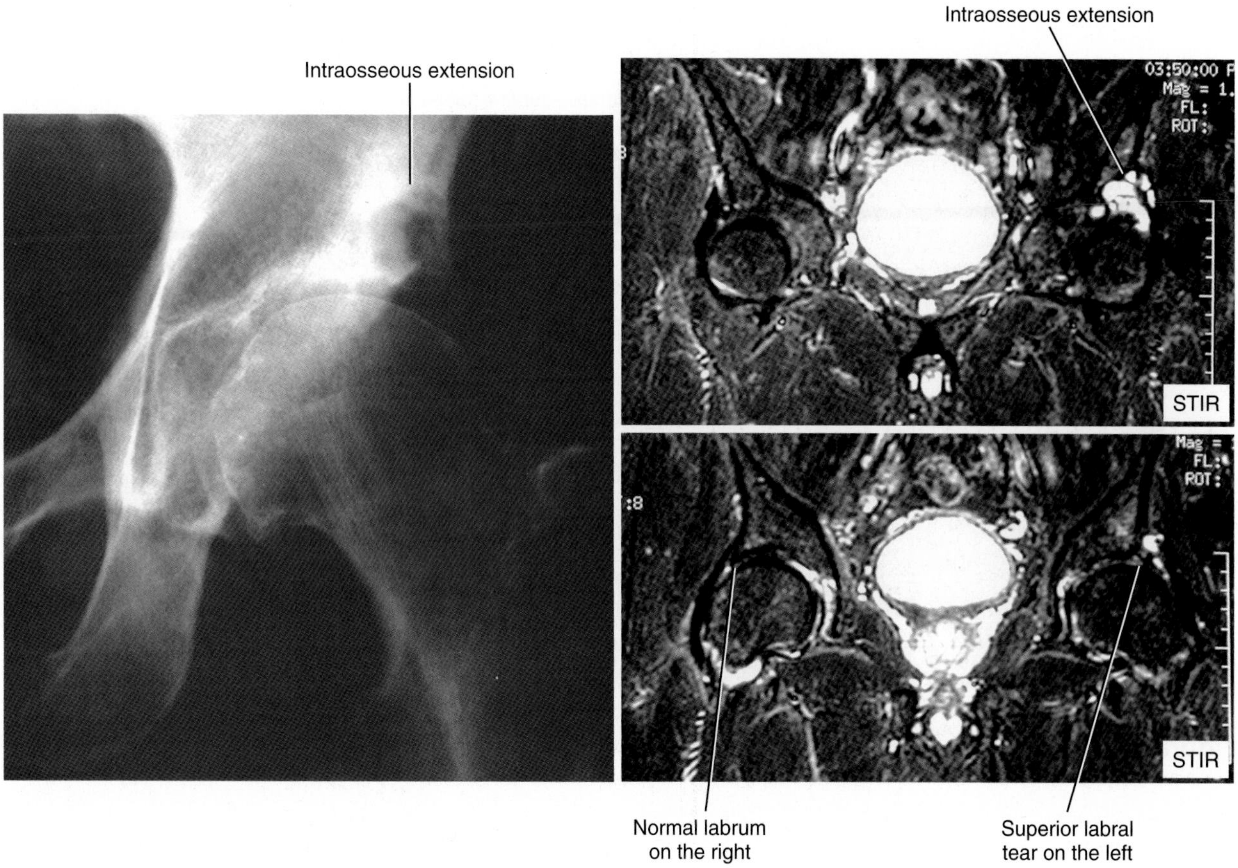
Intraosseous extension
Intraosseous extension
STIR
STIR
Normal labrum on the right
Superior labral tear on the left

Figure 11-60 Paralabral cyst/intraosseous ganglion. Labral tear resulting in formation of a lobulated paralabral cyst. The cyst is eroding into the adjacent bone.

as with the glenoid, acetabular labral tear location and extent can be classified in terms of a clock face, in which the most superior aspect of the acetabular rim is 12:00, and 3:00 is directly anterior by convention. Using this convention, the labrum ends and the transverse ligament extends from 4:30–5:00 to 7:00–7:30.

Osteoarthritis at the hip is seen on radiographs as joint narrowing; location can suggest the underlying etiology. Normally, the medial joint is about two times wider than the superolateral and superomedial joints, the latter two zones being uniform in width. Diffuse narrowing is associated with inflammatory arthropathies; these conditions can also lead to protrusio acetabuli. Later, these patients can get secondary osteoarthritis due to cartilage destruction and are also predisposed to pincer impingement. Superomedial joint narrowing is typical for osteoarthritis; this aspect of the joint is along the line of force. However, such a pattern does not exclude impingement as a cause. Superolateral or anterior joint narrowing should arouse suspicion of impingement or dysplasia. At the hip, subchondral degenerative cysts can become large and simulate a tumor radiographically (called an Egger cyst). CT can be used to document the thin sclerotic margin characteristic of a cyst, or MRI can depict the cystic nature of the lesion and associated joint pathology (Fig. 11-61).

Other arthropathies and infection are discussed in other chapters.

LIGAMENTUM TERES PATHOLOGY (Figs. 11-62 and 11-63)

Although incidence of ligamentum teres pathology in patients with hip pain is debatable, the structure should always be inspected. The normal ligamentum teres is a linear structure with slight curvature,

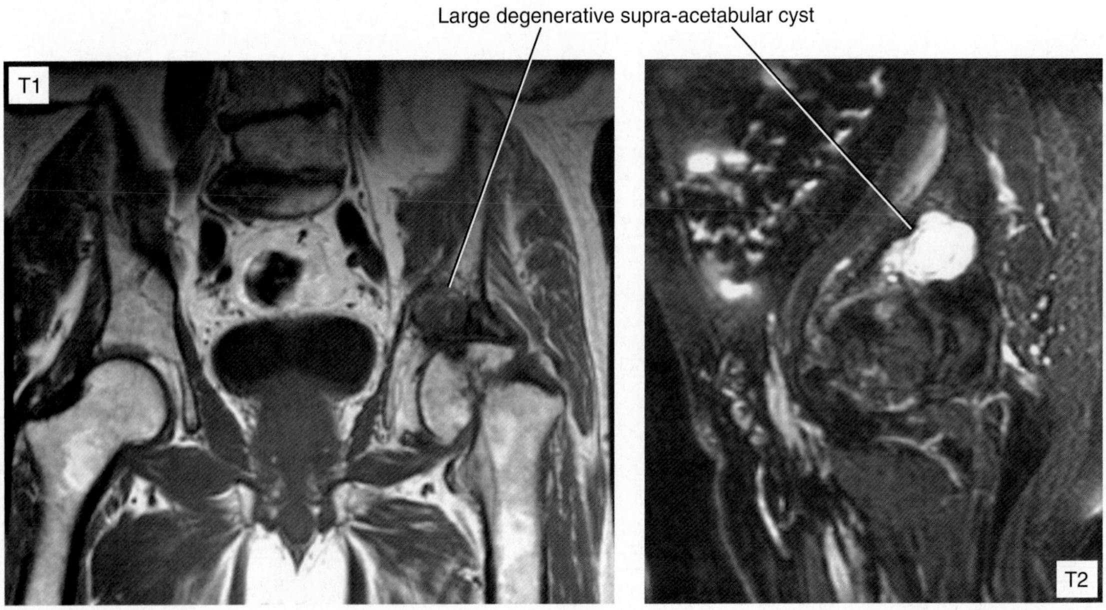
Large degenerative supra-acetabular cyst
T1
T2

Figure 11-61 Osteoarthritis of the hip can be associated with a large supra-acetabular cyst (Egger cyst) that may simulate tumor.

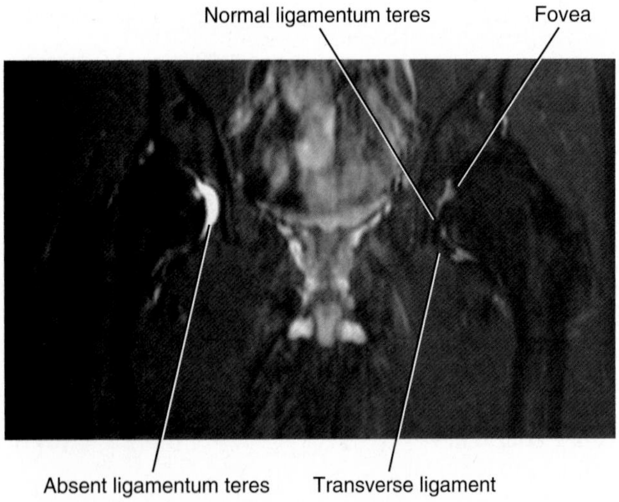
Normal ligamentum teres
Fovea
Absent ligamentum teres
Transverse ligament

Figure 11-62 Professional hockey player with prior ligamentum teres debridement on the right. The ligament normally arises at the fovea and extends inferiorly through the medial aspect of the joint, inserting onto the capsule at the transverse ligament.

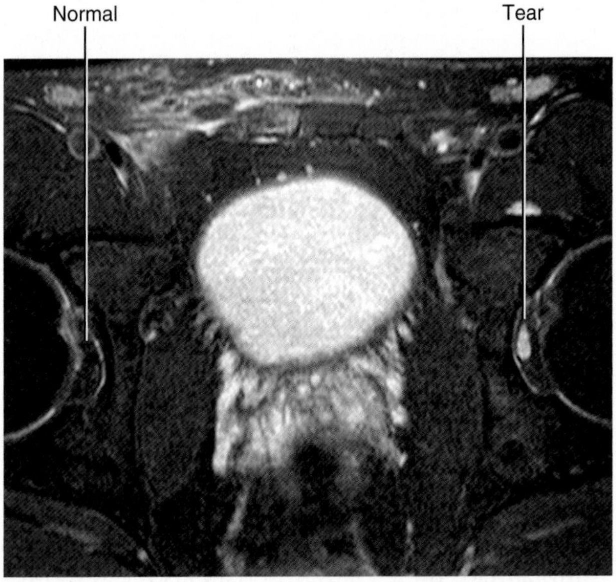
Normal
Tear

Figure 11-63 Ligamentum teres tear on axial images.

extending from the fovea centralis of the femoral head inferiorly through the joint, inserting on the transverse ligament inferiorly. The ligament is normally dark on all sequences. Tearing can cause chronic hip pain and can be seen as asymmetric thickening or internal fluid signal (or contrast on MR arthrography). Symptomatic tears are treated with debridement.

BURSITIS

There are many bursas around the hip and pelvis; virtually every tendon attachment is associated with a bursa. Therefore, a small amount of fluid next to a tendon attachment (especially common at the hamstring origin) may have little clinical significance. However, if asymmetric and on the side of symptoms, bursitis is suggested. In this case, it is important that the radiologist should carefully inspect the tendon itself since bursal fluid may merely be a sign of adjacent pathology, most commonly tendinosis or tear (the same is true for bursal fluid in other areas of the body). The following discussion includes the two most common forms of symptomatic bursitis at the hip—iliopsoas and greater trochanteric bursitis. Young athletic patients can have symptomatic iliopsoas bursitis, whereas elderly and/or obese patients tend to get greater trochanteric bursitis. Pain is the common presenting complaint, often with a snapping sensation during leg range of motion or other activity (Box 11-10).

BOX 11-10 DIFFERENTIAL DIAGNOSIS OF COXA SALTANS (SNAPPING HIP)

Labral tear
Intra-articular bodies
Bursitis

Iliopsoas Bursitis (Fig. 11-64)

The iliopsoas bursa is more of a potential space, extending from the anterior margin of the iliacus muscle in the pelvis to the insertion of the common iliopsoas tendon at the lesser trochanter. Along its course the tendon passes anterior to the acetabular rim and the hip joint. Normally this space contains no detectable fluid on MRI. However, in some patients the space communicates with the hip joint and can fill with fluid in the presence of an effusion or following an arthrogram. Repetitive friction of the iliopsoas tendon along the bony ridge of the anterior

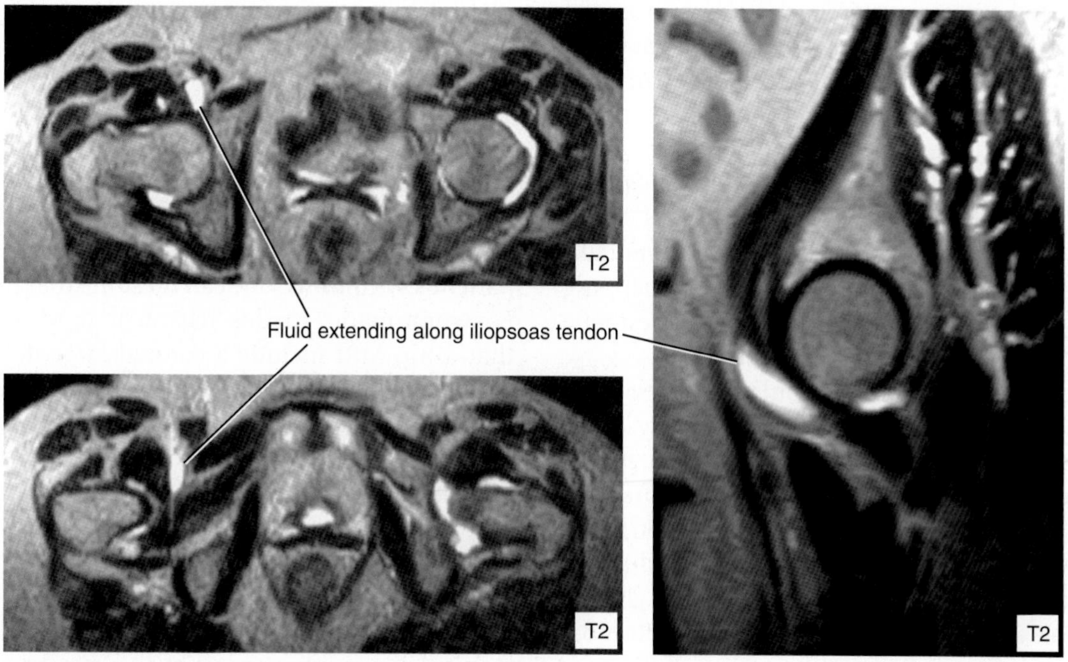
T2
Fluid extending along iliopsoas tendon
T2
T2

Figure 11-64 Iliopsoas bursitis. Note that the fluid does not extend to the labral margin as does a paralabral cyst.

acetabulum is the presumed etiology of iliopsoas bursitis in the athletic population. A bony prominence in this location may predispose to this process. Documentation of iliopsoas bursitis can be achieved by MRI, ultrasound, or CT. MRI provides best visualization of the fluid and differentiation from ganglion cysts and paralabral cysts; however, ultrasound can directly visualize the tendon during leg motion and dynamically visualize the tendon snapping over the acetabulum resulting in characteristic symptoms of pain and snapping. Alternatively, bursography can be useful; the technique is described in the arthrography chapter. After opacification of the bursa with iodinated contrast, range of motion can be performed by the patient with fluoroscopic observation; as the patient attempts to reproduce the motion that causes the sensation, the tendon (seen as a radiolucent line surrounded by contrast) is monitored for sudden deflection associated with reproduction of symptoms. During injection a long-acting anesthetic and/or steroid can be injected to document for subsequent temporary resolution of symptoms.

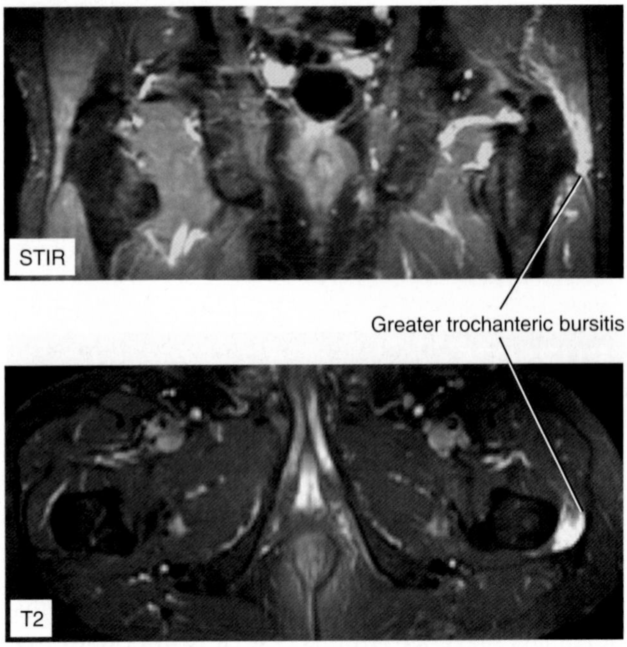
STIR
Greater trochanteric bursitis
T2

Figure 11-65 Greater trochanteric bursitis. Edema or a small amount of fluid is often observed in the region of the bursa in obese patients but is not necessarily symptomatic. If the fluid is asymmetric and on the side of pain, it is more likely to be significant. When such a finding is present, the radiologist should look closely for tear at the gluteus medius/minimus insertion on the greater trochanter. Mechanical bursitis in this location can be related to friction from tight lateral fascia (can cause "external snapping" symptoms) or may be inflammatory related to various arthropathies.

Greater Trochanteric Bursitis (Fig. 11-65)

Greater trochanteric bursitis can be seen in young, thin, athletic individuals with tight lateral fascia (which is also the origin of iliotibial band friction syndrome and excessive lateral pressure syndrome at the knee). In this situation, the tensor fascia lata rubs repeatedly against the greater trochanter, inciting inflammation at the anatomic bursa between the structures. Pain and a snapping sensation occur (external snapping as opposed to internal snapping associated with iliopsoas bursitis as well as labral tear). MRI and ultrasound again are the best modalities for visualization. Documentation of the snapping is generally not needed, but injection with anesthetic can establish the bursa as a pain source.

A much more common population presenting with greater trochanteric bursitis is the elderly, especially obese patients. The cause is less clear, but it may be related to trauma or adjacent gluteus medius/minimus insertional pathology. In fact, sudden onset of pain in this population should prompt evaluation of greater trochanteric avulsion fracture or gluteus tendon tear. Confusing the issue is that on MRI most obese patients have edema in the region of the anatomic trochanteric bursa, which is normal and asymptomatic and analogous to prepatellar edema and soft tissue edema at the lower back that is nearly ubiquitous on MRI of the knee and lumbar spine in obese patients. If there is discrete fluid rather than just edema and if the fluid is on the same side as the patient's symptoms, one can presume that the finding is symptomatic. In this regard, it is recommended that a hip MRI include a coronal large field-of-view STIR sequence to establish asymmetry of the finding. Contrast can help as well, with inflammation enhancing brightly. However, if there is fluid in the bursa care should be taken to follow up the gluteus medius and miminus as well as the obturator insertions on the greater trochanter to make sure the finding truly represents bursitis and not a reaction to adjacent tendon pathology. In addition, calcific tendinosis or bursitis is not uncommon at the greater trochanter and radiographic or CT correlation (or gradient-echo MR imaging sequences) may be helpful in detecting calcification at the tendon or bursa related to hydroxyapatite deposition (HADD).

SPORTSMAN'S HERNIA (ATHLETIC PUBALGIA) AND THE PUBIC SYMPHYSIS (Figs. 11-66 through 11-69)

Sportsman's hernia is a misnomer; only rarely is the cause an actual hernia. In athletic patients with groin pain (a better term is athletic pubalgia), there is a spectrum of findings based on the particular anatomy of the region. The medially positioned paired rectus abdominis myotendinous junctions pass anteriorly to the pubic symphysis, attaching to bone at a common, broad enthesis composed of the pectineus and adductor origin, extending to the gracilis origin at the inferior ischium. These structures are intimately associated with the thick capsule of the pubic symphysis. MRI is the best modality for evaluation of these structures, but it must be performed with a coil, field-of-view and plane specific to the anterior pelvis (see specialized protocol on the accompanying CD). Ultrasound has also been used to visualize the tendon attachments. The injury is a combination of injuries to this common attachment, resulting in edema (strain) of the rectus abdominis, a "cleft sign" with fluid extending inferolaterally around the pubic bone into the capsule and strain of the pectineus/adductor

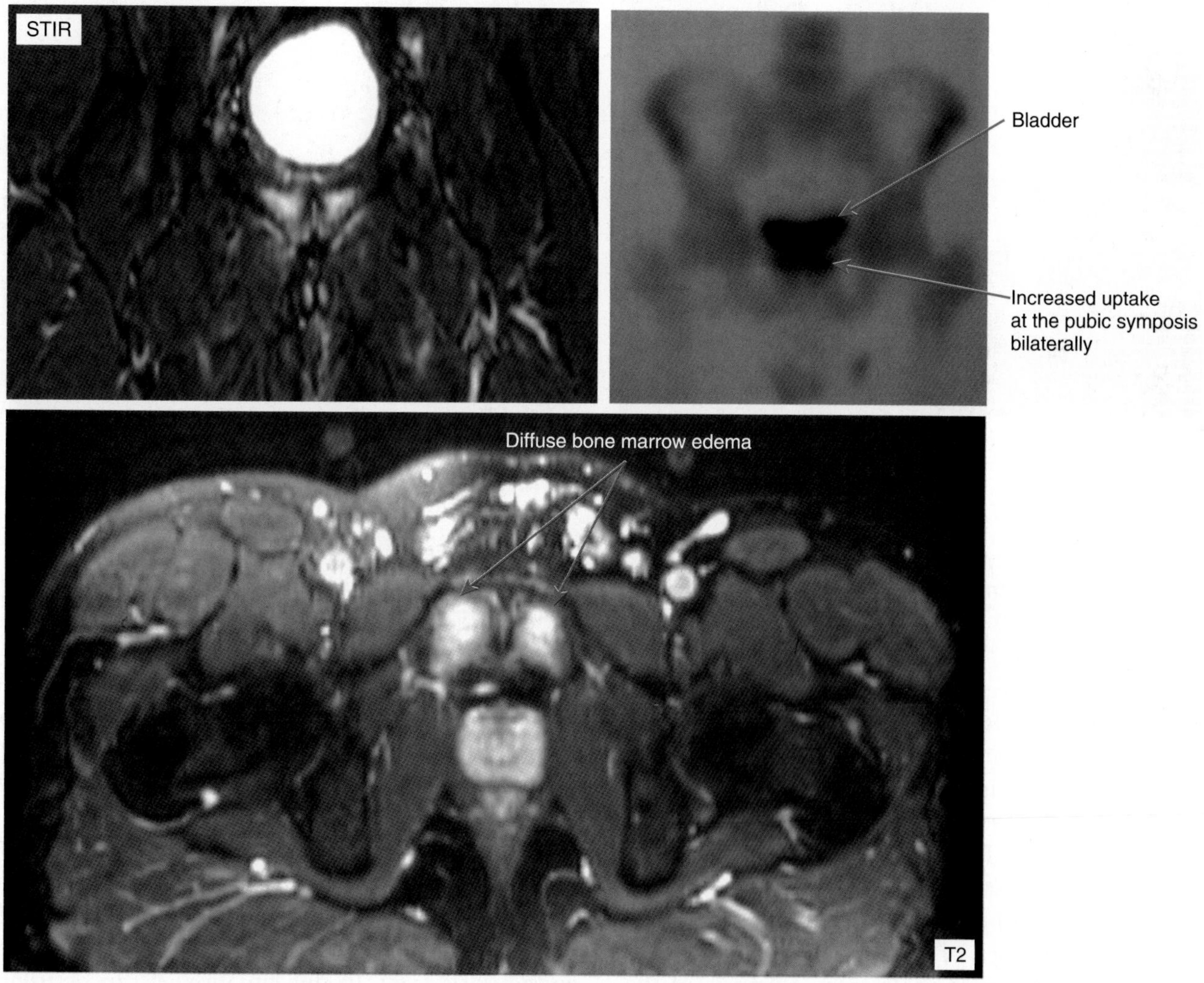
STIR
Bladder
Increased uptake
at the pubic symposis
bilaterally
Diffuse bone marrow edema
T2

Figure 11-66 Osteitis pubis. Diffuse marrow edema across the pubic symphysis may be related to stress response or osteoarthritis.

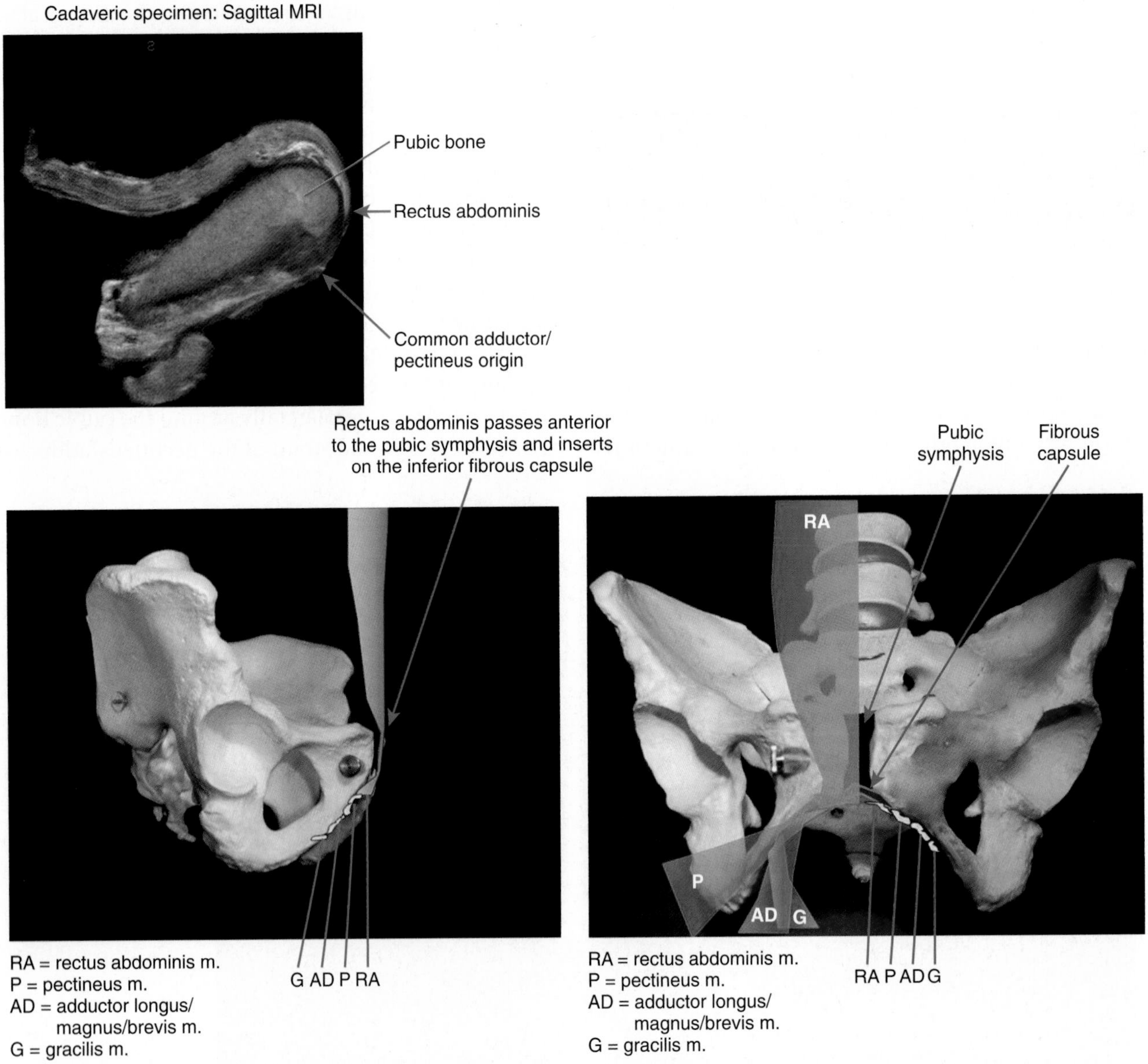
Cadaveric specimen: Sagittal MRI
Pubic bone
Rectus abdominis
Common adductor/
pectineus origin
Rectus abdominis passes anterior
to the pubic symphysis and inserts
on the inferior fibrous capsule
Pubic
symphysis
Fibrous
capsule
RA
P
AD
G
RA = rectus abdominis m.
P = pectineus m.
AD = adductor longus/
magnus/brevis m.
G = gracilis m.
G AD P RA
RA = rectus abdominis m.
P = pectineus m.
AD = adductor longus/
magnus/brevis m.
G = gracilis m.
RA P AD G

Figure 11-67 **Anatomy of the common rectus/adductor aponeurosis. AD, adductor longus/magnus/brevis muscles; G, gracilis muscle; P, pectineus muscle; RA, rectus abdominis muscle.**

origin. In more severe cases, the attachment can tear completely or avulse bone. In this situation, bone resorption can occur, seen radiographically and on CT as focal rarefaction of bone similar to resorption seen in clavicular osteolysis. This can simulate a more aggressive process. The pubic symphysis can alternatively undergo stress response and exhibit symmetric marrow edema, which can be referred to as osteitis pubis, although lack of inflammation makes stress response a more appropriate term. Sclerosis of the pubic symphysis seen on radiographs that is commonly called osteitis pubis is also a poor term, also not due to inflammation, but rather osteoarthritis related to prior injury (especially childbirth, associated with osteitis condensans ilii). It may be related to instability in which case a flamingo view can be helpful for diagnosis. The patient stands on one leg, then the other with AP pelvis images acquired. Offset of the symphysis is seen with instability.

It may not be apparent clinically whether the patient has a problem originating in the hip joint (e.g., labral tear, osteoarthritis) or pubic symphysis/adductors (e.g., stress, osteitis pubis, rectus/adductor aponeurosis tear). In this situation, it can be useful to inject dilute gadolinium into the hip joint along with 3 mL of long-acting anesthetic; then MR arthrography of the hip can be performed as well as MRI of the pubic symphysis region. In addition, after the

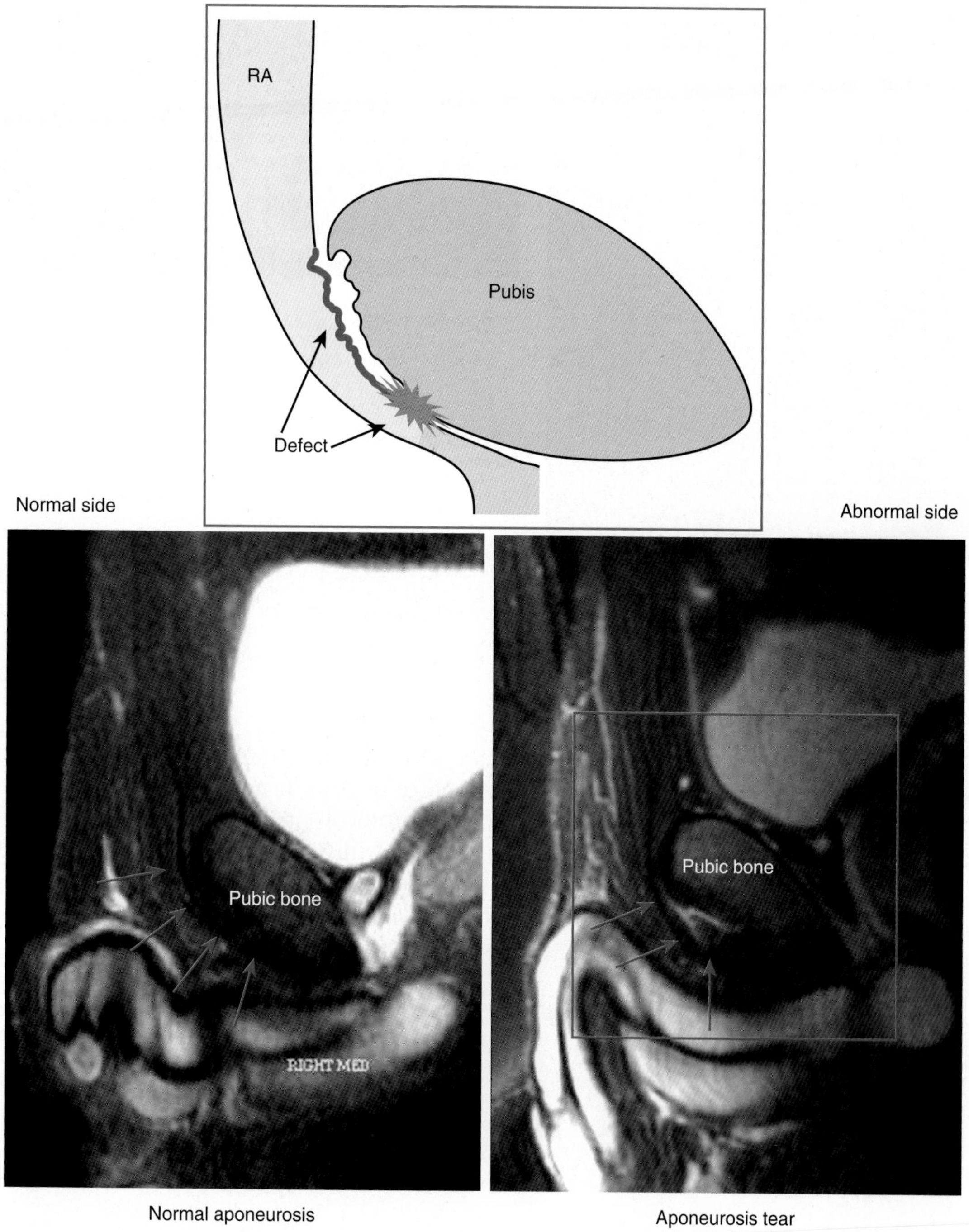
RA
Pubis
Defect
Normal side
Abnormal side
Pubic bone
RIGHT MED
Pubic bone
Normal aponeurosis
Aponeurosis tear

Figure 11-68 Athletic pubalgia. The rectus abdominis tendon (*red arrows*) passes anteriorly over the pubic bone, inserting onto the anteroinferior aspect in a common attachment with the adductor origin. This common rectus-adductor aponeurosis is invested into the capsule of the symphysis. Injuries at this common aponeurosis result in stripping and eventually avulsion from the bone and capsule. RA, rectus abdominis.

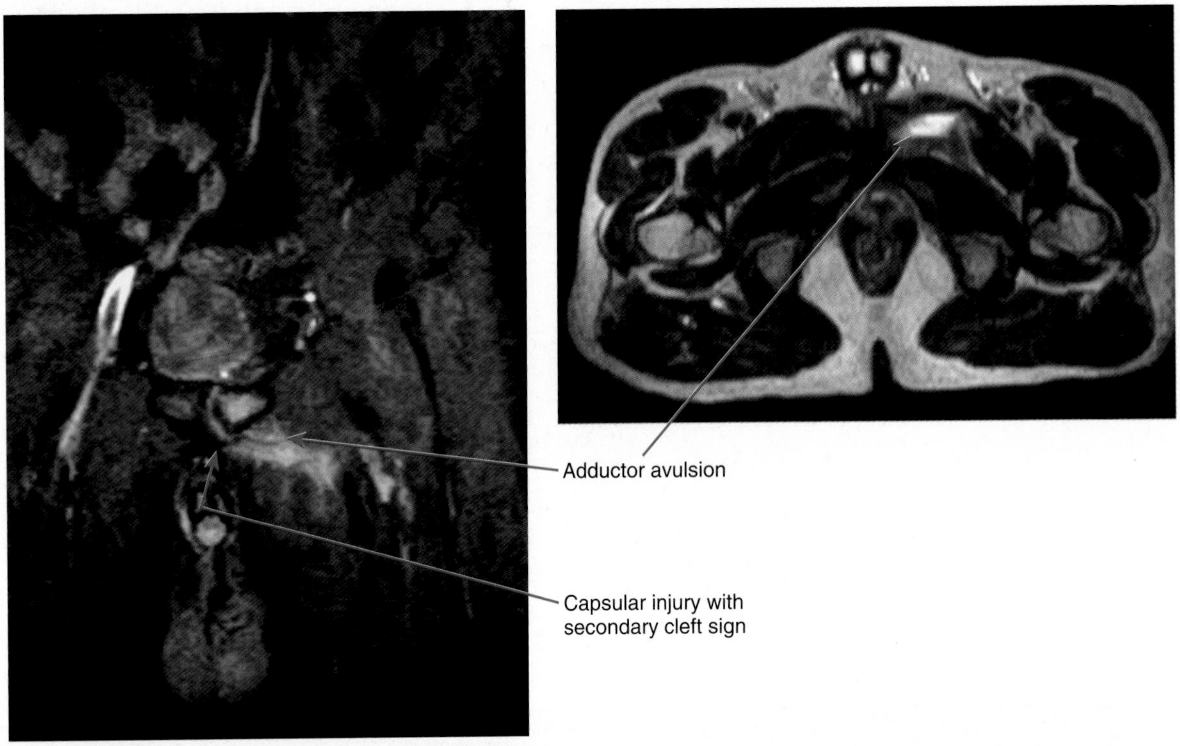
Adductor avulsion
Capsular injury with
secondary cleft sign

Figure 11-69 Adductor avulsion is associated with pubic symphysis capsular injury and formation of a secondary cleft sign.

injection of anesthetic and after walking to the MRI, the patient can be asked about pain relief and the referring clinician will have useful information regarding whether the hip joint is the site of pain generation.

Occasionally (rarely), an actual hernia is the source of pain. If no site of pain can be seen using the protocol previously described, MRI or ultrasound with and without Valsalva maneuver can be useful.

Chapter 12

IMAGING OF THE KNEE

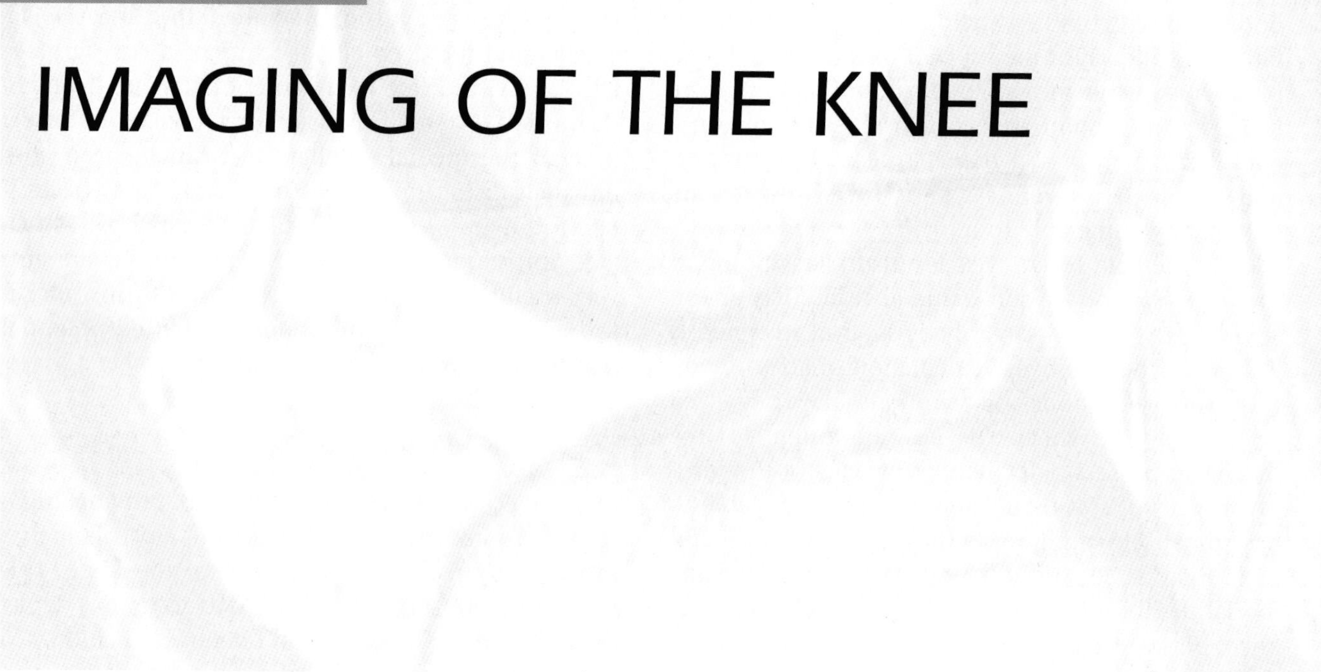

CHAPTER OUTLINE

The knee is the largest synovial-lined joint in the body. It has a complex anatomic design that simultaneously allows for the support of the entire weight of the body while providing maximum mobility. The knee is a hinge joint and as such relies heavily on a complex system of soft tissue structures for support and stability. However, several of these structures are particularly vulnerable to injury.

Over the past several years, our understanding of the intricacies of the soft tissue anatomy has grown significantly, driven primarily by surgical advances as well as by the noninvasive depiction of anatomy on MRI. Surgical options and techniques have advanced to the point at which it is now important for the imager to possess a detailed knowledge of the intricate details of soft tissue anatomy and to be able to describe subtle variations in the injury patterns. Radiography and CT scanning remain the primary imaging modalities for detection of osseous injuries about the knee, but MRI has taken center stage with regard to detecting and describing soft tissue injury patterns.

MODALITIES

Radiography

Radiographs are often the first imaging study obtained on a patient presenting with the chief complaint of knee pain. The standard radiographic series varies depending on the clinical presentation, but in most instances it consists of anteroposterior supine, lateral, and tunnel views. An axial (Merchant) view may be added for evaluation of the patellofemoral joint. These views can be supplemented with oblique views, standing views, or cross-table lateral views, depending on the clinical presentation. Radiographs are best suited for depicting abnormalities of the osseous structures such as fractures, dislocations, and bone lesions. However, most knee injuries affect the soft tissue support structures rather than the osseous structures. Nevertheless, subtle abnormalities are often seen on the radiographs, which can provide helpful hints regarding the type of injury that may be present.

A joint effusion often accompanies internal derangement of the knee and is usually detectable on good-quality radiographs. Detection of a fat-fluid level on a cross-table lateral view indicates a likely intracapsular fracture. Several subtle radiographic abnormalities can be indicators of significant internal derangement. For instance, the Segond fracture (lateral capsular avulsion fracture of the tibia; see Fig. 12-8A) and the deep lateral femoral sulcus sign (see Fig. 12-9A) indicate likely anterior cruciate ligament disruption. A small avulsion fracture of the lower pole of the medial patellar facet can be seen after transient dislocation of the patella and may necessitate followup MRI to delineate the extent of associated soft tissue abnormalities. Radiographs are also very useful for evaluating suspected arthritis, monitoring healing of fractures, and evaluating potential hardware complications after arthroplasty.

Computed Tomography

Multidetector CT with its ability to provide high-resolution reconstructed images in any plane has proved very useful in evaluation of the knee. This modality is most commonly used to accurately depict the location and extent of fractures, including a precise determination of articular incongruity, particularly as it pertains to fractures of the tibial plateau (see Fig. 12-67). The high-resolution multiplanar capability is also ideal for evaluating the status of a healing fracture and is useful for detecting signs of early healing versus nonunion. This can be particularly helpful in evaluating fractures about the knee and the tibial shaft, where fracture nonunion or delayed union is a common complication. Multidetector CT is also very useful for evaluating prosthesis of the knee following arthroplasty for complications such as loosening, infection, and osteolysis. Finally, multidetector CT combined with intra-articular contrast is proving to be very useful in the evaluation of internal derangement, especially in patients who are not able to undergo MRI because of implanted devices such as a pacemaker.

Ultrasound

Ultrasound has only limited usefulness with regard to evaluation of the knee. A few studies have demonstrated the appearance of meniscal tears using ultrasound examination; however, only the peripheral portions of the menisci are typically visualized. MRI remains the modality of choice in evaluation of the menisci primarily because of its increased accuracy and ability to provide more global evaluation of the knee. Ultrasound can accurately depict and classify abnormalities of the collateral ligaments as well as the quadriceps (Fig. 12-1) and patellar tendons (Fig.

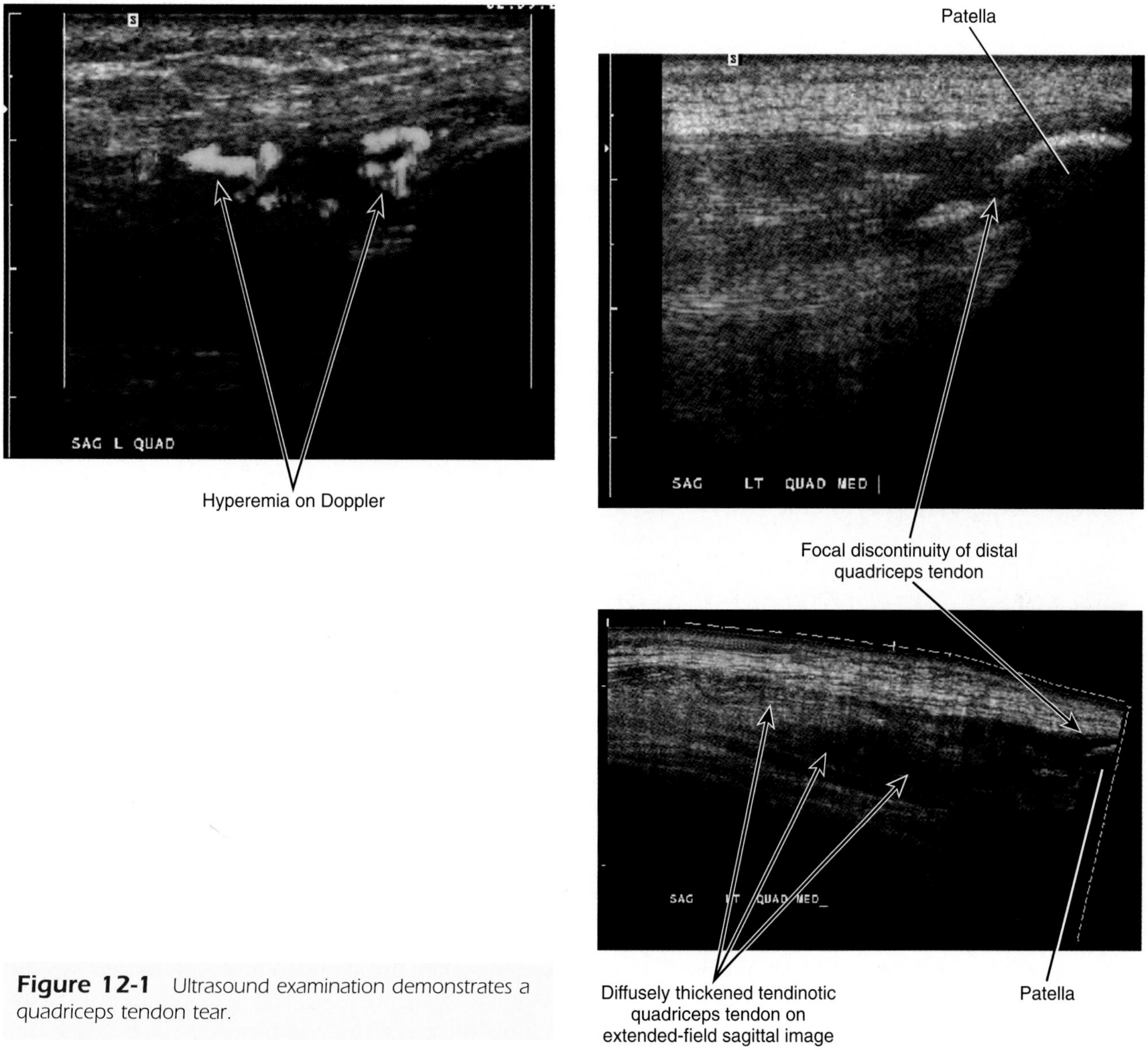
SAG L QUAD
Hyperemia on Doppler
Patella
SAG LT QUAD MED
Focal discontinuity of distal quadriceps tendon
SAG LT QUAD MED
Diffusely thickened tendinotic quadriceps tendon on extended-field sagittal image
Patella

Figure 12-1 Ultrasound examination demonstrates a quadriceps tendon tear.

12-2) and can be useful in a targeted evaluation of these structures, but it is incapable of accurately assessing the anterior or posterior cruciate ligaments. The osseous structures and articular surfaces cannot be adequately evaluated with ultrasound. Probably one of the more common uses of ultrasound with regard to imaging of the knee is to confirm a Baker's cyst, which appears as an anechoic structure along the posterior medial aspect of the knee arising between the medial head of the gastrocnemius and the semimembranosus tendons (Fig. 12-3). The presence of a Baker's cyst has been shown to be associated with an increased incidence of internal derangement of the knee; as a result, MRI may again be the study of choice for providing a more global assessment of the knee with regard to the presence of a Baker's cyst.

Magnetic Resonance Imaging

Magnetic resonance imaging (MRI) is the modality of choice for evaluating the soft tissue structures of the knee, and indeed the knee is the most commonly imaged joint using MRI. MRI accurately depicts abnormalities of the osseous structures and articular cartilage along with all of the soft tissue structures, including the tendons, ligament, and menisci. Direct or indirect MR arthrography is typically reserved for postoperative cases to aid in differentiating

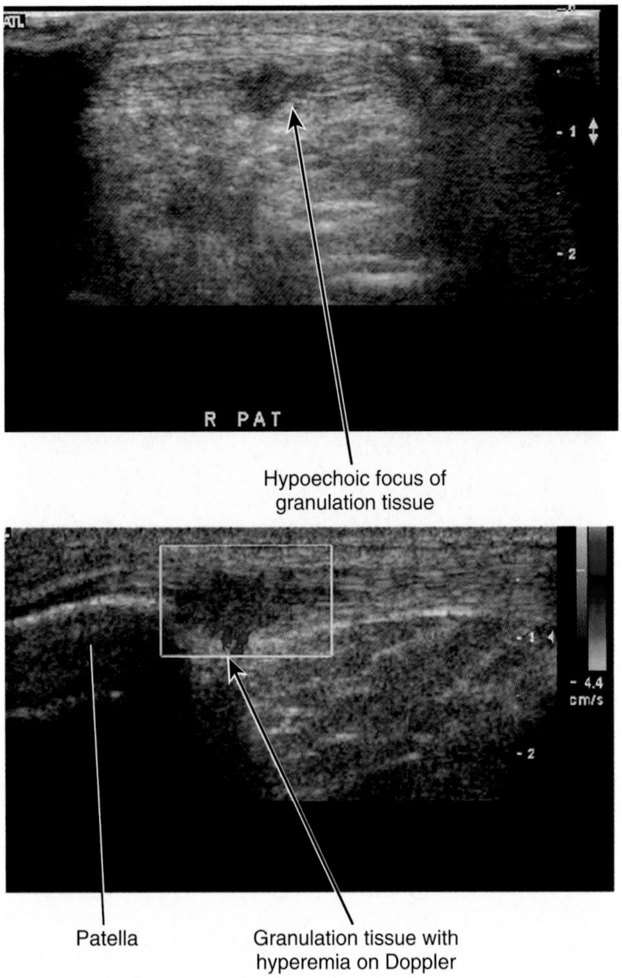
R PAT
Hypoechoic focus of granulation tissue
Patella
Granulation tissue with hyperemia on Doppler

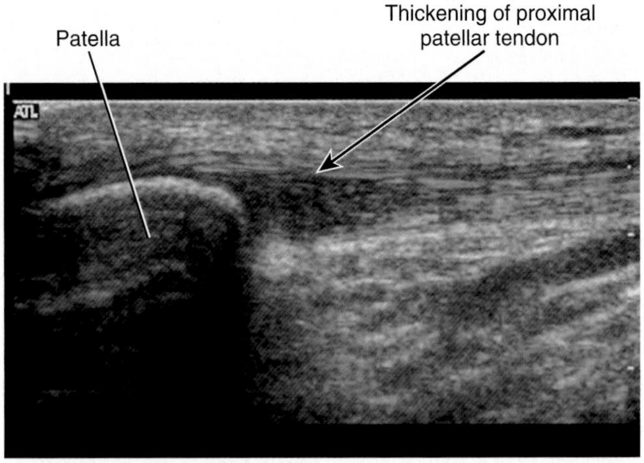
Patella
Thickening of proximal patellar tendon

Figure 12-2 Ultrasound examination demonstrates thickening of the proximal patellar tendon representing focal tendinosis.

postsurgical change from recurrent meniscal tears, but contrast can also be helpful in grading osteochondral lesions and in detecting intra-articular bodies. Intravenous gadolinium may be helpful in selected cases in differentiating solid from cystic lesions and in evaluating soft tissue masses and suspected infection.

Imaging protocols vary widely, depending on the capabilities of the magnet and the preferences of the imager. The standard protocol typically includes a short echo time (TE) sequence (T1 or proton density) in the sagittal and coronal imaging planes. These images are best suited for detecting meniscal pathology. A T2-weighted sequence with some type of fat saturation is typically performed in the axial, sagittal, and coronal imaging planes; however, many imaging centers have substituted proton density fat-saturated images for some of these T2-weighted sequences. High-field-strength magnets most commonly use frequency-selective fat saturation, whereas low-field systems often use short tau inversion recovery (STIR) sequence imaging to achieve fat saturation. Fat saturation increases the conspicuity of soft tissue and osseous injuries by allowing improved detection of water at the site of injury. Of the above imaging sequences, proton density or T2-weighted images with fat saturation are best suited for the evaluation of the articular cartilage. However, gradient-echo (GRE) imaging is occasionally used for this purpose as well.

LIGAMENTS

Cruciate Ligaments

Anterior Cruciate Ligament

The anterior cruciate ligament (ACL) is an intra-articular, extrasynovial structure that is lined by its own synovial sheath separating it from the joint

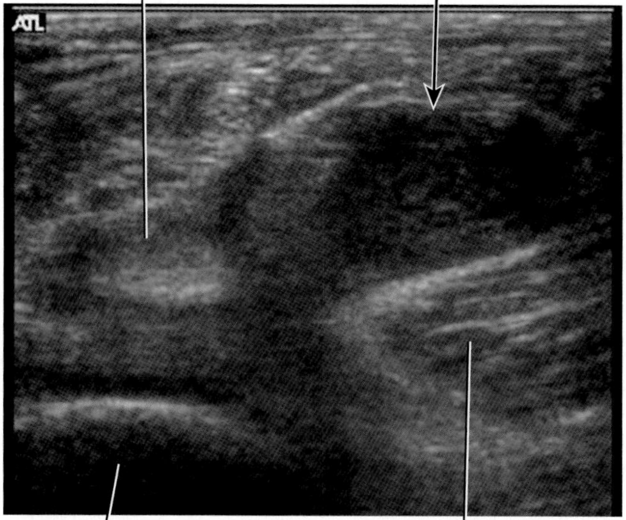
Semimembranosus tendon
Complex fluid collection at the posteromedial knee
ATL
Femoral condyle
Medial head of gastrocnemius muscle

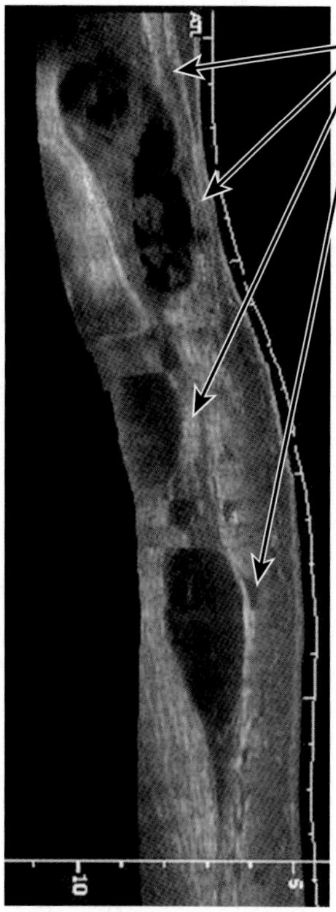
Extended field-of-view image of the calf shows extension of the cyst inferiorly with surrounding fluid representing rupture
ATL
10
5

Figure 12-3 Ultrasound appearance of a large Baker's cyst with rupture; characteristic location between the medial head of the gastrocnemius and semimembranosus and communication with the joint confirm the diagnosis of a Baker's cyst despite internal complexity (which in this case represents synovial proliferation).

space. It is composed of two discrete bundles—the larger posterolateral bundle and the smaller anteromedial bundle—named for their insertion sites on the tibia. The ACL arises proximally from the intercondylar notch of the lateral femoral condyle and inserts distally on the tibial plateau adjacent to the anterior tibial spine. The ACL broadens at both attachment sites to a thickness approximately three times the cross-sectional diameter of the midsubstance of the ligament. The ACL receives its blood supply via a periligamentous plexus contained within the synovial lining of the ligament. Disruption of the periligamentous plexus is primarily responsible for the hemarthrosis that occurs with acute ACL disruption.

The ACL provides the primary restraint to anterior tibial translation and also provides secondary stabilization with regard to rotational forces and varus or valgus stresses applied to the knee. This ligament is commonly injured, and in some series ACL injuries account for nearly half of all ligamentous injuries of the knee. Several mechanisms of injury can lead to disruption of the ACL, but it is most frequently torn as the result of a low-energy noncontact injury during a sporting event. The injury often occurs as the result of internal rotation of the femur against a fixed tibia with the foot planted, as in a sudden deceleration and rotation maneuver. Other mechanisms that can lead to ACL disruption are valgus stress, hyperextension, and direct contact injuries. In the hands of an experienced clinician, disruption of the ACL can be accurately diagnosed on the basis of physical examination in over 95% of patients.

The Lachman test is used clinically to evaluate the status of the ACL. With the patient in the supine position, the test is performed by flexing the knee 20 to 30 degrees and then applying anterior force to the proximal tibia while the femur is stabilized with the opposite hand. The extent of translation of the proximal tibia along with the firmness of the "end point" determines the status of the ACL. Anterior translation of the tibia combined with the lack of a firm end point is the hallmark of a disrupted ACL. As an adjunct to the Lachman test, a variety of devices known as arthrometers (most commonly the KT1000)

BOX 12-1 ROLE OF MRI IN THE EVALUATION OF ANTERIOR CRUCIATE LIGAMENT (ACL) INJURY

Confirm clinical suspicion of ACL injury
Further define extent of ACL injury
- Differentiate partial- from full-thickness tear
- Define location of tear: Midsubstance, femoral avulsion, tibial avulsion

Detect associated abnormalities
- Meniscal tears
- Articular cartilage/osseous abnormalities
- Other ligamentous injuries: Tibial collateral ligament, posteromedial corner, posterolateral corner

can provide an objective measurement of the amount of anterior tibial translation. The role of MRI therefore is to confirm the presence of a suspected ACL injury, to differentiate partial from complete tear, to further define the extent and location of injury as a guide to surgical planning, and finally to detect the presence of associated injuries, including meniscal pathology, articular cartilage injury, and other ligamentous injuries (Box 12-1).

Normal MR Appearance of the ACL The primary evaluation of the ACL is routinely performed using T2-weighted sagittal images. The ACL originates on the intercondylar notch cortex of the lateral femoral condyle and traverses the intercondylar notch to insert onto the tibial plateau. The anteromedial bundle inserts onto the medial tibial spine, whereas the posterolateral bundle inserts between the spines. The proximal ACL demonstrates homogeneous low signal intensity within the substance of the ligament, whereas distally the ligament takes on a more striated appearance with fat and synovium interspersed between the anteromedial and posterolateral bundles as they fan out near their attachment to the tibial plateau. This appearance should not be misinterpreted as a tear (Fig. 12-4A). With the knee in full extension, the course of the normal ligament is usually straight but may demonstrate minimal posterior bowing. With the knee in full extension, the ACL should parallel but not touch the roof of the intercondylar notch (Blumensaat's line). Visualization of both bundles from their origin to insertion indicates an intact ligament.

During evaluation of the ACL in the sagittal imaging plane, partial volume averaging of the proximal fibers of the ACL with the adjacent lateral femoral condyle often limits evaluation of the femoral attachment. The proximal attachment site of the ACL is a common location for injury, and routine evaluation of the ACL should *always* include assessment of the femoral attachment site on both the axial and coronal images. A hurried evaluation of the ACL using only the sagittal imaging plane will undoubtedly result in the occasional embarrassment of a missed proximal ACL tear that is readily apparent on both the coronal and axial imaging planes. Axial images are especially helpful in the evaluation of the femoral attachment site (Fig. 12-4B), whereas the coronal images are complementary in the evaluation of both the femoral and tibial attachments of the ACL (Fig. 12-4C). During our early experience with MRI of the knee, it was often stated that oblique or "tilted" sagittal images were necessary to optimize evaluation of the ACL. However, the proper use of axial and coronal images provides for an adequate evaluation of the ACL, and oblique images are not necessary.

Signs of ACL Disruption Several radiographic signs correlate highly with disruption of the ACL. First, the *deep lateral femoral sulcus sign,* best depicted on lateral radiographs of the knee, is defined as deepening (more than 2 mm) and irregularity of the lateral femoral sulcus. Next, the *Segond fracture* represents a lateral capsular avulsion injury resulting in a small cortical avulsion fracture fragment that arises from the lateral tibial plateau. Avulsion fragments near the proximal or distal attachment of the ACL may also indicate an ACL injury. Other less specific radiographic signs include a large joint effusion following acute trauma and cortical irregularity or fracture of the posterior lip of the lateral tibial plateau.

Direct MRI Signs of ACL Disruption For detection of ACL disruption, MRI is more than 95% sensitive with an overall accuracy ranging between 90% and 95%. There are several direct signs of injury that are very helpful in the evaluation of the ACL (Box 12-2). The most important sign is complete disruption or discontinuity of the fibers. In the acute injury, disruption of the ACL is often associated with thickening, hemorrhage, edema, and distortion of the adjacent fibers. Complete disruption most often occurs in the middle of the ACL and often leads to an abnormal slope (Fig. 12-5A) or posterior bowing of the distal fibers. The proximal fibers appear to "dangle" from the femoral notch while the distal fibers "droop" inferiorly and no longer parallel Blumensaat's line.

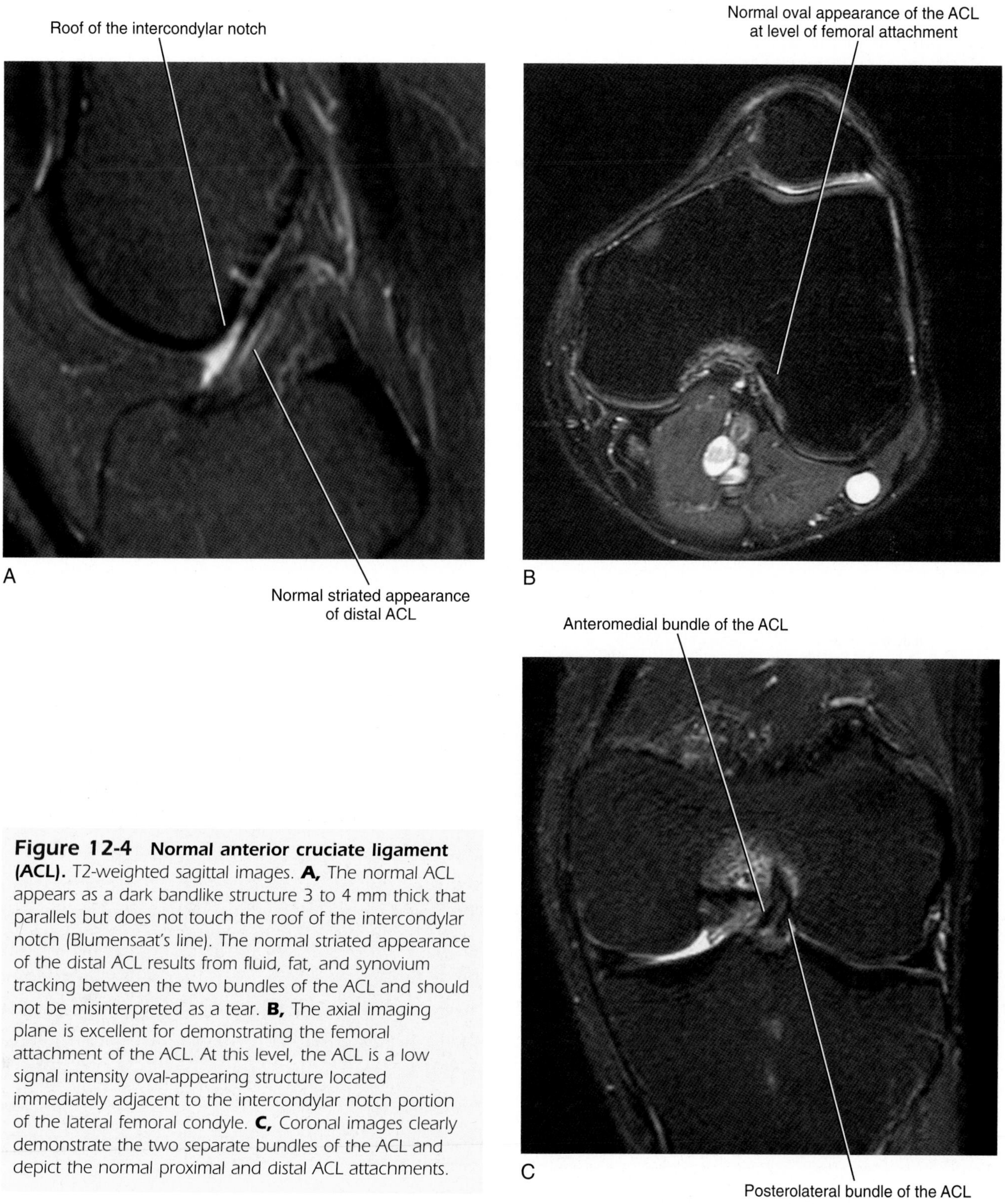
Roof of the intercondylar notch
A
Normal striated appearance of distal ACL
Normal oval appearance of the ACL at level of femoral attachment
B
Anteromedial bundle of the ACL
C
Posterolateral bundle of the ACL

Figure 12-4 Normal anterior cruciate ligament (ACL). T2-weighted sagittal images. **A,** The normal ACL appears as a dark bandlike structure 3 to 4 mm thick that parallels but does not touch the roof of the intercondylar notch (Blumensaat's line). The normal striated appearance of the distal ACL results from fluid, fat, and synovium tracking between the two bundles of the ACL and should not be misinterpreted as a tear. **B,** The axial imaging plane is excellent for demonstrating the femoral attachment of the ACL. At this level, the ACL is a low signal intensity oval-appearing structure located immediately adjacent to the intercondylar notch portion of the lateral femoral condyle. **C,** Coronal images clearly demonstrate the two separate bundles of the ACL and depict the normal proximal and distal ACL attachments.

A complete evaluation of the ACL must also include an assessment of the tibial and femoral attachment sites. The proximal ACL is the second most common site of injury, and a femoral avulsion injury may result in little or no morphologic change in the appearance of the ACL with the exception of the droop. Fluid signal may be seen at the normal ACL attachment site on either axial or coronal images, and this is referred to as the *empty notch sign* (Fig. 12-5B).

Avulsion of the ACL at its distal attachment site usually results in a small osseous fragment that is best visualized on non–fat-saturated sagittal images (Fig. 12-6). The ACL may demonstrate normal morphology but often shows posterior bowing, so if one evaluates only the ACL and not the adjacent tibia, the avulsion fracture can easily be missed. In addition, tibial edema associated with an avulsion fracture is usually minimal, so one's eye is not drawn to this area when evaluating the osseous structures. It is therefore important to specifically evaluate the osseous attachment of the ACL to exclude a tibial avulsion injury. Tibial avulsion injuries of the ACL, though initially reported in adolescent patients, have more recently been described in adult skiers. It is important to accurately detect both femoral and tibial avulsion injuries and to describe the status of the adjacent ligament because these injuries can often be repaired with a direct primary reattachment of the

BOX 12-2 DIRECT MRI SIGNS OF ANTERIOR CRUCIATE LIGAMENT (ACL) DISRUPTION

Discontinuity of fibers
Abnormal slope of ACL: "Dangle" and the "droop"
Nonvisualization of fibers on both the sagittal and coronal images: Chronic injury
Avulsion of the anterior tibial spine
"Empty notch" sign (avulsion of ACL from femoral attachment)

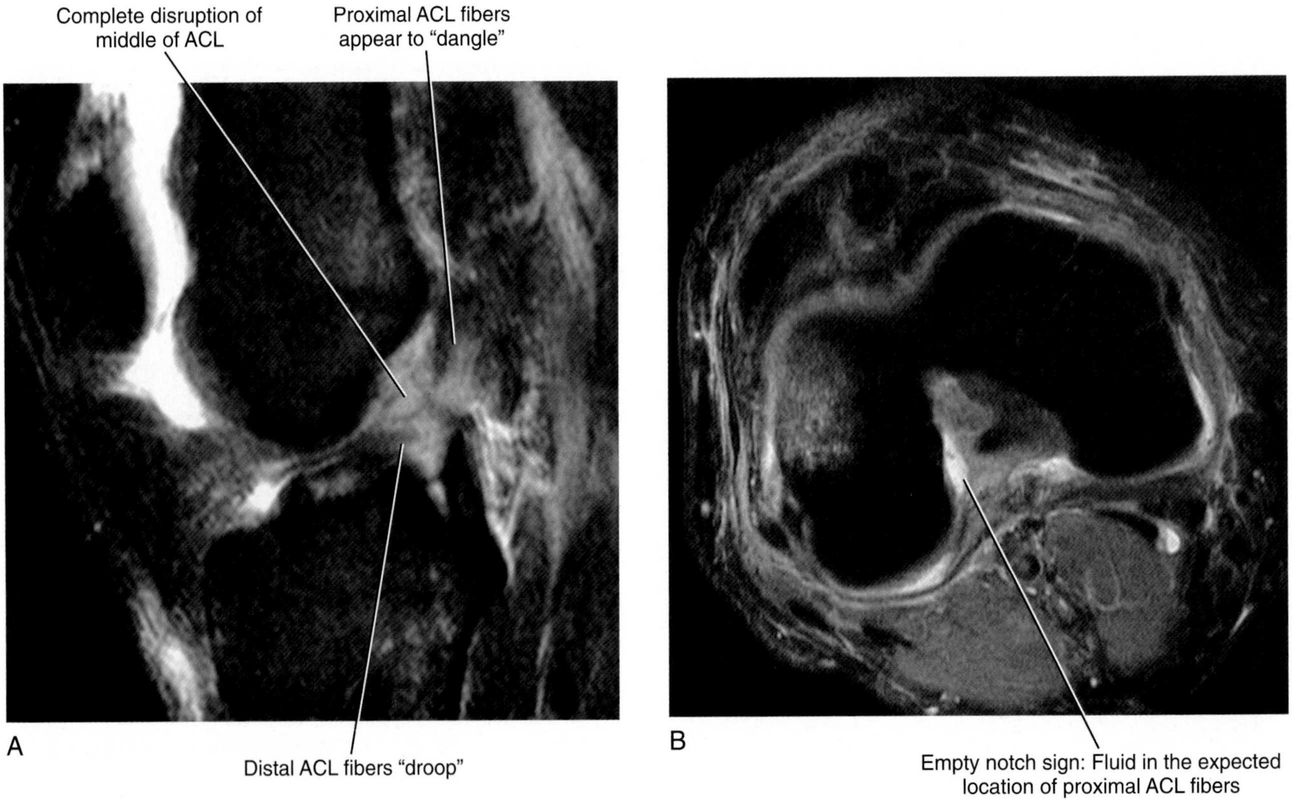
Complete disruption of middle of ACL
Proximal ACL fibers appear to "dangle"
A
Distal ACL fibers "droop"
B
Empty notch sign: Fluid in the expected location of proximal ACL fibers

Figure 12-5 Direct signs of anterior cruciate ligament (ACL) disruption. A, Sagittal T2-weighted image demonstrates complete disruption and discontinuity of the middle of the ACL. **B,** Axial T2-weighted image demonstrates the "empty notch" sign with fluid signal present in the expected location of the proximal ACL. Axial images can be very helpful in confirming the presence of a tear of the proximal ACL.

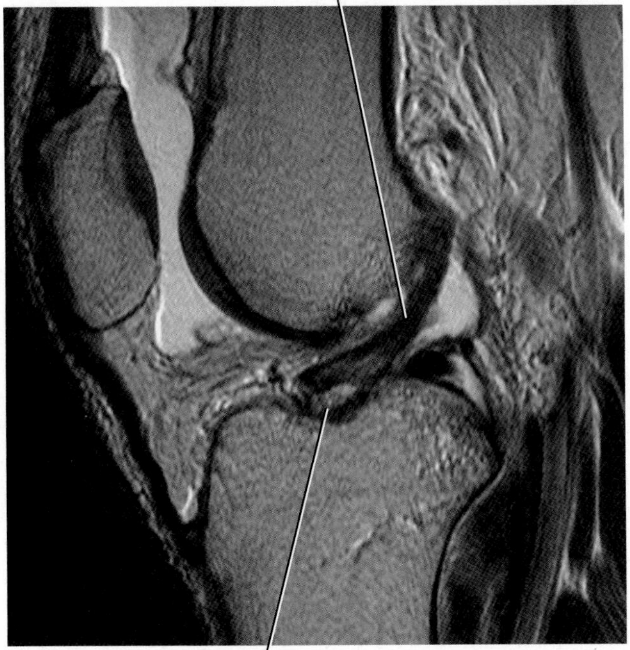
Posterior bowing
of an intact ACL
Tibial avulsion injury at
distal ACL attachment site

Figure 12-6 Tibial avulsion injury of the anterior cruciate ligament (ACL). Sagittal proton T2-weighted image demonstrates an intact ACL ligament but with abnormal posterior bowing. An avulsion fracture is noted at the tibial attachment of the ACL. It is important to distinguish this type of ACL injury from a midsubstance tear because an avulsion fracture may be amenable to direct repair by reattachment of the fracture fragment. The tibial avulsion fracture can be easily overlooked, but abnormal posterior bowing of the ACL, which is clearly evident on the sagittal images, should alert the reader that a problem exists with the ACL, and further evaluation will reveal the avulsion fracture.

ligament proximally or by reattachment of the bone fragment distally rather than necessitating a graft reconstruction, as required with midsubstance tears.

Indirect MRI Signs of ACL Disruption In most instances, the direct MRI signs of ACL disruption are conclusive. However, occasionally the status of the ACL is equivocal on the basis of these direct MRI signs. This is more likely to be true if the images are suboptimal because of patient motion or if the images are obtained on a low field strength magnet or with suboptimal technique. Also, it is occasionally difficult to differentiate a partial-thickness tear or sprain from a complete ACL disruption. In these instances, indirect signs can be especially helpful and can increase the level of confidence in diagnosing ACL disruption (Table 12-1). Most indirect MRI signs are related to osseous abnormalities that occur at the time of acute ACL injury.

Table 12-1 Indirect Signs of ACL Disruption

Specific for ACL disruption	Bone marrow edema sign: lateral femoral condyle and posterolateral tibial plateau (pivot shift injury) Deep notch sign: Lateral femoral sulcus (>2 mm deep) Segond fracture: Capsular avulsion lateral tibial plateau
Associated with but not specific for ACL disruption	Kissing contusions: Anterior tibia and femur (hyperextension injury) Anterior drawer sign: Anterior translation of tibia relative to femur (5 mm) Buckling of the PCL Acute hemarthrosis

ACL, anterior cruciate ligament; PCL, posterior cruciate ligament.

The pivot shift mechanism of injury is one of the most common mechanisms resulting in disruption of the ACL. It is a low-energy noncontact injury that commonly occurs in athletes and is particularly common among American football players and skiers. The injury typically occurs when a valgus load is applied to the knee while the knee is in various states of flexion. At the same time, internal rotation of the tibia or external rotation of the femur takes place while the foot is planted against the ground. This type of injury occurs during maneuvers such as rapid deceleration combined with simultaneous change of direction. These maneuvers load the ACL and can result in its rupture. Once the ACL tears, it allows the tibia to translate anteriorly relative to the femur, and during this first phase of translation the resulting impaction of the tibia against the femur gives rise to the bone bruise pattern described as the "pivot shift" marrow edema pattern (lateral femoral condyle and posterolateral tibial plateau) (Fig. 12-7). The exact location of the bone bruise on the lateral femoral condyle depends on the degree of flexion of the knee at the time of injury. Greater flexion results in a bone bruise located more posteriorly within the femoral

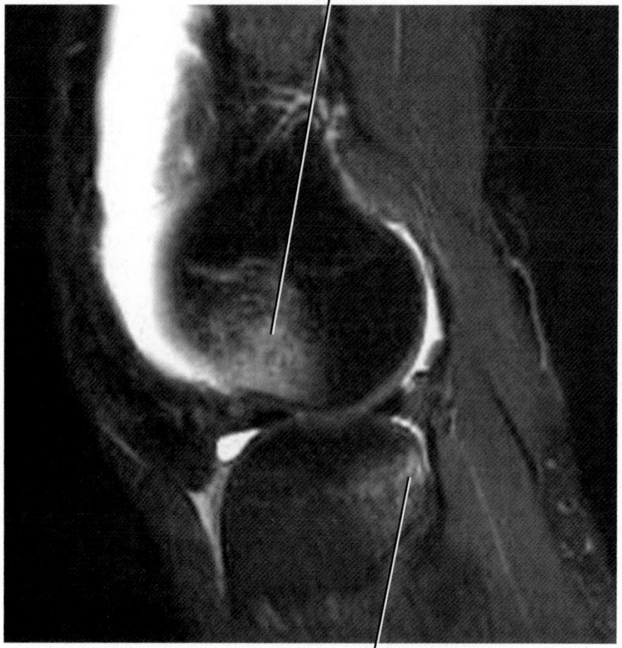
Bone contusion lateral femoral condyle
Bone contusion posterolateral tibial plateau

Figure 12-7 Pivot shift bone marrow edema pattern. Sagittal T2-weighted image demonstrates the classic bone marrow edema pattern involving the lateral femoral condyle and posterior lateral tibial plateau. This contusion pattern is very specific for anterior cruciate ligament disruption.

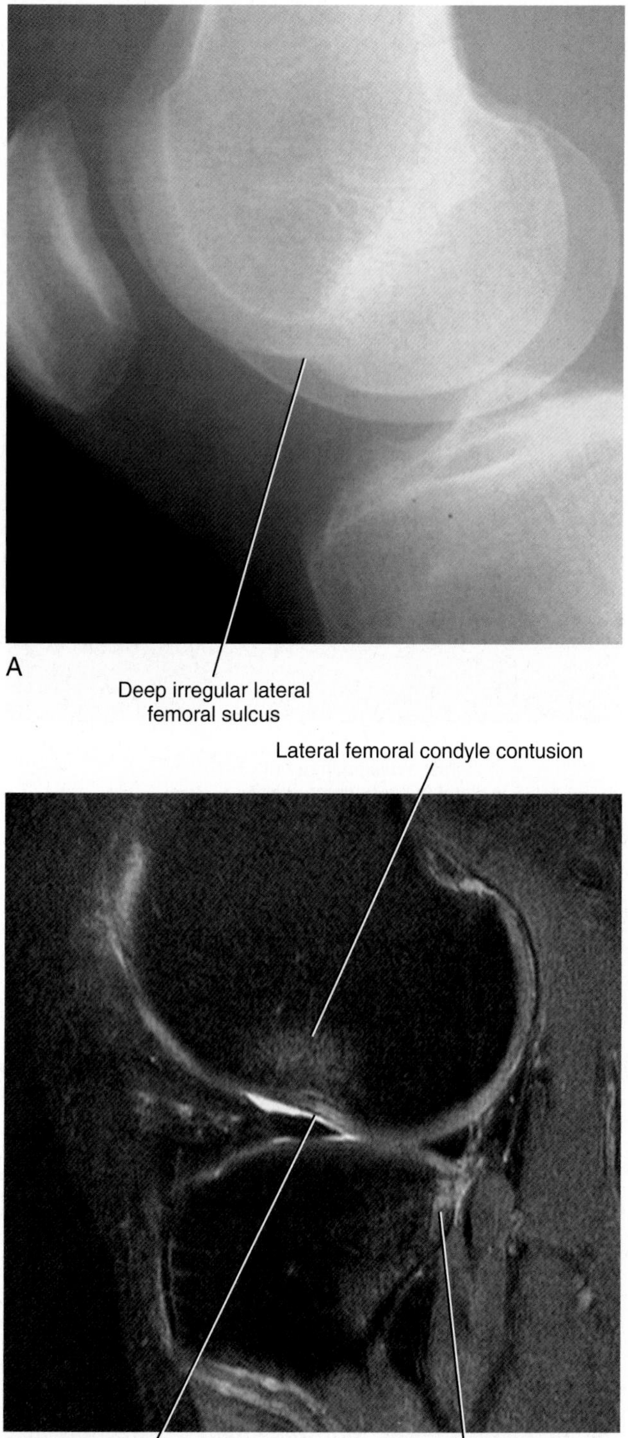
A
Deep irregular lateral femoral sulcus
Lateral femoral condyle contusion
B
Deepening and irregularity of lateral femoral sulcus
Posterior lateral tibial plateau contusion

Figure 12-8 Deep femoral sulcus sign. Lateral radiograph (**A**) and sagittal T2-weighted image with fat saturation (**B**) demonstrate deepening and irregularity of the lateral femoral sulcus. The pivot shift mechanism of injury is responsible for this impaction osteochondral injury of the lateral femoral, and the deep sulcus sign is a very specific secondary imaging sign indicating anterior cruciate ligament disruption.

condyle, whereas less flexion results in a more anteriorly located bone bruise.

Occasionally, a bone contusion is present only in the region of the posterolateral tibial plateau with no associated femoral condyle contusion. Isolated tibial plateau contusions associated with the pivot shift mechanism of injury occur more commonly in the older patient population but carry the same association with ACL injury as the combined femoral and tibial contusion pattern.

Excessive compressive forces at the time of impaction injury can also lead to an osteochondral impaction fracture of the lateral femoral condyle, referred to as the *deep notch* or *deep femoral sulcus sign* of the lateral femoral condyle (Fig. 12-8). This results in an irregular contour of the articular surface of the lateral femoral and deepening of the lateral femoral sulcus, often associated with underlying marrow edema. An impaction injury of the posterior lip of the lateral tibial plateau can also result in a depressed fracture of the posterior articular surface of the tibia. The same mechanism of rotational forces and anterior translation of the tibia can cause a capsular avulsion of the lateral tibial plateau referred to as the Segond fracture (Fig. 12-9). These three injuries all result from abnormal forces at the time of anterior tibial translation. In an adult, the tibia can only translate anteriorly if the ACL is torn. Therefore, these signs (i.e., bone contusions) are specific for ACL disruption and, when present, can be very helpful in confirming the presence of an ACL tear on MRI. There have been reports of the pivot shift bone contusion pattern occurring in children with an intact ACL, and this is thought to be possible because of the increased laxity of the ACL during childhood, which allows anterior translation of the tibia in the face of an intact ACL.

Another bone bruise pattern that has been associated with ACL disruption is the *kissing contusion pattern* (Fig. 12-10). This pattern of injury results from impaction of the anterior tibia against the anterior femur and occurs during a hyperextension injury and is less specific for ACL disruption. It can result in an isolated tear of either the ACL or posterior cruciate ligament (PCL) or a combination injury involving both ligaments. Hyperextension of the knee can also result in extensive soft tissue injury of the posterior medial or lateral capsular structures as well as injury to the posterior neurovascular structures. A combination ACL and PCL injury may indicate previous dislocation or severe hyperextension injury, and the posterior vascular structures should be closely evaluated for evidence of injury. Other less specific signs associated with ACL injury include the anterior drawer sign, buckling of the PCL, and acute hemarthrosis.

Detection of a chronic ACL disruption on MRI is more difficult because the ACL fibers lack the typical edema and thickening that is seen after an acute injury. In addition, most of the indirect signs that are present at the time of acute injury are absent in chronic tears. As a result, MRI is slightly less accurate in the detection of a chronic ACL disruption. Nonvisualization of the ACL in both the sagittal and coronal imaging planes in the absence of edema is a sign of chronic ACL disruption. More commonly, residual fibers are present but demonstrate abnormal morphology (thinning and attenuation) or an abnormal posterior slope. Occasionally, the proximal fibers of the torn ACL scar to the PCL and maintain a relatively normal slope or demonstrate only subtle

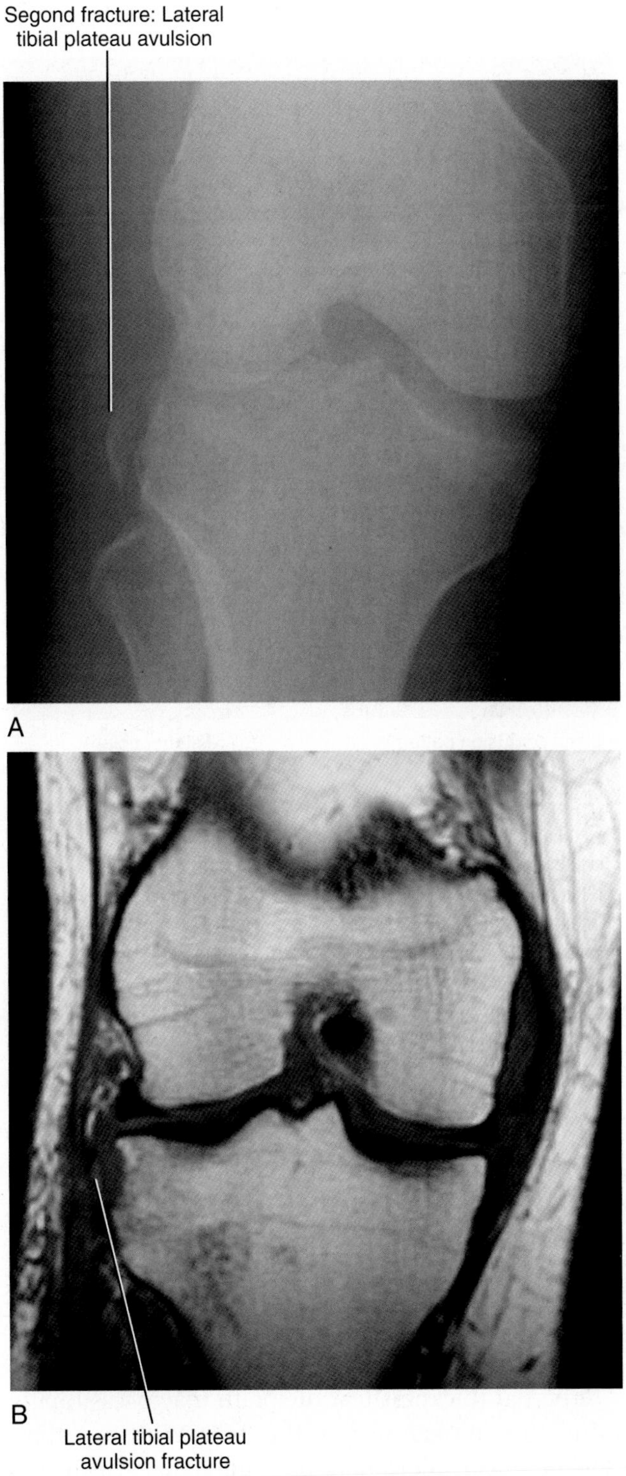
Segond fracture: Lateral tibial plateau avulsion
A
B
Lateral tibial plateau avulsion fracture

Figure 12-9 Segond fracture. Frontal radiograph (**A**) and coronal T1-weighted image (**B**) demonstrate a small cortical avulsion fracture of the lateral tibial plateau resulting from avulsion of the lateral capsule structures. This sign is specific for anterior cruciate ligament disruption.

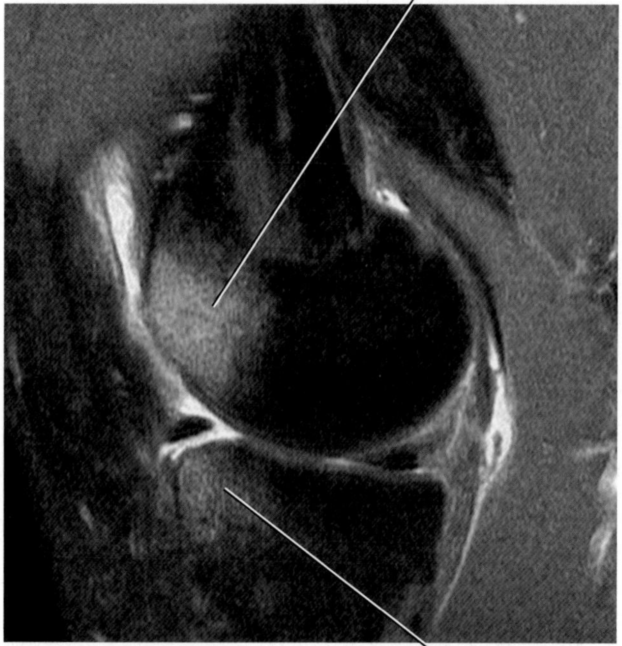
Anterior femoral condyle contusion
Kissing contusion pattern
Anterior tibial plateau contusion

Figure 12-10 Hyperextension marrow edema pattern. Sagittal T2-weighted sagittal image demonstrates the kissing contusion pattern with bone bruises located within the anterior femoral condyle and the anterior tibial plateau. This contusion pattern is less specific for anterior cruciate ligament (ACL) injury and may be associated with injuries of either the ACL or the posterior cruciate ligament.

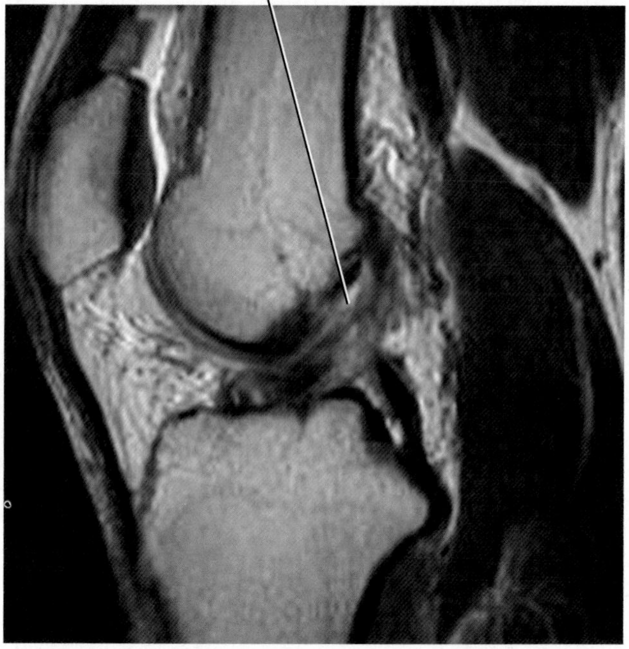
Partial-thickness ACL tear
A

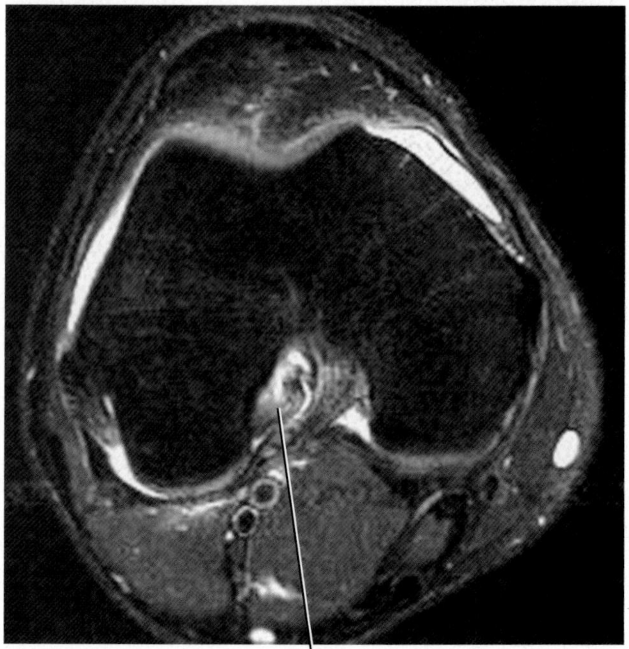
B
Thickened edematous ACL at femoral attachment site representing a partial-thickness tear

Figure 12-11 Partial-thickness anterior cruciate ligament (ACL) tear. Sagittal T2-weighted (**A**) and axial (**B**) images demonstrate a partial-thickness tear of the proximal ACL. High signal and thickening of the proximal fibers of the ACL are seen. However, some fibers do remain intact, and on the basis of the clinical exam the patient had a competent ACL.

posterior bowing. In these instances, the empty notch sign may be helpful in detecting a chronic proximal disruption (see Fig. 12-5B). Other MRI findings that may indicate a chronic ACL disruption include the posterior drawer sign and an old deepened lateral femoral sulcus with no underlying marrow edema.

A partial-thickness tear or sprain may occasionally mimic a complete tear of the ACL. With a partial-thickness tear, there may be fluid signal within the fibers of the ACL, but some fibers remain intact throughout the normal course of the ligament. It is also possible to tear a single bundle of the ACL and see the second bundle intact. If this occurs proximally, the femoral attachment of the ACL demonstrates a round rather than oval appearance on the axial images since one of the bundles will be absent (Fig. 12-11). Typically with a sprain or partial-thickness tear, the secondary signs of injury are absent.

When a partial-thickness tear of the ACL is seen on MRI, it is important to alert the clinician so that correlation can be made with the clinical examination regarding anterior translation of the tibia and the presence or lack of a solid end point. Depending on the extent of the tear, the intact fibers of a partially disrupted ACL may or may not provide functional stability. The presence of the anterior drawer sign on MRI suggests instability associated with a partial-thickness tear of the ACL.

Posterior Cruciate Ligament

The posterior cruciate ligament (PCL) like the ACL is an intra-articular, extrasynovial structure that has its own synovial sheath. It arises along the posterior aspect of the medial femoral condyle and inserts onto the posterior slanted aspect of the tibial plateau. It is roughly twice the diameter of the ACL, but recent studies have shown that it demonstrates more strength only marginally. The PCL comprises three components, with the nomenclature for each referring to its femoral attachment site followed by its tibial attachment site. The anterolateral bundle is the largest and strongest and is taut with the knee in flexion. The smaller posteromedial bundle is taut with the knee in extension. Finally, the meniscofemoral ligaments (Humphry and Wrisberg) arise from the posterior horn of the lateral meniscus and insert onto the posterior aspect of the medial femoral condyle. The meniscofemoral ligaments have been shown to have greater strength than the posteromedial bundle; however, their role in stability of the knee has yet to be precisely defined. Like the ACL, the PCL receives its blood supply from a periligamentous plexus, which is predominantly fed by the middle genicular artery with secondary contributions from the inferior genicular arteries.

The PCL provides the primary restraint to posterior translation of the tibia and is a secondary stabilizer with regard to external rotation of the tibia. It is injured much less commonly than the ACL, and, when injured, the PCL is more likely to suffer a partial-thickness tear. Injuries typically occur when the proximal tibia is forced in a posterior direction relative to the femur. The most common mechanism of injury is referred to as the *dashboard injury*. This injury results in posterior translation of the proximal tibia while the knee is in a flexed position and is so named because it often occurs during a motor vehicle accident as the knee strikes against the dashboard. The dashboard injury can also occur during a fall if the person lands on a flexed knee, thus driving the proximal tibia in a posterior direction. This mechanism commonly occurs during sporting events. A history that is frequently reported for athletes with disruption of the PCL is that of a football player falling on a flexed knee while ending up at the bottom of a pile. Posterior translation of the tibia can also occur while the knee is in full extension, as in a hyperextension injury. MRI plays a crucial role in evaluation of the PCL because unlike in the ACL, injuries of the PCL can be difficult to diagnose on the basis of physical examination, and such injuries frequently go unrecognized at the time of initial clinical evaluation. MRI also plays a role in detecting associated injuries, which can include injuries of the ACL, medial collateral ligament, and menisci.

Normal MRI Appearance of the PCL The PCL is best evaluated on T2-weighted sagittal images of the knee, and although coronal and axial images are complementary, they are rarely necessary to establish the diagnosis of a PCL injury. The PCL is usually visualized in its entirety on one or, at most, two consecutive sagittal images. The PCL is roughly two times the thickness of the ACL, and unlike the ACL typically appears uniformly dark on all pulse sequences. Occasionally, the separate PCL bundles can be seen on MR imaging, giving the PCL a striated appearance, or, on the other hand, intrasubstance degeneration results in intrinsic signal alteration in an intact PCL. With the knee in full extension, the PCL demonstrates an arcuate or curved appearance (Fig. 12-12). The meniscofemoral component of the PCL is best visualized on sagittal or coronal images and can be seen as a small bandlike structure coursing either anterior (Humphry) or posterior (Wrisberg) to the PCL and extending from the posterior horn of the lateral meniscus to attach on the inner aspect of the medial femoral condyle (Fig. 12-13).

Direct MRI Signs of PCL Disruption Most PCL injuries are partial-thickness tears or sprains that involve the posteromedial bundle. MR imaging demonstrates fluid signal partially traversing the PCL with an intact anterolateral bundle (Fig. 12-14A). Complete disruption of the PCL most frequently occurs in the middle of the ligament and in the acute setting demonstrates high T2-weighted signal completely traversing the

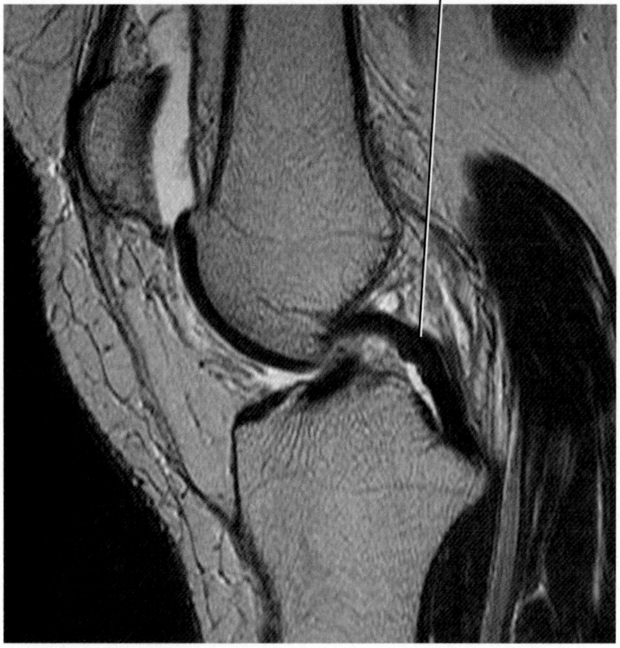
Normal PCL: Arcuate in appearance and dark on all pulse sequences

Figure 12-12 Normal posterior cruciate ligament (PCL). Sagittal T2-weighted image demonstrates the normal MRI appearance of the PCL. It is a thick, uniformly dark bandlike structure that has a curved appearance when the knee is imaged in full extension. It extends from the inner aspect of the medial femoral condyle to the posterior slanted portion of the tibia.

ligament with discontinuity of the fibers (Fig. 12-14B; Table 12-2). Avulsion injuries of the PCL can occur at either the femoral or the tibial attachment site, but most frequently on the tibial side. They are often associated with a large nondisplaced fracture fragment of the posterior tibial plateau and adjacent marrow edema (Fig. 12-14C). An avulsion injury of the PCL at the femoral attachment site has been referred to as a *peel-off injury* and sometimes results in a small fleck of bone being pulled off the femur. Avulsion injuries are important to differentiate from midsubstance tears because they are treated differently. Large tibial avulsion fractures are often treated conservatively if the fracture fragment is not significantly displaced, or, if necessary, the fracture fragment can be reduced and fixed. Primary repair of the PCL may be possible following a peel-off injury at the femoral attachment site. Midsubstance tears require reconstruction with a graft since attempted primary repairs of these tears are usually unsuccessful.

Table 12-2 Direct Signs of PCL Injury

Imaging Finding	PCL Injury
Discontinuity of fibers (fluid signal completely traversing fibers)	Complete tear: Most common in midsubstance
Fluid signal partially traversing ligament	Partial-thickness tear: Most commonly involves posteromedial bundle
Large fracture fragment with edema: PF or MRI	Avulsion of tibial attachment site
Tiny avulsion fragment: PF or MRI	Femoral peel-off injury
Absent PCL fibers or may scar down and appear intact on MRI	Chronic PCL disruption

MRI, magnetic resonance imaging; PCL, posterior cruciate ligament; PF, plain film radiography.

Treatment recommendations for PCL injuries continue to evolve. Whereas once it was very unusual to repair a torn PCL, today they are commonly repaired, especially if the person is in an active occupation such as professional athlethics or is in the military. It is also recommended that a torn PCL be repaired when combined with other injuries such as an ACL tear or with multiple other ligamentous injuries. It has been learned that an unstable PCL in these specific situations will result in premature osteoarthritis of the knee if left untreated.

Identification of a chronic PCL disruption on MRI can be challenging because the ligament often scars back down and may appear intact, even though the ligament is functionally incompetent. Secondary signs of PCL disruption, such as associated soft tissue and marrow edema, are often absent in the setting of a chronic PCL disruption.

Indirect MRI Signs of PCL Disruption As with ACL injuries, most secondary imaging signs associated with PCL injuries represent osseous abnormalities that occur at the time of injury (Table 12-3). The dashboard mechanism of injury can lead to a bone contusion pattern that is isolated to the anterior aspect of the proximal tibia (Fig. 12-15). This pattern of marrow edema has a high association with PCL injury, and it results from a direct impact of the bone against the dashboard or against the ground if secondary to a fall. The kissing contusion pattern (described previously in the section, Indirect MRI Signs of ACL Disruption) may also be seen in association with PCL injuries resulting from a

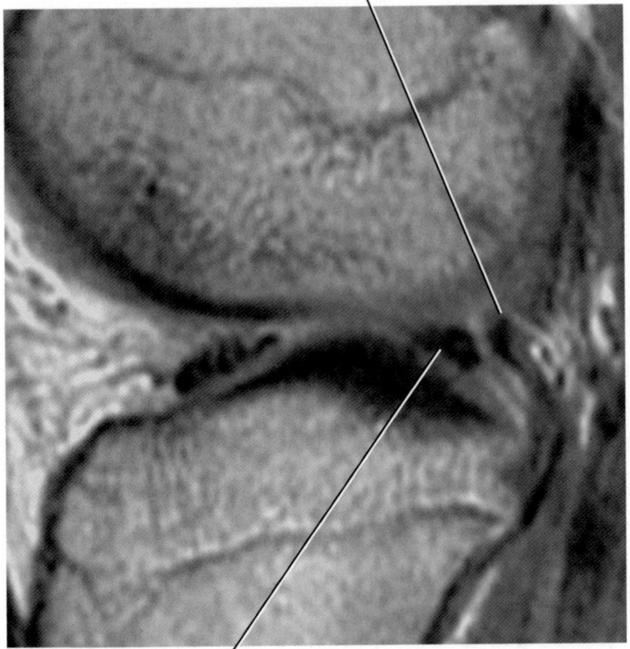
Meniscofemoral ligament just before its insertion on the lateral meniscus
A
Posterior horn of lateral meniscus

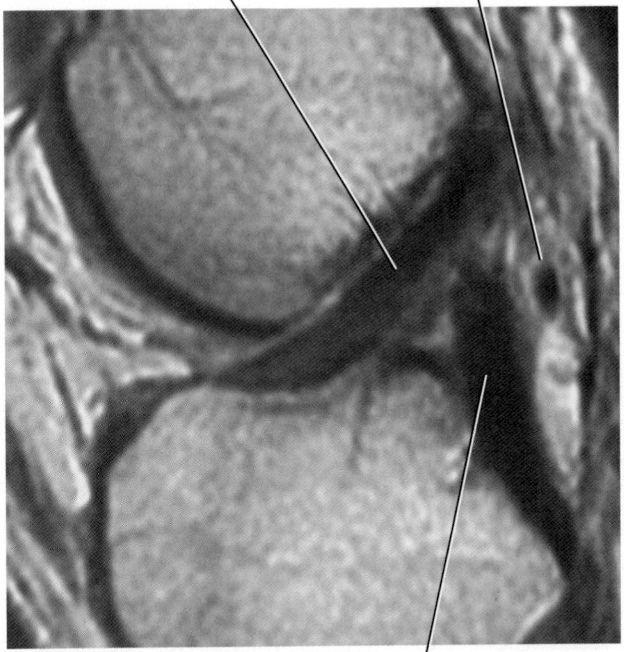
ACL
Meniscofemoral ligament
B
PCL

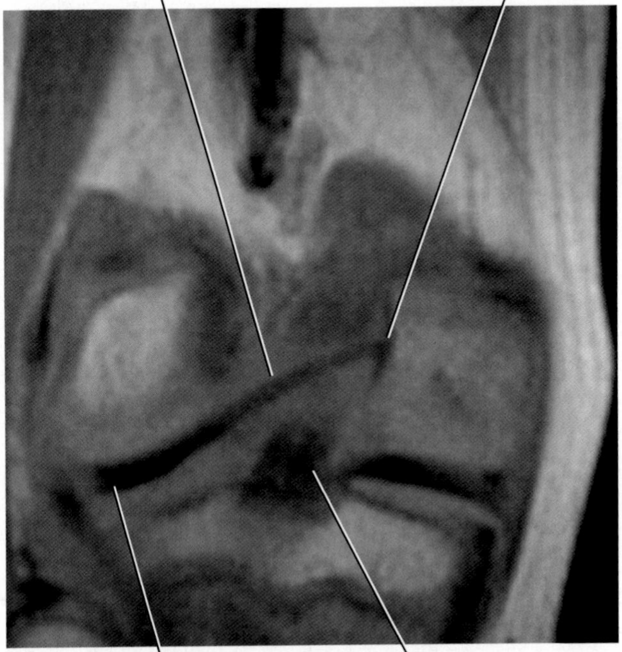
Meniscofemoral ligament
Femoral attachment
C
Posterior horn of lateral meniscus
PCL

Figure 12-13 Meniscofemoral portion of the posterior cruciate ligament (PCL) (meniscofemoral ligament). A, Sagittal T1-weighted image demonstrates the meniscofemoral ligament near its attachment to the posterior horn of the lateral meniscus. This meniscal attachment of the meniscofemoral ligament can mimic a meniscal tear. **B,** The meniscofemoral ligament of Wrisberg extending posterior to the PCL. **C,** The normal course of the meniscofemoral ligament as it extends from the posterior horn of the lateral meniscus to attach on the inner aspect of the medial femoral condyle. ACL, anterior cruciate ligament.

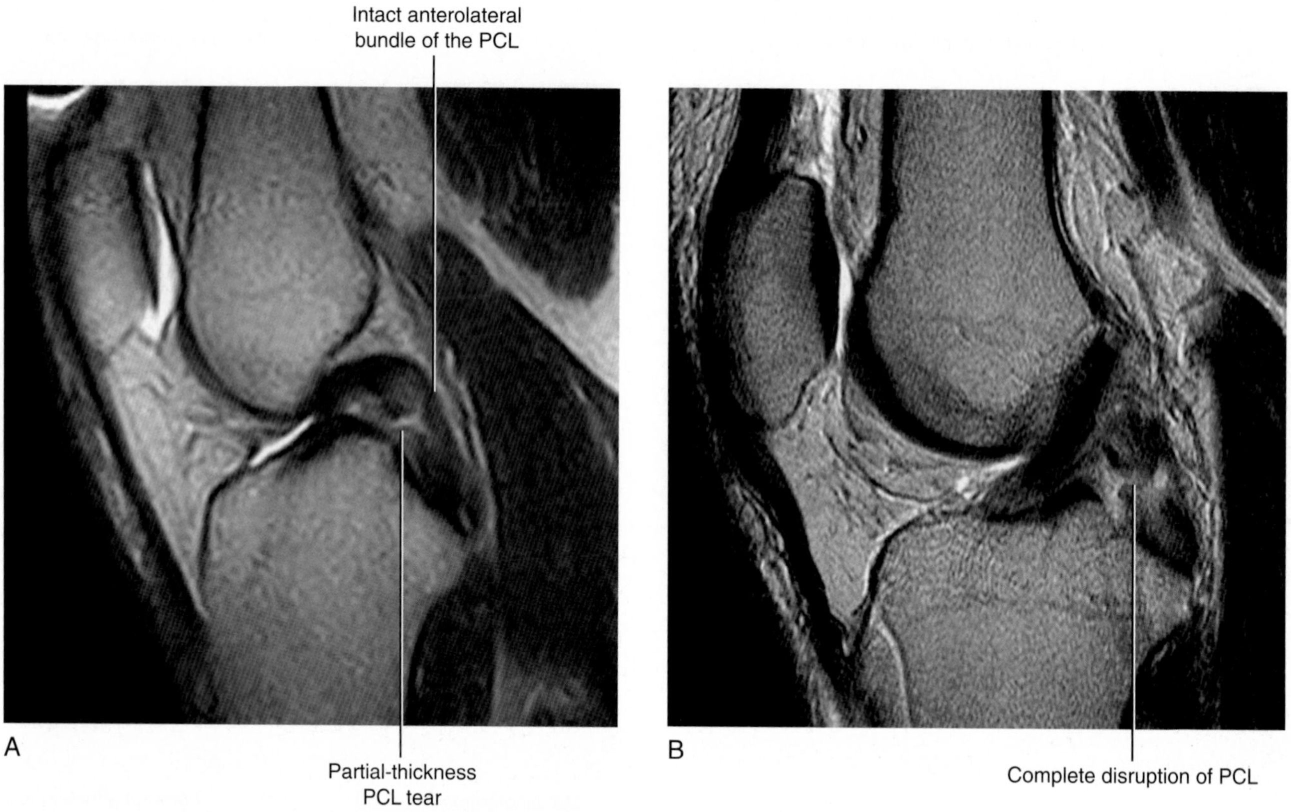
Intact anterolateral bundle of the PCL
A
Partial-thickness PCL tear
B
Complete disruption of PCL

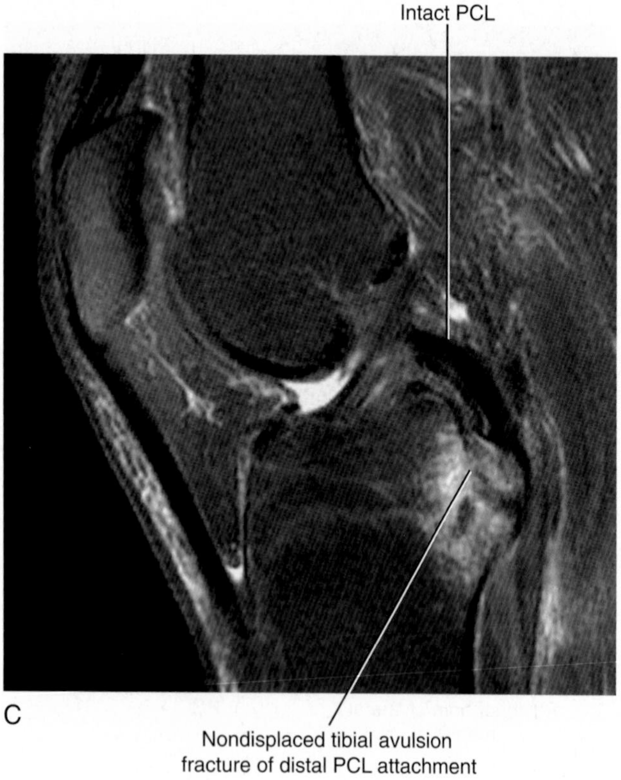
Intact PCL
C
Nondisplaced tibial avulsion fracture of distal PCL attachment

Figure 12-14 Spectrum of posterior cruciate ligament (PCL) injuries. A, Sagittal T2-weighted image demonstrates a partial-thickness tear of the midsubstance of the PCL with fluid signal extending only partially through the thickness of the ligament. **B,** Sagittal T2-weighted image demonstrates fluid signal intensity completely traversing the midsubstance of the PCL consistent with a full-thickness tear. **C,** Sagittal T2-weighted image with fat saturation shows a nondisplaced avulsion fracture of the PCL at its tibial insertion site with extensive surrounding marrow edema. Notice that the PCL demonstrates a normal MRI appearance.

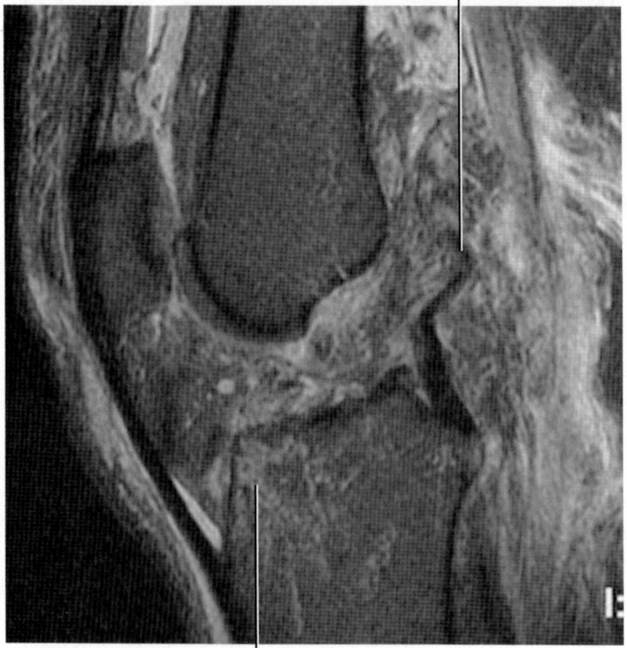
Disrupted PCL
Dashboard contusion pattern
anterior proximal tibia

Figure 12-15 Dashboard injury. Sagittal T2-weighted image demonstrates a bone contusion located within the anterior aspect of the proximal tibia and a complete disruption of the posterior cruciate ligament (PCL).

Table 12-3 Indirect MRI Signs of PCL Injury

Osseous Abnormality	Mechanism of Injury
Dashboard bone contusion pattern	Results from direct impaction injury to anterior aspect of the proximal tibia
Kissing bone contusions	Hyperextension injury
Fibular head avulsion fracture	Avulsion of conjoined tendon
Gerdy's tubercle avulsion	Avulsion of iliotibial band
Medial Segond fracture	Avulsion of medial capsular structures

hyperextension of the knee (see Fig. 12-10). Other osseous abnormalities that have been associated with PCL injury include avulsions of the tibial or femoral attachments of the PCL, often visible on radiographs and on MRI. Avulsion fractures of the fibular head, Gerdy's tubercle, and a medial capsular avulsion injury have also been described as potential secondary signs that can be associated with PCL injury.

Miscellaneous Abnormalities of the Cruciate Ligaments

Mucoid degeneration of the cruciate ligaments is a common finding in the older patient population with osteoarthritis but it can also occur in the younger population as isolated mucoid degeneration. Mucoid degeneration is often mistaken for disruption or a partial-thickness tear of the ACL or PCL. It is not associated with instability of the knee. Histologically, the cruciate ligaments demonstrate distortion of the collagen fibers, multifocal mucoid degeneration, and mutilocular fibrous-walled cysts. This entity appears to be on a continuum with cruciate ganglion cysts, which are described in further detail in the text that follows. On MRI, the ligaments demonstrate an ill-defined appearance with increased girth compared with the normal ligament (Fig. 12-16). There is typically intermediate signal intensity within the substance of the ligament on all pulse sequences. The fibers of the cruciate ligament are usually well visualized and run in the normal orientation but are splayed, revealing what has been described as a "celery stalk" appearance. Mucoid degeneration can also result in reactive marrow edema, erosion, or subchondral cyst formation of the adjacent tibia or femur. The key to differentiating mucoid degeneration from a cruciate tear is that the fibers of the ligament are continuous, demonstrate a normal orientation, and are splayed rather than disrupted. With mucoid degeneration, both bundles of the ACL can usually be identified, whereas with an old partial-thickness tear the bundles may be nonvisualized or indistinct.

As previously described, the cruciate ligaments are enveloped within a synovial fold; as a result, ganglia formation can occur on either the surface or within the substance of the ACL or PCL (Fig. 12-17). Cysts that arise within the substance of the ligament demonstrate an MR appearance similar to that of mucoid degeneration with increased girth of the ligament and splaying of the fibers. Intracruciate ganglia, however, demonstrate more sharply demarcated T2-weighted signal with characteristic cyst morphology. Cruciate ganglia that arise on the surface of the ligament are referred to as pericruciate ganglia and can become large and extend into various recesses about the knee. They can extend into Hoffa's fat pad anteriorly or dissect along the posterior horn of either the medial or lateral meniscus posteriorly. On occasion, they may even penetrate the joint capsule posteriorly or erode into adjacent bone.

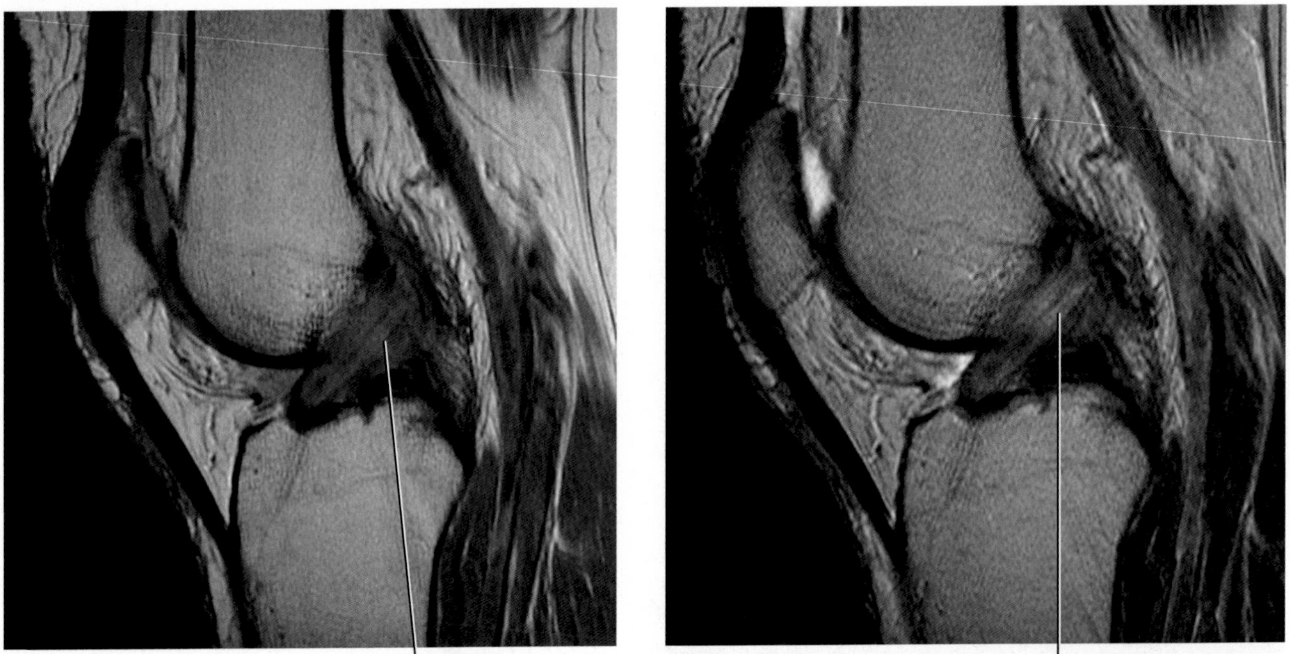
A
Mucoid degeneration of ACL fibers
B
Mucoid degeneration: Celery stalk appearance of ACL

Figure 12-16 Mucoid degeneration of the anterior cruciate ligament (ACL). Sagittal proton density (**A**) and T2-weighted (**B**) images demonstrate a thickened ACL with splaying of its fibers and intermediate signal abnormality described as a celery stalk appearance.

The ganglia are well defined, septated, oval, or lobular, and they follow water signal on all pulse sequences. Ganglia can be differentiated from fluid within a recess of the knee because there is typically a fluid collection separate from the rest of the joint fluid, and they can result in mass effect on the adjacent structures. Ganglia are often incidentally identified on MRI exams performed for other reasons. However, if they are large enough, they may cause symptoms of catching, locking, and pain. Ganglia arising within the substance of the ligament may mimic a tear, whereas those arising on the surface of the ligament may mimic a meniscal cyst. Pericruciate ganglia can be particularly difficult to distinguish from meniscal cysts arising from the anterior horn of the lateral meniscus and adjacent to the posterior horn of the medial meniscus. Clear depiction of a horizontal cleavage tear of the adjacent meniscus with extension of the tear into the cyst is diagnostic of a meniscal cyst rather than a cruciate ganglion. The absence of an adjacent meniscal tear would be more supportive of the diagnosis of a pericruciate ganglion.

MEDIAL SOFT TISSUES OF THE KNEE

Historically, anatomic descriptions of the medial soft tissue support structures of the knee have been oversimplified in MRI literature. Over the past few years, however, the orthopedic community has begun to gain a more thorough understanding of the role of several of the specific soft tissue structures of the medial aspect of the knee and to better understand the importance of their repair when attempting to maximize surgical outcomes after injury. No longer is it adequate for the radiologist to collectively refer to the anteromedial soft tissue support structures as the medial retinaculum or to collectively refer to the medial support structures of the knee as the medial collateral ligament. Increasingly, the surgeon wants to know the status of a specific soft tissue structure such as the medial patellofemoral ligament, the meniscotibial ligament, or the capsular arm of the semimembranosus tendon. The radiologist should possess a detailed knowledge of the anatomy of the

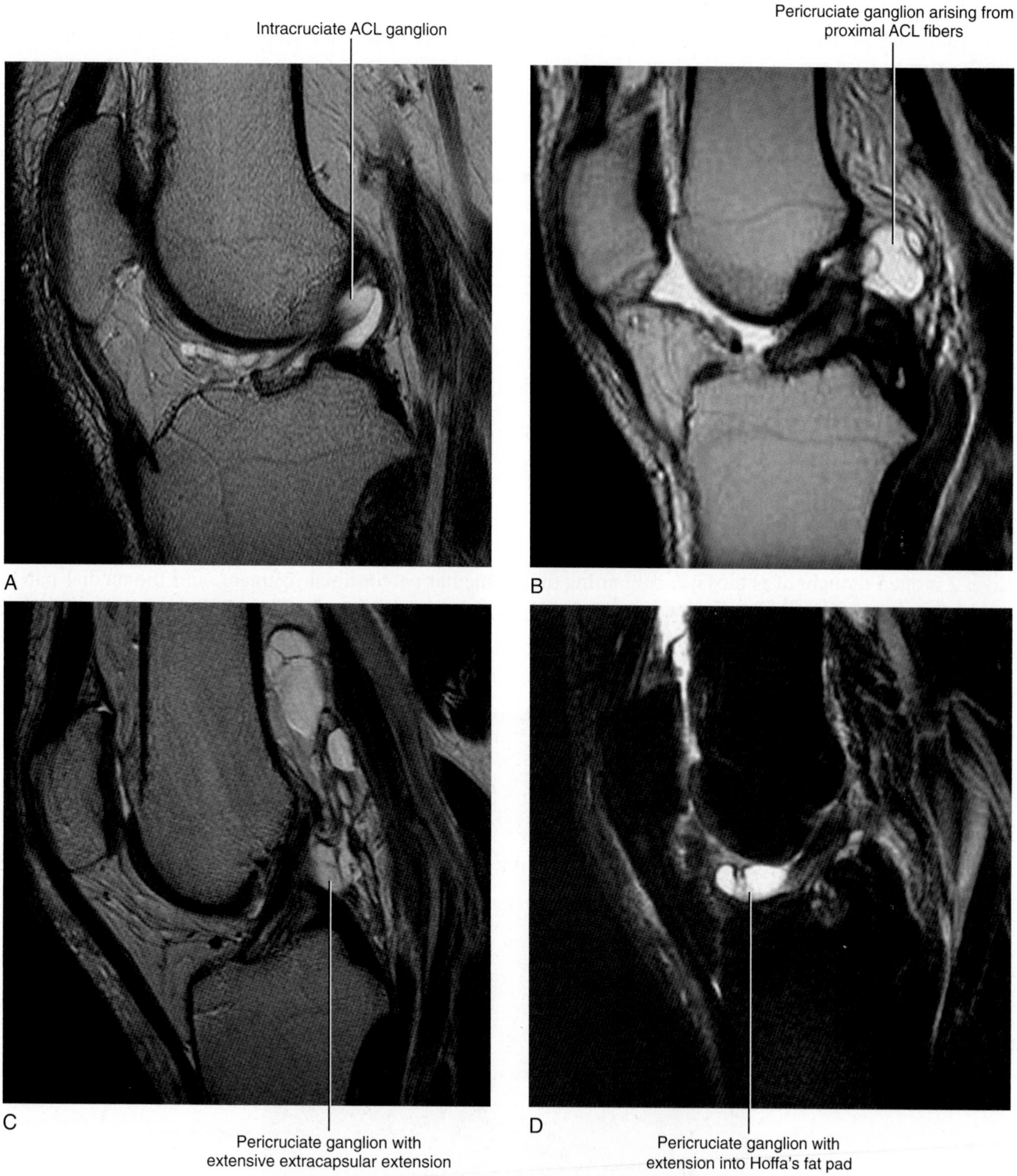
Intracruciate ACL ganglion
Pericruciate ganglion arising from proximal ACL fibers
A
B
C
D
Pericruciate ganglion with extensive extracapsular extension
Pericruciate ganglion with extension into Hoffa's fat pad

Figure 12-17 **Cruciate ganglia. A,** Sagittal T2-weighted image demonstrates a lobulated multiseptated cystic structure within the substance of the anterior cruciate ligament (ACL) consistent with an intracruciate ganglion. **B,** A pericruciate ganglion arising along the posterior margin of the ACL. **C,** A large pericruciate ganglion that has penetrated the posterior joint capsule and has dissected into the posterior soft tissues of the knee. **D,** A large pericruciate ganglion arising from the distal ACL fibers and dissecting into Hoffa's fat pad anteriorly.

medial soft tissues structures of the knee, have an understanding of the specific injury patterns that involve these structures, and finally should be able to recognize the MRI appearance of these specific injuries.

Medial Soft Tissue Anatomy

The medial soft tissues of the knee are divided into three layers according to their depth. The most superficial layer (layer 1) is composed of the deep fascia. This layer invests the sartorius posteriorly and then extends in an anterior direction superficial to the tibial collateral ligament. As it continues anteriorly, it is continuous with the fascia of the vastus medialis muscle and finally merges with the deeper layers to insert onto the medial aspect of the patella as the medial retinaculum. This superficial layer has little importance with regard to injury patterns and stability of the knee. Most of the important stabilizing structures are found in the deeper layers 2 and 3. Layer 2 is often thought of as the layer containing the superficial fibers of the tibial collateral ligament, and layer 3 comprises the joint capsule.

For the purposes of better understanding the anatomy of layers 2 and 3, it is helpful to divide the medial aspect of the knee into anterior, middle, and posterior thirds (Fig. 12-18). A thorough knowledge of the anatomy in each compartment allows the radiologist to accurately describe injuries that are currently of clinical importance to the orthopedic surgeon and it also builds a foundation for the radiologist to expand descriptions of injuries as surgical techniques evolve and additional structures become clinically and surgically relevant.

Anterior Third Anatomy

In the anterior aspect of the knee, layers 2 and 3 cannot be clearly differentiated because they fuse anteriorly to form the medial soft tissue restraint of the patella. The anterior medial soft tissue restraint of the patella is composed of four distinct structures. These include the medial patellofemoral ligament (MPFL), the medial parapatellar retinaculum, the medial patellotibial ligament, and the medial patellomeniscal ligament. The MPFL is the most important of these four structures regarding stabilization of

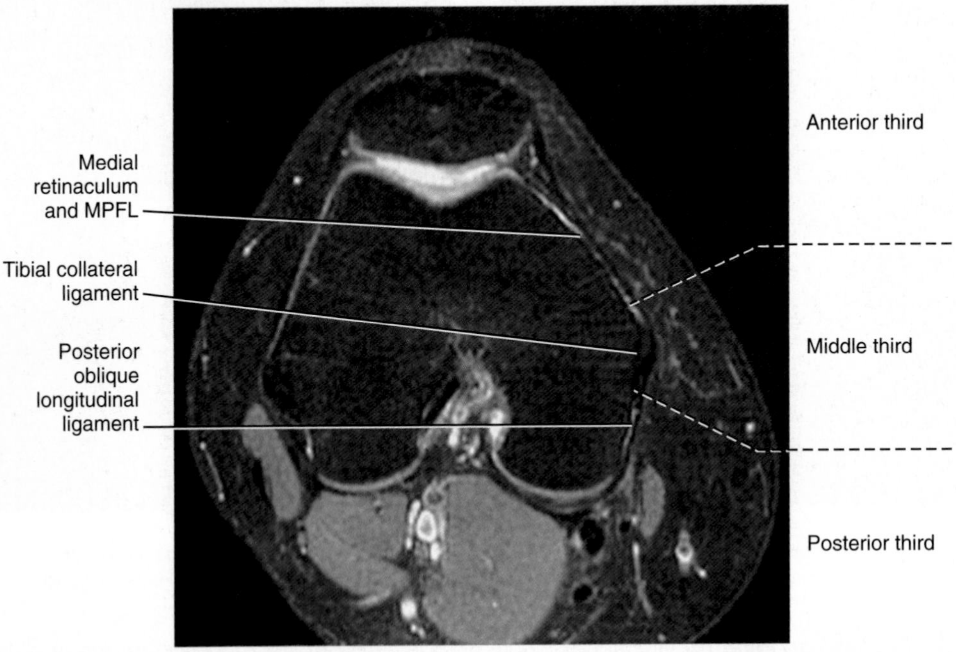
Medial retinaculum and MPFL
Tibial collateral ligament
Posterior oblique longitudinal ligament
Anterior third
Middle third
Posterior third

Figure 12-18 The medial soft tissue restraints of the knee. For ease of understanding the anatomy of the medial aspect of the knee, the knee can be divided into thirds from anterior to posterior. The soft tissue restraints in the anterior third of the knee include the medial patellofemoral ligament (MPFL), medial retinaculum, and medial patellotibial ligament. The tibial collateral ligament is located in the middle third of the knee. The posterior oblique longitudinal ligament is located in the posterior third of the medial aspect of the knee.

the patella. Although it varies in size and thickness, it remains constant in location. The MPFL originates on the adductor tubercle proximal to the origin of the superficial fibers of the medial collateral ligament and then extends distally to insert on the undersurface of the vastus medialis obliquus (VMO) muscle and on the medial aspect of the upper pole of the patella. The parapatellar or "medial" retinaculum originates as a condensation of the fascia and aponeurosis of the VMO muscle and inserts onto the middle third of the medial aspect of the patella. It allows the VMO muscle to insert directly onto the medial aspect of the patella, thereby allowing the VMO muscle to serve as an active stabilizer of the patella. The patellotibial ligament arises from the tibia near the distal attachments of the gracilis and semitendinosus tendons and then courses cephalad to insert onto the medial aspect of the lower pole of the patella. Finally, the patellomeniscal ligament lies deep to the patellotibial ligament running in a similar direction and plane but inserting onto the meniscus rather than the tibia. Some consider this to be a separate ligament, and others consider this structure to be a deep component of the patellotibial ligament.

Injury Patterns of the Anterior Third of the Medial Soft Tissue Structures (MPFL)

Why does any of this anatomy matter? I have always referred to these structures collectively as the medial retinaculum, and no one has ever challenged me. Is there a clinical reason to be more specific when describing these structures, and, if so, how can I differentiate them on MRI? The answer is yes. The MPFL has been shown to be the most important soft tissue stabilizer preventing lateral subluxation of the patella (Table 12-4). It provides most of the restraining force, whereas the other three structures provide minimal restraint toward the prevention of lateral patellar subluxation. Many orthopedic surgeons now repair a torn MPFL to minimize the rate of recurrence of patellar dislocation, whereas disruption of the other three structures does not routinely warrant surgical repair. It is therefore important to comment specifically on the integrity of the MPFL after transient dislocation of the patella and to distinguish between a tear of the MPFL and a tear of the parapatellar or "medial" retinaculum (Table 12-5).

The MPFL and the medial retinaculum are best depicted on axial MR images and are simple to differentiate from one another. These two structures are located at the same depth; however, the MPFL is a more proximal structure. The key to distinguishing the MPFL from the medial retinaculum is its relation to the overlying VMO muscle. The MPFL extends from the adductor tubercle on the medial femoral condyle to the medial aspect of the superior pole of the patella and lies deep to the VMO muscle, whereas the medial retinaculum attaches to the mid-pole of the patella and is located distal to the VMO muscle (Fig. 12-19). Therefore, on axial images if the VMO muscle is present on the image, then the underlying ligamentous structure represents the MPFL. Absence

Table 12-4 Anatomy of the Medial Patellofemoral Ligament

Origin	Adductor tubercle of medial femoral condyle
Insertion	Superior pole of patella
Location on axial MRI	Sits deep to the vastus medialis obliquus muscle
Function	Primary stabilizer of patella (prevents lateral subluxation)
Injury location	Adductor tubercle (80%) Patellar attachment/midsubstance (20%)
Mechanism of injury	Lateral patellar dislocation

Table 12-5 MRI Findings after Transient Lateral Dislocation of the Patella

Bone contusion pattern	Lower pole medial patellar facet Nonarticular surface anterior lateral femoral condyle
Articular surfaces	Describe osteochondral defects or injury Lower pole patella Mid–weight-bearing surface of the lateral femoral condyle Loose bodies
Medial soft tissue restraint injuries	Sprain, partial tear, complete tear MPFL Adductor tubercle (80%) Patellar attachment or middle of ligament (20%) Medial retinaculum—usually at patellar attachment site
Miscellaneous	Joint effusion

MPFL, medial patellofemoral ligament.

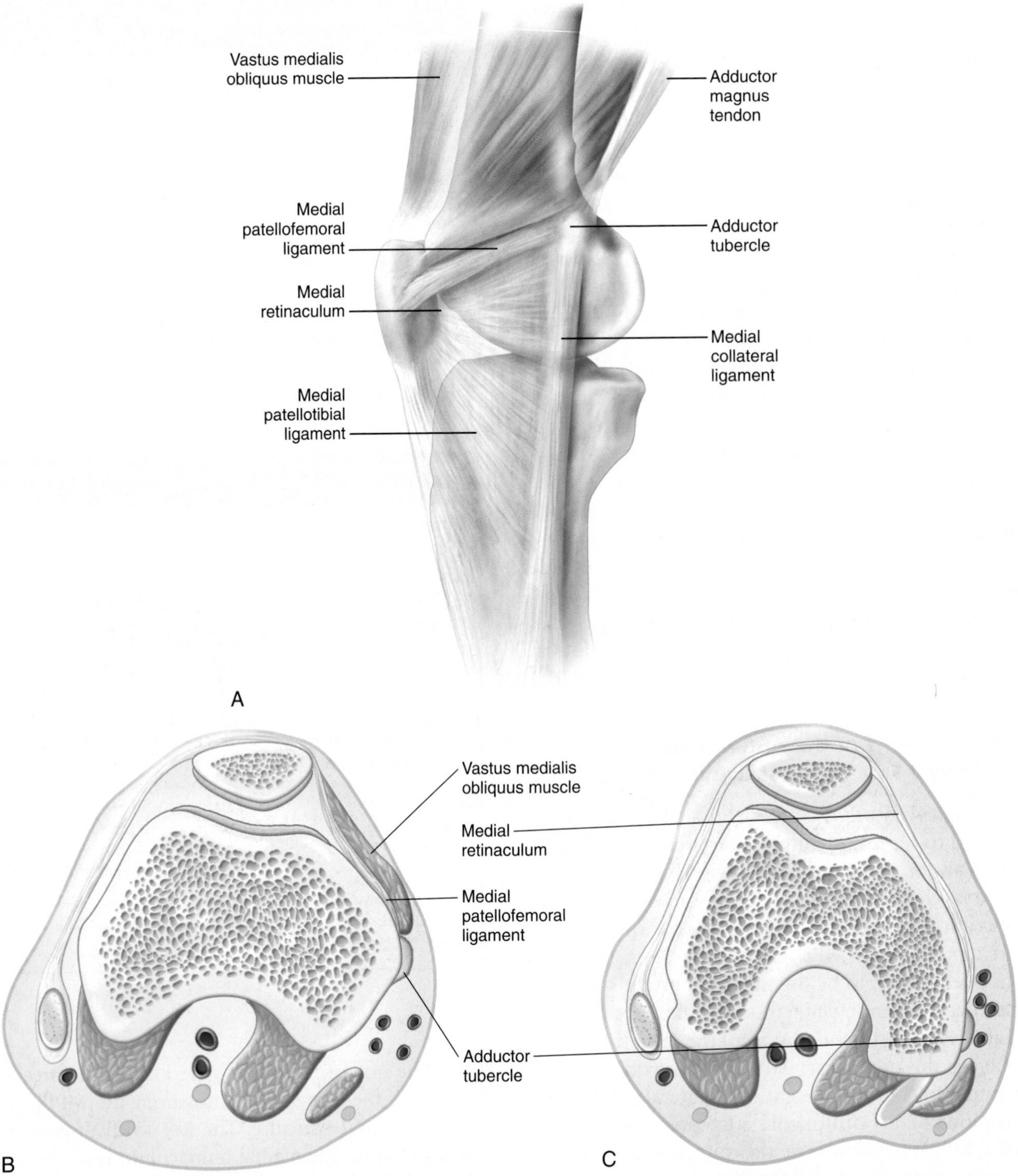
Vastus medialis obliquus muscle
Adductor magnus tendon
Medial patellofemoral ligament
Adductor tubercle
Medial retinaculum
Medial collateral ligament
Medial patellotibial ligament
A
Vastus medialis obliquus muscle
Medial retinaculum
Medial patellofemoral ligament
Adductor tubercle
B
C

Figure 12-19 Artwork shows the medial patellofemoral ligament (MPFL) and the medial retinaculum and its association with the overlying vastus medialis obliquus (VMO) muscle. **A,** Sagittal projection shows the MPFL arising from the medial aspect of the superior pole of the patella and inserting onto the adductor tubercle. The MPFL is located deep to the VMO muscle. **B,** Axial image through the level of the VMO muscle shows the MPFL extending from the superior pole of the patellar to insert onto the adductor tubercle. **C,** Axial image below the level of the VMO muscle shows the medial retinaculum rather than the MPFL. The VMO muscle acts as a landmark on axial images to determine whether the structure arising along the medial aspect of the patella represents the MPFL or the medial retinaculum.

of the VMO muscle on axial images indicates that the image was obtained distal to the level of the VMO muscle, and the medial soft tissue restraint of the patella at these levels represents either the medial patellar retinaculum or the medial patellotibial ligament (Fig. 12-20).

On MRI, the MPFL is visualized in the axial or sagittal imaging planes as a thin linear structure located deep to the VMO, extending from the superior pole of the patellar to the adductor tubercle. As it approaches the adductor tubercle, it blends with the deep fibers of the VMO and is not always clearly differentiated from the deep fascia of the VMO (see Fig. 12-20A). Injury of the MPFL can be classified as a sprain, partial-thickness tear, or complete tear. Approximately 80% of MPFL injuries occur at the femoral attachment site, whereas the remaining 20% occur in either the middle of the ligament or at the patellar attachment site. Disruption of the MPFL at its patellar attachment site or in the middle of the ligament is depicted on MRI as discontinuity and laxity or retraction of the fibers. At the femoral attachment site, the ligament is not clearly differentiated from the fascia of the VMO muscle, and disruption at this level is demonstrated as displacement or uplifting of the VMO muscle away from the adductor tubercle secondary to fluid or hematoma (Fig. 12-21). This can be identified in either the axial or sagittal imaging planes. A sprain or partial-thickness tear appears as edema adjacent to the adductor tubercle, but the VMO muscle is not displaced away from the adductor tubercle.

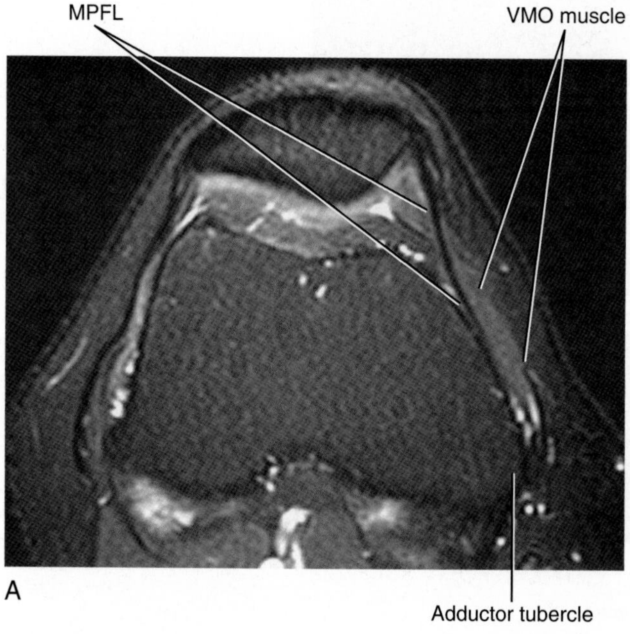
MPFL
VMO muscle
A
Adductor tubercle

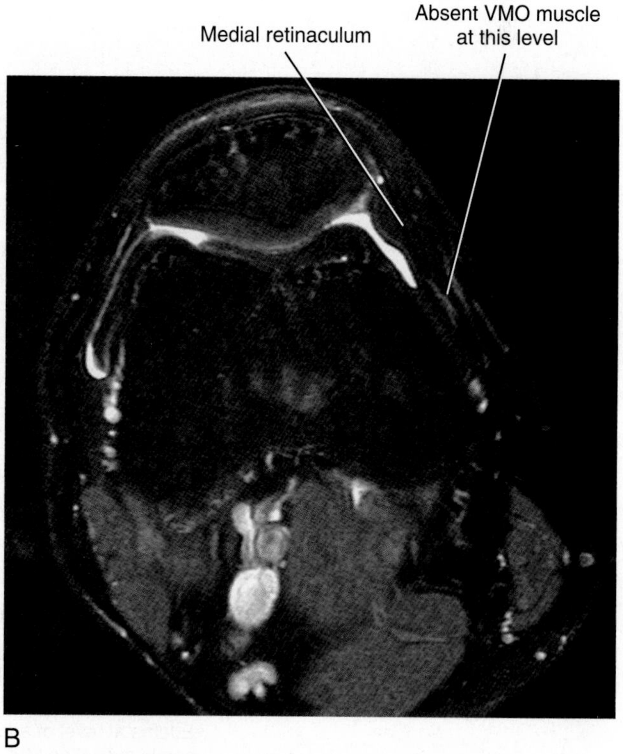
Medial retinaculum
Absent VMO muscle at this level
B

Figure 12-20 Differentiating the medial patellofemoral ligament (MPFL) from the medial retinaculum in the axial imaging plane. If there is muscle present superficial to the medial soft tissue restraints of the patella, then the axial image is at the level of the MPFL. If there is no muscle present, then the image is at the level of the medial retinaculum. **A,** Axial T2-weighted image demonstrates the normal appearance of the MPFL originating on the adductor tubercle of the medial femoral condyle and extending deep to the vastus medialis obliquus (VMO) muscle to insert on the superior pole of the patella. The structure is easily identified as the MPFL in the axial plane, because the VMO muscle is in the field of view and lies directly on top of the MPFL. **B,** Axial T2-weighted image at the level of the medial retinaculum. The medial retinaculum can be differentiated from the MPFL because the image is more distal and there is no overlying muscle at this level.

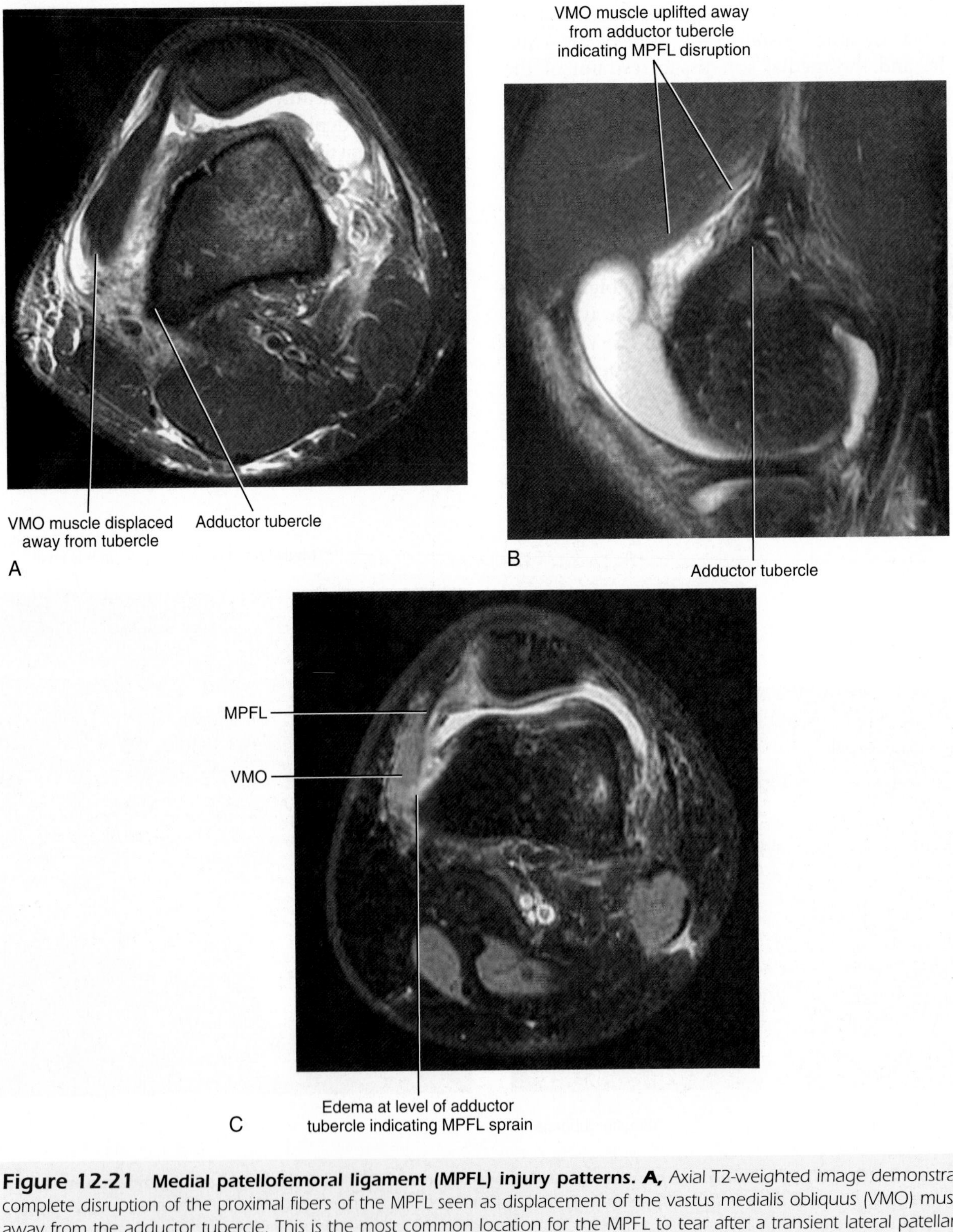
VMO muscle displaced away from tubercle
Adductor tubercle
A
VMO muscle uplifted away from adductor tubercle indicating MPFL disruption
B
Adductor tubercle
MPFL
VMO
Edema at level of adductor tubercle indicating MPFL sprain
C

Figure 12-21 Medial patellofemoral ligament (MPFL) injury patterns. A, Axial T2-weighted image demonstrates complete disruption of the proximal fibers of the MPFL seen as displacement of the vastus medialis obliquus (VMO) muscle away from the adductor tubercle. This is the most common location for the MPFL to tear after a transient lateral patellar dislocation. The typical MRI appearance is that of fluid situated deep to the VMO muscle, separating it from the underlying adductor tubercle. **B,** Sagittal T2-weighted image also demonstrates fluid deep to the fibers of the VMO muscle, uplifting it away from the adductor tubercle having the appearance of a disrupted MPFL in the sagittal plane. Normally, the VMO muscle sits in direct contact with the underlying adductor tubercle in this imaging plane. **C,** Axial T2-weighted image shows a sprain of the MPFL near its origin on the adductor tubercle. There is mild adjacent edema but no uplifting or displacement of the adjacent VMO muscle. This is the appearance of a sprained MPFL and does not require surgical repair.

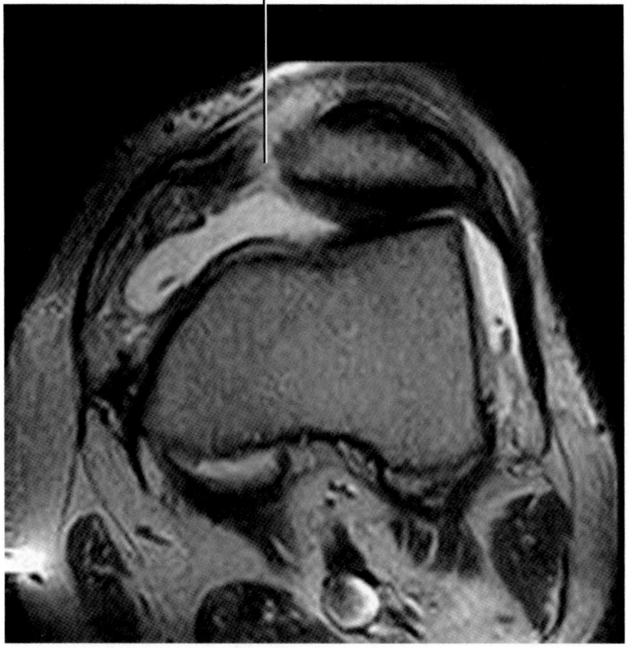
Complete disruption of MPFL and medial retinaculum at patellar attachment site
D

Figure 12-21, cont'd **D,** Axial T2-weighted image demonstrates complete disruption of the MPFL and medial retinaculum at the patellar attachment site.

Middle Third Anatomy

Layer 2 of the middle third of the knee is made up of the superficial fibers of the medial collateral ligament (MCL). The superficial component of the MCL is often thought of as a single unit, but it is actually composed of two separate bundles. The *tibial collateral ligament* refers to a more anteriorly located group of vertically oriented fibers, whereas a separate group of obliquely oriented fibers, referred to as the *posterior oblique ligament,* is located in the posterior third of the knee.

The superficial fibers of the tibial collateral ligament originate on the adductor tubercle of the medial femoral condyle adjacent to the origin of the MPFL and extend in a vertical fashion to an area of broad insertion on the tibia approximately 5 cm below the level of the joint line and deep to the insertion of the pes anserinus tendon. The ligament measures approximately 1.5 cm in anterior to posterior width, and the anterior edge of the tibial collateral ligament often demonstrates a rolled appearance. The ligament is best visualized on coronal images along the medial joint line as a continuous low signal intensity band (Fig. 12-22). The ligament is also seen on axial images as a thin oval structure, which measures approximately 1. 5 cm anterior to posterior and is located superficial to the medial joint line. The rolled appearance of the anterior aspect of the ligament is easily seen on axial images and may give the false impression of thickening of the tibial collateral ligament when imaging through the most anterior aspect of the ligament in the coronal plane.

The deep fibers of the tibial collateral ligament are separated from the superficial fibers by a potential space referred to as the tibial collateral ligament bursa. The deep fibers of the tibial collateral ligament form the medial joint capsule (layer 3) and can be divided into three distinct components. The first part directly overlies the medial meniscus and is firmly attached to the adjacent meniscus. The more inferior component is referred to as the meniscotibial ligament and represents a short ligamentous structure that extends from the inferior aspect of the medial meniscus to the adjacent tibia. The more superior component is the longer meniscofemoral ligament, which provides the femoral attachment of the medial meniscus. The deep fibers of the tibial collateral ligament (meniscotibial and meniscofemoral ligaments) are best evaluated on coronal and sagittal MR images (see Fig. 12-22).

Injury Patterns of the Middle Third of the Medial Soft Tissue Structures (Tibial Collateral Ligament)

Injuries of the tibial collateral ligament usually occur as the result of a valgus injury to the knee and can result from a direct contact injury to the lateral aspect of the knee (clipping injury in football) or as a noncontact twisting mechanism of injury. With complex twisting injuries, tibial collateral ligament tears are often seen in conjunction with ACL or PCL injuries or with meniscal tears.

A three-point grading system is used to describe tibial collateral ligament injuries; grade I indicates a sprain, grade II a partial-thickness tear, and grade III a complete tear (Fig. 12-23). Injuries are best depicted on T2-weighted coronal images, and the use of fat-saturation techniques improves conspicuity of the injury. The axial plane is complementary in the evaluation of tibial collateral ligament injuries.

A sprain is demonstrated on MRI as edema superficial to the tibial collateral ligament. Thickening and

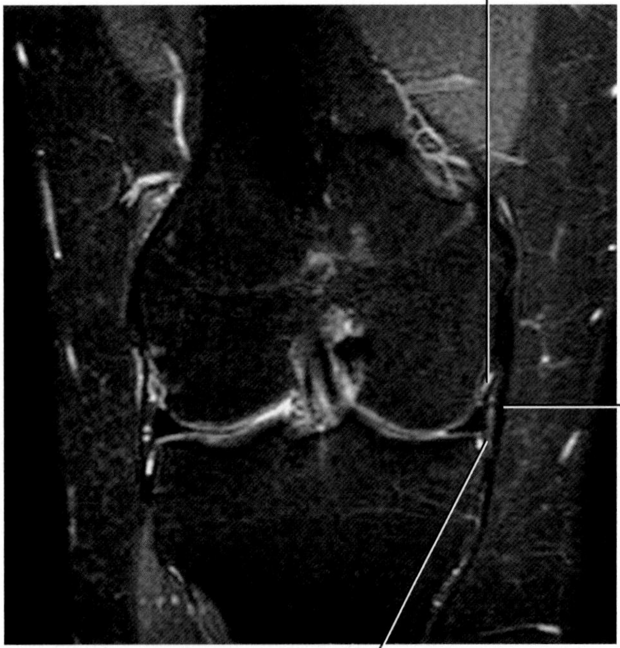
Meniscofemoral ligament
Superficial fibers of the tibial collateral ligament
Meniscotibial ligament

Figure 12-22 Normal MRI appearance of the MCL. Coronal T2-weighted image demonstrates the superficial fibers of the MCL arising proximally from the adductor tubercle of the medial femoral condyle. The ligament inserts distally on the tibia approximately 5 cm below the level of the joint line. The components of the deep fibers of the MCL are shown, the meniscotibial ligament and the longer meniscofemoral ligament.

edema may also be seen within the substance of the ligament, but there should not be fluid signal intensity within the substance of the ligament or disruption of the fibers (see Fig. 12-23). There are a several potential pitfalls with regard to diagnosing a sprain of the tibial collateral ligament (Table 12-6). First, edema isolated to the soft tissues *deep* to the collateral ligament is often seen in association with an intra-articular process, and this pattern of edema does not indicate collateral ligament injury. Second, it is not uncommon to see edema *superficial* to the collateral ligament as a reactive phenomenon secondary to an intra-articular process such as a meniscal tear or osteoarthritis. Therefore, one should use caution in diagnosing a sprain of the tibial collateral ligament purely on the basis of superficial edema in the absence of a history of trauma, especially if an adjacent intra-articular pathologic process is present (Box 12-3). Another potential pitfall that can mimic a sprain of the MCL is the presence of a geniculate vessel paralleling the MCL. This can occasionally give the appearance of a small linear collection of fluid superficial to the MCL, but should not be mistaken for an MCL injury. Finally, a tear of the MPFL at the level of the adductor tubercle results in edema at the level of the proximal MCL attachment and can mimic injury of the MCL.

Table 12-6 Mimics of MCL Injury

MR Finding	Source of MRI Finding
Edema deep to MCL	Intra-articular process
Edema superficial to MCL	May be reactive to intra-articular process/must correlate with clinical history
Edema at level of adductor tubercle	MPFL injury
Fluid signal superficial to MCL	Geniculate vessels
Thick anterior fiber of MCL on coronal image	Anterior edge of MCL has a rolled appearance

BOX 12-3 COMMON CAUSES OF EDEMA ADJACENT TO THE MEDIAL COLLATERAL LIGAMENT (MCL)

MCL injury
Baker's cyst rupture
Osteoarthritis
Medial meniscal tear
Spontaneous osteonecrosis
Patellar dislocation and MPFL injury

MPFL, medial patellofemoral ligament.

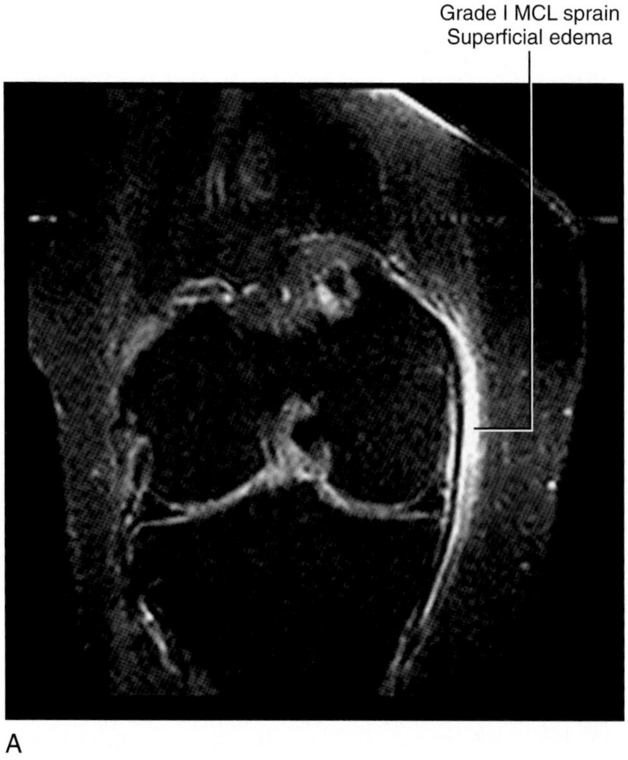
Grade I MCL sprain
Superficial edema
A

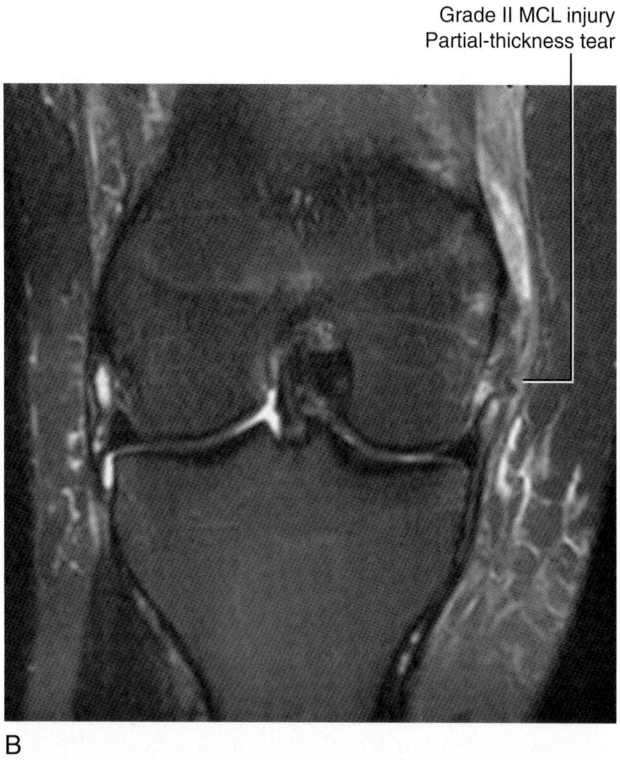
Grade II MCL injury
Partial-thickness tear
B

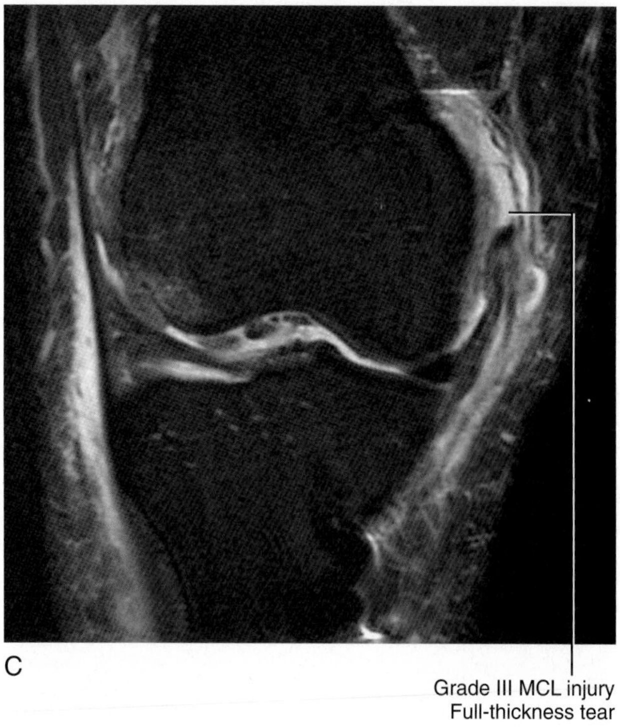
C
Grade III MCL injury
Full-thickness tear

Figure 12-23 Acute medial collateral ligament (MCL) injury patterns. A, Grade I injury. Edema superficial to the MCL represents a mild sprain but no partial- or full-thickness tear. The MCL fibers appear intact. **B,** Grade II injury. Mild thickening and edema are seen within the substance of the MCL and superficial soft tissue edema consistent with a partial-thickness tear. **C,** Grade III injury. There is a complete tear of the proximal MCL fibers with mild retraction of the more distal fibers and adjacent soft tissue edema.

On MRI, a partial-thickness tear appears as a partial-thickness disruption of the fibers with surrounding edema and fluid. These injuries most commonly involve the proximal aspect of the MCL proximal to the level of the joint line. A complete tear is diagnosed when the fibers are completely disrupted with surrounding edema and hemorrhage. Once again these injuries most commonly occur proximal to the joint line. Chronic injury of the tibial collateral ligament results in thickening of the fibers best seen on the coronal images but with a lack of adjacent soft tissue edema. A chronic injury of the tibial collateral ligament may demonstrate ossification within the ligament and is referred to as Pellegrini-Stieda syndrome (Fig. 12-24). A potential pitfall for diagnosing chronic tibial collateral ligament injury is that the most anterior fibers of the normal MCL may appear rolled and as a result, the coronal image through the most anterior portion of the ligament may demonstrate apparent thickening. True thickening resulting from an old injury can be seen on several sequential coronal images and not solely on the most anterior coronal image.

The deep fibers of the tibial collateral ligament can also be disrupted, which usually results from significant trauma to the knee and is often associated with other injuries such as an ACL tear. Disruption of the meniscotibial ligament results in a "floating" meniscus or an avulsed meniscus. This injury has long been recognized in the orthopedic community and requires reattachment or suturing of the meniscus to the tibia. The meniscofemoral ligament usually remains intact. Unlike the meniscotibial ligament, a torn meniscofemoral ligament does not result in a free-floating meniscus and does not require surgical repair. An avulsed meniscus may be minimally displaced but typically demonstrates no other signs of injury and no evidence of a meniscal tear such as surfacing signal. Injury resulting in meniscal avulsion involves the meniscotibial attachment. It is therefore important to evaluate the meniscotibial attachment in patients with evidence of significant knee trauma to alert the surgeon to the possibility of an avulsed meniscus. Two signs of medial meniscal avulsion are (1) discontinuity of the meniscotibial ligament and (2) the "floating" meniscus, which is defined as fluid

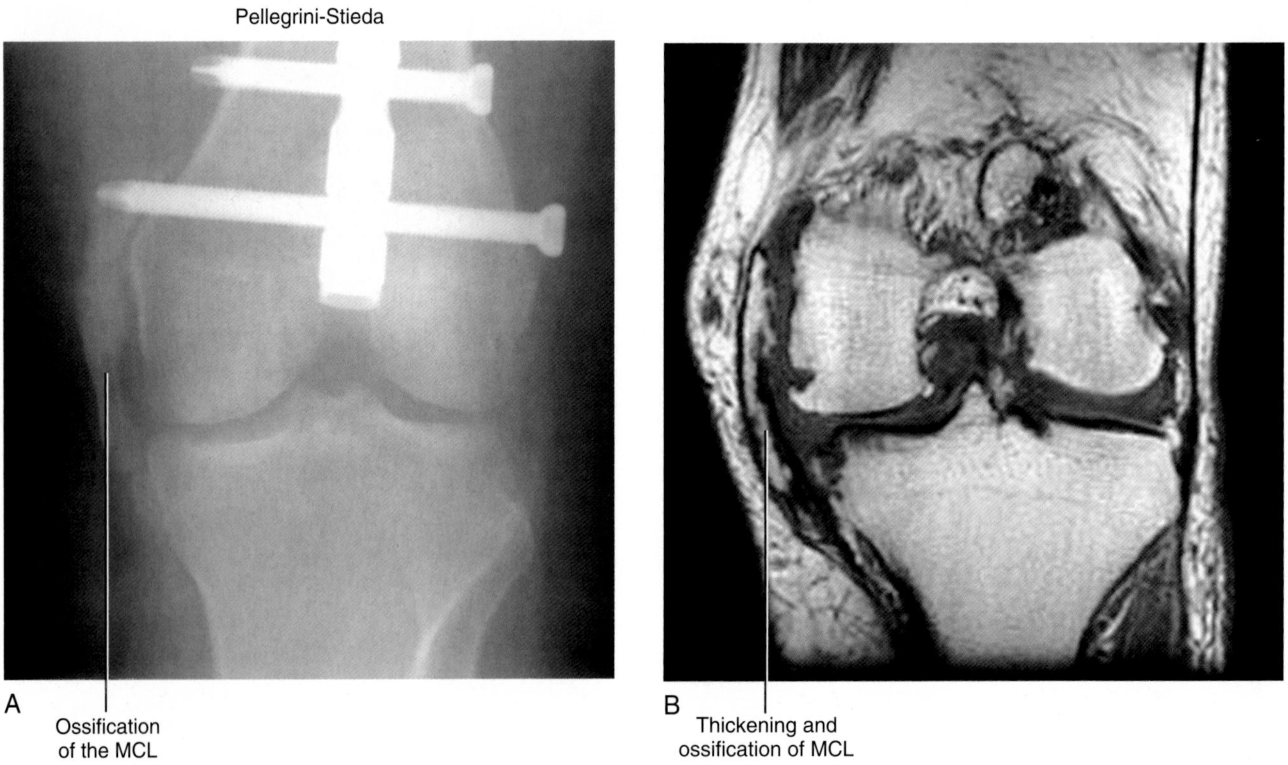
Pellegrini-Stieda
A
Ossification of the MCL
B
Thickening and ossification of MCL

Figure 12-24 Pellegrini-Stieda syndrome. *A,* Anteroposterior radiograph shows extensive ossification within the medial collateral ligament (MCL). Coronal T1-weighted ***B,*** Image in a different patient shows thickening and ossification within the MCL representing an old injury.

completely surrounding the meniscus best seen on T2-weighted sagittal or coronal images (Fig. 12-25).

The potential space between the superficial and deep fibers of the tibial collateral ligament is often referred to as the *tibial collateral bursa* or *MCL bursa* (although this is not a true bursa). This potential space may become inflamed (tibial collateral bursitis) and demonstrate fluid within the space, which is best seen on T2-weighted coronal and axial images of the knee (Fig. 12-26). A meniscal cyst arising from the medial meniscus can dissect into the tibial collateral bursa and may mimic tibial collateral bursitis. A meniscal cyst can be differentiated from a bursitis when the fluid collection is in direct contact with a tear of the medial meniscus and when the meniscal cyst is more lobulated or mass-like in appearance than the fluid collection associated with bursitis.

Posterior Third Anatomy

The oblique fibers of the MCL are referred to as the *posterior oblique ligament* (POL), and this portion of the MCL is located within the posterior third of the knee (see Fig. 12-18). The posterior oblique ligament comprises three separate arms: superficial, tibial, and capsular. All three arms originate on the adductor tubercle immediately posterior to the origin of the superficial fibers of the tibial collateral ligament. The superficial arm is located superficial to the distal semimembranosus tendon and inserts onto the fascia of the distal pes anserinus tendon. The tibial arm extends deep to the semimembranosus tendon and inserts firmly to the tibia. As it crosses the joint line, the tibial arm is also firmly attached to the adjacent posterior horn of the medial meniscus. There is a small triangular gap between the tibial collateral ligament and the anterior edge of the posterior oblique ligament. This gap can be palpated on physical examination and is used as a guide for arthrotomy incisions along the posteromedial joint line. The capsular arm of the posterior oblique ligament also arises from the adductor tubercle and extends deep to the medial head of the gastrocnemius tendon, where it merges with the oblique

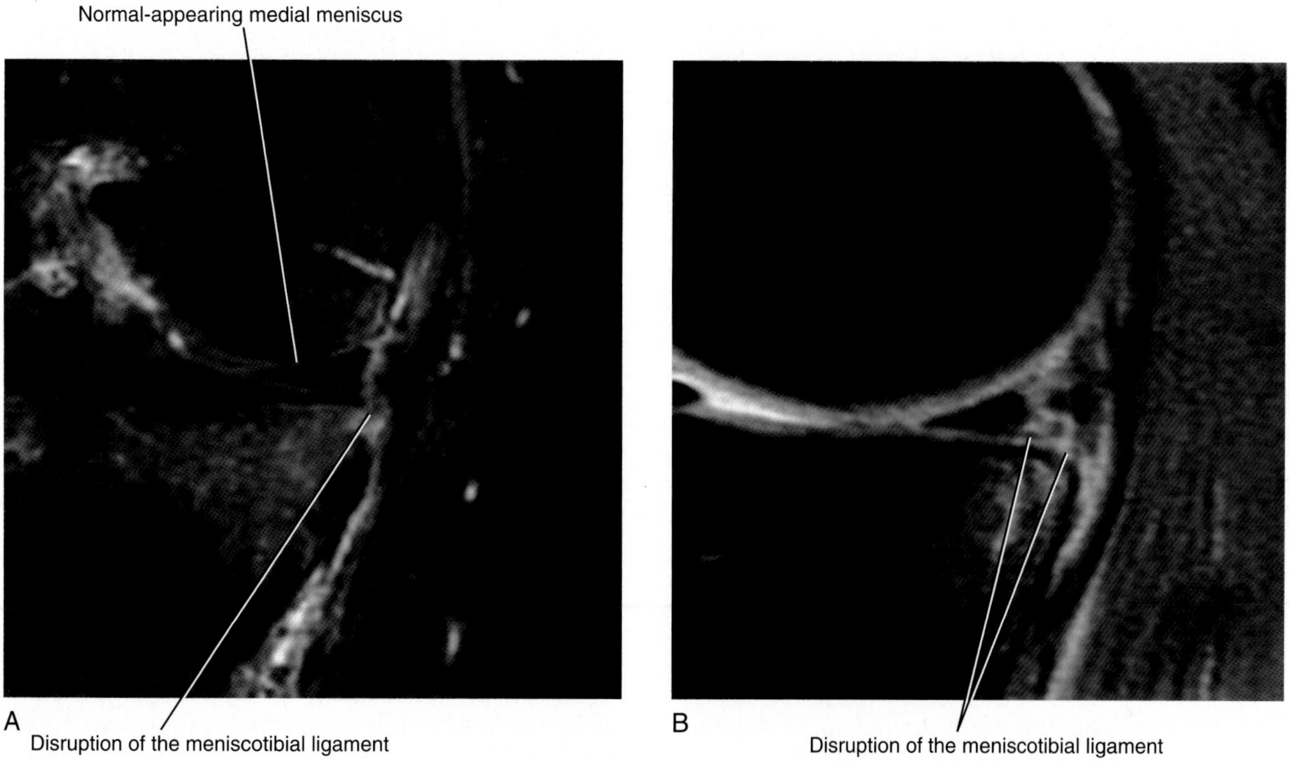
Normal-appearing medial meniscus
A
Disruption of the meniscotibial ligament
B
Disruption of the meniscotibial ligament

Figure 12-25 Disruption of the meniscotibial ligament. Coronal (**A**) and sagittal (**B**) images demonstrate disruption of the meniscotibial ligament. This represents an avulsion of the medial meniscus from its tibial attachment site and requires surgical reattachment of the medial meniscus to the tibia.

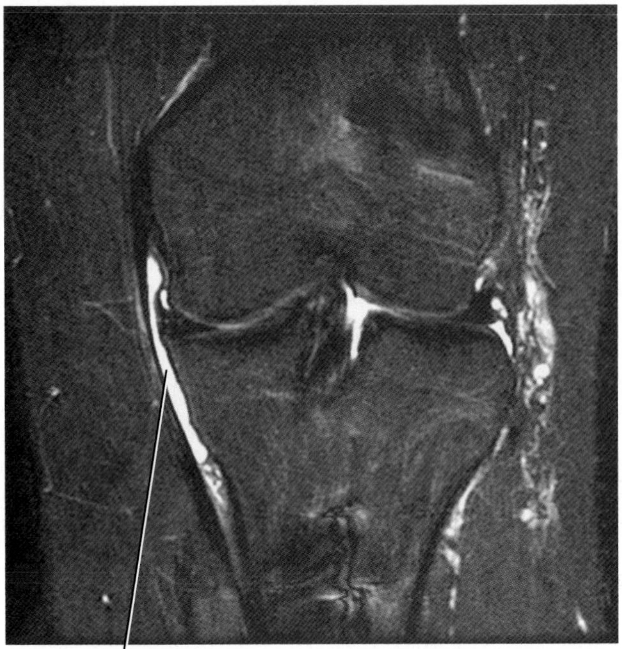
Tibial collateral bursitis
(Fluid between deep and superficial fibers of MCL)

Figure 12-26 Tibial collateral bursitis. Coronal T2-weighted image shows a fluid collection within the tibial collateral bursa between the deep and superficial fibers of the tibial collateral ligament. MCL, medial collateral ligament.

popliteal ligament to form the posterior capsule of the knee.

The distal semimembranosus tendon, one of the hamstring tendons, demonstrates a complex multi-arm insertion along the posterior medial aspect of the knee (Fig. 12-27). It inserts onto the tibia as well as directly into the posterior capsule. Although the primary function of the semimembranosus tendon is knee flexion, its complex insertion also makes it an important stabilizer of the posteromedial corner of the knee during flexion. The distal semimembranosus tendon has five separate arms or attachments. Three of these arms extend deep to the superficial fibers of the oblique popliteal ligament and the tibial collateral ligament to insert directly on the medial aspect of the tibia just below the level of the joint line. These attachments are evaluated on T2-weighted sagittal and coronal images of the knee (Fig. 12-28). The two remaining arms attach directly onto the posterior capsule. The capsular arm of the semimembranosus blends with the capsular arm of the posterior oblique ligament to form a portion of the posterior capsule of the knee. This arm is best seen on T2-weighted axial images of the knee and is best visualized when the knee is distended with fluid. The fifth arm referred to as the oblique popliteal ligament is a broad attachment that blends with the posterior capsule more centrally and crosses the midline to intermingle with the fibers of the arcuate ligament.

Little attention has been paid in the radiology literature to describing injuries of the distal semimembranosus tendon and its complex attachments to the tibia and posterior capsule. Injury to the distal attachment of the semimembranosus tendon is referred to as *posteromedial corner injury*. The mechanism thought to be most often associated with injury to the distal attachment is traction placed on the distal attachments during the valgus stress that results in ACL disruption and impaction injury of the posterolateral compartment of the knee. The spectrum of injury includes partial- or full-thickness tear of the tibial attachment of the semimembranosus tendon or avulsion of a small fragment of bone from the posteromedial tibial plateau (Fig. 12-29). The orthopedic literature suggests that injuries that result in the combination of an ACL and medial meniscal tears are frequently associated with tears of the capsular attachments of the semimembranosus tendon. Some surgeons advocate the surgical repair of a lax capsular arm or oblique popliteal arm of the distal semimembranosus tendon when associated with a tear of the posterior horn of the medial meniscus to recover stability of the knee during flexion. Injuries of the capsular attachments are best evaluated on T2 axial and sagittal images of the posterior knee.

Pes Anserinus Tendons The pes anserinus tendons are situated superficial to the semimembranosus tendon along the posteromedial aspect of the knee. From medial to lateral, they include the sartorius, gracilis, and the semitendinosus tendons. They attach distally along the medial aspect of the tibia approximately 5 cm below the joint line. The pes anserinus tendons are best evaluated on T2-weighted axial and sagittal images. Tenosynovitis, tendinosis, and tears of the pes anserinus tendons rarely occur. Two bursae are located in close proximity to the pes anserinus tendons. Either can become inflamed, and patients can present with posteromedial knee pain, mimicking internal derangement. The *pes anserinus bursa* is located deep to the pes anserinus tendons and located

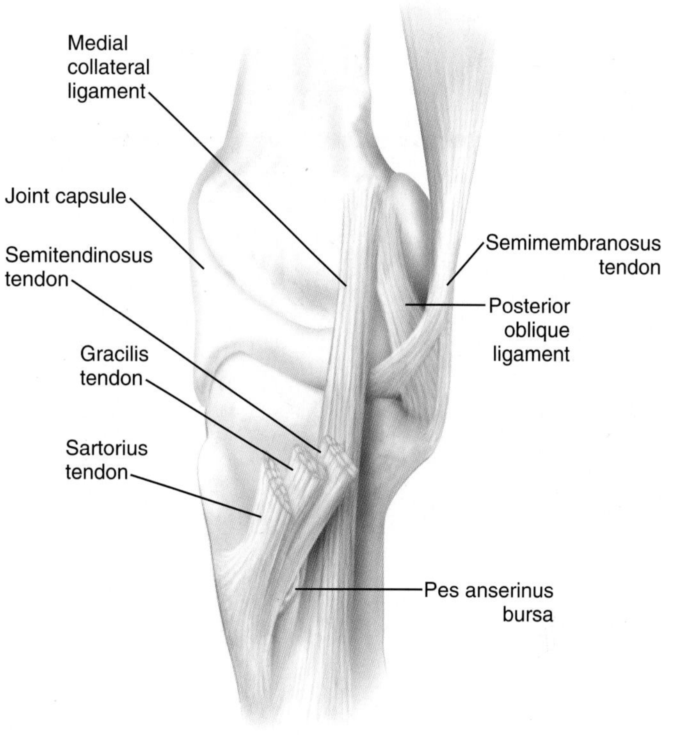

Medial collateral ligament
Joint capsule
Semitendinosus tendon
Gracilis tendon
Sartorius tendon
Semimembranosus tendon
Posterior oblique ligament
Pes anserinus bursa

Figure 12-27 The posterior medial corner of the knee shows the complex distal attachments of the semimembranosus tendon with both capsular and tibial attachments.

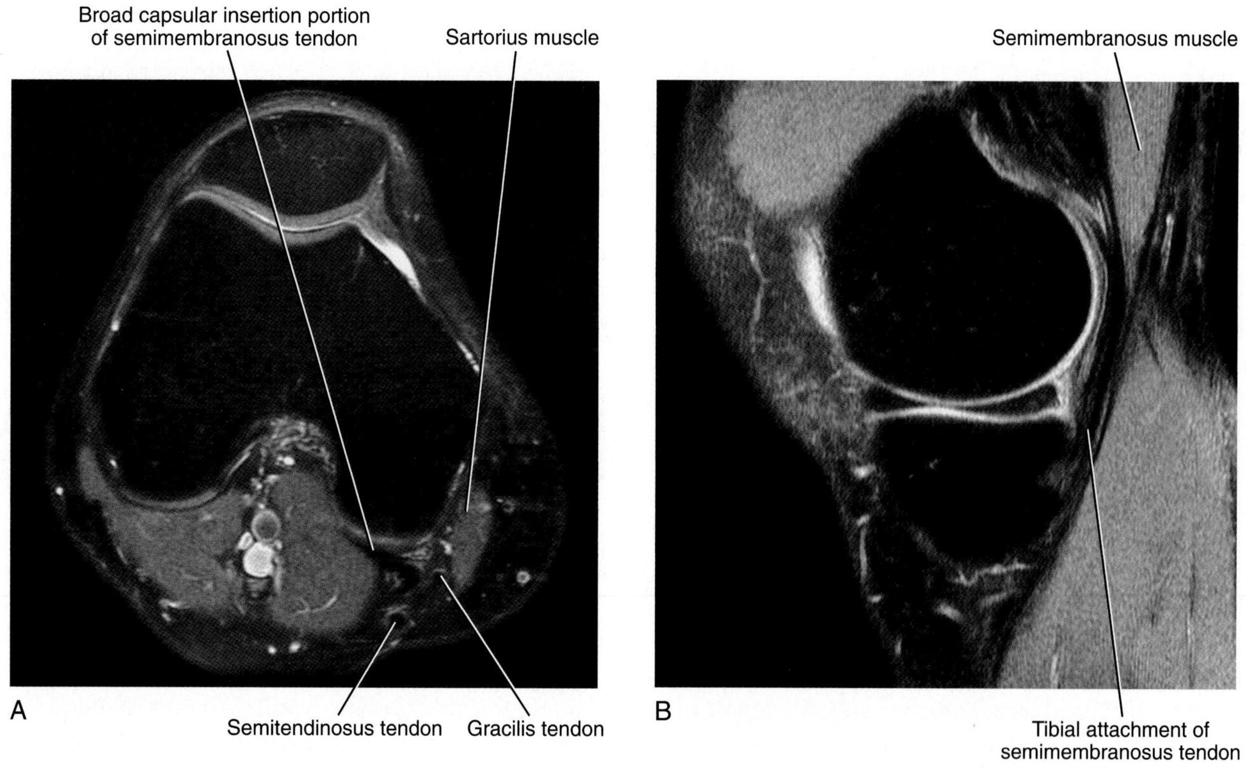

Broad capsular insertion portion of semimembranosus tendon
Sartorius muscle
A
Semitendinosus tendon
Gracilis tendon
Semimembranosus muscle
B
Tibial attachment of semimembranosus tendon

Figure 12-28 **MRI of the normal distal semimembranosus tendon attachment. *A,*** Axial T2-weighted image shows the broad capsular attachment of the distal semimembranosus tendon along the posteromedial joint line. The capsular attachment is best evaluated on the axial T2-weighted images. The capsular attachment sits deep to the pes anserinus tendons. ***B,*** T2-weighted sagittal image shows the distal tibial attachment site of the semimembranosus tendon.

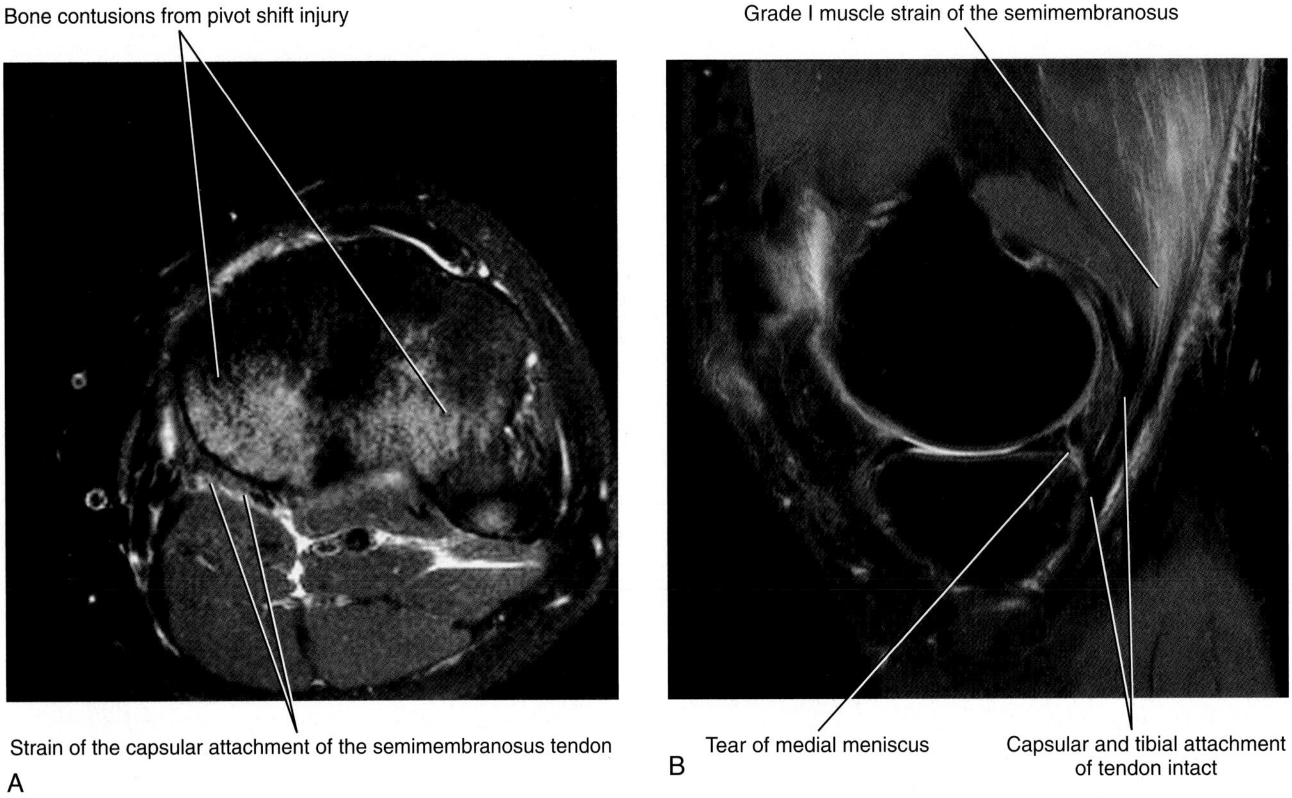
Bone contusions from pivot shift injury
Grade I muscle strain of the semimembranosus
Strain of the capsular attachment of the semimembranosus tendon
A
B
Tear of medial meniscus
Capsular and tibial attachment of tendon intact

Figure 12-29 Semimembranosus injury. A, Axial T2-weighted image shows edema within the substance of the capsular attachment of the semimembranosus tendon with surrounding edema representing a strain and partial-thickness tear of the capsular attachment. This patient experienced a pivot shift mechanism of injury with bone contusions involving the posterior tibial plateau and disruption of the anterior cruciate ligament (not shown). **B,** Sagittal T2-weighted image shows edema within the distal semimembranosus muscle representing a grade I muscle injury. The distal capsular and tibial attachments of the semimembranosus tendon remain intact. A vertical tear of the posterior of the medial meniscus is also present.

distal to the joint line (Fig. 12-30A). The second bursa referred to as the *semimembranosus-tibial collateral ligament bursa* is located slightly proximal to the pes anserinus bursa at the level of the joint line. When it becomes inflamed and fluid filled, it demonstrates a characteristic C-shaped appearance on both coronal and sagittal MR images (Fig. 12-30B). These two bursae can occasionally mimic a meniscal cyst, but knowledge regarding their location and typical appearance should help avoid this pitfall.

The gracilis and semitendinosus tendons can be harvested and used as a *hamstring graft* for repair of a torn ACL or PCL. The distal 10 to 12 cm of the tendons are harvested, and the distal muscles are just left unattached in the posteromedial aspect of the knee. It has been shown on MRI and with histologic studies that these tendons regenerate over time and demonstrate a normal MR appearance on postoperative imaging within 12 to 18 months after tendon harvest.

LATERAL SOFT TISSUES OF THE KNEE

Iliotibial Band Syndrome

The iliotibial band friction syndrome occurs primarily in long-distance runners and results from the iliotibial band repetitively rubbing against the adjacent lateral femoral condyle, leading to anterolateral knee pain. On MRI, this entity presents as soft tissue edema located deep to the iliotibial band at the level of the lateral femoral condyle (Fig. 12-31). Additional MRI findings that are occasionally seen include focal thickening of the iliotibial band and marrow edema

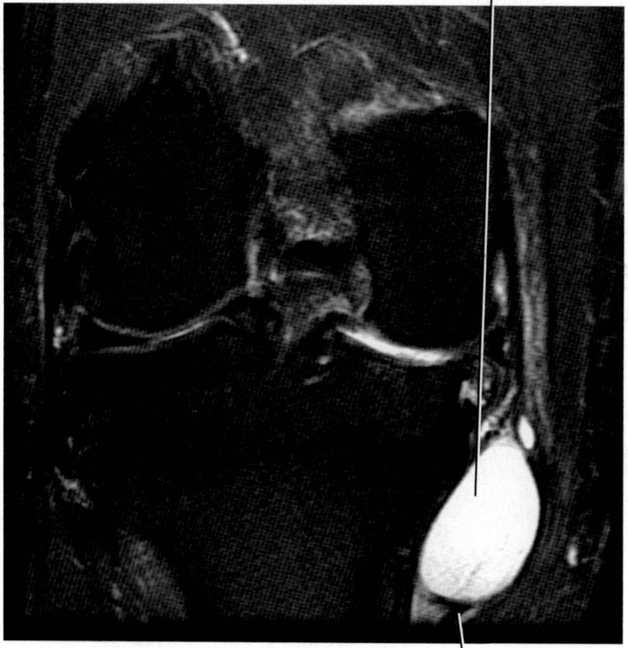
Pes anserinus bursitis
Distal pes anserinus tendon

A

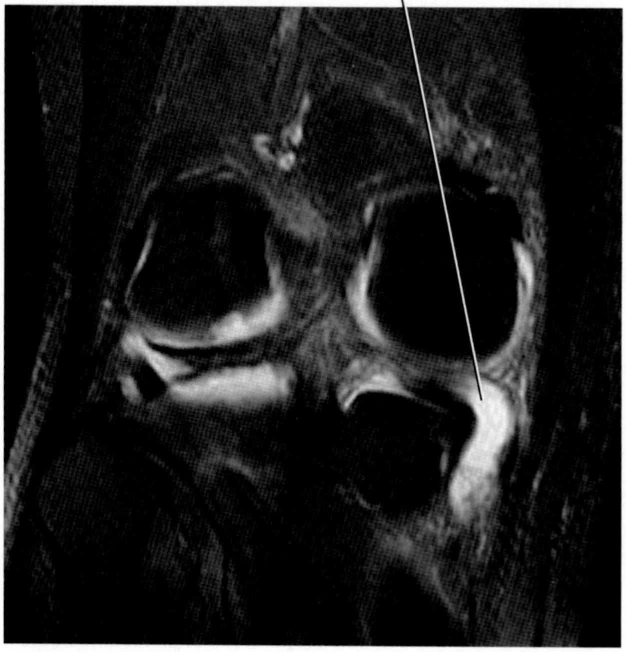
Semimembranosus-tibial collateral ligament bursa

B

Figure 12-30 **A,** Pes anserinus bursa. Fluid-filled mass deep to the distal pes anserinus tendons below the level of the joint line representing pes anserinus bursitis. **B,** Semimembranosus-tibial collateral ligament bursitis. Typical C-shaped appearance of the semimembranosus-tibial collateral ligament bursa at the level of the joint line.

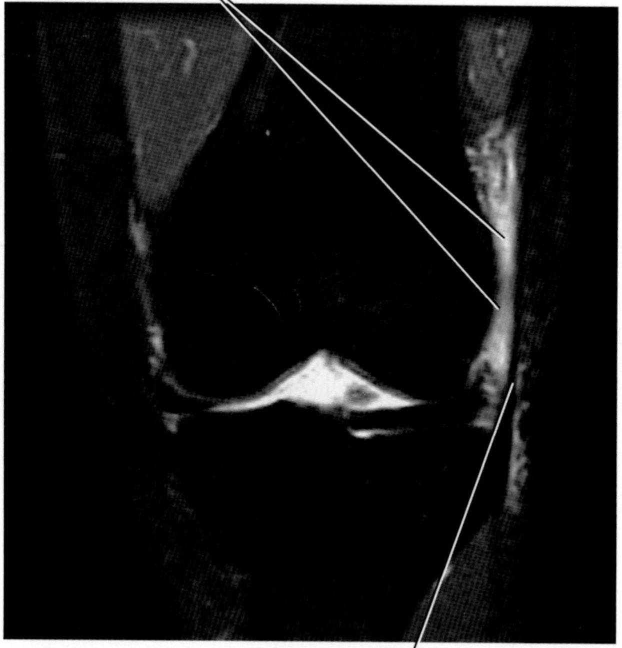
Edema deep to the iliotibial band indicating iliotibial band friction syndrome
Iliotibial band

Figure 12-31 **Iliotibial band syndrome.** Coronal T2-weighted image demonstrates edema deep to the distal iliotibial band.

within the underlying lateral femoral condyle. A potential pitfall is the presence of a recess of the joint, which extends deep to the iliotibial band. Fluid within this recess may mimic soft tissue edema, especially on the T2-weighted coronal images. This pitfall can be avoided by cross-referencing this area of fluid on the axial images to determine whether the fluid is located within the joint space or within the adjacent soft tissues. Fluid deep to the iliotibial band but outside the joint is indicative of iliotibial band syndrome.

Posterolateral Corner Injuries

The posterolateral corner stabilizers are a complex group of anatomic structures that contribute to the stability of the posterolateral corner of the knee. The more superficial structures are the lateral head of the gastrocnemius muscle and tendon, the distal biceps tendon, the fibular collateral ligament, and conjoined tendon. Deeper structures include the posterior capsule, popliteal muscle and tendon, arcuate ligament, popliteofibular ligament, and the fabellofibular ligament. Posterolateral corner injuries usually result from a hyperextension-varus type mechanism of injury and are usually associated with ACL disruption. Bone contusion patterns that often accompany posterolateral corner injuries include *kissing contusions* of the anteromedial femoral condyle and anteromedial tibia or a small avulsion fracture and the presence of marrow edema within the medial aspect of the fibular head, referred to as the *arcuate sign*. Marrow edema in these locations should raise concern for a possible posterolateral corner injury, and any soft tissue abnormality in the posterolateral corner of the knee should be viewed with suspicion.

On MRI, a thorough evaluation of the posterolateral corner structures requires all three imaging planes, and T2-weighted images with fat saturation usually increase conspicuity of injuries. The fibular collateral ligament, conjoined tendon, and biceps femoris tendon are best visualized in the coronal imaging plane, and injuries are described as a partial-thickness tear or complete disruption. Disruption or avulsion of the lateral head of the gastrocnemius tendon usually indicates a severe posterolateral corner injury (Fig. 12-32). Grade I strain of the popliteus musculotendinous junction is a common injury and slightly less specific for posterolateral instability, whereas a complete tear is less common but indicates a more severe injury. Finally, the integrity of the posterolateral capsule and the arcuate and popliteofibular ligaments are usually best assessed on axial and sagittal images. Soft tissue edema adjacent to the posterolateral corner of the knee in the presence of an ACL injury should lead to a thorough evaluation and description of each of these anatomic structures.

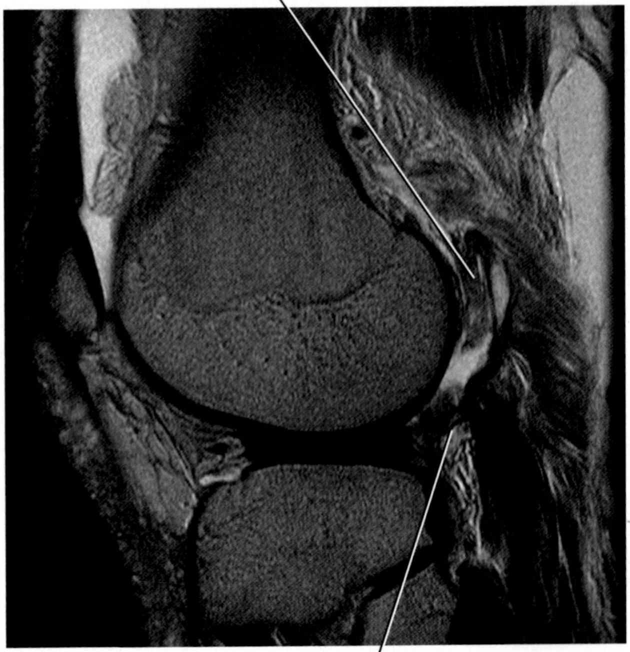
Avulsed retracted lateral head of gastrocnemius tendon
Lax posterolateral capsule with adjacent soft tissue edema

Figure 12-32 Posterolateral corner injury. T2-weighted sagittal image shows a complete avulsion with retraction of the lateral head of the gastrocnemius tendon. This finding is indicative of a severe posterolateral corner injury. The posterior capsule is lax and redundant, indicating complete disruption, and there is extensive surrounding soft tissue edema. The patient experienced a severe hyperextension-valgus injury with kissing contusions involving the anteromedial femoral condyle and anteromedial tibia and had multiple other soft tissue injuries including complete disruption of the anterior cruciate ligament and the fibular collateral ligament (not shown).

MENISCI

Normal Anatomy and MRI Appearance

The menisci are semilunar fibrocartilaginous structures that are interposed between the articular surfaces of the distal femur and the proximal tibia. They serve as shock absorbers to lessen the forces that are transmitted across the joint. They also serve to deepen the tibial plateau and help the femur to glide across the articular surface of the tibia. The medial meniscus is semilunar in shape and larger than the more circular-shaped lateral meniscus. The menisci are thick peripherally and taper centrally to a thin free edge. Both menisci demonstrate firm anterior attachments to the tibial plateau centrally and are also attached to each other anteriorly via the *anterior transverse meniscal ligament*. The medial meniscus is firmly attached to the capsule and deep fibers of the tibial collateral ligament at the level of the mid-body, whereas the body of the lateral meniscus is more mobile and is attached to the capsule via superior and inferior struts. Posteriorly, the medial meniscus attaches firmly to the medial tibial plateau via the *meniscal root*, a structure that is very important for stability of the medial meniscus. The posterior horn of the lateral meniscus is grooved for the adjacent popliteal tendon, which is situated between the peripheral aspect of the posterior horn of the lateral meniscus and the capsule. Finally, the posterior horn of the lateral meniscus attaches to the medial femoral condyle via the *meniscofemoral ligaments* (Humphry and Wrisberg).

The menisci are composed of fibrocartilage and therefore demonstrate low signal intensity on all MRI pulse sequences. The sagittal imaging plane is the primary plane for evaluating the anterior and posterior horns of the menisci, whereas the coronal plane is the primary plane for evaluating the mid-body of the menisci. However, for completeness the menisci must be evaluated in their entirety using both the sagittal and coronal planes; the axial imaging plane is often very useful as well. On sagittal images, the peripheral aspect of the menisci demonstrates a tapering configuration with the anterior and posterior horns connected centrally. While on sagittal images obtained through the central aspect of the menisci, the anterior and posterior horns demonstrate a triangular appearance (Fig. 12-33). The anterior and posterior horns of the lateral meniscus are nearly equal in size, whereas the posterior horn of the medial meniscus is nearly twice the size of the anterior horn.

Although the normal meniscus should be dark on all pulse sequences, nonsurfacing intrameniscal signal is often present. In the adult, this is usually representative of intrasubstance degeneration; in the child or young adult, intrasubstance signal is usually reflective of prominent or persistent meniscal vascularity. The two appear identical and can be differentiated only by knowing the age of the patient (Fig. 12-34). More important, the anterior horn of the lateral meniscus may appear fasciculated with surfacing signal near its central attachment, which often simulates a tear. If surfacing signal within the anterior horn extends toward the body or if there is an associated parameniscal cyst or adjacent reactive subchondral marrow edema, then the appearance most likely represents a tear rather than the normal fasciculated appearance. Otherwise, surfacing signal involving the anterior horn of the lateral meniscus immediately adjacent to the anterior central attachment site should be viewed cautiously and in most instances represents the normal fasciculated appearance of the meniscus.

Meniscal Tears: Evaluation with MRI

Description of a meniscal tear should include the location, plane, shape, completeness, and length of the tear. The location should be described as involving the anterior horn, body, or posterior horn of the meniscus. The location of the tear should be further described as involving the inner two thirds or the outer third of the meniscus (corresponding to the avascular white zone or the vascular red zone of the meniscus, respectively). Tears involving the avascular zone or central two thirds of the meniscus often require partial meniscectomy, but tears isolated to the red zone may be amenable to arthroscopic repair.

The plane of a meniscal tear can be described as vertical, horizontal, or oblique in orientation. A vertical tear can be further described as a radial tear if its orientation is perpendicular to the long axis of the meniscus, or it can be described as longitudinal if it is oriented parallel to the long axis of the meniscus. A single tear may demonstrate more than one orientation, and then it is important to describe all components of the tear. For example, a complex tear demonstrates both a vertical and a horizontal

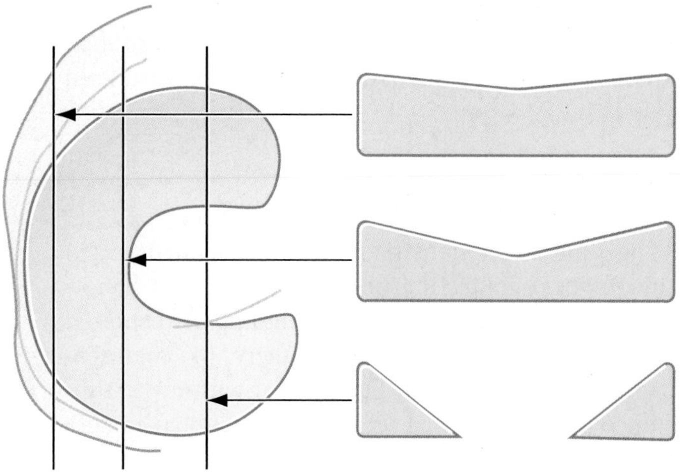

Figure 12-33 Normal sagittal MRI appearance of the meniscus. Line drawing demonstrates the normal morphology and appearance of the meniscus in the sagittal imaging plane as the images move from the peripheral to the central aspect of the meniscus.

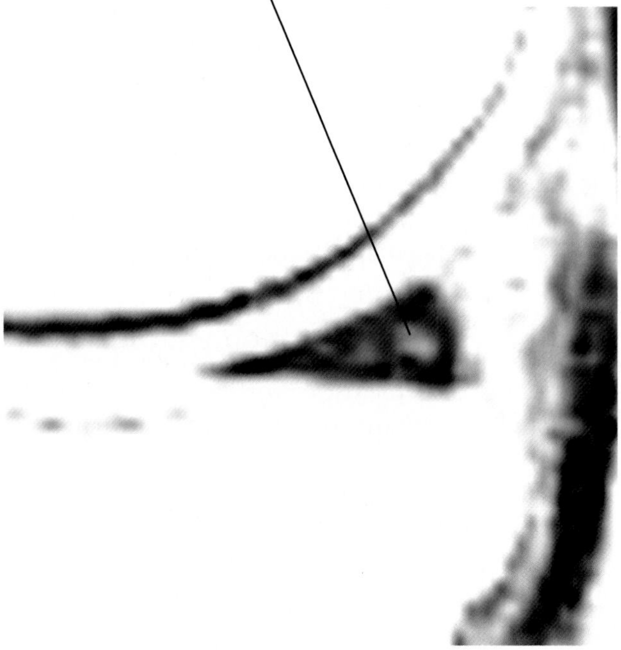
Nonsurfacing intrasubstance signal in an adult representing intrasubstance degeneration
A

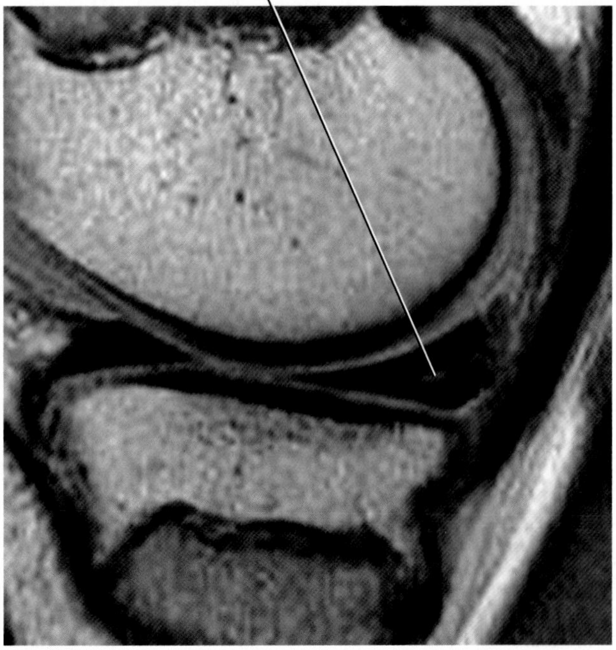
Nonsurfacing intrasubstance signal in a pediatric meniscus representing prominent residual vascularity
B

Figure 12-34 Intrasubstance signal of the meniscus. A, Nonsurfacing intrasubstance signal in the posterior horn of the medial meniscus in this adult patient represents intrasubstance degeneration and not a tear. **B,** Nonsurfacing intrasubstance signal in the meniscus of a child represents prominent vascularity of the meniscus and should not be interpreted as intrasubstance degeneration.

component whereas a parrot-beak tear has both a radial and a longitudinal component. A bucket-handle tear is a specific type of longitudinal tear that results in the inner fragment being displaced into the intercondylar notch or the anterior compartment, or both. Finally, the length and completeness of the meniscal tear should be described. An incomplete tear extends to only a single articular surface of the meniscus whereas a complete tear extends to both the superior and inferior articular surfaces and results in an unstable flap fragment that may become displaced (Fig. 12-35).

Direct Signs of a Meniscal Tear

The four direct signs of meniscal tear include (1) unequivocal grade III (surfacing signal), (2) abnormal meniscal morphology, (3) missing or displaced meniscal tissue with no prior surgery, (4) meniscocapsular injury, and (5) fluid signal within the substance of the meniscus seen on T2-weighted images (Fig. 12-36; Box 12-4).

Intrameniscal signal that extends to the articular surface is indicative of a meniscal tear. Unequivocal surfacing signal present on two images, either on sequential images in the same plane or on both the sagittal and coronal planes, is approximately 94% sensitive for a meniscal tear, whereas sensitivity drops to around 50% if the surfacing signal is seen on only a single image and in a single plane. "Nonsurfacing" signal is unlikely to represent a tear unless there is fluid signal on the T2-weighted images within the substance of the meniscus. In this case, there is a *high* likelihood of a tear even if the signal is nonsurfacing.

Abnormal meniscal morphology is also a direct sign of meniscal tear and is often seen as blunting or truncation of the free edge of the meniscus or as a "too small" meniscus. Differential diagnosis for a truncated meniscus includes prior partial meniscectomy, flipped or displaced meniscal fragment, or a chronic tear with resorption of a portion of the meniscus. The contour of the meniscal surface must also be evaluated for deformities. A focal steplike or

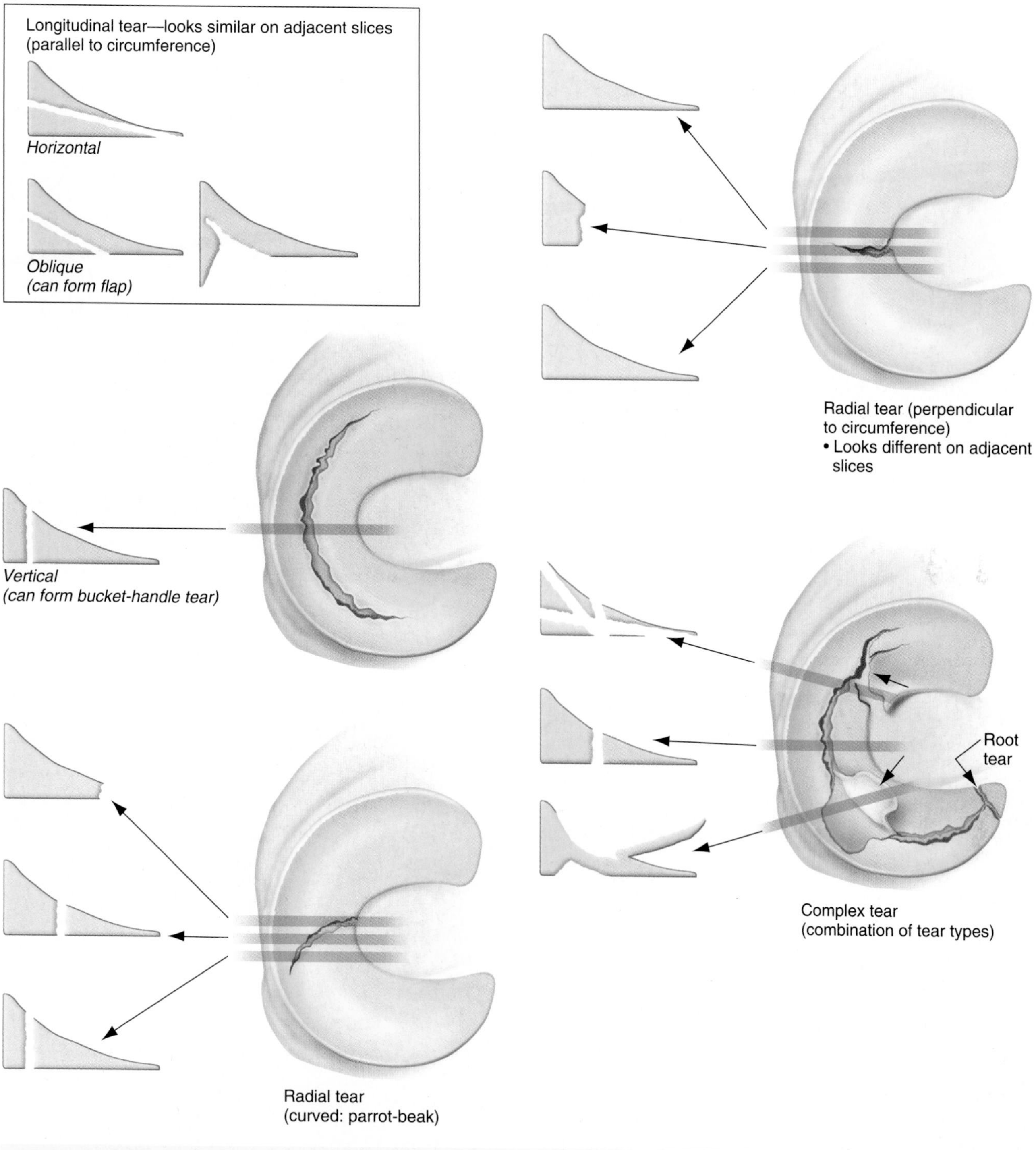

Longitudinal tear—looks similar on adjacent slices
(parallel to circumference)
Horizontal
Oblique
(can form flap)
Vertical
(can form bucket-handle tear)
Radial tear
(curved: parrot-beak)
Radial tear (perpendicular
to circumference)
• Looks different on adjacent
slices
Complex tear
(combination of tear types)
Root
tear

Figure 12-35 **MRI appearance of various meniscal tear patterns.**

wedge-shaped deformity of the meniscal surface is referred to as the notch sign, and when adjacent to intrameniscal signal, it is highly suggestive of a meniscal tear.

Absent or displaced meniscal tissue with no history of meniscal surgery is diagnostic of a tear. A displaced meniscal fragment can result in alterations of meniscal size and shape. A displaced meniscal fragment is usually described as a flap tear or as a flipped fragment. The bucket-handle tear is a specific type of flap tear in which the inner aspect of the meniscus is displaced. Several MRI signs have been described in

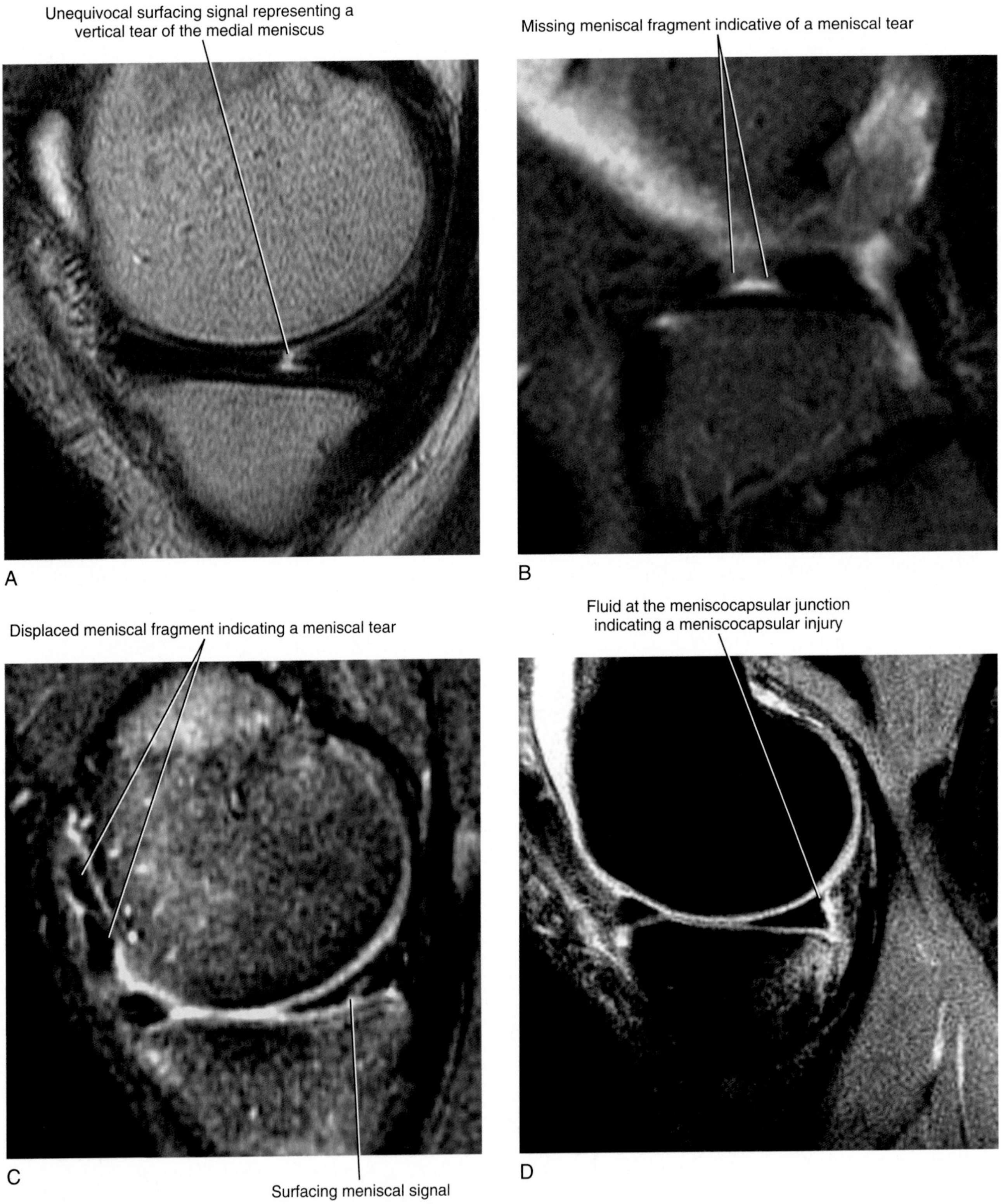
Unequivocal surfacing signal representing a vertical tear of the medial meniscus
A
Missing meniscal fragment indicative of a meniscal tear
B
Displaced meniscal fragment indicating a meniscal tear
C
Surfacing meniscal signal
Fluid at the meniscocapsular junction indicating a meniscocapsular injury
D

Figure 12-36 Direct MRI signs of meniscal tear. A, Surfacing signal extending to both the superior and inferior articular surfaces in a vertical fashion. **B,** A missing fragment, which represents abnormal meniscal morphology. **C,** An anteriorly displaced meniscal fragment. Note surfacing extending to the inferior articular surface of the posterior horn of the medial meniscus. **D,** Fluid intensity signal extending in a vertical fashion between the posterior body of the meniscus and the capsule, representing meniscocapsular separation of the medial meniscus.

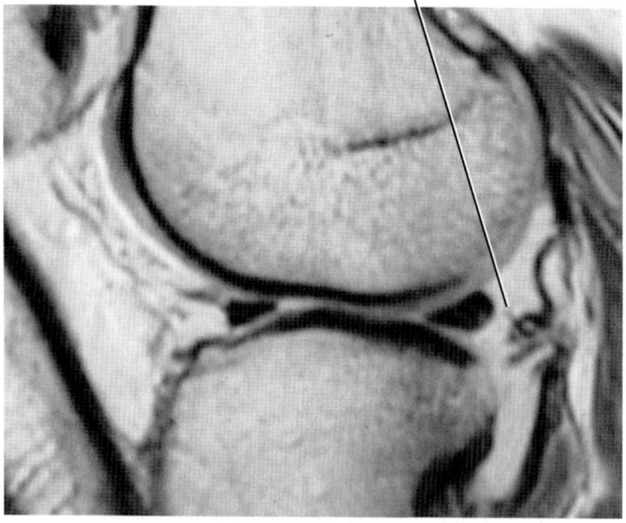
Disruption of meniscal struts lateral meniscus indicating a meniscocapsular injury
E

Figure 12-36, cont'd **E,** Complete disruption of the meniscal fascicles that connect the posterior horn of the lateral meniscus to the capsule, indicating meniscocapsular injury or disruption.

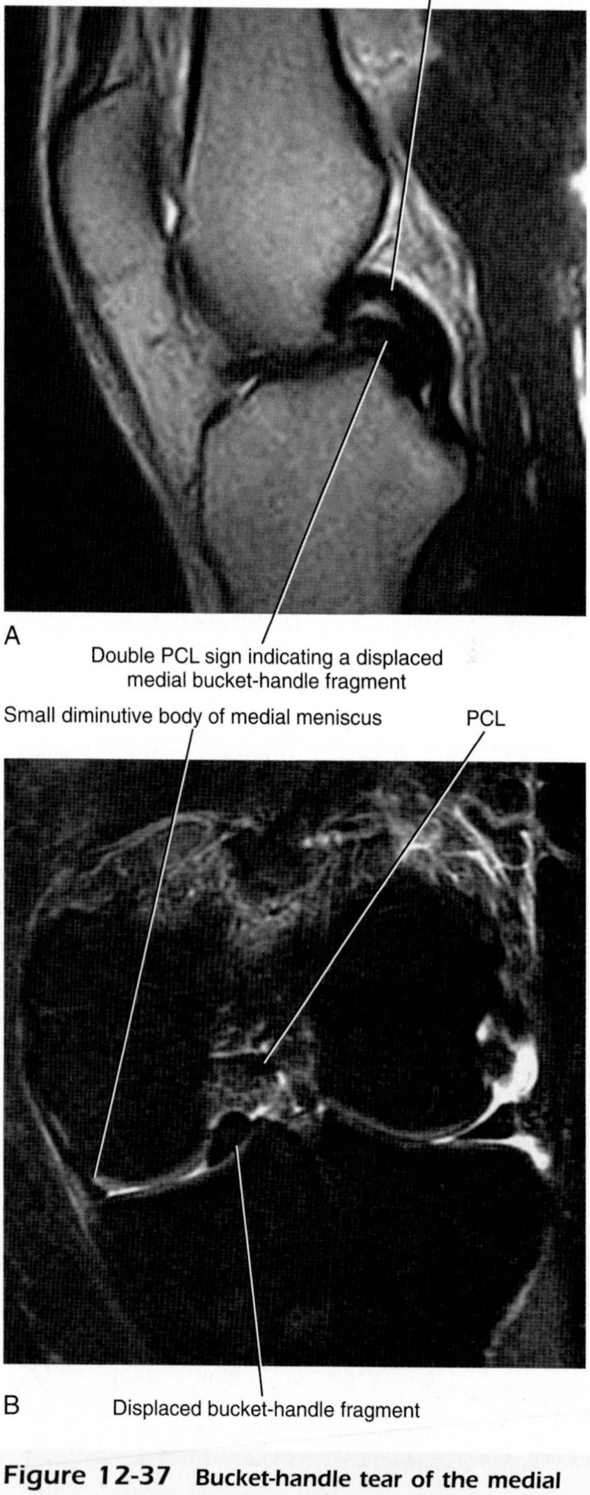
PCL
A
Double PCL sign indicating a displaced medial bucket-handle fragment
Small diminutive body of medial meniscus
PCL
B
Displaced bucket-handle fragment

Figure 12-37 **Bucket-handle tear of the medial meniscus. A,** The double posterior cruciate ligament (PCL) sign with displacement of the bucket-handle fragment into the intercondylar notch. The bucket-handle fragment sits just beneath the PCL. **B,** The displaced bucket-handle fragment sitting beneath the PCL in the coronal imaging plane with a "too small" diminutive body of the medial meniscus.

BOX 12-4 DIRECT SIGNS OF MENISCAL TEAR

Unequivocal surfacing signal on two images
Abnormal meniscal morphology
Displaced or missing meniscal tissue
Meniscocapsular injury or disruption
Intrameniscal fluid on T2-weighted image

association with bucket-handle tears. The *double PCL sign* describes a bucket-handle tear of the medial meniscus in which meniscal tissue is displaced into the intercondylar notch. A linear band of tissue is seen sitting within the intercondylar notch paralleling and just inferior to the PCL and gives the appearance of a double PCL (Fig. 12-37). This sign is often seen in conjunction with a diminutive posterior horn and body of the medial meniscus. Differential diagnosis for the double PCL sign includes an osteophyte extending into the intercondylar notch, a torn displaced ACL, and a prominent meniscal root. The *fragment-in-notch sign* describes a centrally displaced bucket-handle fragment of the medial meniscus that is not seen in the same sagittal imaging plane as the

PCL. The *flipped meniscus sign* describes a bucket-handle fragment that is displaced into the anterior compartment of the knee. Although this is more common in the lateral compartment, the flipped meniscus sign can also be seen with a medial meniscus bucket-handle tear. Bucket-handle tears are 10 times more common medially than laterally. However, when a bucket-handle tear does involve the lateral meniscus, it does not usually result in the double PCL sign because the ACL blocks the bucket-handle fragment from entering the notch. As a result, the displaced fragment usually displaces into the anterior compartment of the knee and sits on top of or adjacent to the anterior horn of the lateral meniscus, giving the appearance of a *large anterior horn* or *double anterior horn*, and an absent or diminutive posterior horn (Fig. 12-38). The reverse, although very uncommon, can also occur in which a fragment from the anterior horn displaces posteriorly to result in a large-appearing posterior horn. In the presence of a bucket-handle tear, the peripheral aspect of the meniscus often appears small or diminutive on sagittal and coronal images (see Fig. 12-37).

Meniscocapsular separation is a special type of meniscal tear in which the meniscus itself demonstrates normal morphology but has been avulsed or torn from its capsular attachment, resulting in a free-floating meniscus. These tears are often subtle because the morphology and appearance of the meniscus remain normal, but the meniscus may be slightly displaced. The meniscus is unstable and may require surgical repair or reattachment. This injury most commonly affects the medial meniscus and is often associated with other significant injuries of the knee including ACL and tibial collateral ligament injury.

MRI may lack sensitivity in detecting a meniscocapsular type of tear, but special attention to the capsular attachments improves diagnostic accuracy. Meniscocapsular separation of the medial meniscus may be seen on MRI as fluid signal extending in a

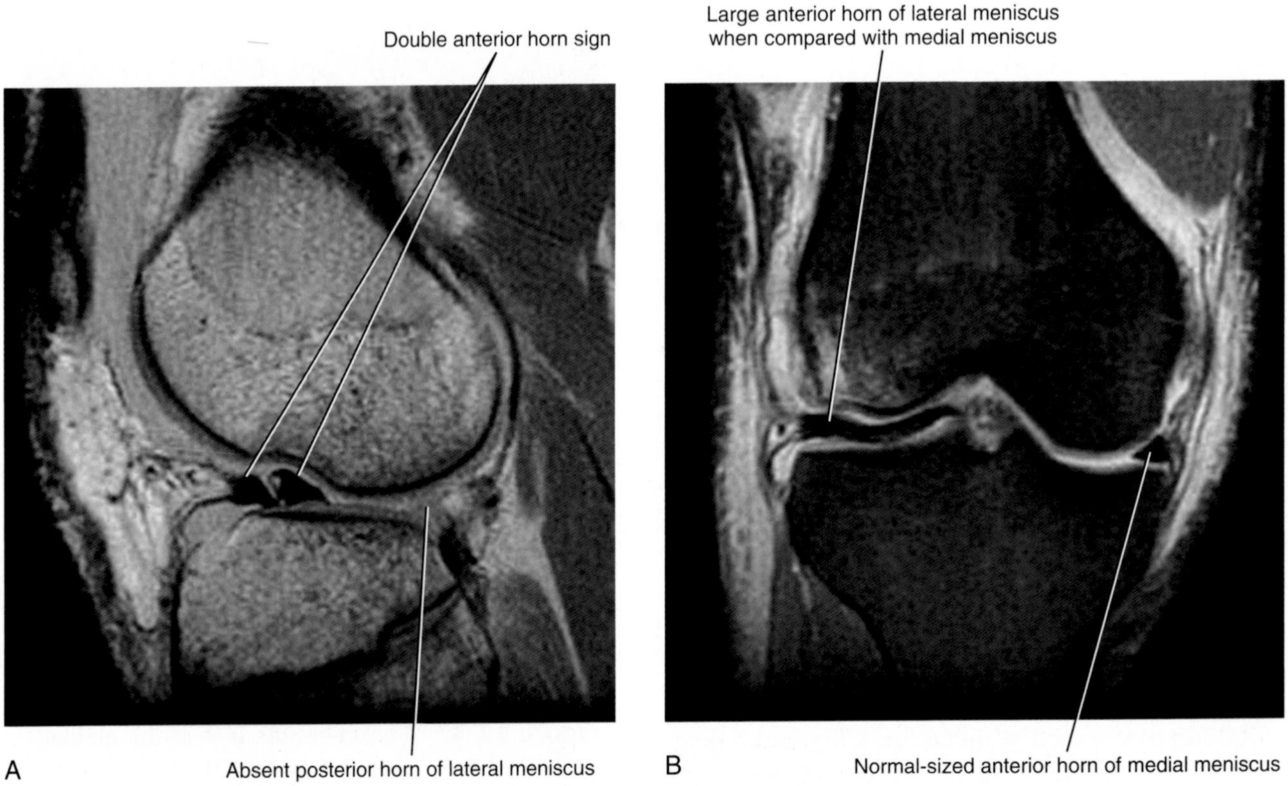
Double anterior horn sign
Large anterior horn of lateral meniscus
when compared with medial meniscus
A
Absent posterior horn of lateral meniscus
B
Normal-sized anterior horn of medial meniscus

Figure 12-38 Bucket-handle tear of the lateral meniscus. Sagittal (**A**) and coronal images (**B**) demonstrate the large anterior horn sign. A bucket-handle fragment of the lateral meniscus is blocked by the anterior cruciate ligament from displacing into the intercondylar notch and instead usually flips anteriorly, creating the appearance of a large or double anterior horn.

vertical orientation between the peripheral aspect of the meniscus and the adjacent capsule (see Fig. 12-36D). It may also be seen as avulsion or disruption of the meniscotibial ligament from the tibial attachment. Lateral meniscocapsular separation may appear as disruption of both the superior and inferior meniscal struts (see Fig. 12-36E). The inferior strut is often absent, and this finding alone does not indicate a disruption of the lateral meniscocapsular attachment. Another sign that has been described is the *floating meniscus sign* seen as fluid completely surrounding the meniscus.

Indirect Signs of Meniscal Tear

Most meniscal tears are easy to detect on MRI, and approximately 80% of tears are "no-brainers" using the standard MRI diagnostic criteria. The rest are debatable, such as fasciculations of the anterior horn lateral meniscus and surfacing signal seen on only a single image. It is these difficult cases in particular in which the secondary imaging signs can be very important and can help improve accuracy with regard to detecting meniscal pathology. The following is a summary of the most commonly encountered indirect MRI signs (Table 12-7).

Table 12-7 Indirect MRI Signs Associated with Meniscal Tears

Imaging Sign	Meniscal Tear
Double PCL sign	Displaced bucket-handle tear of medial meniscus (MM)
Large anterior horn	Displaced bucket-handle tear of lateral meniscus (LM)—fragment displaced anteriorly
Too small or diminutive meniscus	Missing meniscal tissue Prior partial meniscectomy Displaced bucket-handle tear Flipped fragment Chronic tear with resorption of meniscus
Large meniscus	Discoid meniscus Discoid meniscus, usually LM Higher incidence of MM than LM tears
Notch sign	Small notch articular surface of meniscus—high association with meniscal tear
Subchondral edema	Focal subchondral reaction marrow edema directly underlying meniscal tear (nonspecific)
Extruded meniscus (>3 mm)	Seen in association with osteoarthritis—high association with complex tear, radial tear and meniscal root tear

LM, lateral meniscus; MM, medial meniscus; PCL, posterior cruciate ligament.

Medial Meniscal Extrusion Peripheral extrusion of the medial meniscus has been shown to have a high association with (1) a large radial tear or complex tear of the medial meniscus, (2) a tear of the root of the posterior horn of the medial meniscus, and (3) severe degeneration of the medial compartment of the knee. Once the medial meniscus extrudes peripherally, it is no longer capable of distributing the load to protect the medial compartment of the knee, and medial meniscus extrusion has been shown to be a precursor to medial compartment osteoarthritis and spontaneous osteonecrosis (SONC) or insufficiency fracture of the medial femoral condyle or medial tibial plateau. Extrusion of the medial meniscus measuring more than 3 mm at the level of the mid joint line as seen on coronal MR images should prompt a thorough search for either a radial tear of the medial meniscus or especially a tear of the posterior horn meniscal root (Fig. 12-39).

Meniscal Cyst A meniscal cyst is a lobulated fluid collection located within the soft tissues at the level of the joint line that abuts the meniscus. These cysts are nearly always associated with a horizontal cleavage tear or a complex tear of the adjacent meniscus (Fig. 12-40). Meniscal cysts have a very high association with meniscal tears, even if you don't see the tear. This can be especially true when there is a tear in the region of the anterior horn of the lateral meniscus, where a meniscal cyst may be the only sign of a tear. The normal fasciculations of the anterior horn of the lateral meniscus can be difficult to distinguish from a tear, and the presence of a meniscal cyst can help in this regard. In some instances, it may be very difficult to differentiate between a cruciate ganglion and a meniscal cyst arising from the anterior horn of the lateral meniscus.

Cysts can range from a few millimeters in diameter to several centimeters and may be an incidental finding at the time of MRI, or the patient may present clinically with a palpable mass. MRI evaluation for a knee mass should always begin with the standard MRI protocol of the knee to ensure adequate evalua-

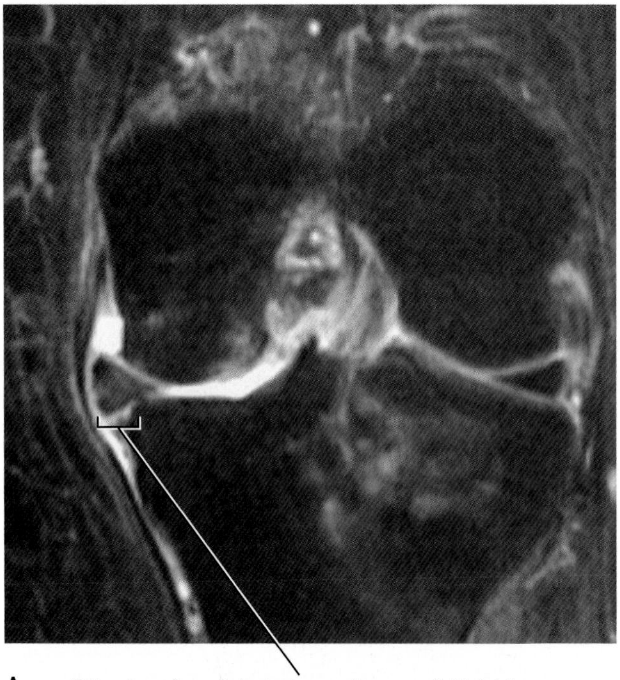
A
Extrusion of medial meniscus along medial joint line

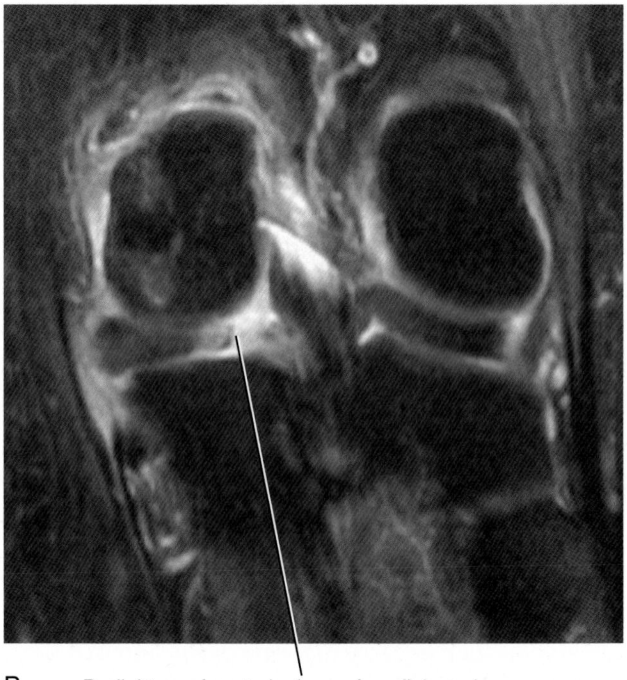
B
Radial tear of posterior horn of medial meniscus associated with meniscal extrusion

Figure 12-39 Extrusion of the medial meniscus. Extrusion of the medial meniscus has been shown to be associated with a tear of either the meniscal root or a vertical tear of the central aspect of the posterior horn of the medial meniscus. Meniscal extrusion is a known precursor of osteoarthritis of the medial compartment of the knee. **A,** Extrusion of the medial meniscus. **B,** A more posterior coronal image from the same patient demonstrates a vertical tear of the medial meniscus immediately adjacent to the meniscal root.

tion of the meniscus, since a palpable mass often turns out to be a meniscal cyst with an associated meniscal tear. A common mistake that is made when developing an MRI protocol for a palpable mass around the knee is to exclude adequate pulse sequences to evaluate the meniscus.

On MRI, a meniscal cyst appears as a lobulated, fluid-filled mass that demonstrates water signal intensity on both T1- and T2-weighted pulse sequences and is usually in direct contact with an adjacent meniscal tear. The cyst can dissect along the joint line for several centimeters and usually takes the path of least resistance. These cycsts can dissect into various recesses within the joint including Hoffa's fat pad anteriorly. Cysts arising from the posterior horn of the medial meniscus can wrap around the PCL and mimic a cruciate ganglion. They can also penetrate the joint capsule and dissect into the subcutaneous tissues of the knee. Occasionally, a meniscal cyst demonstrates intraosseous extension. It is important to alert the orthopedic surgeon to the presence of a meniscal cyst because adequate surgical treatment should address both the meniscal tear and the cyst to prevent recurrence or persistence of symptoms.

Reactive Edema A common MRI finding associated with meniscal tears is reactive soft tissue edema along the joint line or in the adjacent subchondral bone (Fig. 12-41). These are both nonspecific MRI findings but can help draw one's eye to an area of abnormality and should prompt a more thorough evaluation of the adjacent meniscus. This MRI finding may be especially helpful when evaluating the meniscus on a low field strength unit or when the images are limited by artifact or some technical difficulty.

Other Secondary Signs

Other secondary MRI signs that are associated with meniscal tear include focal articular cartilage loss next to the meniscal tear, perimeniscal edema, perivascular edema, and fluid within the substance of the MCL or within the MCL bursa. These findings are all nonspecific but often accompany meniscal pathology.

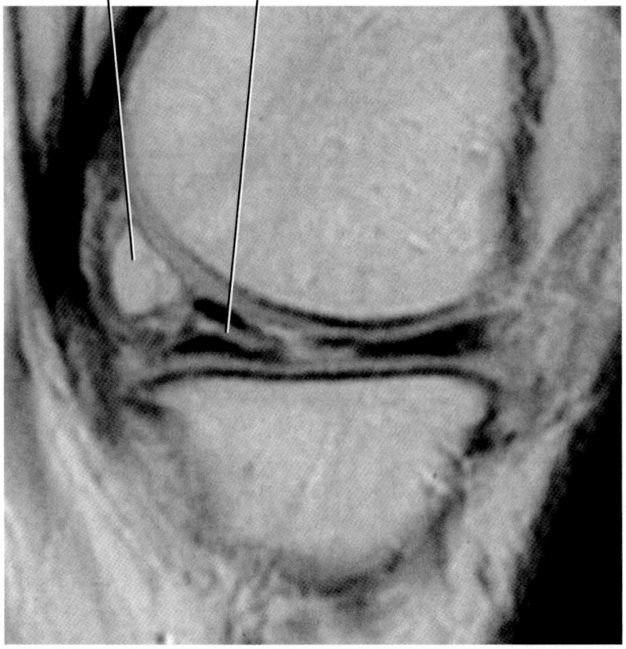
Meniscal cyst
Meniscal cyst

Figure 12-40 Meniscal cysts. Sagittal proton density image demonstrates a lobulated fluid collection at the level of the joint line abutting the posterior horn of the medial meniscus. An extensive horizontal cleavage tear is also present.

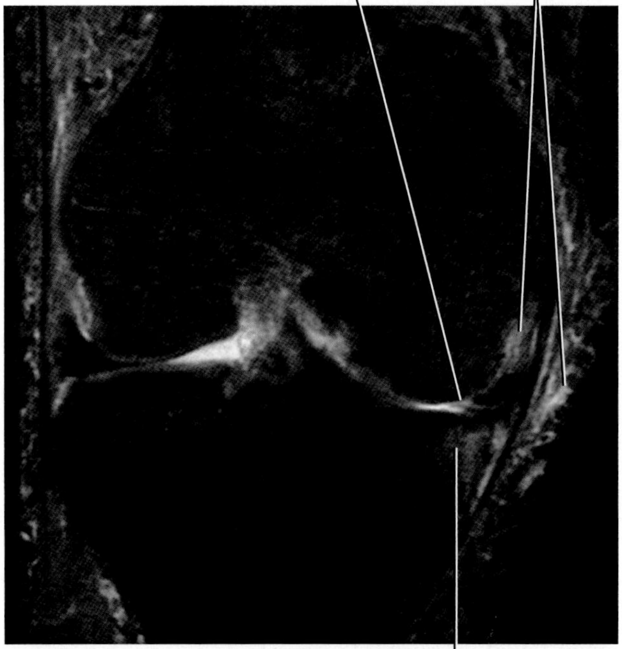
Meniscal tear
Soft tissue edema
Subchondral marrow edema

Figure 12-41 Reactive edema associated with meniscal tears. Coronal T2-weighted image shows reactive subchondral marrow edema in the peripheral aspect of the medial tibial plateau and reactive soft tissue edema both deep and superficial to the medial collateral ligament. These findings are commonly seen in association with a meniscal tear.

Discoid Meniscus A discoid meniscus is an abnormally tall and elongated meniscus that is discoid rather than semilunar in appearance. The etiology appears to be developmental, resulting from variations in the meniscal attachments (deficient). Many discoid menisci also have prominent meniscofemoral ligaments. Although there is some disagreement regarding this point, it is believed by many as well as by the authors that discoid menisci occur only in the lateral meniscus. A classification scheme has been developed based on the amount of meniscal tissue, the degree of tibial plateau coverage, and variations in the attachment of the meniscus. Discoid menisci are clinically significant because their abnormal morphology predisposes them to increased stress on the meniscus, resulting in a higher incidence of meniscal tears. Although discoid menisci occur laterally, there is an increased incidence of both medial and lateral meniscal tears secondary to altered biomechanics of the knee.

Affected persons may present in childhood or early adolescence with an audible click and a palpable snap during flexion and extension of the knee, the Wrisberg variant. Many, however, are first discovered in adults as an incidental finding, and the true incidence in adults is unknown, which may represent a different subset. On MRI, the discoid meniscus is best detected on coronal images, where the meniscus covers more than 50% of the weight-bearing aspect of the femoral condyle or measures more than 14 mm in transverse diameter (Fig. 12-42). Discoid meniscus can also be detected on sagittal MR images, where the meniscus is seen with a continuous connection between the anterior horn and the posterior horn on four or more consecutive images.

Potential Pitfalls in Detecting Meniscal Tears

Although the overall accuracy of MRI for the detection of meniscal tears is in the range of 92% to 95%, discrepancies are occasionally noted between MRI

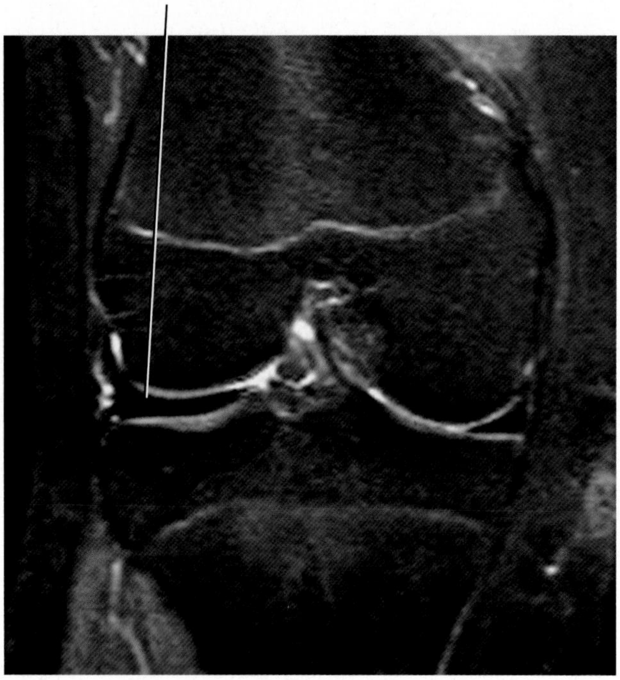
Lateral discoid meniscus covering more than 50% of the lateral femoral condyle articular surface

Figure 12-42 Discoid meniscus. Coronal T2-weighted image shows a large lateral meniscus covering the entire articular surface of the lateral femoral condyle. Lateral discoid menisci are associated with an increased incidence of both medial and lateral meniscal tears.

Table 12-8 Pitfalls in Detecting Meniscal Tears

Category	Specific Pitfall
Normal anatomic structures in close proximity to the meniscus	Anterior transverse meniscal ligament Meniscofemoral ligament Oblique meniscomeniscal ligament Popliteal tendon and hiatus
MRI artifact	Motion Magic angle (PHLM)
Miscellaneous conditions of the meniscus	Intrasubstance degeneration Prominent meniscal vascularity (pediatric age group) Chondrocalcinosis Meniscal ossicle Meniscal flounce Gas within the joint (vacuum phenomenon versus iatrogenic) Adjacent cartilage abnormality
Postsurgical meniscus	Surfacing signal on low TE image Abnormal morphology Missing meniscal tissue

PHLM, posterior horn of the lateral meniscus; TE, echo time.

findings and surgical findings. Potential sources of error include tears that are not visible on the MR images, tears that are missed by the arthroscopist, and interpretation errors made by the MRI reader. It has been shown that the experience level of the reader is one of the most important factors in maximizing the accuracy of MRI interpretation, and knowledge of potential imaging pitfalls helps to prevent many of these interpretation errors. Interpretation errors with regard to meniscal tears can be divided into four broad categories: normal anatomic structures that lie in close proximity to the meniscus, thus simulating grade III signal; pathologic conditions of the meniscus; MRI artifacts; and postsurgical changes of the meniscus (Table 12-8).

Normal Anatomic Structures That Can Mimic Meniscal Pathology

Normal anatomic structures that lie in close proximity to the meniscus often demonstrate MR signal characteristics that are similar to the adjacent meniscus and can be misinterpreted as a tear when they mimic a displaced meniscal fragment or when they mimic surfacing signal at the interface of the meniscus and the adjacent structure. Knowledge of these anatomic structures and their normal MRI appearance can help to avoid these imaging pitfalls.

The attachment of the *anterior transverse meniscal ligament* to the anterior horn of the lateral meniscus can mimic a tear of the anterior horn of the lateral meniscus. This ligament arises from the anterior horn of the lateral meniscus and courses through Hoffa's fat pad to insert onto the anterior horn of the medial meniscus. Its attachment to the anterior horn of the lateral meniscus often mimics surfacing signal and, when combined with the normal fasciculated appearance of the anterior horn lateral meniscus, can be difficult to differentiate from a tear (Fig. 12-43). This pitfall can be avoided by following the ligament on multiple sequential sagittal images from its lateral meniscal to its medial meniscal attachment site. Other principles that help differentiate a tear of the anterior horn lateral meniscus from normal variations include the following

1. Isolated tears of the anterior horn of the lateral meniscus are uncommon.

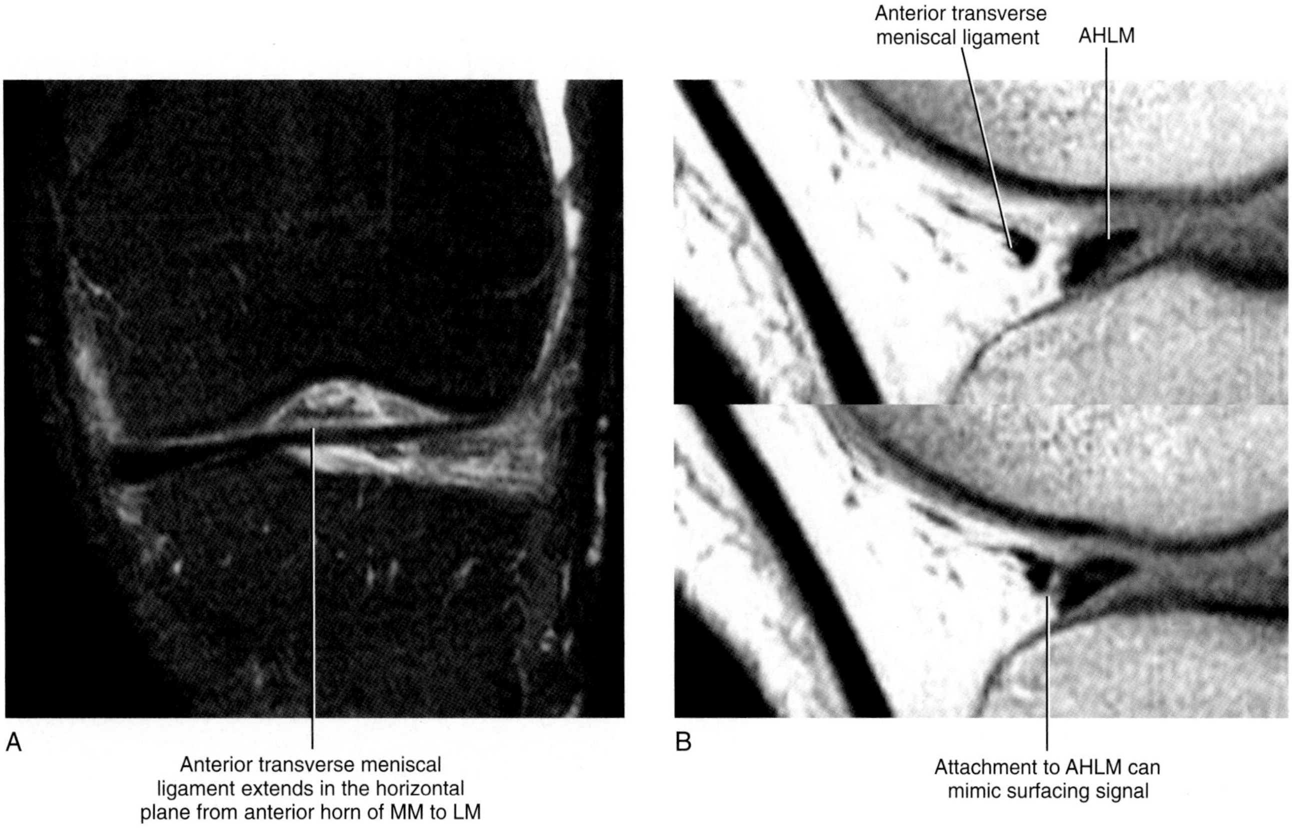
Anterior transverse
meniscal ligament
AHLM
A
Anterior transverse meniscal
ligament extends in the horizontal
plane from anterior horn of MM to LM
B
Attachment to AHLM can
mimic surfacing signal

Figure 12-43 Anterior transverse meniscal ligament. Coronal T2-weighted (**A**) image and sequential sagittal T1-weighted (**B**) images show the anterior transverse meniscal ligament as it extends through Hoffa's fat pad. At the level of attachment to the anterior horn of the lateral meniscus (AHLM), it can mimic a meniscal tear by mimicking surfacing meniscal signal. LM, lateral meniscus; MM, medial meniscus.

2. Follow sequential images peripherally; surfacing signals resulting from a tear usually extend peripherally to at least the junction of the anterior horn and body.
3. Look for secondary signs associated with a meniscal tear (i.e., meniscal cyst, subchondral marrow edema, and so on).

The *meniscofemoral ligament* arises along the central aspect of the posterior horn of the lateral meniscus and extends obliquely to insert onto the inner aspect of the medial femoral condyle. The ligament is composed of two separate bundles: the ligament of Humphry, which is located anterior to the PCL, and the ligament of Wrisberg, which is located posterior to the PCL. In any given patient, one or both ligaments may be present. These ligaments can mimic a tear at their attachment site to the central aspect of the posterior horn of the lateral meniscus or can mimic a displaced meniscal fragment (Fig. 12-44). On occasion, the attachment can be lengthy along the posterior horn of the lateral meniscus and mimic a tear on several sequential sagittal images. This appearance of a lengthy attachment can be problematic, but the pitfall can be avoided by tracing the ligament on sequential sagittal images from its origin along the posterior horn of the lateral meniscus to its insertion on the medial femoral condyle.

The medial and lateral *oblique meniscomeniscal* ligaments are an uncommon source of diagnostic difficulty with a reported incidence of between 1% and 4%. These ligaments extend obliquely from the anterior horn of one meniscus to the posterior horn of the opposite meniscus and are named for their anterior attachment site. As the ligament traverses the intercondylar notch, it passes between the ACL and PCL and can mimic the appearance of a double PCL sign on sagittal MR images, mimicking a displaced

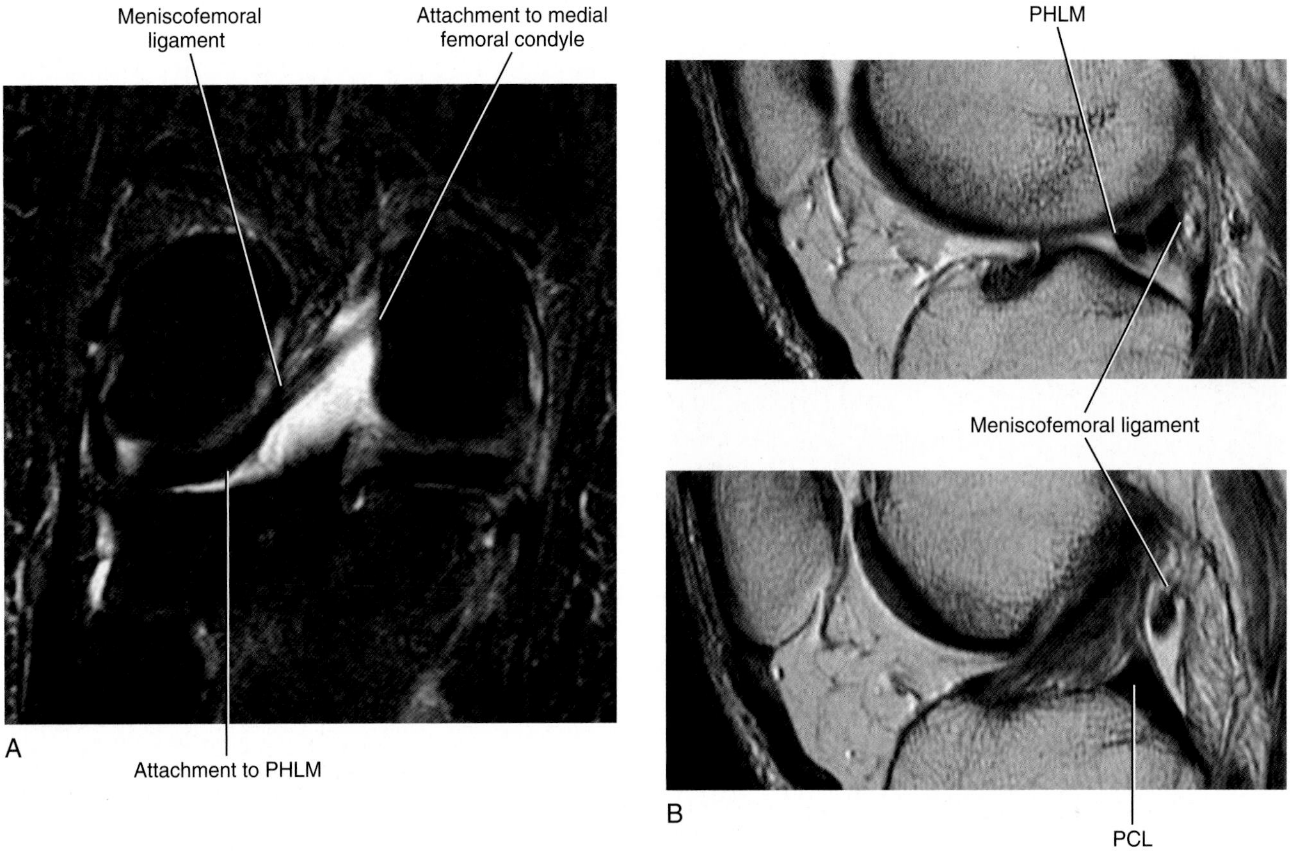
Meniscofemoral ligament
Attachment to medial femoral condyle
A
Attachment to PHLM
PHLM
Meniscofemoral ligament
B
PCL

Figure 12-44 Meniscofemoral ligament. A, Coronal T2-weighted image shows the normal course of the meniscofemoral ligament from the posterior horn of the lateral meniscus (PHLM) to its attachment on the inner aspect of the medial femoral condyle. **B,** Sagittal images show the normal course of the ligament of Wrisberg as it courses posterior to the posterior cruciate ligament. The attachment of the ligament to the PHLM can mimic a tear or a displaced meniscal fragment. PCL, posterior cruciate ligament.

meniscal fragment or bucket-handle tear (Fig. 12-45). Knowledge of the existence of this ligament, its normal anatomic course, and MRI appearance will help prevent the misdiagnosis of a displaced meniscal fragment. The ligament usually mimics a displaced meniscal fragment in the sagittal imaging plane, whereas in the coronal or axial imaging plane the ligament can be traced from the anterior horn of one meniscus through the intercondylar notch to its attachment on the posterior horn of the opposite meniscus.

The *popliteal tendon* sits within the popliteal bursa, which lies in close proximity to the posterior horn of the lateral meniscus. Fluid within the bursa can be mistaken for a meniscal tear (Fig. 12-46). This structure typically mimics a vertical or slightly diagonal tear of the posterior horn of the lateral meniscus.

Artifacts That Can Mimic a Meniscal Tear

Motion artifact is the most common MRI artifact that can result in the misinterpretation of a meniscal tear. Movement of the knee during acquisition of the images can cause blurring and give the false appearance of surfacing signal extending to the articular surface of the meniscus and thus mimicking a tear (Fig. 12-47). One should use extreme caution in diagnosing a meniscal tear on the basis of surfacing signal if motion is present on the images, unless the surfacing signal can be confirmed on other pulse sequences or in additional imaging planes in the absence of motion. If motion is present, the surfacing signal should be ignored and the patient should be brought back for repeat imaging without motion before making the diagnosis of a meniscal tear. Alternatively,

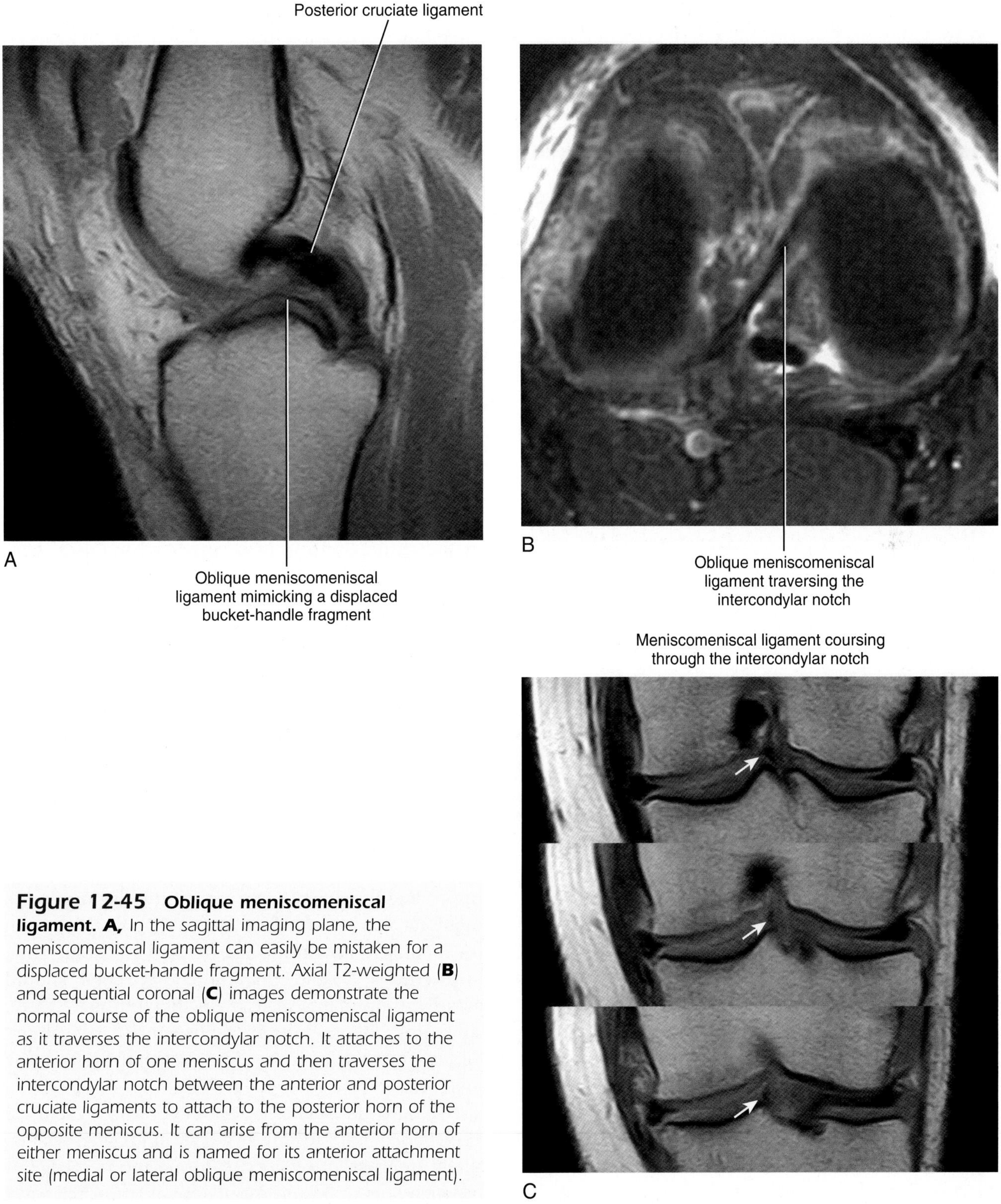
Posterior cruciate ligament
A
Oblique meniscomeniscal ligament mimicking a displaced bucket-handle fragment
B
Oblique meniscomeniscal ligament traversing the intercondylar notch
Meniscomeniscal ligament coursing through the intercondylar notch
C

Figure 12-45 Oblique meniscomeniscal ligament. A, In the sagittal imaging plane, the meniscomeniscal ligament can easily be mistaken for a displaced bucket-handle fragment. Axial T2-weighted (**B**) and sequential coronal (**C**) images demonstrate the normal course of the oblique meniscomeniscal ligament as it traverses the intercondylar notch. It attaches to the anterior horn of one meniscus and then traverses the intercondylar notch between the anterior and posterior cruciate ligaments to attach to the posterior horn of the opposite meniscus. It can arise from the anterior horn of either meniscus and is named for its anterior attachment site (medial or lateral oblique meniscomeniscal ligament).

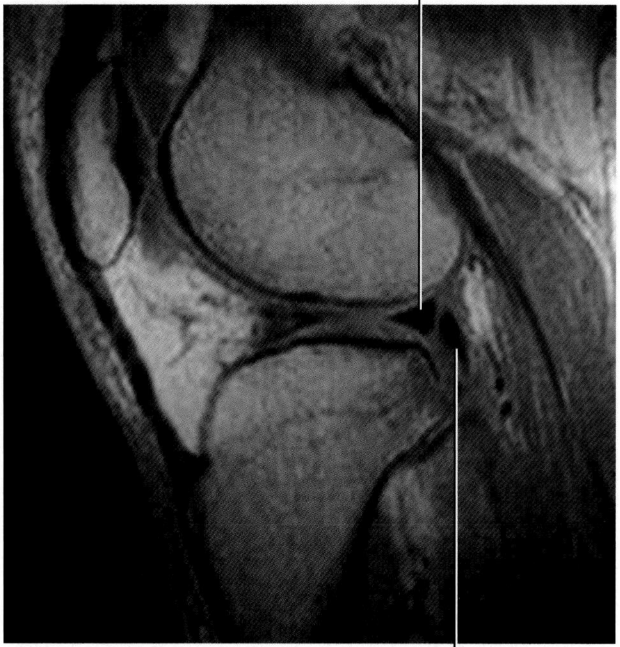
Posterior horn of LM
Popliteal tendon
can mimic a tear

Figure 12-46 Popliteal tendon. Proton density sagittal image shows the popliteus tendon located just posterior to the posterior horn of the lateral meniscus (LM). The space separating the two structures can be misinterpreted as a tear. Following the popliteal tendon on several sequential sagittal images and comparison with T2-weighted images helps to avoid this pitfall.

if the exam is being monitored and motion continues to be a problem, it may be useful to swap the frequency and phase encoding to confirm or refute the presence of surfacing signal.

Magic angle phenomenon may result in areas of intermediate signal intensity on short TE sequences when the structure being imaged is oriented obliquely rather than parallel or perpendicular to the static magnetic field. With regard to the menisci, magic angle phenomenon classically occurs in the central segment of the posterior horn of the lateral meniscus. As viewed in the coronal plane, this portion of the meniscus makes an abrupt upward turn near its posterior central tibial attachment. In this location, increased signal can be seen within the substance of the meniscus on the short TE sequences, mimicking either a meniscal tear or degeneration (Fig. 12-48). Imaging the knee in slight abduction can alter the orientation of the fibers in the posterior aspect of the lateral meniscus and eliminate this artifact. However, simply the knowledge of this potential pitfall is usually sufficient to recognize the increased signal as artifact rather than true meniscal pathology.

Other Meniscal Pathology That Can Mimic a Meniscal Tear

The most problematic mimic of meniscal tear in clinical practice is the presence of *intrasubstance signal,* particularly in the posterior horn of the medial meniscus. Intrasubstance degeneration or prominent vascularity within the posterior horn of the medial meniscus can result in extensive intrasubstance signal that approaches the surface of the meniscus or occasionally extends to the surface of the meniscus on a single image. This appearance can be a source of considerable difficulty and frustration when trying to determine the presence of a meniscal tear, especially in the clinical setting of a suspected meniscal tear. Use of a low field strength system can accentuate the intrasubstance signal within the posterior horn of the medial meniscus. In these instances, the best approach is to accurately describe the MRI findings and to use strict imaging criteria for the diagnosis of a tear. Definite surfacing signal should be identified on two sequential images in the same imaging plane, or if seen on only a single image in one plane, it should be confirmed in the other imaging plane before making the diagnosis of a tear.

In difficult cases, the secondary imaging signs described in a previous section can be very helpful in improving the overall accuracy of the diagnosis of a meniscal tear. A word of caution in working with the pediatric age group in particular is that strict MRI criteria should be applied and one should avoid calling meniscal tears in indeterminate cases, since this often results in a false-positive diagnosis because of prominent residual vascularity within the meniscus.

The *meniscal flounce* is an uncommon meniscal appearance that can mimic a tear and is seen when a single symmetric fold occurs along the free edge of the meniscus. A flounce results in an abnormal wavy S-shaped appearance of the free edge of the meniscus on sagittal images and demonstrates a truncated appearance of the free edge of the meniscus on coronal images. The wavy contour can result in a magic angle phenomenon on the short TE images along the free edge of the meniscus and mimic a

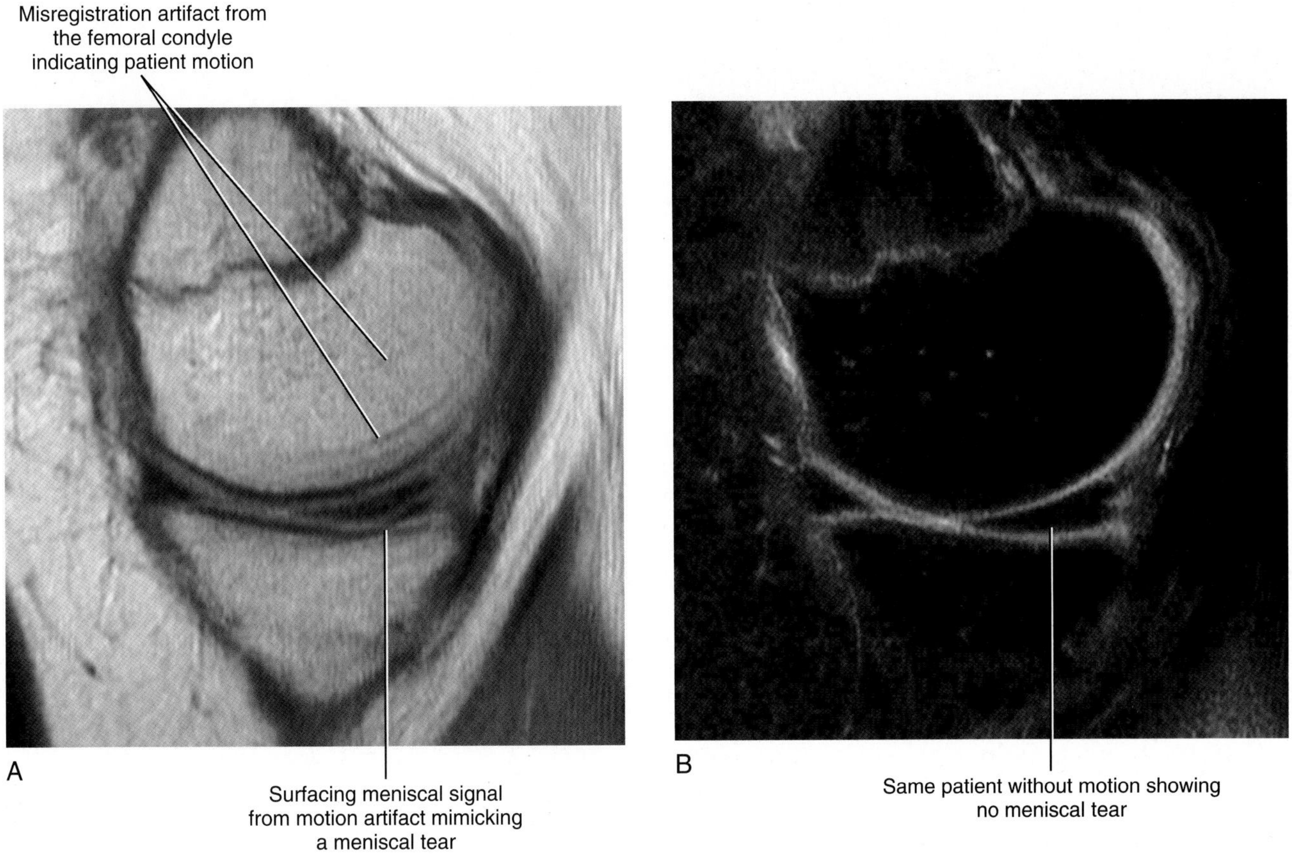
Misregistration artifact from the femoral condyle indicating patient motion
A
Surfacing meniscal signal from motion artifact mimicking a meniscal tear
B
Same patient without motion showing no meniscal tear

Figure 12-47 Motion artifact mimicking a meniscal tear. A, Sagittal proton density image without fat saturation shows surfacing signal mimicking a meniscal tear. Note the misregistration artifact propagated across the image indicating the presence of motion. **B,** Sagittal proton density image with fat saturation obtained without patient motion during the same study shows a normal medial meniscus with no surfacing signal or evidence of a meniscal tear.

meniscal tear or degeneration (Fig. 12-49). The T2-weighted images usually demonstrate the wavy contour of the free edge of the meniscus and help to distinguish a meniscal flounce from a true tear.

The radiographic or pathologic presence of calcification within the fibrocartilage of the meniscus is referred to as *chondrocalcinosis*. The presence of calcification within the meniscus can result in increased signal, mimicking a tear. Correlation with radiographs helps prevent a false-positive diagnosis of a meniscal tear in the presence of chondrocalcinosis (Fig. 12-50). Another potential source of error in the evaluation of the meniscus is the presence of ossification within the meniscus. This is referred to as a *meniscal ossicle* and most commonly occurs in the central aspect of the posterior horn of the medial meniscus (Fig. 12-51). Various theories have suggested that meniscal ossicles are either developmental or are possibly the result of prior trauma to the meniscus. Radiographs demonstrate an intra-articular ossified body in the expected location of the central aspect of the posterior horn of the meniscus. MRI confirms the location of the ossicle as intrameniscal. The ossicle usually demonstrates fat signal intensity seen as high signal on T1-weighted images secondary to the presence of marrow elements. Occasionally, a meniscal tear occurs adjacent to a meniscal ossicle, but the marrow elements of the ossicle should not be misinterpreted as a tear. A meniscal ossicle can be associated with localized pain even without a tear and may require a partial meniscectomy of the affected portion of the meniscus for pain relief.

Gas within the joint can occur as the result of a vacuum phenomenon or iatrogenically from installation of gas during an aspiration or injection of the joint or during an arthrogram. If the gas collects next to the meniscus, the low magnetic susceptibility of gas can produce a discrete signal void on T1-weighted

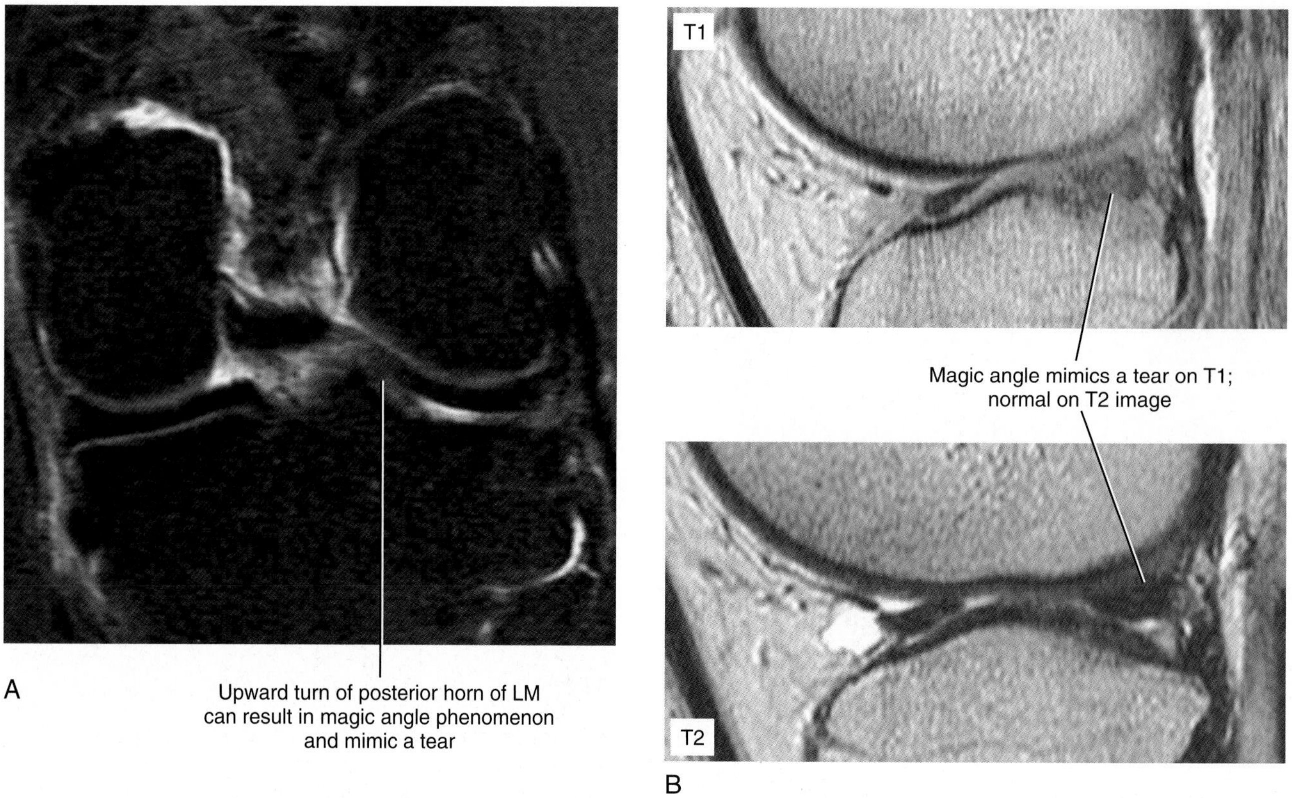
T1
Magic angle mimics a tear on T1; normal on T2 image
T2
A
Upward turn of posterior horn of LM can result in magic angle phenomenon and mimic a tear
B

Figure 12-48 Magic angle posterior horn lateral meniscus mimicking a tear. A, Coronal T2-weighted image shows the normal upward slope of the central aspect of the posterior horn of the lateral meniscus (LM). This upward curvature can result in magic angle phenomenon on short echo time sequence images through this region of the meniscus. **B,** Sagittal T1-weighted and T2-weighted images through the curved portion of the posterior horn of the lateral meniscus shows extensive signal within the meniscus on the short TE sequence but normal intrinsic signal on the T2-weighted image. One should be cautious in calling a tear when signal is isolated to this area of the lateral meniscus, especially if the T2-weighted image shows normal signal and morphology.

images that can simulate a tear or a displaced meniscal fragment. Careful technique during performance of an arthrogram and once again radiographic correlation can help one avoid this pitfall. Finally, articular cartilage abnormalities are another source of error when evaluating the meniscus. There are case reports of chondral flap tears or chondral fragments being misinterpreted as displaced meniscal fragments. Evaluation of the cartilage-sensitive techniques in addition to evaluation of short TE sequence images should help to prevent this pitfall.

Postoperative changes of the meniscus can also be a source of considerable difficulty when evaluating the meniscus for evidence of tear. This topic is discussed in detail later in the section, Imaging of the Postoperative Knee.

EXTENSOR MECHANISM

The extensor mechanism is composed of the quadriceps and patellar tendons, the medial and lateral retinacular structures, the patella and the trochlear groove portion of the distal femur, the suprapatellar and infrapatellar (Hoffa's) fat pads, and several bursae. A wide variety of pathologic processes, injuries, and anatomic variations can affect these structures and result in anterior knee pain. The next section summarizes the various abnormalities that can affect the extensor mechanism and describes some of the common pitfalls that mimic pathology.

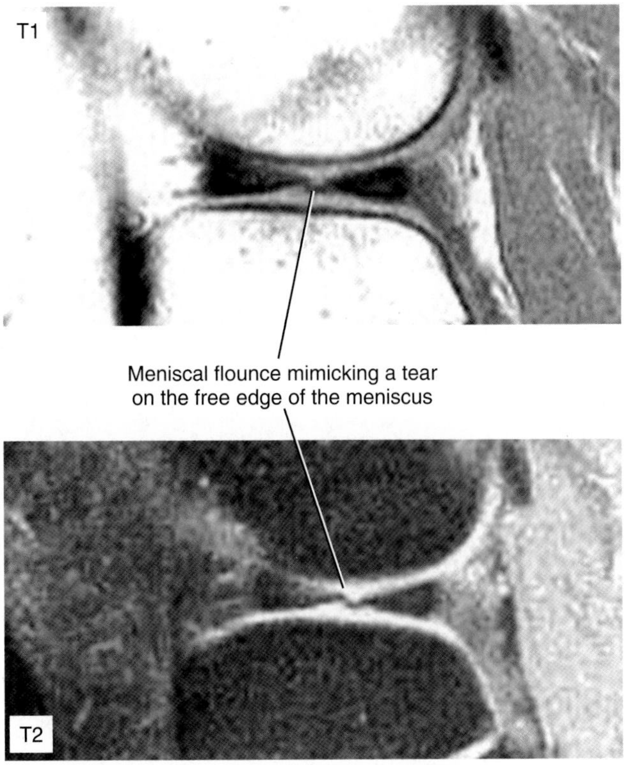
T1
Meniscal flounce mimicking a tear
on the free edge of the meniscus
T2

Figure 12-49 Meniscal flounce. Sagittal T1- and T2-weighted images demonstrate a wavy or undulating contour of the free edge of the lateral meniscus. This represents a normal variant buckling of the free edge of the meniscus and is usually positional in etiology. A meniscal flounce should not be misinterpreted as an abnormal morphology or tear of the meniscus.

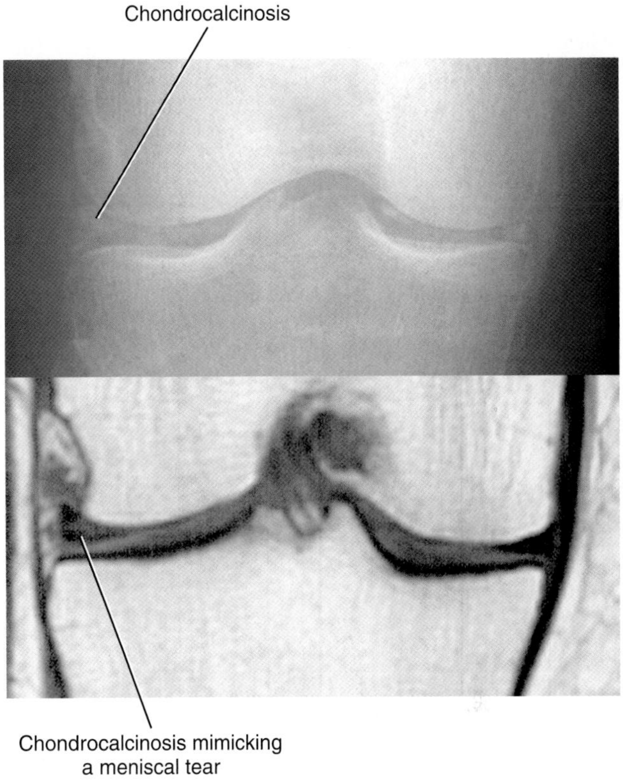
Chondrocalcinosis
Chondrocalcinosis mimicking
a meniscal tear

Figure 12-50 Chondrocalcinosis. Anteroposterior radiograph of the knee and coronal T1-weighted of same patient reveals areas of chondrocalcinosis within the meniscus on the radiograph. Chondrocalcinosis is seen as surfacing signal on the T1-weighted image, mimicking a meniscal tear. This pitfall can be avoided by comparing the MR image with radiographs.

Patella

Articular Cartilage Abnormalities

Abnormalities of the patellar articular cartilage are the most common source of anterior knee pain, and several cartilage-specific sequences have been developed to aid in the evaluation of articular cartilage. GRE imaging is highly accurate in the detection and description of articular cartilage abnormalities. However, it is of little value when evaluating other structures of the knee such as marrow, tendons, and ligaments. In addition, GRE sequences are lengthy and significantly increase the overall exam time. Moreover, they are prone to artifacts (magnetic susceptibility).

Promising research is also being performed in the area of T2 relaxation time mapping, and this MRI technique appears capable of identifying areas of early breakdown of the collagen component of the matrix and identifying areas of early cartilage abnormality prior to morphologic changes demonstrated on conventional MRI. This area requires additional study but may one day be used in standard clinical practice for detection of early chondral changes.

In current clinical practice, the T2-weighted fast spin-echo and proton density sequences with fat saturation are most commonly used in the evaluation of the articular cartilage. These sequences provide adequate signal-to-noise ratio and contrast to differentiate the articular cartilage (intermediate signal intensity) from the underlying cortex (low signal intensity). The presence of joint fluid, which appears bright on these sequences, increases the conspicuity of patellar cartilage abnormalities.

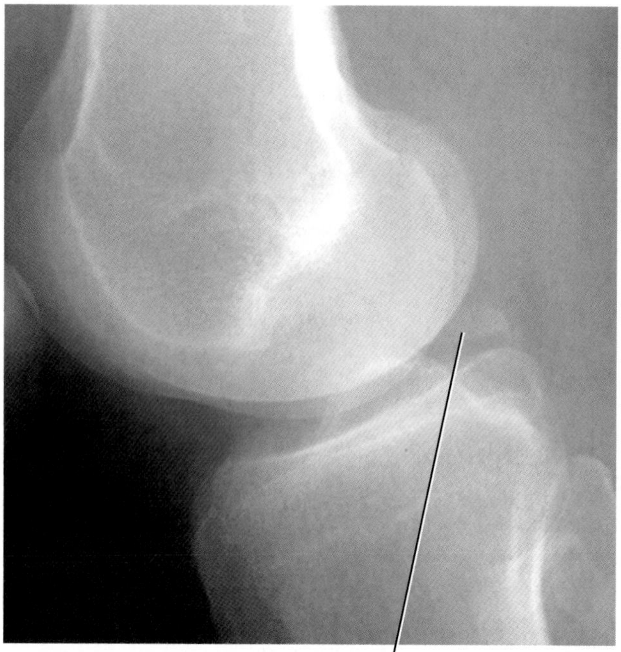
A
Meniscal ossicle located in posteromedial aspect of knee

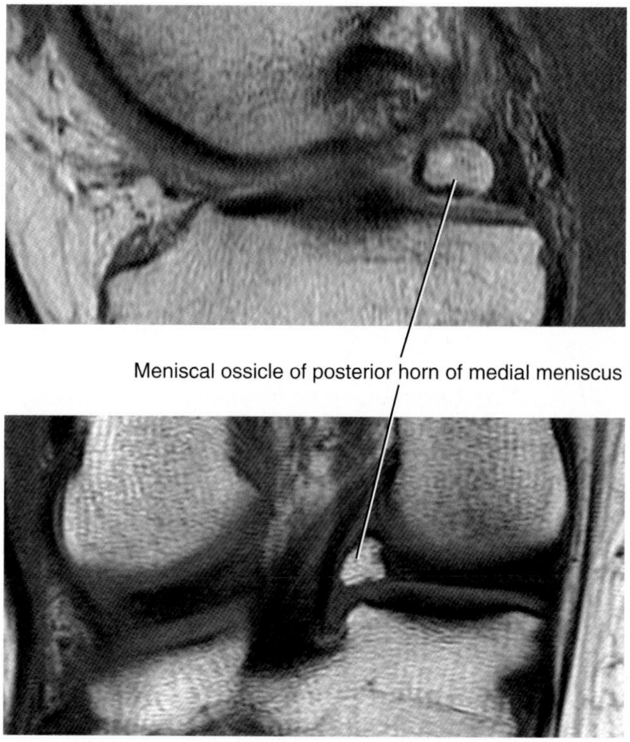
Meniscal ossicle of posterior horn of medial meniscus
B

Figure 12-51 Meniscal ossicle. A, Lateral radiograph of the knee shows the meniscal ossicle in the posterior aspect of the knee. **B,** Sagittal and coronal T1-weighted images confirm the location of the meniscal ossicle within the posterior horn of the medial meniscus. The high signal intensity within the ossicle is indicative of fatty marrow elements. There is no surfacing signal or evidence of a meniscal tear.

The term "chondromalacia" is a clinical term used to describe patellar cartilage degeneration resulting in pain associated with the extensor mechanism. A four-point grading system has been developed and widely used to describe the extent of articular cartilage abnormality (Table 12-9). Recently however, several new cartilage repair techniques have been developed, and as a result an even more precise method of describing lesions of the articular cartilage is required when evaluating the preoperative MRI. It is best to use descriptive terms (Table 12-10) to precisely describe articular cartilage abnormalities within the body of the report. Then if necessary, the four-point grading system can be used as a method of summarizing the extent of articular cartilage abnormality (Fig. 12-52). The patellar articular cartilage is best evaluated on MRI using the axial and sagittal imaging planes.

There are a few potential pitfalls that can mimic an abnormality of the patellar articular cartilage. Perhaps the most troubling is the presence of motion artifact that results from flowing blood in the popliteal vessels. This artifact occurs in the phase-encoding direction and results in a "ghosting" or replication of the appearance of the popliteal vessels in a predictable frequency (Fig. 12-53). To the unsuspecting, this artifact can mimic the appearance of a focal cartilage

Table 12-9 Grading System for Describing Articular Cartilage Abnormalities

Grade	MR Findings
Grade I (low grade)	Swelling, abnormal signal, surface irregularity/thinning (<50% of articular cartilage thickness)
Grade II (intermediate grade)	Thinning of articular cartilage (>50%, but less than full thickness)
Grade III (high grade)	Full-thickness cartilage loss but no underlying marrow signal change
Grade IV (high grade)	Full-thickness articular cartilage loss with underlying marrow signal abnormalities

defect. It can be easily differentiated as artifact because it repeats itself at regular intervals across the entire image. This pitfall is easily eliminated by changing the direction of the phase encoding from the anteroposterior direction to the transverse direction on axial images of the knee or by applying out-of-plane saturation bands above and below the area of interest.

Table 12-10 Descriptive Terms for Articular Cartilage Abnormalities

Diffuse abnormalities	Diffuse low signal (T2-weighted)—degeneration/dehydration Diffuse thinning Diffuse loss—denuded of articular cartilage Diffuse surface irregularity—fraying
Focal lesions	Describe specific location (medial/lateral patellar facet, lateral trochlear groove, etc.) Size of defect Partial-versus full-thickness defect Subchondral marrow signal change/subchondral cysts Cartilage flap tear

The posterior surface of the patella is composed of four components: the medial patellar facet, lateral patellar facet, median eminence, and odd facet. The *odd facet* is a vertically oriented non–load-bearing facet located along the most peripheral aspect of the medial patella, which lacks articular cartilage (Fig. 12-54). The lack of articular cartilage on the odd facet can mimic a focal chondral defect, and this is most likely to occur in the presence of a large joint effusion, which accentuates the absence of articular cartilage on this facet.

Patellar fractures typically occur as a result of direct trauma but may also result from avulsion of either the patellar or quadriceps tendon or from avulsion of the medial soft tissue restraints after a transient dislocation of the patella. Fractures usually appear as a focal area of linear low-signal abnormality on both T1- and T2-weighted images, and in the acute or subacute phase they demonstrate adjacent marrow edema (Fig. 12-55). Fractures may be oriented in either the vertical or horizontal plane or may be comminuted and complex in appearance. All three image planes can be helpful in identifying fractures of the patella. The coronal imaging plane is of particular help in

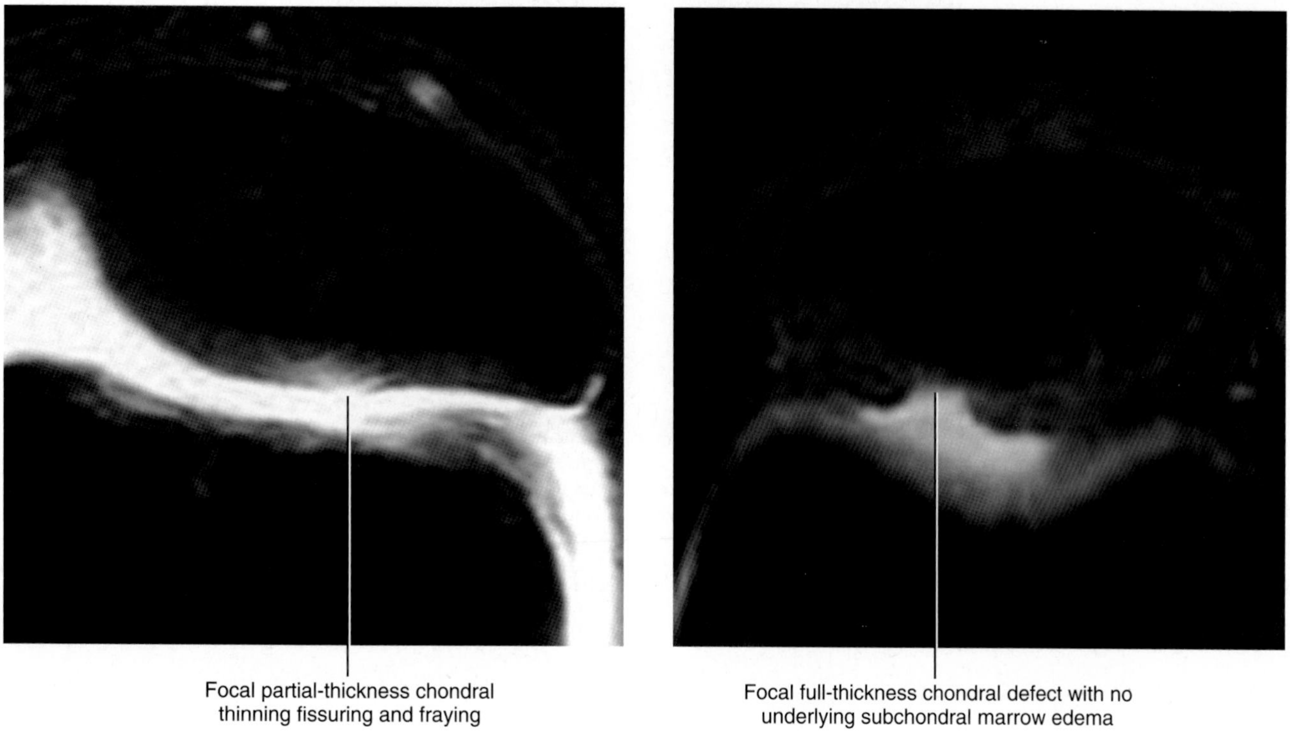
Focal partial-thickness chondral thinning fissuring and fraying
Focal full-thickness chondral defect with no underlying subchondral marrow edema

Figure 12-52 Descriptive terms for articular cartilage abnormalities. *Continued*

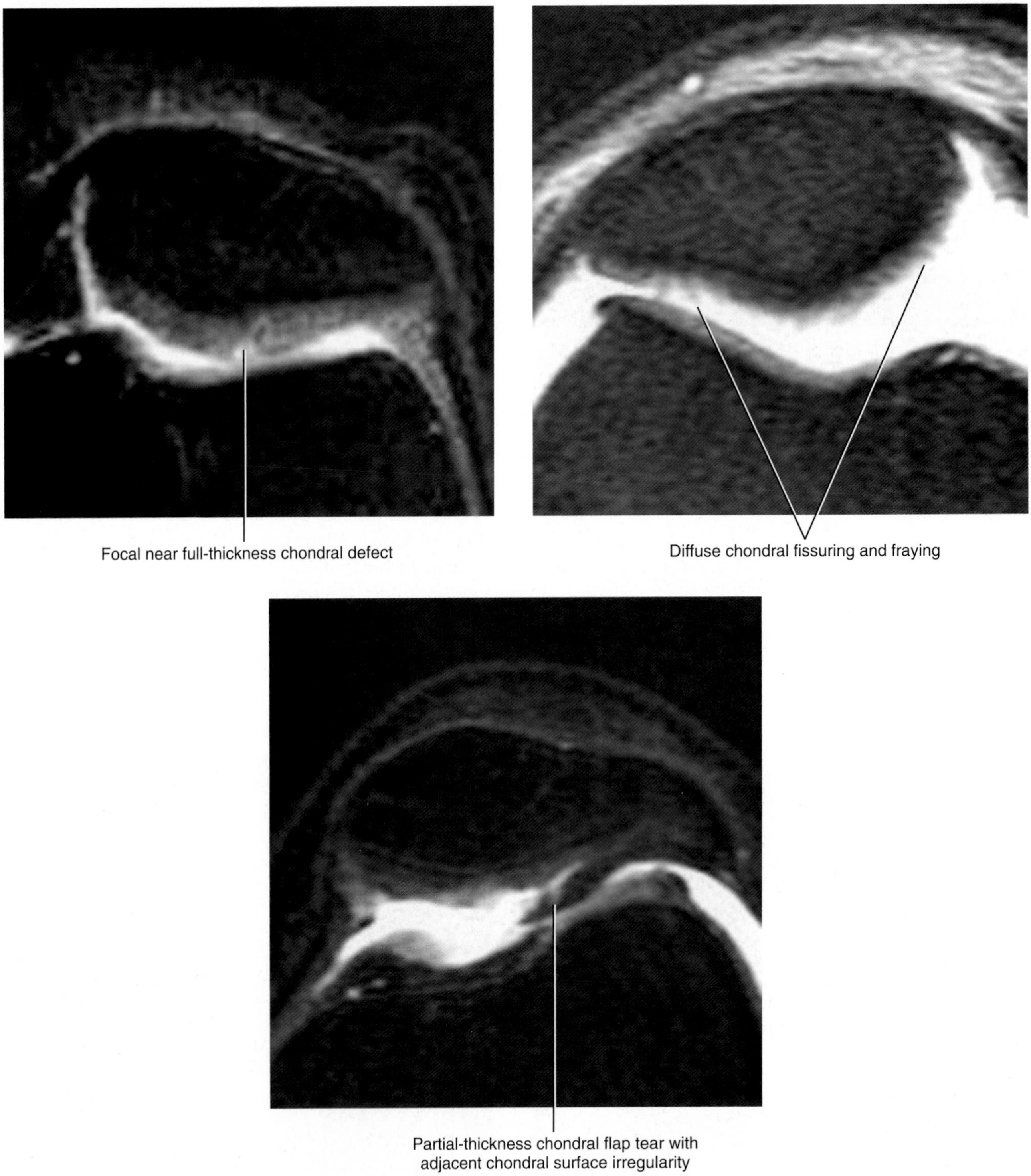
Focal near full-thickness chondral defect
Diffuse chondral fissuring and fraying
Partial-thickness chondral flap tear with adjacent chondral surface irregularity

Figure 12-52, cont'd Descriptive terms for articular cartilage abnormalities.

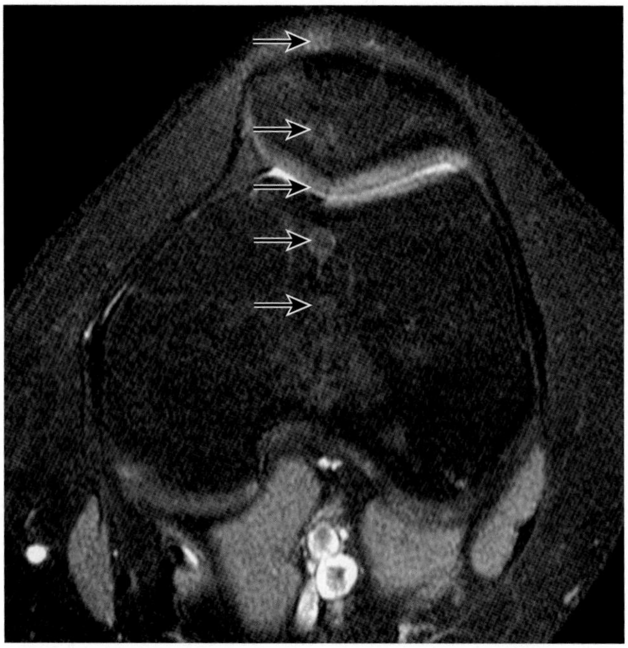

Phase-encoding artifact propagated across image can mimic a chondral defect of the trochlear groove and patellar surface

Figure 12-53 Phase-encoding artifact mimicking a chondral lesion. Axial T2-weighted image shows pulsation artifact from the popliteal vessels propagated across the patella in the axial imaging plane mimicking a focal chondral lesion.

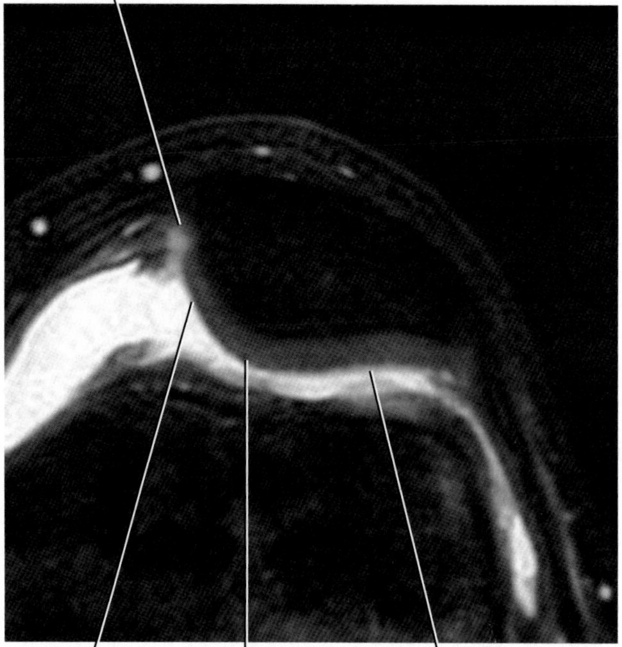
Odd facet
Medial patellar facet
Median eminence
Lateral patellar facet

Figure 12-54 **Odd facet.** The posterior patella is composed of four components: lateral patellar facet, median eminence, medial patellar facet, and odd facet. The odd facet is a vertically oriented nonload-bearing facet located along the medial aspect of the patella. Because it is non–weight-bearing, it has no articular cartilage. This normal nonarticular portion of the medial patella is often misinterpreted as a focal osteochondral defect. This area may be especially problematic when there is a large joint effusion or focal subcortical marrow edema in this area such as after a transient dislocation of the patella.

identifying these fractures, and the standard coronal images of the knee should cover the entire patella. The axial and sagittal images are best suited for defining the extent of articular surface step-off. Axial imaging through the patella with CT can be very helpful in determining the precise orientation of the fracture and in determining the extent of articular surface step-off.

Bipartite Patella

A common pitfall that can mimic a patellar fracture is a bipartite patella. Typically regarded as a developmental anomaly, the bipartite patella results from the failure of fusion of separate ossification centers. It has been suggested that this failure of fusion may be related to chronic tension placed on the skeletally immature patella. The unfused ossification center is nearly always located in the superolateral aspect of the patella and is often bilateral. MRI demonstrates an oval or rounded well-corticated ossification center located in the superolateral aspect of the patella with intact articular cartilage overlying the junction. The gap should demonstrate low signal on both T1- and T2-weighted images. The location and typical MRI appearance are usually sufficient to differentiate a bipartite configuration from a patellar fracture.

A bipartite patella is usually an incidental finding, but a patient may occasionally present with symptoms of anterior knee pain. When symptomatic, MRI usually shows marrow edema on either side of the synchondrosis, and fluid may be within the synchondrosis. There may also be fragmentation or irregularity of the ossification center. Separation or a gap in the overlying articular cartilage is also associated with a symptomatic bipartite configuration (Fig. 12-56).

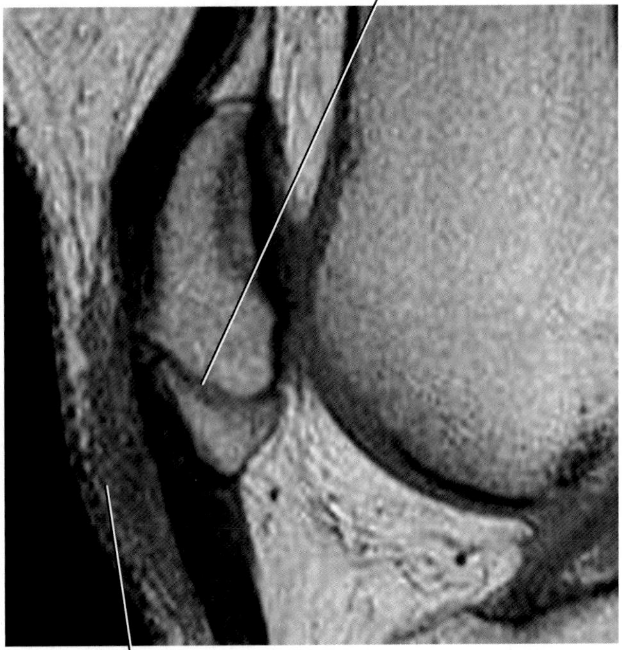
Transverse fracture of lower pole of patella
Overlying soft tissue edema

Figure 12-55 Patellar fracture. Sagittal T1-weighted image demonstrates a transverse fracture through the lower pole of the patella resulting from direct trauma. Note the overlying soft tissue edema resulting from direct trauma to the knee.

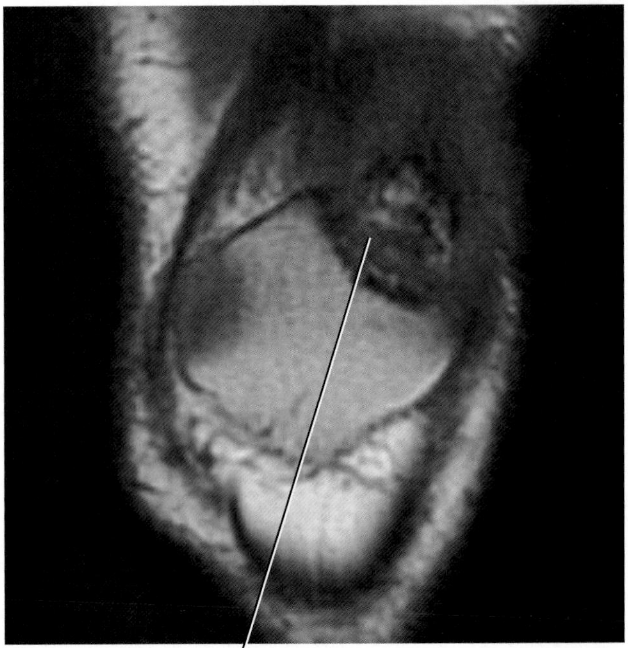
A
Bipartite patella: Separation and irregularity of ossification center

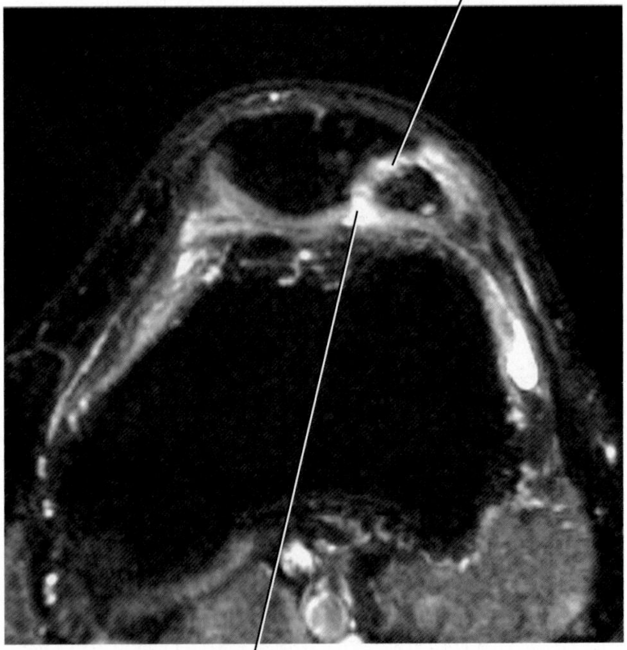
Fluid within synchondrosis
B
Cartilage defect overlying gap

Figure 12-56 Symptomatic bipartite patella. Coronal T1-weighted (**A**) and T2-weighted axial (**B**) images show a bipartite patella with widening of the synchondrosis, irregularity of the bipartite ossification center, fluid within the synchondrosis, and a cartilage defect overlying the junction. These changes indicate instability at the level of the synchondrosis and can be associated with anterior knee pain.

Findings on CT examination that are associated with symptoms are subcortical cysts and arthritis at the junction. A bone scan reveals no uptake in the asymptomatic patient, but may be warm or hot in the patient with a symptomatic bipartite configuration.

Dorsal Patellar Defect

The dorsal patellar defect is another anatomic variant that is thought to result from abnormal ossification. Like the bipartite patella, it typically occurs in the superolateral pole of the patella and may be related to traction forces resulting from the insertion of the vastus lateralis. The defect appears as a well-defined oval or round lesion in the subchondral bone of the superolateral aspect of the patella. It can be easily detected on radiographs or CT imaging. Although the defect can mimic an osteochondral injury or articular cartilage defect, MRI most often reveals a well-defined oval area of signal alteration in the subchondral bone of the superolateral aspect of the patella with normal overlying articular cartilage. The defect is occasionally difficult to detect on MRI, but at times the overlying articular cartilage may demonstrate surface irregularity or fissuring, in which case the defect may be symptomatic (Fig. 12-57).

Patellar Tendinopathy

The patellar tendon extends from the lower pole of the patella to insert onto the anterior tibial tuberosity. On MRI, the normal tendon demonstrates homogeneous dark signal. Injury can range from tendinopathy to partial or complete disruption of the tendon. Patients with patellar tendinopathy typically present with anterior knee pain, and the condition has been referred to as jumper's knee because of its prevalence in athletes participating in sports that require frequent jumping such as basketball. Patellar tendinopathy is seen on MRI as increased intrinsic signal and thickening of the tendon, and cases of moderate to marked tendinopathy are easily diagnosed with MRI. However, early or subtle changes can present a diagnostic challenge.

Commonly, the earliest changes of patellar tendinopathy manifest as subtle changes that typically occur first along the medial aspect of the tendon immediately adjacent to its attachment on the lower pole of the patella. MRI signs of early tendinosis include focal thickening of the tendon and globular signal alteration within the proximal aspect of the tendon. Patellar tendinopathy is often associated with edema in the underlying Hoffa's fat pad (Fig. 12-58). Subtle striations, intermediate in signal intensity and located within the substance of the tendon at the proximal attachment site, are considered a normal MRI appearance of the patellar tendon. Mild thickening and increased T2 signal are diagnostic of tendinopathy. Fluid signal within the substance of the tendon indicates a partial-thickness tear, whereas complete disruption of the tendon (Fig. 12-59) appears as discontinuity and retraction of the tendon fibers and proximal migration of the patella—*patella alta*.

There may be variations in the appearance of the normal patellar tendon, and several of these variations can mimic tendinopathy. First, the patellar

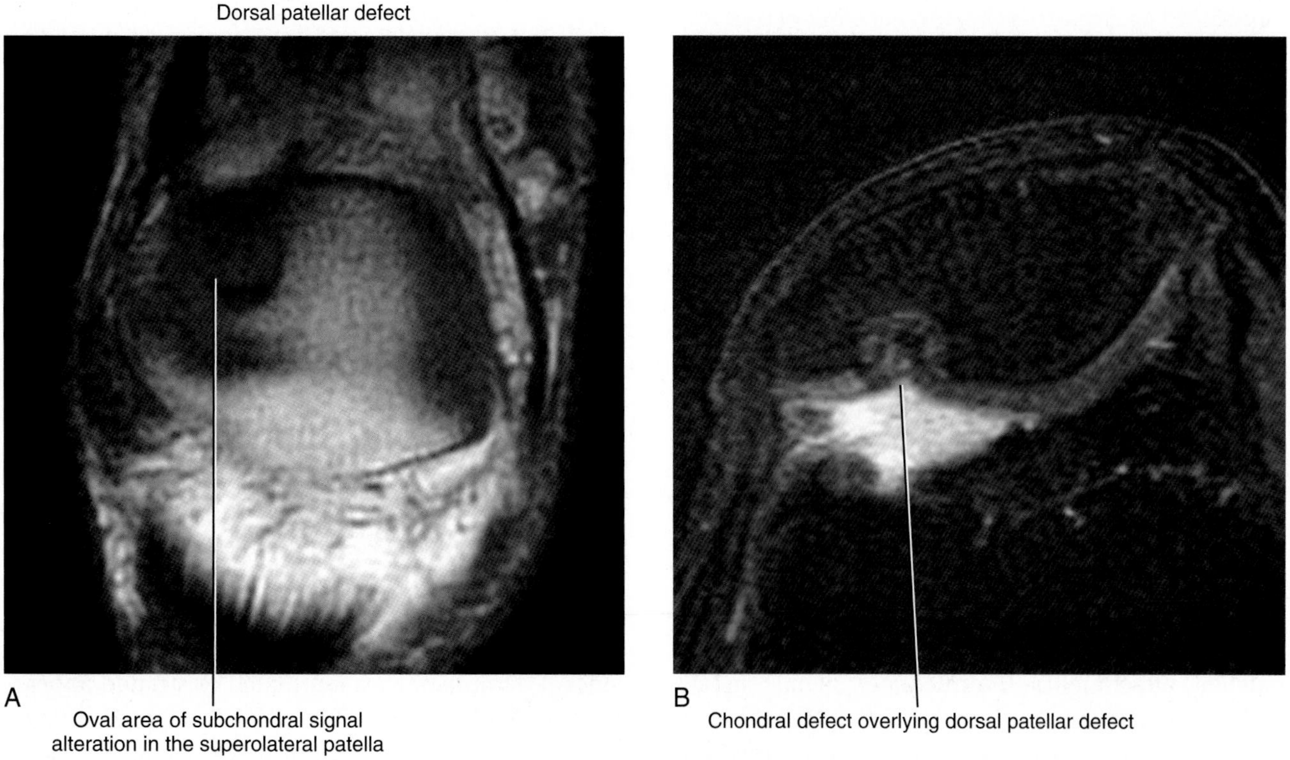
Dorsal patellar defect
A
Oval area of subchondral signal alteration in the superolateral patella
B
Chondral defect overlying dorsal patellar defect

Figure 12-57 Symptomatic dorsal patellar defect. Coronal T1-weighted (**A**) and axial T2-weighted (**B**) images demonstrate a dorsal patellar defect with an overlying articular cartilage defect. Although most dorsal patellar defects are incidental lesions and asymptomatic, overlying articular cartilage abnormality may result in associated symptoms.

SECTION IV

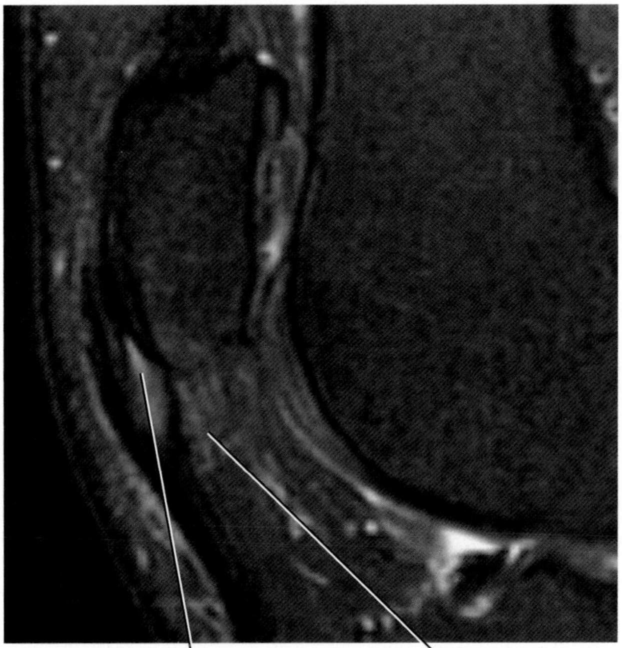
Patellar tendinosis
Subtle thickening and edema in proximal patellar tendon
Minimal edema Hoffa's fat pad

Figure 12-58 Patellar tendinopathy. Sagittal T2-weighted image demonstrates mild thickening and increased T2-weighted signal within the proximal patellar tendon consistent with patellar tendinopathy. There is also subtle edema in underlying Hoffa's fat pad.

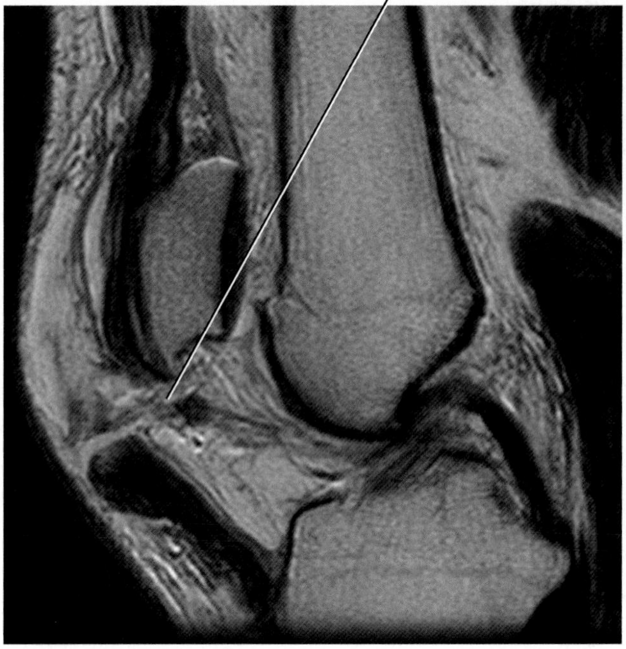
Complete disruption of patellar tendon

Figure 12-59 Patellar tendon rupture. T2-weighted sagittal image shows complete disruption of the patellar tendon at the level of attachment to the lower pole of the patella.

tendon occasionally demonstrates a lax or buckled appearance (Fig. 12-60). This normal variant results from laxity of the tendon that occurs when the knee is fully extended. On T1-weighted sagittal images, this wavy appearance may result in focal areas of intermediate signal intensity within the substance of the tendon secondary to magic angle artifact. On T2-weighted sagittal images, however, the normal tendon demonstrates homogeneous low signal throughout the length of the tendon.

Another potential pitfall is the presence of increased T1 signal, which commonly occurs within the substance of the tendon immediately adjacent to the patellar attachment. Intermediate signal streaks within the substance of any tendon at the level of attachment are usually normal findings. However, increased T2 signal at the same location is usually evidence of early tendinopathy. Finally, at the level of the distal attachment of the patellar tendon, the anterior tibial tuberosity may appear fragmented with associated thickening of the distal fibers of the patellar tendon. In the adult patient, this appearance usually represents the sequela of old Osgood-Schlatter disease, and in most instances it is asymptomatic. In the adolescent or young adult patient, increased T2 signal and thickening of the distal patellar tendon in association with fragmentation of the anterior tibial tuberosity, adjacent soft tissue, and marrow edema indicate acute Osgood-Schlatter disease (Fig. 12-61).

Quadriceps Tendinopathy

The distal quadriceps tendon is formed by the coalescence of four separate tendons arising from the vastus lateralis, vastus medialis, vastus intermedius, and the rectus femoris muscles. As a result, the normal tendon demonstrates a laminated or striated appearance on MRI. On both T1- and T2-weighted images, the tendon demonstrates linear streaks of intermediate signal oriented longitudinally within the substance of the distal quadriceps tendon. This appearance can present a source of diagnostic difficulty when evaluating the distal quadriceps tendon.

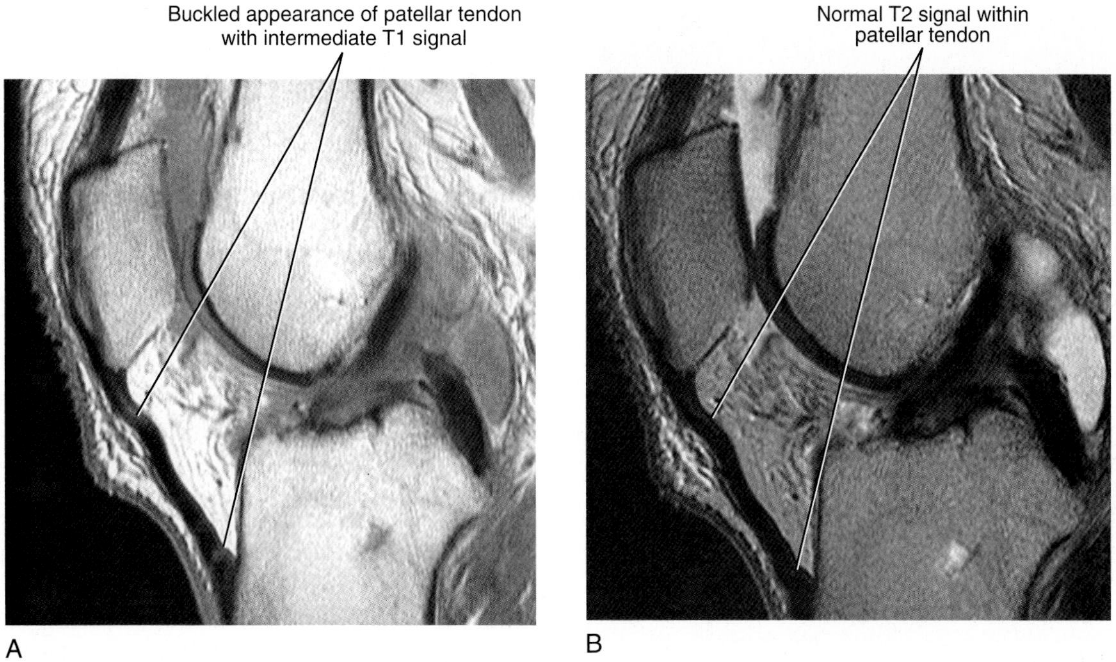
Buckled appearance of patellar tendon with intermediate T1 signal
Normal T2 signal within patellar tendon
A
B

Figure 12-60 Alterations in the appearance of the patellar tendon that can mimic tendinopathy. Sagittal T1-weighted (**A**) and T2-weighted (**B**) images show a buckled or lax appearance of the patellar tendon. On the T1-weighted image, there is increased signal in the region of buckling of the tendon resulting from magic angle artifact. These areas demonstrate normal low signal intensity on the T2-weighted image, which is a normal appearance of the patellar tendon and does not represent tendinopathy.

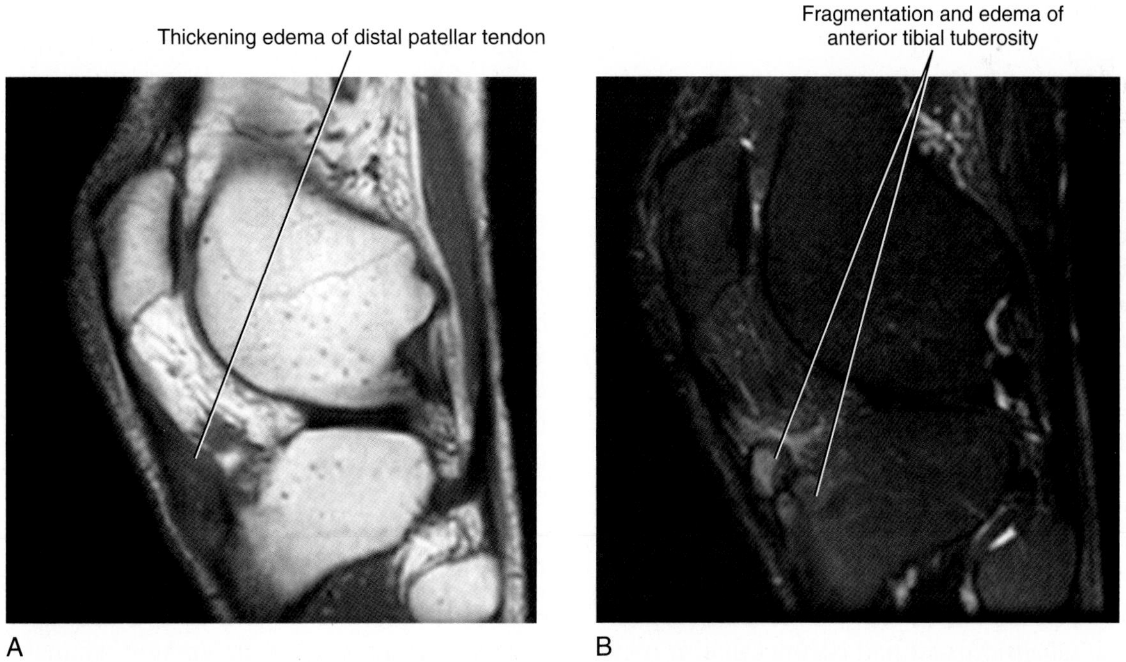
Thickening edema of distal patellar tendon
Fragmentation and edema of anterior tibial tuberosity
A
B

Figure 12-61 Osgood-Schlatter disease. A, Sagittal T1-weighted image shows marked thickening and signal alteration involving the distal attachment of the patellar tendon. **B,** Sagittal T2-weighted image shows marked thickening of the distal patellar tendon, fragmentation, and marrow edema of the anterior tibial tuberosity. The marrow edema within the area of fragmentation indicates acute Osgood-Schlatter disease.

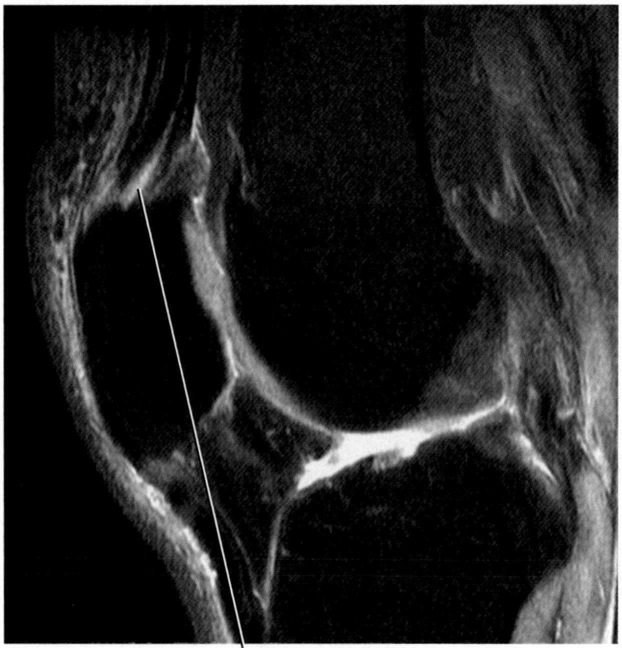
Linear high T2 signal within distal
quadriceps tendon—focal thickening

Figure 12-62 Mild quadriceps tendinopathy. Sagittal T2-weighted image shows minimal thickening of the distal quadriceps tendon with fluid tracking between the individual strands of the distal tendon. There is minimal reactive soft tissue edema superficial to the quadriceps tendon.

Tendinopathy of the quadriceps tendon is usually the result of chronic overuse of the tendon and occurs most commonly in middle-aged men, but it can also be related to collagen vascular disease or the use of exogenous steroids. The MRI appearance is that of a thickened tendon with high-signal tracking either between the separate stands of the tendon or within the substance of one or more of the strands (Fig. 12-62). Quadriceps tendinopathy is often associated with soft tissue edema located in the suprapatellar fat pad just deep to the distal fibers of the quadriceps tendon. Edema just deep to the distal quadriceps tendon is a secondary sign that can help clinch the correct diagnosis, especially if the appearance of the distal fibers of the quadriceps tendon is borderline abnormal. Quadriceps fat pad edema can also occur as an isolated MRI finding and is associated with anterior knee pain and may occur separate from quadriceps tendinopathy (Fig. 12-63). Causes of quadriceps isolated fat pad edema include trauma, inflammation, and possible entrapment.

A partial- or full-thickness tear of the quadriceps tendon can also occur and appears as partial or complete disruption of the tendon with retraction noted of the proximal fibers following complete disruption (Fig. 12-64). A complete tear of the quadriceps tendon requires urgent surgical repair, preferably accomplished within the first 24 hours after injury. Delayed treatment allows further retraction of the proximal fibers of the tendon and requires a more extensive surgical procedure. Often the MRI examination is ordered to differentiate partial from complete tear of the tendon and should be performed as soon as possible to expedite diagnosis and timely repair.

Extensor Mechanism Bursa

Several bursae are located in close proximity to the extensor mechanism, any of which may become inflamed and fluid-filled resulting in anterior knee pain or a palpable mass (Fig. 12-65). These bursae include the prepatellar bursa (housemaid's knee), superficial infrapatellar (pretibial) bursa, and the deep infrapatellar bursa. The deep infrapatellar bursa normally communicates with the knee joint, and a small fluid collection within this bursa is a normal finding in the presence of a knee effusion. A large isolated fluid collection within this bursa or fluid that results in mass effect on the adjacent Hoffa's fat pad is indicative of bursitis. Prepatellar and pretibial bursitis usually results from repetitive trauma to the anterior knee. Fluid within these two bursae is often complex in appearance, and bursal linings are often thick and irregular in appearance. The suprapatellar pouch, though not considered a true bursa, can also present with a large loculated fluid collection. Although rare, this occurs as a result of a thickened obstructing plica. Affected patients present clinically with a painful mass in the superior aspect of the anterior knee. Arthroscopic debridement of the plica is usually necessary to reestablish communication between the suprapatellar pouch and the remainder of the knee joint.

Hoffa's Disease

Hoffa's disease is a term that has been used to describe symptomatic inflammatory changes occurring in the infrapatellar fat pad. These changes are usually post-traumatic and result from entrapment of the fat pad between the patella and the femoral condyle. They typically occur in young athletes. The pain is usually longstanding and exacerbated by full

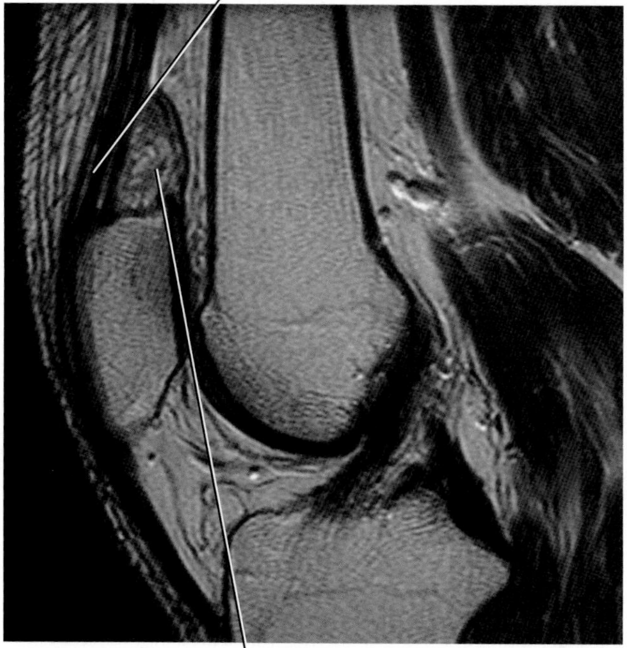
Normal distal quadriceps tendon
A
Focal masslike area of fibrosis and edema in suprapatellar fat pad

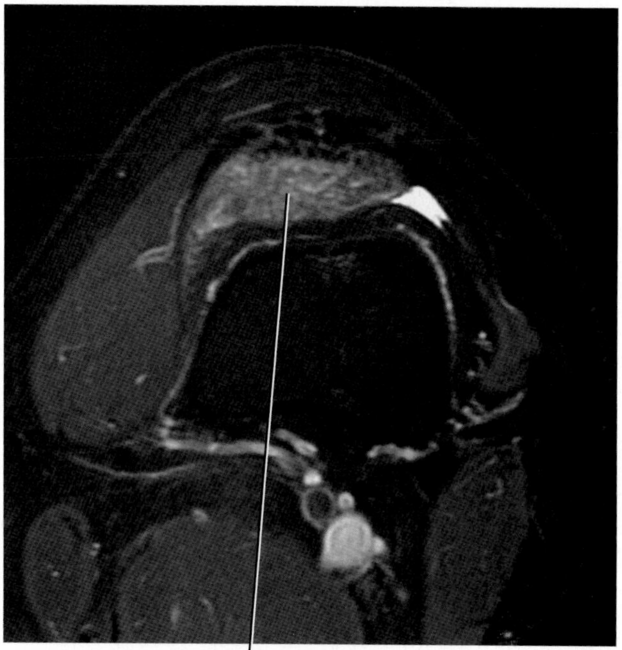
B
Isolated masslike area of focal edema in suprapatellar fat pad

Figure 12-63 Suprapatellar fat pad edema. Sagittal T2-weighted (**A**) and axial T2-weighted (**B**) images demonstrate a focal area of fibrosis and edema located with the suprapatellar fat pad just deep to the distal quadriceps tendon. This finding can be associated with quadriceps tendinopathy; however, when seen as an isolated finding as in this case, it can also result in anterior knee pain. Isolated suprapatellar edema may result from trauma, from an inflammatory process, or from entrapment of the fat pad. The edema is best seen on fat-saturated images as shown on the axial images. It may also result in mass effect as seen in the sagittal images.

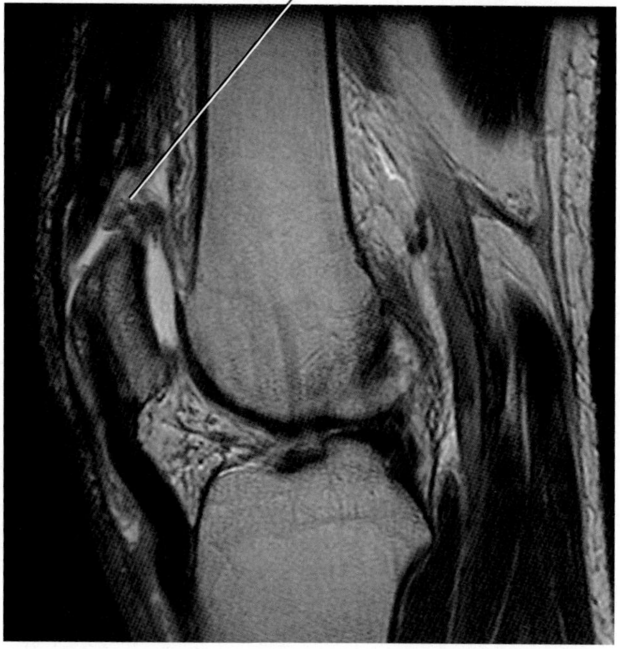
Complete disruption of distal quadriceps tendon

Figure 12-64 Quadriceps tendon disruption. Sagittal T2-weighted image shows complete disruption of the quadriceps tendon at the level of attachment to the superior pole of the patella. A fluid-filled gap is seen on the T2-weighted image, but there is no significant retraction of the quadriceps tendon.

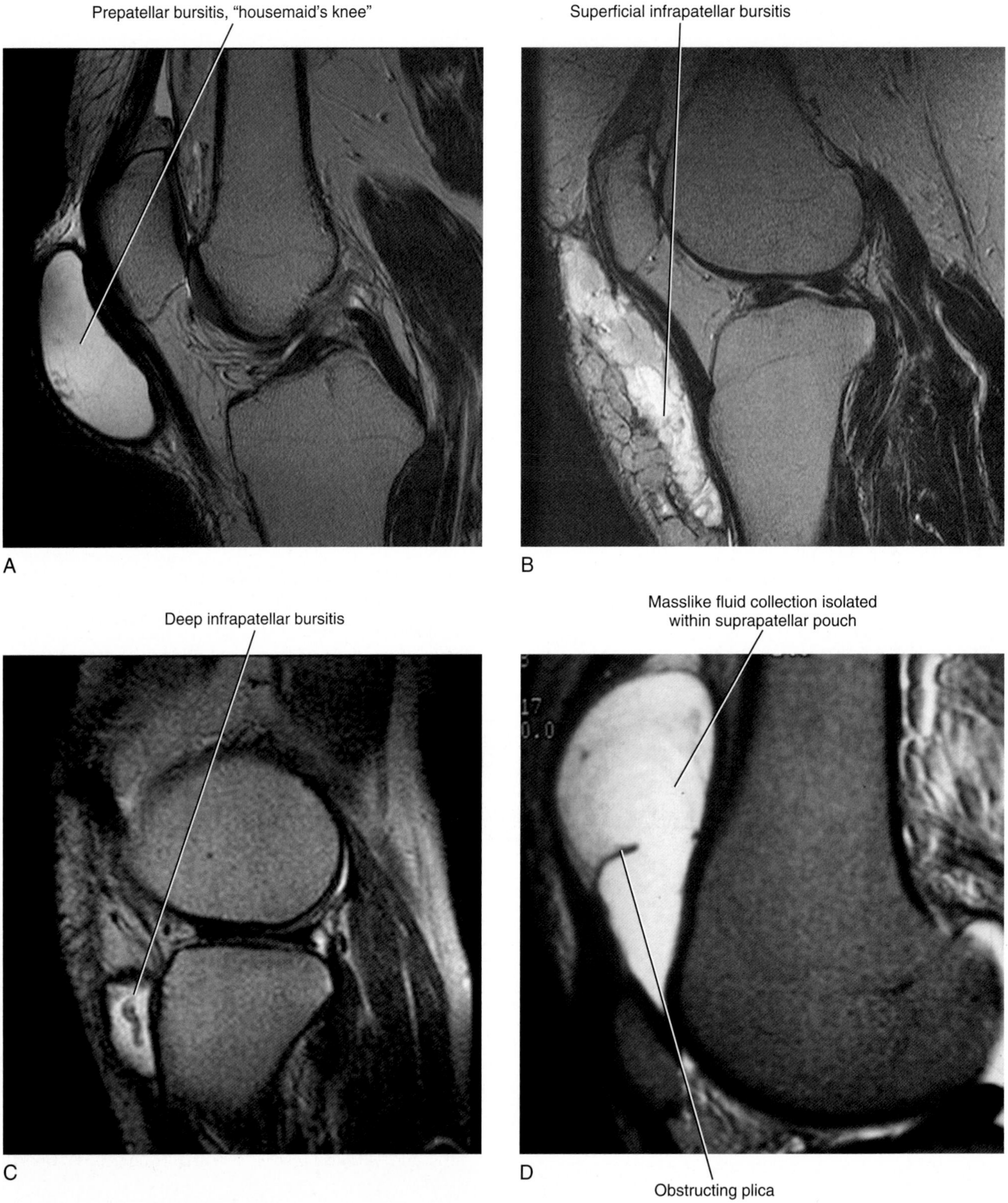
Prepatellar bursitis, "housemaid's knee"
Superficial infrapatellar bursitis
A
B
Deep infrapatellar bursitis
Masslike fluid collection isolated within suprapatellar pouch
C
D
Obstructing plica

Figure 12-65 Extensor mechanism bursae. A, Prepatellar bursitis. **B,** Superficial infrapatellar bursitis. **C,** Deep infrapatellar bursitis. **D,** A large loculated fluid collection is seen within the suprapatellar pouch in this patient who presented with a palpable mass and anterior knee pain. Note the thickened obstructing plica. The plica was subsequently resected and the fluid-filled suprapatellar pouch decompressed.

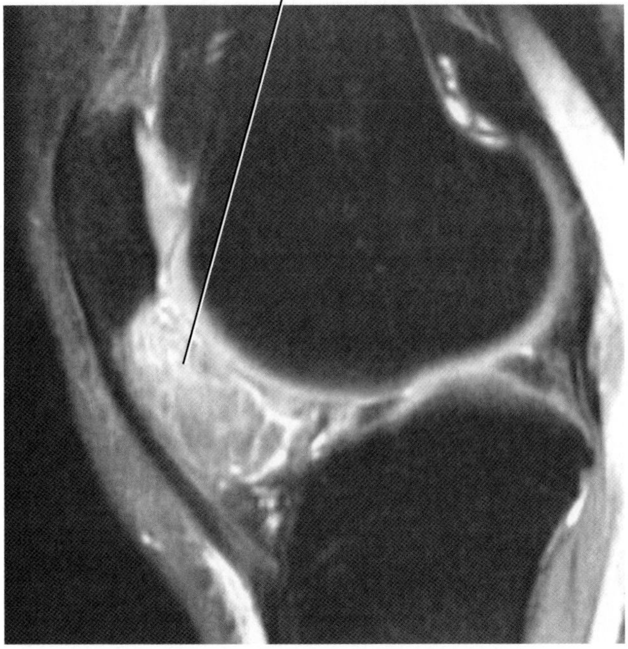
Hoffa's disease—diffuse increased T2 signal within Hoffa's fat pad

Figure 12-66 Hoffa's disease. Sagittal T2-weighted image with fat saturation shows diffuse increased T2 signal isolated to Hoffa's fat pad representing the diffuse inflammatory process of Hoffa's disease.

extension of the knee. In mild cases, MRI typically demonstrates focal edema within Hoffa's fat pad just below the inferior pole of the patella (Fig. 12-66). In more severe cases, edema is present diffusely throughout the entire fat pad. Treatment is usually conservative, but in refractory cases it may require resection of the fat pad. Focal inflammatory change or arthrofibrosis of Hoffa's fat pad is a complication of arthroscopy and is discussed in the section, Imaging of the Postoperative Knee.

OSSEOUS STRUCTURES AND ARTICULAR SURFACES

Normal Anatomy

The normal marrow signal about the knee is bright on T1-weighted images and dark on T2-weighted images with fat saturation. The cortex appears as a dark structure on all pulse sequences. MR imaging is very sensitive for detecting abnormalities of the bone marrow. Marrow abnormalities usually present as low signal on T1-weighted images and bright signal on T2-weighted fat-saturated images. Common abnormalities include fracture, bone marrow edema or contusions, tumor, infection, and avascular necrosis. Prominent or patchy hematopoietic marrow can sometimes simulate other marrow abnormalities. Muscle can be used as an internal standard with signal alteration within the marrow that is darker than muscle, which usually indicates disease, whereas marrow signal brighter than adjacent muscle on T1-weighted images usually indicates normal hematopoietic marrow.

Fractures

On MRI, a fracture typically appears as an area of linear low-signal abnormality within the marrow; cortical disruption and articular surface incongruity may also be detected. Depending on the location of the fracture, all three imaging planes are often useful in fully delineating the extent of fracture. Acute fractures usually demonstrate surrounding marrow edema, whereas a subacute or old fracture may demonstrate very minimal adjacent marrow edema. A cortical avulsion fracture may be very difficult to detect on MRI, since the small cortical avulsion fragment is usually dark and similar in appearance to the adjacent capsular or ligamentous structure that caused the avulsion. Minimal adjacent subcortical marrow edema or overlying soft tissue edema may be the only clue that an avulsion fracture is present. If fracture is suspected on the basis of these criteria, then further evaluation can be performed with radiographs or CT through the area of concern. MRI can be very useful for determining the amount of articular surface step-off. Multidetector CT examination with reconstructed images in the sagittal and coronal imaging planes is very useful in delineating the full extent of fractures about the knee especially with regard to the location and extent of articular surface step off (Fig. 12-67).

Stress-Related Osseous Changes

There is a wide spectrum of stress-related osseous changes that occur about the knee. On one end of the spectrum is early reactive marrow edema; on the other end of the spectrum is a completed fracture resulting in cortical disruption. Osseous stress changes occur when repetitive stresses on the bone result in osteoclastic activity that outpaces the bone's ability

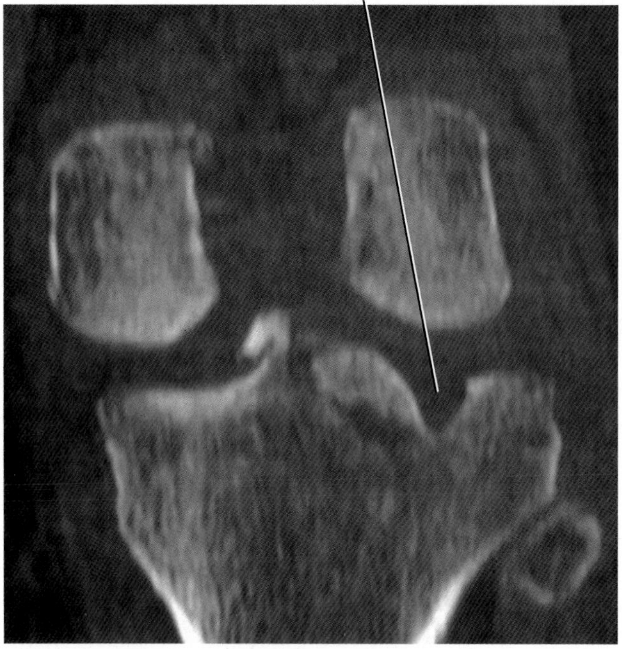
Lateral tibial plateau fracture
and articular surface step-off

Figure 12-67 Lateral tibial plateau fracture. A three-dimensional reconstructed coronal image shows a significantly displaced lateral tibial plateau fracture.

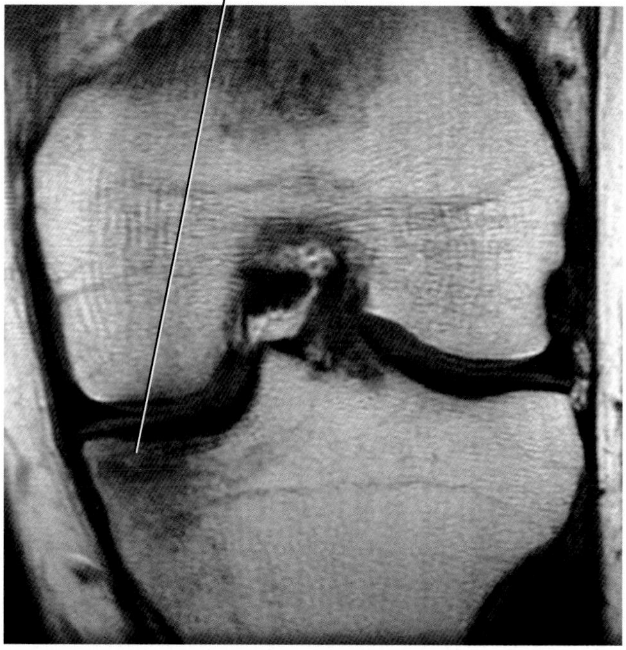
Subtle ill-defined subchondral line with adjacent
marrow edema representing early stress fracture

Figure 12-68 Tibial plateau stress fracture. Coronal T1-weighted image shows a subtle ill-defined subchondral linear area of low-signal abnormality with surrounding marrow edema representing an early stress fracture. T2-weighted image (not shown) demonstrates extensive increased signal within the surrounding marrow.

to repair itself (osteoblastic activity). Although the changes begin at the cellular level, if the stresses persist, they eventually lead to a macroscopic fracture. A *stress fracture* is defined as a fracture in normal bone that is exposed to repeated abnormal stress and typically occurs in the young active athlete. An *insufficiency fracture* is defined as a fracture in abnormal or weakened bone that is exposed to the normal stresses of daily life. Insufficiency fractures typically occur in the older patient population with weakened or demineralized bones.

The tibia is the common location for stress-related changes in the runner, and the proximal tibia is a common location of abnormality. On MRI, early stress-related changes result in diffuse marrow edema, most often located in the subchondral region of the medial tibial plateau. An early stress fracture is seen as a subtle indistinct linear area of low signal abnormality usually oriented perpendicular to the long axis of the bone with adjacent marrow edema (Fig. 12-68). More advanced stress fractures result in a more extensive area of ill-defined low-signal linear abnormality and eventually cortical disruption. Subacute post-traumatic fractures with partial healing can appear very similar to a stress fracture and may require clinical correlation to differentiate the two. An uncommon type of stress fracture that involves the tibia is the longitudinal stress fracture, which typically occurs in the mid tibial shaft. This unusual type of stress fracture can mimic other osseous pathology such as infection and bone tumors. The appropriate diagnosis of stress-related osseous change is usually established if a linear area of signal abnormality is present in the mid tibial shaft with adjacent marrow edema. Typically, either the anterior or the posterior cortex is disrupted.

Other stress fractures that occur about the knee include proximal fibular shaft fractures, which are rare and typically seen in jumpers. Patellar stress fractures can occur in either the transverse or the longitudinal plane. Some consider symptomatic bipartite patella configuration to be a stress-related injury. It is rare for a stress fracture to occur at the level of the distal femoral diaphysis or the distal femoral condyles.

Bone Contusion Patterns

Bone contusions frequently occur at the time of knee injury and are clearly depicted on MRI. They often result from a direct blow to the knee or from the compressive forces of two bones impacting each another. At the cellular level, bone contusions represent a combination of edema, microtrabecular injury, and hemorrhage. On MRI, marrow contusions appear as focal areas of decreased signal intensity on T1-weighted images and increased signal intensity on T2-weighted images. Five specific bone contusion patterns of the knee have been described. With each pattern, the distribution of marrow edema is like a "footprint" that can be used to understand the mechanism of injury, which in turn will allow an accurate prediction of the likely associated soft tissue injuries (Table 12-11).

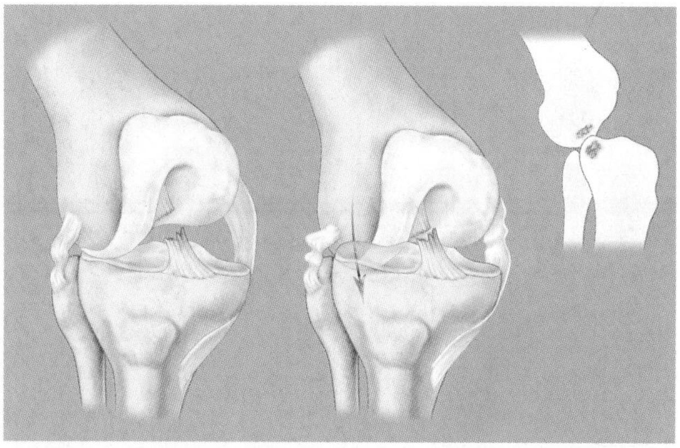

Figure 12-69 Pivot shift injury, a noncontact injury commonly seen in American football players and skiers. With the foot planted, a combination of valgus stress applied to the knee and internal rotation of the femur results in disruption of the anterior cruciate ligament. The tibia then translates anteriorly relative to the distal femur, allowing impaction of the lateral femoral condyle against the posterolateral tibial plateau and resulting in the pivot shift bone contusion pattern *(far right image)*. Increasing degrees of flexion at the time of injury result in a more posteriorly located contusion on the femur.

Table 12-11 Bone Contusion Patterns and Associated Soft Tissue Injuries

Mechanism of Injury	Marrow Edema Location	Primary Soft Tissue Injury	Other Associated Injuries
Pivot-shift injury (Figs. 12-69 and 12-70)	Lateral femoral condyle Posterior tibial plateau	ACL disruption	Posterior capsular structures Medial/lateral meniscus Medial collateral ligament (MCL) Osteochondral injury of the posterolateral tibia and lateral femoral condyle
Dashboard injury (Figs. 12-71 and 12-72)	Anterior proximal tibia +/− Inferior pole patella	PCL disruption	Posterior capsule disruption Patellar fracture/osteochondral injury Hip fracture/posterior dislocation
Hyperextension injury (Figs. 12-73 and 12-74)	"Kissing contusions" Anterior tibia and anterior femoral condyle	ACL/PCL disruption	Posterior capsule disruption Popliteal neurovascular injury Meniscal injury Gastrocnemius injury
Clip injury (Figs. 12-75 and 12-76)	Lateral femoral condyle Lateral tibial plateau	MCL sprain/disruption	ACL tear Medial meniscal injury
Lateral patellar dislocation (Figs. 12-77 and 12-78)	Anterolateral femoral condyle Inferomedial patella	Medial patellofemoral ligament	Patellar/lateral femoral condyle osteochondral injury Intra-articular body Medial retinaculum injury Vastus medialis obliquus muscle injury

ACL, anterior cruciate ligament; PCL, posterior cruciate ligament.

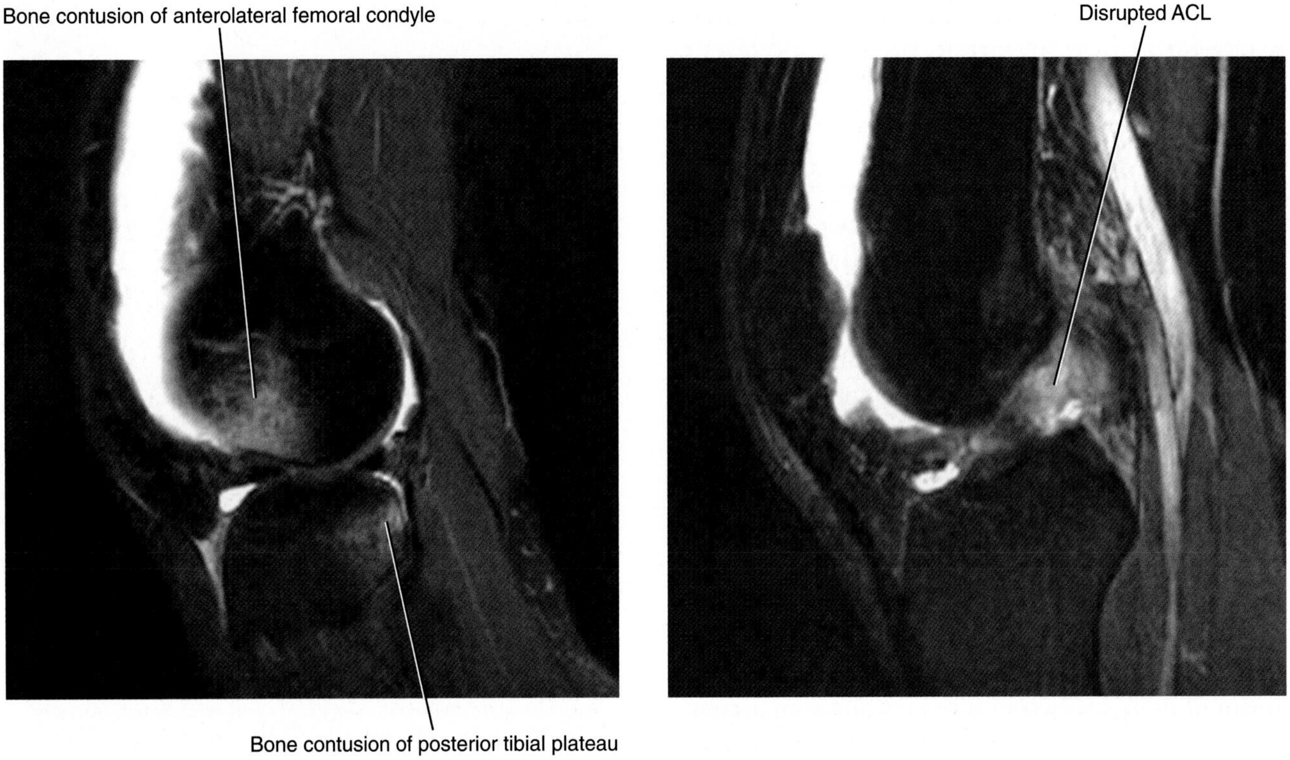
Bone contusion of anterolateral femoral condyle
Disrupted ACL
Bone contusion of posterior tibial plateau

Figure 12-70 Pivot shift bone contusion pattern. T2-weighted sagittal images demonstrate the typical appearance of the pivot shift bone contusion pattern with anterior cruciate ligament (ACL) disruption.

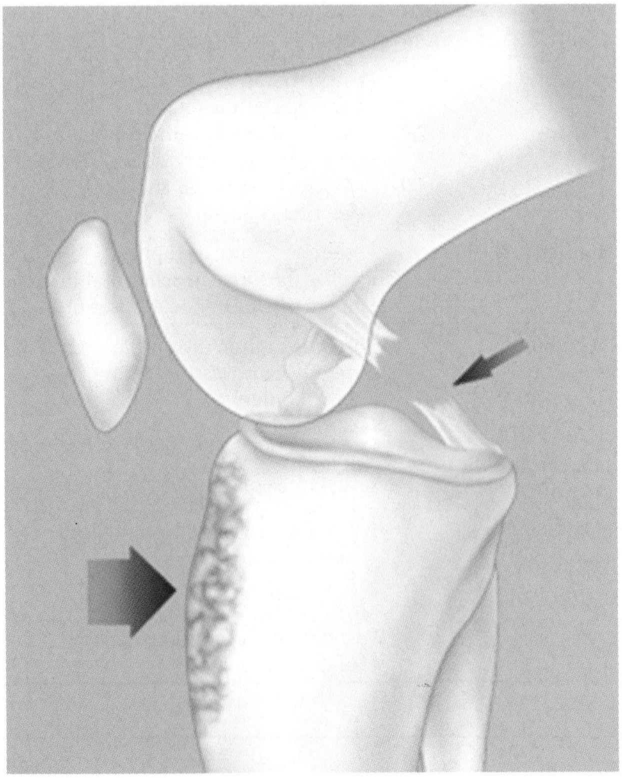

Figure 12-71 Dashboard injury. The bone contusion results from the application of an external force to the proximal anterior tibia of the flexed knee. The impact results in the posterior translation of the tibia relative to the femur. With the knee in 90 degrees of flexion, the posterior cruciate ligament is taut and at risk for disruption, whereas the anterior cruciate ligament is lax and usually spared injury.

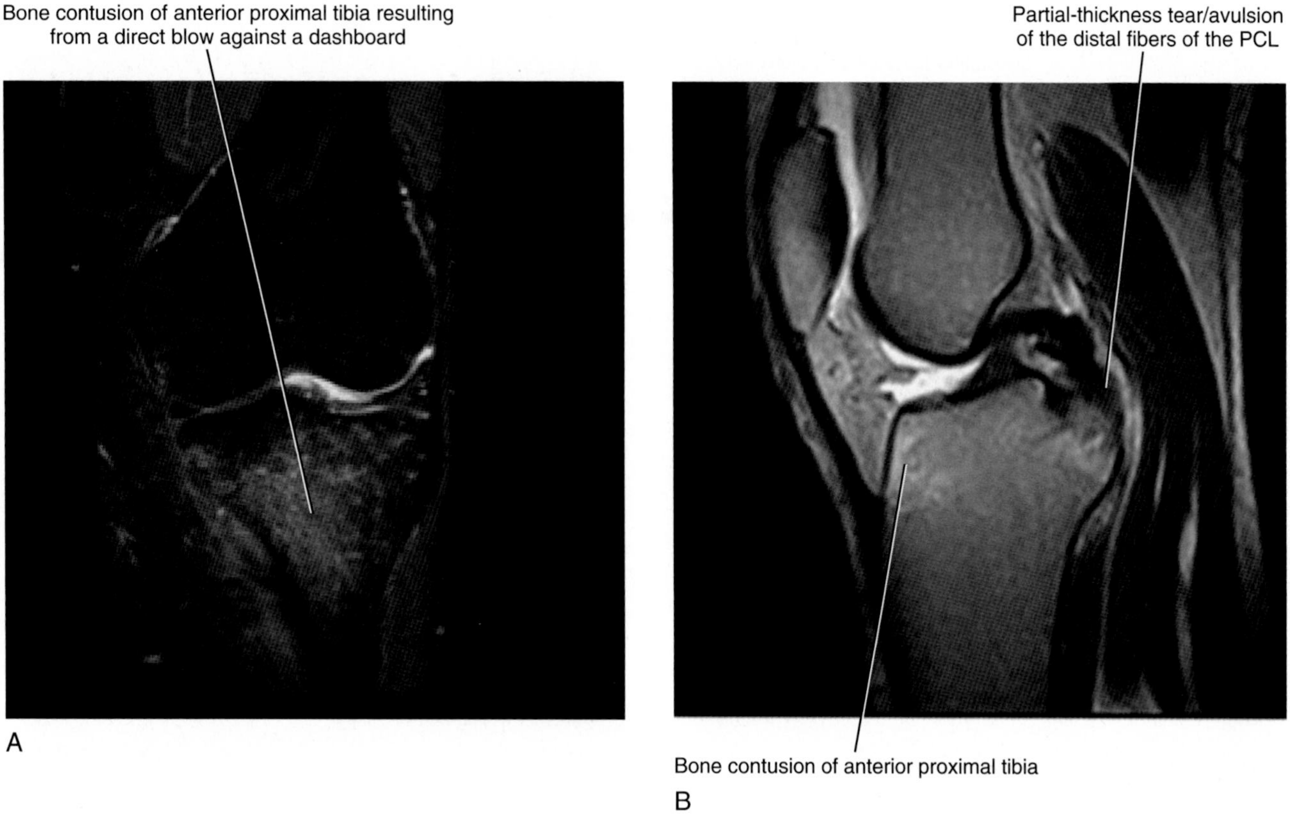
Bone contusion of anterior proximal tibia resulting from a direct blow against a dashboard
Partial-thickness tear/avulsion of the distal fibers of the PCL
Bone contusion of anterior proximal tibia
A
B

Figure 12-72 Dashboard bone contusion pattern. A, Coronal STIR image shows a bone contusion involving the anterior aspect of the proximal tibia. **B,** Sagittal T2-weighted image shows the bone contusion and partial disruption of the distal attachment of the posterior cruciate ligament (PCL).

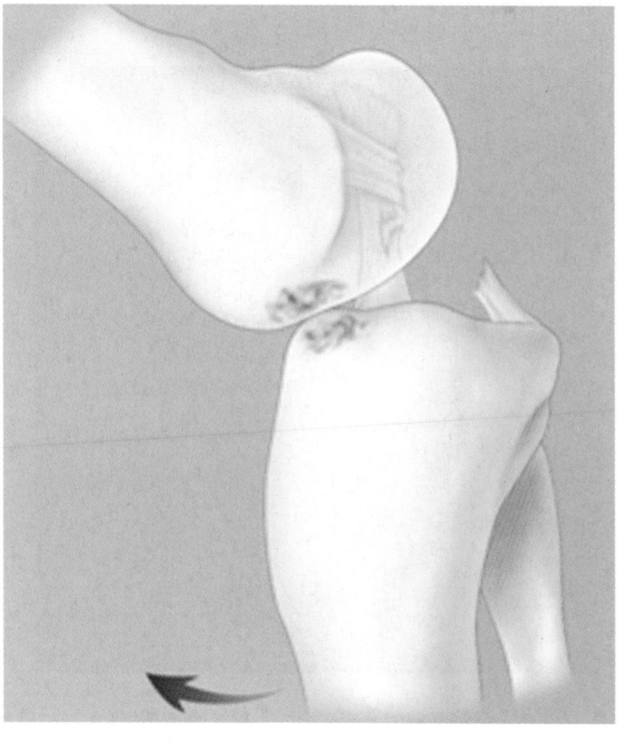

Figure 12-73 Hyperextension injury. A kissing contusion bone edema pattern occurs from impaction of the anterior tibia against the anterior femur. This injury can occur from a forceful kicking motion, but the most severe injuries often occur as the result of the bumper of a car making impact against the anterior tibia.

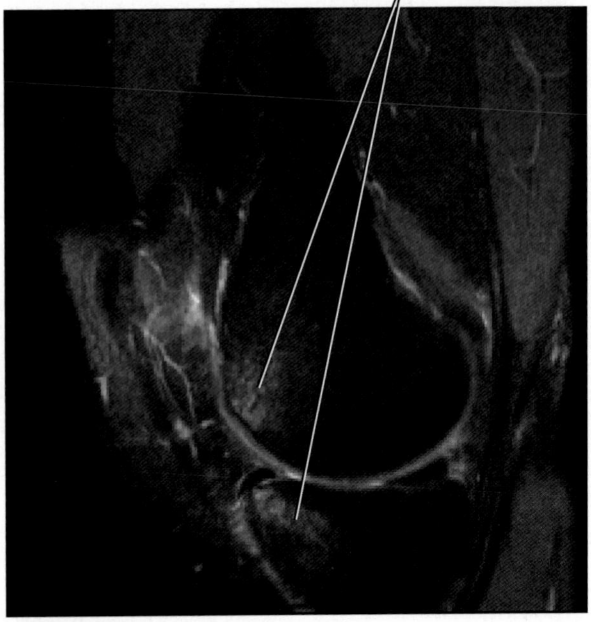
Kissing contusion pattern of edema within the anterior femur and tibia secondary to hyperextension injury

Figure 12-74 Hyperextension bone contusion pattern. Sagittal T2-weighted image shows the kissing contusion pattern often associated with injury of the anterior and posterior cruciate ligaments. When a severe force is applied, soft tissue injuries may also include disruption of the posterior capsular structures and injury of the popliteal neurovascular bundle.

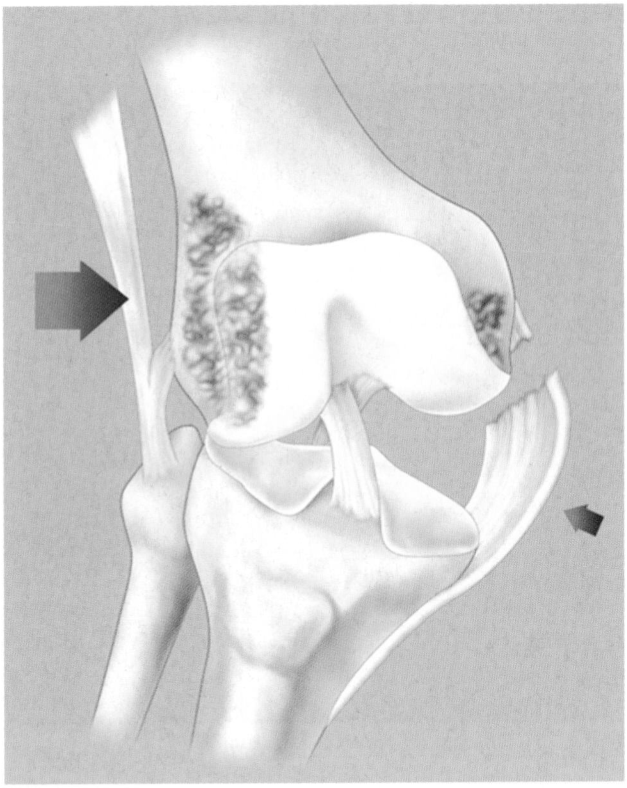

Figure 12-75 Clip injury. The bone marrow contusion *(large arrow)* results form a direct blow to the lateral aspect of the knee. This is a common injury in American football. The valgus force results in an injury to the medial collateral ligament *(small arrow)*.

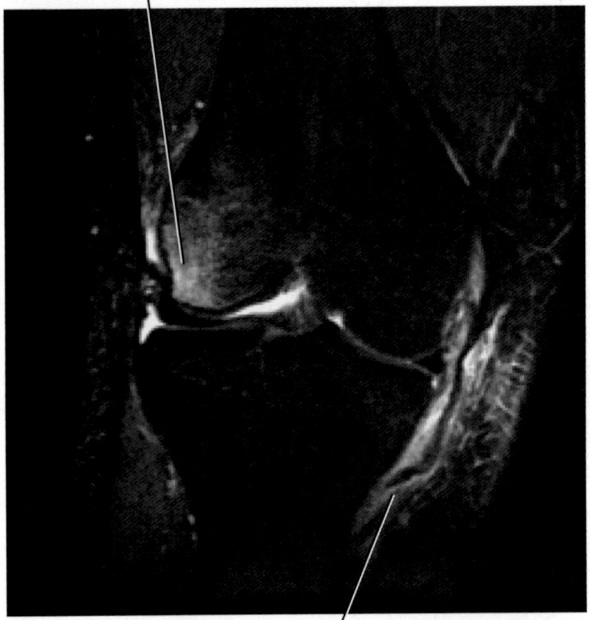
Bone marrow contusion of lateral femoral condyle resulting from direct impact injury
Complete disruption of distal MCL fibers

Figure 12-76 Clip injury bone contusion pattern. Coronal T2-weighted image shows a bone contusion of the lateral femoral condyle resulting from a direct impaction injury. There is complete disruption of the distal fibers of the medial collateral ligament (MCL), resulting from the valgus stress applied across the knee at the time of injury.

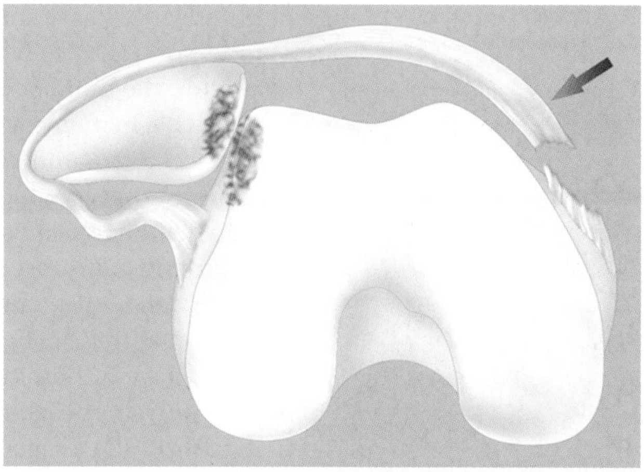

Figure 12-77 Lateral patellar dislocation. This injury is most frequently seen in adolescent female athletes. The injury classically occurs with the person standing while the knee is slightly flexed and the femur internally rotated. The person attempts to straighten the knee by firing the quadriceps, but rather than straightening the knee, the contracting quadriceps pulls the patella laterally. The impact of the patella against the lateral femoral condyle produces the classic bone contusion pattern. Disruption of the medial patellofemoral ligament (MPFL) *(arrow)* may occur. The dislocation is usually transient because the associated pain causes the person to fall to the ground, often leading to spontaneous reduction of the patella.

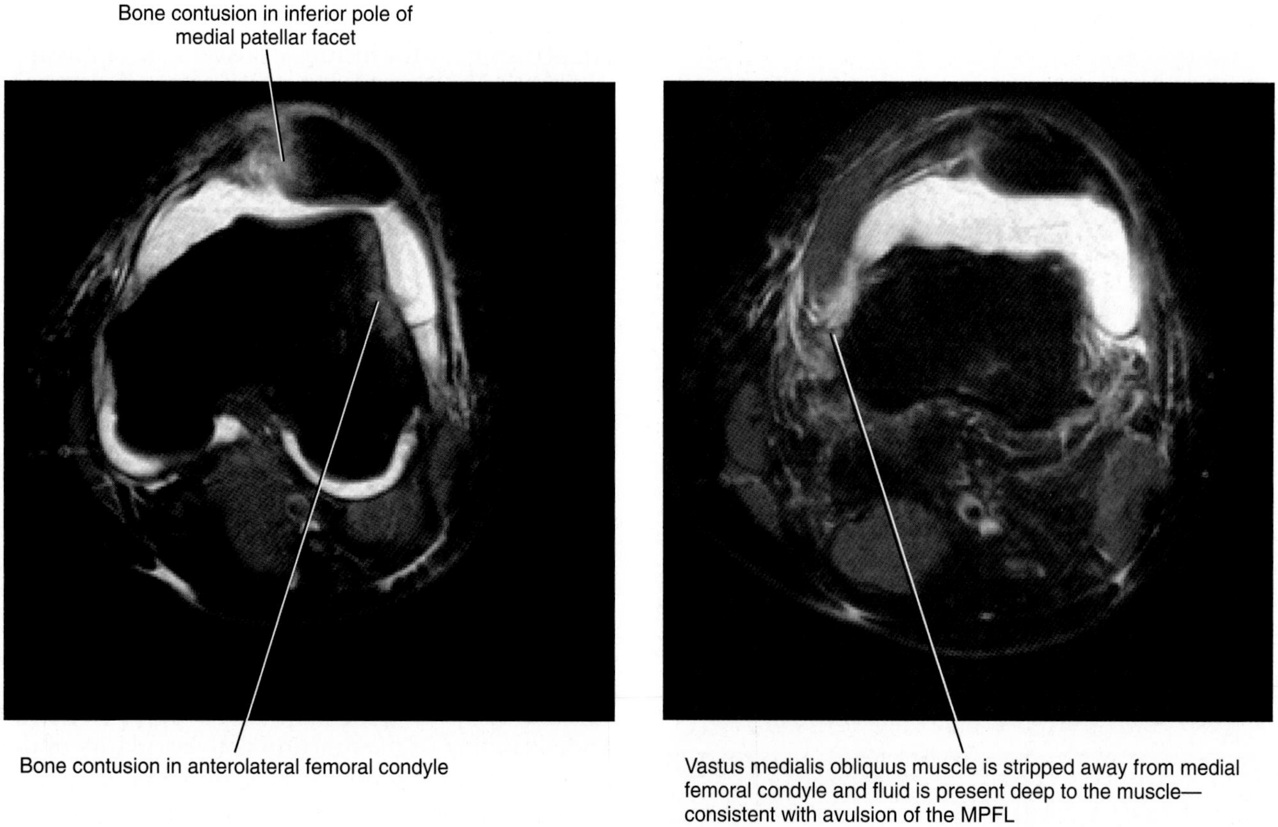
Bone contusion in inferior pole of medial patellar facet
Bone contusion in anterolateral femoral condyle
Vastus medialis obliquus muscle is stripped away from medial femoral condyle and fluid is present deep to the muscle—consistent with avulsion of the MPFL

Figure 12-78 Lateral patellar dislocation bone contusion pattern. Axial T2-weighted images show the typical bone contusion pattern involving the inferior pole of the medial patellar facet and anterolateral femoral condyle and avulsion of the medial patellofemoral ligament (MPFL) from the adductor tubercle. Surgical indications include disruption of the MPFL or a displaced osteochondral fragment from the patella or lateral femoral condyle.

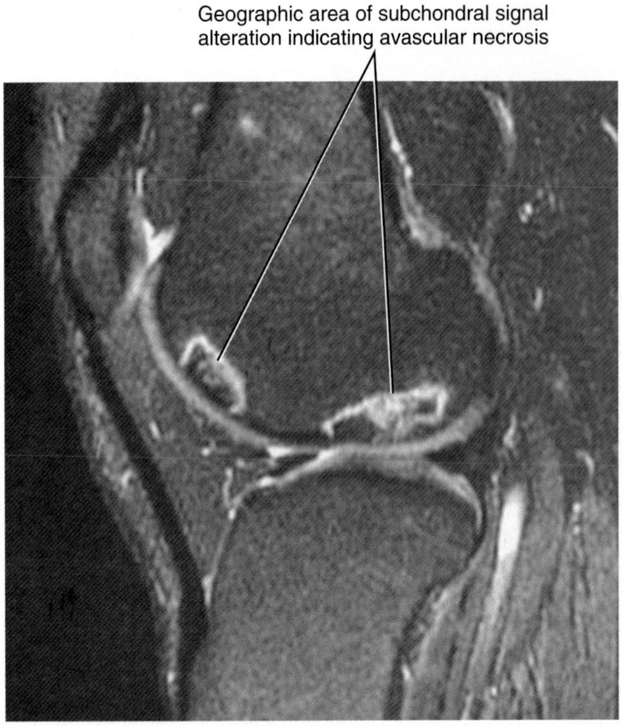
Geographic area of subchondral signal alteration indicating avascular necrosis

Figure 12-79 Avascular necrosis. Sagittal T2-weighted image with fat saturation reveals two areas of geographic signal alteration in the subchondral region of the distal femur representing avascular necrosis. This patient had a long history of steroid use.

Avascular Necrosis

Avascular necrosis involving the osseous structures about the knee is usually associated with steroid use or one of the collagen vascular diseases. The MRI appearance of avascular necrosis about the knee is similar to its appearance in other areas such as the femoral head and the humeral head. The classic appearance is that of a geographic area of signal alteration in the subchondral region of the bone. A *double-line sign* on T2-weighted images is diagnostic of avascular necrosis (Fig. 12-79).

IMAGING OF THE POSTOPERATIVE KNEE

Over the past decade many technical advances have been achieved with regard to knee surgery, including several new meniscal and cartilage repair techniques and improved fixation devices for ACL and PCL grafts. These advances have made it possible for increasing numbers of people to benefit from surgical treatment; as a result, the number of knee surgeries has been on a steady rise. In many radiology practices, the number of patients who undergo MRI of the knee with a history of surgery now constitute up to 5% of all those who undergo knee MR examinations. Persistent or recurrent pain after knee surgery is a common problem, and MRI can play a pivotal role in the evaluation of these patients. However, the radiologist needs to have a thorough knowledge of the normal postoperative appearance and the MRI criteria used to establish the diagnosis of recurrent disease or injury.

Imaging of the Postoperative Meniscus

When evaluating the MR appearance of the menisci, it is important to know whether there has been prior meniscal surgery because the MRI criteria for diagnosing a tear change in the setting of prior surgery. This information is often provided in the clinical history or in a patient's response to a questionnaire, but occasionally the history is unavailable or missing. In such instances, the MR images can provide the evidence of prior surgery. The presence of a linear or rounded scar in Hoffa's fat pad represents the portal of the arthroscopist's cannula (scope scar) and indicates that the patient has undergone prior arthroscopy (Fig. 12-80). The scope scar is usually seen within Hoffa's fat pad on either side of the patellar tendon. The presence of susceptibility artifact from microscopic metal fragments or from suture material, especially on GRE imaging, may also be an indication of prior surgery. The routine evaluation of the knee MRI should include a search for these clues, indicating prior surgery, and, when present, the MR images should be interpreted accordingly.

Meniscal surgery is one of the most common procedures performed on the knee. In the past, the meniscus was freely excised with little understanding of the long-term consequences. More recently, a better understanding of the function and vascularity of the meniscus has led to the practice of meniscal-sparing surgery in an attempt to maintain the function of the knee to as close to normal as possible. The complication rate after meniscal surgery is under 10% and includes laceration of the popliteal artery, peroneal and saphenous nerve palsies, deep infection, instrument breakage, deep vein thrombosis, pulmonary

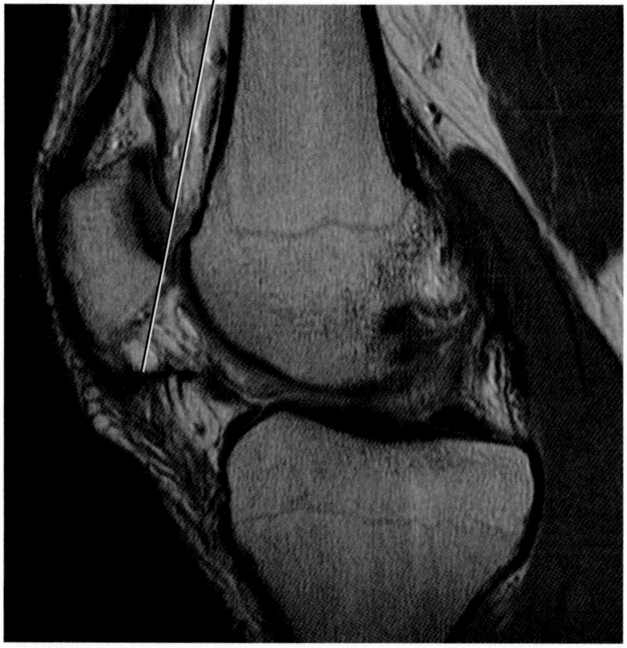
Linear arthrofibrosis in Hoffa's fat pad representing the "scope scar"

Figure 12-80 **Scope scar in Hoffa's fat pad.** Sagittal proton density image shows a focal area of linear low signal scar tissue in Hoffa's fat pad indicating prior arthroscopic cannula placement.

BOX 12-5 PERSISTENT OR RECURRENT KNEE PAIN IN THE POSTMENISCECTOMY PATIENT

Persistent tear or re-tear of the meniscus
Articular cartilage abnormality
Osteoarthritis
Intra-articular bodies
Spontaneous osteonecrosis/insufficiency fracture

embolism, meniscal cysts, arthrofibrosis, and spontaneous osteonecrosis of the adjacent osteochondral surfaces.

The most common role for MRI following meniscal repair, however, is in the evaluation of persistent or recurrent knee pain. Possible causes of persistent pain in the postmeniscectomy patient include persistent or recurrent meniscal tear, chondromalacia of the adjacent articular surface, osteoarthritis of the involved compartment, loose bodies, and spontaneous osteonecrosis of the adjacent femoral condyle or tibial plateau (Box 12-5).

MRI Criteria for a Recurrent Meniscal Tear

The normal postoperative appearance of the meniscus will differ, depending on the type and extent of tear and whether meniscal tissue was resected or repaired. Using conventional MRI, a meniscus that demonstrates blunting or truncation of its free edge but no surfacing signal can be interpreted as a normal postoperative meniscus. The meniscal remnant may show minimal surface irregularity or fraying, but there should be no surfacing signal and no displaced or unstable meniscal fragment. Studies have shown that after partial meniscectomy, if less than 25% of the meniscus was resected, the MRI should be read using the same criteria as for a nonoperative meniscus. In patients in whom more than 25% of the meniscus was resected, surfacing signal seen only on the short TE sequence is indeterminate for a re-tear.

To diagnose a recurrent tear after a partial meniscectomy in which more than 25% of the meniscus was resected requires the detection of surfacing fluid signal on T2-weighted images or surfacing gadolinium signal on MR arthrography. In clinical practice, it is often difficult to determine the precise amount of meniscus that has been resected, and often the amount of meniscal resection is unknown at the time of prescribing the protocol to use on a particular patient. There are many ways to approach the evaluation of the postoperative meniscus, but the following sections try to provide a rational approach for the evaluation of the postoperative meniscus.

On conventional MRI, the appearance of the postoperative meniscus can be classified as (1) normal postoperative appearance with no evidence of a re-tear, (2) indeterminate for re-tear, or (3) torn (Table 12-12). Conventional MRI has a reported accuracy of 65% to 82%, and sensitivities range from 60% to 86% in the detection of recurrent tears in the postoperative setting. The criteria for a persistent or recurrent tear of the meniscus using conventional MRI include (1) surfacing fluid signal seen on T2-weighted image (Fig. 12-81), (2) a tear in a new location (requires a detailed surgical history regarding the location of meniscal surgery), (3) a displaced meniscal fragment, such as a bucket-handle tear or flipped fragment, and (4) abnormal morphology of the meniscal remnant including notching or a radial defect.

The presence of surfacing signal seen solely on the short TE sequence of a conventional MRI and not on

SECTION IV

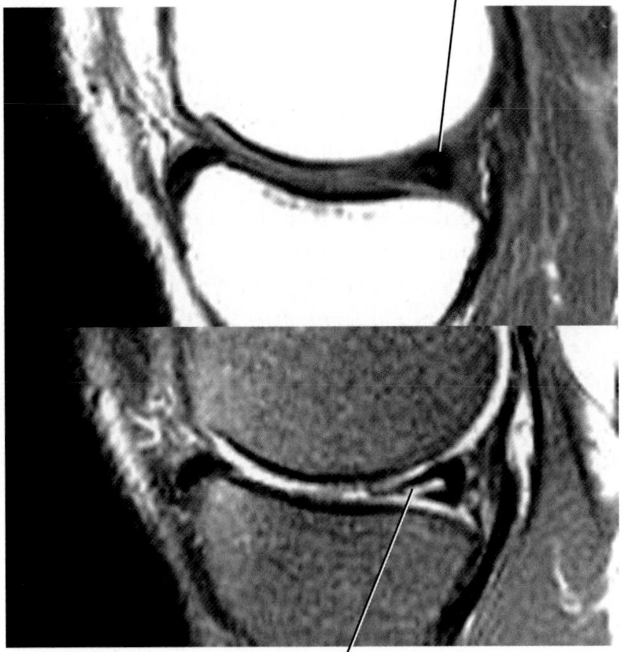
Surfacing T1 signal in postoperative meniscus
Surfacing fluid signal on T2 indicating re-tear of the postop meniscus

Figure 12-81 Recurrent meniscal tear on conventional MRI in the postoperative meniscus. Figure shows surfacing signal on T1-weighted (*top*) image and surfacing fluid signal on T2-weighted (*bottom*) image. This represents a recurrent tear in this patient after partial medial meniscectomy. Surfacing fluid signal seen on a T2-weighted image is specific for a recurrent tear following meniscal surgery.

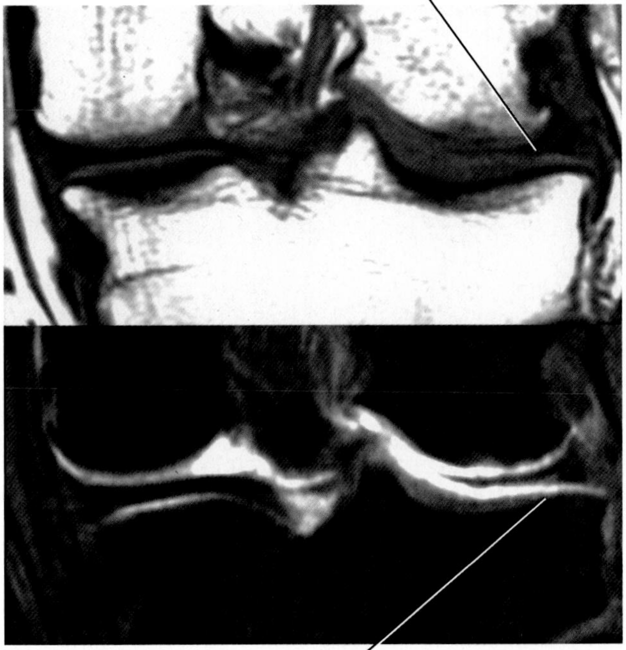
Surfacing T1-weighted signal on conventional MRI is indeterminate for a recurrent tear
Follow-up direct MR arthrogram demonstrates no surfacing gadolinium, representing the normal postoperative appearance with no evidence of a recurrent tear

Figure 12-82 Postoperative meniscus indeterminate for re-tear on conventional MRI. Conventional MRI examination demonstrates surfacing signal on short echo time sequence only coronal T1-weighted image (*top*). This finding was considered indeterminate for tear and required additional evaluation. A follow-up direct MR arthrogram was performed and coronal T1-weighted image with fat saturation image (*bottom*) shows intermediate surfacing signal with no surfacing gadolinium signal. This finding represents the normal appearance of the postoperative meniscus with no evidence of a recurrent tear.

Table 12-12 Postoperative Meniscus on Conventional MRI

Meniscal Appearance	Diagnosis
Small truncated meniscus Minimal surface irregularity No surfacing signal	Normal postoperative appearance
Surfacing signal seen only on short echo time sequence (>25% of meniscus resected) No surfacing signal on T2	Indeterminate for tear
Surfacing fluid signal on T2 Tear in a new location Displaced meniscal fragment Abnormal morphology (i.e., notching or radial defect)	Persistent tear or re-tear of meniscus

the T2-weighted sequence (or intermediate surfacing signal on T2, without fluid in the surfacing signal) in the setting of prior partial meniscal resection is indeterminate for a persistent or recurrent tear and may indicate the presence of a re-tear of the meniscus, postoperative granulation tissue in the region of repair, or persistent surfacing signal that was stable to probing at the time of surgery (Fig. 12-82). In some series, the finding of surfacing signal seen only on the short TE sequence (and thus indeterminate for a tear) is present in up to 30% to 40% of menisci without re-tear. If a re-tear of the meniscus is suspected clinically, then this MRI finding requires additional evalu-

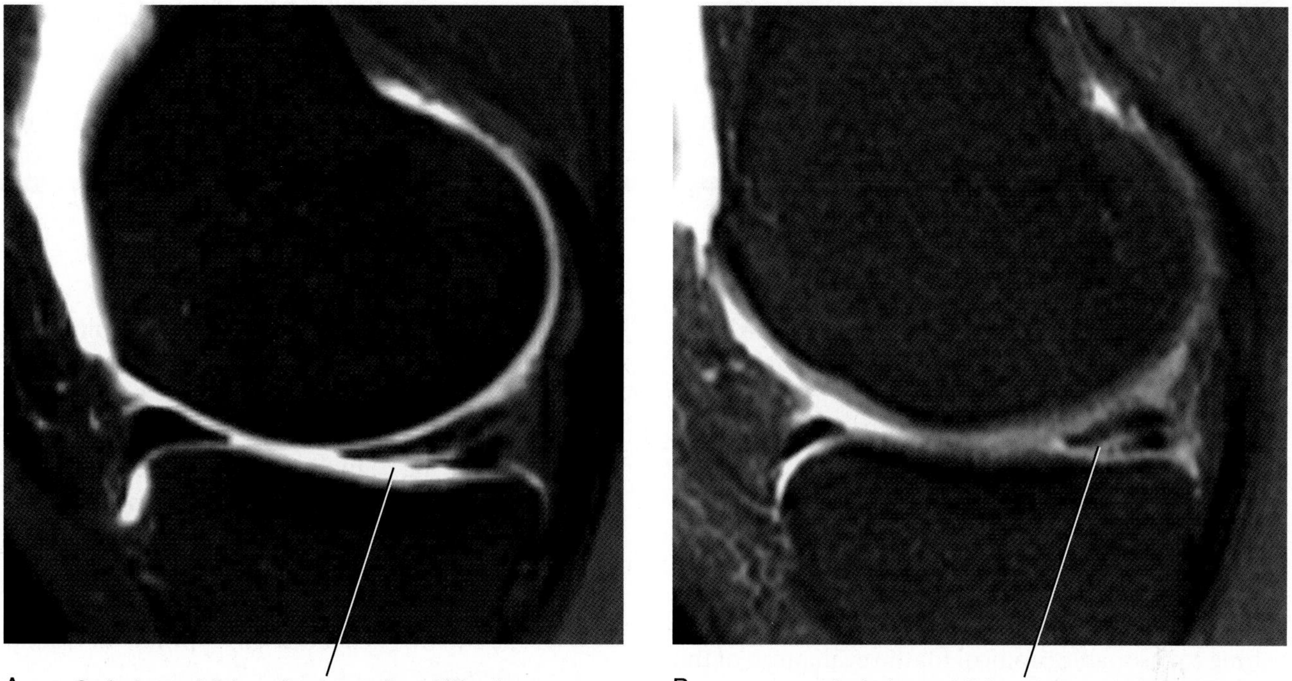

A Surfacing gadolinium signal on a direct MR arthrogram indicating a recurrent meniscal tear

B Surfacing gadolinium signal on indirect MRI in the same patient indicating a recurrent meniscal tear

Figure 12-83 Recurrent meniscal tear on direct and indirect MR arthrography. Direct MR arthrogram (**A**) and indirect MR arthrogram (**B**) images from the same patient after partial medial meniscectomy demonstrate surfacing gadolinium signal extending to the inferior articular surface of the meniscus representing a recurrent meniscal tear. Notice the distention effect with a larger volume of joint fluid present on the direct MRI.

ation of the meniscus by performing either a follow-up MR arthrogram or arthroscopy.

MR Arthrography of the Postoperative Meniscus

Both direct and indirect MR arthrography have been shown to improve accuracy in the detection of recurrent meniscal tears when compared with conventional MRI. The menisci are evaluated using T1-weighted images with fat saturation in both the sagittal and coronal imaging planes. The distention effect created by the injection of contrast directly into the joint forces fluid into the meniscal tears and improves the detection rate of a meniscal tear (Fig. 12-83). Furthermore, with MR arthrography, high signal-to-noise T1-weighted images are used to detect tears rather than relying on the lower signal-to-noise T2-weighted images as with the conventional MRI in the postoperative patient. The disadvantage of direct MR arthrography is that it requires the presence of a physician and is more invasive than a conventional MRI or indirect MR arthrogram.

Using either direct or indirect MR arthrography, meniscal tears are detected by the presence of surfacing gadolinium signal on the T1-weighted images. Surfacing signal that does not reach gadolinium signal intensity represents either postoperative scar tissue or stable grade III signal persisting from the time of surgery and does not represent a re-tear. Using either direct or indirect MR arthrography, the overall accuracy in the evaluation of postoperative menisci can be improved to more than 90%, but there does not appear to be a statistically significant difference between the two techniques. One potential pitfall in using MR arthrography is that during the first year, scar tissue in the area of a repaired meniscus may demonstrate enhancement and give a false-positive for recurrent meniscal tear, but after the first year scar tissue does not typically enhance. Because of this potential pitfall, it is probably best to avoid indirect MRI during the first year immediately after meniscal resection or repair.

After meniscal repair (suturing of the meniscus), surfacing T1-weighted signal may persist indefinitely, and it is not always clear at the time of MR imaging that the patient underwent meniscal suturing, since the operative report is often unavailable. This is another reason why T2-weighted images are so critical in the evaluation of the postoperative meniscus. Surfacing short TE signal in the sutured meniscus is a normal postoperative appearance, whereas surfacing fluid signal on T2 is never a normal appearance, regardless of the type of meniscal procedure that was performed. Surfacing gadolinium into an area of meniscal suturing is abnormal on direct MR arthrography. With indirect MR arthrography, enhancement may occur in the region of suturing during the first year, but the area of repair does not usually enhance after the first year.

Guidelines for Imaging of the Postoperative Meniscus

Many different approaches can be used when establishing a reasonable protocol for the evaluation of the postoperative meniscus, and many factors must be considered in each practice to determine what imaging strategy will be appropriate in a given set of circumstances. Factors include the type of MRI equipment (high versus low field strength magnet), the availability of a physician to perform an injection for direct MR arthrography, and access to surgical reports to determine the type and location of meniscal surgery. All these factors can play a role in determining the best protocol for postoperative imaging in a particular patient. The key is to understand the benefits and limitations of conventional MRI and indirect and direct MR arthrography, and then to develop a protocol that fits within the limitations of a particular practice. The following is a suggested set of options or guidelines that can be used in the evaluation of the postoperative meniscus.

Options

1. Option 1. Start the evaluation of all postoperative menisci with a conventional MRI.

   This is a totally acceptable approach and is used in many radiology practices. With this approach the radiologist needs to be aware of the limitations of conventional MR in the evaluation of the postsurgical meniscus and understand that sensitivities and specificities will be slightly lower than with MR arthrography in certain subsets of patients.

   When beginning the evaluation of the postoperative meniscus with conventional MRI, the following algorithm should be used.

   a. If the meniscus appears normal on conventional MRI, then the meniscus is normal and no additional workup is required
      - i. Normal meniscal morphology (or slightly blunted or truncated meniscus if prior partial meniscectomy)
      - ii. No surfacing signal
      - iii. No displaced fragment

   b. A tear (re-tear or persistent tear) can be diagnosed on conventional MRI using the following criteria:
      - i. Surfacing fluid signal on T2-weighted sequence
      - ii. Surfacing signal on short TE sequence if less than 25% of the meniscus has been resected
      - iii. Displaced meniscal fragment
      - iv. Abnormal morphology of the meniscal remnant (i.e., notched appearance, radial defect)
      - v. Tear in a new location (requires detailed surgical history)

   c. Indeterminate for tear using conventional MRI
      - i. Surfacing signal seen only on short TE sequence (T1, PD) with more than 25% of meniscus resected
      - ii. No fluid present on the T2-weighted images within the surfacing signal

   d. Presence of a meniscal cyst
      - i. A meniscal cyst in the postoperative setting does not necessarily indicate a recurrent tear because the cyst is not always resected or completely decompressed

   When using this approach, if the meniscus is definitely *torn* or *normal*, then the workup is complete. If the meniscus is *indeterminate* for recurrent tear, additional workup is required. This may include bringing the patient back for direct or indirect MR arthrography or taking the patient to arthroscopy if there is a high clinical suspicion of recurrent tear in the face of an indeterminate result on conventional MRI.

   e. *Advantages*: High patient acceptance, rapid throughput of patients, noninvasive procedure for most patients

   f. *Disadvantages*: Up to 25% to 30% of patients may demonstrate an indeterminate finding on conventional MRI and require a second study. However, this does limit the number of invasive procedures to only 25% of the original patient population.

2. Option 2. Perform direct MR arthrography as the first exam on all patients with the history of meniscal surgery.
   a. Criteria for a recurrent meniscal tear
      i. Surfacing gadolinium signal
      ii. Displaced meniscal fragment
      iii. Abnormal morphology of the meniscal remnant (i.e., notched appearance, radial defect)
   b. *Advantages*: When evaluating all patients with prior meniscal surgery, option 2 achieves the highest sensitivities and specificities for recurrent meniscal tear. No patients need to return for additional imaging.
   c. *Disadvantages*: MR arthrography requires the highest number of invasive procedures and requires scheduling the patient when a physician is available to inject the joint. Patient acceptance is poor, and MR arthrography is more costly than conventional MRI.
3. Option 3. Perform indirect MR arthrography as the first exam on all patients
   a. Criteria for a recurrent meniscal tear
      i. Surfacing gadolinium signal
      ii. Displaced meniscal fragment
      iii. Abnormal morphology of the meniscal remnant (i.e., notched appearance, radial defect)
   b. *Advantages*: Sensitivities and specificities are statistically similar to those with direct MR arthrography. In many practices, intravenous injections can be performed by the technician and do not require the immediate presence of a physician.
   c. *Disadvantages*: Indirect MR arthrography requires intravenous injection for all postoperative patients, thus increasing costs. Scan time is longer because of the injection and waiting time after injection. It may increase false-positive results during the first 12 months after meniscal surgery.

Any of the latter three approaches is acceptable as long as the limitations, advantages, and disadvantages of each option are understood. In many practices, it is actually a combination of these three options that are used, depending on available resources and the specific situation for an individual patient.

MRI Evaluation of Meniscal Transplant

Meniscal transplantation surgery is increasing in frequency and is typically reserved for people under 40 years of age who have minimal osteoarthritis and who are unresponsive to more conservative treatment options for a torn meniscus, demonstrating persistent pain and swelling of the knee. The telltale bone plugs or sutures that are used to attach the meniscal transplant to the tibia make it easy to identify when a meniscal transplant has been used (Fig. 12-84). Evaluation of the meniscal transplant should include an evaluation of the appearance and location of the meniscus using the same criteria that is used to evaluate the native meniscus (Table 12-13). Special attention should be paid to the meniscal root or osseous attachment sites. The transplant should be evaluated for the presence of surfacing signal, meniscal morphology, and displaced meniscal fragments. Artifact is often present from suture material used to stabilize the meniscus. Although this may occasionally limit the evaluation of the meniscus, it should not be misinterpreted as surfacing signal (see Fig. 12-84).

Table 12-13 MRI Evaluation for Complications of Meniscal Transplant (Recurrent Pain)

Complication	MR Finding
Tear of meniscal transplant	Surfacing signal on T1 or T2 Displaced meniscal fragment Abnormal meniscal morphology
Shrinkage of meniscal transplant	Should be similar in size to contralateral meniscus
Displaced meniscal transplant	Position and location
Arthrofibrosis	Scar tissue adjacent to meniscus
Articular cartilage	Thinning, surface irregularity, chondral defects, loose bodies

Specific abnormalities unique to the meniscal transplant include abnormal position of the meniscal tissue and shrinkage of the meniscal tissue (Fig. 12-85). The meniscus should be similar in size to the contralateral native meniscus; shrinkage as much as 30% has been reported and can result in decreased effectiveness of the meniscal tissue in cushioning the adjacent articular surfaces (Fig. 12-86). Extensive arthrofibrosis can also occur, which can lead to pain and decreased range of motion of the knee. Finally, the overlying articular cartilage should be evaluated for abnormalities or defects.

Other Sources of Pain after Meniscal Surgery

Articular Cartilage Damage

Articular cartilage abnormalities occur in up to 40% of patients after meniscal repair or resection and are the most common cause of persistent or recurrent knee pain after meniscal surgery (Fig. 12-87). The

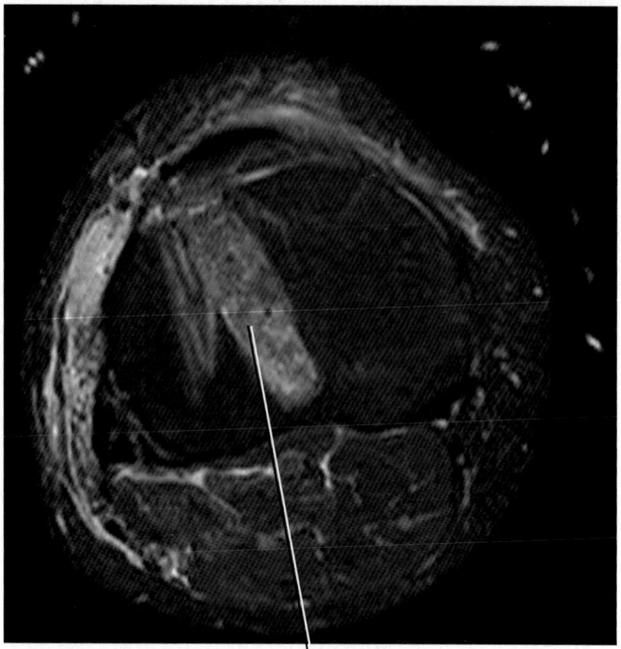
Tibial bone plug used to suture the meniscal transplant to the tibia
A

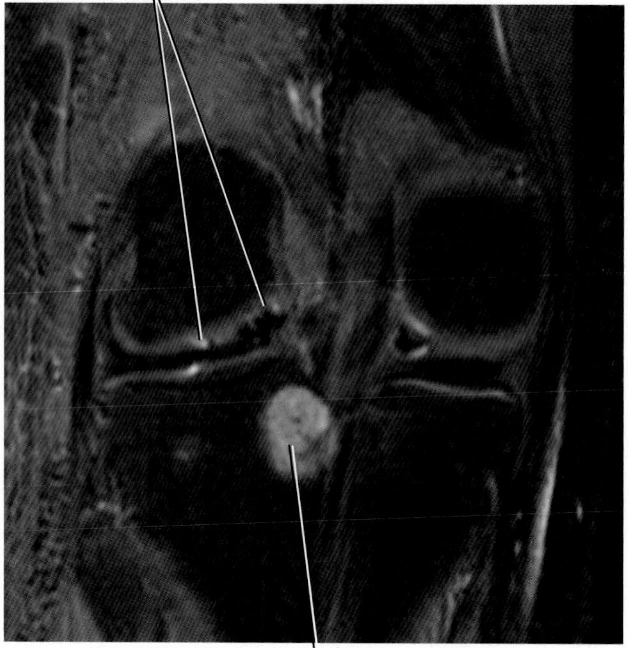
Suture artifact
Tibial bone plug used to suture the meniscal transplant to the tibia
B

Figure 12-84 Normal MRI appearance of a meniscal transplant. A, Normal appearance of the bone plug used to attach the meniscal transplant to the tibia. **B,** Normal appearance of the bone plug as well as small focal areas of susceptibility artifact from suture material used to stabilize the transplanted meniscus. This signal clearly extends off of the meniscus and should not be misinterpreted as surfacing signal or a meniscal tear.

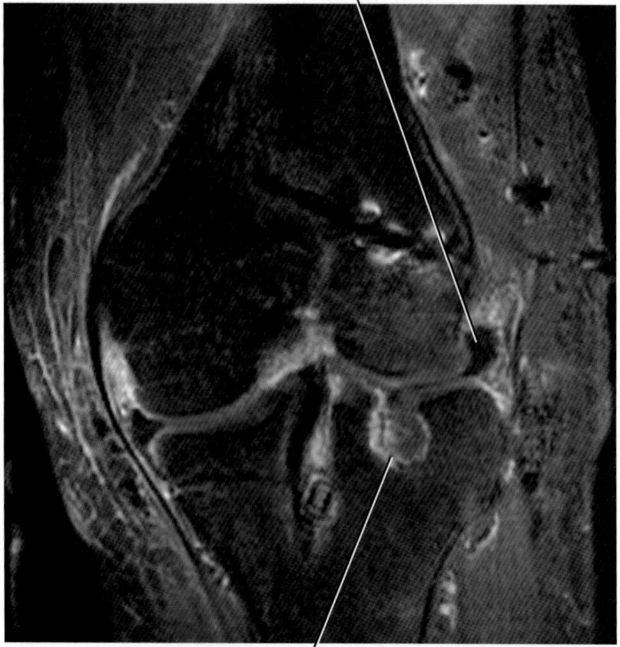
Extrusion of the meniscal transplant
Bone plug indicating meniscal transplant

Figure 12-85 Abnormally positioned meniscal transplant. Coronal T2-weighted image shows extrusion of the meniscal graft resulting in the lack of the normal cushioning effect of the meniscus. The bone plug is seen near the anterior attachment of the meniscal tissue.

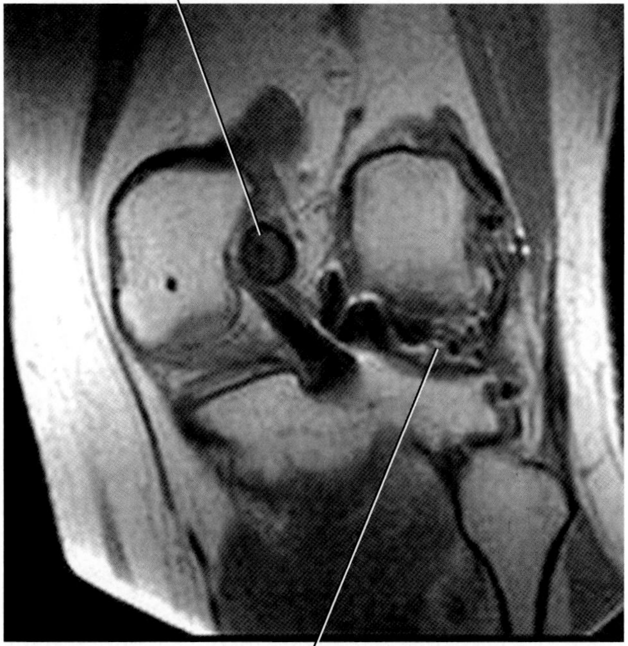

Intra-articular body
A
Suture artifact from meniscal transplant

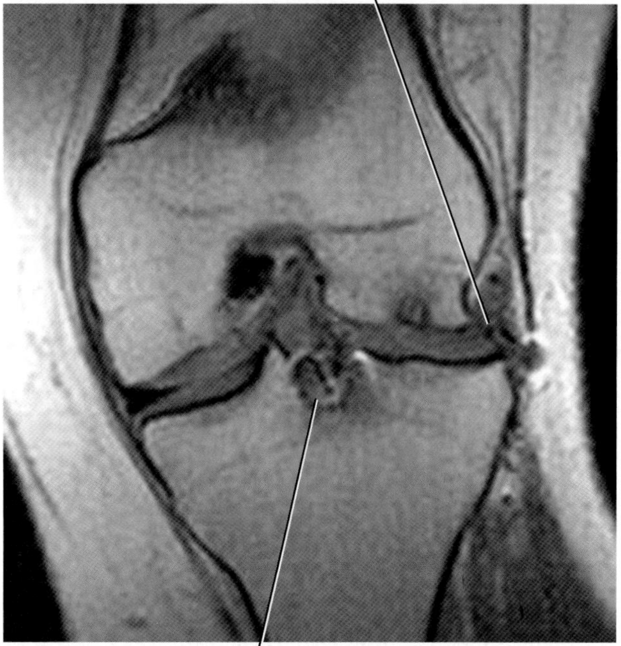

Shrinkage of meniscal transplant and surfacing signal indicating a tear
B
Bone plug indicating prior meniscal transplant

Figure 12-86 Shrinkage and tear of a meniscal transplant. A, Extensive artifact resulting from suture material along the posterior horn of the meniscal transplant limiting the evaluation of the posterior horn. Also note a large intra-articular body within the intercondylar notch. **B,** Shrinkage of the body of the meniscal transplant and surfacing signal representing a tear of the meniscus; osseous changes from an osteochondral allograft in the lateral femoral condyle.

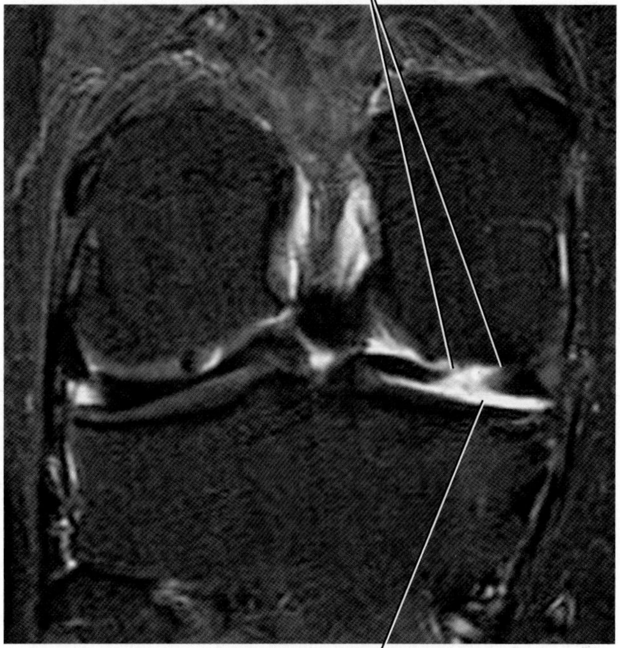

Chondral defect resulting in recurrent knee pain after meniscal surgery
Postsurgical changes indicating prior partial medial meniscectomy

Figure 12-87 Chondral abnormality as a source of recurrent knee pain after meniscal surgery. Coronal T2-weighted image with fat saturation shows a significant chondral defect directly overlying the area of previous partial meniscectomy. This defect occurred as a result of altered weight-bearing forces and was the source of recurrent knee pain after meniscal surgery. No recurrent meniscal tear was present.

appearance of the overlying articular cartilage should be carefully evaluated. Articular cartilage damage may be sustained at the time or the original meniscal injury, or it may occur as a late complication secondary to altered weight-bearing forces after meniscal resection or possibly as a result of destabilization of the knee associated with the meniscal tear and partial meniscal resection. A broad range of chondral injuries can be seen following meniscal surgery, such as diffuse chondral thinning, fissuring or fraying, and a discrete partial- or full-thickness chondral defect. These chondral abnormalities can be a source of considerable pain.

Osteoarthritis

Osteoarthritis is a well-documented long-term complication of meniscal surgery. The development of osteoarthritis appears to be related to the amount of meniscal tissue resected, with up to 40% of patients developing osteoarthritis following complete or near-complete meniscal resection. MRI findings include articular cartilage loss or thinning, subchondral sclerosis, reactive marrow edema, and marginal osteophyte formation. Although the chondral abnormalities and subchondral marrow signal changes are best depicted on T2-weighted or proton density images with fat saturation, the marginal osteophytes are usually best depicted on T1-weighted images (Fig. 12-88).

Intra-articular Bodies

Intra-articular bodies can occur as a result of fragmentation of articular cartilage occurring at the time of original injury or from altered weight-bearing after meniscal surgery. As they are bathed in the normal synovial fluid, they may grow and over time may ossify and develop into ossified intra-articular bodies. Patients with these bodies may present clinically with pain, catching, or locking of the knee. On MRI, purely cartilaginous intra-articular bodies may be difficult to detect unless a joint effusion is present. However, once ossified they are easier to detect and usually

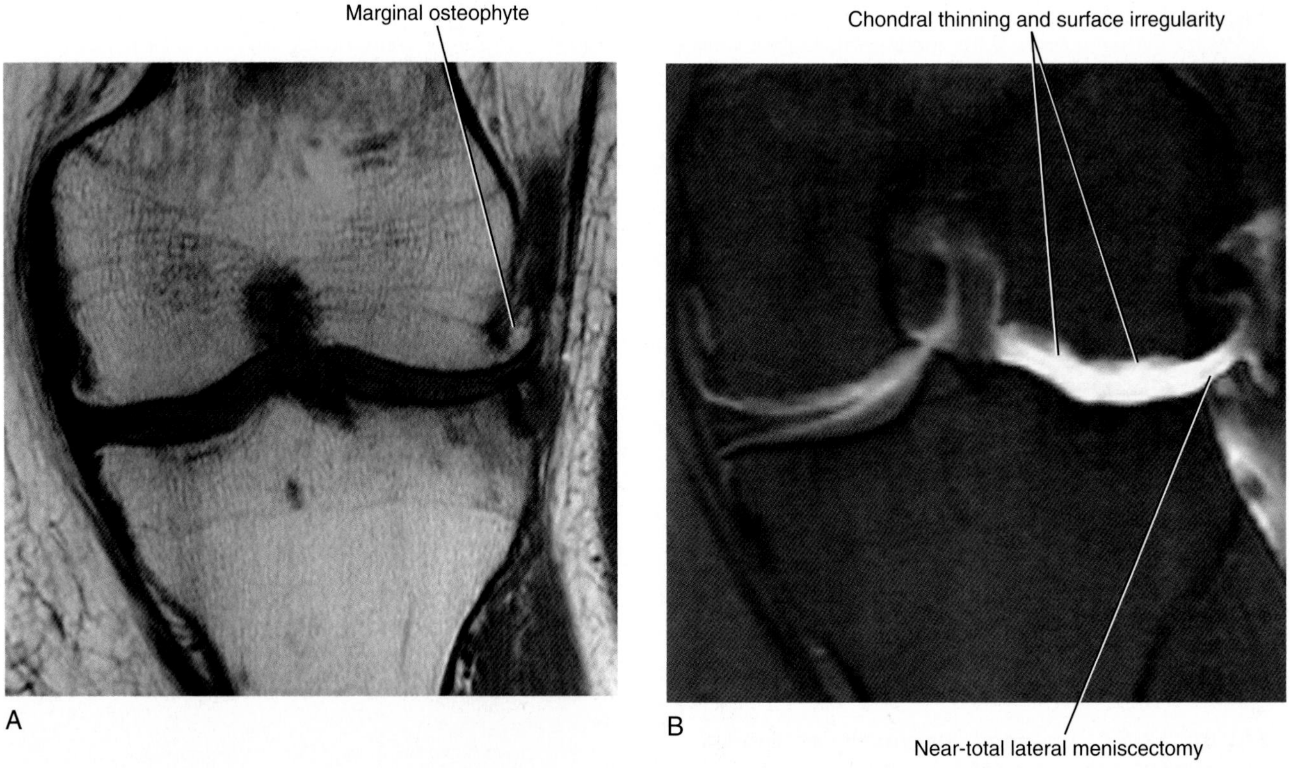
Marginal osteophyte
A
Chondral thinning and surface irregularity
B
Near-total lateral meniscectomy

Figure 12-88 Osteoarthritis as a source of recurrent knee pain after extension lateral meniscal resection. Coronal T1-weighted (**A**) and T2-weighted (**B**) images demonstrate marked osteoarthritis of the lateral compartment of the knee following near-total lateral meniscectomy. Extensive chondral thinning and surface irregularity and large bulky marginal osteophytes are present.

demonstrate a well-corticated margin and marrow signal within the central aspect of the intra-articular body (see Fig. 12-86A).

Subchondral Insufficiency Fracture (Previously SONC)

Subchondral insufficiency fracture is an uncommon postoperative complication that occurs primarily in the middle-aged to elderly patient population, appearing to be more common in women. In the typical clinical scenario, an elderly patient with little or no preexisting osteoarthritis is doing fine after meniscal surgery; then 2 to 18 months after surgery, the patient develops acute-onset knee pain. MRI demonstrates a small subchondral dark line representing a small subchondral fracture with extensive surrounding marrow edema (Fig. 12-89). The medial femoral condyle is most often involved, but spontaneous osteonecrosis can also involve the lateral femoral condyle or either tibial plateau (see Fig. 12-89B). The fracture is usually seen in the mid weight-bearing aspect of the involved articular surface.

In the past, this entity has been referred to as spontaneous osteonecrosis (SONC), but most cases are now thought to represent a focal insufficiency fracture secondary to altered weight-bearing forces that occur as a result of the removal of meniscal tissue. These insufficiency fractures can also occur after a meniscal tear without meniscal surgery and in these cases are thought to occur as a result of destabilization of the meniscus, resulting from the meniscal tear especially if the tear is present at the level of the meniscal root. MRI criteria for these insufficiency fractures include a linear or crescent-shaped subchondral fracture line with extensive adjacent subchondral marrow edema. In the acute setting, this marrow edema may extend all the way to the femoral notch or to the level of the tibial spines when the tibia is involved. Noted that there continues to be considerable debate regarding the proper terminology for describing this entity, and many

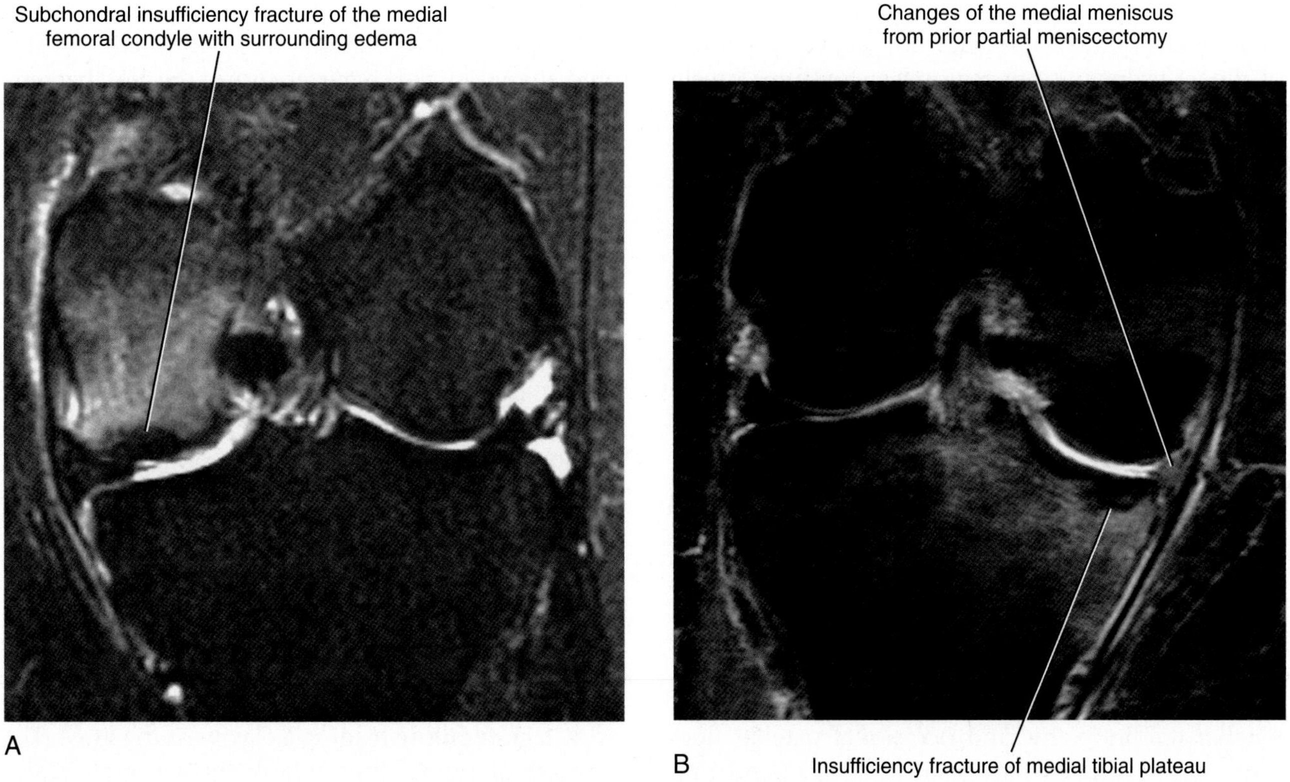
Subchondral insufficiency fracture of the medial femoral condyle with surrounding edema
A
Changes of the medial meniscus from prior partial meniscectomy
B
Insufficiency fracture of medial tibial plateau

Figure 12-89 Insufficiency fracture as a source of pain after partial meniscectomy. A, Coronal T2-weighted image shows a subchondral insufficiency fracture of the medial femoral condyle with extensive surrounding edema following meniscal surgery. **B,** Coronal T2-weighted image from a different patient shows an insufficiency fracture involving the medial tibial plateau with extensive surrounding edema following partial medial meniscectomy.

in the orthopedic community still use the term spontaneous osteonecrosis (SONC) to describe these changes.

MRI of the Reconstructed Anterior Cruciate Ligament

Although many graft options are available for repair of a torn ACL, most often one of the two following types of graft material is used. The *bone-patellar tendon-bone (BTB) graft* is harvested from the central third of the patient's own patellar tendon and contains a bone plug harvested from the patellar attachment on one end of the graft and from the tibial attachment on the other end of the graft. The bone plugs are used to fix the graft in place in the femoral and tibial tunnels. The *hamstring graft* comprises the gracilis and semitendinosus tendons typically harvested from the ipsilateral knee. The hamstring graft does not include bone plugs and therefore requires a different type of fixation device to secure the graft within the osseous tunnels. Graft selection is usually based on surgeon preference. Surgeons can also make a selection between autografts (graft taken from the same patient) or allografts (grafts harvested from cadavers). The use of allografts remains very regional and again is largely dependent on the surgeon's experience and biases. Autografts are still considered the "gold standard" with bone-patellar tendon-bone and hamstring grafts used with about equal frequency. There are some significant risks associated with the use of allografts including HIV, bacterial infection, and delayed integration.

The two types of grafts provide similar long-term outcomes with regard to knee stability. However, the bone-patellar tendon-bone graft may provide slightly stronger fixation early in the course of recovery and is therefore more often used in competitive athletes who are attempting to return to full strength as quickly as possible. The length of rehabilitation, however, may be slightly longer as a result of problems associated with the extensor mechanism. There is increased harvest site morbidity associated with the patellar tendon graft such as anterior knee pain, patellar tendinopathy, and occasional patellar fracture complicating the harvest site. Use of a hamstring graft results in similar long-term outcomes, but because the graft lacks bone plugs, the strength of the graft is slightly diminished during the first year. There is little harvest site morbidity associated with the hamstring tendons because the hamstring muscle strength typically returns to within 80% of normal during the first year after harvest.

The MRI appearance of the normal graft varies based on the time interval from surgery as well as on the type of graft used. The patellar tendon graft is a solid structure and initially demonstrates homogeneous low signal on all pulse sequences, whereas the hamstring graft is composed of either two or three strands and typically demonstrates linear striations within the graft, representing the separate bundles of the graft. During the first 3 months, the grafts are avascular and demonstrate signal intensity similar to the native harvest site. Between 4 and 8 months, the grafts undergo a revascularization process as tiny vessels penetrate the graft and a synovial lining develops. This leads to an MRI appearance of intermediate intrinsic signal within the graft. This appearance should not be misinterpreted as a partial- or full-thickness graft disruption.

The continuity of the fibers should remain intact, and no fluid signal abnormality should be present within the graft. By 12 months, both types of grafts undergo a process referred to as "ligamentization," in which the graft actually undergoes histologic change and appears more like the native ligament. By this time, the MR signal characteristics of the graft become very similar to the native ACL. Various fixation devices are available for use and some of the newer devices are bioabsorbable and may appear radiolucent on radiographs.

After ACL reconstruction, patients with graft complications usually present with one of two clinical scenarios—either with a sensation of laxity (unstable knee) or with a complaint of decreased range of motion (lack of full extension; Table 12-14). Patients with an unstable knee either demonstrate graft disruption, which is seen on MRI as complete discontinuity of the graft fibers (Fig. 12-90), or with a stretched graft, which may appear on MRI as a normal-appearing graft or as an intact graft but with buckling or posterior bowing (Fig. 12-91). The type and age of the graft should be taken into consideration when evaluating the integrity of the graft.

Tunnel lysis or *expansion* is another potential source of ACL graft failure leading to laxity of the knee. The etiology of tunnel lysis following ACL graft placement is thought to be multifactorial but results in inadequate fixation of the graft fibers within the osseous tunnel. Tunnel lysis results in a higher incidence of graft failure over the long term owing primarily to abnormal graft motion. The expanded

Table 12-14 MRI of Anterior Cruciate Ligament Graft Complications

Complaint	Graft Abnormality	MRI Findings
Lax (unstable) knee	Graft disruption	Discontinuity of graft fibers
	Stretched graft	Posterior bowing or buckling
	Tunnel lysis (expansion)	Tunnel enlargement High signal within tunnel surrounding graft
Decreased range of motion	Graft impingement	Anteriorly placed tibial tunnel Increased intrasubstance signal Kinking of graft Posteriorly placed tibial tunnel—vertically positioned graft
	Loose intra-articular bodies	Loose bodies in joint
	Arthrofibrosis	Diffuse or focal spiculated soft tissue Low signal T1/T2

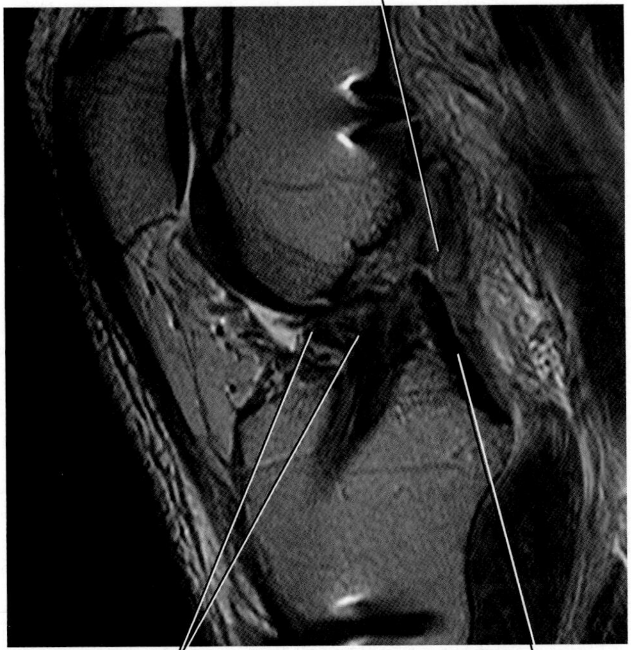
Proximal fibers of disrupted ACL graft
Distal fibers of disrupted ACL graft
Normal PCL

Figure 12-90 Disrupted anterior cruciate ligament (ACL) graft. Sagittal T2-weighted image shows a complete disruption and discontinuity of the ACL graft. PCL, posterior collateral ligament.

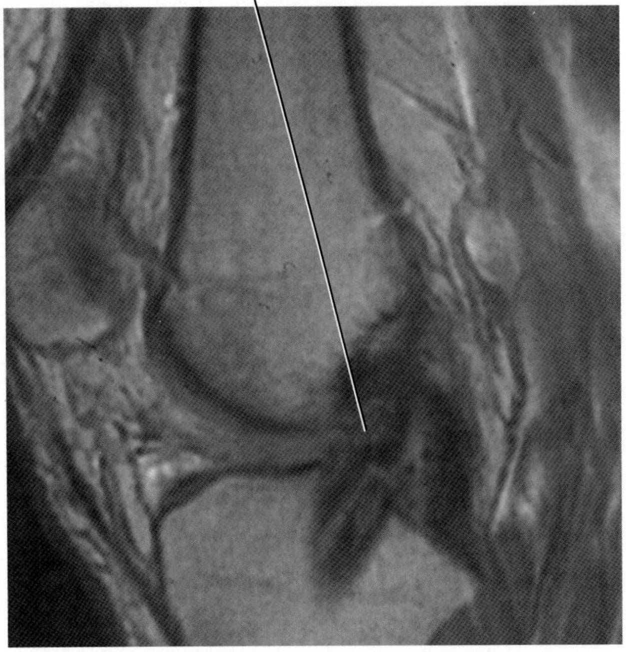
Buckling of the ACL graft indicating a lax stretched graft

Figure 12-91 Stretched graft resulting in increased laxity of the knee after anterior cruciate ligament (ACL) reconstruction. Sagittal T2-weighted image shows buckling of the ACL graft consistent with a stretched graft. Stretching of the ACL graft is more likely to occur when a hamstring-type graft has been used and results in the clinical presentation of a lax knee, mimicking graft disruption.

tunnel complicates graft revision, which must be accomplished in two stages. That is, bone grafting of the enlarged tunnel must first be accomplished; then a delayed graft revision is carried out after the tunnel has filled in with new bone. MRI demonstrates enlargement of the tunnel with either fluid or granulation tissue surrounding the ACL graft (Fig. 12-92). Tunnel lysis typically occurs within the first 3 months after graft placement. Small collections of fluid are normally seen within the osseous tunnels during the first 12 to 18 months when a hamstring graft is used for ACL reconstruction (Fig. 12-93). The fluid collects within the osseous tunnel and between the fibers of the hamstring graft at the time of surgery, and then slowly resorbs over the next 12 to 18 months. These fluid collections are a normal finding and should not be misinterpreted as tunnel expansion. They can be differentiated from tunnel expansion because these small fluid collections do not result in expansion or enlargement of the tunnel.

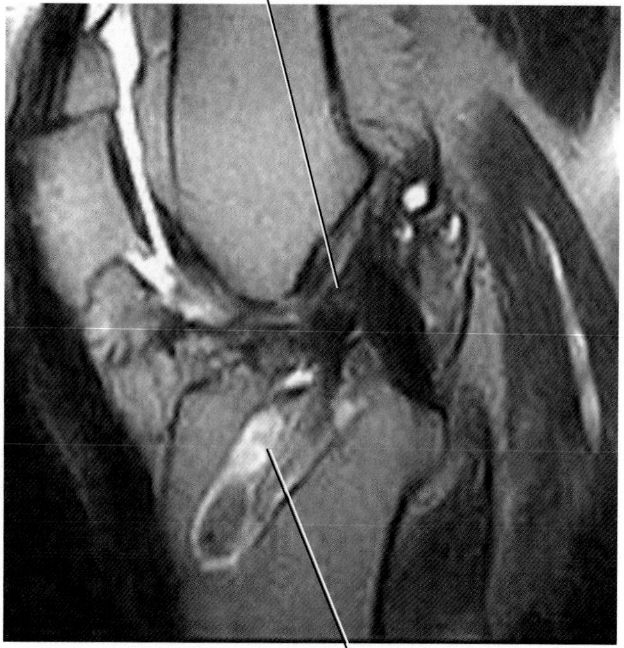
ACL graft normal in region of intercondylar notch
Tibial tunnel expansion with granulation tissue

Figure 12-92 Tunnel lysis (expansion). Sagittal T2-weighted image shows marked expansion of the tunnel and high-signal granulation tissue surrounding the anterior cruciate ligament (ACL) graft fibers within the osseous tunnel.

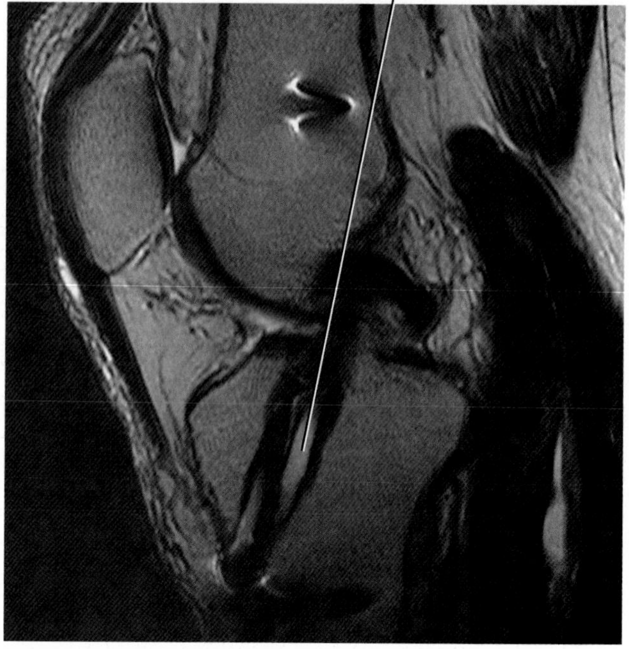
Fluid collection within the tibial tunnel during the first postoperative year is a normal finding; note the lack of tunnel expansion

Figure 12-93 Normal postoperative fluid in tibial tunnel. Sagittal T2-weighted image demonstrates a small normal fluid collection within the tibial tunnel after anterior cruciate ligament reconstruction with a hamstring graft. This is a normal postoperative appearance during the first 18 months. There is no tunnel expansion, and over time this fluid will resorb. The small amount of fluid within the tibial tunnel during the first 18 months is not associated with an increased risk of ganglion formation or tunnel expansion.

Decreased range of motion of the knee following ACL reconstruction usually results from graft impingement, loose intra-articular bodies, or arthrofibrosis. Graft impingement occurs as a result of an improperly positioned tibial tunnel or as a result of regrowth of bone at the level of the roof of the intercondylar notch following notchplasty. If the tibial tunnel is placed too far anteriorly at the time of surgery, the graft impacts the roof of the intercondylar notch when the patient attempts to fully extend the knee, thus preventing full extension of the knee and eventually resulting in disruption of the graft at the site of impingement. MRI findings of graft impingement include (1) an anteriorly placed tibial tunnel (no part of the tunnel should be anterior to an extension of the line drawn along the roof of the intercondylar notch), (2) increased signal within the intercondylar portion of the ACL graft, (3) a change in the course (kinking or posterior bowing) of the graft as it contacts the roof of the intercondylar notch, and (4) fraying or partial-thickness tearing of the anterior margin of the graft at the level of the intercondylar notch (Fig. 12-94). Graft impingement can also occur during extreme flexion of the knee if the ACL graft is positioned too vertically. The normal ACL graft should parallel but not touch the roof of the intercondylar notch. Positioning of the tibia tunnel either too far anterior or too far posterior can result in impingement of the graft.

Patients with intra-articular bodies can present with locking, catching, or decreased range of motion. Loose bodies may arise from articular cartilage damage that occurred at the time of initial injury or may result from hardware failure after ACL graft placement (Fig. 12-95). *Arthrofibrosis* is a term used to describe intra-articular scar tissue that develops after surgery and can present as either as a focal (cyclops lesion) or diffuse area of scar tissue (Fig. 12-96). Diffuse arthrofibrosis is usually seen on MRI as an area of spiculated ill-defined low T2-weighted

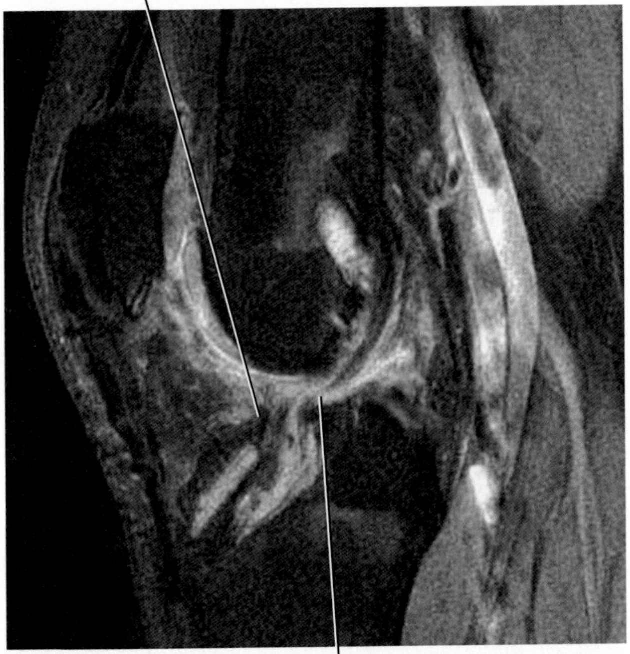
Anteriorly positioned tibial tunnel
Buckling and high signal within the substance of the ACL graft

Figure 12-94 Anterior cruciate ligament (ACL) graft impingement. Sagittal T2-weighted image with fat saturation shows that the anterior portion of the tibial tunnel is positioned anterior to an extension of the line drawn along the roof of the intercondylar notch. This results in impingement of the graft against the roof of the notch when the knee is in full extension. There is kinking of the graft and high signal within the substance of the graft as it passes the roof of the intercondylar notch and enters the tibial tunnel, indicating graft impingement.

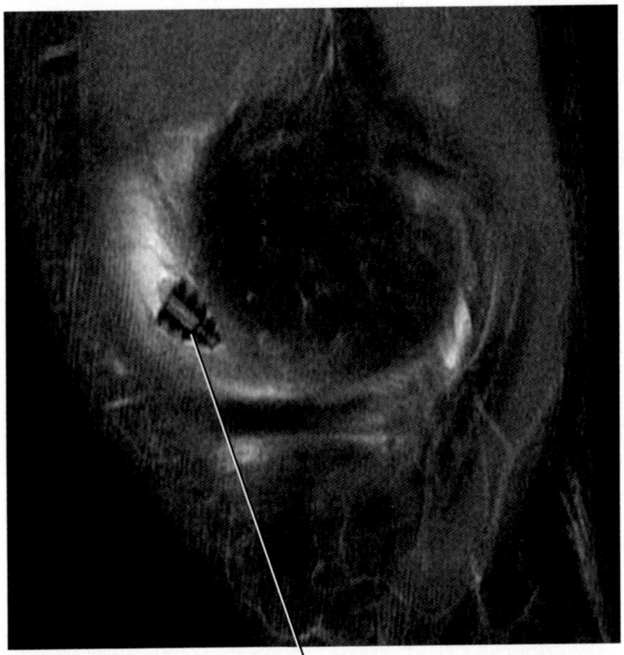
Broken piece of hardware resulting in an intra-articular body following ACL reconstruction

Figure 12-95 Hardware complication following anterior cruciate ligament (ACL) reconstruction. A broken screw fragment in seen within the joint following ACL reconstruction resulting in locking and catching of the knee and decreased range of motion.

signal intensity within Hoffa's fat pad or occasionally as diffuse thickening of the synovium, again dark on T2-weighted images. Focal arthrofibrosis (cyclops lesion) presents as a small focal nodule of scar tissue located just anterior to the intra-articular portion of the ACL graft. Both focal and diffuse forms of arthrofibrosis can result in pain and limitation of motion. Arthrofibrosis is usually initially treated with aggressive physical therapy in an attempt to break up the scar tissue. If this fails, repeat arthroscopy can be performed to resect the scar tissue.

MRI of the Reconstructed Posterior Cruciate Ligament

The PCL is injured less commonly than the ACL, and when injured, it is usually only partially torn. As a result, repair of the PCL is uncommon. Recently, however, it has been shown that a PCL-deficient knee will progress to premature osteoarthritis if left untreated, especially in certain subgroups of patients such as high-performance athletes, military members, or patients with multiple concurrent ligamentous injuries. PCL reconstructions are therefore becoming more common in an attempt to prevent premature osteoarthritis in these subsets of patients. The bone-patellar tendon-bone graft and the hamstring graft are the two most common graft materials used to reconstruct the PCL. The typical MRI of a PCL graft is that of a markedly thickened graft with diffuse intermediate intrasubstance signal during the first year (Fig. 12-97A). This appearance can mimic graft disruption if the knee is imaged during the first year after PCL reconstruction. Graft disruption should not be diagnosed unless discontinuity of the fibers or fluid signal is noted traversing the fibers of the graft. By the end of the first year, the graft becomes better defined and begins to demonstrate low signal throughout (Fig. 12-97B). Extensive arthrofibrosis is commonly seen and is considered a normal finding

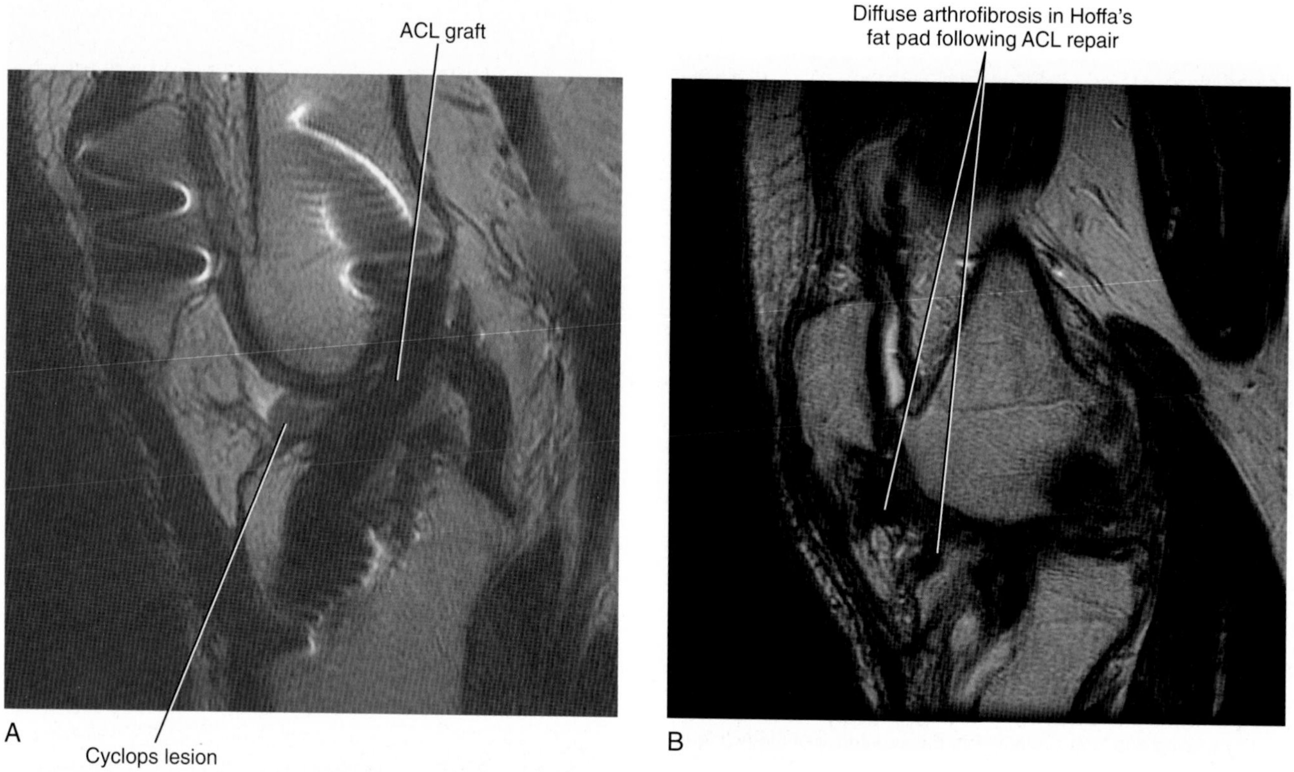
ACL graft
Cyclops lesion
A
Diffuse arthrofibrosis in Hoffa's fat pad following ACL repair
B

Figure 12-96 Arthrofibrosis—focal and diffuse forms following anterior cruciate ligament (ACL) reconstruction. A, Sagittal T2-weighted image shows a focal low-signal mass in the intercondylar notch immediately anterior to the ACL graft representing focal arthrofibrosis (cyclops lesion). **B,** Sagittal T2-weighted image shows diffuse low-signal intensity within Hoffa's fat pad representing a diffuse form of arthrofibrosis.

adjacent to the PCL graft within the posterior aspect of the knee.

Another potential complication of ACL or PCL reconstruction is the formation of an intraosseous tunnel ganglion. If the ganglion protrudes through the nonarticular opening of the tunnel, it will manifest as a palpable mass beneath the surface of the skin (Fig. 12-98). Extrusion of the ganglion through the intra-articular opening of the tunnel and into the intercondylar notch can result in impingement and lead to pain, decreased range of motion, or locking of the knee. Formation of a ganglion within the intraosseous tunnel is associated with graft degeneration and usually indicates impending graft failure. However, note that when a hamstring graft is used for ACL/PCL reconstruction, it is a normal postoperative finding to see small fluid collections located between the separate bundles of the graft during the first year after graft placement. This fluid apparently seeps into the tunnel at the time of graft placement and is easily seen on T2-weighted axial or sagittal images; it should not be misinterpreted as ganglion formation (see Fig. 12-93). This fluid typically resorbs during the first 12 to 18 months and does not lead to ganglion formation.

MRI Evaluation of the Graft Harvest Site

Complications are more likely to occur at the graft harvest site when the patellar tendon graft is used. Anterior knee pain is a common clinical complaint after patellar tendon harvest. Complications include patellar tendinopathy, tendon rupture, or patellar fracture (Fig. 12-99). During the first 2 years after graft harvest, the patellar tendon normally demonstrates moderate to marked thickening and diffuse abnormal signal on MRI. A defect can be seen within the central third of the patellar tendon, but this often fills in with scar tissue and regenerated tendon during the first 2 years after graft harvest (Fig. 12-100). By the end of the second year, the patellar tendon should return to its normal thickness and demonstrate

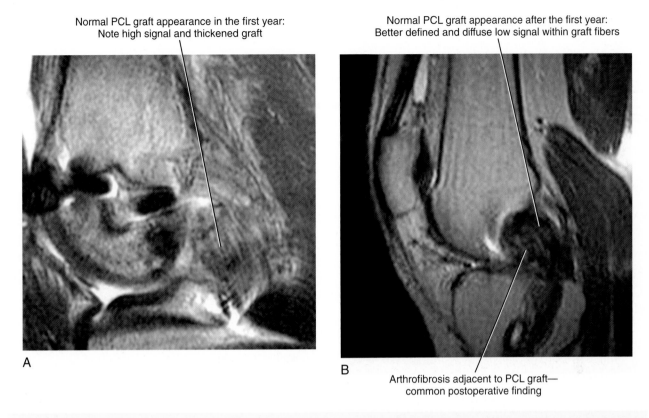

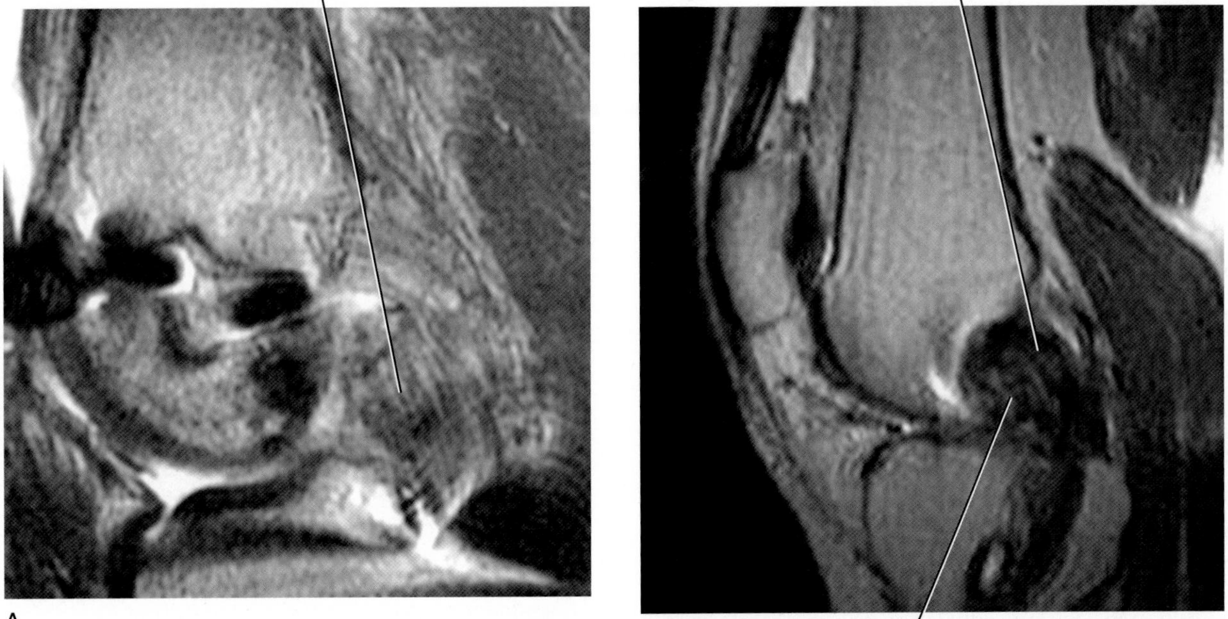
Normal PCL graft appearance in the first year:
Note high signal and thickened graft
A
Normal PCL graft appearance after the first year:
Better defined and diffuse low signal within graft fibers
B
Arthrofibrosis adjacent to PCL graft—
common postoperative finding

Figure 12-97 MRI appearance of a posterior cruciate ligament (PCL) graft. A, Normal appearance of an intact PCL graft within the first year after repair. The graft is thickened and demonstrates extensive intrasubstance signal. This should not be misinterpreted as graft disruption. **B,** A PCL graft in a different patient more than 1 year after surgery. The graft shows low signal throughout and is better defined than during the first year. Note the extensive arthrofibrosis anterior to the graft. This is a common finding following PCL reconstruction and is thought to be partially responsible for the improved stability of the knee after PCL reconstruction.

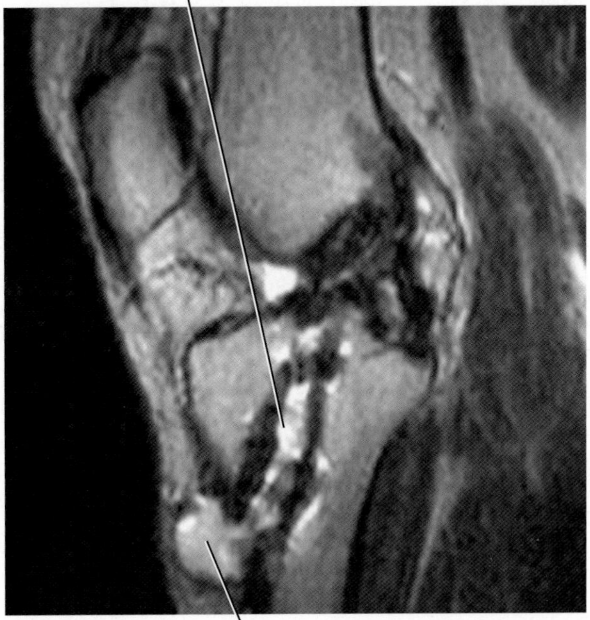
Osseous tunnel ganglion usually
indicates impending graft failure
Extraosseous component presented as a palpable mass

Figure 12-98 Osseous tunnel ganglion. Sagittal T2-weighted image shows a large intraosseous ganglion with extraosseous extension of the ganglion through the distal opening of the tunnel into the anterior soft tissues of the leg. This ganglion presented as a palpable mass and usually indicates degeneration of the graft and impending graft failure.

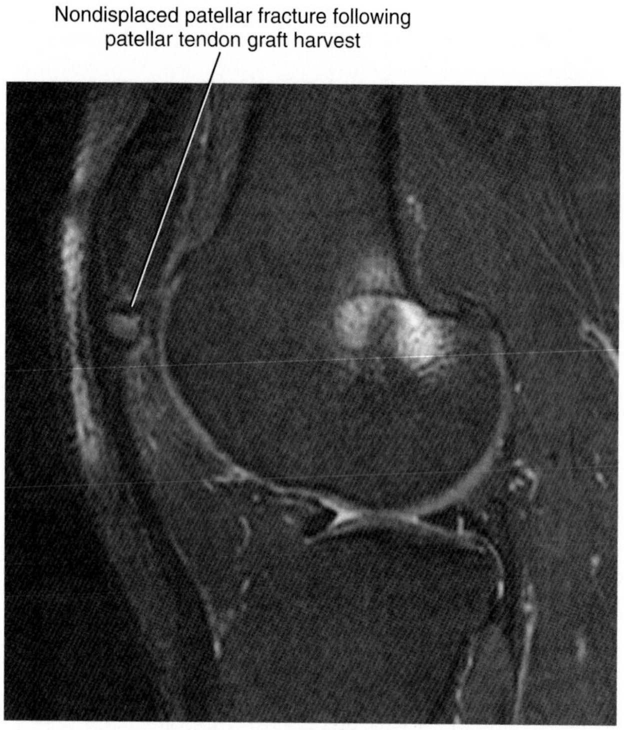
Nondisplaced patellar fracture following patellar tendon graft harvest

Figure 12-99 Patellar fracture complicating graft harvest. Sagittal T2-weighted image shows a nondisplaced fracture of the lower pole of the patella with adjacent marrow edema complicating a patellar tendon graft harvest, which was the source of persistent anterior knee pain in this patient following anterior cruciate ligament reconstruction with a bone-patellar tendon-bone graft.

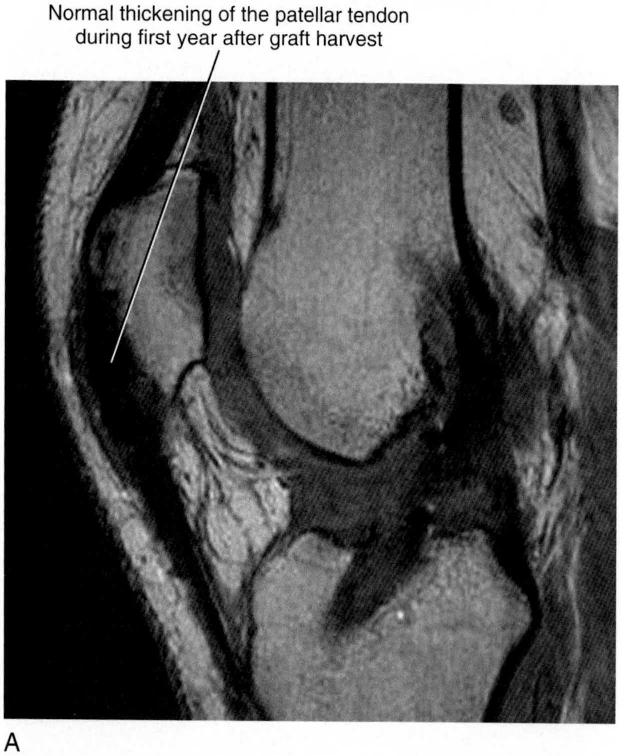
Normal thickening of the patellar tendon during first year after graft harvest
A

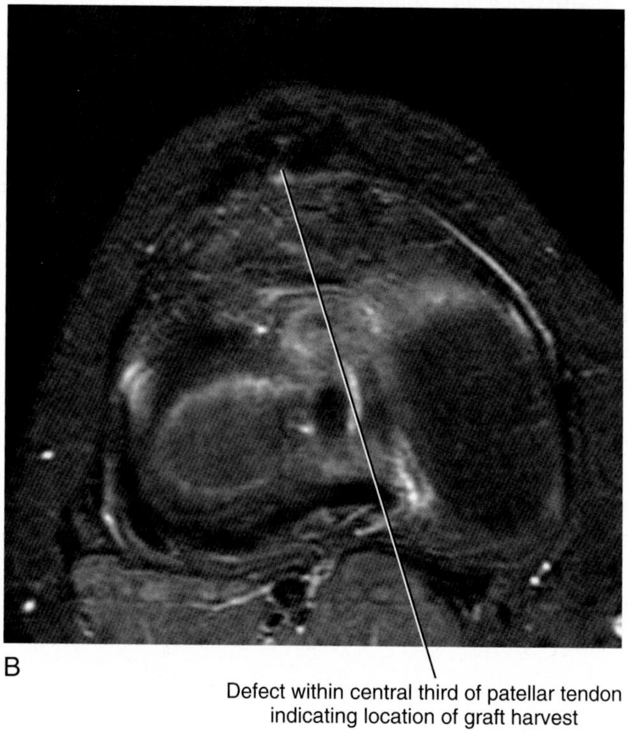
B
Defect within central third of patellar tendon indicating location of graft harvest

Figure 12-100 Normal postoperative appearance of the patella within the first 2 years after graft harvest. **A,** Sagittal T2-weighted image shows marked thickening of the proximal aspect of the patellar tendon—a normal postoperative appearance during the first 2 years after patellar tendon graft harvest. **B,** Axial T2-weighted image shows a defect within the central third of the patellar tendon indicating the location of the patellar graft harvest. This defect typically fills in completely with regenerated patellar tendon and scar tissue and will no longer be evident on MRI by the end of the second year after graft harvest.

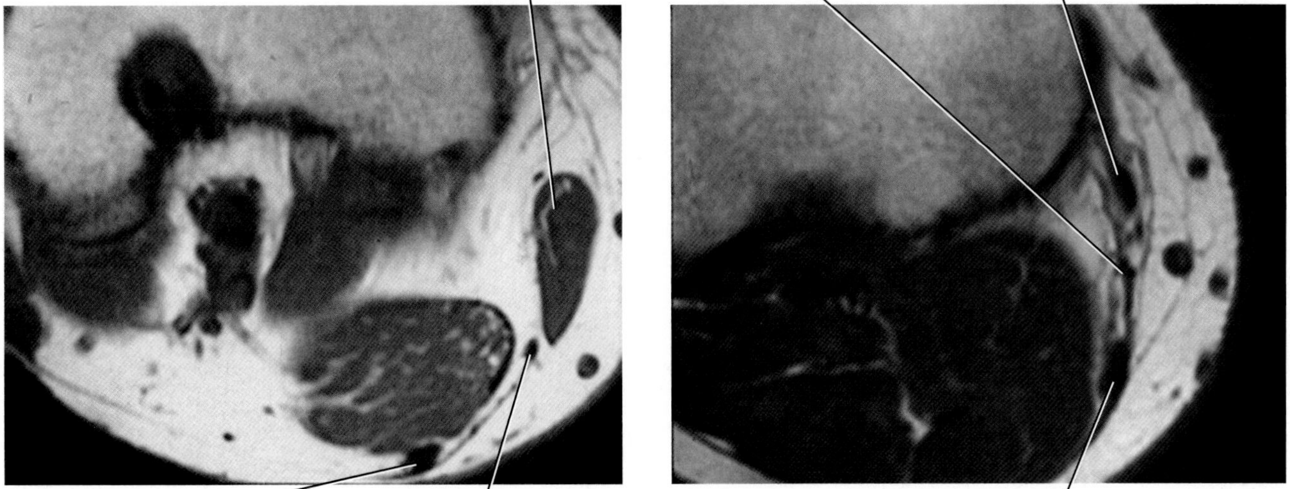
Sartorius muscle
A
Regenerated
semitendinosus tendon
Regenerated gracilis tendon
Regenerated
gracilis tendon
Semimembranosus tendon
B
Regenerated semitendinosus tendon

Figure 12-101 Normal MRI appearance of the hamstring tendon harvest site after 1 year. Axial T2-weighted images at the level of the joint line (**A**) and below the level of the joint line (**B**) show reconstitution of the gracilis and semitendinosus tendons by 1 year after surgical harvest of these tendons.

normal intrinsic signal intensity. It is difficult to diagnose patellar tendinopathy solely on the basis of MRI findings during the first 2 years after graft harvest, and one must rely heavily on the clinical evaluation. During this time frame, the main role of MRI is to detect other complications including patellar tendon rupture and patellar fracture. A patellar tendon more than 1 cm thick 2 or more years after surgery usually indicates patellar tendinopathy.

Hamstring harvest site complications are unusual, and by the end of the first year, the hamstring strength typically returns to more than 80% of its original strength. Immediately after harvest of the hamstring tendons, the tendons are absent and MRI demonstrates fluid in the expected location of the tendons. However, the hamstring tendons have been shown to regenerate over time and usually demonstrate a normal MRI appearance by 8 to 12 months after resection, often making it difficult to even determine that they were previously harvested (Fig. 12-101).

Suggested Readings

Anderson MW. MR imaging of the meniscus. Radiol Clin North Am 2002;40:1081–1094.

Beltran J, Matityahu A, Hwang K, et al. The distal semimembranosus complex: normal MR anatomy, variants, biomechanics and pathology. Skeletal Radiol 2004;32:435–445.

Christian SR, Anderson MB, Workman R, Conway WF, Pope TL. Imaging of anterior knee pain. Clin Sports Med 2006;25: 681–702.

De Smitt AA. MR imaging and MR arthrography for diagnosis of recurrent tears in the postoperative meniscus. Semin Musculoskelet Radiol 2005;9:116–24.

Elias D, White LM. Imaging of patellofemoral disorders. Clin Radiol 2004;59:543–557.

Harish S, O'Donnell P, Connell D, Saifuddin A. Imaging of the posterolateral corner of the knee. Clin Radiol 2006;61: 457–466.

Hayes CW, Coggins CA. Sports-related injuries of the knee: an approach to MRI interpretation. Clin sports Med 2006;25:659–679.

Lerer DB, Umans HR, Hu MX, Jones MH. The role of meniscal root pathology and radial meniscal tear in medial meniscal extrusion. Skeletal Radiol 2004;33:569–574.

Mohana-Borges AV, Resnick D, Chung CB. Magnetic resonance imaging of knee instability. Semin Musculoskelet Radiol 2005; 9:17–33.

Mosher TJ. MRI of osteochondral injuries of the knee and ankle in the athlete. Clin Sports Med 2006;25:843–866.

Naraghi A, White L. MRI evaluation of the postoperative knee: special considerations and pitfalls. Clin Sports Med 2006;25: 703–725.

Sanders TG. MR imaging of postoperative ligaments of the knee. Semin Musculoskelet Radiol 2002;6:19–33.

Sanders TG, Medynski MA, Feller JF, Lawhorn KW. Bone contusion patterns of the knee at MR imaging: footprint of the mechanism of injury. RadioGraphics 2000;20:S135–151.

White LW, Miniaci A. Cruciate and posterolateral corner injuries in the athlete: clinical and magnetic resonance imaging features. Semin Musculoskelet Radiol 2004;8:111–131.

Yao L, Stanczak J, Boutin RD. Presumptive subarticular stress reactions of the knee: MRI detection and association with meniscal tear patterns. Skeletal Radiol 2004;33:260–264.

Chapter 13

IMAGING OF THE ANKLE

CHAPTER OUTLINE

MODALITIES

Radiography

Imaging of the ankle nearly always begins with radiographs, whether in the setting of trauma, arthritis, infection, or suspected mass. The routine radiographic evaluation of the ankle typically includes an anteroposterior view, lateral view (to include the base of the fifth metatarsal) and a mortise view. On the anteroposterior view, the ankle mortise is usually partially obscured by the overlapping fibula. The mortise view is obtained by internally rotating the ankle approximately 15 to 20 degrees, thus eliminating the overlap of the fibula and providing an unobstructed view of the talar dome and the tibial plafond.

Several additional views are available and may be useful in answering specific questions about stability of the ankle or about better delineating the complex anatomy of the hindfoot and the subtalar joint. Anteroposterior views of the ankle may be obtained with inversion or eversion stress to show ligamentous laxity. The unstable ankle demonstrates asymmetry of the mortise (widening or narrowing) when stressed. The contralateral ankle is often imaged for comparison of "normal" laxity. Lateral stress views may also demonstrate an anterior drawer sign indicating ligamentous and capsular injury. Several variations of oblique views are available and may help detect subtle fractures of the ankle or hindfoot. For example, the Harris-Beath (skier's) view is an axial oblique view obtained with the foot in dorsiflexion and provides an additional view of the posterior calcaneal tubercle and the sustentaculum tali.

Computed Tomography

Computed tomography (CT) is often used to assess complex fractures of the ankle and hindfoot. In particular, multislice axial CT examination with sagittal and coronal reconstructions is very helpful in defining the extent of fracture and in delineating the extent of articular surface involvement, particularly in regard to the subtalar joint. CT examination can also be very helpful in detecting fractures that are difficult to visualize on radiographs. These include fractures of the talar dome or neck, fractures of the anterior calcaneal process, fractures of the lateral talar process, and stress fractures of the tarsonavicular bone. CT examination is also very helpful in the evaluation of fracture healing to assess for evidence of delayed union or nonunion and to evaluate for potential complications of fracture fixation hardware such as loosening or infection. Suspicion of tarsal coalition is also an indication for CT examination of the ankle.

Ultrasound

Ultrasound is most often used as a targeted study to answer a specific clinical question about the ankle. Ultrasound has been shown to be very useful in the evaluation of the tendons about the ankle, in particular the Achilles tendon, where ultrasound can accurately detect tendinopathy and partial- and full-thickness tears. The plantar fascia is a superficial structure that can be accurately evaluated with sonography. Ultrasound can accurately differentiate between cystic structures such as a ganglion and soft tissue masses, and it has been shown to be useful in the evaluation of the plantar fascia. Ultrasound is the study of choice to accurately detect and localize foreign bodies with the soft tissues of the ankle and hindfoot. Dynamic evaluation can demonstrate abnormalities such as intermittent subluxation of the peroneal tendons.

Magnetic Resonance Imaging

Magnetic resonance imaging (MRI) is the modality of choice for evaluation of most suspected soft tissue abnormalities of the ankle. MRI accurately depicts abnormalities of the tendons, ligaments, and adjacent musculature. Neurovascular bundles can be evaluated with regard to entrapment syndromes. Moreover, soft tissue and osseous masses can be characterized and their extent described in relation to the adjacent anatomy with the use of MRI. Finally, MRI is very useful in depicting radiographically subtle or occult osseous abnormalities, such as osteochondral injuries of the talar dome, stress fractures of the ankle and hindfoot, and stress-related marrow edema and bone contusions.

PATHOLOGY

Tendons

The tendons of the ankle can be divided into three compartments, anterior, lateral, and posterior, with the posterior compartment further subdivided into deep and superficial compartments (Fig. 13-1). A

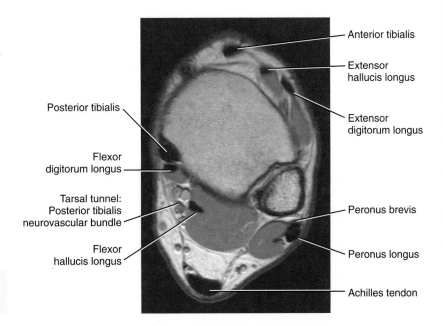

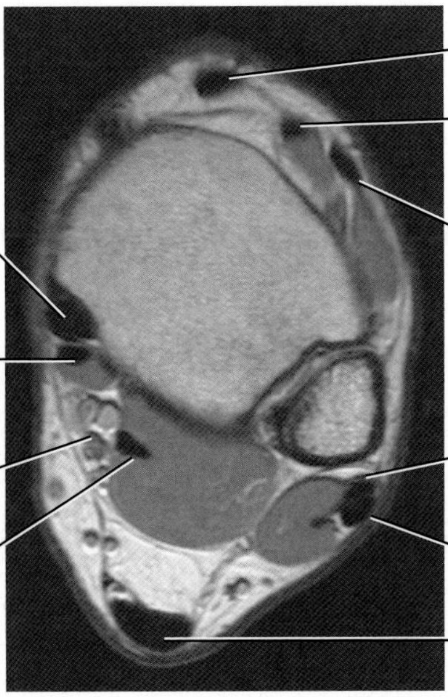
Anterior tibialis
Extensor hallucis longus
Extensor digitorum longus
Posterior tibialis
Flexor digitorum longus
Tarsal tunnel: Posterior tibialis neurovascular bundle
Flexor hallucis longus
Peronus brevis
Peronus longus
Achilles tendon

Figure 13-1 Normal tendon anatomy in the axial MRI plane.

BOX 13-1 RANGE OF TENDON PATHOLOGY

- Tenosynovitis
- Tendinopathy
- Tethering/stenosing tenosynovitis
- Subluxation/dislocation
- Tear
  - Partial/longitudinal split
  - Complete
- Tumor/ganglion
- Ossification
- Congenital anomalies

wide array of disorders can affect these tendons, including tenosynovitis, tendinopathy, tethering, subluxation or dislocation, partial and complete tears, tumors, ossification, and congenital abnormalities (Box 13-1). A thorough understanding of the normal anatomy and MR appearance along with knowledge of the common pitfalls is necessary to accurately evaluate the tendons of the ankle.

In general, tendons are best evaluated using MRI. Axial T1-weighted or proton density images are best suited for demonstrating tendon anatomy, whereas axial T2-weighted images with fat saturation are best suited for demonstrating tendon pathology. Each tendon, however, should be assessed along its entire course in all three imaging planes to ensure normal signal characteristics, morphology, and position. The normal tendon should appear dark on all pulse sequences with the exception of increased T1 signal resulting from magic angle artifact.

A small amount of fluid can occur within any of the tendon sheaths of the ankle in an asymptomatic patient, with the exception of the Achilles tendon, which does not have a surrounding sheath. Small asymptomatic fluid collections can be difficult to differentiate from symptomatic fluid because the precise volume of fluid indicative of disease has not been determined. A good rule of thumb to follow when evaluating the quantity of fluid within a tendon sheath is that any fluid collection smaller in diameter than the adjacent tendon is likely a normal physiologic finding and clinically insignificant, whereas a fluid collection that is equal to or greater in diameter than the adjacent tendon or a fluid collection containing complex debris (synechiae) is probably indicative of tenosynovitis (Fig. 13-2A). The one exception is the flexor hallucis longus (FHL) tendon sheath, which communicates freely with the ankle joint and can contain large quantities of fluid in asymptomatic patients. The diagnosis of FHL tenosynovitis should be considered when a fluid collection within the tendon sheath is large and out of proportion to the volume of the ankle effusion or when synechiae or debris are present.

Tenosynovitis usually results from repetitive overuse, but it may occur in association with an inflammatory arthropathy or may be infectious in origin. Differentiating between an infectious and an inflammatory tenosynovitis may not always be

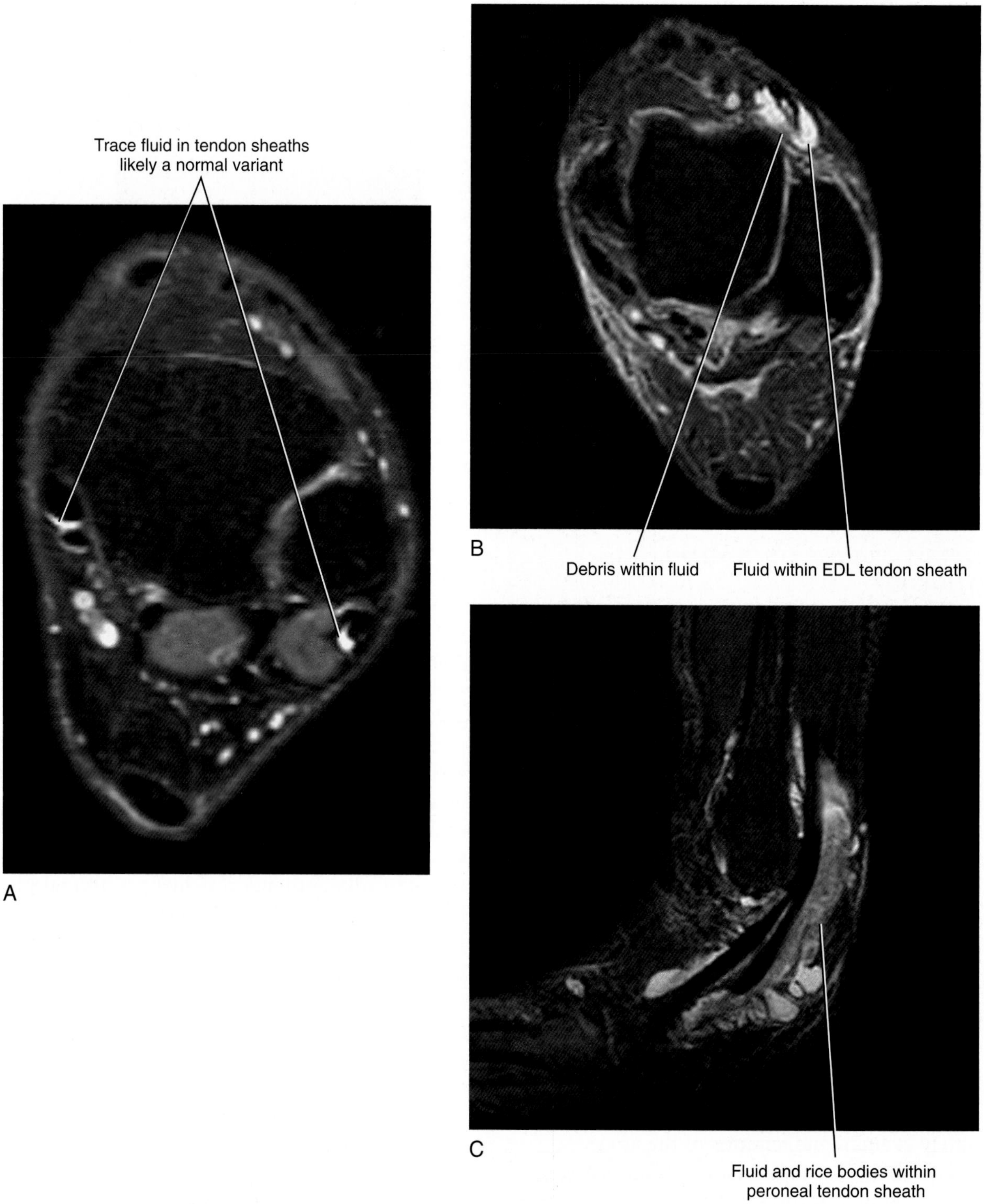
Trace fluid in tendon sheaths
likely a normal variant
A
B
Debris within fluid
Fluid within EDL tendon sheath
C
Fluid and rice bodies within
peroneal tendon sheath

Figure 13-2 Tenosynovitis. ***A,*** Axial T2-weighted image demonstrates minimal fluid within the posterior tibialis and peroneal tendon sheaths likely a normal asymptomatic finding. ***B,*** Axial T2-weighted image shows moderate fluid and debris within the extensor digitorum longus (EDL) tendon sheath consistent with tenosynovitis. ***C,*** Sagittal T2-weighted image with fat saturation show extensive fluid and rice bodies in the peroneal tendon sheath in this patient with rheumatoid arthritis.

possible on the basis of MRI; however, infectious tenosynovitis often contains debris or appears complex and may demonstrate inflammatory changes, edema, and enhancement of the surrounding soft tissues. These signs, however, are not specific and can be seen with noninfectious tenosynovitis as well. Tenosynovitis associated with a chronic inflammatory arthropathy may contain rice bodies, which represent fibrinous exudative debris and often occur in conjunction with inflammatory changes of the adjacent joint, such as synovial thickening, erosions, and subchondral reactive marrow edema (Fig. 13-2C).

Abnormalities of the tendons occur along a continuum beginning with mild tendinosis; more significant disease includes moderate tendinosis with or without partial-thickness tearing and finally complete disruption. Tendinosis usually appears as thickening or thinning/attenuation of the tendon with associated intermediate intrinsic signal abnormality on both T1- and T2-weighted images. Subtendinous bone marrow edema often occurs in association with overlying tendon pathology and may be symptomatic. Chronic tendinosis or an old partial-thickness tear of the Achilles tendon may result in calcific tendinitis or even ossification of the affected tendon, but this finding is rarely seen in other tendons of the ankle. Radiographs can be of great value in confirming calcific tendinitis or heterotypic bone formation. A partial-thickness tear of the tendon may present as an interstitial tear, which can be seen on MRI as linear fluid signal within the substance of the tendon or as a focal area of tendon thinning and attenuation. Finally, a complete tear appears as discontinuity of the tendon with a gap between the torn tendon ends. The gap may be filled with fluid or granulation tissue, depending on the chronicity of the injury.

Several MRI pitfalls can potentially mimic tendon pathology (Box 13-2). Magic angle phenomenon is a common artifact resulting in increased signal within the substance of the tendon seen only on the T1-weighted images. It most commonly occurs in the posterior tibialis and peroneal tendons as they transition from the ankle into the foot, and it should not be misinterpreted as tendinosis. Phase-encoding artifact resulting from patient motion or from pulsation of blood within adjacent vessels can result in intrinsic signal within the substance of the tendon mimicking tendinosis. Finally, unfamiliarity with certain normal anatomic configurations or anatomic variations of the tendons can mimic disease. The posterior tibialis tendon normally broadens and splays and then splits just before its insertion on the tubercle of the navicular bone with the largest portion of the tendon inserting on the tubercle and several smaller slips extending into the midfoot to attach more distally. The appearance of the posterior tibialis tendon just proximal to its navicular insertion site can mimic focal tendinosis. With regard to normal anatomic structures mimicking pathology of the peroneal tendons, the presence of an accessory peroneus quartus tendon can mimic a split peroneus brevis tendon, and the calcaneofibular ligament, which is normally located just deep to the peroneal tendons below the distal tip of the fibula, can also mimic a split of the peroneus brevis tendon.

BOX 13-2 PITFALLS MIMICKING TENDON PATHOLOGY

Magic angle artifact
Phase-encoding artifact
Anatomic variations

Anterior Compartment

The tendons of the anterior compartment are responsible for dorsiflexion of the foot with the tibialis anterior tendon functioning as the primary dorsiflexor. From medial to lateral, the tendons include the anterior tibialis tendon, the extensor hallucis longus (EHL), and the extensor digitorum longus (EDL) tendons (see Fig. 13-1). Rupture of the anterior tibialis tendon is rare, occurring most commonly in people over 45-years of age and in athletes who participate in downhill running or marching and soccer kicking (Fig. 13-3). Injury also occasionally occurs as a result of direct trauma or laceration since the extensor tendons are superficial structures along the dorsal aspect of the foot and ankle. Unlike most tendons of the foot, which have dual blood supplies, the anterior tibialis tendon has a singular blood supply derived from the anterior tibial artery and as such is at increased risk for ischemia and injury in older persons with peripheral vascular disease. Ischemic changes of the anterior tibialis muscle and tendon classically manifest as a tender anterior soft tissue mass above the level of the ankle in the elderly patient with peripheral vascular disease.

It is less common to see physiologic fluid in the extensor compartment than in the flexor

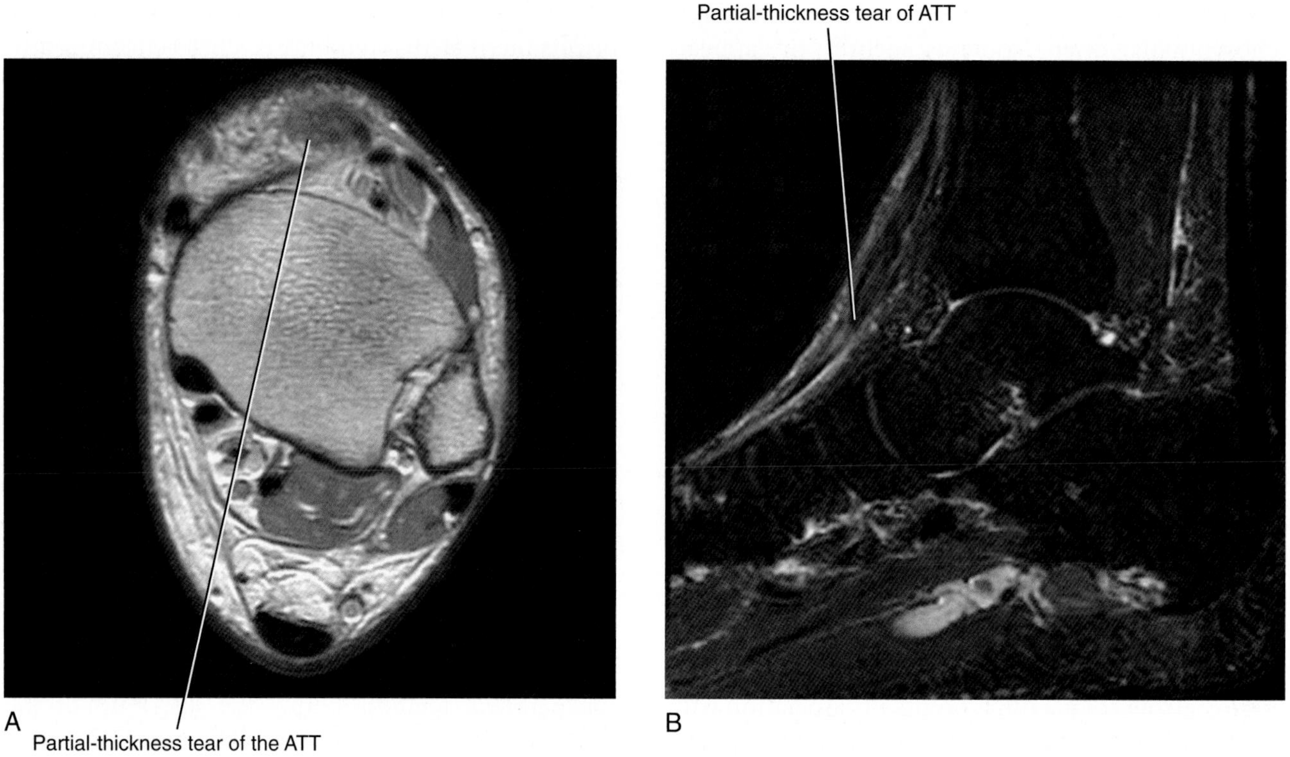
Partial-thickness tear of ATT
A
Partial-thickness tear of the ATT
B

Figure 13-3 Partial-thickness tear of the anterior tibialis tendon (ATT). Axial proton density (**A**) and sagittal (**B**) STIR images show marked thickening and abnormal intrinsic signal within the proximal aspect of the ATT consistent with marked tendinosis; slightly more distal there is marked attenuation and thinning of the tendon representing a partial-thickness tear.

compartment tendon sheaths, and, as a result, any fluid—even a small quantity seen within an extensor tendon sheath—is more likely to be associated with symptoms (see Fig. 13-2A). Occasionally, an accessory tendon, the peroneus tertius, is present within the anterior compartment positioned lateral to the extensor digitorum tendon and should not be misinterpreted as a tear or split tendon. When present, the peroneus tertius tendon is seen as the "fourth extensor tendon" and is located lateral to the extensor digitorum longus tendon and inserts on the base of the fifth metatarsal.

Posterior Compartment

The tendons within the deep aspect of the posterior compartment are primarily responsible for plantar flexion and inversion of the foot. From medial to lateral are the posterior tibialis tendon, the flexor digitorum longus (FDL) and the flexor hallucis longus (FHL) tendons (see Fig. 13-1). The tarsal tunnel is a confined space along the posterior medial aspect of the ankle that is bound superficially by the flexor retinaculum and deep by the posterior border of the tibia and talus. It contains the posterior tibialis tendon, FDL and FHL tendons and the posterior tibialis neurovascular bundle.

Posterior Tibialis Tendon The posterior tibialis (PT) tendon is the primary inverter of the foot and also provides important stability to the arch of the midfoot. Posterior tibialis tendon dysfunction refers to a spectrum of abnormalities ranging from mild tendinosis to complete tendon rupture resulting in medial sided ankle pain. Although complete rupture is rare, it is a devastating injury that leads to progressive collapse of the arch of the foot and a painful degenerative midfoot arthritis that often requires a triple arthrodesis for stabilization and pain relief. Posterior tibialis tendon dysfunction most commonly occurs in women over age 50, but other predisposing factors include prior flatfoot deformities, diabetes, renal failure, rheumatoid arthritis, and seronegative arthropathies. Acute disruption can also occur in young athletes participating in sports that require rapid change of direction, and it has been reported in ballet dancers and soccer and basketball players.

The normal posterior tibialis tendon is roughly twice the diameter of the adjacent FDL tendon and sits within a shallow retromalleolar groove along the posterior margin of the distal tibia, held in place by the flexor retinaculum as it transitions from the ankle to the foot. Just prior to the level of the tarsonavicular bone, the tendon broadens and splits with the majority of the tendon inserting onto the medial tubercle of the tarsonavicular bone with several smaller tendon slips extending distally into the midfoot to insert on the cuneiforms and the base of the second through fourth metatarsals. The focal area of transition of the posterior tibialis tendon just before its insertion on the tarsonavicular bone can easily be misinterpreted as a focal area of tendinosis because the tendon broadens immediately before insertion onto the navicular tubercle.

Signs associated with focal tendinosis at this level include abnormal intrinsic signal within the tendon, fluid and synechiae adjacent to the tendon and peritendinous soft tissue edema, or adjacent reactive subcortical marrow edema within the navicular tubercle. The presence of fluid adjacent to the distal 1 to 2 cm of the posterior tibialis tendon just prior to insertion on the navicular bone is a good sign of pathology because there is no tendon sheath at this level.

The os naviculare is a common normal variant accessory ossification center located at the level of the navicular tubercle. Os naviculare can be classified as type 1—small accessory ossicle contained with the posterior tibialis tendon with no articulation to the navicular; type 2—large accessory ossicle with an articular facet (synchondrosis); and type 3—a cornuate bony navicular tuberosity. Types 2 and 3 are often associated with an increased incidence of posterior tibialis tendon dysfunction and medial-sided ankle pain. MRI signs that are associated with a symptomatic os naviculare include marrow edema within the accessory ossification center and adjacent soft tissue edema. An unstable synchondrosis can also be associated with medial-sided ankle pain. The presence of fluid within the synchondrosis, subcortical cysts, sclerosis, and marrow edema on either side of the synchondrosis are MR and CT imaging signs, thus suggesting instability of the os naviculare, and indicate a potential unstable attachment of the posterior tibialis tendon (Fig. 13-4).

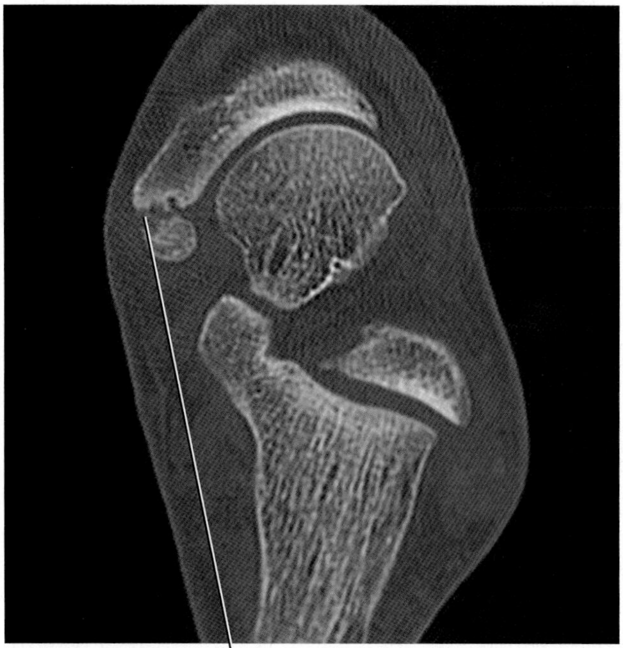
A
Sclerosis and medullary cystic change involving synchondrosis indicates an unstable os naviculare

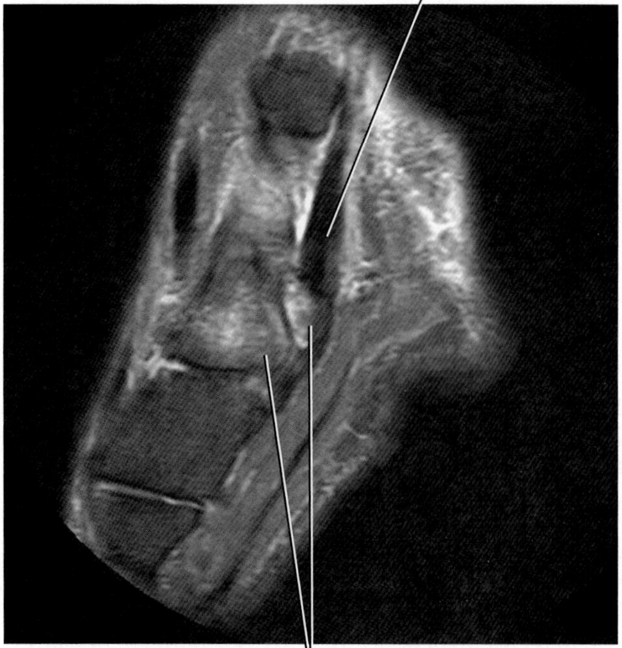
Posterior tibialis tendon
B
Marrow edema on either side of synchondrosis indicates instability

Figure 13-4 Os naviculare. A, Axial CT section through the midfoot shows an os naviculare with sclerosis and cystic change on both sides on the synchondrosis indicative of instability. **B,** Sagittal T2-weighted image with fat saturation shows marrow edema on both sides of the synchondrosis also indicative of instability of the os naviculare.

SECTION IV

Table 13-1 Posterior Tibialis Tendon Dysfunction: MRI Grading System

Type	Description of Tendon	Treatment
I	Hypertrophic (thickened)	Conservative
II	Atrophic (thinned/attenuated)	Surgical
III	Complete tear	Surgical

Table 13-2 Posterior Tibialis Tendon Dysfunction: Surgical Grading System

Stage	Clinical Findings	Treatment Options
I	Tendinosis/tenosynovitis	Conservative
II	Tendinopathy/flexible	Brace: Low risk, lifelong, does not correct deformity
	Correctible	Surgery: Corrects deformity, long recovery
III	Fixed/midfoot arthritis	Brace Surgery: Triple arthrodesis
IV	Fixed/midfoot and ankle arthritis/ankle varus deformity	Surgery: Triple arthrodesis with calcaneal osteotomy; triple arthrodesis with deltoid repair

An MRI grading system has been described, which can be used to quantify abnormalities of the posterior tibialis tendon. The various grades have surgical implications (Table 13-1). A type I tear is seen as thickening of the tendon with intrinsic signal alteration and is referred to as hypertrophic tendinosis (Fig. 13-5). Partial-thickness interstitial longitudinal tears often accompany hypertrophic tendinosis and appear on MRI as fluid signal intensity streaks within the substance of the tendon. A type I tear is usually treated conservatively. A type II tear is considered atrophic with thinning and attenuation of the tendon. The tendon is usually thinner than the adjacent FDL tendon, and this type of tear typically requires surgical repair. A type III tear is complete seen on MRI as disruption of the tendon with a fluid-filled gap and retraction of the torn tendon ends. Types II and III tears lead to progressive midfoot collapse and osteoarthritis, resulting in chronic midfoot pain.

Failure of the posterior tibialis tendon is referred to clinically as posterior tibialis tendon dysfunction and leads to anatomic changes of the hindfoot. It is often associated with stretching or disruption of the spring ligament. Radiographic changes associated with posterior tibialis tendon dysfunction include pes planus, arch collapse, hindfoot valgus, overpronation, and forefoot abduction. On MRI, changes that can be seen are hindfoot valgus, uncovering of the medial talar head, calcaneofibular abutment, and pes planus deformity.

A four-point classification system is used for clinical staging of posterior tibialis dysfunction (Table 12-2), which deals more with the clinical presentation than with the extent of posterior tibialis tendon pathology. Stage I is tenosynovitis in which the patient presents with medial ankle pain and swelling. At this stage, the tendon remains normal and there is no arthritis of the midfoot. Stage II is a tendinopathy with flexibility of the ankle and midfoot. There may be early arthritis of the midfoot, but the midfoot remains flexible and the deformity is passively correctible. Stage III is tendinosis with fixed arthritic changes of the midfoot. At this stage, the deformity of the midfoot is no longer passively correctible. This stage of disease is most commonly seen in patients over 60 years of age. Stage IV is tendinopathy with rigid arthritis of the midfoot and ankle. At this stage, radiographs or MRI demonstrate arthritis of the tibiotalar joint and ankle valgus in addition to the arthritic changes of the midfoot. Surgical treatment of stage IV disease usually consists of triple arthrodesis, possibly with deltoid repair or calcaneal osteotomy. Ultrasound examination with power Doppler can also accurately detect and classify abnormalities of the posterior tibialis tendon (Fig. 13-6).

Flexor Digitorum Longus Tendon At the level of the ankle, the flexor digitorum longus (FDL) tendon is positioned between the posterior tibialis tendon and the flexor hallucis longus (FHL) tendon (see Fig. 13-1). As the FDL tendon extends into the midfoot, it crosses superficial to the FHL tendon (an anatomic landmark called Henry's knot) and then gives off a tendon slip to each of the second through fifth digits. Isolated abnormalities of the FDL tendon are rare, but it is not uncommon to have tenosynovitis of the FDL tendon sheath in conjunction with tenosynovitis of the adjacent posterior tibialis or FHL tendons. Tenosynovitis of the FDL tendon is most likely to occur in the midfoot at the level of intersection with the FHL tendon, and MRI will demonstrate the presence of fluid within the tendon sheath at the level of Henry's knot (Fig. 13-7).

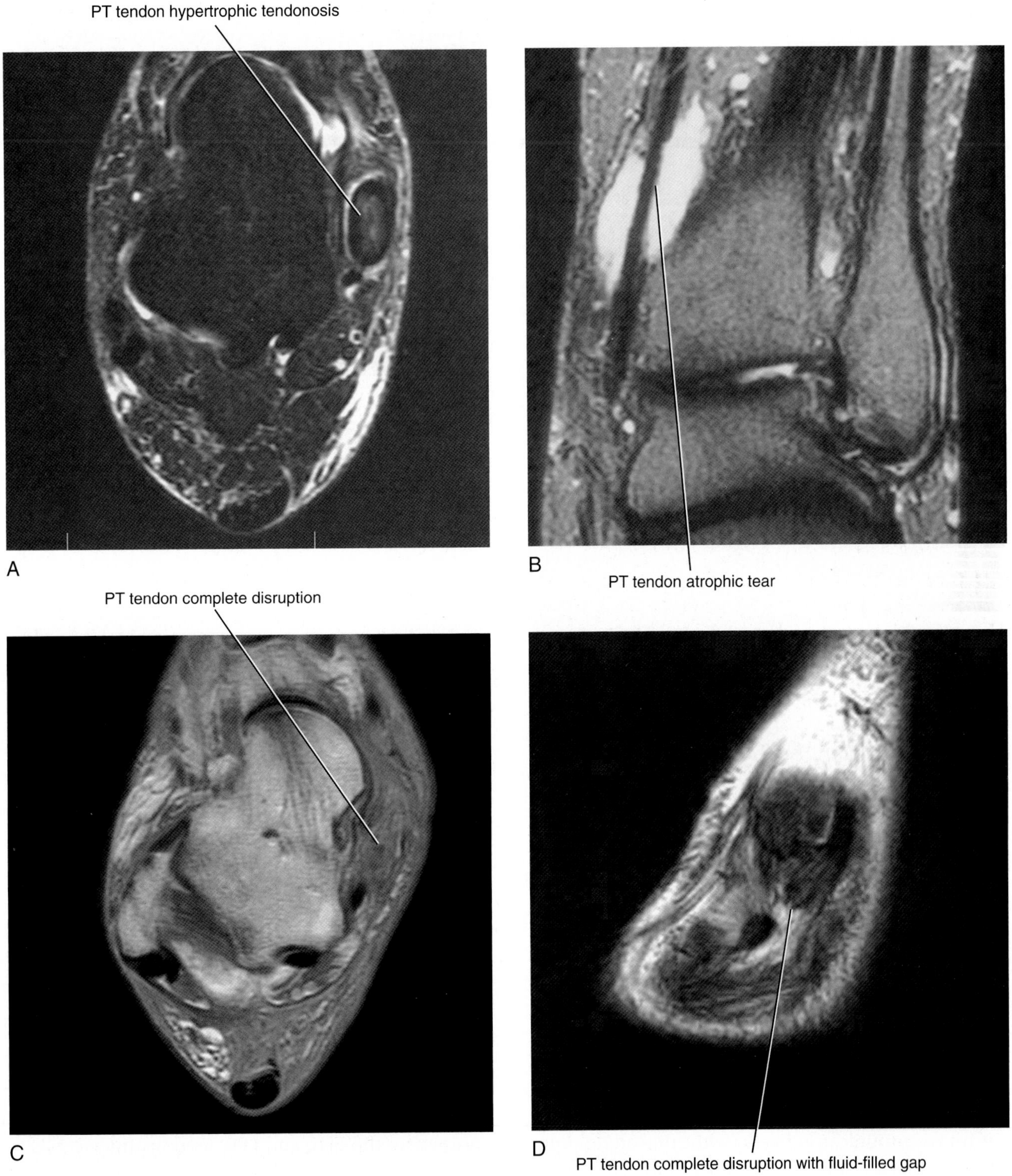
PT tendon hypertrophic tendonosis
A
B
PT tendon atrophic tear
PT tendon complete disruption
C
D
PT tendon complete disruption with fluid-filled gap

Figure 13-5 Grading system for posterior tibialis (PT) tendon tears. A, Type I tear is referred to as hypertrophic tendinosis and shows thickening and abnormal intrinsic signal of the PT tendon. **B,** Type II tear is referred to as an atrophic tendinosis and reveals thinning, attenuation, and partial-thickness tearing of the tendon. **C** and **D,** Type III tear is complete with a full-thickness disruption and retraction of the torn tendon ends. PTT, posterior tibialis tendon.

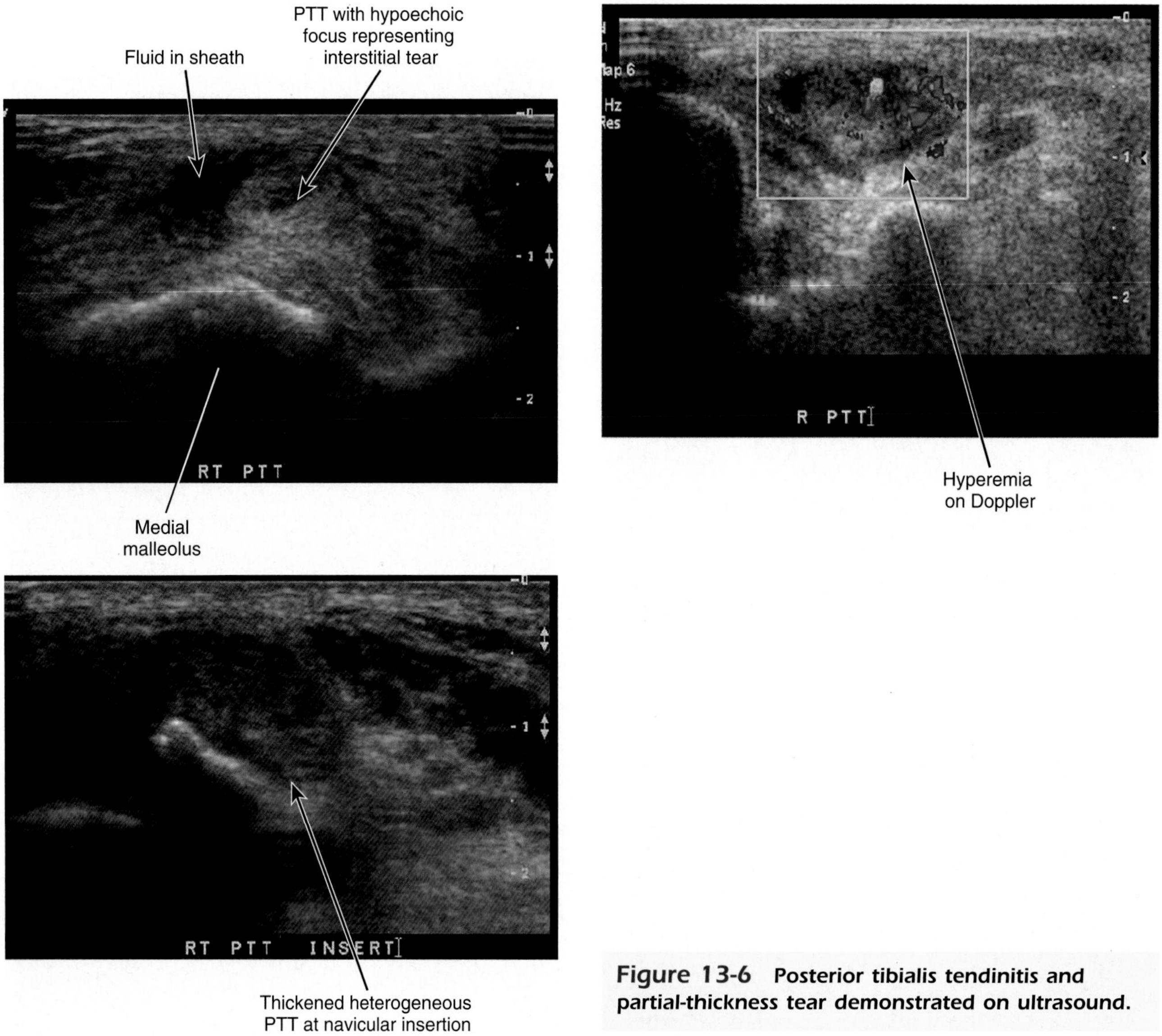
Fluid in sheath
PTT with hypoechoic focus representing interstitial tear
RT PTT
Medial malleolus
R PTT
Hyperemia on Doppler
RT PTT INSERT
Thickened heterogeneous PTT at navicular insertion

Figure 13-6 Posterior tibialis tendinitis and partial-thickness tear demonstrated on ultrasound.

Flexor Hallucis Longus Tendon At the level of the ankle, the FHL tendon is positioned between the medial and lateral talar tubercles and then passes beneath the sustentaculum tali as it extends to the level of the midfoot. It then crosses deep to the FDL tendon at Henry's knot before inserting onto the base of the distal phalanx of the great toe. The FDL tendon sheath communicates freely with the ankle joint space and as a result, considerable fluid can be seen within the tendon sheath even in asymptomatic individuals. To diagnose tenosynovitis of the FHL, a large amount of fluid out of proportion to the ankle effusion or the presence of synechiae or complex debris within the fluid should be present.

Tendinosis of the FHL most commonly occurs in athletes who perform extreme plantar flexion and push-off from a plantar-flexed position. It can also occur in association with an os trigonum, or an unfused posterior lateral tubercle of the talus, which has been referred to as the os trigonum syndrome (Fig. 13-8). Tendinosis of the FHL most commonly occurs at the level of the tibiotalar joint, but another common location includes the midfoot at Henry's knot where the FHL and FDL tendons intersect.

Achilles Tendon The Achilles tendon is the most superficial of the flexor tendons at the level of the ankle and is formed by a confluence of fibers arising from the soleus and the gastrocnemius muscles and attaches distally to the posterior calcaneus. The Achilles tendon differs from most tendons in that it lacks a sheath and is instead covered by a thin membrane

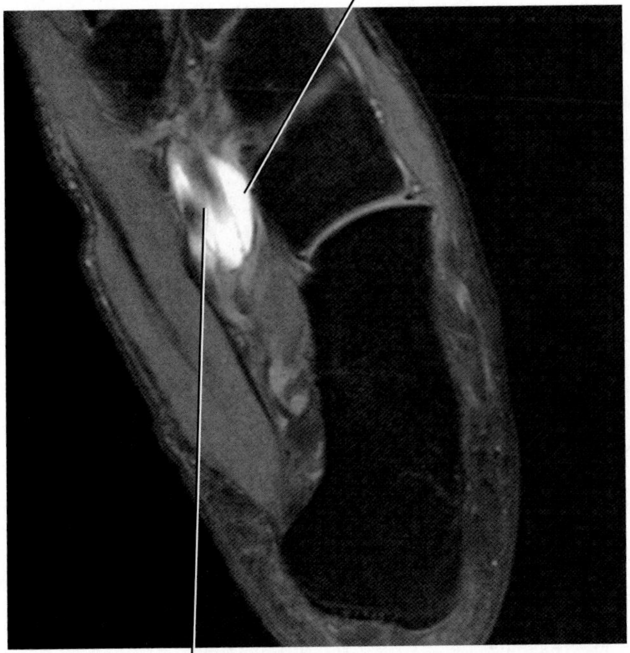
Fluid within the tendon sheath
Henry's knot: Cross-over of the FHL and FDL tendons

Figure 13-7 Tenosynovitis of flexor hallucis longus (FHL) and flexor digitorum ligament (FDL) tendon sheath. Axial T2-weighted image at the level of the midfoot demonstrates a large fluid collection within the common flexor tendon sheath at the level of crossover of the FDL and FHL tendons consistent with tenosynovitis.

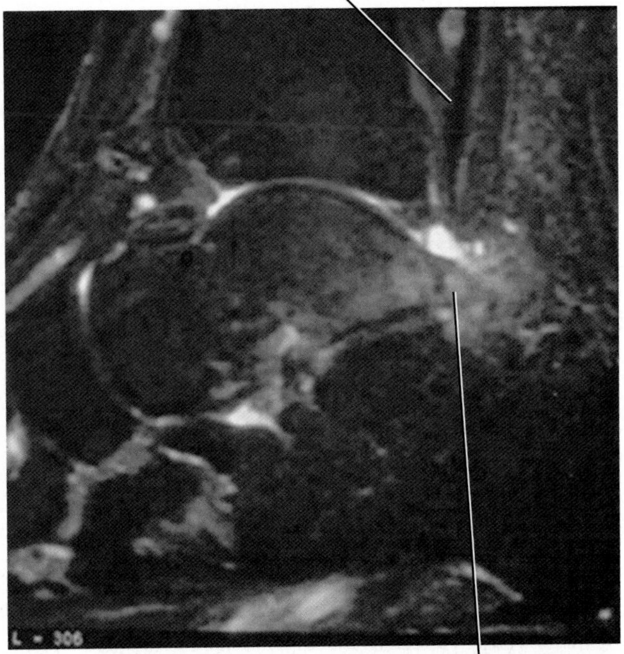
Flexor hallucis longus tendon
Edematous os trigonum

Figure 13-8 Os trigonum syndrome. Sagittal T2-weighted image with fat saturation shows a large edematous os trigonum. There is fluid within the adjacent flexor hallucis longus (FHL) tendon sheath. These findings are consistent with a posterior impingement syndrome and tenosynovitis of the adjacent FHL tendon sheath.

and a delicate network of blood vessels referred to as a paratenon (see Fig. 13-1). Injury is usually secondary to chronic overuse and is most prevalent in middle-aged men. Achilles tendinosis can also be associated with chronic steroid use and numerous systemic diseases such as rheumatoid arthritis, diabetes, gout, chronic renal failure, collagen vascular disease, and fluoroquinolone therapy.

Injuries of the Achilles tendon are classified as either insertional or noninsertional. The noninsertional injuries most often occur at the watershed vascular zone approximately 4 to 6 cm above the distal insertion or at the musculotendinous junction. Noninsertional injuries also include proximal myotendinous junction strains of the Achilles tendon. These injuries can be classified as peritendinitis, tendinosis, or partial- or full-thickness tear (Fig. 13-9). Peritendinitis is the mildest form of injury, and on MRI, the Achilles tendon is normal in appearance; however, fluid and edema can be seen surrounding the tendon and within the pre-Achilles fat (Kager's fat pad). A small fluid collection may also be present within the retrocalaneal bursa.

Tendinosis is usually seen as thickening of the tendon and may also demonstrate abnormal intrinsic signal representing intrasubstance myxoid degeneration. Sagittal MRI shows fusiform thickening of the tendon, and axial images demonstrate a rounded or convex anterior margin. Hypoxic tendinosis shows low signal on both T1- and T2-weighted images and thickening of the Achilles tendon. Calcific tendinosis is a rather common finding associated with chronic Achilles tendinosis. Ossification of the Achilles tendon, on the other hand, is an uncommon complication that has been reported after trauma to the Achilles tendon, resulting in either a partial- or full-thickness tear of the tendon or in surgery (Fig. 13-10). Calcific tendinosis may be difficult to detect on MRI

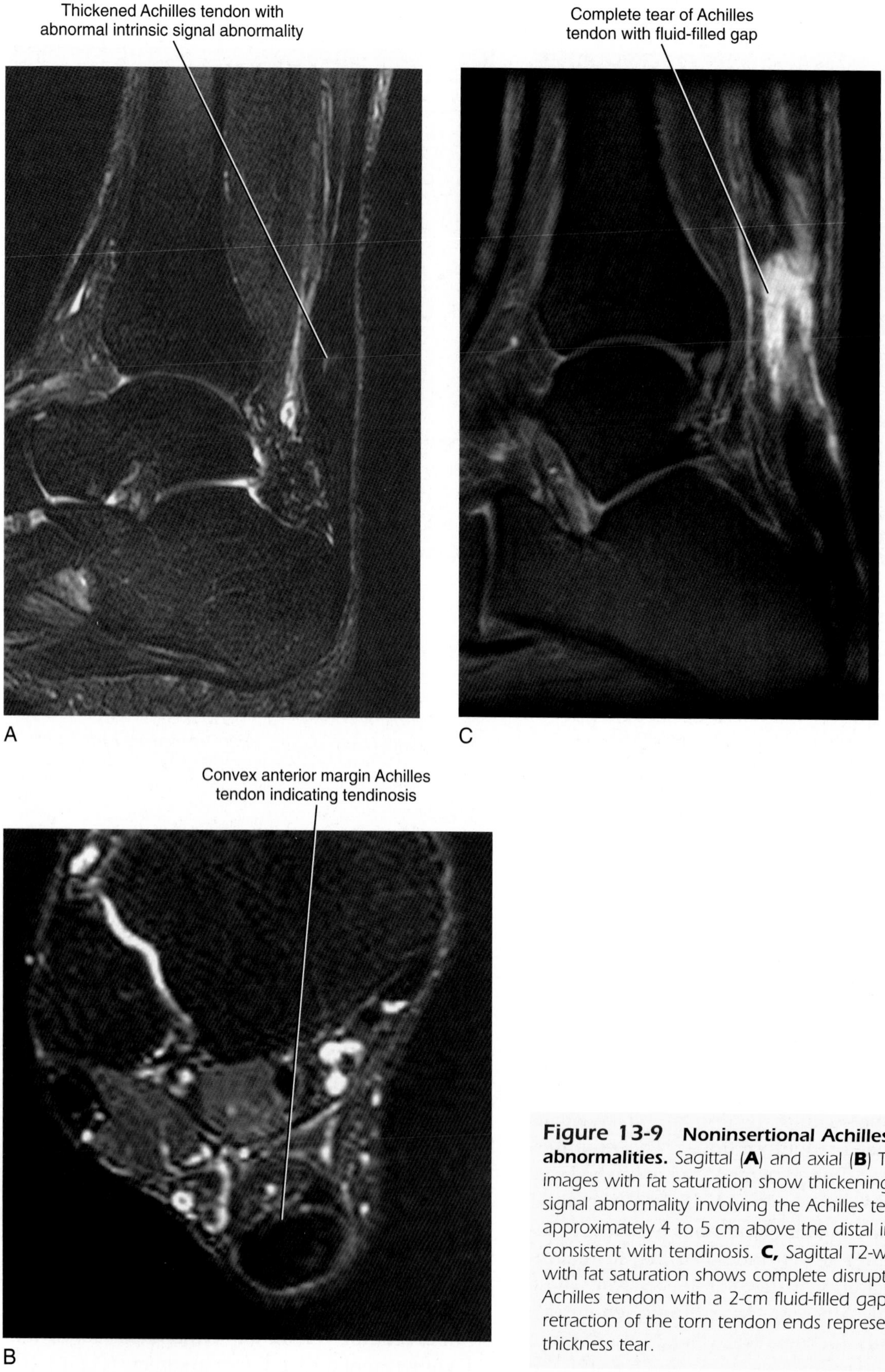
Thickened Achilles tendon with abnormal intrinsic signal abnormality
A
Complete tear of Achilles tendon with fluid-filled gap
C
Convex anterior margin Achilles tendon indicating tendinosis
B

Figure 13-9 Noninsertional Achilles abnormalities. Sagittal (**A**) and axial (**B**) T2-weighted images with fat saturation show thickening and intrinsic signal abnormality involving the Achilles tendon approximately 4 to 5 cm above the distal insertion site consistent with tendinosis. **C,** Sagittal T2-weighted image with fat saturation shows complete disruption of the Achilles tendon with a 2-cm fluid-filled gap and mild retraction of the torn tendon ends representing a full-thickness tear.

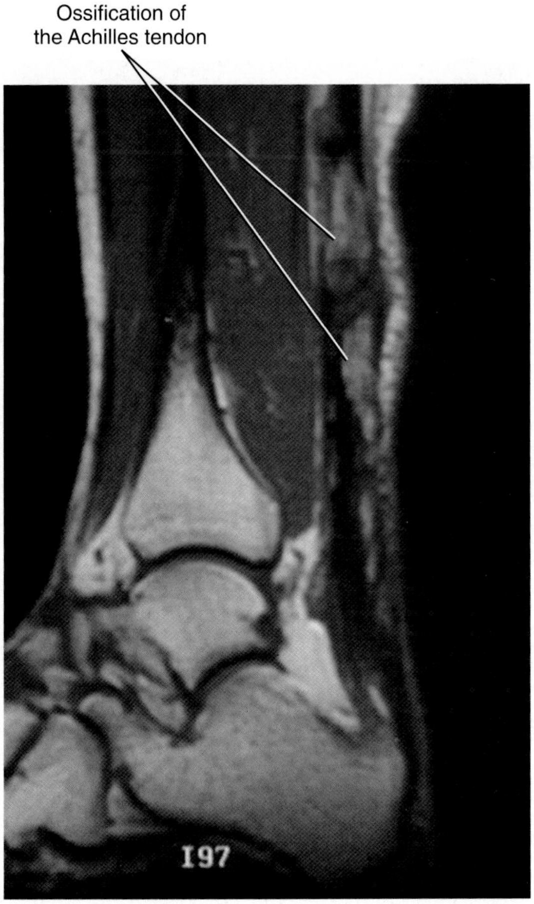
Ossification of
the Achilles tendon
I97

A

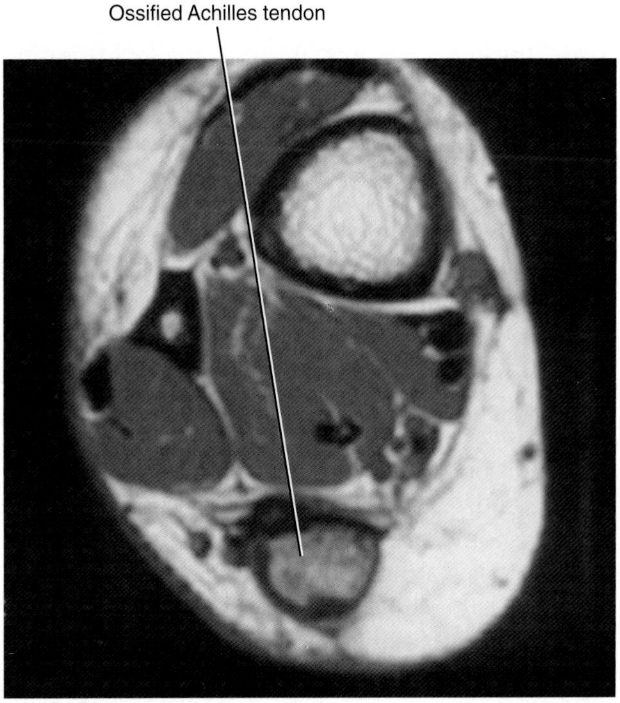
Ossified Achilles tendon

B

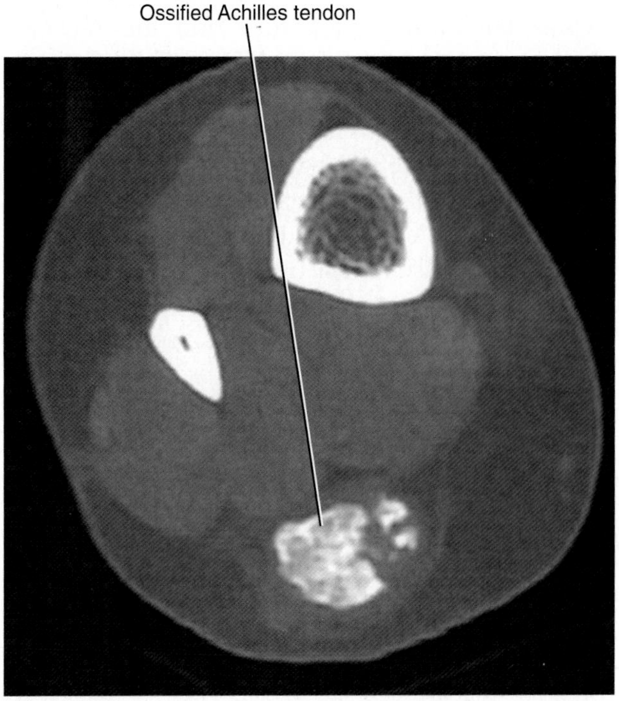
Ossified Achilles tendon

C

Figure 13-10 Ossification of the Achilles tendon. *Sagittal (**A**) and axial (**B**) T1-weighted images show a markedly thickened Achilles tendon indicating chronic tendinosis. Areas of bright T1 signal followed fat signal on all pulse sequences and indicate marrow fat within areas of ossification of the Achilles tendon.* **C,** *Axial CT image confirms the presence of mature bone within the substance of a markedly thickened area of chronic Achilles tendinosis.*

but is easily seen on radiographs of the ankle. Ossification of the Achilles tendon demonstrates as areas of high T1-weighted signal representing areas of fat within mature marrow surrounded by dark-rimmed cortex within the substance of a thickened Achilles tendon. Ossification at the level of distal insertion of the Achilles tendon usually represents enthesopathy and is of no clinical significance.

Fluid signal within the substance of the tendon indicates a partial-thickness tear. This is often seen initially as linear longitudinal streaks of fluid signal indicating longitudinal interstitial tearing. Intermediate signal streaks, however, within the substance of the tendon distally can be a normal finding. A high-grade partial-thickness tear may result in marked thinning and attenuation of the tendon and in partial retraction of the torn portion of the tendon. A full-thickness tear demonstrates complete discontinuity of the fibers with a fluid-filled gap and retraction of the torn tendon ends. A complete description should include the location of the tear as it relates to the level of distal attachment, the extent of retraction of the proximal tendon end, and the length of the gap between the torn tendon ends. The status of the torn tendon end is also important for presurgical planning, and a complete description should indicate the presence of thickening, edema, fraying, or irregularity of the torn tendon ends. A description of an intact plantaris tendon should also be described because this can lead to a false-negative clinical exam in the presence of a complete Achilles tendon tear.

Insertional Achilles tendon abnormalities occur at the distal attachment site and are often associated with enthesiophyte formation and calcification within the distal tendon. Insertional abnormalities include tendinosis and partial- and full-thickness tear. Inflammatory changes and fluid are often present within the superficial adventitial (retro-Achilles) bursa as well as within the deep retrocalcaneal bursa (Fig. 13-11). Subcortical marrow edema is commonly seen in the posterior calcaneal tubercle in association with insertional Achilles tendinosis. Marrow signal in this situation is usually reactive in etiology and should not be mistaken for osteomyelitis.

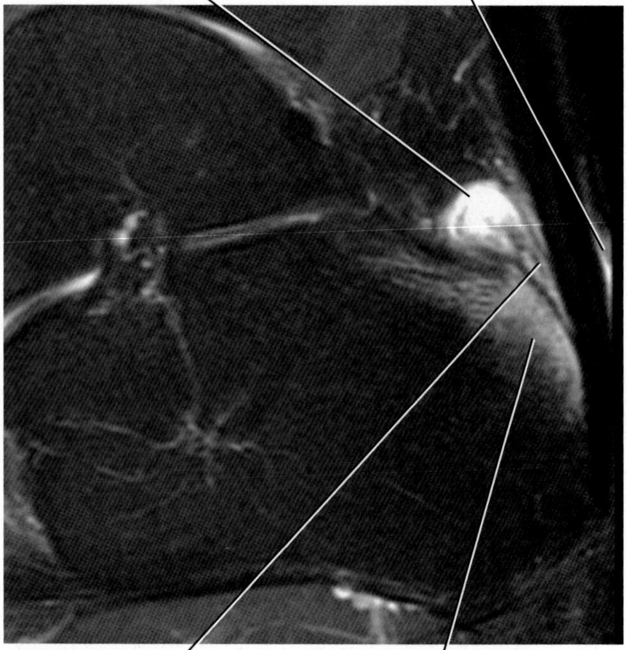
Retrocalcaneal bursitis
Tendo-Achilles bursa
Peritendinitis
Reactive marrow edema

Figure 13-11 **Retrocalcaneal bursitis.** Sagittal T2-weighted image with fat saturation demonstrates a large fluid collection within the retrocalcaneal bursa representing bursitis. Fluid surrounding the distal Achilles tendon represents peritendinitis as well as associated reactive subcortical marrow edema involving the posterior calcaneal tubercle.

Haglund syndrome describes a specific type of insertional Achilles tendinosis that is associated with a bony prominence (a Haglund deformity) extending off of the superior aspect of the posterior calcaneus, which results in impingement of the deep fibers of the Achilles tendon just above the level of distal attachment (Fig. 13-12). This may be exacerbated by certain footwear, especially pumps (e.g., "pump bump"). Repetitive impingement results in fraying and irregularity of the deep fibers of the Achilles tendon and eventually leads to a partial- or full-thickness tear. Treatment includes not only debridement or repair of the tendon abnormality but also an osteotomy of the bony prominence to prevent recurrent impingement.

Peroneal Tendons The peroneus longus and brevis tendons are the primary evertors of the foot and ankle. They share a common tendon sheath at the level of the ankle with the peroneus brevis tendon positioned anterior or medial to the peroneus longus tendon (see Fig. 13-1). The muscle of the peroneus brevis extends more distal than the peroneus longus muscle with the former visible on axial images at the level of the ankle. The peroneal tendons sit within a shallow retrofibular groove located along the posterior margin of the distal tip of the fibula and are maintained within the groove by the superior peroneal retinaculum. Below the level of the distal tip of the fibula, the peroneal tendons are held in place against the lateral aspect of the calcaneus by the inferior peroneal retinaculum. The brevis tendon then inserts onto the base of the fifth metatarsal while the peroneus longus tendon inserts onto the plantar aspect of the medial cuneiform and the base of the first metatarsal.

Pathology of the peroneal tendons is often associated with repeated inversion injuries or severe ankle

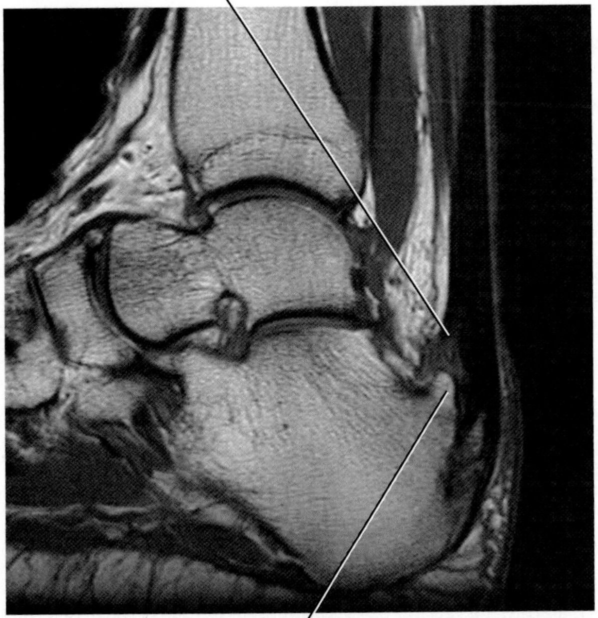
Insertional Achilles tendinosis
A
Bony prominence of posterior calcaneus

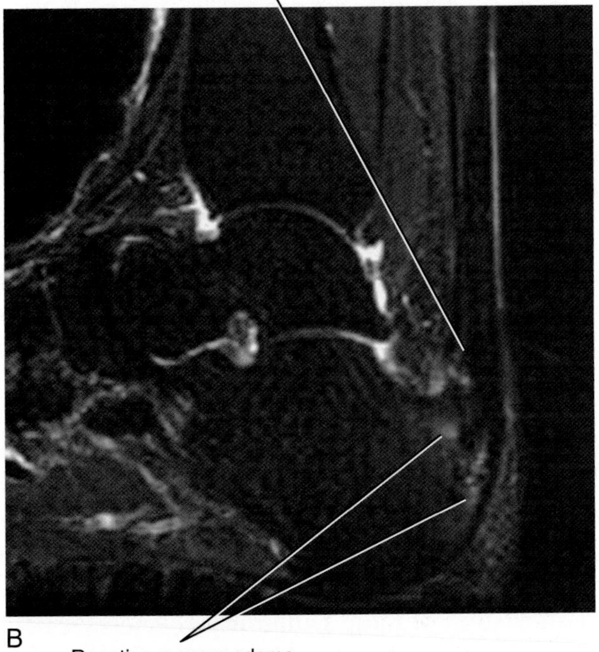
Thickened distal Achilles tendon with fraying
B
Reactive marrow edema

Figure 13-12 Haglund's deformity with insertional tendinosis. A, Sagittal T1-weighted image shows a large bony prominence along the superior margin of the posterior calcaneus resulting in impingement against the adjacent Achilles tendon. **B,** The distal Achilles tendon shows thickening and abnormal intrinsic signal indicating tendinosis. Adjacent reactive marrow edema is common and should not be misinterpreted as osteomyelitis.

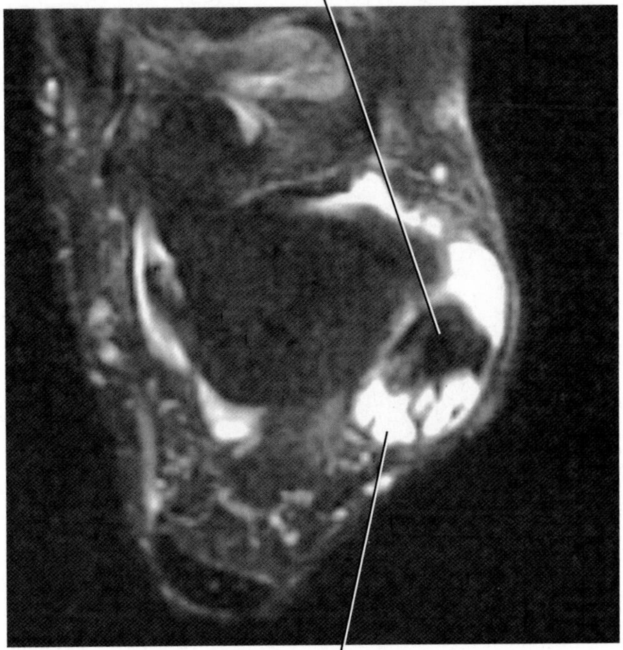
Peroneal tendons markedly thickened with adjacent fibrosis
Fluid within peroneal tendon sheath

Figure 13-13 Stenosing tenosynovitis. Axial T2-weighted image shows thickening of the peroneus longus and brevis tendons with adjacent scarring and fibrosis representing stenosing tenosynovitis. There is extensive fluid within the tendon sheath representing tenosynovitis.

sprains. Tenosynovitis is the most common abnormality and on MRI is seen as fluid within the tendon sheath. Although a small amount of fluid may be seen in the tendon sheath of an asymptomatic individual, more fluid than tendon or the presence or debris or synechiae is abnormal. Stenosing tenosynovitis describes the condition in which scarring, fibrosis, and adhesions occur within the tendon sheath and result in the two tendons scarring to one another, thus preventing the tendons from gliding smoothly over one another (Fig. 13-13). On MRI, the presence of debris or complexity within the tendon sheath is suggestive of stenosing tenosynovitis and is often associated with tendinosis seen as thickening and signal abnormality involving the peroneal tendons. As with other tendons, tendinosis and partial- and full-thickness tear can occur (Fig. 13-14).

Mucinous degeneration occasionally occurs within the substance of the peroneal tendons, which can

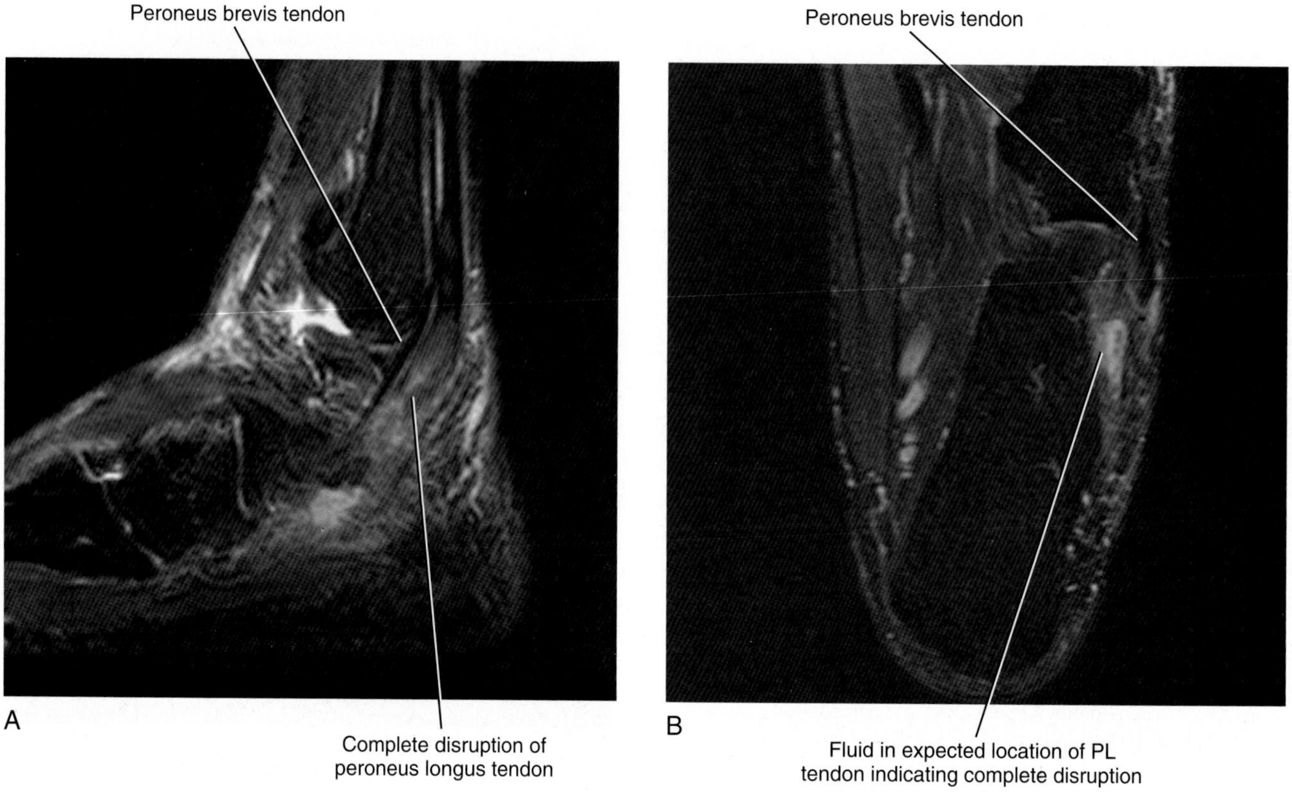
Peroneus brevis tendon
A
Complete disruption of peroneus longus tendon
Peroneus brevis tendon
B
Fluid in expected location of PL tendon indicating complete disruption

Figure 13-14 Peroneus longus (PL) tendon disruption. A, Sagittal T2-weighted image shows marked thickening of the peroneus longus tendon to the level of the distal fibula with complete disruption and retraction of the torn thickened tendon end. **B,** Axial T2-weighted image shows fluid in the expected location of the peroneus longus tendon and absence of the tendon below the level of the lateral malleolous consistent with a complete disruption.

lead to intratendinous ganglion formation. A ganglion arising within the tendon sheath appears as a water-signal intensity mass, often with septations. The mass is located within the tendon sheath resulting in mass effect on the adjacent tendon (Fig. 13-15).

Partial-thickness tears of the peroneus brevis tendon often present as a longitudinal tear or a "split" tendon. This occurs because of the unique arrangement of the peroneus brevis tendon sandwiched between the fibula and the peroneus longus tendon. After repeated ankle inversion injuries, the peroneus longus tendon can migrate into the substance of the brevis tendon, initially resulting in flattening of the peroneus brevis tendon. Over time, the peroneus brevis tendon develops a convex posterior margin, and this appearance has been described as a boomerang or crescent shape and is considered a precursor to a full-thickness longitudinal split (Fig. 13-16). Finally, a longitudinal split of the brevis tendon develops. The peroneus longus tendon then becomes insinuated between the two tendon slips of the split peroneus brevis tendon. On axial MR images, there appears to be three tendon slips rather than two just below the level of the distal tip of the fibula (Fig. 13-17). The longitudinal split usually begins as a short segment but can extend over time to several centimeters in length. The patient with a split brevis tendon usually presents with chronic retromalleolar pain, snapping, and occasionally with symptoms of lateral ankle instability and requires surgical repair for alleviation of these symptoms.

The peroneus quartus is an accessory peroneal muscle that gives rise to a separate tendon slip, which inserts distally on the peroneal tubercle along the lateral margin of the body of the calcaneus (Fig. 13-18) and on axial MRI gives the appearance of three tendon slips in the retrofibular groove. A split peroneus brevis tendon must be differentiated from a peroneus quartus tendon to prevent unnecessary surgery. A split tendon can be easily differentiated from an accessory quartus tendon by following the

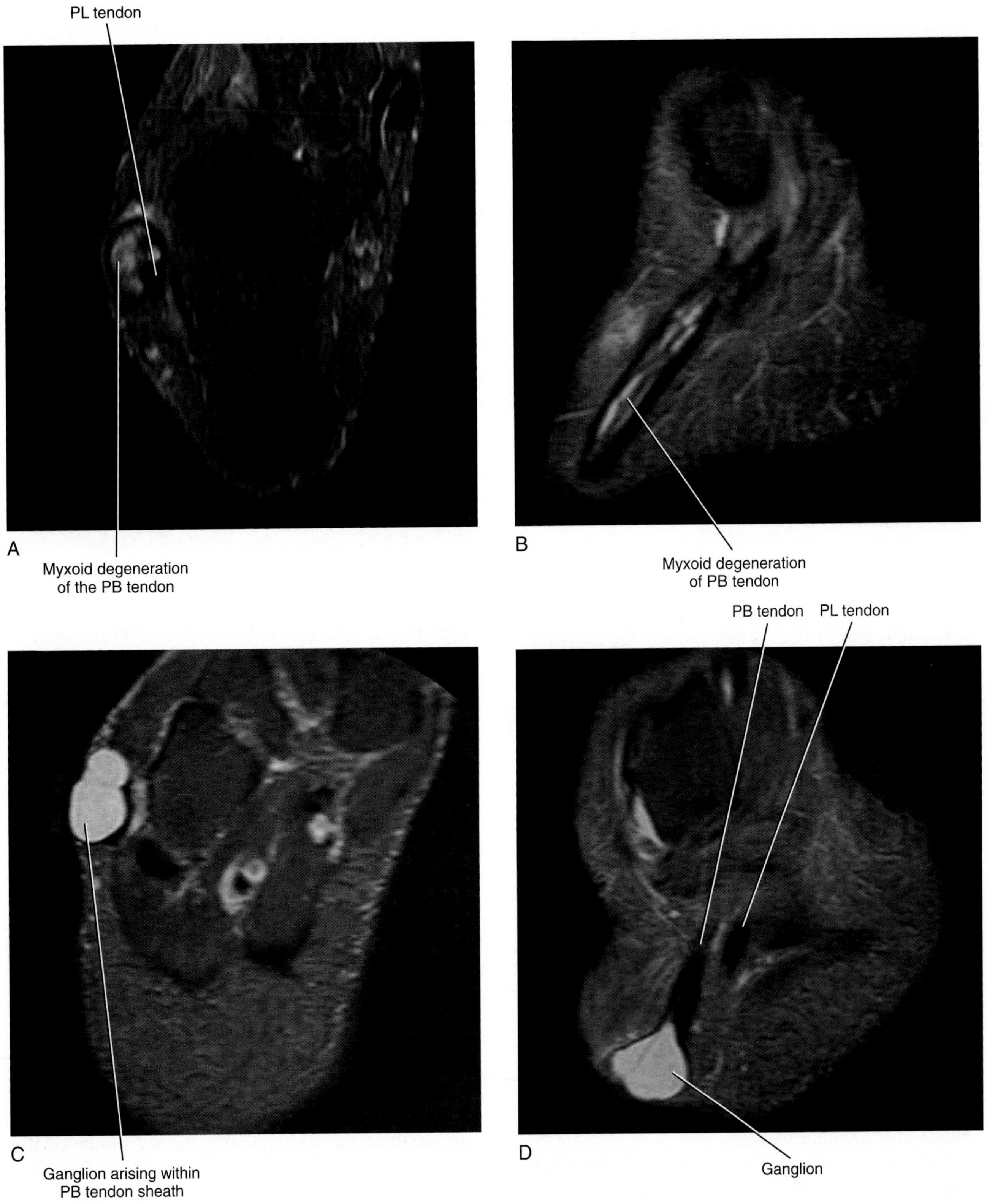
PL tendon
A
Myxoid degeneration of the PB tendon
B
Myxoid degeneration of PB tendon
PB tendon
PL tendon
C
Ganglion arising within PB tendon sheath
D
Ganglion

Figure 13-15 Myxoid degeneration and ganglion formation of peroneus brevis (PB) tendon. A and **B,** Axial and sagittal T2-weighted images with fat saturation show intrasubstance myxoid degeneration and longitudinal partial-thickness interstitial tearing of the PB tendon with linear areas of fluid signal within the substance of the tendon. **C** and **D,** A ganglion arising out of the substance of the PB tendon and contained within the peroneal tendon sheath.

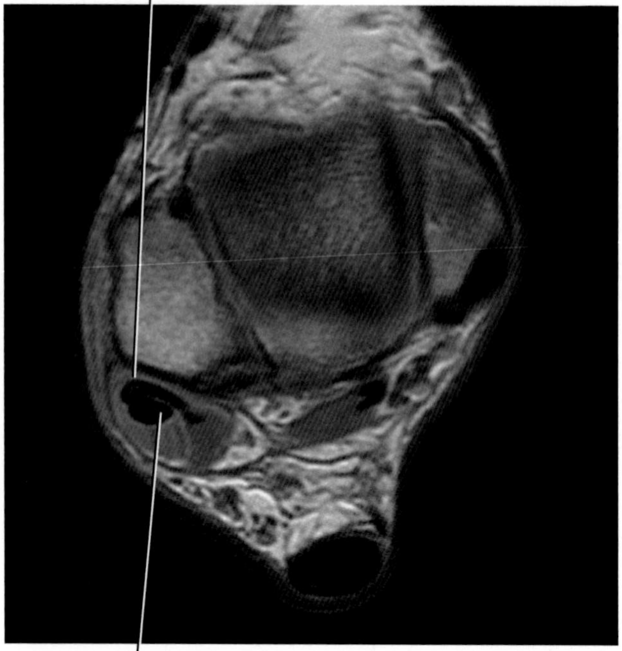
Boomerang-shaped PB tendon
Peroneus longus tendon

Figure 13-16 Boomerang-shaped peroneus brevis (PB) tendon. Proton density axial image shows a concave border to the posterior margin of the PB tendon and a boomerang appearance, indicative of a partial-thickness longitudinal tear. This appearance represents a precursor to a full-thickness longitudinal split of the PB tendon.

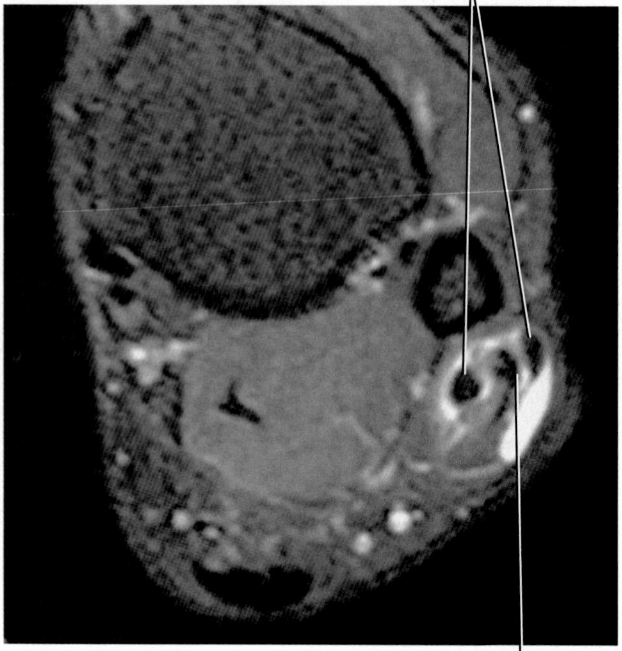
Slips of the split PB tendon
PL tendon

Figure 13-17 Split peroneus brevis (PB) tendon. Axial T2-weighted image shows a split PB tendon with the peroneus longus (PL) tendon insinuated between the separate tendon slips of the split peroneus brevis tendon. Note the appearance of three rather than two tendon slips at the level of the distal fibula.

tendon slips proximally and distally on sequential axial sections. A split brevis tendon reconstitutes both proximally and distally into a single tendon slip, whereas a peroneus quartus tendon arises from a separate muscle belly proximally and inserts onto the lateral aspect of the calcaneus distally. With a peroneus quartus, the two tendon slips never merge. It is important to accurately identify the presence of the peroneus quartus since there are case reports of surgery being performed to repair a split peroneus brevis tendon only to identify a peroneus quartus tendon at the time of surgery.

Lateral subluxation of the peroneal tendons usually occurs secondary to disruption or injury of the superior peroneal retinaculum. This diagnosis is best made on axial MRI, which can demonstrate the peroneal tendons lateral to the distal fibula rather than within the retrofibular groove (Fig. 13-19). Lateral subluxation usually occurs after repeated ankle inversion injuries or after a forced inversion injury of the ankle, and it results in a snapping sensation in the lateral ankle as the tendon subluxes in and out of the retrofibular groove. Repeated subluxations result in eventual tenosynovitis and or tendinosis of the peroneal tendons. Dynamic ultrasound examination is well suited for detecting subluxation of the peroneal tendons, which may be intermittent and may be detected only when putting the ankle through full range of motion (Fig. 13-20).

An os peroneum refers to the presence of an accessory ossification center within the substance of the peroneus longus tendon. When present, this ossification center is usually located at approximately the level of the proximal cuboid. The os peroneum can be associated with a focal area of tendinosis with focal thickening and edema of the peroneus longus tendon (Fig. 13-21). In addition to the changes of the tendon, in many cases MRI imaging also demon-

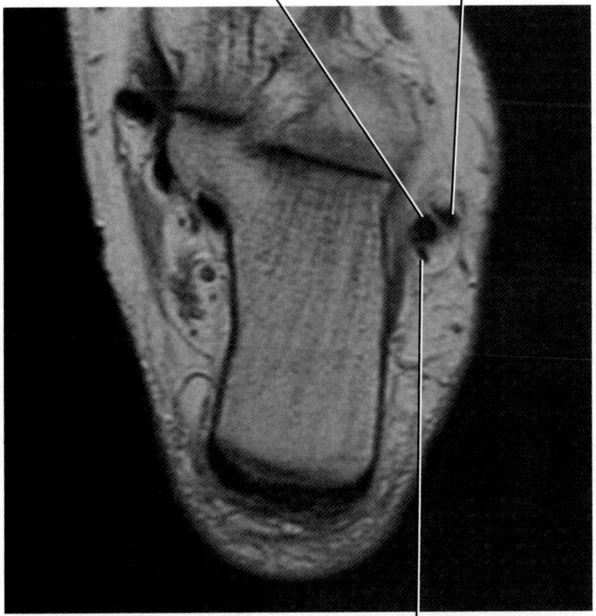
PL tendon
PB tendon
PQ tendon

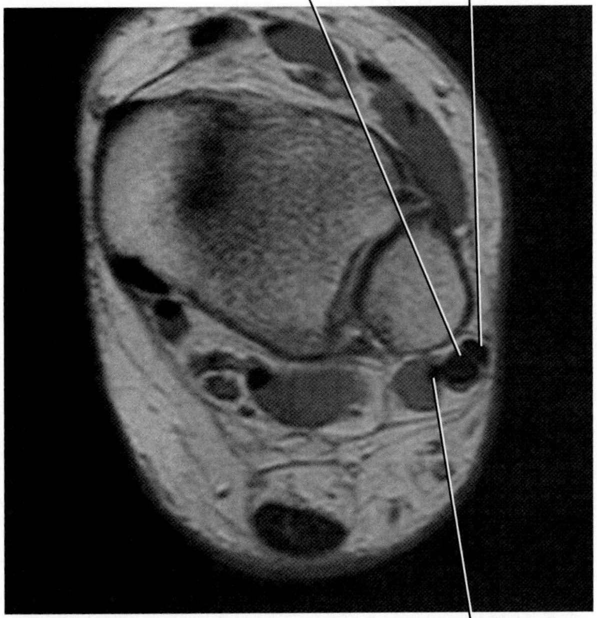
PL tendon
PB tendon
PQ muscle and tendon

Figure 13-18 Peroneus quartus (PQ) tendon. Axial images through the level of the ankle. The peroneus quartus is an accessory muscle and tendon that can mimic a split peroneus brevis (PB) tendon. The PQ tendon can be differentiated from a split PB tendon because it arises out of a separate muscle belly and rather than reconstituting with the PB tendon distally, it has a separate insertion site on the peroneal tubercle along the lateral aspect of the calcaneus. PL, peroneus longus.

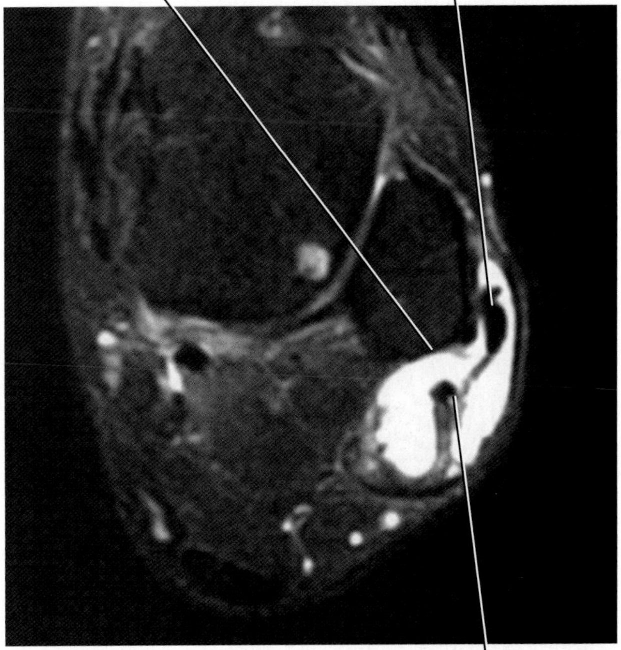
Retrofibular groove
Laterally subluxed PB tendon
PL tendon

Figure 13-19 Lateral subluxation of the peroneus brevis (PB) tendon. Axial T2-weighted image with fat saturation shows extensive fluid within the peroneal tendon sheath representing tenosynovitis. There is lateral subluxation of the PB tendon out of the retrofibular groove indicating disruption of the superior peroneal retinaculum, which is responsible for holding the peroneal tendons in their normal location within the retrofibular groove. PL, Peroneus longus.

strates reactive marrow edema within the adjacent cuboid. Radiographically, the symptomatic os peroneum may demonstrate sclerosis and fragmentation. If the peroneus longus tendon disrupts distally, radiographs will show proximal migration of the os peroneum to the level of the calcaneocuboid joint. When symptomatic this is referred to as a painful os peroneum syndrome or POPS. Surgical removal of the os peroneum may be required for alleviation of symptoms.

The peroneal tubercle is located along the lateral margin of the calcaneus. It is the normal insertion site for the calcaneofibular ligament and is also situated between the peroneus longus and brevis tendons along the lateral aspect of the calcaneus. A prominent peroneal tubercle can result in impingement of the

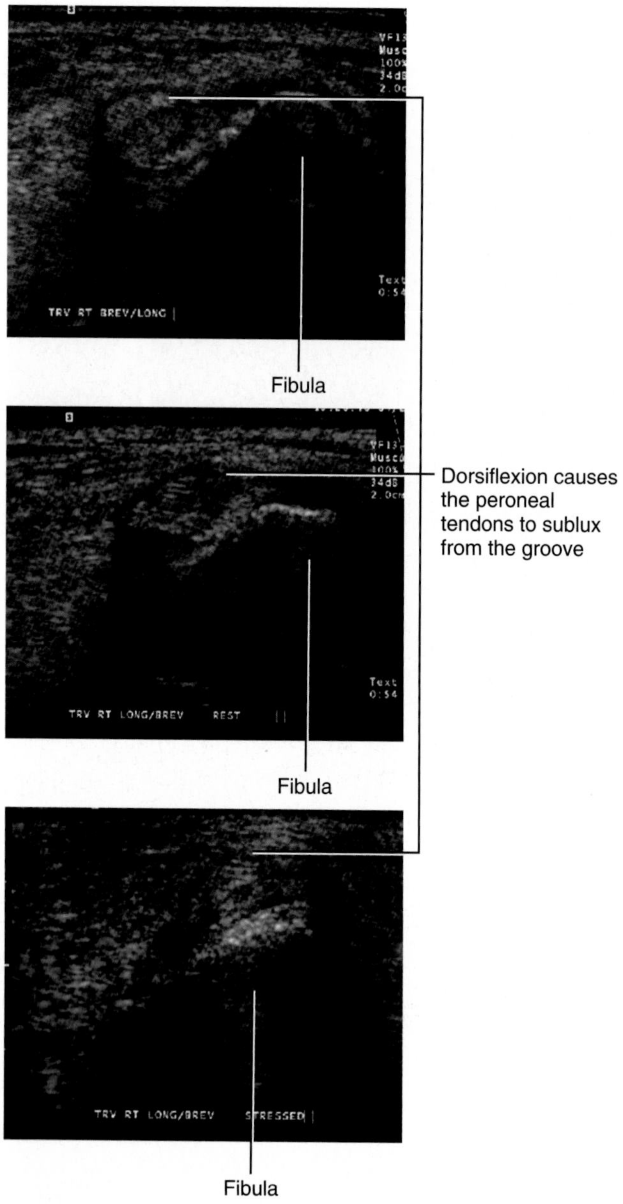
Fibula
Dorsiflexion causes the peroneal tendons to sublux from the groove
Fibula
Fibula

Figure 13-20 Ultrasound examination demonstrating subluxation of the peroneal tendons. Dynamic scan of the ankle demonstrates peroneal tendon subluxation only during dorsiflexion of the ankle.

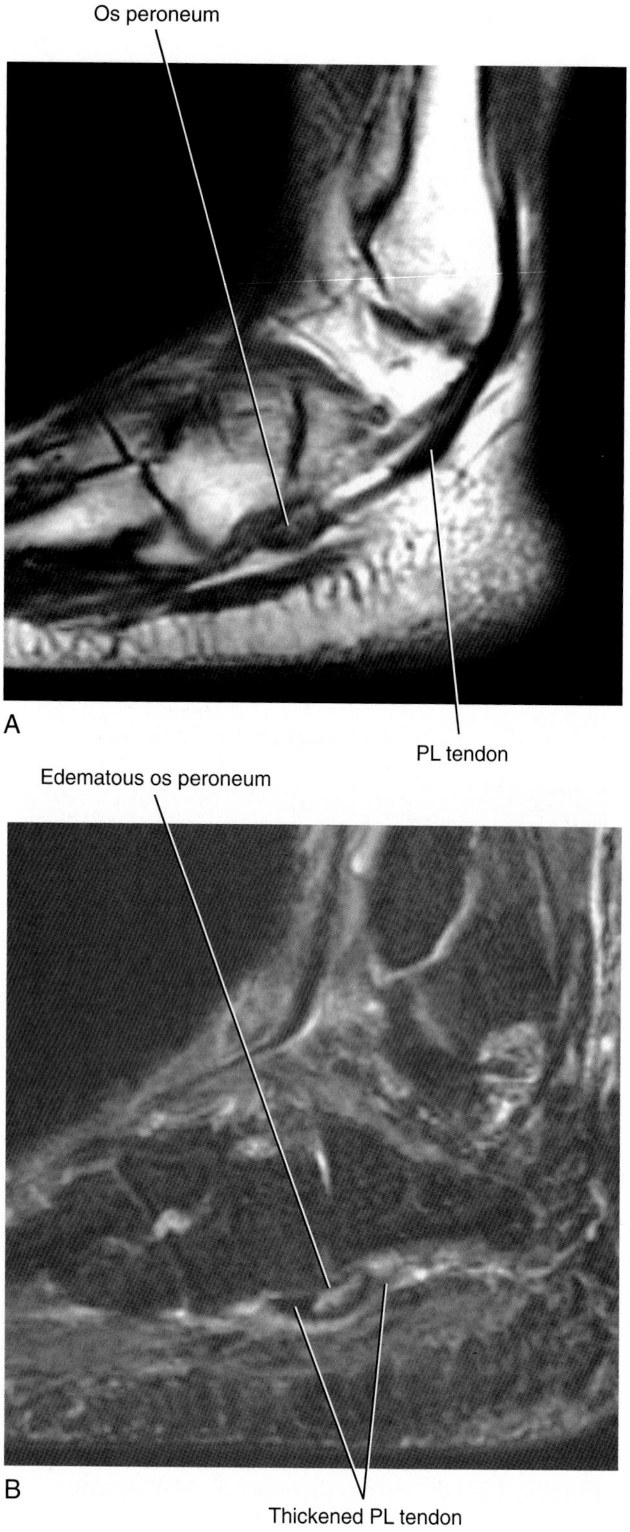
Os peroneum
A
PL tendon
Edematous os peroneum
B
Thickened PL tendon

Figure 13-21 Painful os peroneum. Sagittal T1- (**A**) and T2-weighted (**B**) images demonstrate an edematous os peroneum representing an accessory ossification center within the substance of the peroneus longus (PL) tendon at the level of the distal calcaneus. Edema within the os peroneum usually indicates a symptomatic or painful os peroneum.

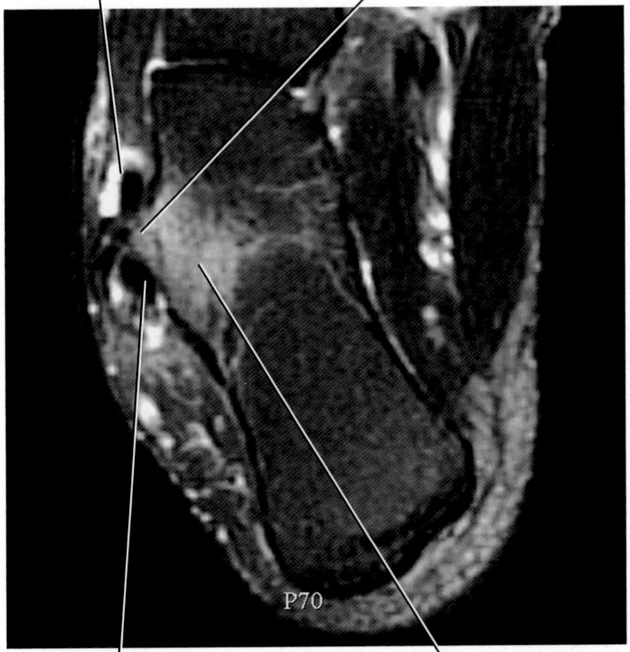
PB tendon
Prominent peroneal tubercle
P70
PL tendon
Subtendinous reactive marrow edema

Figure 13-22 Prominent peroneal tubercle. Axial T2-weighted image with fat saturation shows a prominent peroneal tubercle along the lateral aspect of the calcaneus. This tubercle is normally positioned between the peroneus longus (PL) and peroneus brevis (PB) tendons as seen in this image. A prominent peroneal tubercle has been shown to be associated with tendinosis and tenosynovitis of the peroneal tendons. Also note the fracture and marrow edema located within the peroneal tubercle.

peroneal tendons and can be a potential source of peroneal tendinosis (Fig. 13-22). Various peroneal tendon pathologies can be associated with subtendinous reactive marrow edema in several locations along the course of the peroneus brevis tendon including the posterior distal fibula, lateral calcaneus, and inferior cuboid. Subtendinous reactive marrow edema is an important secondary imaging sign of peroneal tendon pathology.

MRI of Postoperative Tendons

Numerous surgical procedures are available for tendon repair depending on the nature and location of the tendon abnormality. Symptoms associated with tendinosis or tenosynovitis may respond to simple debridement or synovectomy. Partial- and full-thickness tendon tears are often repaired using either a tendon-to-bone or a tendon-to-tendon repair technique. Tendon tears associated with extensive abnormality of the underlying tendon may require a tendon transfer. The flexor hallucis longus and flexor digitorum longus tendons are often used as grafts to repair a torn tendon. Tendon-lengthening procedures and osseous realignment procedures can also be performed.

An accurate surgical history can be helpful in the proper evaluation of the postoperative MRI appearance. Tendon-to-tendon or tendon-to-bone procedures often result in suture artifact at the site of repair. Tendon thickening and abnormal intrinsic signal often persist for long periods of time following repair and do not necessarily indicate recurrent tendinosis or tear (Fig. 13-23A). Tendon transfer procedures, such as a transfer of the FHL tendon to repair a torn adjacent Achilles tendon, result in altered anatomy. The most common complication following tendon repair is a recurrent partial- or full-thickness tear (Fig. 13-23B). On MRI, a recurrent partial-thickness tear manifests as attenuation and thinning of the postoperative tendon, and fluid signal may be seen extending partially through the thickness of the tendon. An acute recurrent full-thickness tear demonstrates discontinuity of the repaired tendon and a fluid-filled gap with retraction of the torn tendon ends.

Ligaments

Ankle sprain is the most common athletic injury, and the symptoms of ankle pain are usually self-limiting and resolve with conservative therapy. Evaluation of the ankle with MRI is usually reserved for patients with persistent ankle pain or instability following a single episode or multiple episodes of ankle inversion. The differential diagnosis for persistent lateral ankle pain after inversion injury includes ligamentous injury as well as abnormalities of the peroneal tendons, as described in the previous section. Other injuries that can result in persistent lateral ankle pain are osteochondral injury of the talar dome, lateral talar process fracture, sinus tarsi syndrome, anterior impingement, anterolateral ankle impingement, synovial cysts, and subtalar ankle instability (Box 13-3).

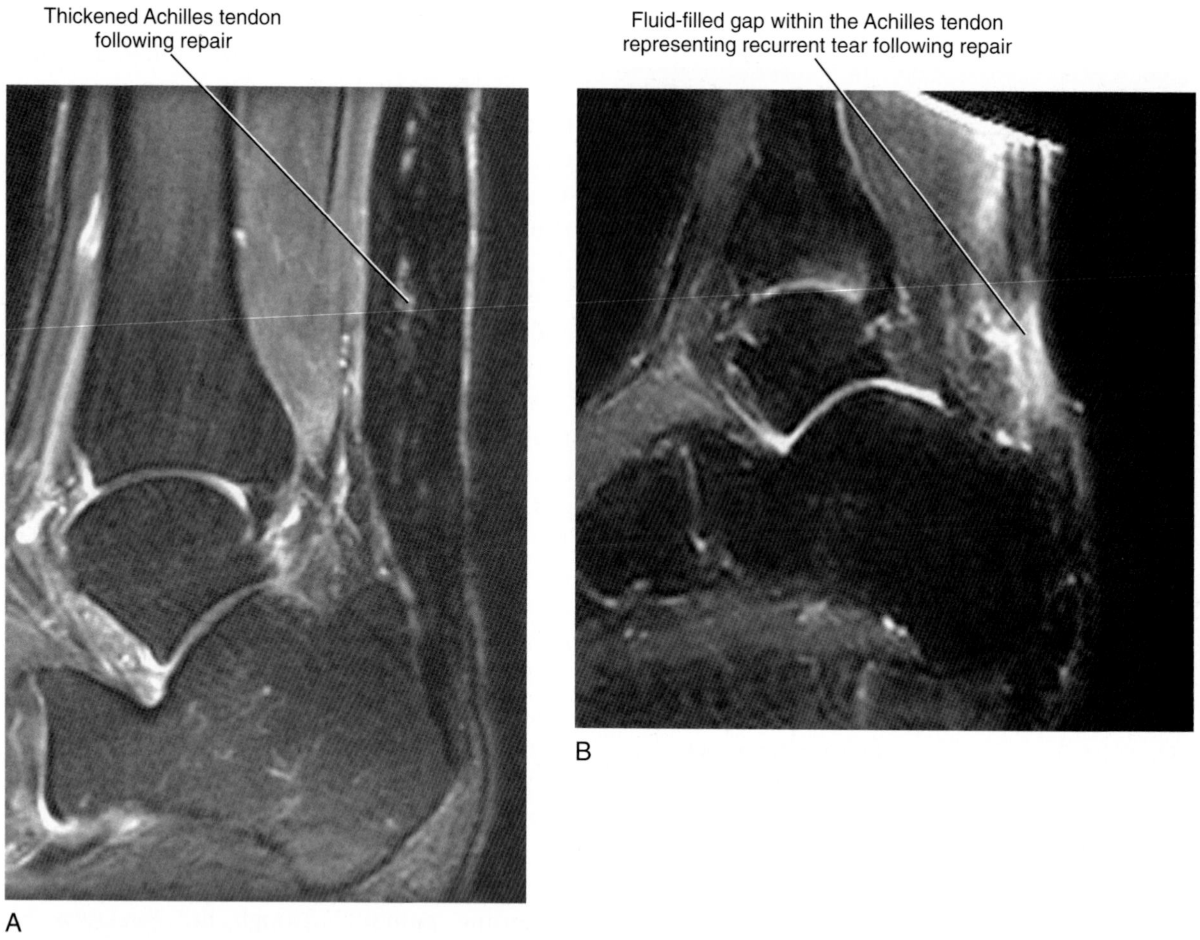
Thickened Achilles tendon following repair
Fluid-filled gap within the Achilles tendon representing recurrent tear following repair
B
A

Figure 13-23 Postoperative appearances of the Achilles tendon. A, Sagittal T2-weighted image shows marked thickening and intrinsic signal abnormality within the substance of the Achilles tendon. This appearance can persist for several years after repair of the Achilles tendon. **B,** Sagittal STIR image shows a complete re-tear with retraction of the torn tendon ends after repair of the Achilles tendon.

BOX 13-3 CAUSES OF PERSISTENT LATERAL ANKLE PAIN AFTER INVERSION INJURY

Ligamentous injury
Peroneal tendon abnormalities
Osteochondral injury to talar dome
Lateral talar process fracture
Sinus tarsi syndrome
Impingement syndromes (anterior, anterolateral)
Synovial ganglion
Subtalar instability

Lateral Collateral Ligament Complex

The lateral collateral ligament complex is composed of the anterior and posterior talofibular ligaments and the calcaneofibular ligament (Fig. 13-24). The anterior and posterior talofibular ligaments are best seen on axial MRI, and the coronal imaging plane is complementary in their evaluation. The anterior talofibular ligament appears as a thin bandlike structure extending from the anterior tip of the distal fibula to the lateral talar process and is usually seen on axial images through the most distal tip of the fibula or at the level of the C-shaped fossa located along the medial aspect of the fibula. The posterior talofibular ligament is seen at the same level but it appears thicker than the anterior ligament and contains numerous internal striations. The calcaneofibular ligament extends from the inferior tip of the distal fibula to insert onto the lateral cortex of the calcaneus and is positioned deep to the peroneal tendons. It is usually well seen on both axial and coronal MRI.

The lateral collateral ligament complex demonstrates a predictable pattern of injury depending on the severity of the ankle inversion. The anterior talofibular (ATF) ligament is injured first, followed by injury to the calcaneofibular (CF) ligament. Increasing severity of injury may also result in involvement of the syndesmotic ligaments; however, the posterior talofibular ligament is rarely involved. A three-point grading system is used to describe acute injuries of the anterior talofibular ligament (Table 13-3 and Fig. 13-25). Grade I injury is seen on MRI as superficial lateral ankle soft tissue edema around the anterior talofibular ligament. A grade II injury is a partial-thickness tear and on MRI shows thickening and internal signal alterations within the substance of the ligament. Finally, grade III injury is a complete tear, with MRI showing complete disruption or avulsion of the anterior talofibular ligament (Fig. 13-26). Ultrasound examination also accurately depicts the normal appearance of the components of the lateral

Table 13-3 Acute Anterior Talofibular Ligament Injury: MRI Grading System

Grade	Definition	MRI Findings
I	Mild sprain	Superficial soft tissue edema around ligament
II	Partial-thickness tear	Thickening/edema of ligament with intrinsic signal abnormality
III	Complete tear	Complete disruption or avulsion of ligament

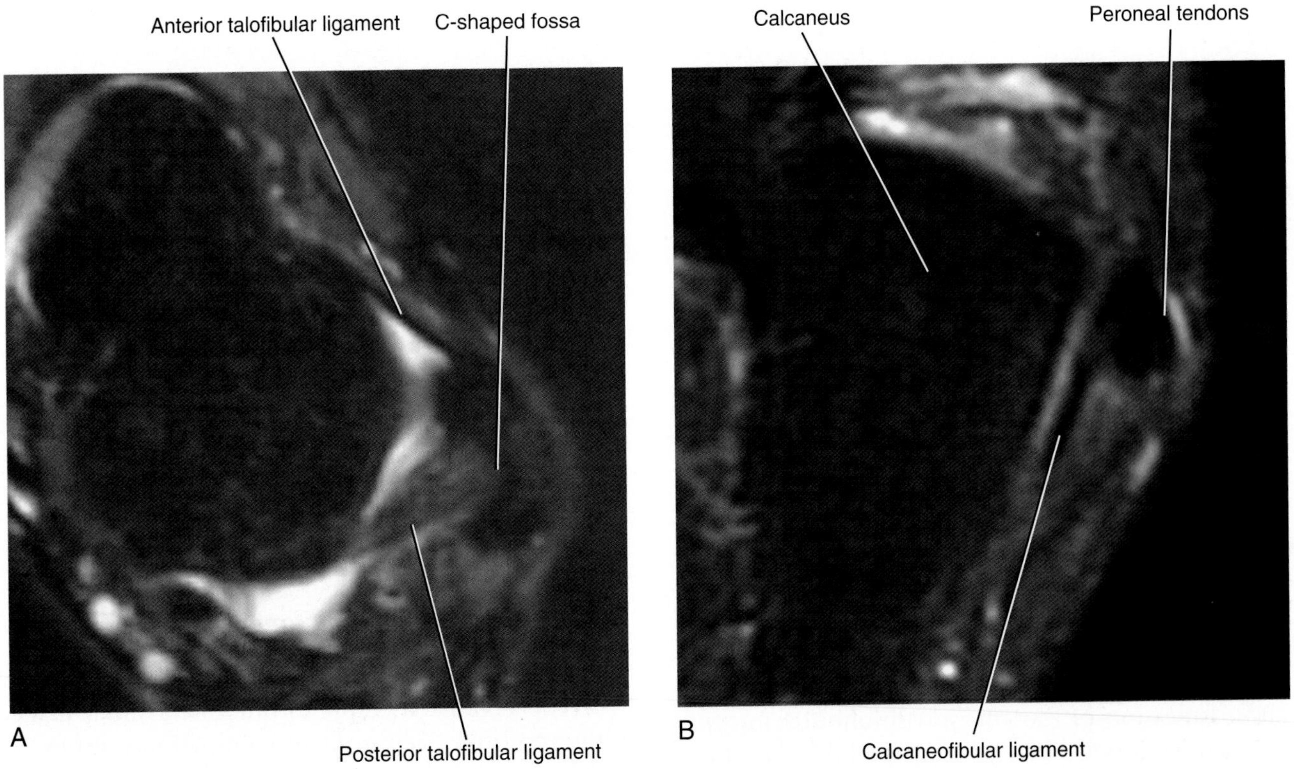
Anterior talofibular ligament
C-shaped fossa
A
Posterior talofibular ligament
Calcaneus
Peroneal tendons
B
Calcaneofibular ligament

Figure 13-24 Normal MRI appearance of the lateral collateral ligament complex. A, Axial T2-weighted image with fat saturation shows the anterior and posterior talofibular ligaments, which can always be located on the image demonstrating the C shaped fossa along the medial border of the distal fibula. The anterior talofibular ligament is a thin bandlike structure, whereas the normal posterior talofibular ligament is thicker and contains internal intermediate signal striations. **B,** Axial T2-weighted image with fat saturation shows the calcaneofibular ligament as a thin linear structure located deep to the peroneal tendons extending from the inferior tip of the fibula to insert on the lateral aspect of the calcaneus.

Continued

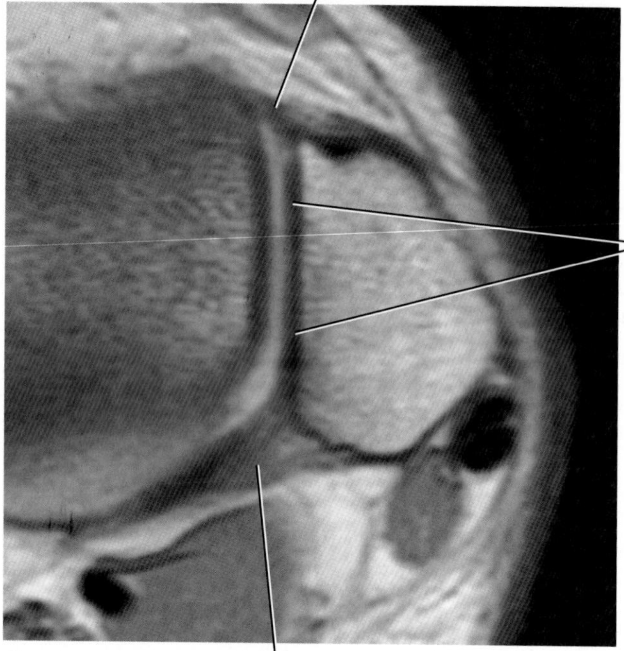
Anterior tibiofibular ligament
Flat surface medial aspect of fibula
C
Posterior tibiofibular ligament

Figure 13-24, cont'd **C,** Axial proton density image shows the normal appearance of the anterior and posterior tibiofibular ligaments. The anterior tibiofibular ligament appears as a thin bandlike structure and is usually seen on two to three consecutive axial images as it courses in a superior direction from the fibula to insert on the tibia. The posterior tibiofibular ligament is thicker than the anterior ligament and contains striations. The anterior and posterior tibiofibular ligaments can always be identified by finding the one image of the distal fibula that demonstrates a flat medial border, as seen in this image. Axial images at other levels demonstrate a more rounded appearance of the distal fibula.

collateral ligament and can accurately grade partial- and full-thickness tears (Fig. 13-27).

Progression from an acute to a chronic ligamentous injury often results in either thickening of the involved ligament representing fibrosis and scarring or a chronic tear with complete absence of the ligament (Fig. 13-28; see also Fig. 13-26).

A high ankle sprain refers to a syndesmotic injury involving the anterior and less commonly the posterior tibiofibular ligament (Fig. 13-29). The high ankle sprain may occur as an isolated injury or in association with anterior talofibular and calcaneofibular ligament injuries. This is a more severe type of ankle sprain, and if the injury goes unrecognized, it may result in chronic pain and instability of the ankle and late ossification of the anterior tibiofibular interval. The acute injury is often associated with bone contusions of the posterior aspect of the distal tibia and is reported commonly among American football players.

Deltoid Ligament Complex

The deltoid or medial collateral ligament is a strong thick ligament with both superficial and deep fibers. The deltoid ligament complex may be sprained or partially torn as the result of an eversion injury, but it rarely disrupts completely. It is more likely for an injury of the deltoid complex to result in a small avulsion fragment of the distal tibia than in a full-thickness tear of the deltoid ligament. On MRI, a sprain appears as thickening and edema within the fibers of the ligamentous complex, whereas a complete tear demonstrates complete discontinuity and fluid traversing the substance of the ligamentous complex.

MRI of Postoperative Ligaments

Although most ankle sprains are successfully treated with conservative therapy, chronic lateral ankle instability resulting from numerous inversion injuries or following a severe ankle sprain may require surgical treatment. Several surgical options are available to reestablish ankle stability, and most procedures use the peroneus brevis tendon or a portion of it repositioned to provide ankle stability, often via a fibular tunnel. Direct ligamentous repair is less commonly performed but may be attempted after an avulsion of the anterior talofibular or calcaneofibular ligament

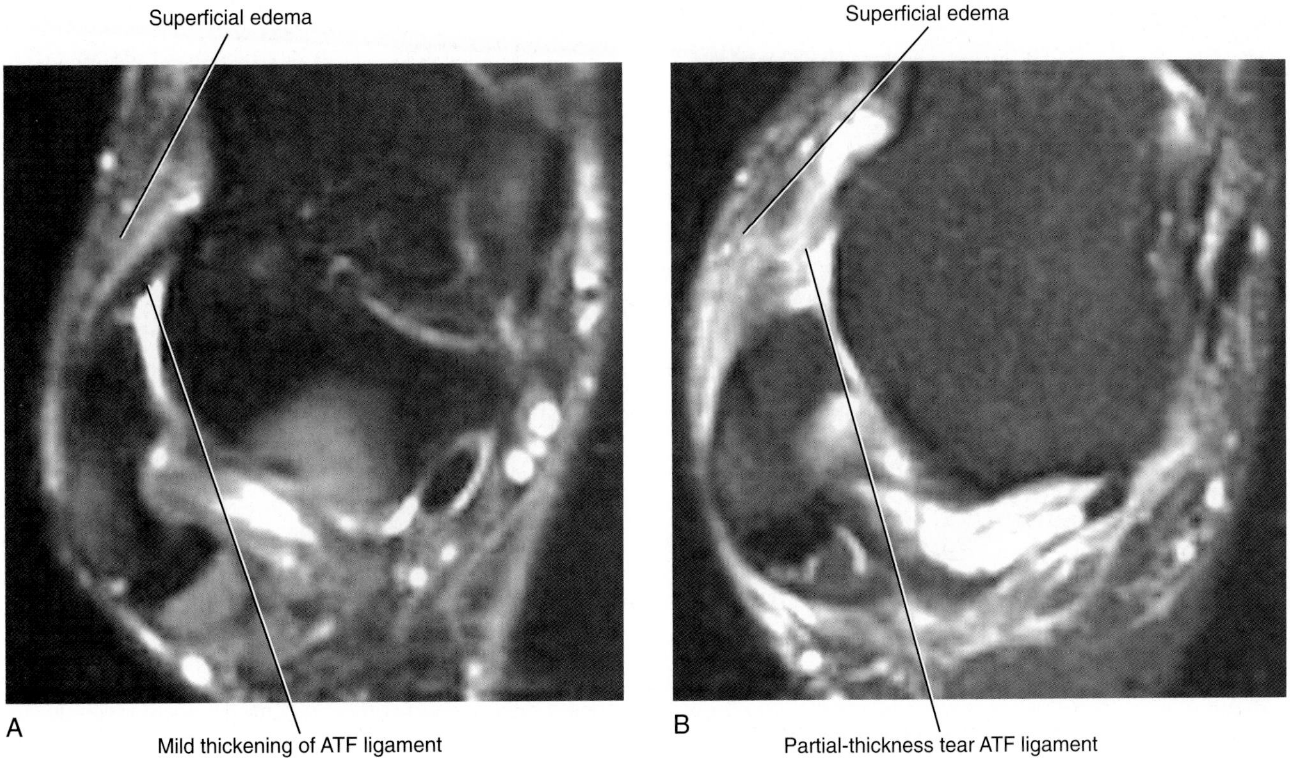
Superficial edema
A
Mild thickening of ATF ligament
Superficial edema
B
Partial-thickness tear ATF ligament

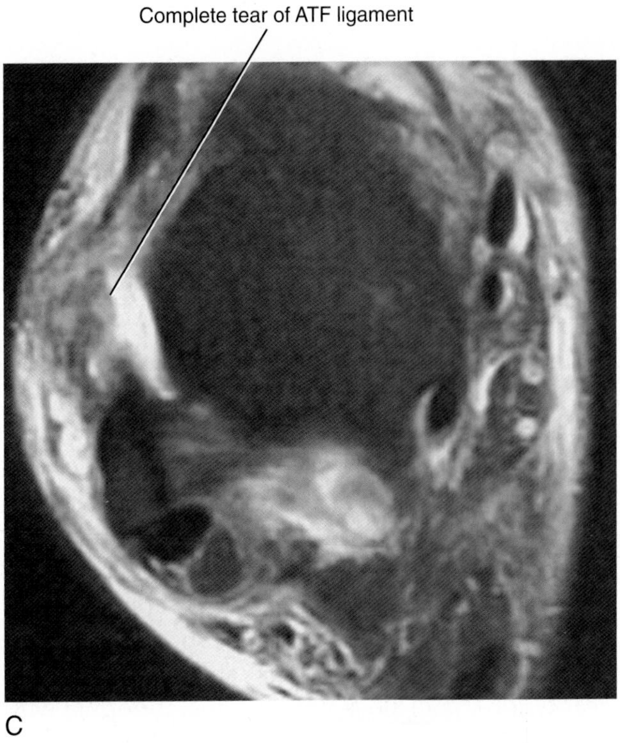
Complete tear of ATF ligament
C

Figure 13-25 Grading system of acute anterior talofibular (ATF) ligament sprains. A, Grade I. Superficial edema and minimal thickening and edema of the ATF ligament. **B,** Grade II. Superficial edema and a partial-thickness tear of the ATF ligament. **C,** Grade III. C complete disruption of the ATF ligament.

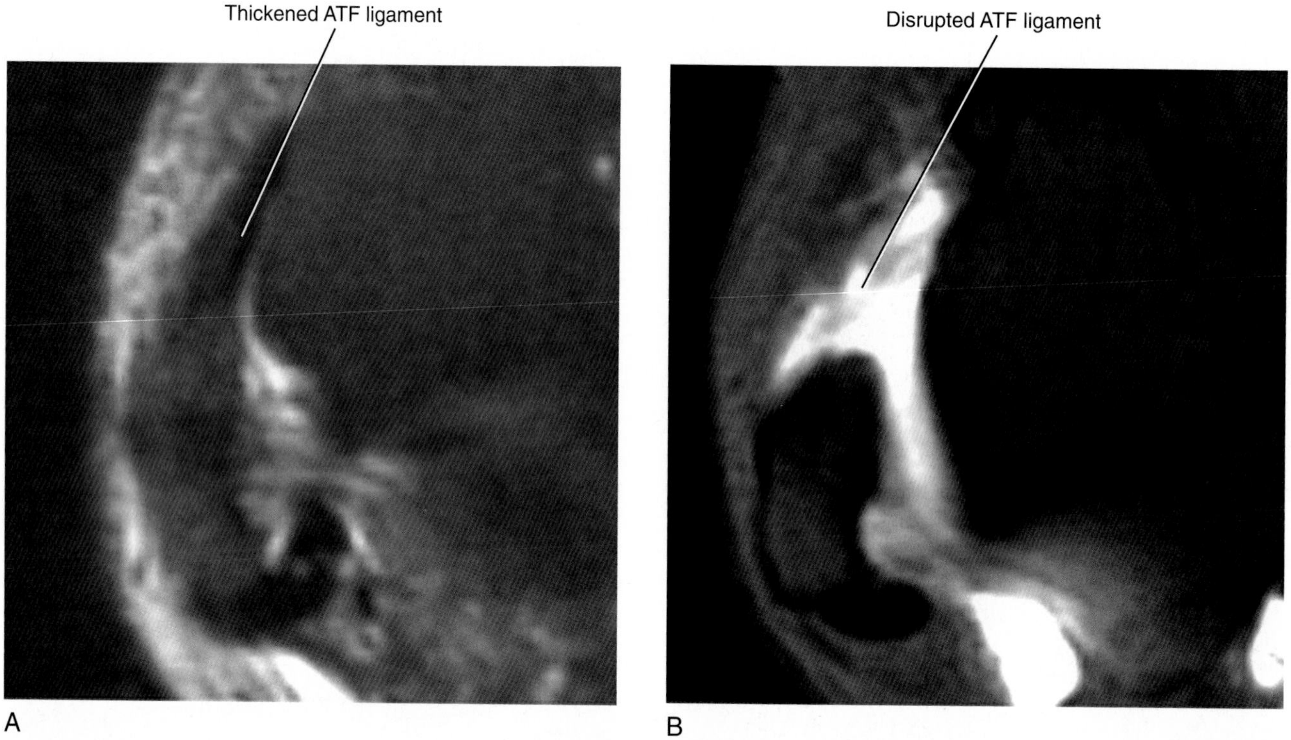
Thickened ATF ligament
A
Disrupted ATF ligament
B

Figure 13-26 Chronic anterior talofibular (ATF) ligament injuries. A, Axial T2-weighted image with fat saturation shows marked thickening of the ATF ligament with no overlying edema, representing chronic scarring associated with an old inversion injury. **B,** Axial T1-weighted image with fat saturation and intra-articular gadolinium shows complete absence of the ATF ligament representing a chronic tear.

from their osseous attachment sites. The normal postoperative appearance of the ankle depends on the specific procedure performed.

Direct repair of the ligament demonstrates chronic thickening of the ligament with suture artifact at the site of reattachment to the fibula. Discontinuity or disruption of the repaired ligament seen on MRI is evidence of either a failed repair or a recurrent injury. Ankle reconstruction using the peroneus brevis tendon demonstrates altered peroneal tendon anatomy on MRI, and depending on the specific procedure performed, the peroneus brevis tendon may pass through an intraosseous tunnel of the distal fibula. The peroneal graft should appear intact without evidence of disruption. A successful stabilization procedure of the lateral ankle using a peroneal tendon graft does not alter the abnormal MRI appearance of the lateral collateral ligament complex, which may demonstrate persistent thickening or even disruption of the involved ligamentous components.

Spring Ligament Complex (Calcaneonavicular Ligament)

The spring ligament complex originates on the anteromedial aspect of the calcaneus and inserts on the medioplantar aspect of the navicular bone. It is also referred to as the calcaneonavicular ligament complex. This ligamentous complex serves two functions. First, it acts as a sling to support the plantar and medial aspect of the talar head. Second, it acts synergistically with the posterior tibialis tendon and the plantar fascia to support the arch of the midfoot. The spring ligament rarely disrupts as a result of acute trauma. Chronic disruption may occur as a part of a degenerative process in conjunction with posterior tibialis tendon dysfunction and has been shown to be associated with acquired flatfoot deformity. Because of its important role in providing stability of the midfoot arch, repair of an abnormal spring ligament often accompanies repair of the posterior tibialis tendon.

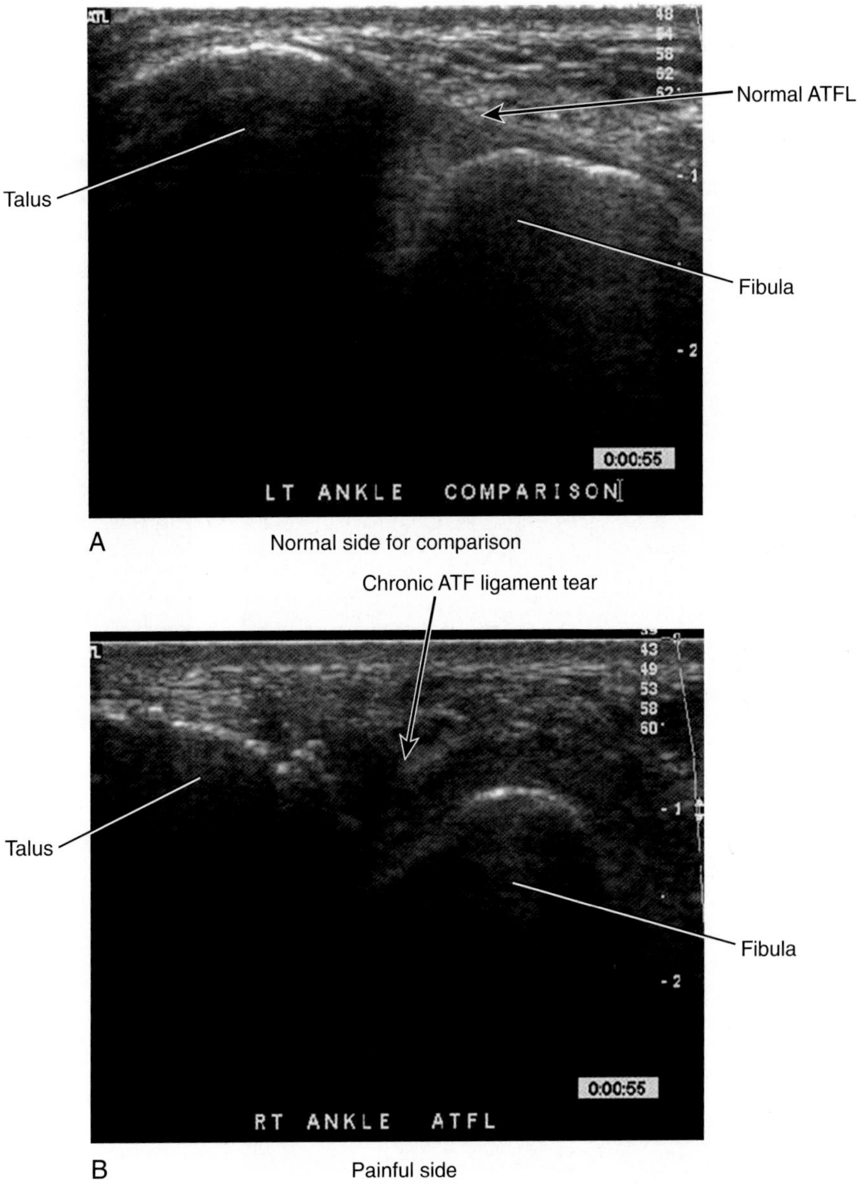
Normal ATFL
Talus
Fibula
LT ANKLE COMPARISON
0:00:55
A
Normal side for comparison
Chronic ATF ligament tear
Talus
Fibula
RT ANKLE ATFL
0:00:55
B
Painful side

Figure 13-27 Normal and disrupted anterior talofibular (ATF) ligament on ultrasound examination. A, The normal ultrasound appearance of the ATF. **B,** Complete disruption of the ligament.

Several different anatomic descriptions of the spring ligament complex are found in the literature, but the most accepted description is that of three separate bundles arising along the medial aspect of the anterior calcaneus. Each bundle extends distally along the medial and plantar aspect of the talar head to insert onto the navicular bone. MRI may demonstrate edema and disruption of the spring ligament components after an acute injury, but this is rare. More frequently, chronic degenerative disruption is depicted on MRI as thickening and heterogeneity of the ligamentous components without adjacent edema (Fig. 13-30). The spring ligament should be thoroughly evaluated in a patient with findings of posterior tibialis tendon dysfunction, since injuries of these two structures often occur in conjunction with one another.

IMPINGEMENT SYNDROMES

Impingement is defined as a progressive abnormality resulting from mechanical encroachment of one anatomic structure upon another. With regard to the ankle, most cases of impingement are associated with prior ankle inversion injury and are associated with chronic ankle pain and instability. Five types of ankle impingement have been described (Box 13-4).

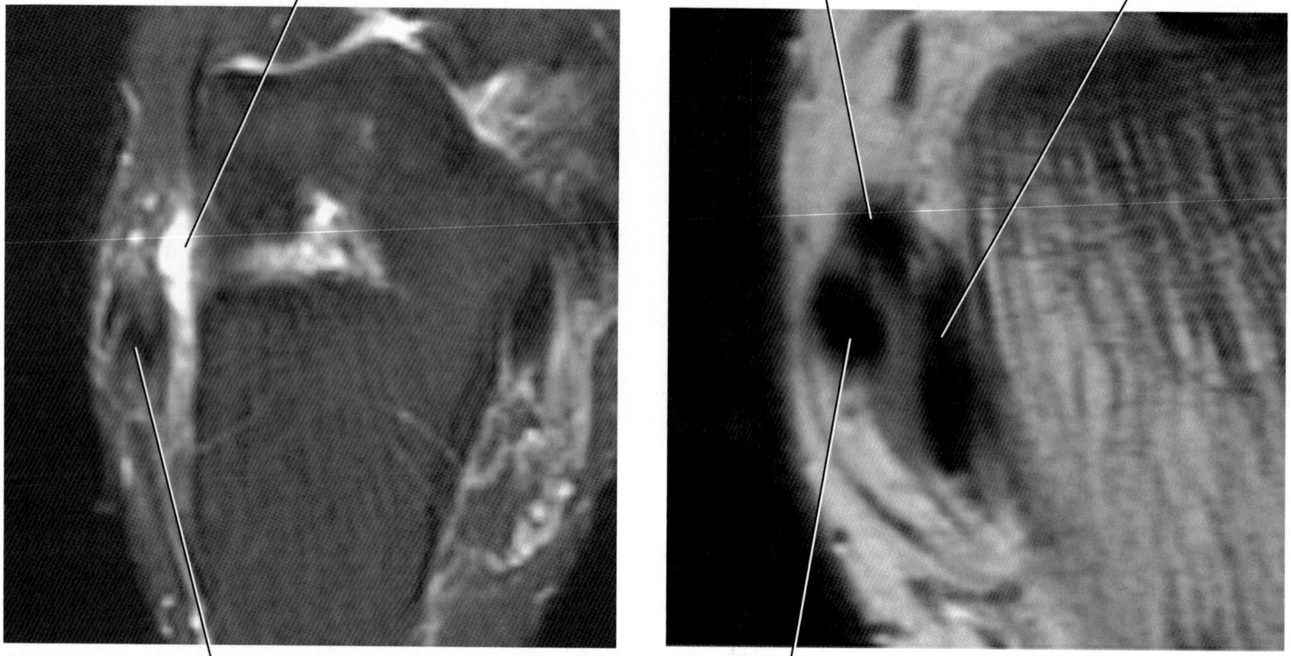
Fluid in expected location of CF ligament representing a complete tear
Peroneal tendons
A
PB tendon
Thickened CF ligament
PL tendon
B

Figure 13-28 Calcaneofibular (CF) ligament injury patterns. A, Axial T2-weighted image with fat saturation shows fluid in the expected location of the CF ligament consistent with an acute tear. **B,** Axial proton density image shows marked thickening of the CF ligament consistent with a chronic injury. PB, peroneus brevis; PL. peroneus longus.

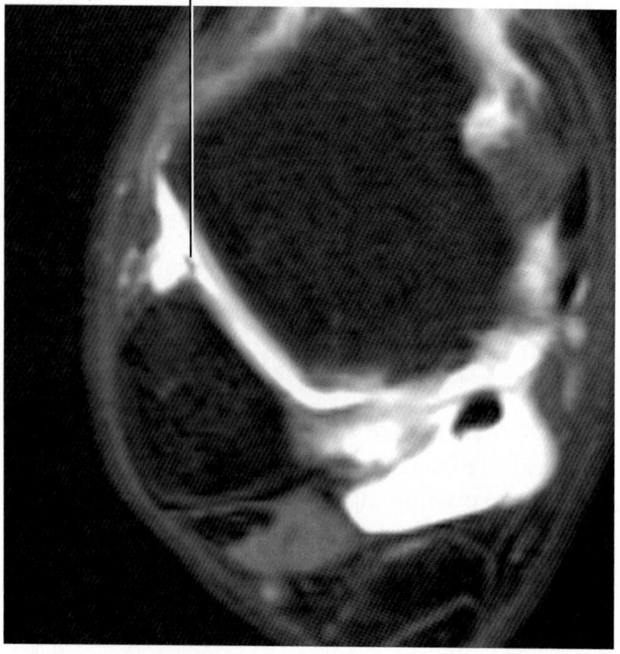
Torn anterior tibiofibular ligament

Figure 13-29 High ankle sprain. Axial T1-weighted image with fat saturation and intra-articular gadolinium shows complete disruption of the anterior tibiofibular ligament consistent with a high ankle sprain. Note the flat surface of the medial border of the distal fibula. This appearance of the fibula indicates that the tibiofibular ligaments should be present at this level.

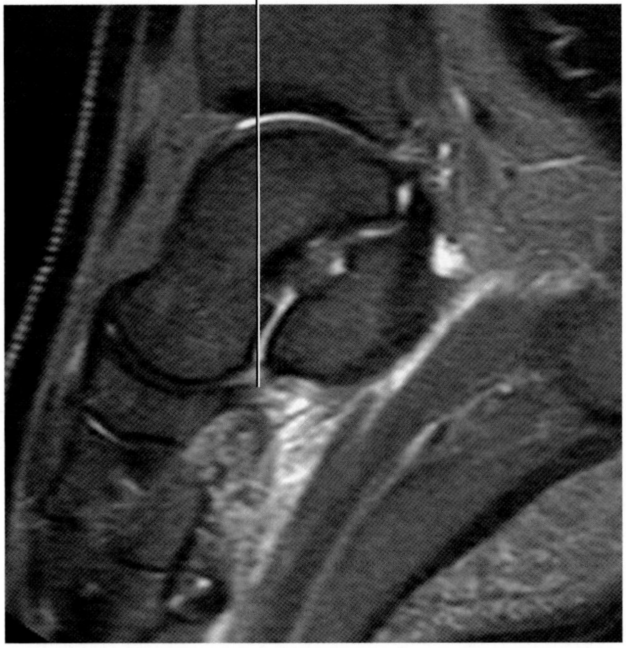
Partial tear of the spring ligament

Figure 13-30 Spring ligament injury. Sagittal T2-weighted image shows thickening and edema involving the spring ligament with adjacent soft tissue edema inferior to the ligament.

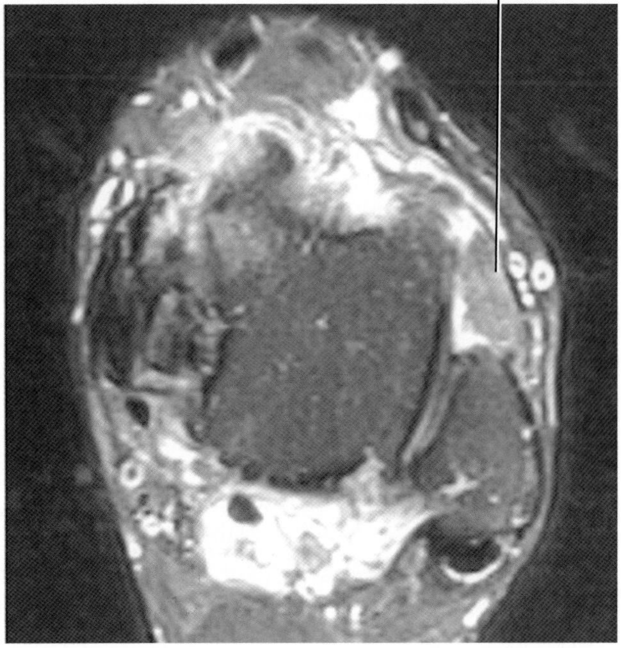
Meniscoid lesion (scarring and fibrosis) within the anterolateral gutter

Figure 13-31 Anterolateral impingement syndrome. Axial T2-weighted image with fat saturation shows thinning and attenuation of the anterior talofibular ligament consistent with a partial-thickness tear from an old inversion injury. A moderate-sized joint effusion outlines the diskoid lesion in the anterolateral gutter.

BOX 13-4 TYPES OF ANKLE IMPINGEMENT

Anterolateral
Anterior
Syndesmotic
Posterior
Medial

Treatment for each form of ankle impingement typically includes nonsteroidal anti-inflammatory medications for pain relief and debridement of the hyperplastic synovium or scar tissue. Finally, if indicated, ankle stabilization may be performed.

Anterolateral Impingement

Anterolateral impingement is the most common form of ankle impingement, accounting for 30% to 40% of all cases, and it is usually a sequela of ankle inversion injury. Patients present with persistent lateral ankle pain and instability. The impingement results from entrapment of the synovial membrane between the anterior talus and the adjacent tibia or fibula, leading to the formation of scar tissue or fibrosis within the anterolateral gutter, which has been described as a meniscoid lesion (Fig. 13-31). The patient typically presents with anterolateral ankle pain, swelling, and limited dorsiflexion of the ankle. Physical examination reveals tenderness to palpation and sometimes a palpable mass in the region of the anterior lateral gutter.

On MRI, a focal masslike area of low T1 and T2 signal representing fibrosis and scar tissue is identified within the anterolateral gutter just deep to the anterior talofibular ligament with an associated ankle effusion. There is nearly always abnormality of the anterior talofibular ligament, which may demonstrate thickening, nodularity, or complete disruption/absence.

Anterior Impingement

Anterior ankle impingement, also known as anteromedial impingement, refers to an osseous impingement that results from repetitive impact of the anterior tibia against the talar neck and is associated with longstanding ankle instability from previous ankle inversion injury. Over time, this repetitive impingement leads to osteophyte formation along the anteromedial margin of the distal tibia and anterior talar neck. Reactive subchondral marrow edema and adjacent synovitis of the anterior ankle may also occur. The patient presents with anterior ankle pain and limited painful dorsiflexion of the foot.

MRI findings include osteophyte formation involving the anteromedial aspect of the distal tibia and adjacent talar neck, reactive subcortical sclerosis, and marrow edema accompanied by adjacent synovial thickening and joint effusion (Fig. 13-32). Abnormalities of the lateral collateral ligament complex are often seen in conjunction with this type of impingement. Treatment may include osteotomy of any significant osteophyte and possibly a stabilization procedure of the lateral ankle.

Syndesmotic Impingement

Syndesmotic impingement is the sequela of a high ankle sprain and typically occurs after disruption of the inferior anterior tibiofibular ligament with or without adjacent soft tissue injury. This type of impingement has been most commonly reported in football and hockey players. After disruption of the syndesmotic ligament, the torn fascicle of the ligament abrades the lateral dome of the talus, resulting in synovitis of the anterior and posterior syndesmotic ligaments. Chronic impingement can lead to chondromalacia, osteophyte formation, and loose body formation. The patient complains of tenderness over the region of the syndesmosis and describes pain with bimalleolar compression of the syndesmosis. MRI demonstrates injury of the anterior tibiofibular ligament, adjacent high signal, and synovitis (Fig. 13-33).

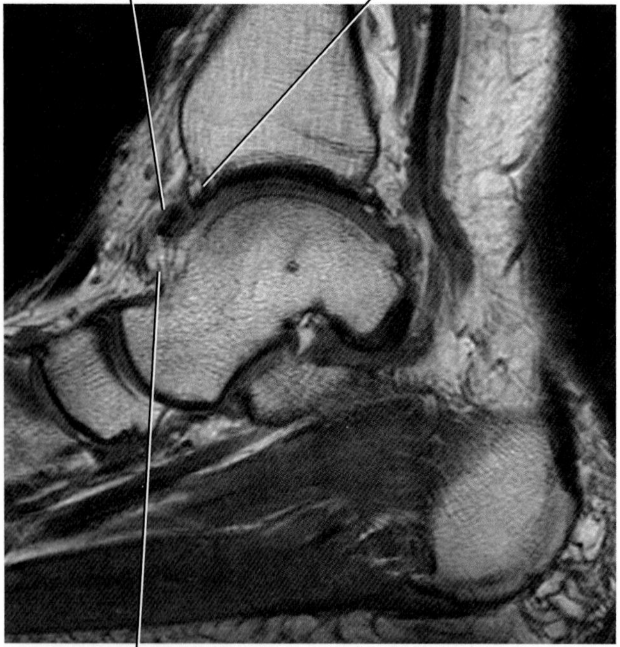
Synovitis with loose body
Anterior spur distal tibia
Spur neck of talus

Figure 13-32 Anterior impingement. Sagittal T1-weighted image shows anterior osteophyte formation involving the anterior aspect of the distal tibia and the adjacent talar neck. There is also adjacent synovitis and loose body formation.

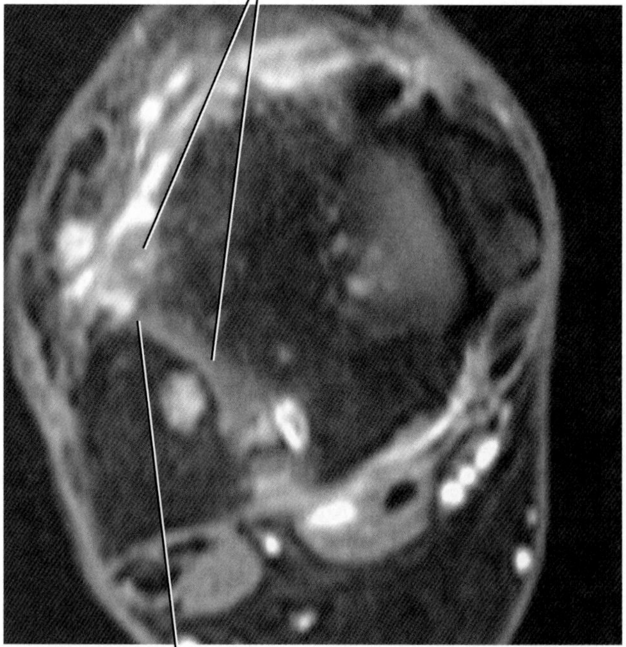
Extensive synovitis at the level of the syndesmosis
Injury of anterior tibiofibular ligament

Figure 13-33 Syndesmotic impingement. Axial T2-weighted image shows injury to the anterior tibiofibular ligament associated with a previous high ankle sprain. There is extensive intermediate signal abnormality in the region of the syndesmosis representing synovitis. Note the subchondral cyst of the distal fibula associated with osteoarthritis of the distal tibiofibular joint.

Posterior Impingement

Posterior ankle impingement was first described in ballet dancers, but it has also been described in jumping athletes. It results from the painful compression of the posterolateral aspect of the talus between the posterior margin of the tibia and the adjacent calcaneus. The symptoms of posterior ankle impingement are exacerbated with forceful plantar flexion of the ankle or with repetitive full weight-bearing in the extreme plantar-flexed position, as performed by ballet dancers. MRI findings may demonstrate edema involving the posterior talus as well as soft tissue edema and evidence of synovitis involving the posterior aspect of the ankle joint and subtalar joint.

Other potential causes predisposing a person to posterior ankle impingement include disruption or injury involving the posterior tibiofibular ligament, thickened posterior capsule, and ankle instability. An enlarged or prominent os trigonum or Stieda process can also predispose an individual to posterior impingement, and this form of impingement has also been described as os trigonum syndrome, which is a subset of posterior impingement of the ankle. Posterior ankle impingement is often associated with tethering and tendinosis of the flexor hallucis longus tendon and tenosynovitis of its tendon sheath. In each of these forms of posterior ankle impingement, the patient presents with posterior ankle pain, exacerbated by plantar flexion. MRI demonstrates edema within or adjacent to the prominent os trigonum and edema and thickening of the adjacent posterior soft tissues (Fig. 13-34). Findings of tendinosis and tenosynovitis of the flexor hallucis longus may or may not be present. In the setting of ankle instability, posterior impingement may coexist with anterior impingement.

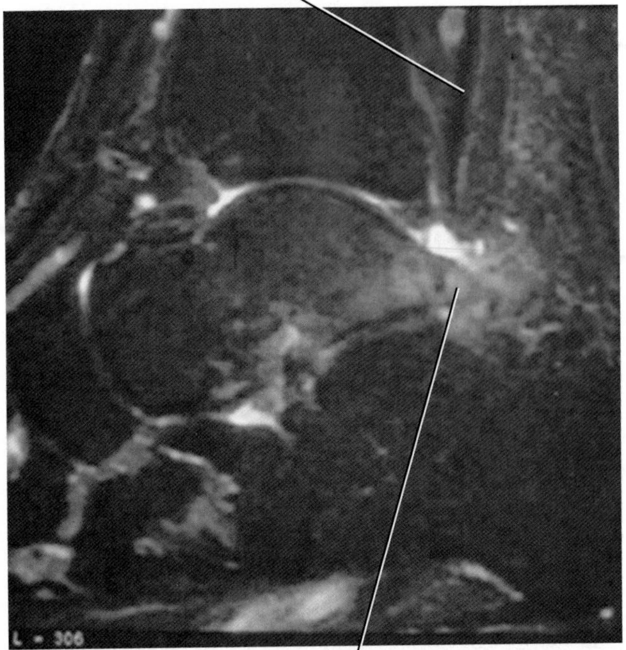
FHL tendon
Edema within os trigonum

Figure 13-34 Os trigonum syndrome (posterior impingement). Sagittal T2-weighted image with fat saturation shows extensive edema within a prominent os trigonum and extensive adjacent soft tissue edema. There is also moderate tendinosis of the flexor hallucis ligament (FHL) tendon at this level (not seen on this image) in this patient with posterior ankle pain.

Medial Impingement

Medial impingement of the ankle can occur after an ankle inversion injury and disruption of the deltoid ligament complex. The deep fibers of the deltoid ligament are compressed between the medial malleolous and the medial aspect of the talus, resulting in medial-sided ankle pain. The patient complains of medial-sided ankle pain, and MRI demonstrates soft tissue edema and synovitis along the medial joint line (Fig. 13-35).

OSSEOUS STRUCTURES

An understanding of the complex osseous anatomy of the ankle and knowledge of the potential abnormalities are essential to ensure an adequate evaluation in the patient with a history of trauma and persistent ankle pain. Cross-sectional imaging using either CT or MRI is often necessary to provide an accurate description of the osseous abnormalities. Injuries range from osteochondral impaction or shearing injuries to fractures, cortical avulsions, and stress-related injuries associated with chronic repetitive stress.

Bone Marrow Edema

Bone marrow edema is commonly detected on MRI of the ankle and is a nonspecific finding. Common

SECTION IV

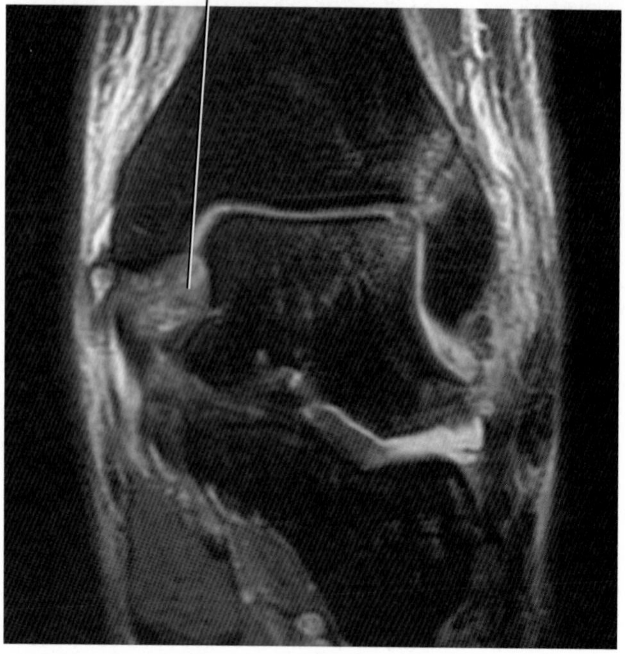
Injury of deep fibers of deltoid ligament with adjacent synovitis

Figure 13-35 Medial impingement. Coronal T2-weighted image with fat saturation shows extensive edema and injury of the deep fibers of the deltoid ligament with adjacent synovitis.

causes of marrow signal alterations include bone contusions, reactive subcortical marrow edema in association with overlying tenosynovitis or tendinosis, and stress-related changes associated with increased activity levels. Altered weight-bearing and abnormal stresses resulting from altered biomechanics as seen in tarsal coalition can also result in abnormal areas of marrow edema. Other less common causes of marrow edema are reflex sympathetic dystrophy, infection, and avascular necrosis and tumor, but other signs and symptoms are often present, which help in establishing these diagnoses. Reactive subcortical marrow edema of the calcaneus is often seen in association with abnormalities of the plantar fascia and the Achilles tendon. Also, immobilization of the foot and ankle can result in extensive subcortical and subarticular marrow edema that resolves after normal weight-bearing resumes. In the pediatric and adolescent age group, the normal osseous structures of the ankle often demonstrate a diffuse patchy, heterogeneous marrow signal that can mimic marrow edema. Familiarity with the normal MRI appearance in this age group of patients helps to prevent misinterpretation of this finding as a pathologic marrow process. Comparison with the contralateral ankle may be helpful in certain situations to determine whether heterogeneous marrow signal in this select group of patients is normal or pathologic.

Fractures

Most ankle fractures are adequately detected and described radiographically. However, if the fracture is nondisplaced, in an unexpected location, or in an area that is difficult to detect on radiographs, CT or MRI may be performed to aid in the evaluation of an individual's persistent symptoms. On MRI, an acute fracture is often seen as a linear area of low signal on T1- and high signal on T2-weighted images with surrounding marrow edema. Often, MRI is delayed in patients following trauma and is used to evaluate individuals with normal radiographs who do not respond to conservative therapy. Subacute fractures typically continue to demonstrate adjacent marrow edema for 6 to 8 weeks and possibly longer if there is repetitive injury, instability, or lack of immobilization. Trabecular callus forms at the fracture line resulting in an ill-defined area of linear low signal intensity on both T1- and T2-weighted images. At this point, the signal characteristics may mimic a stress fracture, although history may help to differentiate between the two entities.

Avulsion injuries often lack edema or demonstrate very minimal edema at the donor site and as a result may be difficult to detect on MRI because the avulsed cortical fragment is often small and obscured by adjacent soft tissue edema. If a small cortical avulsion injury is suspected clinically or on radiographs, then a CT examination is the preferred imaging modality. Common radiographically occult fractures about the ankle include various stress fractures and fractures of the talar neck, talar dome, anterior calcaneal process, and lateral talar process.

Stress Fractures of the Ankle and Hindfoot

Stress fractures in the region of the ankle occur commonly in runners as a result of abnormal repetitive stress on normal bone. The calcaneus is the most frequently involved tarsal bone, but other areas of concern include the distal tibia and fibula, the cuboid, and the navicular bone. Early radiographic findings demonstrate a subtle fluffy-appearing ill-defined sclerotic line oriented perpendicular to the primary trabeculae of the involved bone. This finding represents early endosteal or periosteal new bone formation and occurs in response to the abnormal stresses. If the aggravating activity persists, radiographic findings progress to include an incomplete lucent line representing an incomplete fracture, and it may eventually progress to a complete fracture. Both MRI and nuclear bone scan are more sensitive than radiographs in the detection of early stress fractures, but MRI has been shown to be more specific than nuclear bone scanning and should be considered the imaging modality of choice when a stress fracture is suspected in the setting of normal radiographs (Fig. 13-36).

Navicular Bone Stress fractures of the navicular bone are potentially one of the most devastating stress fractures to occur in the region of the ankle and midfoot. They typically occur in high-performance athletes and long-distance runners. Diagnosis is often delayed because of unfamiliarity with the diagnosis and because early injuries are difficult to detect radiographically. The patient presents with dorsal foot pain over the navicular region, which is exacerbated with activity. The fracture is usually located in the central third of the navicular bone and is oriented in the sagittal plane perpendicular to the long axis of the bone. The fracture usually begins in the region of the proximal articular surface and extends distally to involve the distal articular surface in the more extensive and chronic fractures. The fracture is thought to occur as a result of shearing forces that are transmitted along the shaft of the second metatarsal and deposited in the central third of the navicular bone. A short first metatarsal combined with a long second metatarsal appears to increase the risk of these stress fractures.

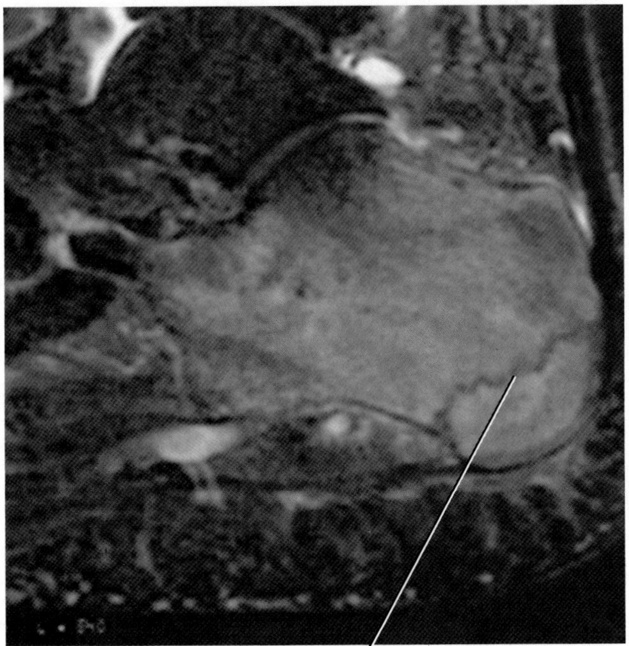
Calcaneal stress fracture
with adjacent marrow edema

Figure 13-36 MRI appearance of a calcaneal stress fracture. Sagittal T2-weighted image with fat saturation shows an extensive stress fracture of the posterior calcaneal process with extensive adjacent marrow edema.

Radiographic findings are often subtle or absent in the early phases of injury but may demonstrate a small focal linear lucency involving the proximal articular surface of the central third of the navicular bone (Fig. 13-37A). Chronic stress fractures demonstrate sclerosis extending across the short axis of the central third of the bone (Fig. 13-37B). A complete fracture may occur across the short axis of the navicular bone often with separation and fragmentation of the fracture fragments. CT and/or MRI are the preferred methods of evaluation, and axial imaging (long axis of the foot) is the preferred imaging plane. MRI can detect marrow edema within the central third of the navicular bone before the fracture line becomes evident. Treatment is conservative if the fracture is identified early. However, an extensive stress fracture or a completed fracture often requires open reduction and fixation. Once a fracture goes on to completion, the patient usually develops debilitating osteoarthritis of the proximal and distal articulations, and the goal should be to identify and successfully treat the fracture before completion. CT and MRI findings typically lag behind the clinical improvement.

Osteochondral Lesion of the Talus

Osteochondral lesion of the talus (OLT) usually occurs as the result of ankle inversion injury and involves the medial and lateral aspects of the talar dome with approximately equal frequency. Medial talar dome lesions result from ankle inversion injury with the foot in plantar flexion, whereas lateral talar dome lesions result from inversion injury with the foot in dorsiflexion. Although a small cortical defect may be identified on radiographs, these lesions can be very subtle and are often occult radiographically.

SECTION IV

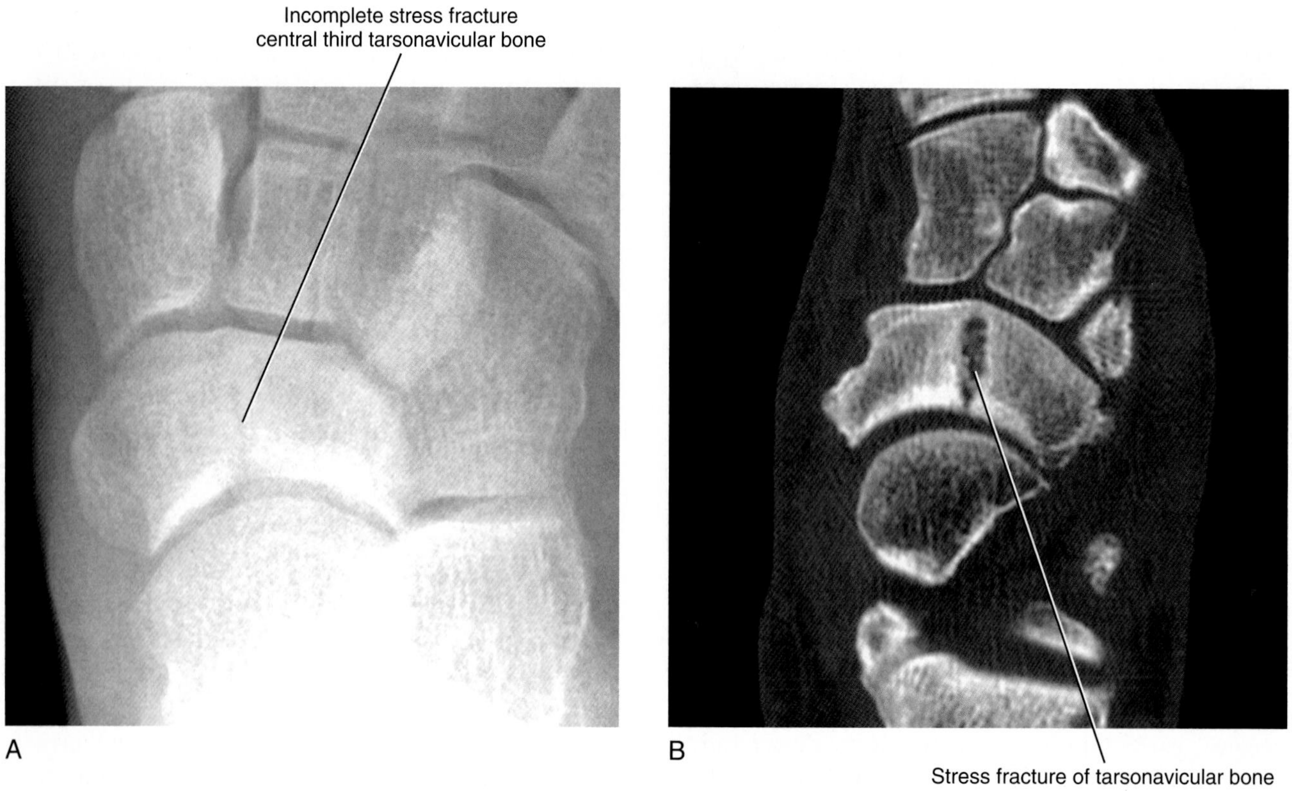
Incomplete stress fracture
central third tarsonavicular bone
A
B
Stress fracture of tarsonavicular bone

Figure 13-37 Stress fracture tarsonavicular bone. A, Anteroposterior radiograph of the midfoot shows a linear area of lucency extending across the short axis of the central third of the tarsonavicular bone representing an acute stress fracture. **B,** Long-axis CT image through the midfoot shows a chronic stress fracture of the tarsonavicular bone with sclerotic margins.

Several classifications schemes have been proposed to aid with the description of osteochondral lesions of the talar dome, and the main goal of each system is to differentiate stable from unstable lesions (Fig. 13-38).

MRI is the modality of choice in evaluation of osteochondral lesion of the talus, as an MR can accurately detect abnormalities of the overlying articular cartilage and cortex (Fig. 13-39). Subchondral marrow edema is common and may be associated with the severity of symptoms. Signs that indicate an unstable lesion include fluid signal partially or completely surrounding a fragment and/or cystic change underneath a fragment, and a displaced fragment. Unstable fragments generally progress and eventually are released into the joint as a loose body. Direct MR arthrography can be useful in classifying osteochondral defects of the talar dome. Contrast extending beneath a fragment is a sign of instability. MR arthrography can be especially useful in differentiating granulation tissue surrounding an osteochondral fragment; this granulation tissue, which can represent a healing response, often appears fluidlike and can be very bright on T2-weighted images, which can simulate a loose osteochondral fragment on conventional MRI.

Differentiation should be made between an osteochondral defect of the talar dome and osteoarthritis. Similar findings on both sides of the joint or diffuse findings of the talar dome often indicate the presence of osteoarthritis. Osteochondral lesions can occur in other locations about the ankle, including the talar head and the navicular bone.

Lateral Talar Process Fracture

Fractures of the lateral talar process are being reported more and more frequently and have been shown to be associated with the sport of snowboarding—hence the recent eponym snowboarder's fracture. The mechanism of injury is thought to be an inversion injury of the ankle with the foot in dorsiflexion, resulting in a shearing force that is transmit-

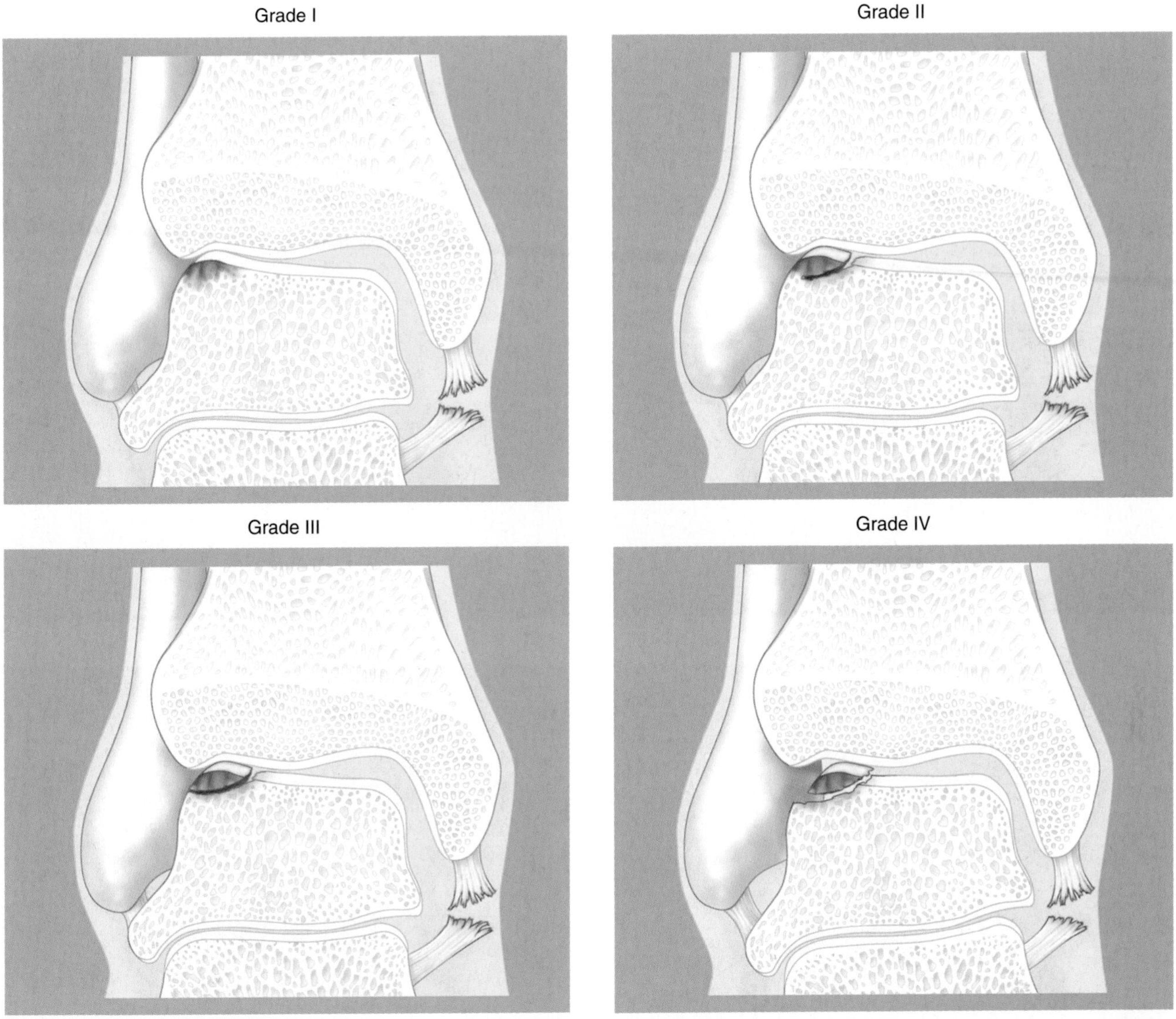
Grade I
Grade II
Grade III
Grade IV

Figure 13-38 Grading system for osteochondral lesions of the talar dome. Grade I. Subchondral marrow edema with an intact overlying cortex and chondral surface. Grade II. Fluid extends partially beneath the osteochondral fragment indicating a partially detached lesion. Grade III. Fluid extends completely beneath the osteochondral fragment indicating an unstable lesion, but the fragment maintains its normal position. Grade IV. Completely detached and displaced osteochondral fragment.

ted across the subtalar joint from the calcaneus to the lateral talar process. A second less common mechanism is a high-speed impaction injury as may occur when the foot slams against the floorboard of a car in an automobile accident. This type of injury is often accompanied by multiple other ankle injuries.

Patients presenting with isolated fractures of the lateral talar process usually demonstrate symptoms indistinguishable from those of the more common lateral ankle sprain. Radiographs may be of little help because series have shown that up to 40% of these fractures are missed on initial radiographs (Fig. 13-40A). The imaging modalities of choice include CT and MRI, since their multiplanar capabilities allow accurate detection and classification of a suspected lateral talar process fracture (Fig. 13-40B). A delay in diagnosis can be devastating, because unrecognized injuries lead to persistent pain, instability, and premature osteoarthritis, requiring subtalar fusion in up to 30% of cases to alleviate symptoms.

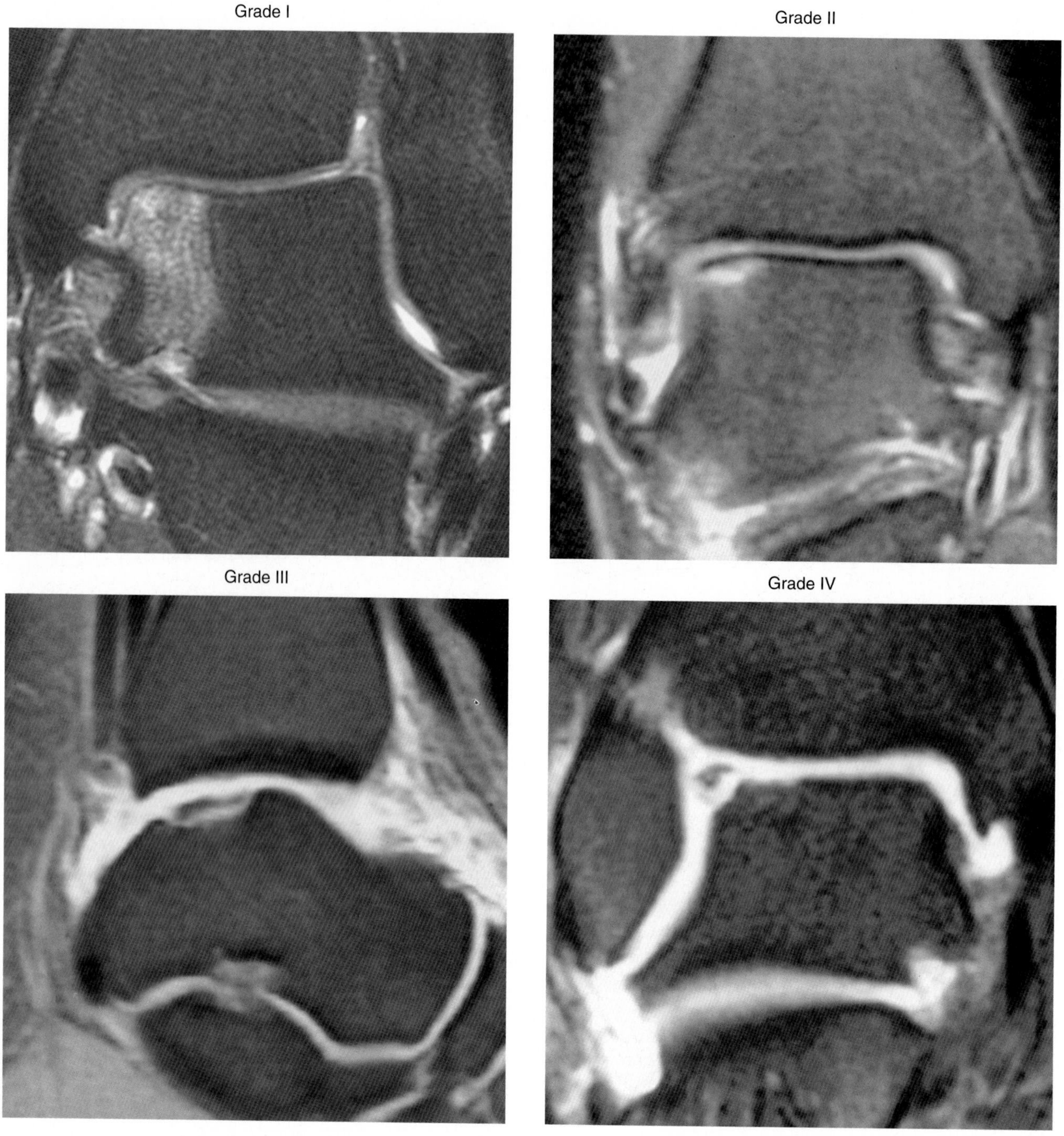
Grade I
Grade II
Grade III
Grade IV

Figure 13-39 Osteochondral lesions of the talar dome. Coronal and sagittal MRI showing grade I through grade IV osteochondral lesions of the talar dome.

The lateral talar process is a broad-based triangular process of the body of the talus and is contiguous with the trochlear surface of the talus. The anterior margin of the lateral talar process has a roughened surface that serves as the attachment site of the anterior talofibular ligament. The superior surface of the lateral talar process articulates with the distal fibula, whereas the inferior surface articulates with the calcaneus, forming the posterior facet of the subtalar joint. Thus, fractures of the lateral talar process are

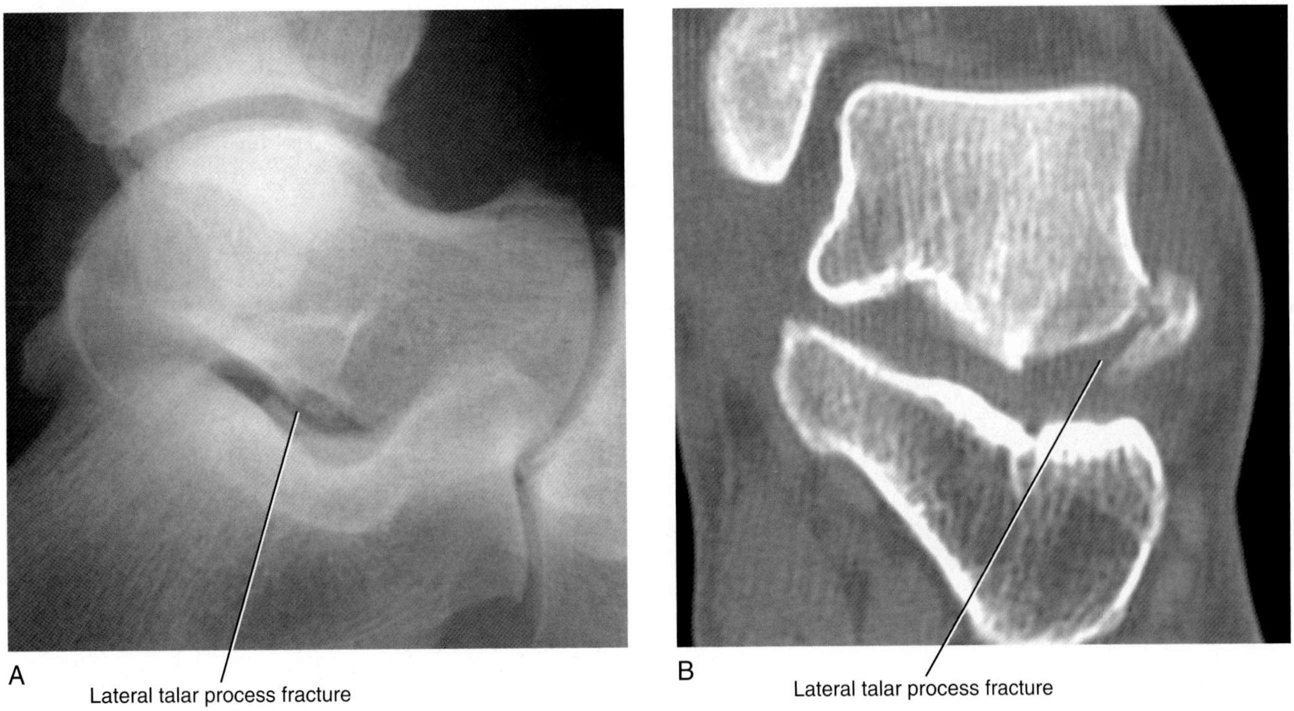
A
Lateral talar process fracture
B
Lateral talar process fracture

Figure 13-40 Lateral talar process fracture. A, Lateral radiograph of the ankle shows disruption of the cortex of the lateral talar process. The lateral radiograph is usually the best projection to detect fractures of the lateral talar process and demonstrate disruption of the triangular-appearing cortex of the lateral process. **B,** Coronal CT image shows the lateral talar process fracture and demonstrates the extent of articular surface step-off involving the subtalar joint.

intra-articular and may involve both the talofibular articulation as well as the posterior facet of the subtalar joint.

Fractures are graded using a three-point system (Table 13-4). Nondisplaced fractures or small cortical avulsion fractures are treated conservatively with a non–weight-bearing cast. If the fracture fragment is larger than 1 cm or if more than 2 mm of articular surface step-off exists, then surgical treatment is indicated. A single large fragment can be treated with open reduction and internal fixation, whereas a comminuted fracture is usually treated with debridement. Delayed diagnosis leads to an incongruent articular surface with rapid onset of subtalar osteoarthritis that may require fusion for symptomatic relief.

Both CT and MRI can accurately detect a fracture of the lateral talar process. The coronal and sagittal imaging planes are best suited for detection of these fractures. In the acute setting, marrow edema is visible on MRI (Fig. 13-41). The size and number of fragments should be described as well as the extent of articular surface step-off involving both the superior and inferior articular surfaces. Small cortical avulsion fractures may be better depicted on CT than on MRI. However, marrow edema seen on MRI in the region of the anterior margin of the lateral talar process at the site of attachment of the anterior talofibular ligament should raise suspicion of a small cortical avulsion fracture.

Table 13-4 Lateral Talar Process Fracture: Grading System

Grade	Findings
I	Simple fracture involving both articular surfaces
II	Comminuted fracture
III	Cortical avulsion fracture

Anterior Calcaneal Process Fracture

The most common avulsion fracture of the foot involves the anterior process of the calcaneus at the level of attachment of the bifurcate ligament. The bifurcate ligament has two bundles that arise from the anterior calcaneal process and extend to the lateral

SECTION IV

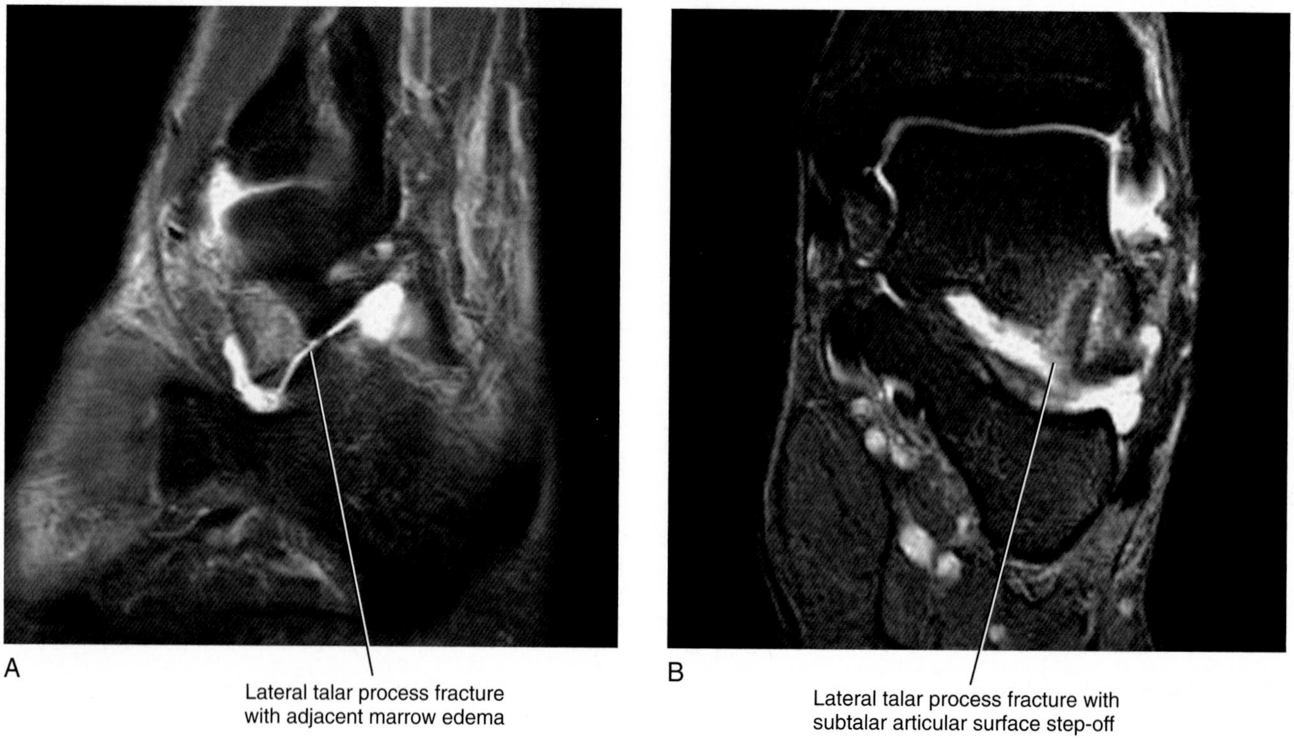
A
Lateral talar process fracture
with adjacent marrow edema
B
Lateral talar process fracture with
subtalar articular surface step-off

Figure 13-41 MRI appearance of a lateral talar process fracture. Sagittal (**A**) and coronal (**B**) T2-weighted images with fat saturation demonstrate a lateral talar process fracture with a single large fracture fragment. There is extensive adjacent marrow edema. The coronal image typically best delineates the extent of articular surface step-off as demonstrated in this case.

aspect of the navicular bone and the adjacent cuboid. Fractures usually result from an adduction injury to the foot and cause lateral ankle pain. These fractures are often radiographically occult. They are clearly depicted on either CT or MRI of the ankle and are usually best visualized in the sagittal imaging plane (Fig. 13-42). MRI also demonstrates edema isolated to the anterior calcaneal process.

Other Difficult-to-Detect Fractures

Numerous other less common fractures can involve the osseous structures of the ankle. The complexity of this anatomic region makes the use of cross-sectional imaging very useful in the detection and accurate description of each of these fractures.

INTRA-ARTICULAR BODIES

Intra-articular bodies of the ankle are often associated with osteochondral lesions of the talar dome, osteoarthritis, or prior injury (see Fig. 13-38). If numerous loose bodies are detected, then the diagnosis of synovial osteochondromatosis should be considered. MRI signal characteristics vary depending on the composition of the bodies, which may contain a combination of cartilage, bone, and fibrous tissue. Intra-articular bodies often collect in recesses of the joint, and in the ankle they are often noted anteriorly or posteriorly (see Fig. 13-32). They are more easily detected in the presence of a joint effusion. Direct MR arthrography can be helpful in the detection of intra-articular bodies by causing joint distention, which results in the intra-articular body being surrounded by fluid. Care must be taken not to confuse synovial folds or ligaments with intra-articular bodies (Fig. 13-43).

TARSAL COALITION

Tarsal coalition represents a developmental abnormality in which there is failure of proper segmentation of the tarsal bones. It may be bilateral in up to

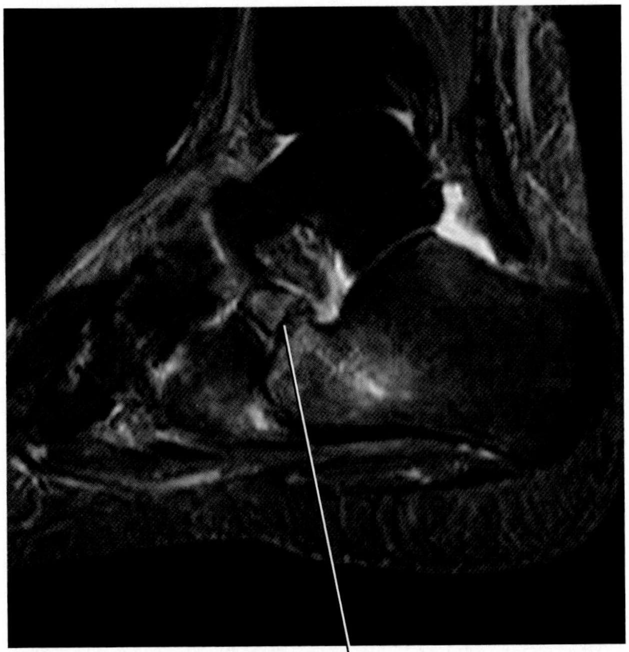
Anterior calcaneal process fracture
with adjacent marrow edema

Figure 13-42 MRI appearance of anterior calcaneal fracture. Sagittal T2-weighted image with fat saturation shows a minimally displaced fracture of the anterior calcaneal process with adjacent marrow edema.

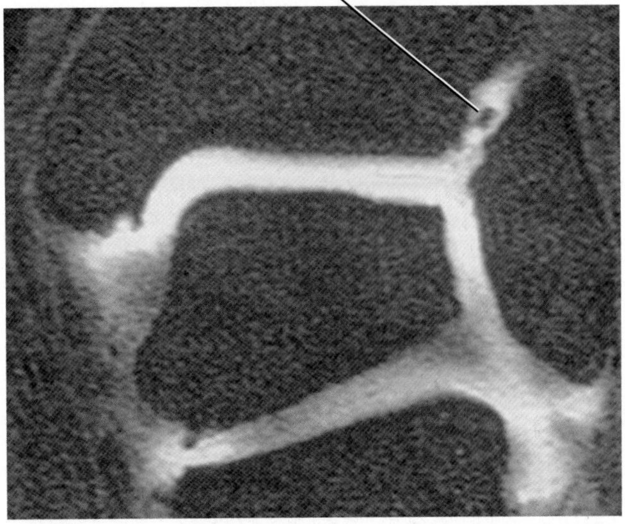
Synovial fold mimicking a
loose intra-articular body

Figure 13-43 Synovial fold mimicking a loose intra-articular body. Coronal T1-weighted image with fat saturation and intra-articular gadolinium shows a synovial fold that mimics an intra-articular body.

50% of cases. As a result, bilateral ankle imaging is often performed when tarsal coalition is suspected. The most common locations for tarsal coalition are the calcaneonavicular interval and the middle facet of the subtalar joint. However, rarely the calcaneocuboid or cuboid-navicular joints may also be involved. The types of tarsal coalition vary and may include areas of osseous, fibrous, and/or cartilaginous coalition. Patients usually present during adolescence with midfoot or hindfoot pain and stiffness. Areas of cartilaginous coalition are usually more flexible until maturity when they undergo ossification.

Tarsal coalition maybe suspected on the basis of physical examination and radiographic findings. Calcaneonavicular coalition is best visualized on a 45-degree oblique view of the foot, and radiographic findings include an osseous bar across the interval with sclerosis, elongation of the anterior calcaneal process (anteater sign), and talar beaking. Talocalcaneal (subtalar) coalition most commonly occurs at the level of the middle facet and only rarely involves either the anterior or posterior fact. The most common radiographic findings in subtalar coalition include nonvisualization of the middle facet subtalar joint and proliferation of the sustentaculum tali (C sign), best depicted on the Harris-Beath view. Talar beaking may also be present.

When tarsal coalition is suspected on the basis of physical examination or radiographs, it is important to complete the evaluation with either a CT or MRI examination. These imaging modalities allow differentiation between osseous and fibrous coalition and can estimate the extent of coalition, which is important for preoperative planning (Fig. 13-44). On MRI, osseous coalition demonstrates marrow continuity across the interval. Fibrous coalition demonstrates low T1 and T2 signal across the interval, whereas cartilaginous coalition demonstrates intermediate T1 and T2 signal across the interval. Hindfoot valgus is usually associated with tarsal coalition and can be demonstrated on either CT or MRI. Surgical treatment includes resection of the coalition with fat interposed within the interval.

AVASCULAR NECROSIS

Avascular necrosis (AVN) of the tarsal bones is not uncommon and, when present, usually involves the

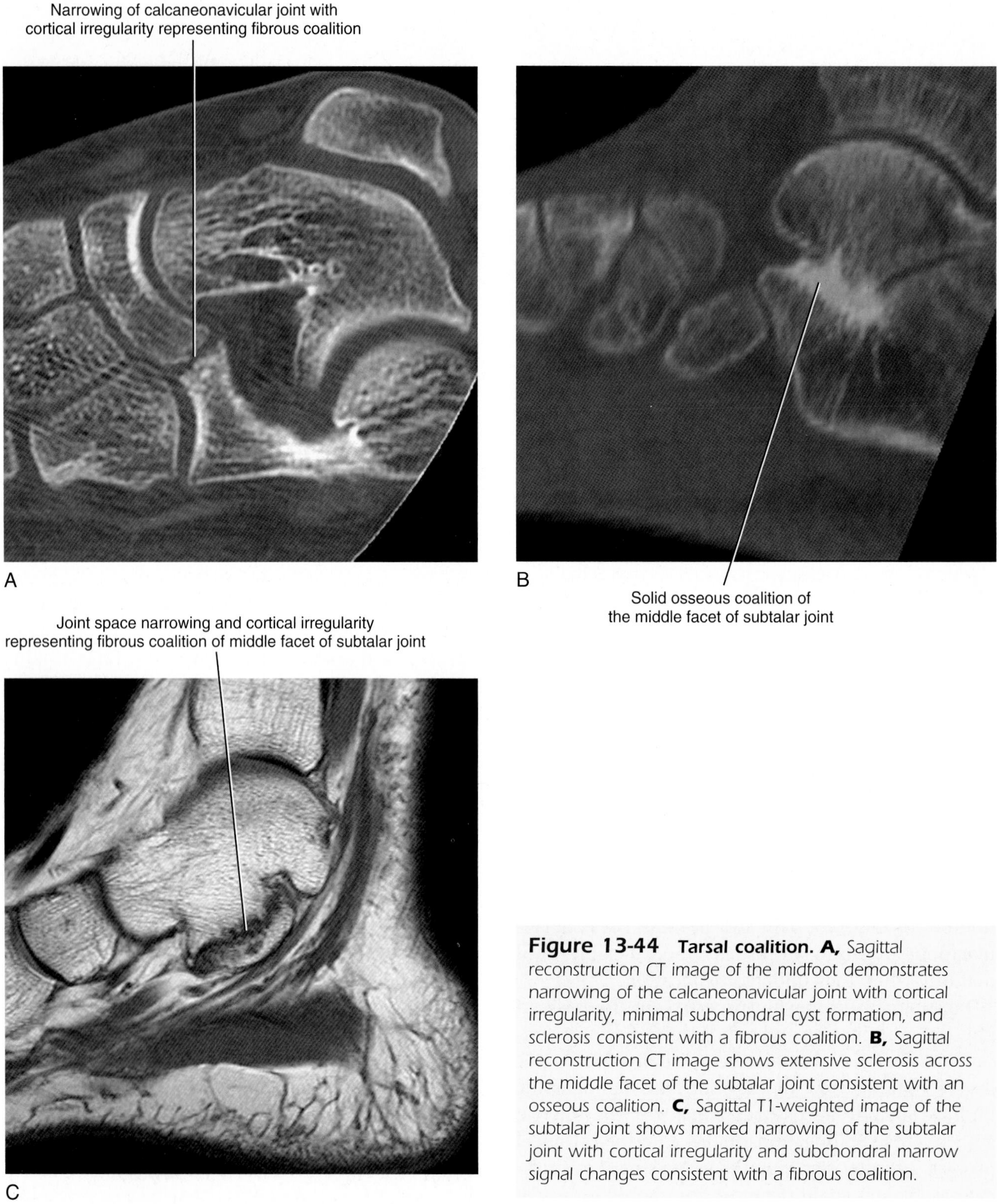
Narrowing of calcaneonavicular joint with
cortical irregularity representing fibrous coalition
A
B
Solid osseous coalition of
the middle facet of subtalar joint
Joint space narrowing and cortical irregularity
representing fibrous coalition of middle facet of subtalar joint
C

Figure 13-44 Tarsal coalition. A, Sagittal reconstruction CT image of the midfoot demonstrates narrowing of the calcaneonavicular joint with cortical irregularity, minimal subchondral cyst formation, and sclerosis consistent with a fibrous coalition. **B,** Sagittal reconstruction CT image shows extensive sclerosis across the middle facet of the subtalar joint consistent with an osseous coalition. **C,** Sagittal T1-weighted image of the subtalar joint shows marked narrowing of the subtalar joint with cortical irregularity and subchondral marrow signal changes consistent with a fibrous coalition.

subchondral region of the talar dome. A fracture of the talar neck, resulting in disruption of the blood supply to the talar dome is the most common cause of AVN of the talus. However, metabolic causes may also be responsible for AVN of the talus. Conventional radiographs may help predict the likelihood of talar AVN following trauma. The presence of a subchondral linear lucency involving the subtalar dome is referred to as the Hawkins sign and indicates normal blood supply and post-traumatic osteopenia (Fig. 13-45). Absence of this sign during the first 6 weeks after trauma to the talus may be an indicator that AVN is likely to occur, whereas the presence of Hawkins sign is an indicator of good blood supply to the talar dome. MRI can accurately evaluate the presence and extent of talar AVN. The appearance of subchondral AVN of the talus is similar to that seen in either the femoral or humeral head. A geographic area of subchondral signal alteration is noted. A double-line sign on T2-weighted images is very specific for AVN (Fig. 13-46). The double-line sign is seen more commonly in cases of metabolic AVN, whereas post traumatic cases of AVN are less likely to result in the double-line sign in the region of the talus. A complete description should include the extent of subchondral involvement and a description of associated cortical or articular surface collapse.

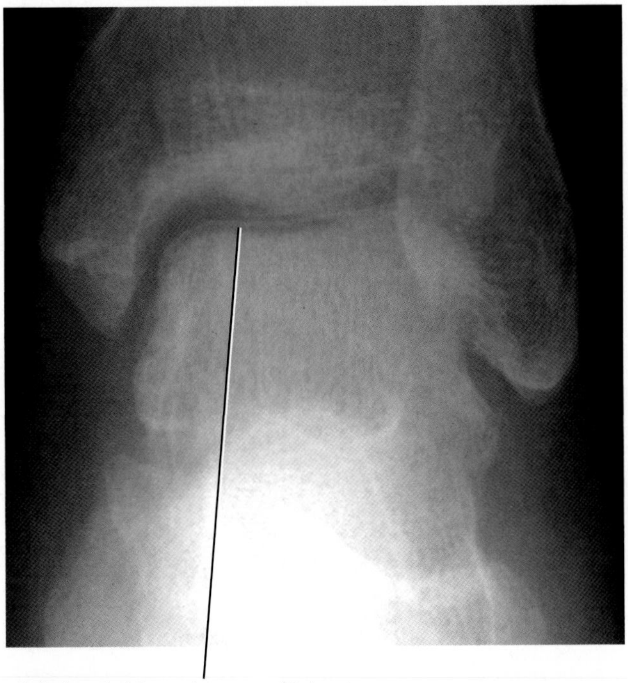
Subchondral linear lucency of talar dome

Figure 13-45 Hawkins sign. Anteroposterior radiograph of the ankle shows a subchondral linear lucency involving the talar dome within the first 6 weeks after injury. This indicates hyperemia and is a sign that avascular necrosis is unlikely to occur.

SINUS TARSI SYNDROME

The sinus tarsi is a cone-shaped area located between the talus and the calcaneus in the anterolateral aspect of the subtalar joint, with the base (wide portion) located laterally. The contents of the sinus tarsi include abundant fat surrounding a venous plexus, arterial branches arising from the lateral malleolar artery, and the lateral tarsal artery and nerve branches arising from the deep peroneal nerve, which play an important role in hindfoot proprioception. The inferior extensor retinaculum is the most superficial structure of the sinus tarsus, and there are two ligaments—the cervical ligament at the level of the mid cone and the interosseous ligament at the level of the apex of the cone (anterior margin of the posterior facet). These ligaments help to stabilize the subtalar joint (Fig. 13-47).

Sinus tarsi syndrome is a clinical syndrome characterized by lateral ankle pain and a sensation of hindfoot instability. It typically results from a severe ankle inversion injury and is nearly always associated with damage to the lateral collateral ligamentous complex. Alternative causes of sinus tarsi syndrome are ganglion formation within the sinus tarsi and post-traumatic venous fibrosis resulting in venous outflow obstruction and disorders of nociception and proprioception of the nerve endings of the sinus tarsi. Treatment options include arthroscopic subtalar joint synovectomy, denervation of the subtalar joint, and corticosteroid injection.

Sinus tarsi syndrome is considered a clinical diagnosis (pain over the sinus tarsi and lateral ankle instability) and cannot be established solely on the basis of MRI findings. Nevertheless, certain MRI findings are associated with the sinus tarsi syndrome. The sinus tarsi is best evaluated on T1- and T2-weighted sagittal MR images. The normal sinus tarsi demonstrates bright fat signal on T1-weighted images, and the ligamentous structures previously described are clearly outlined by the bright fat. After disruption of the sinus tarsi, the fat signal is replaced with low signal on T1- and bright fluid signal on

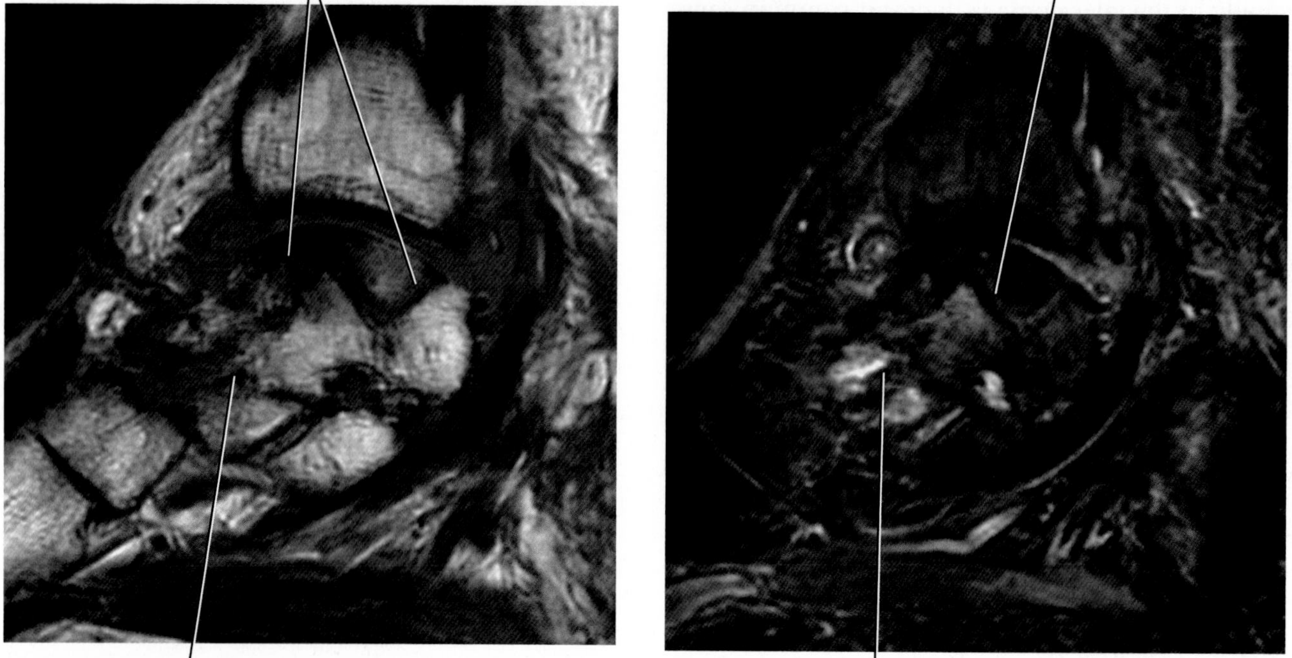
Geographic area of signal alteration in subchondral region of talar dome
Talar neck fracture
Double-line sign representing talar dome AVN
Talar neck fracture

Figure 13-46 Avascular necrosis (AVN) of the talus. An extensive area of marrow edema involving the subchondral region of the talar dome with a double-line sign representing AVN of the talus. A fracture of the talar neck is also present.

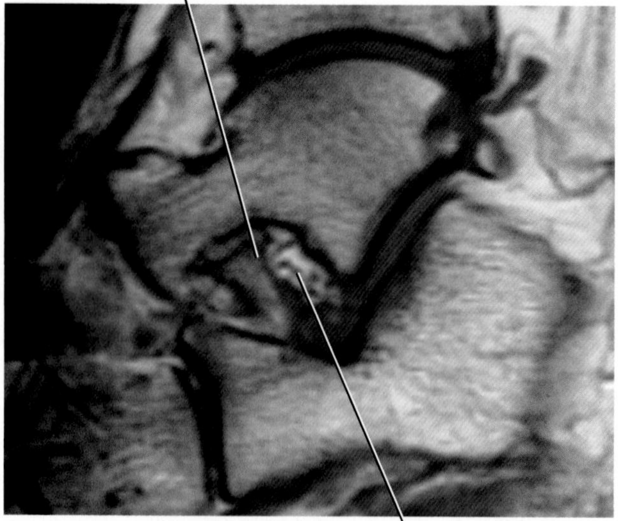
Cervical ligament
Normal fat signal in the sinus tarsi

Figure 13-47 Normal MRI imaging appearance of the sinus tarsi. Sagittal T1-weighted image shows the normal fat signal filling the sinus tarsi with the normal appearance of the cervical ligament.

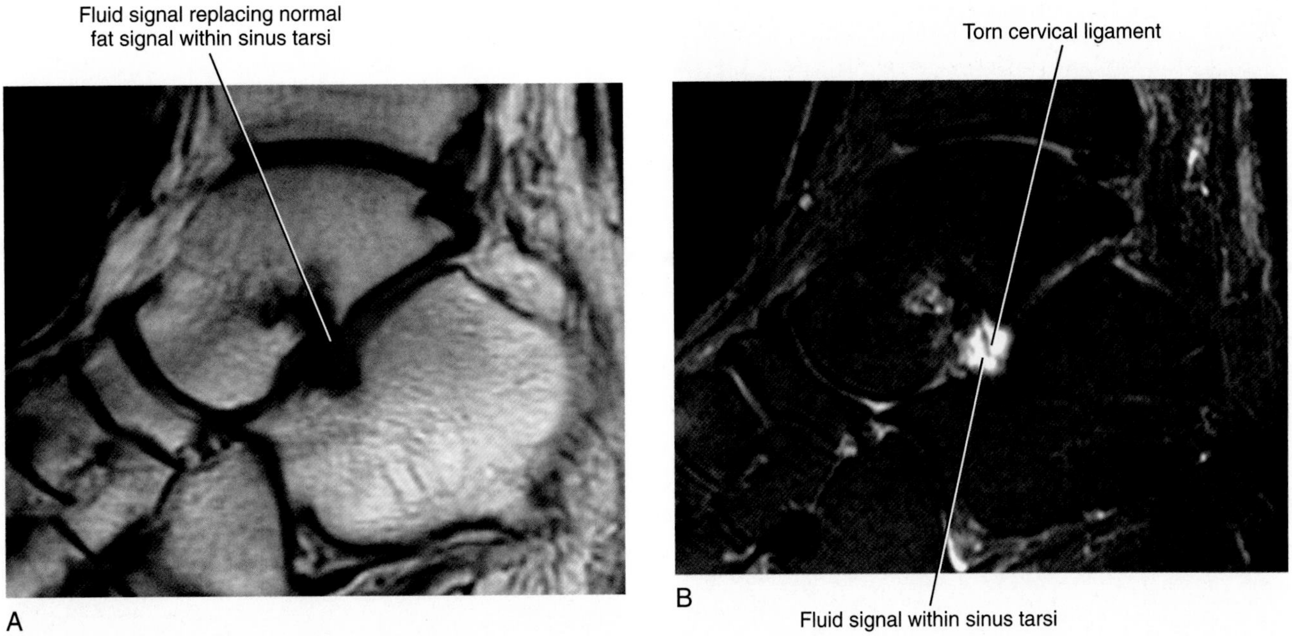
Fluid signal replacing normal fat signal within sinus tarsi
A
Torn cervical ligament
B
Fluid signal within sinus tarsi

Figure 13-48 **Sinus tarsi syndrome.** Sagittal T1- (**A**) and T2-weighted (**B**) images show fluid signal, completely replacing the normal fat signal within the sinus tarsi with complete disruption of the cervical ligament.

T2-weighted images with disruption or indistinctness of the cervical and interosseous ligaments (Fig. 13-48).

The major pitfall in the diagnosis of sinus tarsi syndrome on the basis of MRI is the fact that fluid signal is often seen within the sinus tarsi as a normal MRI finding. The combination of lateral collateral ligamentous injury, fluid within the sinus tarsi, and disruption or indistinctness of the ligaments of the sinus tarsi in conjunction with the clinical findings of hindfoot instability and lateral ankle pain must be used to establish the diagnosis of sinus tarsi syndrome.

TARSAL TUNNEL

The tarsal tunnel is a fibro-osseous tunnel located within the posteromedial aspect of the ankle and contains the posterior tibial vein, artery, and nerve. The flexor retinaculum forms the superficial boundary of the tunnel, whereas the medial aspect of the talus forms the floor of the tunnel. The medial boundary includes the flexor digitorum longus and posterior tibialis tendons, and the lateral boundary is formed by the flexor hallucis longus tendon (see Fig. 13-1). Any mass or other process that results in entrapment of the tunnel contents can lead to paresthesias in the distribution of the posterior tibialis nerve or one of its branches. MRI can be useful in the evaluation of tarsal tunnel syndrome, which most often results from entrapment of the posterior tibialis nerve by a ganglion within the tarsal tunnel (Fig. 13-49). Other potential sources of nerve entrapment include focal soft tissue mass, varicosities, accessory muscles, scar tissue, and alteration in the osseous anatomy resulting from an adjacent fracture.

PLANTAR FASCIA

Plantar Fasciitis

The plantar fascia is a strong fibrous aponeurosis originating along the plantar aspect of the calcaneus and coursing along the plantar margin of the flexor digitorum brevis muscle. The plantar fascia fans out at the level of the metatarsal heads where it gives off five slips, one attaching to the base of the proximal phalanges of each toe. The plantar fascia provides support to the longitudinal arch of the foot, preventing collapse and providing support during the lift-off phase of gait. Although the plantar fascia can be acutely disrupted in an athlete, most abnormalities

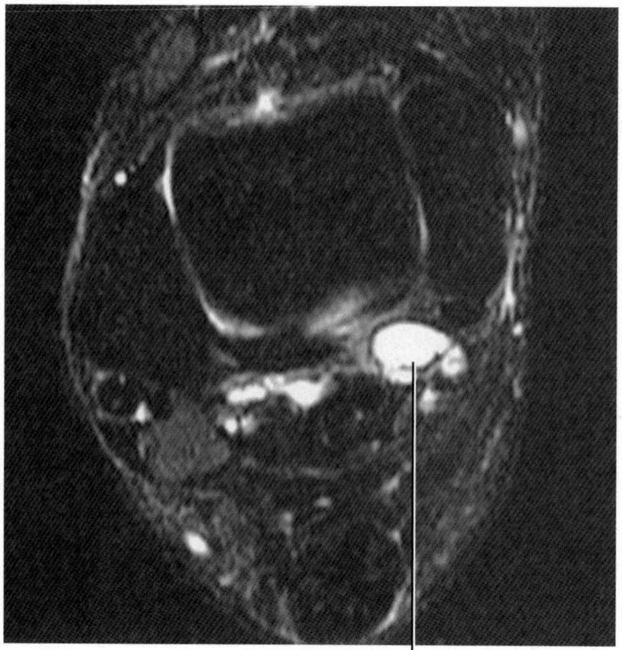
Ganglion within the tarsal tunnel

Figure 13-49 MRI appearance of tarsal tunnel syndrome. Axial T2-weighted image with fat saturation shows a large ganglion within the tarsal tunnel compressing the posterior tibialis nerve and resulting in the symptoms of tarsal tunnel syndrome.

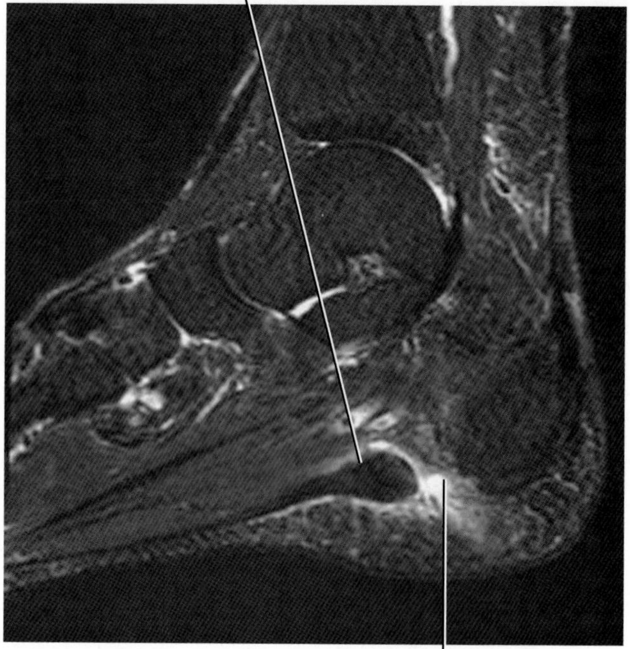
Marked thickening of the plantar fascia with adjacent edema
Full-thickness tear of proximal fibers of plantar fascia

Figure 13-50 Plantar fasciitis. Sagittal T2-weighted image with fat saturation shows marked thickening of the medial bundle of the plantar fascia and a complete tear near its calcaneal attachment. There is surrounding soft tissue edema.

of the plantar fascia result from chronic degeneration of the plantar fascia secondary to poor biomechanics of the foot. Most abnormalities of the plantar fascia are located near the calcaneal insertion and usually involve the medial bundle. MRI may demonstrate thickening and heterogeneous signal within the substance of the plantar fascia. Adjacent reactive soft tissue edema, enthesiophyte formation involving the plantar aspect of the calcaneus, and subcortical marrow edema of the calcaneus are also common findings (Fig. 13-50). Because of the superficial nature of the plantar fascia, ultrasound is ideally suited for demonstrating abnormalities of the fascia, such as signs of plantar fasciitis and partial- or full-thickness tears (Fig. 13-51). Conservative treatment methods are preferred and include nonsteroidal anti-inflammatory medications, physical therapy, and orthotics. Surgical release of the medial attachment and spur resection may be required for pain relief, but these can lead to and instability and eventual collapse of the arch of the foot.

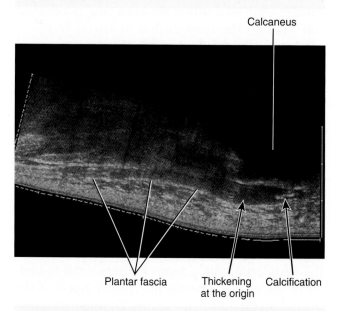

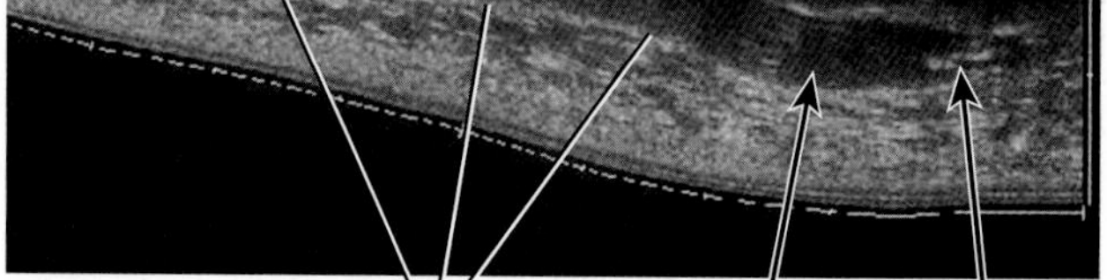
Calcaneus
Plantar fascia
Thickening at the origin
Calcification

Figure 13-51 Plantar fasciitis on longitudinal ultrasound image. Note thickening of the plantar fascia and calcification at its insertion site on the inferior aspect of the calcaneus.

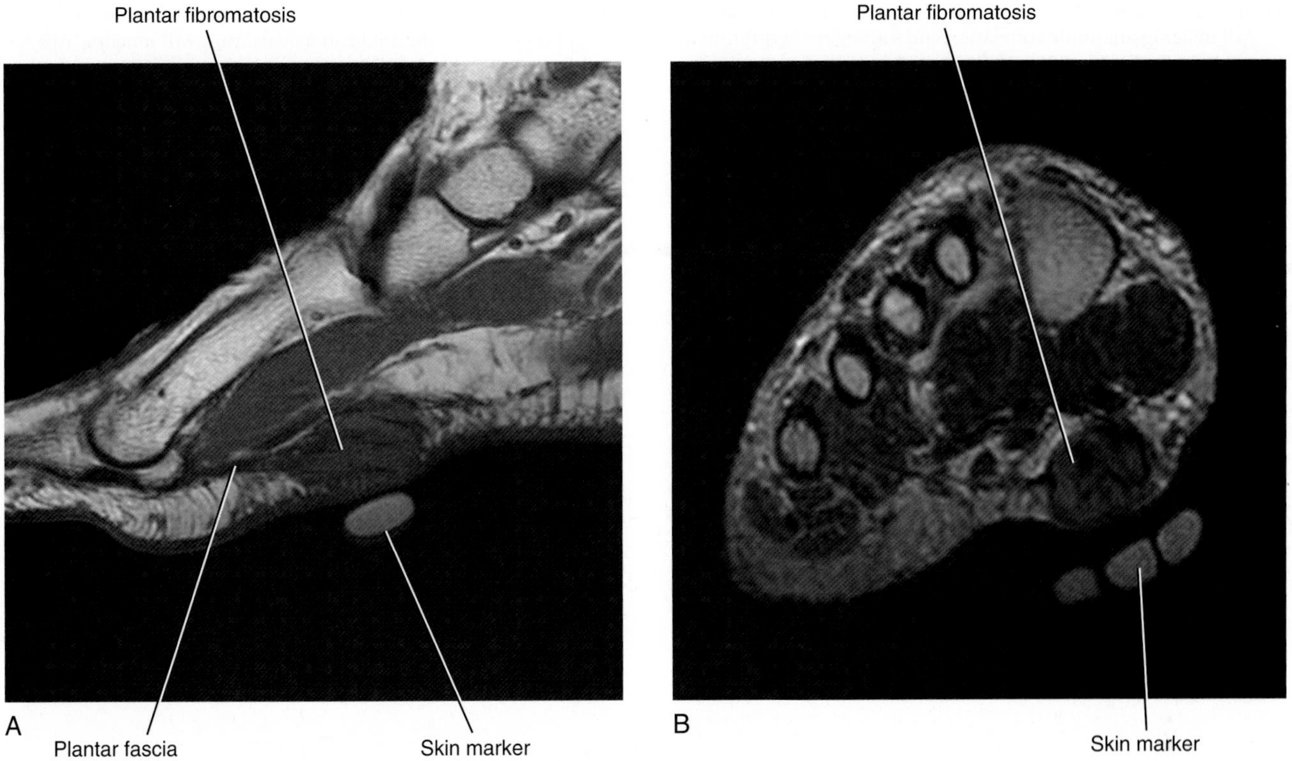
Plantar fibromatosis
A
Plantar fascia
Skin marker
Plantar fibromatosis
B
Skin marker

Figure 13-52 **Plantar fibromatosis.** Sagittal T1-weighted (**A**) and axial T2-weighted (**B**) images show a large oblong-shaped mass with low T1 and T2 signal. The mass is located along the plantar aspect of the medial bundle of the plantar fascia and is nicely outlined by the adjacent fat.

Plantar Fibromatosis

Plantar fibromatosis represents a benign fibrous proliferation of the planar aponeurosis. Plantar fibromatosis is most commonly seen along the medial aspect of the plantar fascia and is more common in men than women. Patients usually present with a painless mass along the plantar aspect of the midfoot. Conservative treatment is preferable, but surgical resection may be required. Incomplete resection may lead to aggressive recurrence, resulting in a larger lesion that invades adjacent soft tissue structures. On MRI, the mass shows intermediate to low signal T1 and T2 signal and often demonstrates intense enhancement (Fig. 13-52). The mass is usually located along the plantar aspect of the medial bundle of the plantar fascia at the level of the midfoot. Use of fat saturation techniques may partially obscure the lesion as the low signal intensity of the lesion may blend with the saturated fat signal, whereas the adjacent bright signal of the subcutaneous fat will improve conspicuity of the lesion.

Suggested Readings

Bencardino JT, Rosenberg ZS, Serrano LF. MR imaging features of diseases of the peroneal tendons. Magn Reson Imaging North Am 2001;9:493–505.

Bencardino JT, Rosenberg ZS, Serrano LF. MR imaging of tendon abnormalities of the foot and ankle. Magn Reson Imaging North Am 2001;9:475–492.

Bergin D, Morrison WB. Postoperative imaging of the ankle and foot. Radiol Clin North Am 2006;44:391–406.

Brown KW, Morrison WB, Schweitzer ME, et al. MRI findings associated with distal tibiofibular syndesmosis injury. AJR Am J Roentgenol 2004;182:131–136.

Campbell SE. MRI of sports injuries of the ankle. Clin Sports Med 2006;25:727–762.

Lektrakul N, Chung CB, Lai Y, et al. Tarsal tunnel: arthrographic, MR imaging, MR arthrographic and pathologic findings in cadavers and retrospective study data in patients with sinus tarsi syndrome. Radiology 2001;219:802–810.

Linklater J. Ligamentous, chondral, and osteochondral ankle injuries in athletes. Semin Musculoskelet Radiol 2004;8:81–98.

Mengiardi B, Pfirrmann CW, Zanetti M. MR imaging of tendons and ligaments of the midfoot. Semin Musculoskelet Radiol 2005; 9:187–198.

Mengiardi B, Zanetti M, Schottle, et al. Spring ligament complex: MR imaging-anatomic correlation and findings in asymptomatic subjects. Radiology 2005;237:242–249.

Muthukumar T, Butt SH, Cassar-Pullicino VN. Stress fractures and related disorders in the foot and ankle: plain films, scintigraphy, CT, and MR imaging. Semin Musculoskelet Radiol 2005;9: 210–226.

Robinson P, White L. Soft-tissue and osseous impingement syndromes of the ankle: role of imaging in diagnosis and management. RadioGraphics 2002;22:1457–1469.

Rubin DA, Tishkoff NW, Britton CA, et al. Anterolateral fibrous impingement of the ankle: diagnosis using MR imaging. AJR Am J Roentgenol 1997;95:293–297.

Schweitzer ME, Karasick D. MR imaging of the Achilles tendon. AJR Am J Roentgenol 2000;175:613–625.

Yu JS. Pathologic and post-operative conditions of the plantar fascia: review of MR imaging appearances. Skeletal Radiol 2000;29: 491–501.

Zoga AC, Schweitzer ME. Imaging sports injuries of the foot and ankle. Magn Reson Imaging North Am 2003;11:295–310.

Chapter 14

IMAGING OF THE FOREFOOT AND MIDFOOT

CHAPTER OUTLINE

MODALITIES

Radiography

Radiographs are very useful in the initial evaluation of most conditions affecting the forefoot and midfoot. Acute fractures, stress fractures, arthritis, sesamoid pathology, and malalignment can be assessed. For the forefoot and midfoot, anteroposterior, lateral, and external oblique views are usually satisfactory. For the forefoot, a sesamoid view is useful to evaluate sesamoid position and articular surfaces. This can be obtained by centering the x-ray beam as if to acquire an anteroposterior ankle image, but centered lower over the metatarsophalangeal joints. Dorsiflexion of the toes removes superimposed density.

Computed Tomography

CT (especially multidetector CT) offers the ability to more precisely evaluate the articular surfaces and cortical margins for fractures, arthritis, as well as increased bone density, which can indicate avascular necrosis. Images are obtained at 1-mm intervals through the forefoot and midfoot in the axial plane, and sagittal and coronal reformatted images are obtained. Alternatively, with the patient's knee flexed, the foot can be positioned flat against the CT table, and direct coronal images can be acquired. This technique was popular with older-generation CT scanners but is not necessary with multidetector CT.

Ultrasound

Ultrasound is excellent for answering specific clinical questions in many circumstances, especially regarding tendinopathy, foreign body localization (Fig. 14-1), ganglion and bursitis evaluation, Morton neuroma (Fig. 14-2), and ligament/plantar plate injury (Fig. 14-3). A distinct advantage of ultrasound is its ability to image while dynamically stressing a structure. Comparison can be made with adjacent normal regions or the contralateral side.

Magnetic Resonance Imaging

MRI is versatile and can be used to answer specific questions, such as ruling out plantar plate injury, or it can be used as a survey exam when the clinical picture is more nebulous. However, it is important to note that the ankle, midfoot, and forefoot are

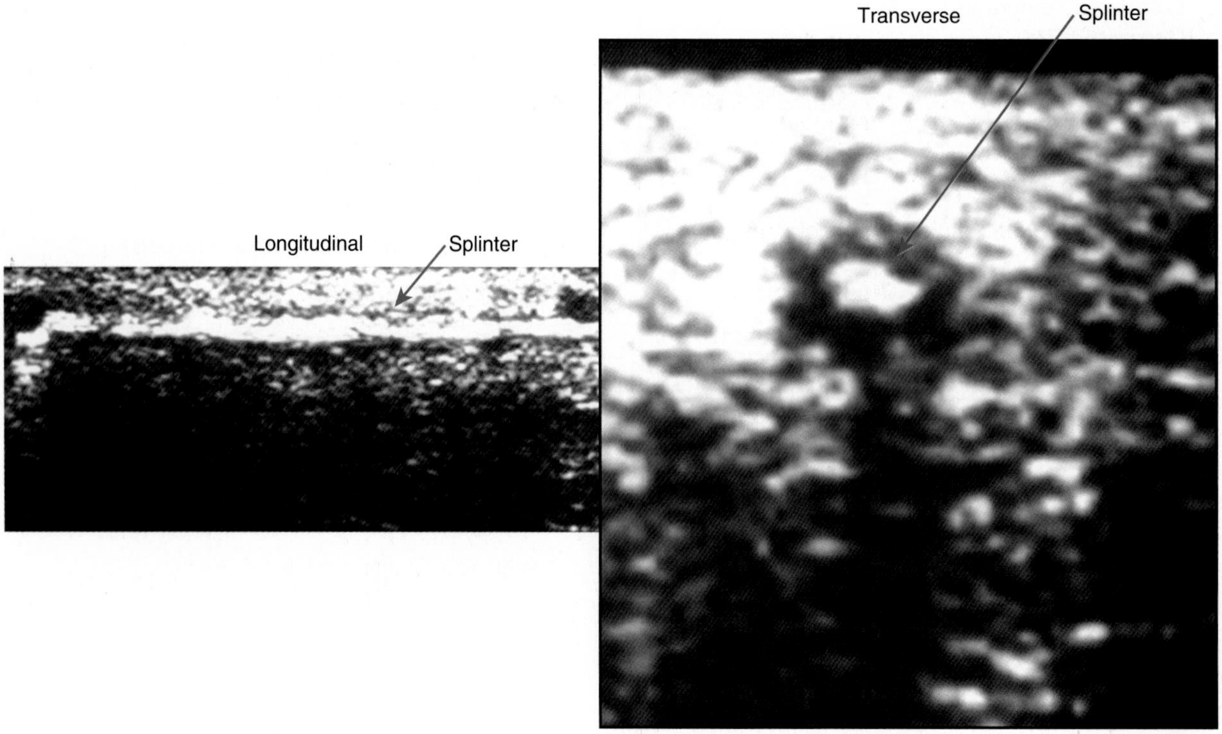
Longitudinal
Splinter
Transverse
Splinter

Figure 14-1 Splinter detected by ultrasound.

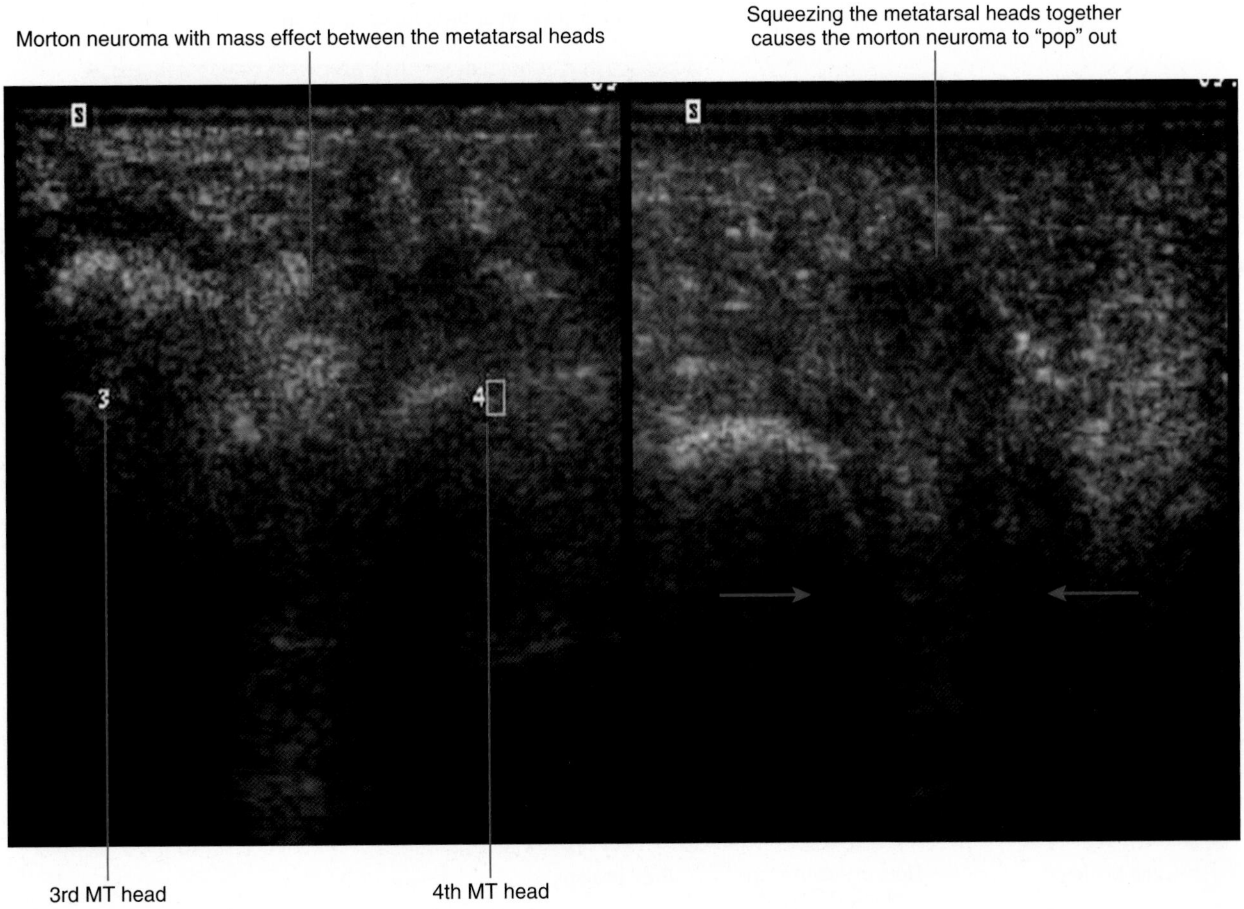
Morton neuroma with mass effect between the metatarsal heads
Squeezing the metatarsal heads together causes the morton neuroma to "pop" out
3rd MT head
4th MT head

Figure 14-2 Morton neuroma in the third intermetatarsal space between the third and fourth metatarsal (MT) heads.

separate MRI exams, and unless there is a global problem such as extensive infection or reflex sympathetic dystrophy, these foot and ankle regions should not be mixed into one exam. Even a very experienced musculoskeletal radiologist can miss findings if the foot and ankle are imaged together with a large field of view.

The small bones of the forefoot, and especially the digits, are subject to volume-averaging effects with thick slices and a large field of view. In the same regard, scanners that cannot acquire a small field of view, such as open scanners, are limited for most forefoot problems. Selection of appropriate coils and imaging planes is essential as well. For the midfoot, an axial (long-axis) plane is essential for evaluating the Lisfranc ligament and joint. This plane is also useful for evaluation of stress fractures of the metatarsals. In the forefoot, coronal (short-axis) images are very useful for assessment of the sesamoids, plantar plates, and Morton neuromas. It is also helpful to identify which sequences are most important for each body part imaged. These sequences should be done first after the scout in case the patient cannot tolerate the entire examination.

MIDFOOT

Anatomy and Mechanics

The midfoot is superbly constructed for ambulation. The tarsal bone articulations have capability of motion that allows for twisting of the foot and pronation/supination. However, during the push-off phase of walking, a stable midfoot column is more important than flexibility. This goal is achieved via the "windlass mechanism" (Fig. 14-4). A windlass is a mechanism commonly used on boats. It is a cylinder,

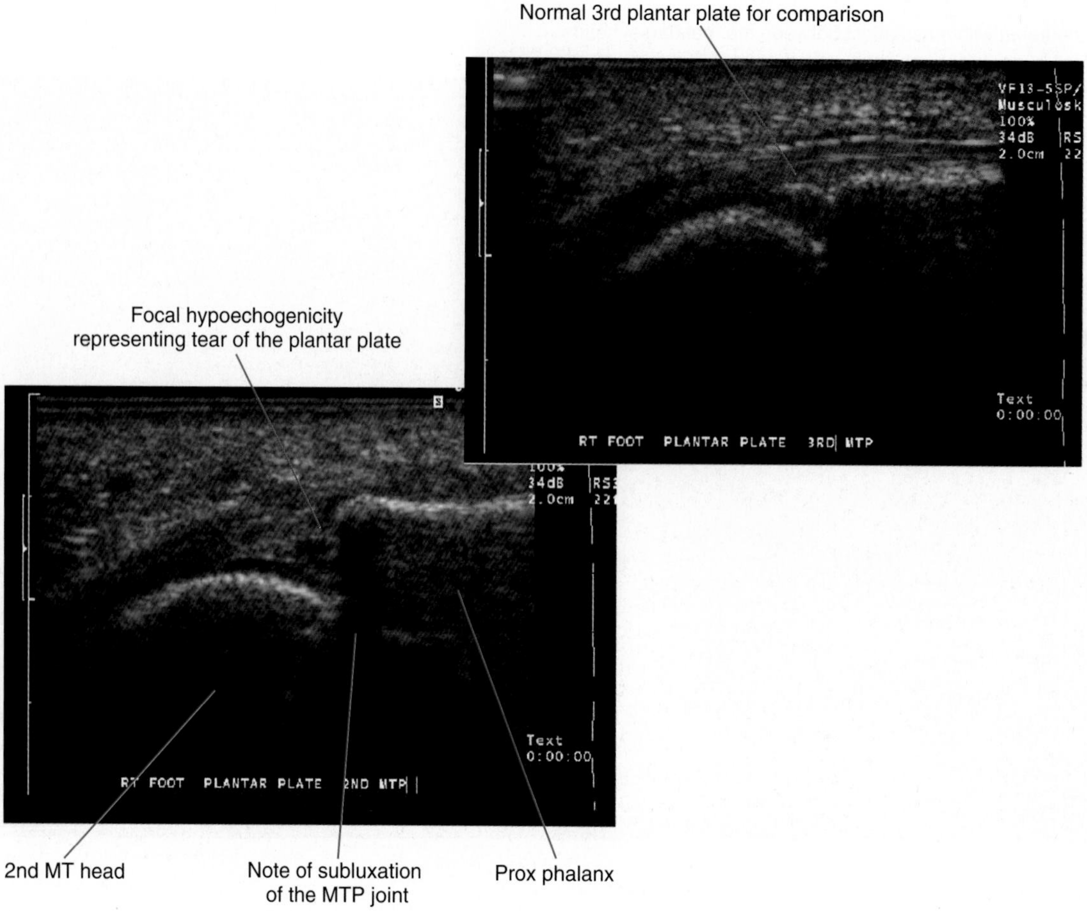
Normal 3rd plantar plate for comparison
Focal hypoechogenicity representing tear of the plantar plate
RT FOOT PLANTAR PLATE 3RD MTP
RT FOOT PLANTAR PLATE 2ND MTP
2nd MT head
Note of subluxation of the MTP joint
Prox phalanx

Figure 14-3 Chronic second plantar plate injury with subluxation of the proximal phalanx at the metatarsophalangeal (MTP) joint. Third MTP joint is shown for comparison.

which, when cranked, tightens a rope attached to a sail, anchor, and so on. The plantar fascia acts as a windlass of the foot. It is connected to the calcaneus and the digits. During the push-off phase of ambulation, dorsiflexion of the toes causes the plantar fascia to wrap around the metatarsal heads (i.e., the cylinder), which tightens the fascia, pulling the tarsal bones together and creating a stable column across the midfoot. Deformity of the arch or plantar fascia disruption, prevents this from working and can lead to pain with walking.

The Lisfranc joint is very important in stabilization of the midfoot and longitudinal arch. The second metatarsal base is inset compared with the other tarsometatarsal joints, and this and the middle cuneiform are shaped like a keystone in the coronal plane (Fig. 14-5). The Lisfranc joint is shaped like a Roman arch, which is well known for its stability. Lisfranc disruption may be seen after acute injury or in the setting of neuropathic disease. In either case, there is usually superior migration of the metatarsal bases and inferior excursion of the tarsal bones. This can create a rocker-bottom deformity with reversal of the longitudinal arch curvature (Fig. 14-6). Intercuneiform and intermetarsal ligaments exist in the midfoot (Figs. 14-7 and 14-8); however, the Lisfranc ligament, running obliquely from the medial cuneiform to the second metatarsal base (Fig. 14-9), is the main structure keeping the midfoot congruent—it is the cement of the Roman arch. There is no intermetatarsal ligament between the first and second metatarsals. Therefore, fracture of the second metatarsal base or disruption of the Lisfranc ligament creates instability of the entire tarsometatarsal axis, destabilizes the

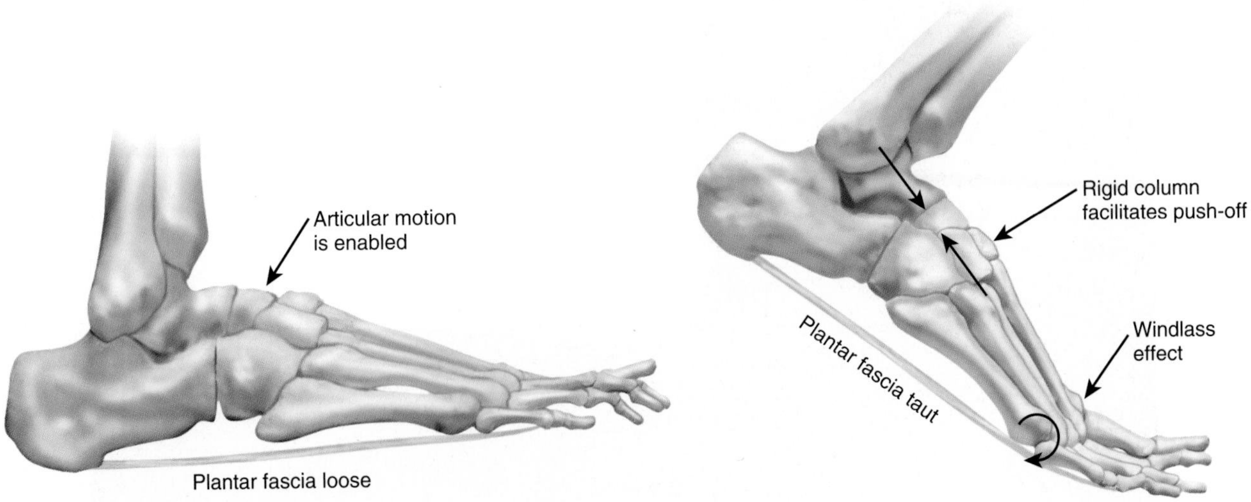
Articular motion is enabled
Plantar fascia loose
Rigid column facilitates push-off
Plantar fascia taut
Windlass effect

Figure 14-4 The windlass mechanism and function of the plantar fascia. When the foot is at rest, there is some mobility between the bones of the midfoot, allowing flexibility. During the push-off phase of gait, this flexibility would be detrimental. The plantar fascia, which inserts distal to the metatarsophalangeal (MTP) joints, tightens as the toes are dorsiflexed, which pulls the tarsal bones together and "locks" them into a rigid column. This effect has been likened to a windlass, which is a rope or chain extending over a drum used to raise and lower sails and anchors on a ship.

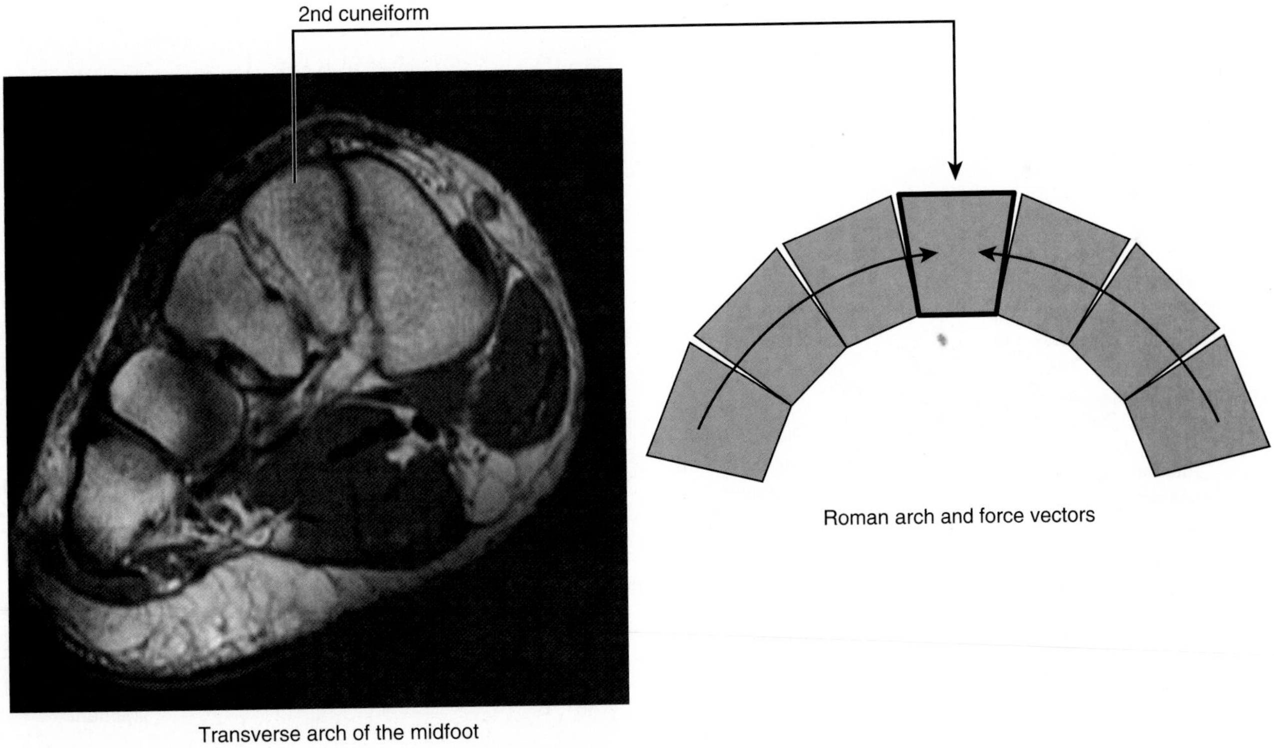
2nd cuneiform
Transverse arch of the midfoot
Roman arch and force vectors

Figure 14-5 The second cuneiform and second metatarsal base are shaped like a keystone in the coronal plane. The Lisfranc joint is shaped like a Roman arch. This anatomy, and stabilization by the Lisfranc ligament, is important for support of the arch of the foot.

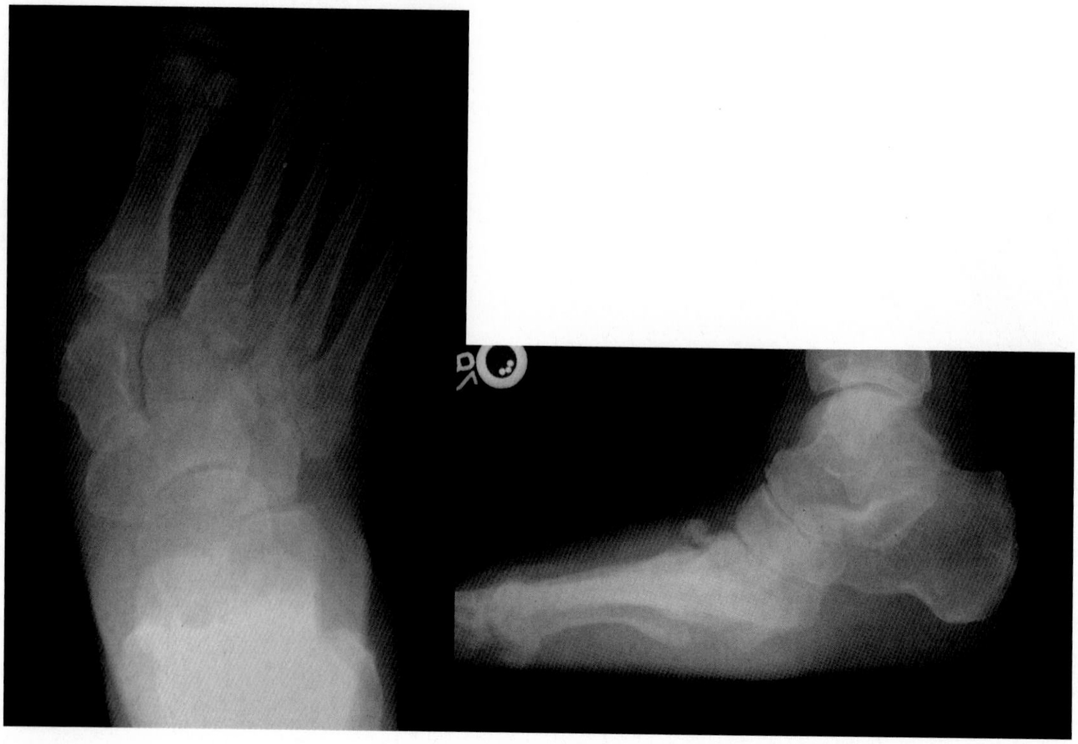

Figure 14-6 Chronic untreated Lisfranc injury seen here in a patient with diabetic neuropathy results in deformity with collapse of the arch and a rocker-bottom configuration.

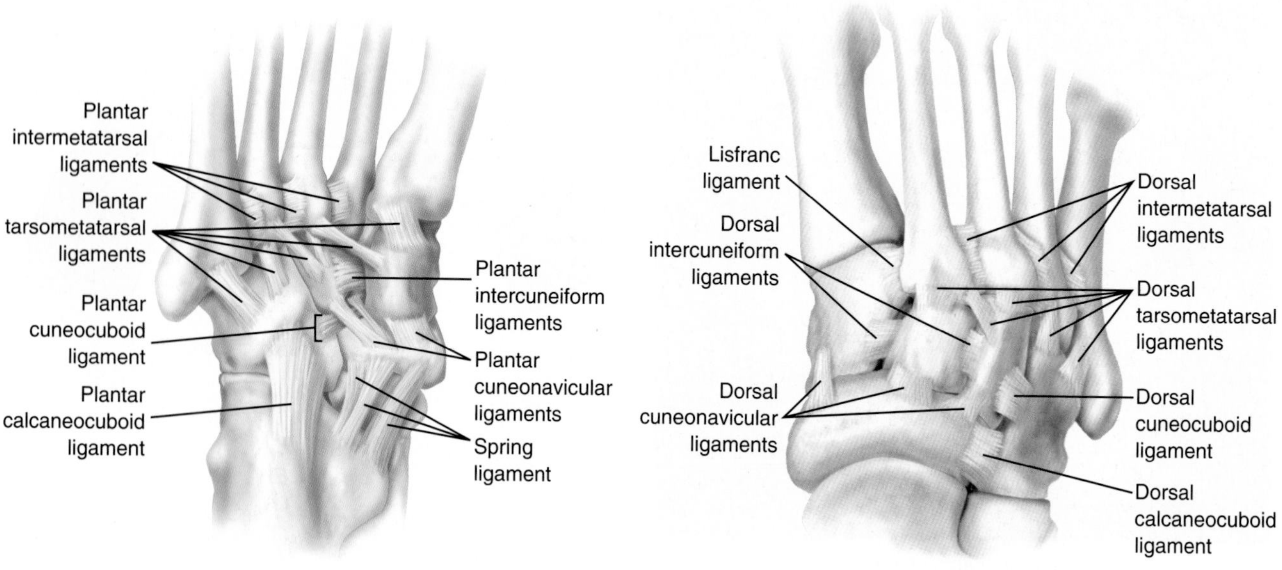
Plantar intermetatarsal ligaments
Plantar tarsometatarsal ligaments
Plantar cuneocuboid ligament
Plantar calcaneocuboid ligament
Plantar intercuneiform ligaments
Plantar cuneonavicular ligaments
Spring ligament
Lisfranc ligament
Dorsal intercuneiform ligaments
Dorsal cuneonavicular ligaments
Dorsal intermetatarsal ligaments
Dorsal tarsometatarsal ligaments
Dorsal cuneocuboid ligament
Dorsal calcaneocuboid ligament

Figure 14-7 **Ligaments of the midfoot.**

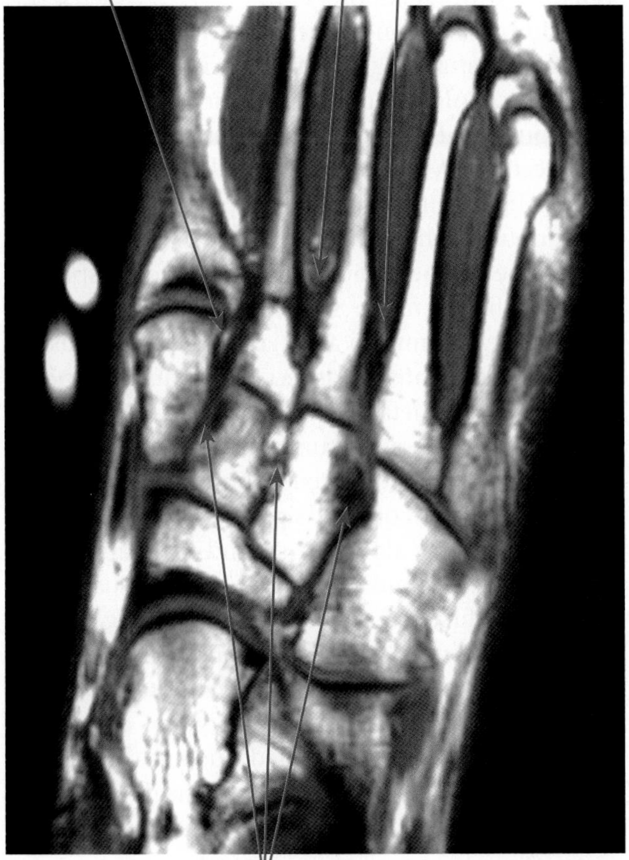
Lisfranc ligament
Intermetatarsal ligaments
Intercuneiform ligaments and cuneocuboid ligament

Figure 14-8 The intercuneiform ligaments and intermetatarsal ligaments are somewhat variable in presence are not consistently seen on routine MRI, but are best evaluated on axial (long-axis) images.

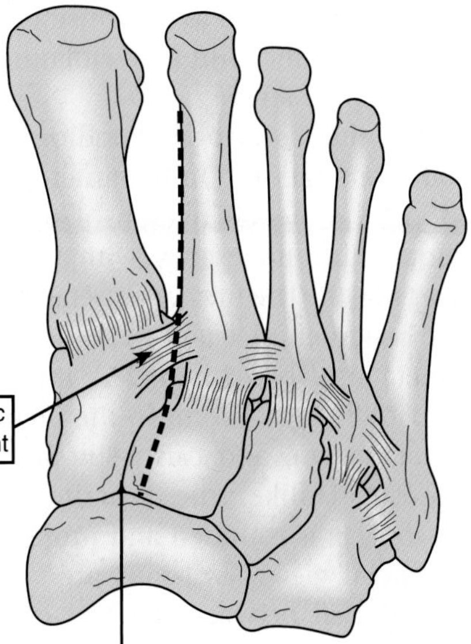
Lisfranc ligament
With intact Lisfranc ligament there should be an unbroken line from the 2nd MT to 2nd cuneiform medially

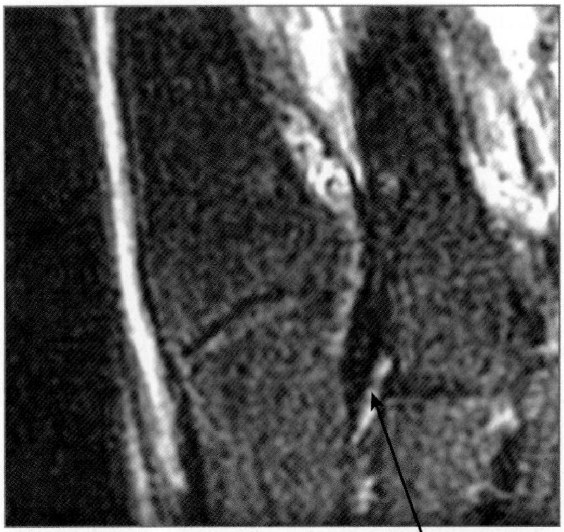
Lisfranc ligament
• Extends from 1st cuneiform to 2nd MT base

Figure 14-9 On an anteroposterior view of the foot the medial margin of the second metatarsal should line up exactly with the middle cuneiform. MT, metatarsal.

midfoot, and results in collapse of the longitudinal arch.

PATHOLOGY

Lisfranc Injury and Associated Pathology

Lisfranc injuries occur from twisting at the midfoot. The classic mechanism of falling from a horse with the foot twisted in the stirrup is not seen frequently. More commonly, the patient twists the foot in a pothole or lands wrong after a jump. More extensive injuries are associated with multitrauma patients as well. Lisfranc injuries are common in athletes and may be seen in sports that require pivoting, or when another player steps on their foot immobilizing the forefoot as the body rotates around the midfoot. Clinically, the injury is very painful and patients cannot bear weight on the affected extremity. Therefore, the diagnosis is usually suspected before imaging. If imaging is indeterminate, patients may undergo examination under anesthesia to demonstrate abnormal motion at the Lisfranc joint and widening of the ligament interval under stress.

When Lisfranc injury is suspected, radiographs are the best initial examination. On the anteroposterior view of the foot, the medial margin of the second metatarsal should line up exactly with the second cuneiform (Fig. 14-10). The first tarsometatarsal joint should also be congruent. Distance between the first and second metatarsal bases is of less importance, and can vary; widening can occur in the presence of an os intermetatarseum, and can result in a false-positive diagnosis. Unlike true Lisfranc ligament avulsions, this ossicle is rounded and projects superiorly on the lateral view. Avulsions are very thin, linear, and positioned between the first cuneiform and the second metatarsal base. CT may be needed to confirm the finding (Fig. 14-11). If an injury is detected radiographically, CT is typically required to evaluate the extent of fractures, which is characteristically underestimated on radiographs. MRI is an excellent test to directly evaluate the Lisfranc ligament and other ligaments of the midfoot as well as to diagnose associated fractures and bone bruises, often obviating the need for examination under anesthesia. The best plane is axial (long axis); the best sequence is T2-weighted with fat suppression.

An important concept in interpreting an MRI of suspected Lisfranc ligament injury is that a ligament with a mechanically significant injury may still appear intact on MRI. First, small avulsions can be very hard to detect on MRI; second, the ligament may be stretched and insufficient without appearing discontinuous. In the setting of injury, any edema in or around the ligament should be considered suspicious for a significant injury. Secondary signs are also very useful. A very common association is bone bruise or fracture of the inferior aspect of the middle cuneiform or second metatarsal base (Fig. 14-12). In more severe injuries, bone bruises or fractures are also observed in various other tarsal bones and metatarsal bases. Another secondary sign is soft tissue edema extending distally along the second metatarsal shaft, frequently with strain of the first interosseous muscle between the first and second metatarsals (Fig. 14-13). Resultant feathery edema in the muscle is not significant by itself but is a sign of traumatic separation of the metatarsals. It is helpful to surgeons to identify other ligaments that are injured, such as the intercuneiform ligaments, the intermetatarsal ligaments,

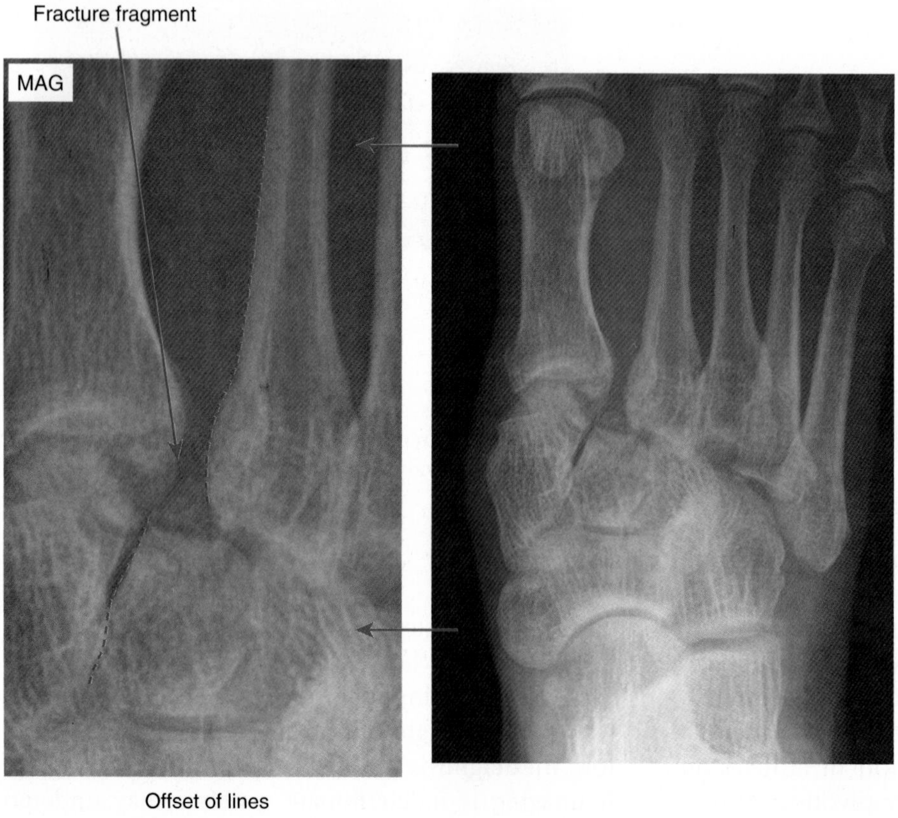
Fracture fragment
MAG
Offset of lines

Figure 14-10 Lisfranc injury on radiographs. Measurement of the interval between the first and second metacarpal bases can vary, but the medial aspect of the second metatarsal shaft should align precisely with the medial aspect of the second cuneiform. If not, consider a Lisfranc injury in a trauma setting.

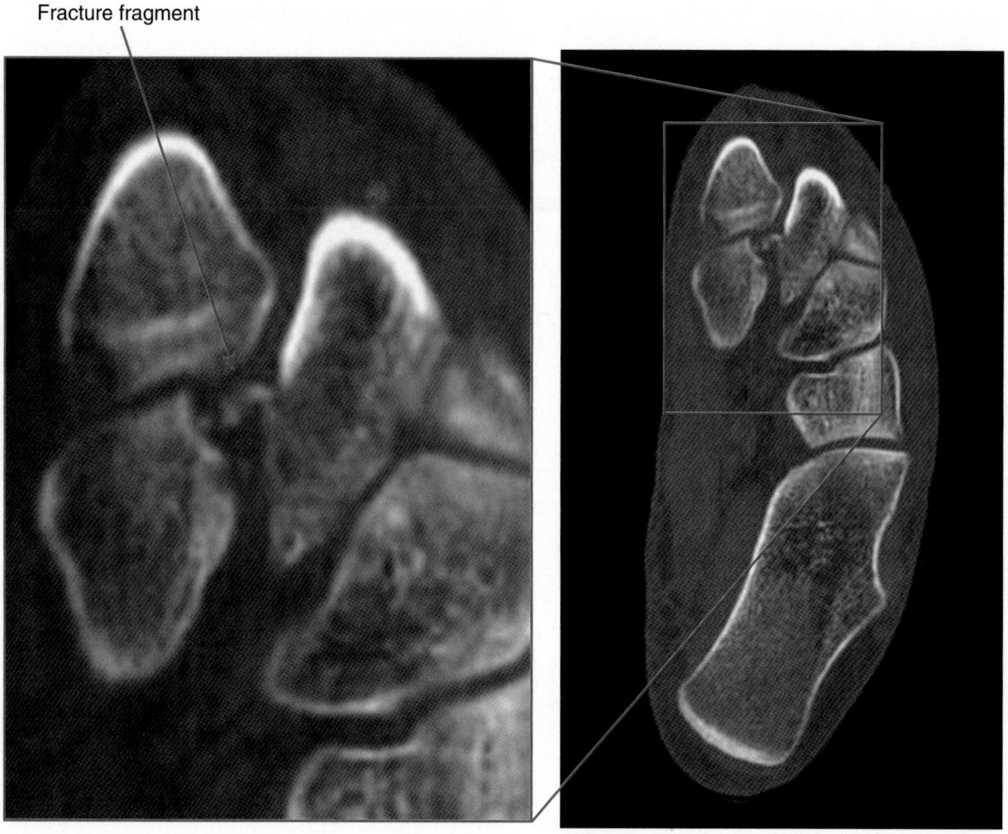
Fracture fragment

Figure 14-11 **Lisfranc injury on CT.** CT is very useful for confirming a fracture suspected clinically, especially if radiographs are negative. CT is also useful for identifying additional fractures. However, a significant Lisfranc injury may exist in the absence of fracture. MRI is the test of choice for evaluation of the ligament itself as well as bone bruises and muscle tears indicative of a more severe injury. Still, CT serves a complementary role, since small fracture fragments may not be visible on MRI.

and the deep plantar ligaments of the midfoot. The intercuneiform ligaments and intermetatarsal ligaments are somewhat variable and are best evaluated on axial (long-axis) images but are not consistently seen on routine MRI (see Fig. 14-8). The deep plantar ligaments are best seen on coronal (short-axis) images (Fig. 14-14), just inferior to the tarsal bones and just deep to the peroneus longus tendon as it courses toward the first metatarsal base. However, prominent veins in this region make it difficult to detect soft tissue edema.

FOREFOOT

Anatomy

The medial (tibial) and lateral (fibular) sesamoid bones articulate on facets at the inferior aspect of the first metatarsal head. Facets are separated by a bony prominence called the "crista" (Figs. 14-15 and 14-16). Articular cartilage is present on the metatarsal head and the sesamoids (the metatarsal-sesamoid, or MTS joint), and synovial fluid communicates with the rest of the first metatarsophalangeal (MTP) joint. Processes that alter the position or tracking of the sesamoids or that result in cartilage loss can cause pain and secondary osteoarthritis. Any articular disease affecting the first MTP joint also affects the MTS joint. The sesamoid bones are stabilized by their capsular location and metatarsal articulation. Additional stabilization is provided by an intersesamoid ligament that extends between them as well as sesamoid-phalangeal ligaments distally. However, this stable position under the first metatarsal head also makes the sesamoid bones—especially the tibial sesamoid—susceptible to compressive force. Loss or migration of the plantar fat pad from callus, from

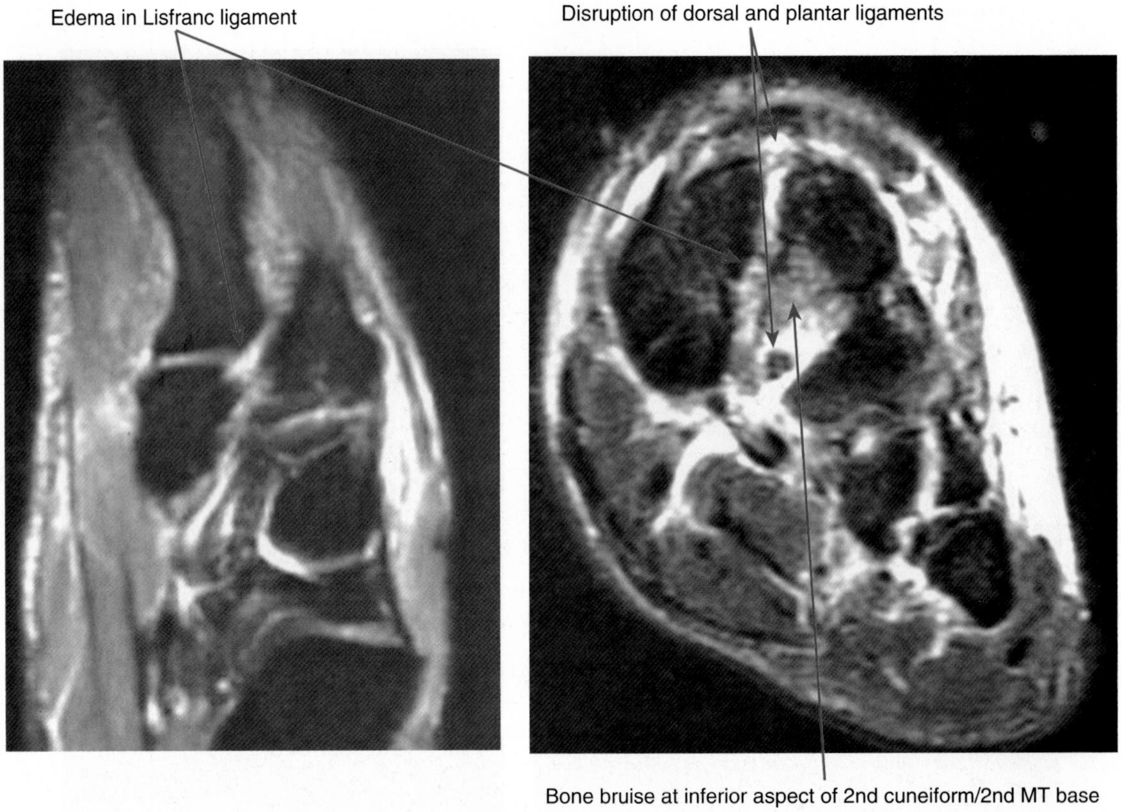
Edema in Lisfranc ligament
Disruption of dorsal and plantar ligaments
Bone bruise at inferior aspect of 2nd cuneiform/2nd MT base

Figure 14-12 **Lisfranc ligament tear.** Classic signs on MRI; axial and coronal T2-weighted fat-suppressed images.

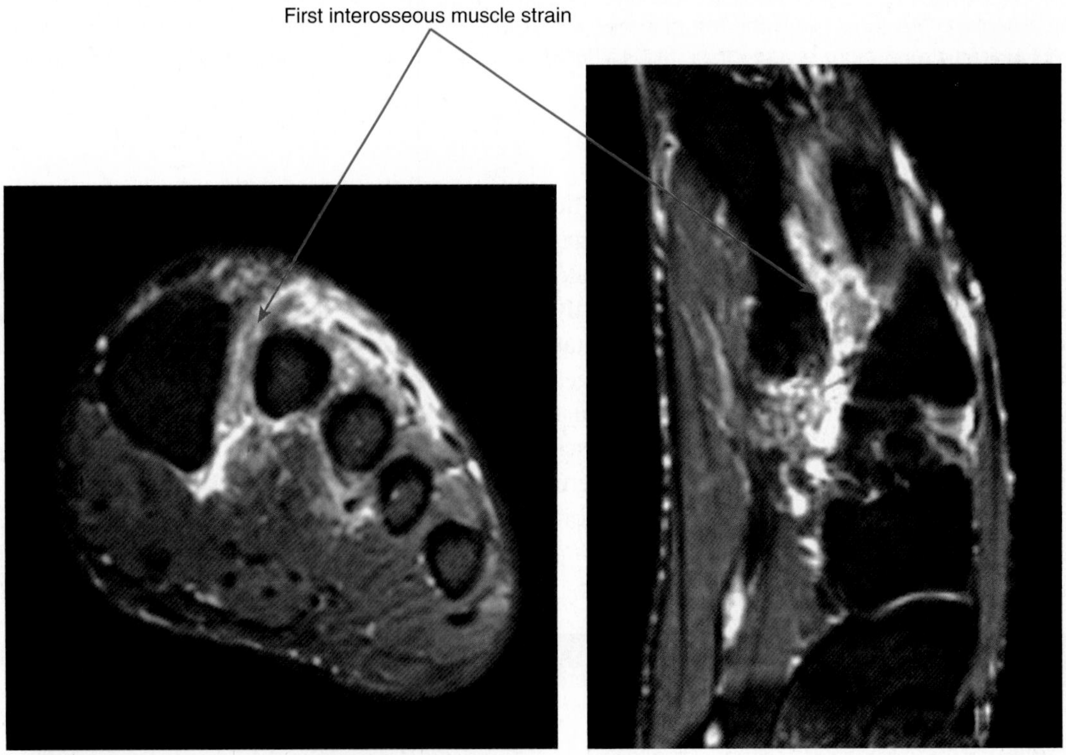
First interosseous muscle strain

Figure 14-13 **Lisfranc injury on MRI.** First interosseous muscle strain is another common association.

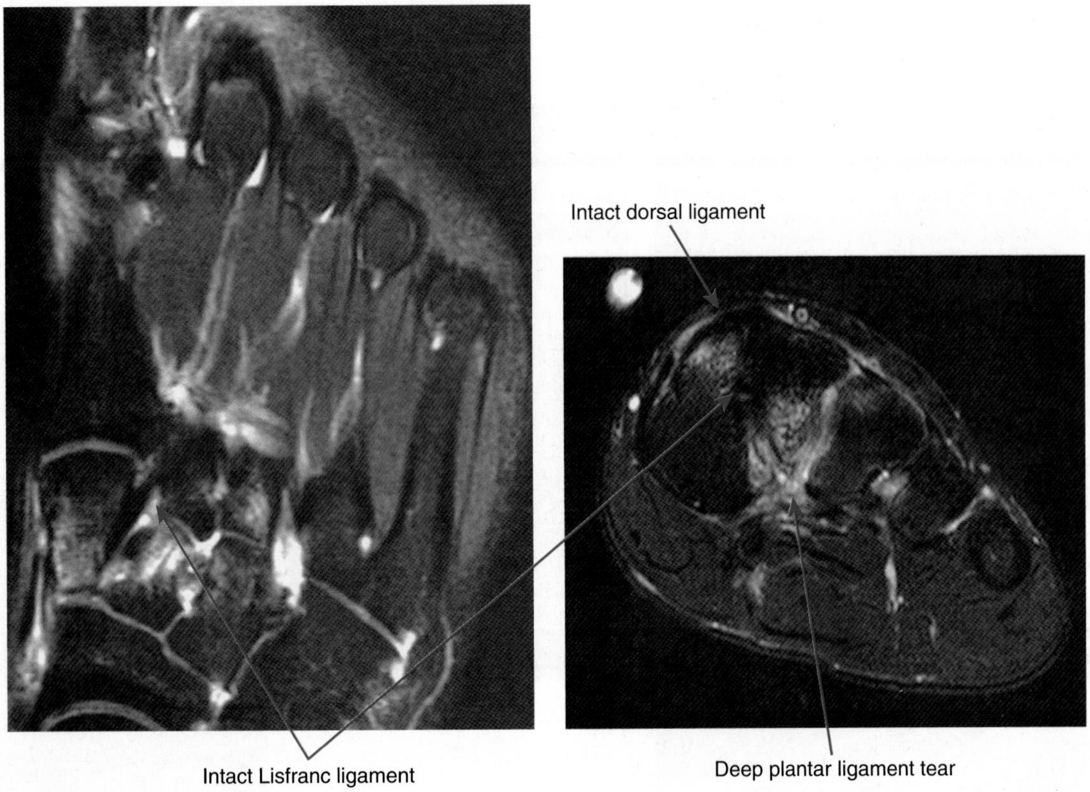
Intact dorsal ligament
Intact Lisfranc ligament
Deep plantar ligament tear

Figure 14-14 Partial Lisfranc injury. Professional football player with intact Lisfranc ligament but tearing of the deep plantar ligaments. The patient was treated conservatively and did well.

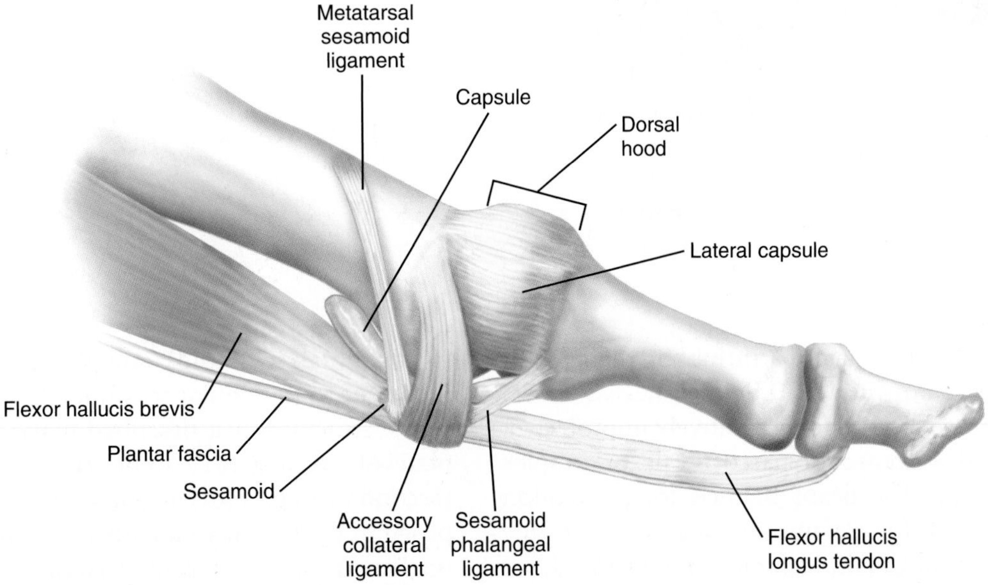
Metatarsal sesamoid ligament
Capsule
Dorsal hood
Lateral capsule
Flexor hallucis brevis
Plantar fascia
Sesamoid
Accessory collateral ligament
Sesamoid phalangeal ligament
Flexor hallucis longus tendon

Figure 14-15 Forefoot anatomy.

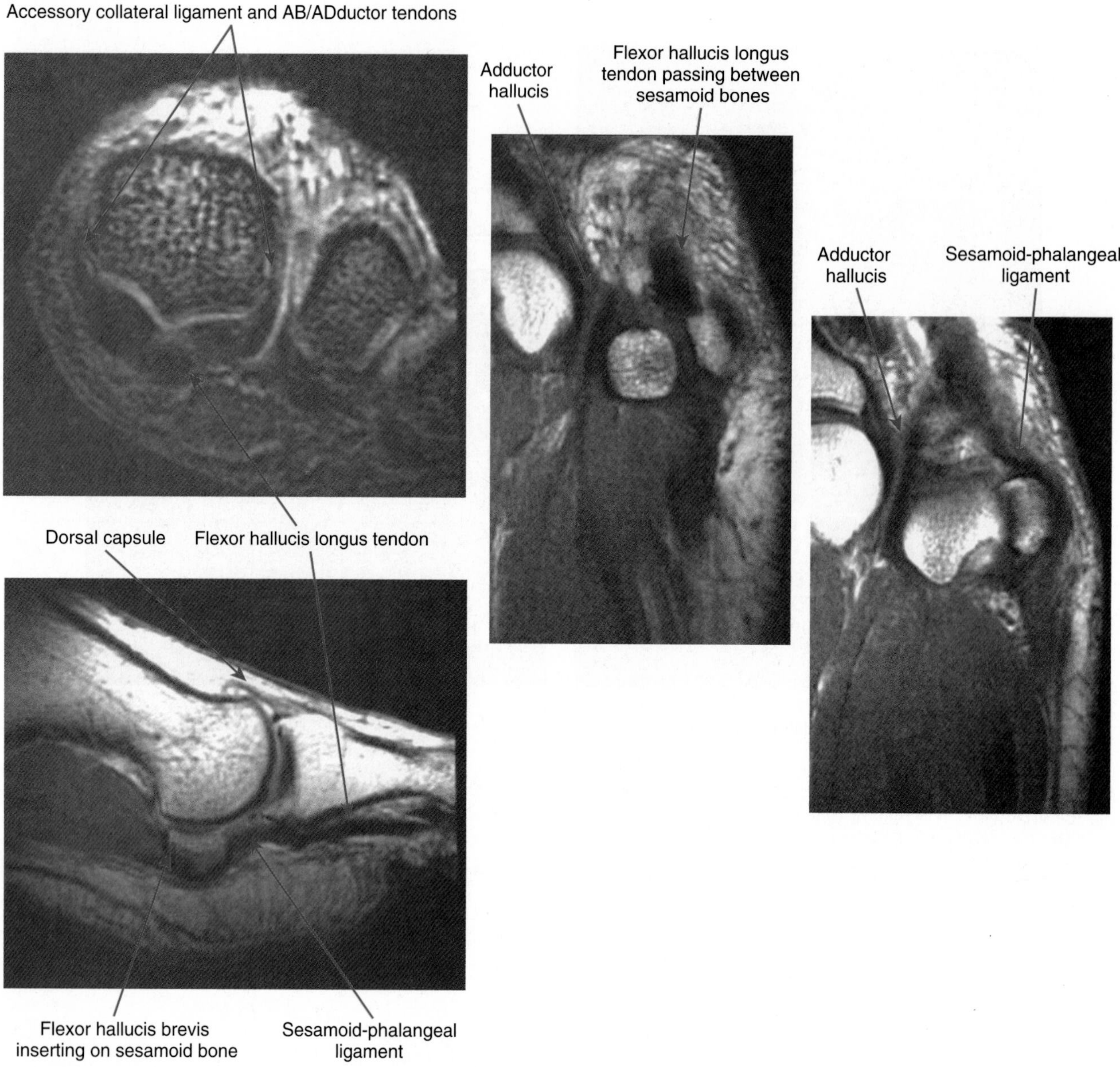
Accessory collateral ligament and AB/ADductor tendons
Dorsal capsule
Flexor hallucis longus tendon
Flexor hallucis brevis inserting on sesamoid bone
Sesamoid-phalangeal ligament
Adductor hallucis
Flexor hallucis longus tendon passing between sesamoid bones
Adductor hallucis
Sesamoid-phalangeal ligament

Figure 14-16 ***Sesamoids–normal anatomy.***

diseases such as rheumatoid arthritis and diabetes, or from excessive dorsiflexion (i.e., high-heeled shoes) can leave the sesamoid bones relatively unprotected. The sesamoid bones are also part of the flexor complex of the first ray. The flexor hallucis longus tendon passes between the sesamoids, superficial to the intersesamoid ligament. Separate slips of the flexor hallucis brevis tendon insert on the tibial and fibular sesamoid bones. The sesamoid bones are also intimately associated with the capsule near the attachment of the tendons of the abductor hallucis (adjacent to the tibial sesamoid) and the adductor hallucis (adjacent to the fibular sesamoid).

The structures just described make up the plantar plate of the first MTP joint. The lesser MTP joints (second through fifth) also have plantar plates, composed of thickening of the inferior joint capsule. This thickened, fibrous capsule makes a dark U-shaped structure on coronal (short-axis) MR images when intact (Fig. 14-17). Flexor and extensor tendons pass by the MTP joints inferiorly and superiorly, on course to insert onto the phalanges. Between the metatarsal

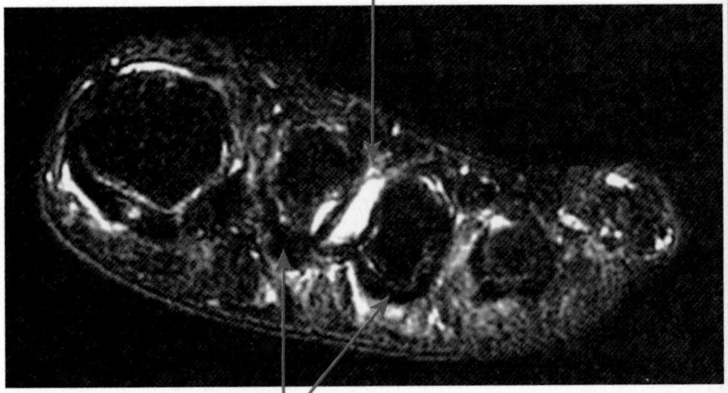
2nd intermetatarsal bursitis
Intact plantar plates
• The "dark U"

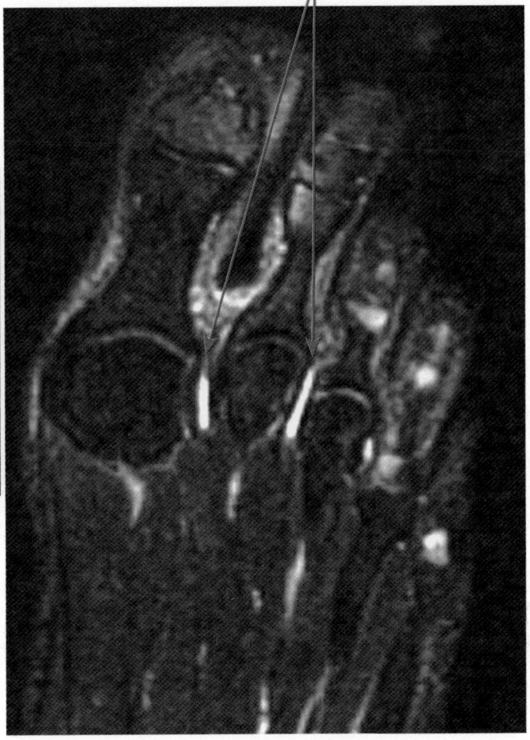
1st and 2nd intermetatarsal bursitis

Figure 14-17 **Intermetarsal bursitis.**

heads there is an anatomic bursa called the intermetarsal bursa, which can fill with fluid. On coronal T2-weighted images, it is seen as a third line of fluid between the bones (joint, bursa, joint), separated by the adjacent joint capsules (see Fig. 14-17). Immediately inferior to this bursa is a fascial arch that extends between the metatarsal heads. Inferior to this courses the interdigital nerve. Using standard protocols at or below 1.5 T, this nerve is not routinely seen unless pathologically enlarged, as in Morton neuroma. Interosseous muscles extend between the metatarsal shafts, thinning distally as they inset on the MTP joint capsules. The flexor muscles are separated into three compartments (medial, central, and lateral), between which are interposed two neurovascular bundles containing the medial and lateral plantar calcaneal branches of the posterior tibial nerve from the tarsal tunnel. The plantar fascia originates from the inferior calcaneus and inserts onto the superficial fascia and the flexor tendons of the toes. It is also intimately associated with fascial arches that bridge the gap between the metatarsal heads inferior to which the neurovascular bundles run.

THE SESAMOIDS

In evaluating the sesamoid bones on MRI, one should review their location, cartilage, and marrow signal as well as the signal of the adjacent first metatarsal head and subcutaneous tissues. If there is malalignment, it is usually because of hallux valgus, in which case there is likely to be osteoarthritis. Equivalent involvement of the metatarsal head also suggests arthritis, which can be degenerative or inflammatory. The capsule and separate ligaments should be inspected in the setting of trauma. If a marrow abnormality is observed that is isolated to a sesamoid, consider a bipartite sesamoid (with or without superimposed injury), fracture/stress response, or avascular necrosis (Table 14-1). Associated signal abnormality in the subcutaneous tissues could represent bursitis, callus, various manifestations of arthropathy, or metabolic disease (e.g., gouty tophus), or transcutaneous spread of infection.

Table 14-1 Summary of Sesamoid Pathology

	Radiographs/CT	Bone Scan	MRI	Comments
Avascular necrosis	–/↑ Density	+	Black T1 +/– Edema T2	Especially tibial; may collapse/ fragment
Stress response/fracture	–/Linear lucency	+	Intermediate T1 Edema T2	Acute: Linear high T2 Subacute/stress: Linear low T2
Sesamoiditis	–	+	Intermediate T1 Edema T2	No fracture line; look for stress Changes elsewhere
Normal bipartite	Rounded; bigger	–	Low at interval	
Bipartite with pseudarthrosis	Rounded; bigger	+	Edema T2 Fluid at junction	
Osteoarthritis	Spurs/↑ density	+	Cysts Edema T2 Spurs Hallux Valgus/subluxation	
Osteomyelitis	–/STS/erosion	+3-phase	Soft tissue edema/enhancement Ulcer Low T1 Edema T2 Effusion Thick rim enhancement	

Acute Fracture, Stress, and Sesamoiditis

Acute sesamoid fracture can generally be detected radiographically like other acute fractures (Fig. 14-18), but they are often overlooked on initial inspection because of the high incidence of bipartite sesamoids. However, the bipartite sesamoid has rounded edges, whereas an acute fracture has sharp edges. Also, the pieces of a bipartite are larger in total than the other sesamoid. Finally, bipartite sesamoids do not change over time. A short follow-up period of 5 to 7 days will show evolution of a fracture; if old exams are available, ambiguity may be removed. Because sesamoid fractures are often overlooked on initial radiographs, patients are occasionally referred for MRI to explain the persistent pain. Because of the delay in referral to MRI, the injury is nearly always subacute when imaging is performed. As previously noted, the MRI appearance of subacute sesamoid fracture is virtually indistinguishable from stress fracture (Fig. 14-19) except for a history of a single traumatic episode. Both can show sesamoid marrow edema and intermediate to low T1 signal, with a discrete low-signal fracture line.

To detect the fracture line, multiple imaging planes should be acquired. However, the optimal plane is difficult to plan ahead of time, since the fracture line can be oriented in a variety of obliquities (although most frequently the fracture line is oriented in the coronal plane). Small field-of-view images (10 to 12 cm) and/or thin sections facilitate detection of the fracture line.

Sesamoiditis is a painful condition of the hallux sesamoid complex and surrounding soft tissues. The term *sesamoiditis* is a nonspecific clinical term (like metatarsalgia). Sesamoid pain has a differential, the underlying pathology of which can best be distinguished on MRI. Most cases of clinical sesamoiditis are likely to be in the spectrum of stress response. Radiographs and CT are generally normal. On MRI, sesamoiditis is seen as diffuse high signal on T2-weighted or STIR images (Fig. 14-20). Diffuse enhancement may be seen in the same distribution. This can be useful for distinguishing sesamoiditis from avascular necrosis, which would show little to no enhancement. On T1-weighted images, sesamoiditis may show intermediate to low signal, but if the signal is black, consider avascular necrosis. Stress changes can also occur at a bipartite sesamoid. These normal variants can thereby be a source of pain (Fig. 14-21).

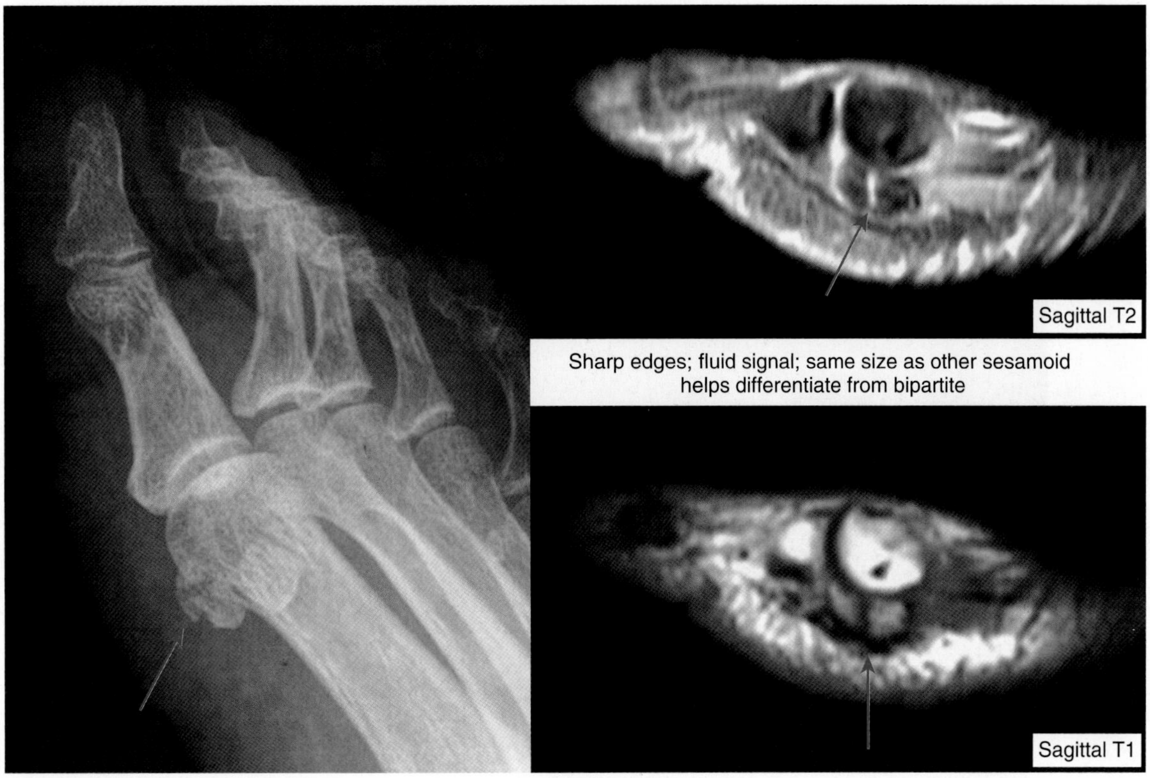
Sagittal T2
Sharp edges; fluid signal; same size as other sesamoid helps differentiate from bipartite
Sagittal T1

Figure 14-18 **Acute tibial sesamoid fracture.**

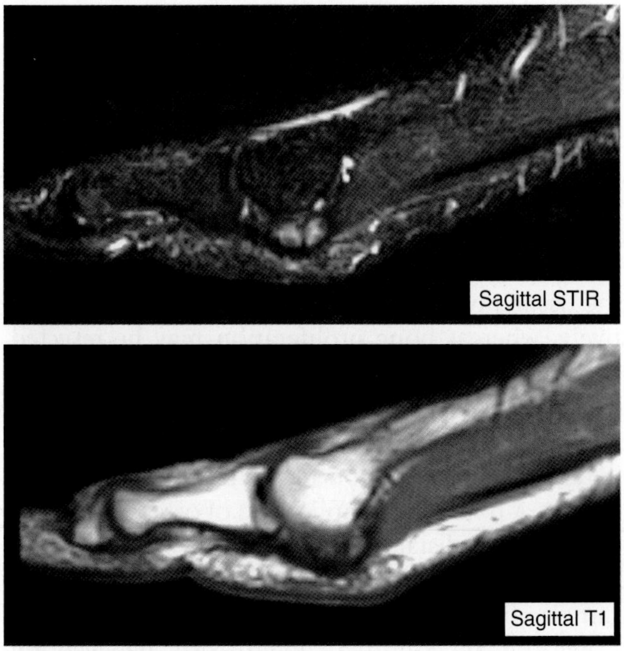
Sagittal STIR
Sagittal T1

Figure 14-19 **Sesamoid fracture—subacute versus stress.** Low signal on T2; size is the same as the other sesamoid.

Nonunion and Pseudarthrosis

Occasionally a sesamoid fracture does not heal. On radiographs, there is persistence of the fracture line. The edges may become rounded and sclerotic like a bipartite. A similar situation can occur at a developmentally bipartite sesamoid, where acute trauma or chronic stress ruptures the normal fibrous connection. This is undetectable on radiographs apart from the presence of an apparently innocuous bipartite. On MRI, a synovial nonunion (or pseudarthrosis) is characterized by fluid signal between the sesamoid fragments or bipartite elements. If the intervening tissue is dark on fluid-sensitive sequences, it may represent a fibrous union of a prior fracture or a normal developmental bipartite sesamoid. If edema is in the adjacent marrow, there is likely ongoing stress response.

Avascular Necrosis

On radiography and CT, avascular necrosis is seen as increased sesamoid density; typically only one sesamoid bone is involved (Fig. 14-22). The sclerosis

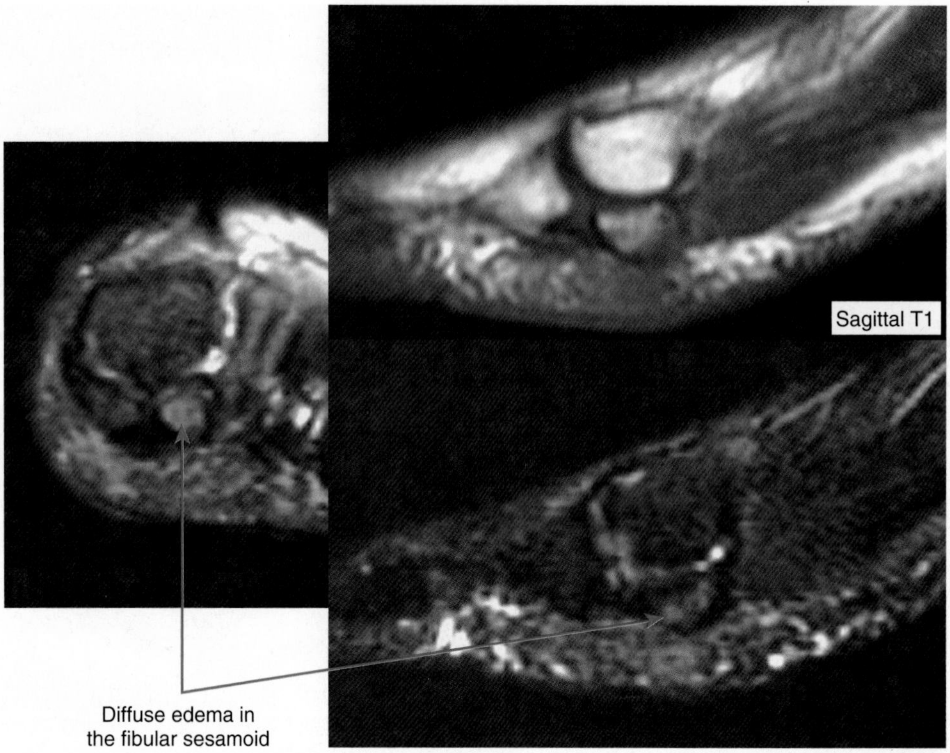
Sagittal T1
Diffuse edema in
the fibular sesamoid

Figure 14-20 **Sesamoiditis.** Diffuse edema without a discrete fracture line, likely representing stress response.

is generally more extensive than would be expected from osteoarthritis and is not present on the metatarsal side of the joint. On MRI, T2 signal can vary from low to high; the T1-weighted images help confirm the diagnosis (see Fig. 14-22); the T1 signal of the affected sesamoid is diffusely low in avascular necrosis with replacement of the normal marrow fat. A black sesamoid on T1 is compatible with avascular necrosis; if T1 signal is not black, consider other pathology. Unlike osteomyelitis, there is little to no surrounding soft tissue inflammation in avascular necrosis, although often a joint effusion is present. Avascular necrosis chronically may result in collapse and fragmentation of the sesamoid and secondary osteoarthritis of the MTS joint (see Table 14-1).

HALLUX VALGUS/BUNION/BUNIONETTE

Hallux valgus is angulation of the first MTP joint, usually associated with medial angulation of the first metatarsal shaft (metatarsus primus adductus). This angulation results in poor fitting of shoes and soft tissue friction at the medial eminence of the first metatarsal head; this friction eventually causes bursitis and callus in the soft tissues—which may be exquisitely painful—and proliferation and cystic change of adjacent bone (Fig. 14-23). Therefore, a clinically perceived bunion deformity can be composed of soft tissue, bone, or a combination of pathologic structures. In the report, it is helpful to be specific about the tissue involved. Bursitis can be treated conservatively, whereas bone proliferation may be resected. If the first intermetatarsal angle is over 12 degrees (metatarsus primus adductus), generally a first metatarsal rotational or shifting (chevron) osteotomy is performed in addition to the bunionectomy (Fig. 14-24). A potential complication of osteotomy, especially at the distal shaft where the nutrient vessel courses, is avascular necrosis (Fig. 14-25). Nonunion can also occur (Fig. 14-26).

Because an abnormal angle exists between the metatarsal and phalanges, the associated flexor and extensor tendons bowstring laterally. The flexor hallucis longus forces the sesamoids laterally as well, and they rotate so that the metatarsal sesamoid joints become incongruent. The bony prominence (the

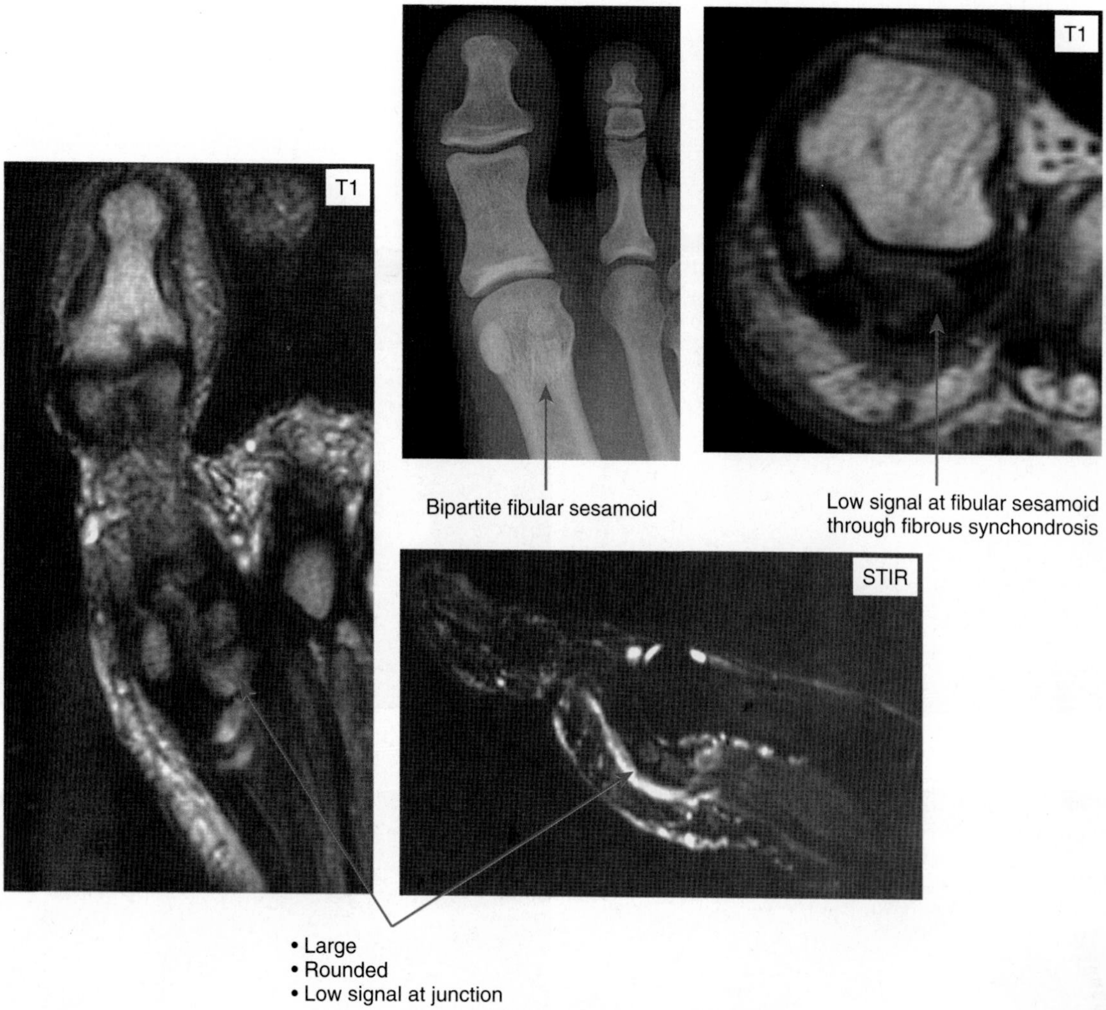
T1
T1
T1
Bipartite fibular sesamoid
Low signal at fibular sesamoid through fibrous synchondrosis
STIR
• Large
• Rounded
• Low signal at junction

Figure 14-21 Bipartite fibular sesamoid with marrow edema on STIR indicating stress response.

crista) between the facets erodes, facilitating lateral sesamoid subluxation and propagation of osteoarthritis with edema and cyst formation on both sides of the joint (see Fig. 14-23). As the sesamoids sublux more, they may abut the second metatarsal head with intervening bursitis. As the great toe deviates laterally, it displaces the second toe dorsally, causing crossover toe deformity.

Hallux valgus and bursitis are usually mechanical but can also be seen in rheumatoid arthritis or gout. It is also common in the setting of diabetes, in which case ulceration may also occur over the medial eminence.

A bunionette is bony prominence of the lateral aspect of the fifth metatarsal head (Fig. 14-27) that maybe associated with bursitis. This is also called a "tailor's bunion" because tailors would cross their legs placing weight on the fifth metatarsal head. The condition may be due to a laterally curving fifth metatarsal or a "splay foot" in which the metatarsal angles are all widened with widening of the forefoot.

BURSITIS

Bursitis generally appears on imaging as a focal, flattened fluid collection. In the foot there are anatomic bursae and adventitial bursae. Anatomic bursae are present in all individuals, in place to cushion areas prone to friction due to natural activities such as walking. Adventitial bursae are acquired and result

Text continued on page 720

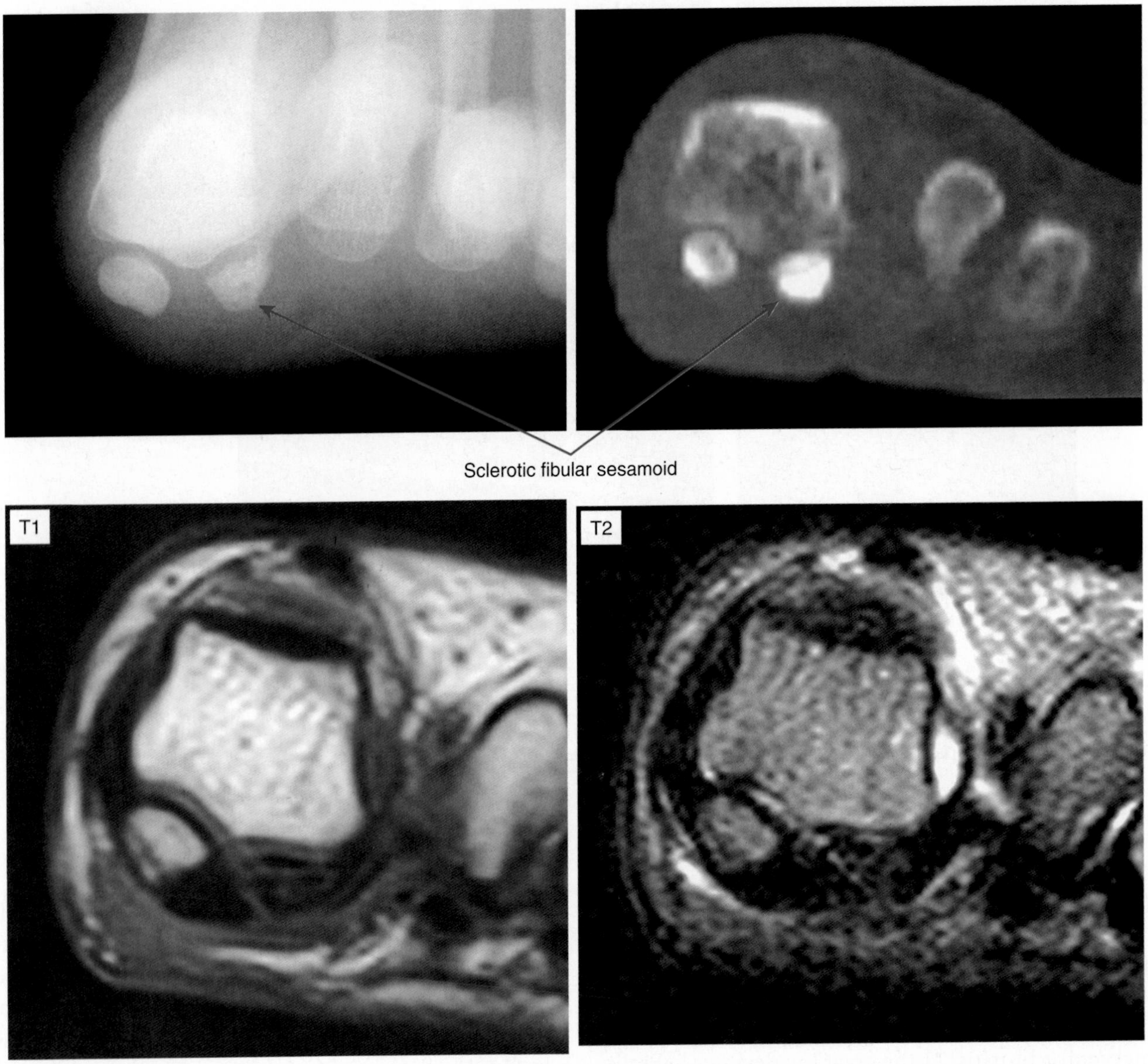
Sclerotic fibular sesamoid
T1
T2

Figure 14-22 Avascular necrosis of the fibular sesamoid. Note sclerosis on CT with low signal on T1- and T2-weighted images.

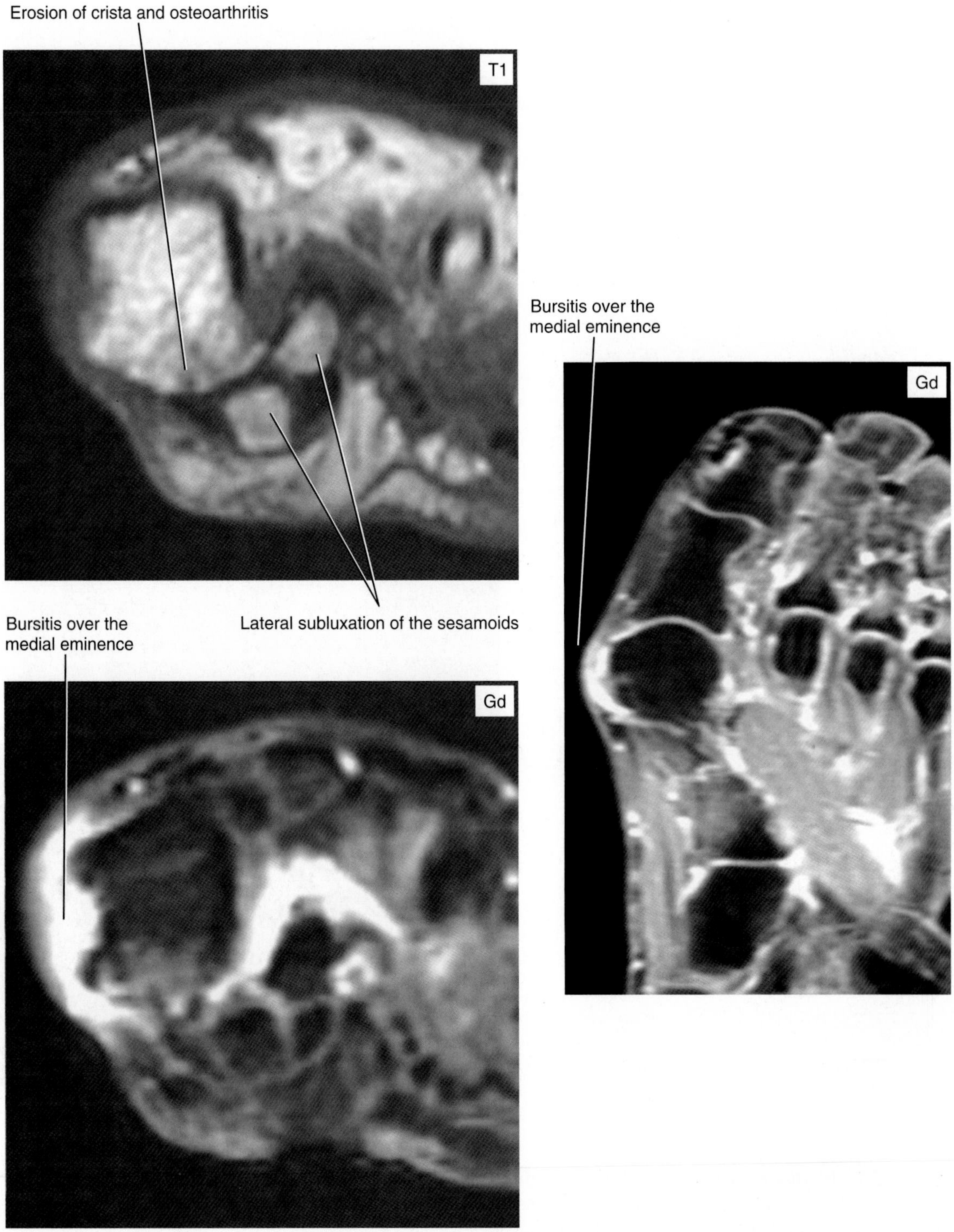
Erosion of crista and osteoarthritis
T1
Lateral subluxation of the sesamoids
Bursitis over the medial eminence
Gd
Bursitis over the medial eminence
Gd

Figure 14-23 Hallux valgus on MRI, with associated osseous proliferation (bunion) at the medial aspect of the first metatarsal head and overlying bursitis.

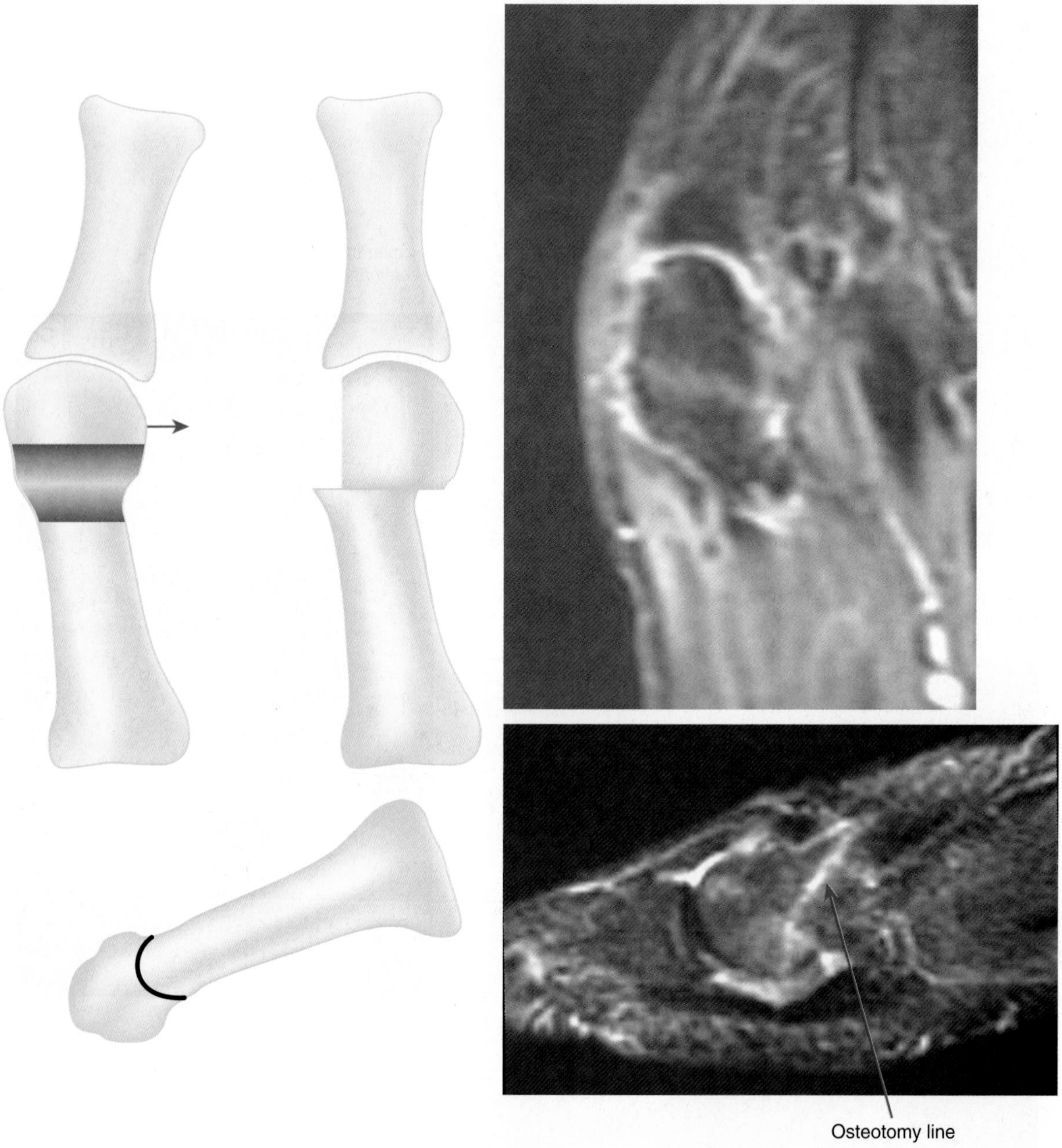
Osteotomy line

Figure 14-24 Medial eminence (bunion) resection and distal metatarsal shaft chevron osteotomy. Alternatively osteotomy can be performed at the proximal shaft. Osteotomy is performed when there is an increase in the first intermetatarsal angle (metatarsus primus adductus).

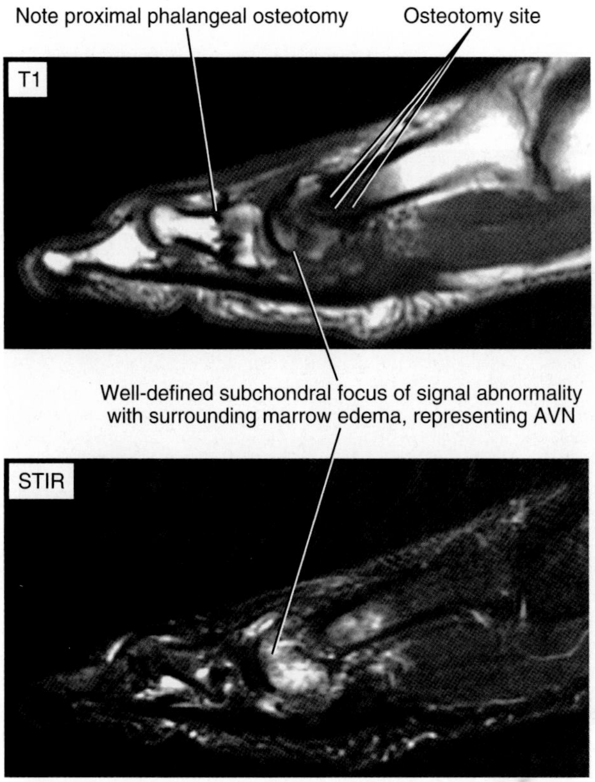
Note proximal phalangeal osteotomy
Osteotomy site
T1
Well-defined subchondral focus of signal abnormality with surrounding marrow edema, representing AVN
STIR

Figure 14-25 Distal first metatarsal osteotomy (chevron osteotomy) with secondary avascular necrosis. Note well-defined subchondral signal abnormality with surrounding marrow edema. Areas of devascularized bone often exhibit entrapped, or mummified fat. AVN, avascular necrosis.

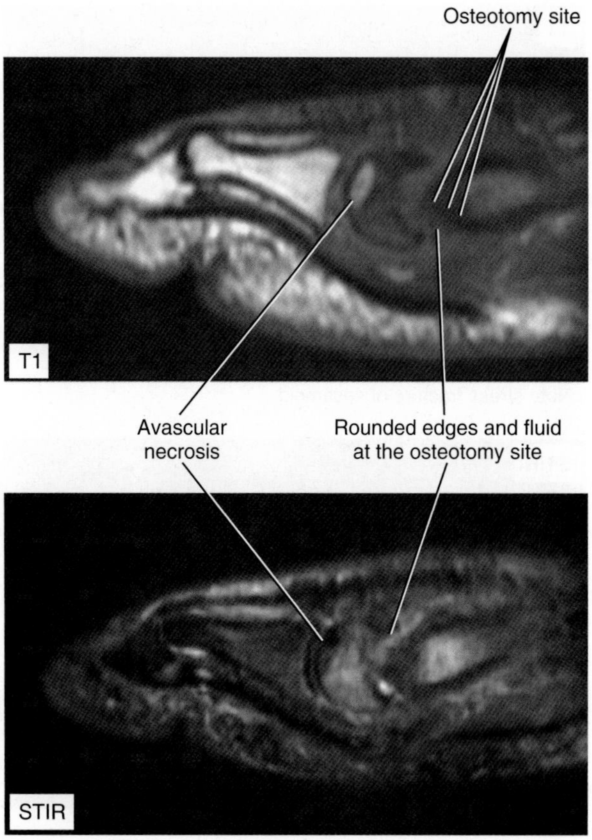
Osteotomy site
T1
Avascular necrosis
Rounded edges and fluid at the osteotomy site
STIR

Figure 14-26 Hallux valgus repair with nonunion at the osteotomy site.

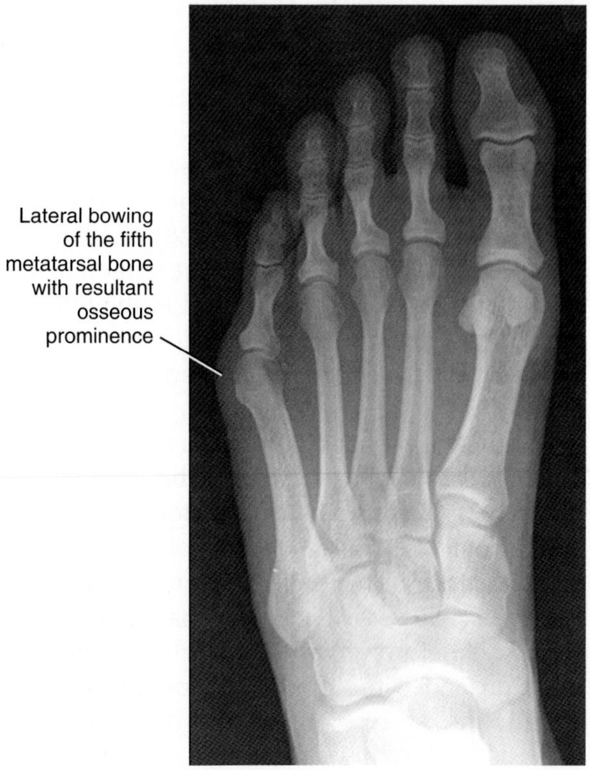
Lateral bowing of the fifth metatarsal bone with resultant osseous prominence

Figure 14-27 Bunionette deformity (Tailor's bunion).

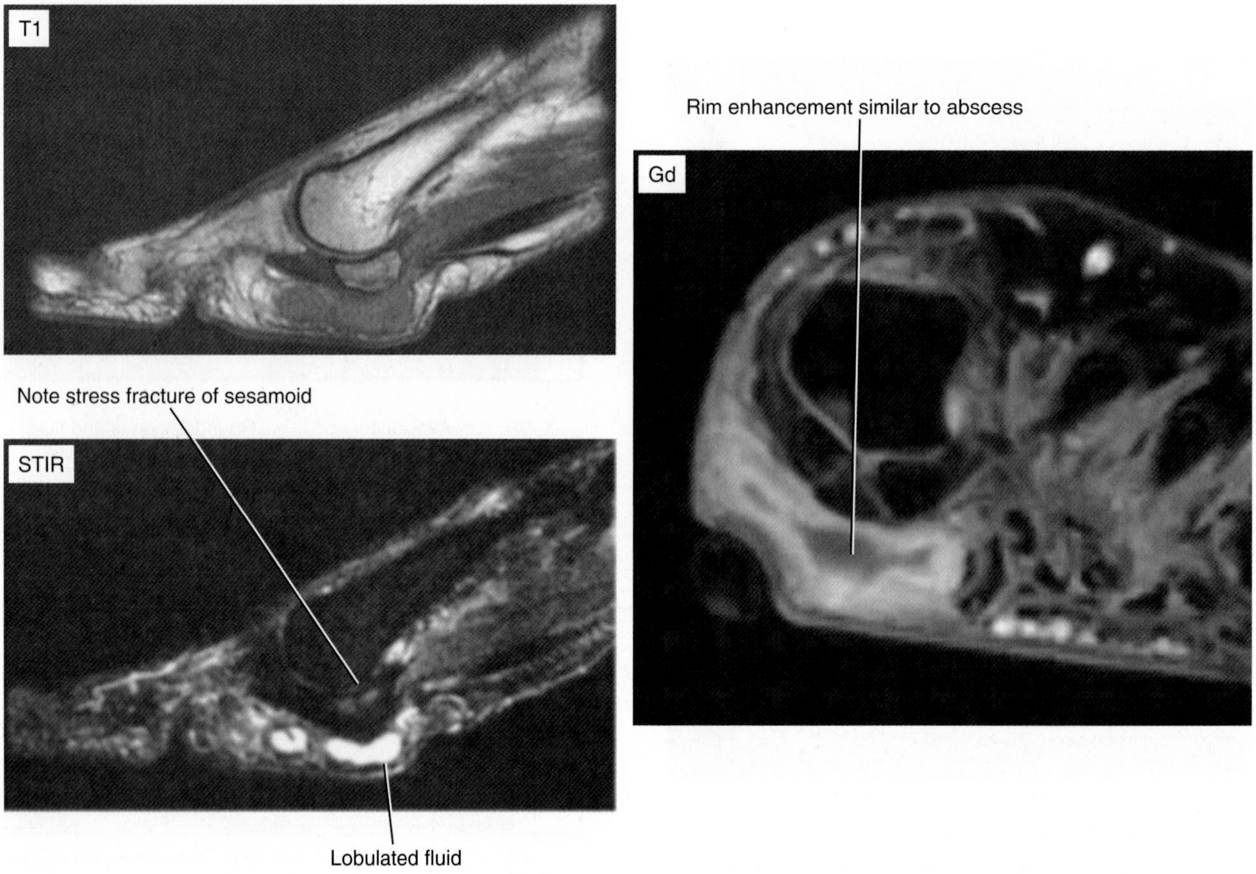
T1
Rim enhancement similar to abscess
Gd
Note stress fracture of sesamoid
STIR
Lobulated fluid

Figure 14-28 Altered stresses in a ballerina. Friction may induce mechanical bursitis.

from atypical friction, such as wearing tight shoes or having foot deformity. An example of an anatomic bursa is the intermetatarsal bursa (see Figs. 14-15 and 14-17). Adventitial bursae commonly occur inferior to the metatarsal heads (Fig. 14-28), medial to the first metatarsal head, that is, over the bunion in hallux valgus (see Fig. 14-23), and lateral to the fifth metatarsal head, that is, over a bunionette deformity. However, bursae can occur at a variety of locations, depending on the areas of friction.

Whether on MRI or ultrasound, a flat subcutaneous fluid collection in the foot should be considered suspicious for bursitis. Even in anatomic bursae, any fluid should be considered pathologic and potentially a source of the patient's pain. Administration of contrast will reveal thick rim enhancement, as with an abscess. However, without clinical suspicion of infection and without adjacent soft tissue findings of cellulitis, abscess can usually be excluded. The morphology and classic location of bursae usually help differentiate them from tumor. Ganglion cysts can occasionally appear like bursal fluid collections, but communication with a joint or tendon sheath helps to make the diagnosis of a ganglion.

When bursitis is seen, a number of associations should be considered. Although most cases of bursitis in the foot are mechanical, bursitis may also be seen in various inflammatory arthropathies, such as gout and rheumatoid arthritis. The key is to look for involvement of joints or tendon sheaths. Bursitis under the first metatarsal head is commonly seen in association with sesamoid pathology (see Fig. 14-28) and can be seen with plantar plate injuries. Bursitis is common in diabetic patients with foot deformity or decreased sensation, which makes them prone to repetitive trauma. Intermetatarsal bursitis has a high association with Morton neuroma.

TURF TOE/LESSER METATARSOPHALANGEAL PLANTAR PLATE INJURIES

Capsular/Ligamentous Injury

In acute trauma, the capsule of the first MTP joint and associated ligaments may be injured. This is especially the case in hyperextension injuries to the MTP joint. The MTP joint and/or sesamoids may even transiently dislocate, resulting in a radiographic finding of soft tissue swelling only. Slight malpositioning or separation of the sesamoids should raise suspicion of a ligamentous injury. MRI is the optimal method for evaluation of the capsular ligamentous complex. The intersesamoid ligament is seen on short-axis coronal images, and disruption is easily observed on T2-weighted images, with fluid penetrating through the normally low signal fibers (Fig. 14-29). Disruption of this ligament results in increased separation of the sesamoids and subluxation from the sulci. Similarly, disruption of the sesamoid phalangeal ligament is detectable especially on T2-weighted images in the sagittal or axial planes (Fig. 14-30). Disruption of this ligament causes the involved sesamoid to migrate proximally. Disruption of the plantar capsule, also known as "turf toe," is a relatively common entity in high-performance athletes involved in sports that require running with rapid change in speed and direction. The injury is accentuated by artificial playing surfaces. Radiographs and CT are normal. MRI shows effusion within the first MTP joint, with synovitis seen as "dirty" fluid, or intermediate signal material within the joint. The synovium enhances brightly with gadolinium contrast. Fluid signal, edema, and enhancement extend into the plantar soft tissues adjacent to the joint, indicating capsular injury. Intravenous contrast is especially useful for diagnosing chronic injuries (Fig. 14-31). Unlike sesamoiditis, the marrow signal is normal. A similar pattern can be seen in inflammatory arthropathies such as rheumatoid arthritis, but trauma history and lack of erosion limit the differential.

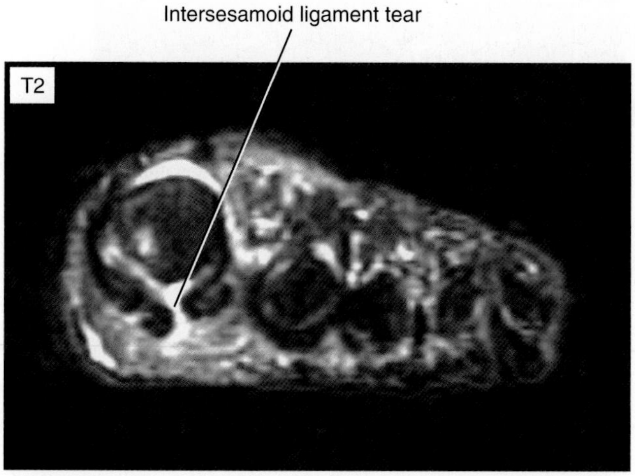
Intersesamoid ligament tear
T2

Figure 14-29 Acute turf toe injury with intersesamoid ligament tear. Sesamoids are displaced away from each other.

Whereas the first MTP joint is acutely injured in athletic patients, the lesser MTP joints (especially the second and occasionally the third) are typically an indolent problem owing to chronic, repetitive injury. This is seen most frequently in women who wear high-heeled shoes, and particularly in people with a relatively long second metatarsal. The combination of dorsiflexion, shifting of the fat pad distally, and pressure on the plantar plate during the push-off phase of ambulation stretches and tears the plantar plate. Similar to chronic plantar fasciitis, as the capsule scars, it is recurrently injured before it heals completely, which leads to chronic pain.

On MRI, the normal lesser MTP plantar plate has a dark, thick linear U-shaped pattern that is easily identified on T2-weighted short-axis (coronal) images (see Fig. 14-17). The first clue that there is a plantar plate problem should be effusion and synovitis at a single MTP joint (Fig. 14-32), usually the second. This pattern would be uncommon in the setting of an inflammatory arthropathy, and osteoarthritis is also relatively uncommon in the second to fifth MTP joints. Therefore, this finding alone should prompt one to inspect the plantar plate. If the dark U is broken, thickened, or edematous, the diagnosis of plantar plate injury can be made. Arthrography can document leakage through the plantar plate if necessary (Fig. 14-33). Especially on routine MR imaging it is helpful to compare with the other MTP joints. Frequently, disruption of the plantar plate results in synovial fluid leaking out of the joint into the adjacent intermetatarsal space,

Text continued on page 726

SECTION IV

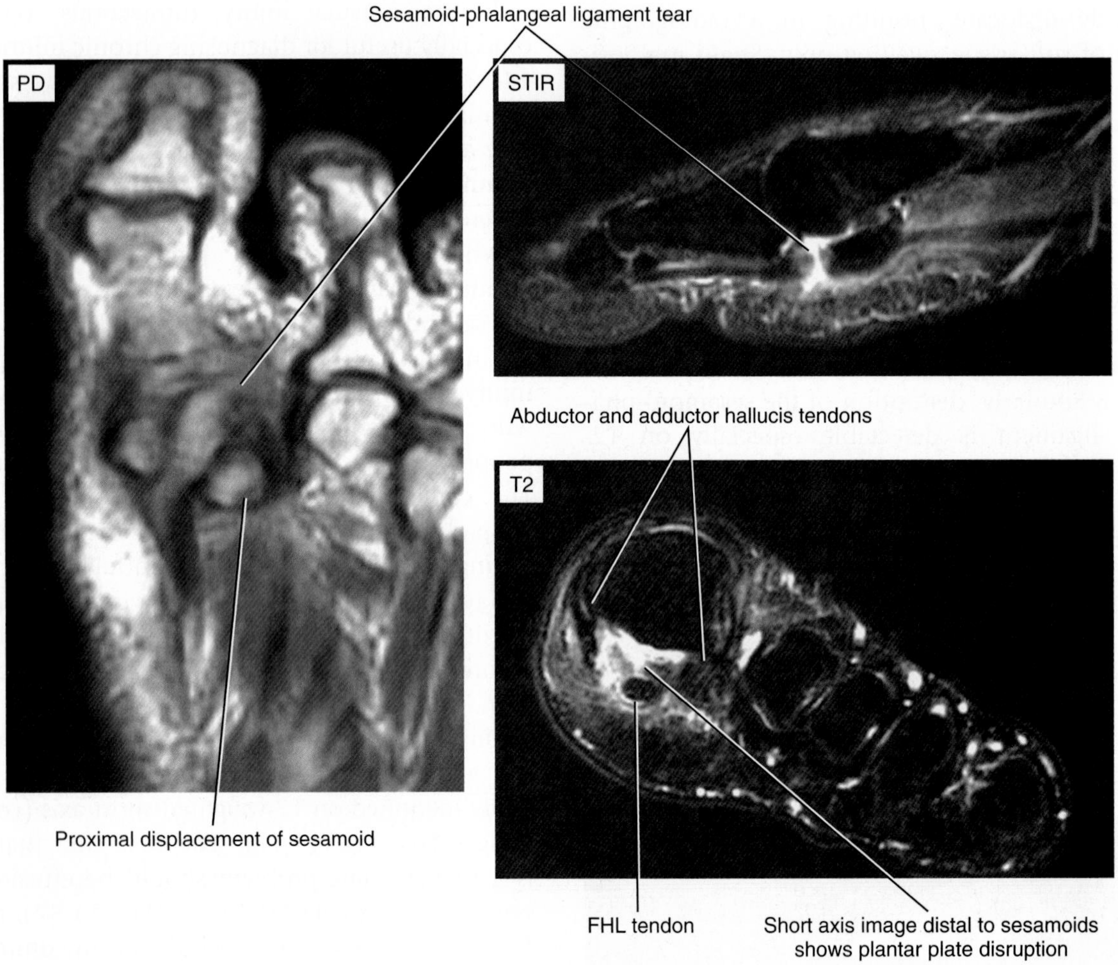
Sesamoid-phalangeal ligament tear
PD
STIR
Abductor and adductor hallucis tendons
T2
Proximal displacement of sesamoid
FHL tendon
Short axis image distal to sesamoids shows plantar plate disruption

Figure 14-30 Acute turf toe injuries. FHL, flexor hallucis longus.

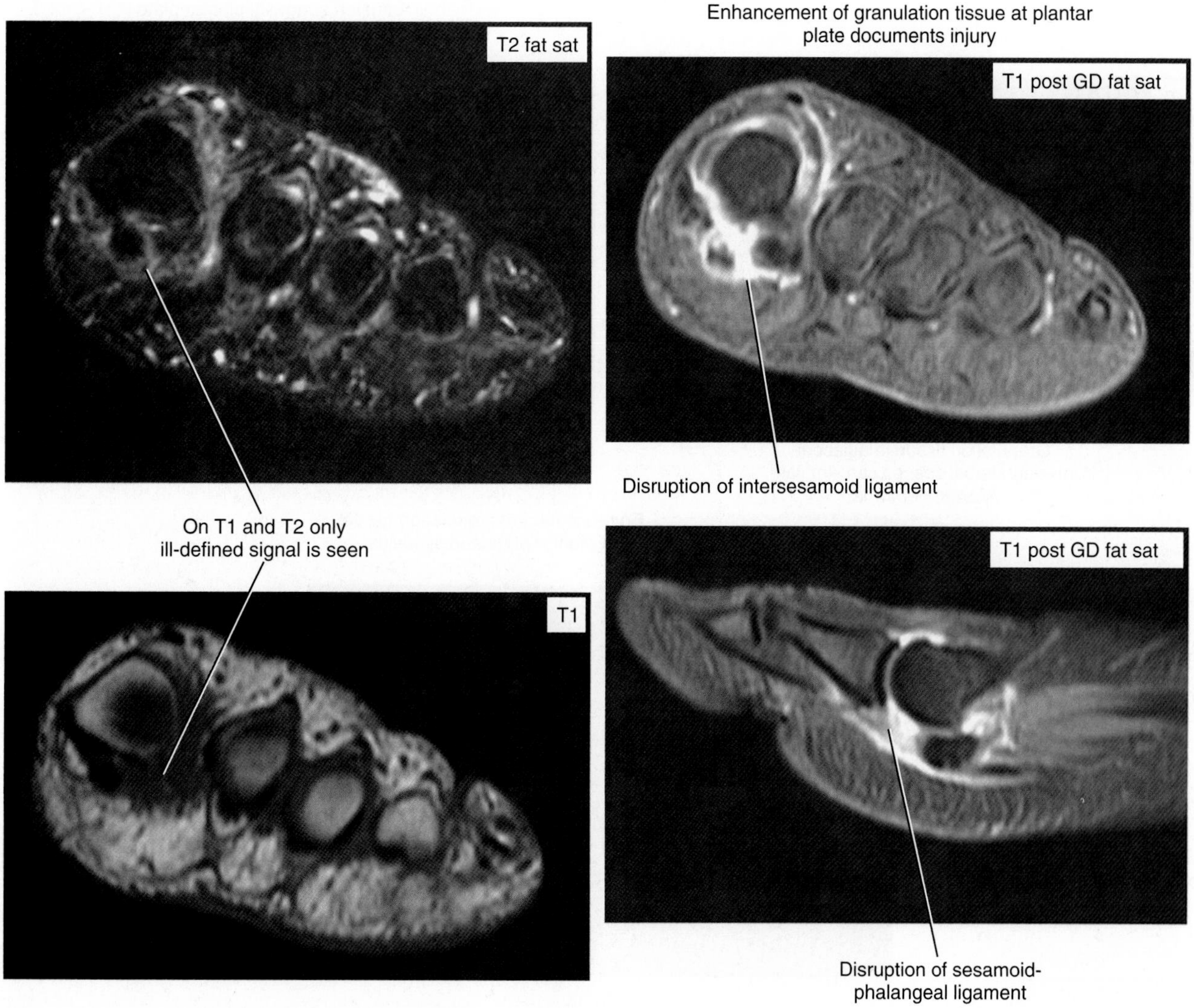
T2 fat sat
Enhancement of granulation tissue at plantar plate documents injury
T1 post GD fat sat
Disruption of intersesamoid ligament
On T1 and T2 only ill-defined signal is seen
T1
T1 post GD fat sat
Disruption of sesamoid-phalangeal ligament

Figure 14-31 **Chronic turf toe injury—value of intravenous contrast.**

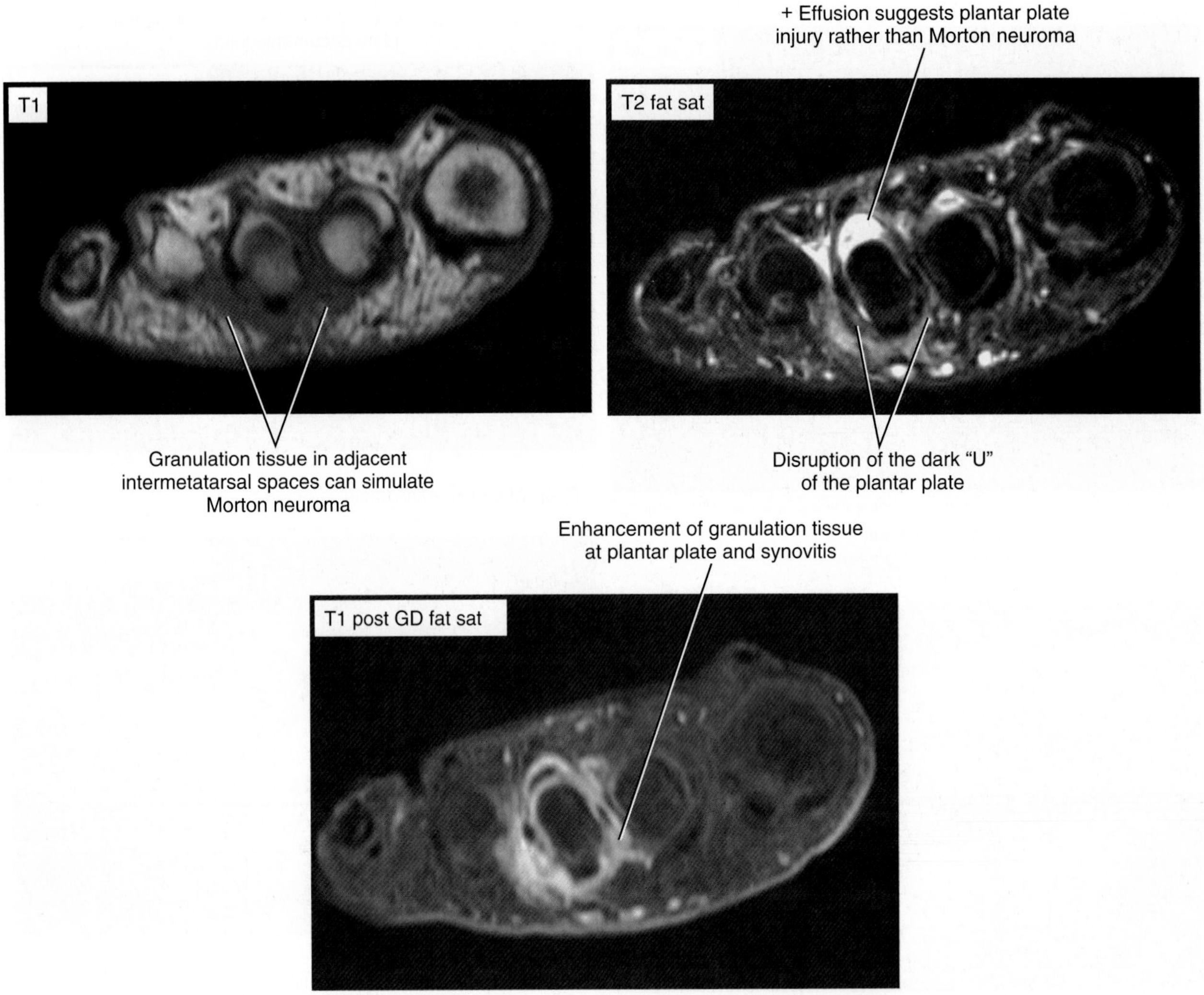
+ Effusion suggests plantar plate injury rather than Morton neuroma
T1
T2 fat sat
Granulation tissue in adjacent intermetatarsal spaces can simulate Morton neuroma
Disruption of the dark "U" of the plantar plate
Enhancement of granulation tissue at plantar plate and synovitis
T1 post GD fat sat

Figure 14-32 Lesser plantar plate injury—value of intravenous contrast. Lesser plantar plate injuries are chronic by nature and can simulate a Morton neuroma. Adjacent metatarsophalangeal (MTP) joint synovitis is the key to diagnosis.

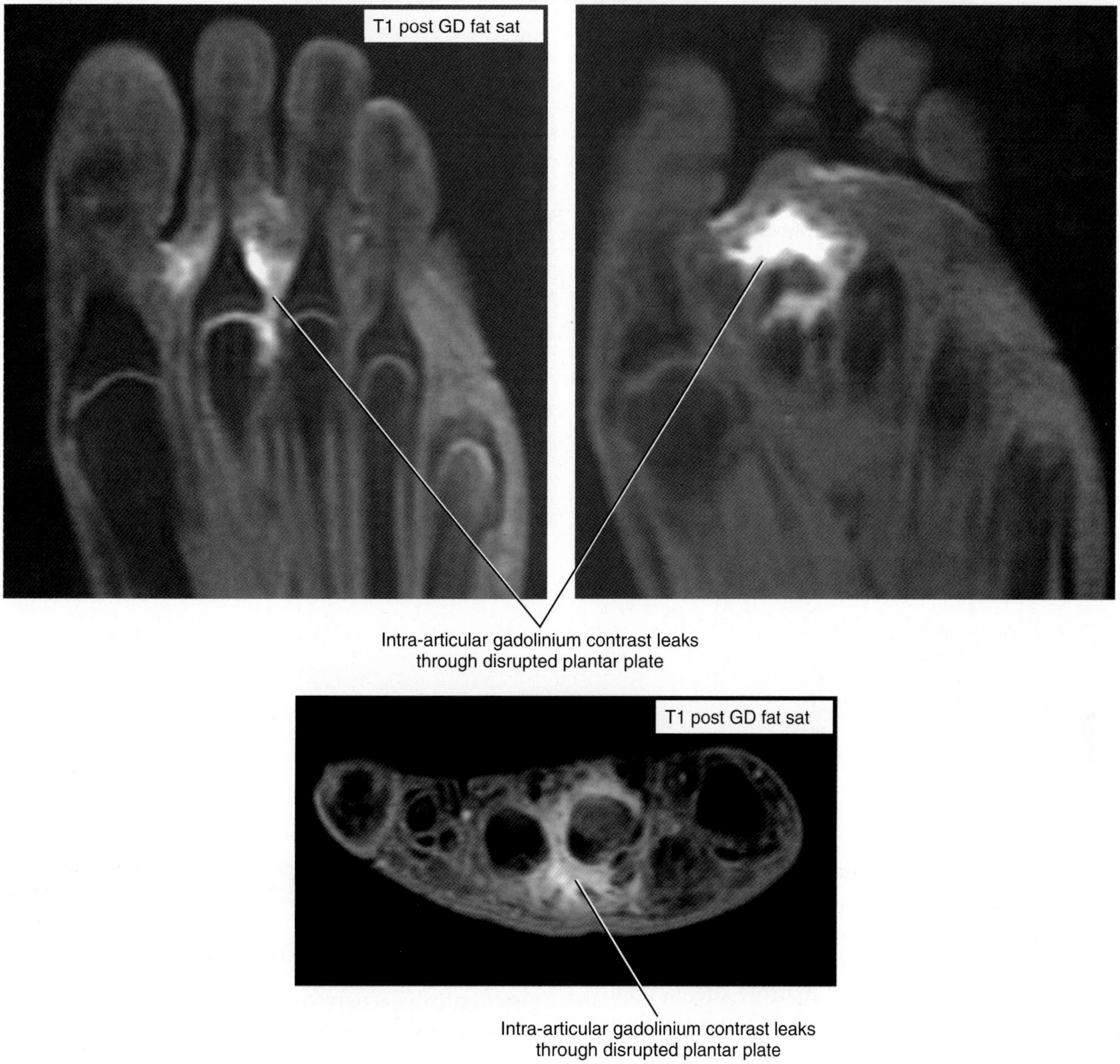
T1 post GD fat sat
Intra-articular gadolinium contrast leaks through disrupted plantar plate
T1 post GD fat sat
Intra-articular gadolinium contrast leaks through disrupted plantar plate

Figure 14-33 **Plantar plate injury documented on MR arthrography.**

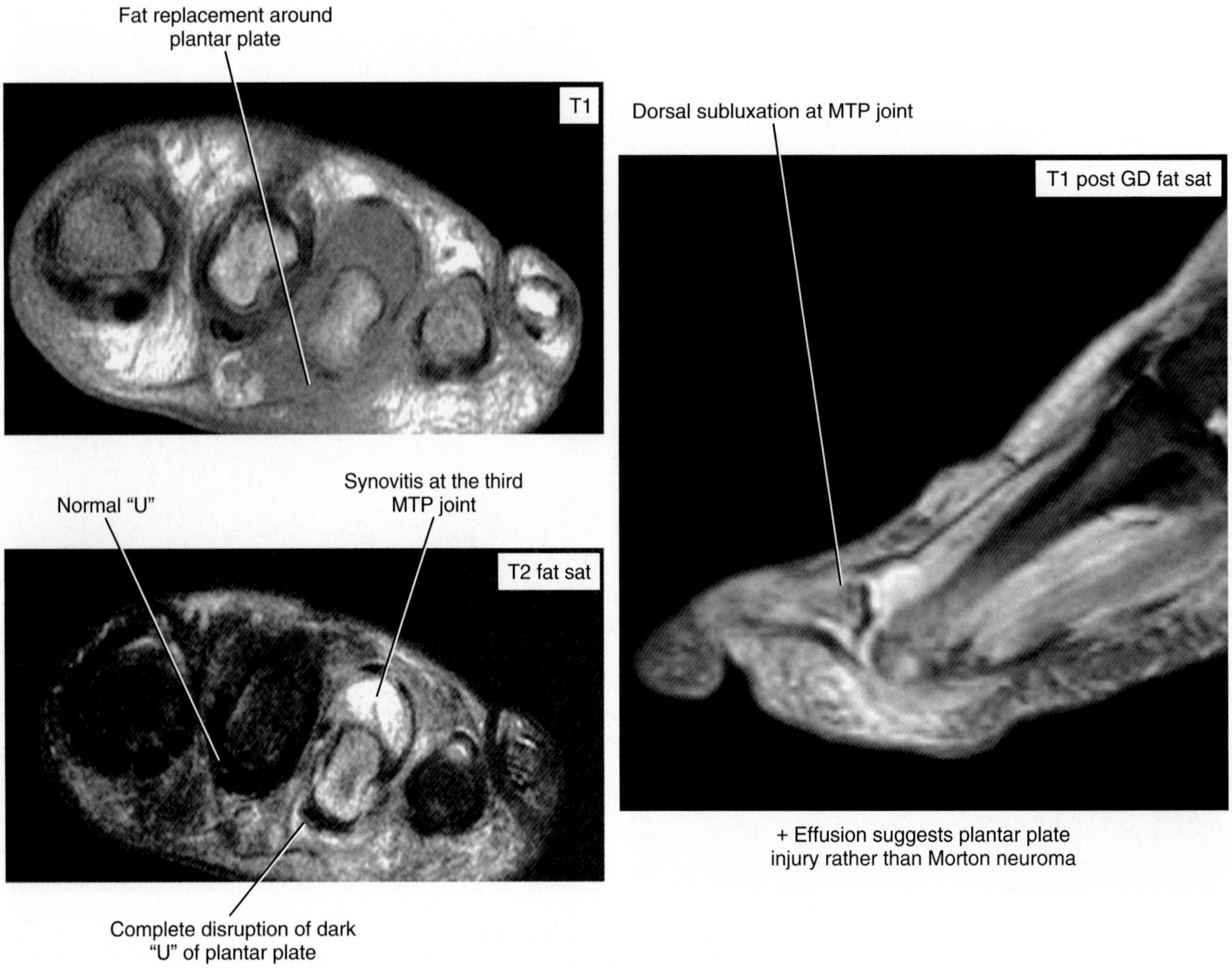
Fat replacement around plantar plate
T1
Normal "U"
Synovitis at the third MTP joint
T2 fat sat
Complete disruption of dark "U" of plantar plate
Dorsal subluxation at MTP joint
T1 post GD fat sat
+ Effusion suggests plantar plate injury rather than Morton neuroma

Figure 14-34 With more advanced chronic plantar plate injury, the proximal phalanx subluxes dorsally. Marrow edema is related to joint instability but can simulate septic arthritis. MTP, metatarsophalangeal.

which can simulate a Morton neuroma (see Figs. 14-32 through 14-34). In more advanced cases, there can be dorsal subluxation of the proximal phalanx, with an appearance suggestive of neuropathic arthropathy (Fig. 14-34). Associated marrow edema related to instability can simulate septic or other inflammatory arthritis.

INFECTION

Infection of the forefoot is discussed in detail in Chapter 5, but it should be considered in the differential diagnosis of a marrow signal abnormality adjacent to which are a skin ulcer and signs of surrounding cellulitis.

ARTICULAR DISEASE

Osteoarthritis/Hallux Rigidus

Osteoarthritis is very common in the forefoot, especially at the first MTP joint, and involvement of the metatarsal-sesamoid (MTS) articulation generally mirrors its severity of disease. At the arthritic MTS joint initially there is loss of cartilage. Associated joint narrowing may be very subtle on radiographs and CT images, but the cartilage loss is directly visualized on MRI. Subchondral cystic change is seen on both sides of the MTS joint, and sclerosis may be present, which radiographically can resemble avascular necrosis. This process can be differentiated from avascular necrosis on MRI. Avascular necrosis dif-

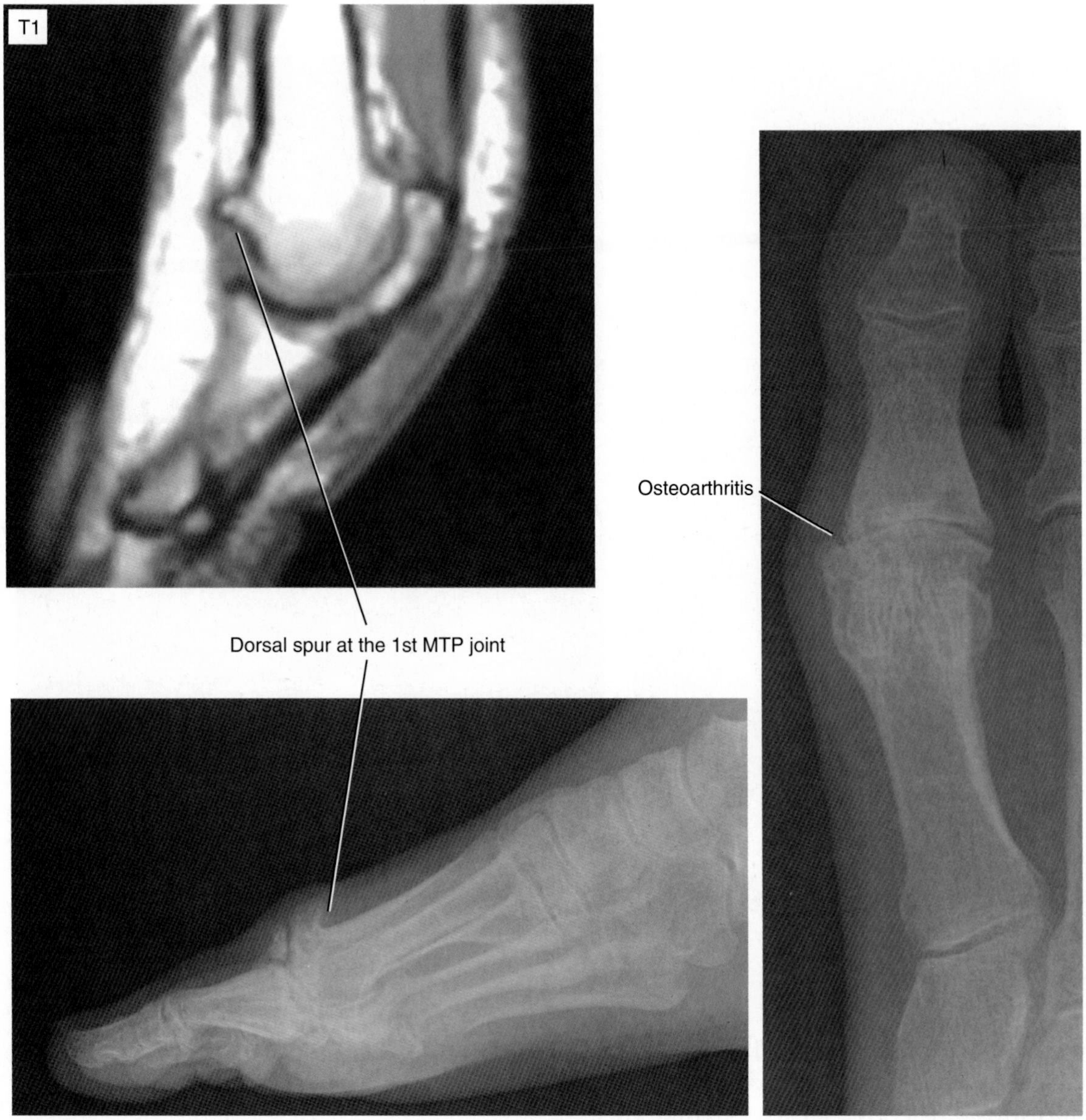
T1
Osteoarthritis
Dorsal spur at the 1st MTP joint

Figure 14-35 **Hallux rigidus.** Osteoarthritis at the first metatarsophalangeal (MTP) joint with dorsal spurring results in pain and limited range of motion especially on dorsiflexion.

fusely replaces the sesamoid bone marrow on T1-weighted images, whereas osteoarthritis preserves at least a portion of marrow fat signal. Osteoarthritis may also occur superimposed upon other etiologies, as an end stage of the disease process. Processes that can accelerate development of osteoarthritis include fracture, inflammatory arthropathy, infection, and avascular necrosis.

Hallux rigidus represents osteoarthritis of the first MTP joint in which prominent spurs extend dorsally (Fig. 14-35), limiting range of motion or causing pain on dorsiflexion. Removal of a spur is called a chielectomy.

Osteochondral Lesions

Osteochondral lesions are uncommon in the forefoot but can be a source of significant pain. Imaging findings are fairly characteristic and similar in appearance to osteochondritis dissecans of the talar dome. On CT and MRI, osteochondral lesions are seen as a crescentic or rounded subchondral abnormality,

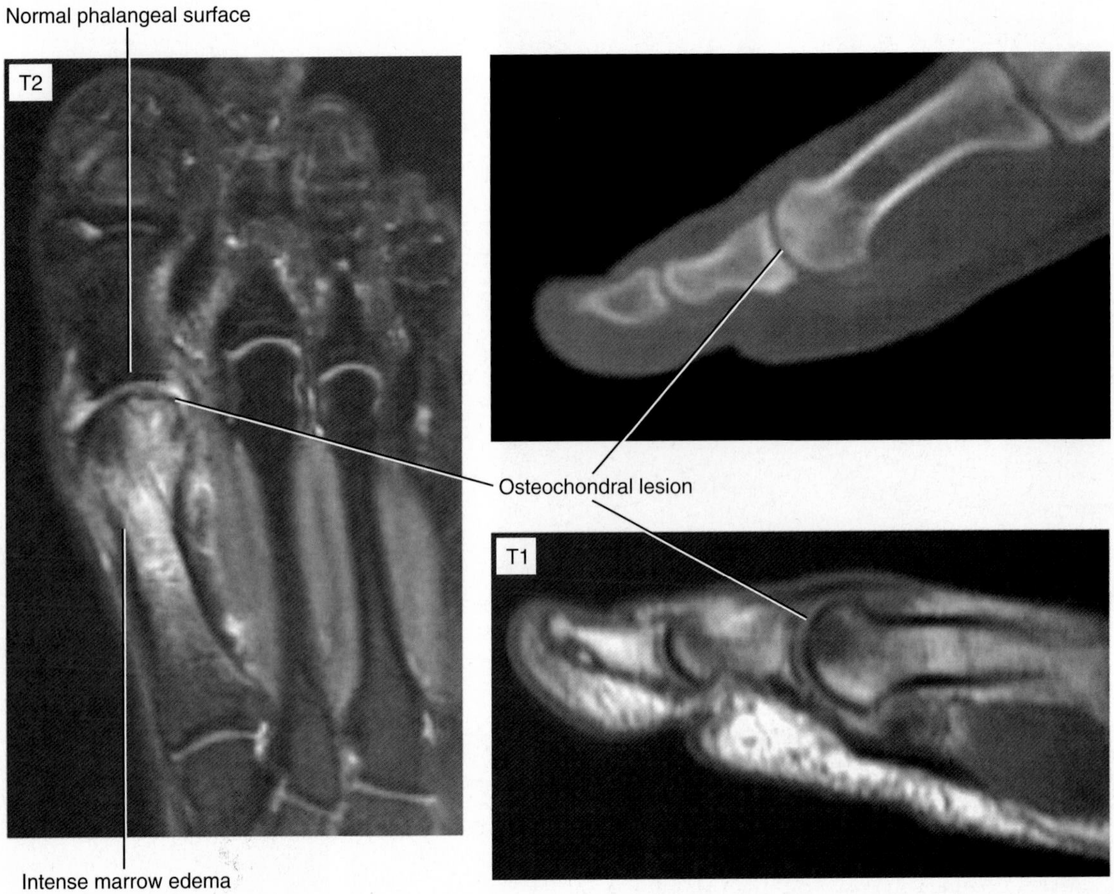
Normal phalangeal surface
T2
Osteochondral lesion
T1
Intense marrow edema

Figure 14-36 Osteochondral lesion of the first metatarsal head.

usually at the first metatarsal head (Fig. 14-36). If high-resolution imaging is used, occasionally an overlying cartilage defect is seen. Surrounding edema is common; it may be intense and is generally a marker of pain response. Lack of change on the phalangeal side of the joint helps to exclude arthritis as an etiology. Avascular necrosis can look similar but is rare in the absence of surgery. However, osteochondral lesions, as in the talar dome, may have a component of osteonecrosis, and avascular necrosis is an end stage of some osteochondral lesions. Freiberg infraction, or avascular necrosis of the second metatarsal head with resultant flattening of the dorsal articular surface, may originate as an osteochondral injury (Fig. 14-37). If necessary, dynamic contrast enhancement can differentiate hyperemic marrow with reactive inflammation from edematous ischemic bone.

Inflammatory Arthropathies

Inflammatory arthropathies such as rheumatoid arthritis, psoriatic arthritis, Reiter disease, and gout may involve the forefoot. All can cause synovitis, with complex effusion and thick, hyperemic synovium, the appearance of which is similar to that of septic arthritis. Inflammatory bursitis can result in the formation of complex fluid collections and rim enhancement that can simulate abscess. Inflammatory tenosynovitis is also common. Synovial inflammation can cause marginal erosions and reactive edema on MRI. Although the pattern of disease and differential diagnosis is facilitated by radiographs, subtle erosion may be more apparent on CT or MRI. Of the inflammatory arthropathies, gout can have a distinct appearance on MRI. Intra-articular tophi produce masslike foci of low signal on T1- and T2-weighted images. Extra-articular tophi are also common adjacent to the first MTP joint and can cause extrinsic

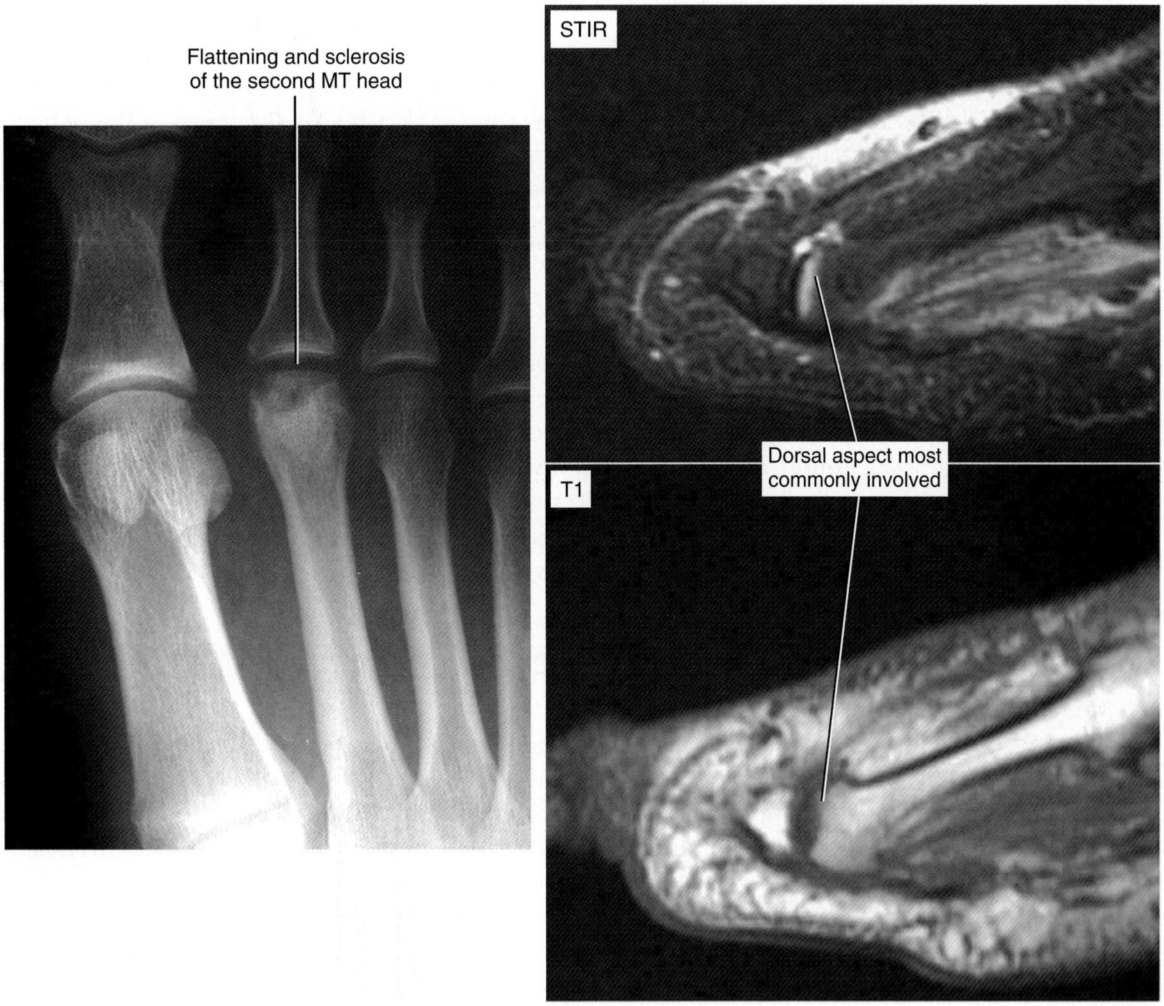
Flattening and sclerosis of the second MT head
STIR
Dorsal aspect most commonly involved
T1

Figure 14-37 Freiberg infraction. Avascular necrosis of the metatarsal head (typically the second, especially in the setting of a long second toe). Dorsal articular surface is most commonly involved and may be related to chronic repetitive stress.

erosion (periarticular erosion). Rheumatoid arthritis in particular causes capsular and ligamentous laxity resulting in joint deformity. Manifestations of inflammatory arthropathies are discussed in detail in Chapter 4.

MORTON NEUROMA (PERINEURAL FIBROSIS)

A Morton neuroma is actually perineural fibrosis, which occurs at the interdigital nerve as it passes beyond the metatarsal heads. The presumptive cause is repetitive injury to or pressure on the nerve, which is in a susceptible location and can become impinged during walking or running, especially with dorsiflexion of the toes in people who wear high-heeled shoes. There is a close association between Morton neuroma and intermetatarsal bursitis, which may be causal. That is, the mass effect from the bursa above the nerve can place added pressure on the nerve. Or, the association may be due to a common etiology. That is, footwear with a narrow toebox may cause pinching of the metatarsal heads and incite bursitis between them. In any case, both intermetatarsal bursitis and Morton neuroma can be a source of pain and should be reported. It is helpful to first look for intermetatarsal bursitis on short-axis T2-weighted fat-suppressed images. When present, one should look for the associated Morton neuroma. It is uncommon to see a Morton neuroma without intermetatarsal bursitis.

Intemetatarsal bursitis hurts when a person wears tight shoes or squeezes the forefoot and metatarsal heads together. Morton neuroma hurts during the push-off phase of ambulation or when pressing focally over the lesion at the plantar aspect of the foot. It is helpful on MRI to place a vitamin E marker at the site of pain, but one should place it at the dorsal aspect to avoid soft tissue distortion in the area of concern. In the case of Morton neuroma, the patient can usually localize the area precisely.

Morton neuroma is most common at the second and third intermetatarsal spaces. At the fourth space it is uncommon; at the first space it is rare. It is common to have two lesions, which may be a source for recurrent or persistent pain after neuroma resection. Size of the lesion is important to describe, since larger lesions are more likely to be a source of pain and are more likely to be treated aggressively. If open surgery is performed, the approach is dorsal, as is most surgery of the forefoot to avoid scarring and pain at the plantar surface. Recently, more lesions are being treated with percutaneous ablation.

On MRI, Morton neuroma is best seen on short-axis (coronal) images. As previously mentioned, one should first look at the T2-weighted fat-suppressed (or STIR) images for vertically oriented, linear or bulbous fluid signal between the joint capsules of adjacent metatarsal heads, representing intermetatarsal bursitis. At that same location, look at the short-axis T1-weighted images, paying attention to the plantar fat. Follow the images distally, and a Morton neuroma will appear as a rounded focus of low to intermediate signal at the distal margin of the metatarsal heads, with mass effect on the adjacent fat (Figs. 14-38 and 14-39). Refer back to the T2-weighted images; a Morton neuroma will appear intermediate to low in signal, helping to differentiate it from prominent bursitis or a ganglion cyst, which will appear as fluid signal. Gadolinium contrast is not necessary to make the diagnosis, but Morton neuromas typically enhance brightly, which makes them very easy to see.

Ultrasound can also effectively visualize a Morton neuroma as a focal mass in the characteristic location as just described (see Fig. 14-2), with tenderness elicited upon increased pressure.

Mass effect between the metatarsal heads may be caused by bursitis or a ganglion cyst. However, a very common mimicker is a plantar plate injury of the adjacent MTP joint. As discussed in the plantar plate injury section of this chapter, chronic injury of the lesser MTP plantar plates, can result in granulation tissue extending into the adjacent soft tissues, the very location where Morton neuromas occur. This tissue also appears intermediate in signal and enhances brightly. The key is to look at the adjacent joints: If one of the adjacent MTP joints (usually the second) has effusion and synovitis, the correct diagnosis may very well be plantar plate injury rather than Morton neuroma. Look closely at the plantar plate of the joint in question on short-axis T2-weighted images. An intact plantar plate will appear as an unbroken low-signal U-shaped line.

MUSCLES AND TENDONS

Muscle atrophy is often clinically important and can be easily detected on MRI. Early atrophy is seen as muscle edema and usually (but not necessarily) decreased muscle bulk (Fig. 14-40). This usually can be differentiated from muscle injury (strain) based on the edema pattern, which is diffuse within the muscle belly. Injury typically creates a feathery pattern of edema, with fluid separating the muscle fibers (Fig. 14-41). Diffusely distributed muscle atrophy may be due to primary (e.g., paralysis) or secondary (e.g., diabetes with neuropathy) neurologic conditions. Focal atrophy patterns should raise concern for nerve impingement at the foot or ankle. A common impingement pattern is the posterior tibial nerve in the tarsal tunnel, resulting in atrophy of the abductor digiti minimi, and lateral forefoot muscles (Fig. 14-42). This pattern is also very common in the setting of posterior tibial tendon dysfunction with arch collapse, possibly owing to stretching of the nerve as the foot overpronates.

Tenosynovitis is not commonly symptomatic in the forefoot, but pathology is often seen with underlying inflammatory arthropathies or diabetes. In these cases multiple tendons are usually involved, with complex fluid in the sheath. In the setting of infection, fluid within a sheath of a tendon traversing the area should be considered suspicious for septic tenosynovitis. A single tendon with sheath fluid is often mechanical, but it may be a sign of associated joint

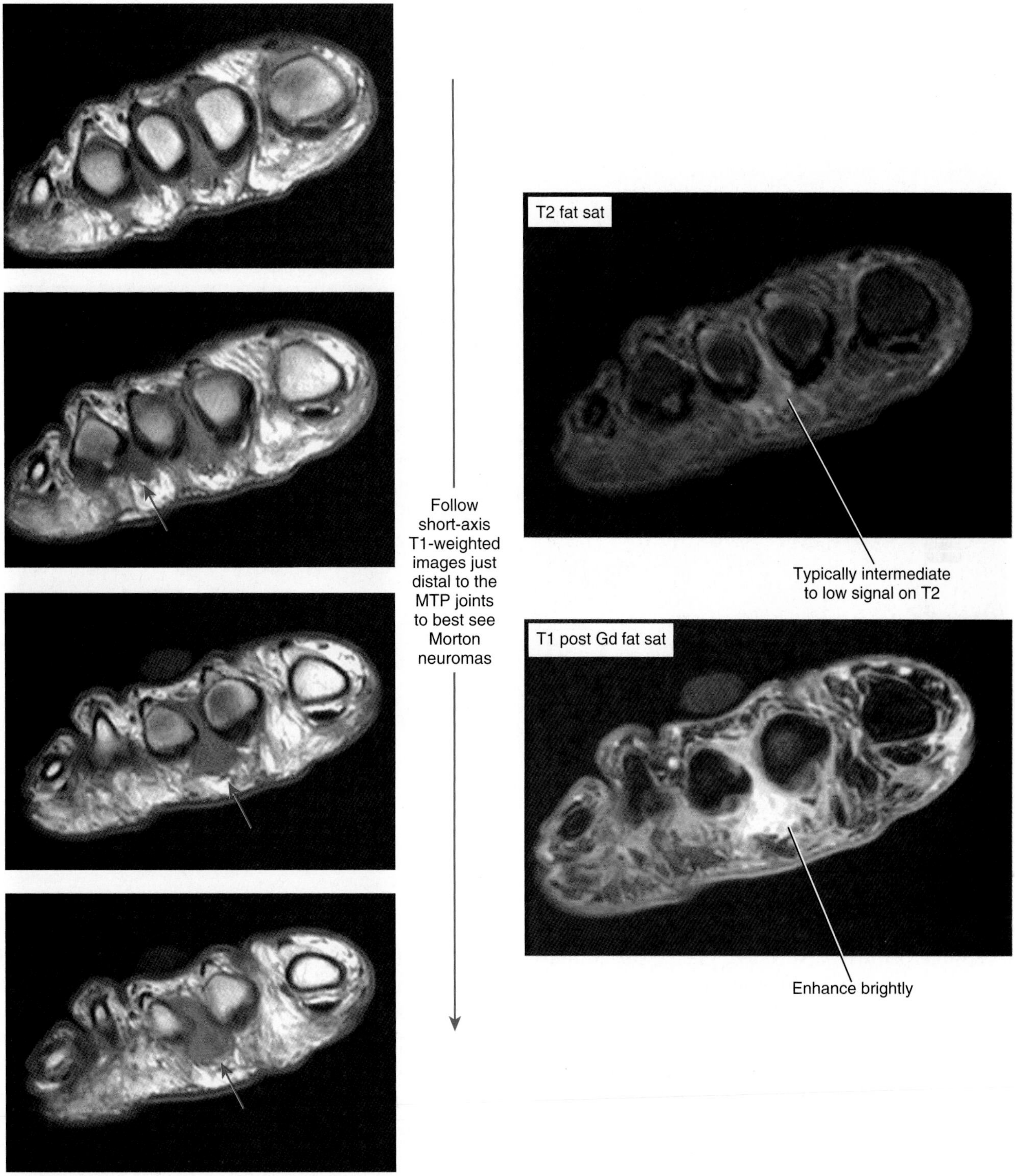
Follow
short-axis
T1-weighted
images just
distal to the
MTP joints
to best see
Morton
neuromas
T2 fat sat
Typically intermediate
to low signal on T2
T1 post Gd fat sat
Enhance brightly

Figure 14-38 Morton neuroma—detection and characteristic features on MRI. MTP, metatarsophalangeal.

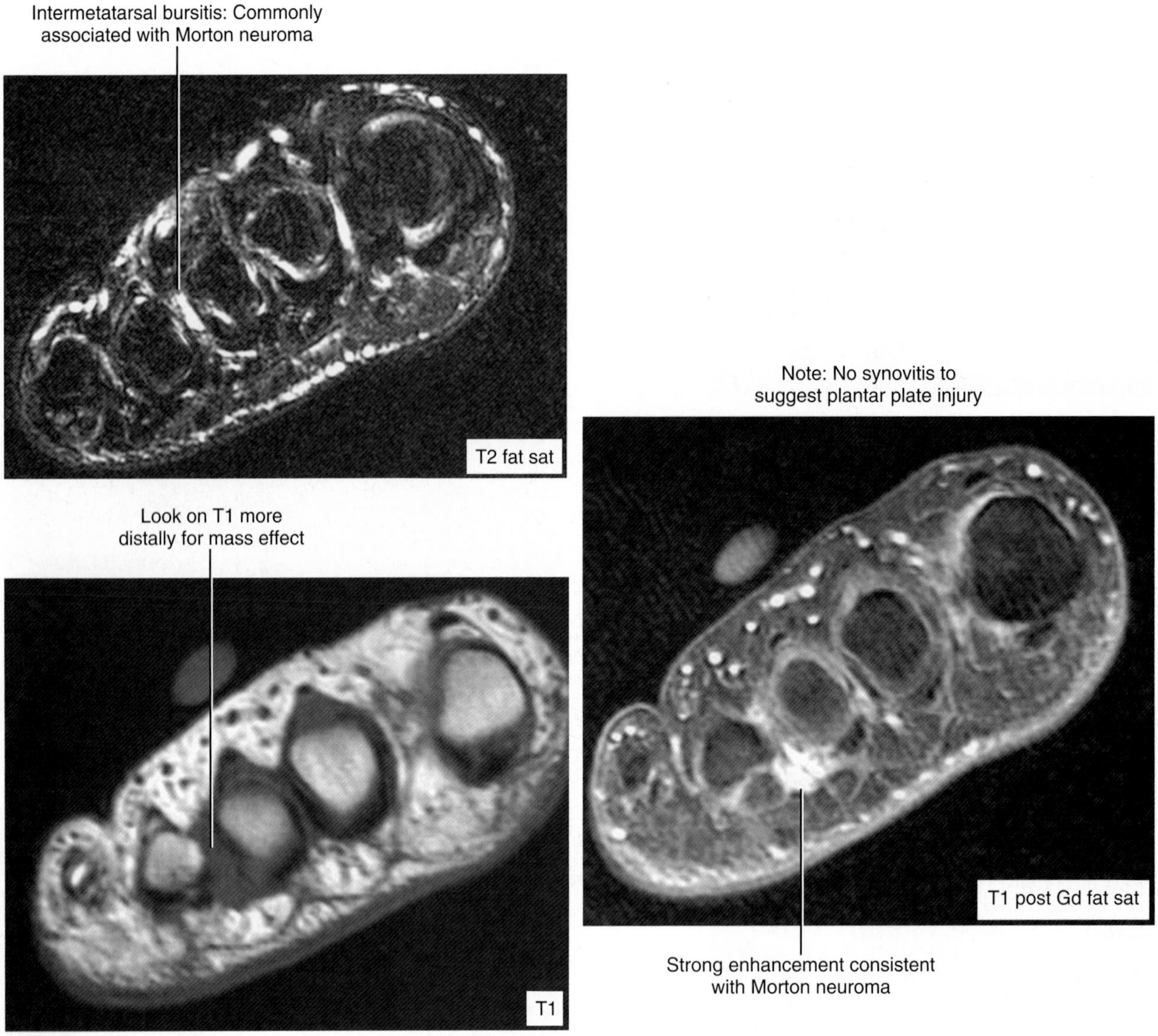
Intermetatarsal bursitis: Commonly associated with Morton neuroma
T2 fat sat
Look on T1 more distally for mass effect
T1
Note: No synovitis to suggest plantar plate injury
T1 post Gd fat sat
Strong enhancement consistent with Morton neuroma

Figure 14-39 **Morton neuroma.**

or capsular pathology, such as a plantar plate injury. Tendon transection is rare but can occur with penetrating injury (Fig. 14-43).

STRESS FRACTURE/RESPONSE

Stress fractures are common at the foot and ankle. In the foot, characteristic locations are the metatarsal necks and bases, and the sesamoid bones. Similar to stress in other locations, radiographs and CT show increased density or periosteal reaction, occasionally with a discrete fracture line. MRI shows marrow edema with a low signal line representing the microcallus forming at the lines of stress (Fig. 14-44). A long-axis plane shows the low signal line best, which may be seen only as a dark notch at the corticomedullary margin. Periosteal reaction is seen on MRI as edema surrounding the bone circumferentially; in the foot, periosteal reaction is not commonly seen other than at the metatarsal bones.

PLANTAR FIBROMATOSIS

Plantar fibromatosis (Ledderhose disease) is one of the superficial fibromatoses (such as Peyronie disease and Duypuytren contracture) and affects the plantar

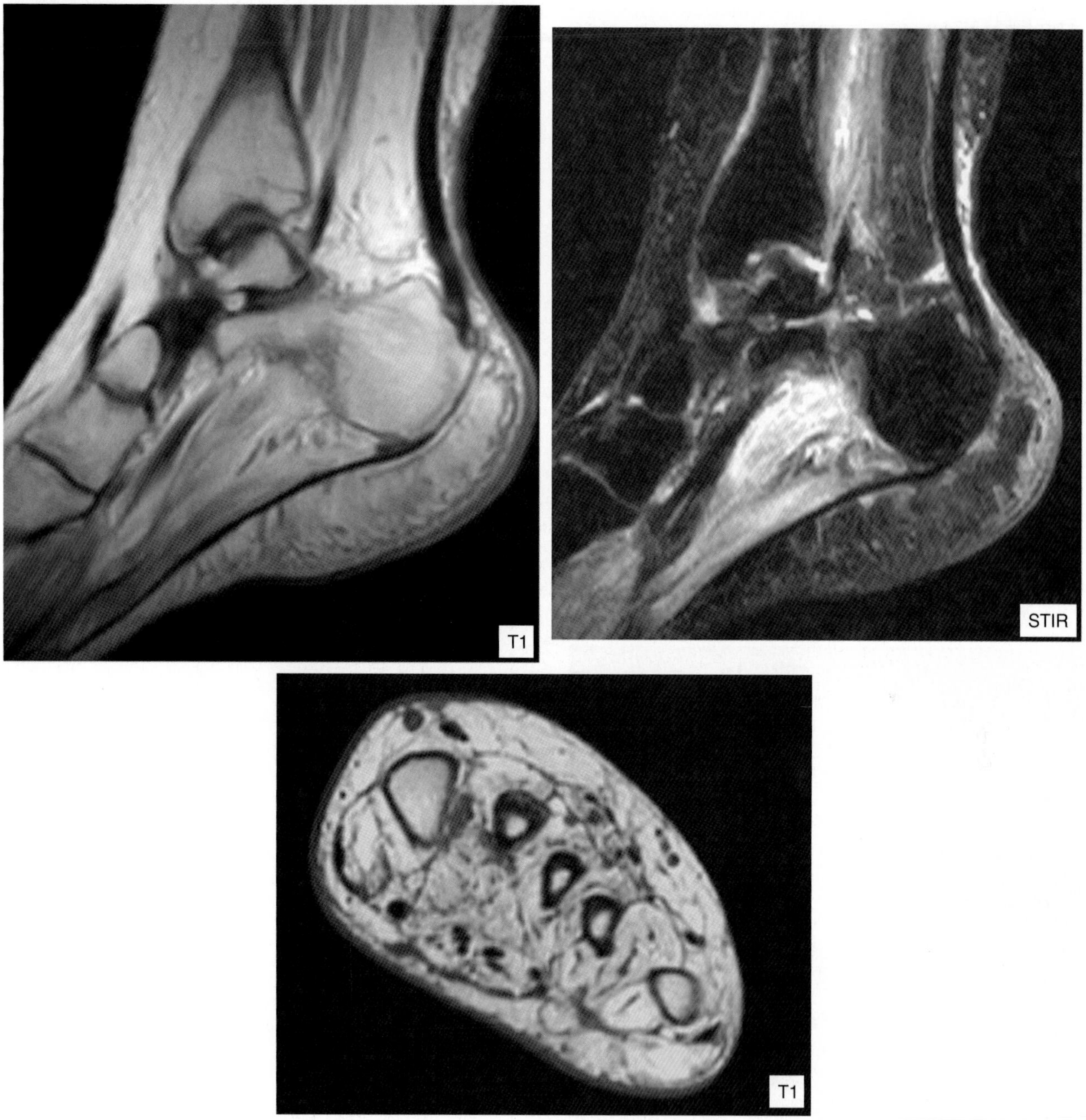
T1
STIR
T1

Figure 14-40 Diffuse muscle atrophy in a diabetic patient. Atrophic muscles typically demonstrate hyperintensity on STIR or fat-suppressed T2-weighted sequences, especially in the early stages.

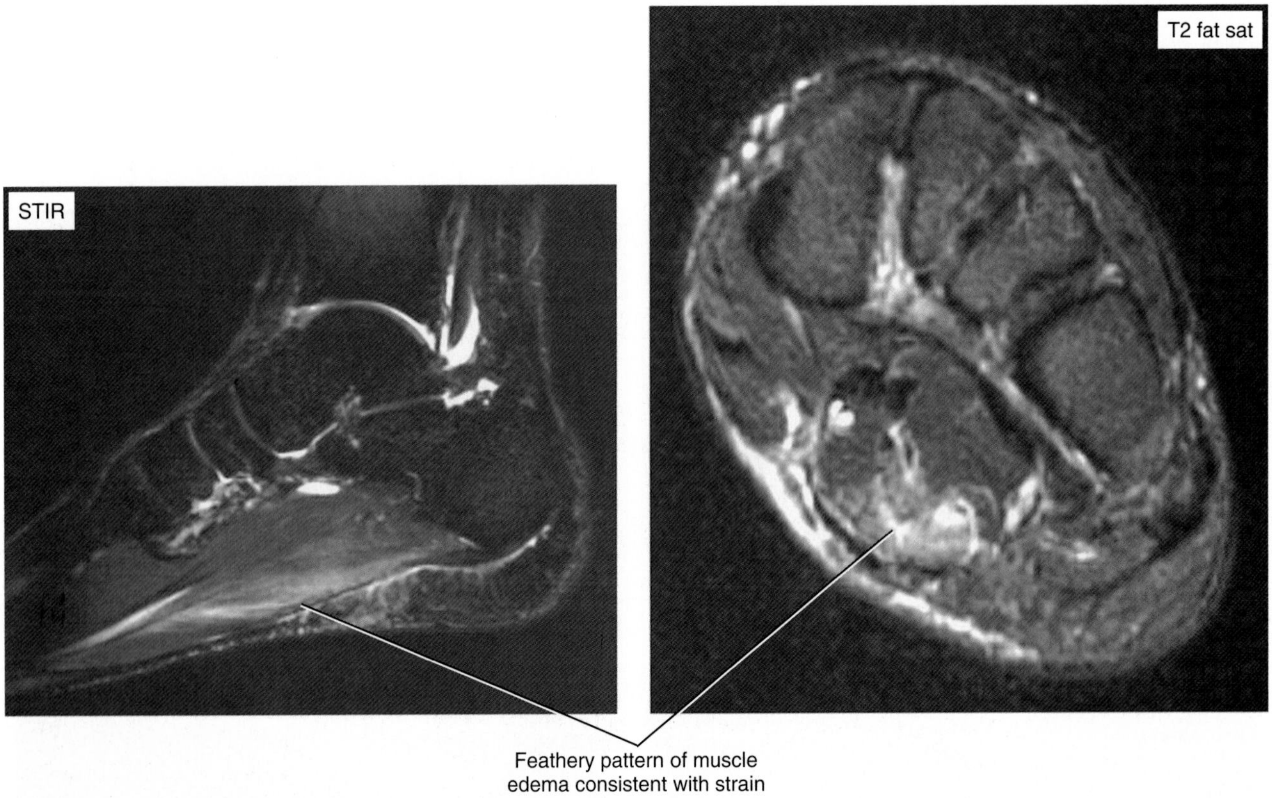
STIR
T2 fat sat
Feathery pattern of muscle edema consistent with strain

Figure 14-41 Professional football player with grade 2 muscle strain (partial tear) of the flexor digitorum brevis.

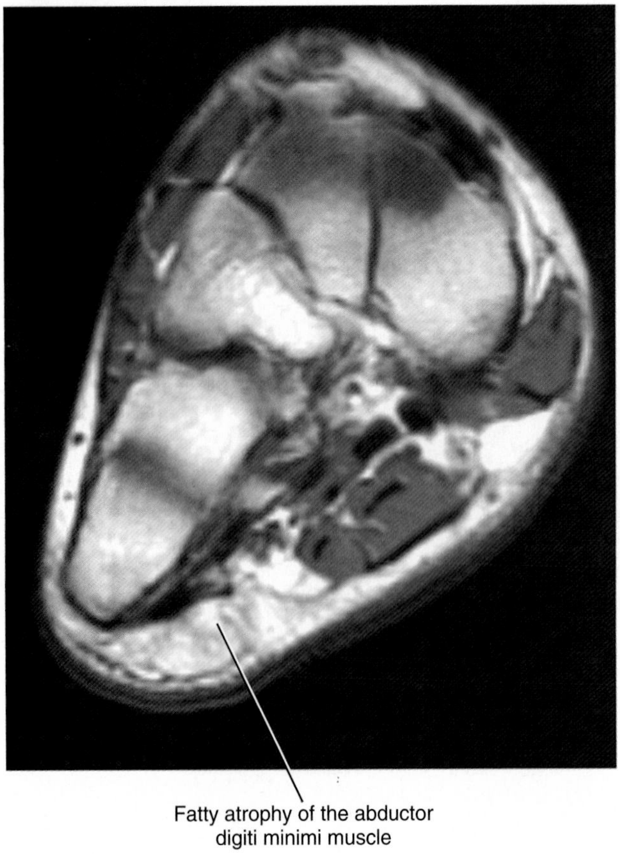
Fatty atrophy of the abductor digiti minimi muscle

Figure 14-42 **Focal atrophy of the abductor digiti minimi muscle.** This pattern is seen with impingement of the posterior tibial nerve in the tarsal tunnel or with posterior tibialis tendon dysfunction.

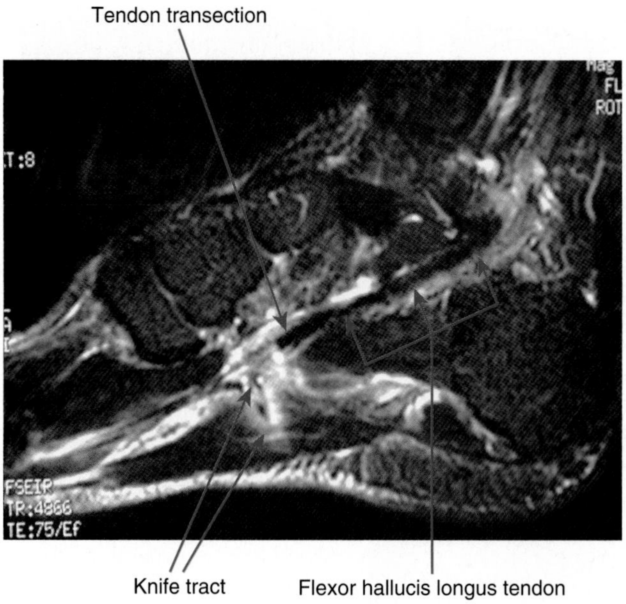
Tendon transection
FSEIR
TR:4866
TE:75/Ef
Knife tract
Flexor hallucis longus tendon

Figure 14-43 Complete transection of the flexor hallucis longus tendon from a stab wound.

fascia, typically at the medial midfoot. Patients with plantar fibromatosis present with plantar pain and nodular mass effect, which creates discomfort at the plantar arch when wearing hard shoes. The lesion is composed of fibroblasts in the active, early phase and collagen in the indolent, late phase. The proportion of cells to collagen largely determines the MRI signal characteristics. Collagen is low signal on T1- and T2-weighted sequences, whereas in the more cellular phase there may be areas of intermediate or even high T2 signal. Enhancement with gadolinium occurs in 60% of lesions with more enhancement seen in the cellular phase, and intravenous contrast may be useful for detecting additional, smaller lesions. Lesions typically grow longitudinally along the superficial margin of the fascia, with fascial tails at each end (Fig. 14-45). Often these lesions are slow growing, and conservative management limited to shoe inserts is all that is required. Surgical management for localized lesions consists of wide debridement; residual tumor can recur aggressively. Extension into adjacent

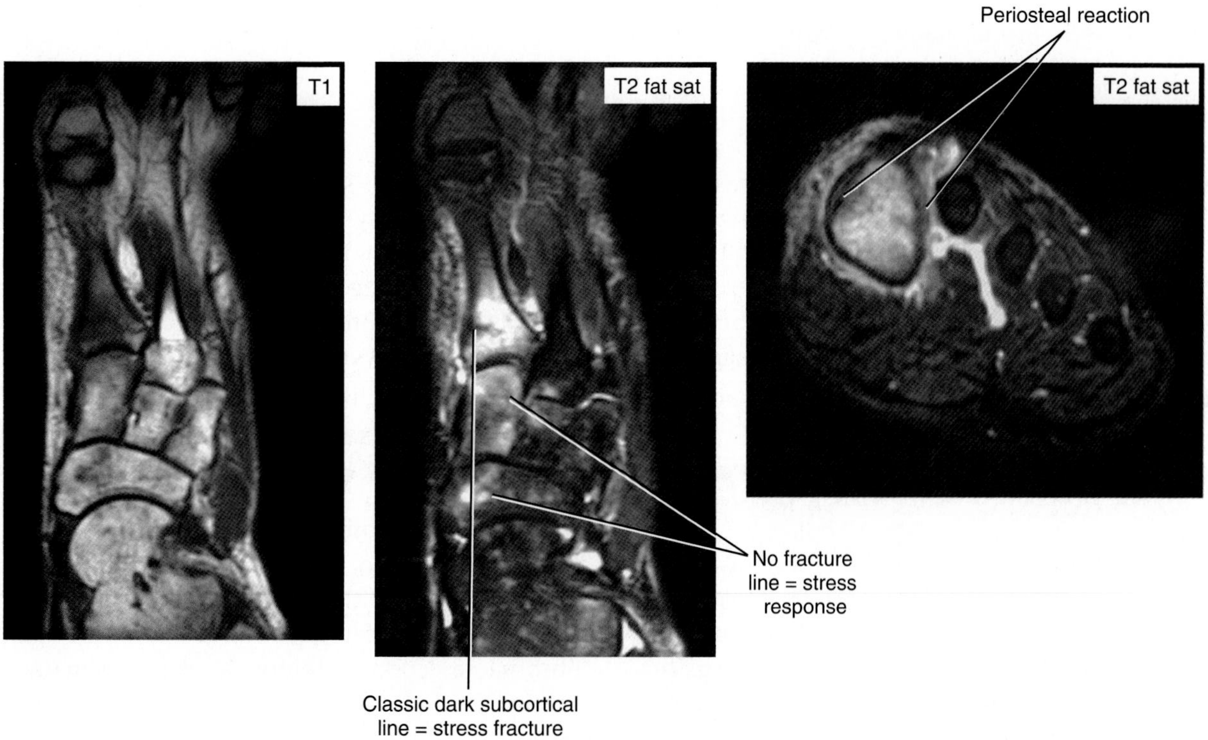
Periosteal reaction
T1
T2 fat sat
T2 fat sat
No fracture
line = stress
response
Classic dark subcortical
line = stress fracture

Figure 14-44 **Stress fracture of the first metatarsal base.** A dark line extending perpendicular to the cortex (representing trabecular callus) with surrounding marrow edema is characteristic. History is important since a subacute fracture can look identical.

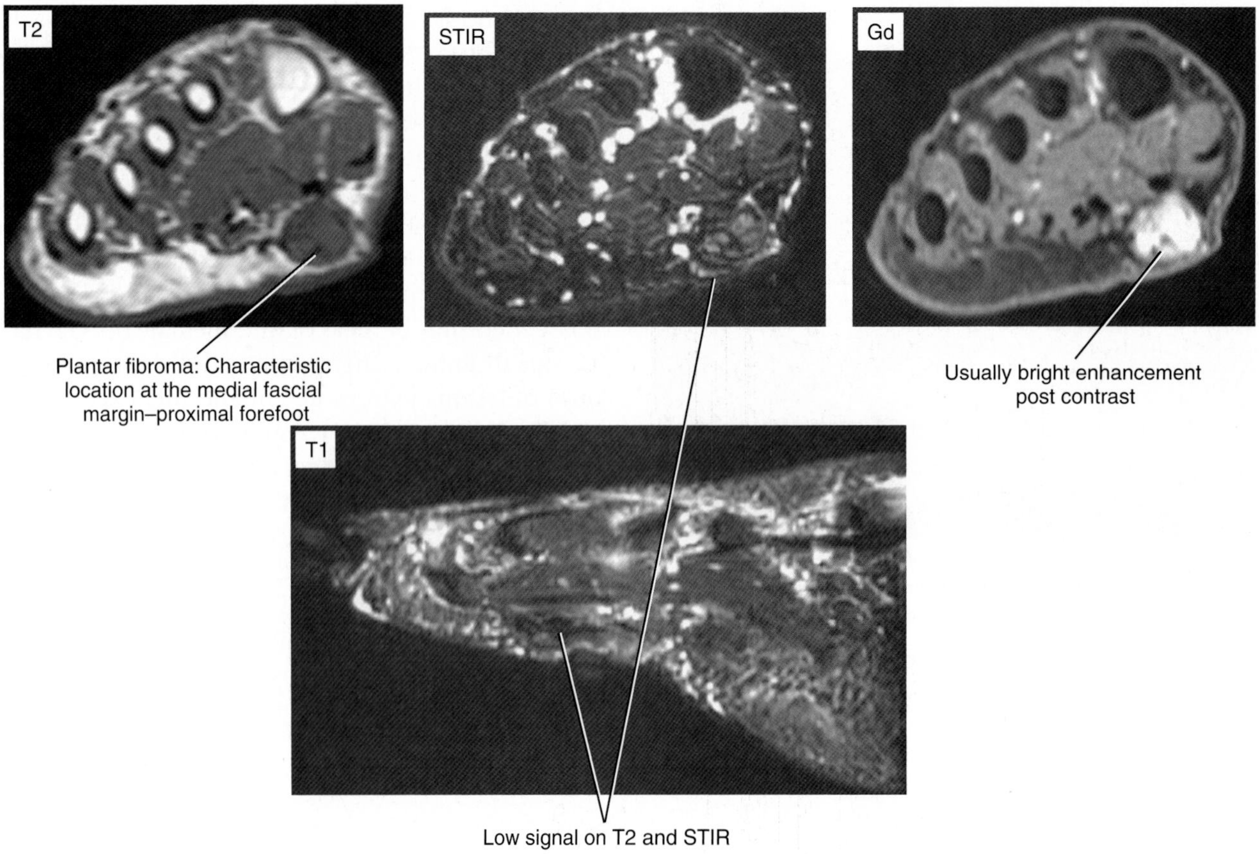
T2
STIR
Gd
Plantar fibroma: Characteristic location at the medial fascial margin–proximal forefoot
Usually bright enhancement post contrast
T1
Low signal on T2 and STIR

Figure 14-45 Plantar fibroma—classic MRI features.

soft tissues tends to be superficial, but occasionally there is deep spread, which is very important to identify. Like fibromatosis elsewhere, lesions can be quite aggressive, ignoring compartmental tissue planes. Deep invasion can result in infiltration of the neurovascular bundles and lead to a need for aggressive surgical management (i.e., amputation).

FOREIGN BODY GRANULOMA

The foot is susceptible to implantation of foreign bodies, especially on the plantar aspect. Most of the time people are aware of the injury, but depending on the size, material, and neurologic status (e.g., diabetes), it may be unrecognized. The material may implant bacteria and generate cellulitis, or incite a sterile inflammatory response (foreign body granuloma). This reactive tissue is intermediate to hyperintense on T2-weighted images and is usually ill defined, unlike a tumor. The edematous region enhances brightly. In the center of this process, the actual foreign body may be obscured. Often contrast assists in detection of a well-defined low signal focus; gradient-echo images are especially useful because the bodies often contain materials that generate magnetic susceptibility artifact (Fig. 14-46).

POSTOPERATIVE APPEARANCES

As mentioned in other chapters, it is helpful to look at a gradient-echo image to detect areas of prior surgery. Based on the location, one can predict the type of surgery. Keep in mind that except for plantar fibroma resection, forefoot surgery is usually performed via a dorsal approach to avoid plantar pain associated with scarring.

Location of Artifact and Common Forefoot Surgeries

Plantar foot—plantar fibroma resection (consider foreign body if no history of surgery)

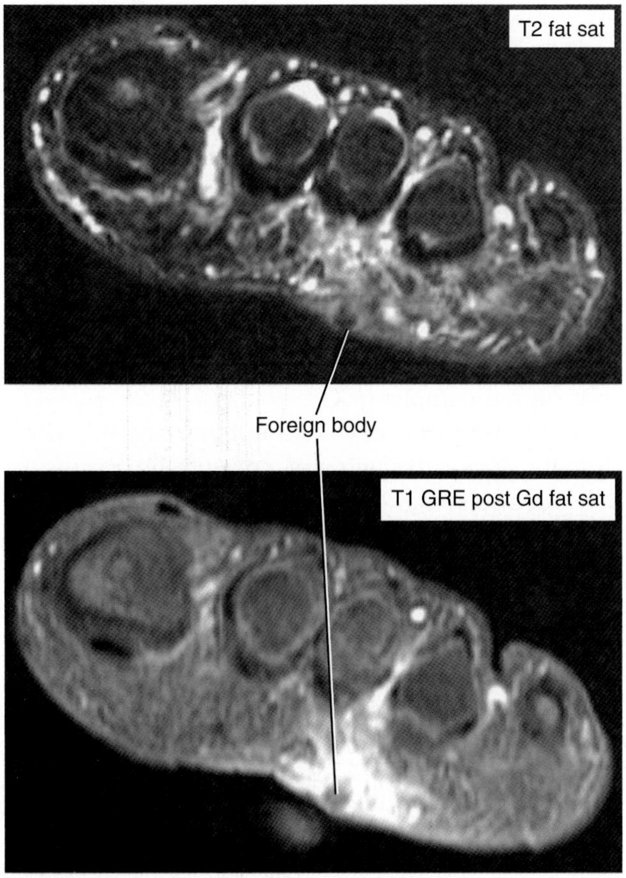
T2 fat sat
Foreign body
T1 GRE post Gd fat sat

Figure 14-46 Foreign body granuloma. Gradient-echo imaging with intravenous contrast can accentuate the foreign body owing to susceptibility artifact, surrounded by enhancing granulation tissue.

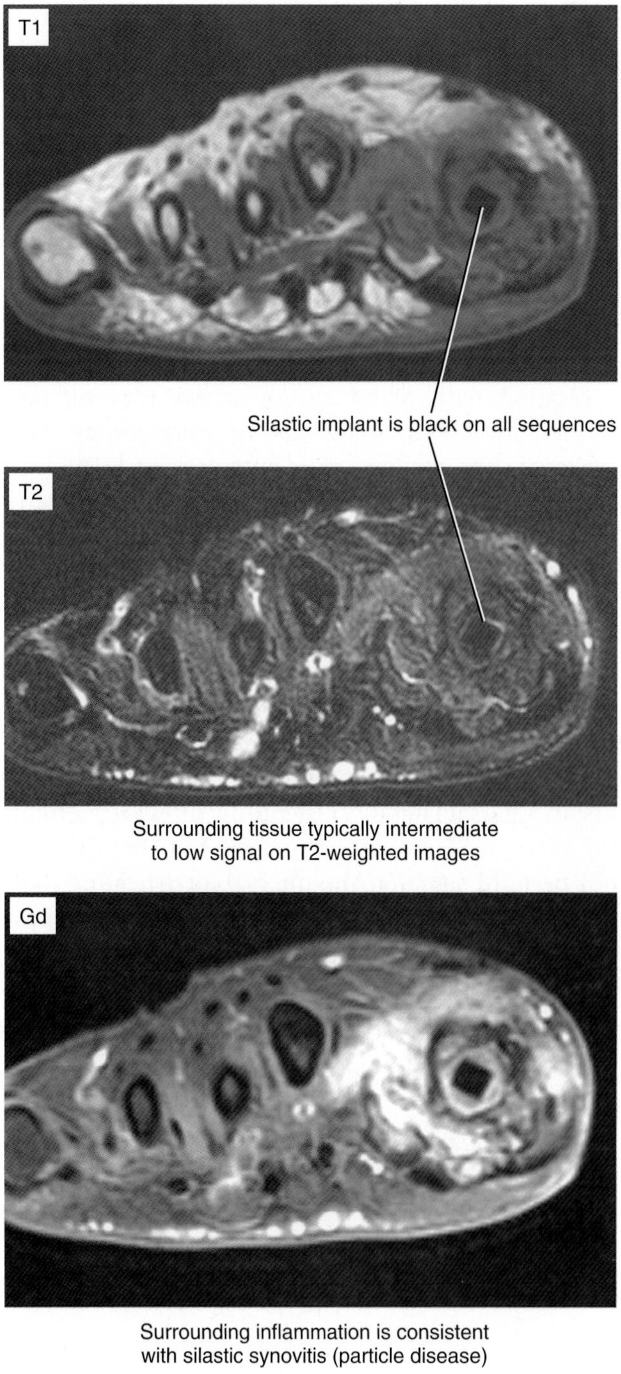
T1
Silastic implant is black on all sequences
T2
Surrounding tissue typically intermediate to low signal on T2-weighted images
Gd
Surrounding inflammation is consistent with silastic synovitis (particle disease)

Figure 14-47 Silastic implant with particle disease.

Medial first metatarsal—bunionectomy
Dorsal first metatarsal—chielectomy (spur removal)
Distal aspect of proximal phalanges—hammertoe repair (resection of the distal aspect of the proximal phalanx)
Between metatarsal heads—Morton neuroma resection
Various locations—tumor resection (check history)

For mass and masslike surgery—such as Morton neuroma, plantar fibroma, and sarcoma—the method for MRI interpretation is very similar. The radiologist should look through the postoperative artifact and scar for any mass effect that could indicate recurrence. Granulation tissue can appear masslike within a few months after surgery but it should become flattened over time. It is very helpful to acquire a baseline postoperative exam 1 or 2 months after surgery for surveillance in cases of sarcoma resection. Contrast is useful for delineating recurrent masses, but scar also enhances. Again, focal mass effect on adjacent structures is an important finding. Alternatively, ultrasound is useful for detection of recurrent mass.

Amputation-type surgeries such as hammertoe repair and amputations related to osteomyelitis generally leave little artifact, and even shortly after surgery the marrow signal should be normal. The abrupt cutoff of the end of the bone with normal marrow can make it difficult to detect minor amputations. In the setting of infection/wound breakdown, any abnormal marrow signal on MRI in the amputated bone should be considered suspicious. However, amputation can also alter weight-bearing, which results in stress response in adjacent bones.

Fixation with plates and/or screws may be performed for fractures, fusions, or osteotomies. This makes it very challenging to interpret on MRI, even with metal artifact-suppression techniques. Therefore, other modalities such as CT may be needed to evaluate the bone next to the metal or to look for fusion under the hardware. One commonly seen osteotomy of the forefoot is hallux valgus repair (see Figs. 14-24 through 14-26). This is performed as a proximal or distal first metatarsal osteotomy, either rotating with a curved osteotomy or shifting with a V-shaped chevron osteotomy the distal aspect of the first metatarsal laterally. Osteotomy lines may remain for years on T1-weighted images, but there should not be fluid signal at the interval after healing. Soft tissue edema and mass effect may be signs of complication such as infection. Bone proliferation on radiographs or CT is also a sign of motion or infection. Always look for lucency around the screws or screws "backing out," indicating loosening and motion. Look for aberrant placement of screws inadvertently across joints. With hallux valgus repair, another potentially devastating complication is avascular necrosis of the first metatarsal head (see Fig. 14-25). This is especially common in distal osteotomies resulting from cutoff of the blood supply that enters through the metaphysis. Look for dark signal on T1-weighted images and lack of enhancement; increased density and later fragmentation may be seen on radiographs or CT.

Silastic (silicone plastic) implants are still occasionally seen, although not commonly because of the osteolysis that often results. Silastic hingelike implants were used to replace the MTP joints (usually the first MTP) in severe arthritis. The implants are faintly radiopaque and can be overlooked on radiographs. On MRI, silastic is black on all sequences with little-to-no artifact, making it very easy to evaluate the tissues surrounding the implant (Fig. 14-47). Granulation tissue representing particle disease, an aggressive granulomatous response, is easily seen on post-contrast MRI as masslike enhancement. On T1-weighted images, the associated osteolysis is seen as loss of marrow fat focally around the implant. Radiographs and CT reveal the osteolysis in later stages, and close observation allows detection of implant fragmentation often associated with complications.

Chapter 15

IMAGING OF MUSCLE

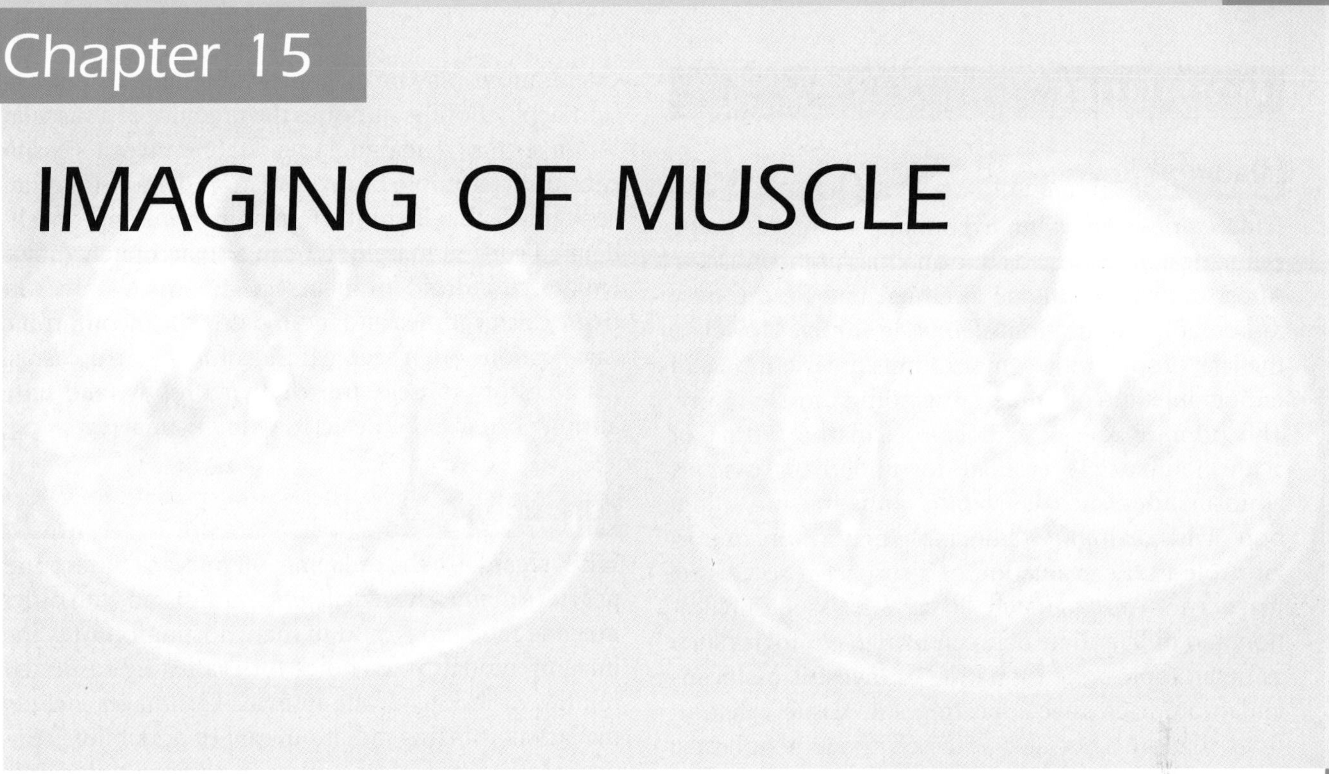

CHAPTER OUTLINE

MODALITIES

Radiography

Radiography plays a limited but important role in the evaluation of suspected abnormalities of the muscles. After trauma, soft tissue swelling may be the only radiographic indication of muscle injury. However, the lack of soft tissue contrast limits the usefulness of radiographs in confirming or grading muscle injury. The primary role of radiography in the setting of acute trauma is to evaluate for underlying osseous abnormalities, such as fracture, stress fracture, and a bony avulsion injury. Radiographs play a more important role in the evaluation of a suspected soft tissue mass. They can accurately detect soft tissue calcification and differentiate between benign etiologies such as heterotopic bone formation or myositis ossificans and more aggressive-appearing soft tissue calcifications that are associated with soft tissue neoplasms. Radiographs can also accurately detect and localize other soft tissue calcifications such as those seen in tumoral calcinosis, postinjection granulomas, dermatomyositis, and scleroderma.

Computed Tomography

Cross-sectional imaging findings of muscle injury were first described using computed tomography (CT), but because of improved soft tissue contrast, ultrasound and MR imaging have largely replaced CT in the evaluation of suspected muscle injury. CT is often used to detect and classify complex fractures; and in these cases the soft tissue should always be evaluated for swelling and indistinctness of fat planes, which can be a sign of associated soft tissue or muscle injury. In addition, CT imaging may demonstrate a small cortical avulsion fracture associated with a musculotendinous abnormality that is not visualized on ultrasound or MR imaging.

CT can be very useful in the evaluation of certain soft tissue masses, such as hematoma and abscess formation. The presence of gas within the soft tissues may be an indication of infection or may be seen following penetrating trauma or surgery. Intravenous contrast improves conspicuity of these lesions. However, if a foreign body is suspected, both pre- and post-contrast images should be obtained because areas of enhancement may mask the detection of a foreign body.

CT demonstrates soft tissue calcifications with greater detail than radiographs, and certain soft tissue calcifications may be diagnostic of lesions. The detection of phleboliths indicates the presence of a vascular lesion such as a hemangioma. Mature myositis ossificans or heterotopic bone formation demonstrates an appearance that is similar to mature bone with a well-defined cortical margin. CT can also accurately differentiate chondroid from osseous matrix within soft tissue calcifications, and it can detect the pleomorphic calcifications often seen within soft tissue neoplasms. An accessory muscle, muscle hypertrophy, and fatty atrophy can also be detected with CT imaging.

Ultrasound

With regard to the imaging of muscle, ultrasound provides many advantages when compared with other imaging modalities, and in many institutions it is the imaging modality of choice for evaluating suspected injuries or lesions of the muscle. Advantages include the lack of ionizing radiation, ease of portability, relatively low cost, and its ability to perform a dynamic examination, whereas the major disadvantage is the significant reliance on operator skill and expertise. Ultrasound provides excellent special resolution, but lacks contrast resolution compared with MRI. As a result, although ultrasound is very accurate in detecting and grading acute muscle injuries, in the subacute and chronic phases of injury as the edema resolves, ultrasound loses its accuracy in the detection and grading of these injuries. Ultrasound is more accurate in the detection of superficial muscle injuries, whereas the deeper structures of the thigh may be difficult to adequately assess. In addition, ultrasound is less accurate in defining underlying osseous abnormalities compared with CT and MR imaging.

Ultrasound is often used in the evaluation of a suspected soft tissue mass, particularly in differentiating a solid from a cystic lesion. Doppler ultrasound can also demonstrate the presence of blood flow indicating the vascularity of an intramuscular lesion. Ultrasound is often used as an adjunct to interventional procedures, guiding aspirations of a suspected intramuscular fluid collection or directing the biopsy of a soft tissue neoplasm. Finally, ultrasound is very accurate in detecting and localizing foreign bodies within the soft tissues.

Magnetic Resonance Imaging

MRI is often considered the imaging modality of choice in the evaluation of a suspected muscle abnormality. This is primarily because of its superior soft tissue contrast, superb spatial resolution, and reproducibility. The standard MRI protocol includes a combination of axial and long axis T1- and T2-weighted images through the area of concern. This combination provides for excellent visualization of both normal compartmental muscle anatomy and for detection of pathologic processes within the muscles. Fat is bright on T1-weighted images, allowing for excellent contrast and depiction of the fat planes against the intermediate signal intensity of normal muscle. T2-weighted images clearly depict the increased water content of most muscle abnormalities, including muscle strain or tear and most soft tissue masses. Fat-saturation techniques or the use of intravenous gadolinium typically increase the conspicuity of lesions.

ANATOMIC VARIATIONS

Anatomic variations of muscle are common and range from complete absence of a specific muscle to hypertrophy and even an accessory muscle. It is also common to identify variations in the attachment, course, and size of a particular muscle. Although these variations are not of themselves pathologic, they occasionally manifest with symptoms such as neurovascular entrapment or post-exercise pain, or even a palpable abnormality mimicking a mass (Fig. 15-1). MRI is particularly well suited to identifying variations in muscular anatomy and can depict the course, size, and shape of a muscle. Accessory muscles can be clearly differentiated from a soft tissue mass and can also be identified as the potential source of neurovascular entrapment (Box 15-1).

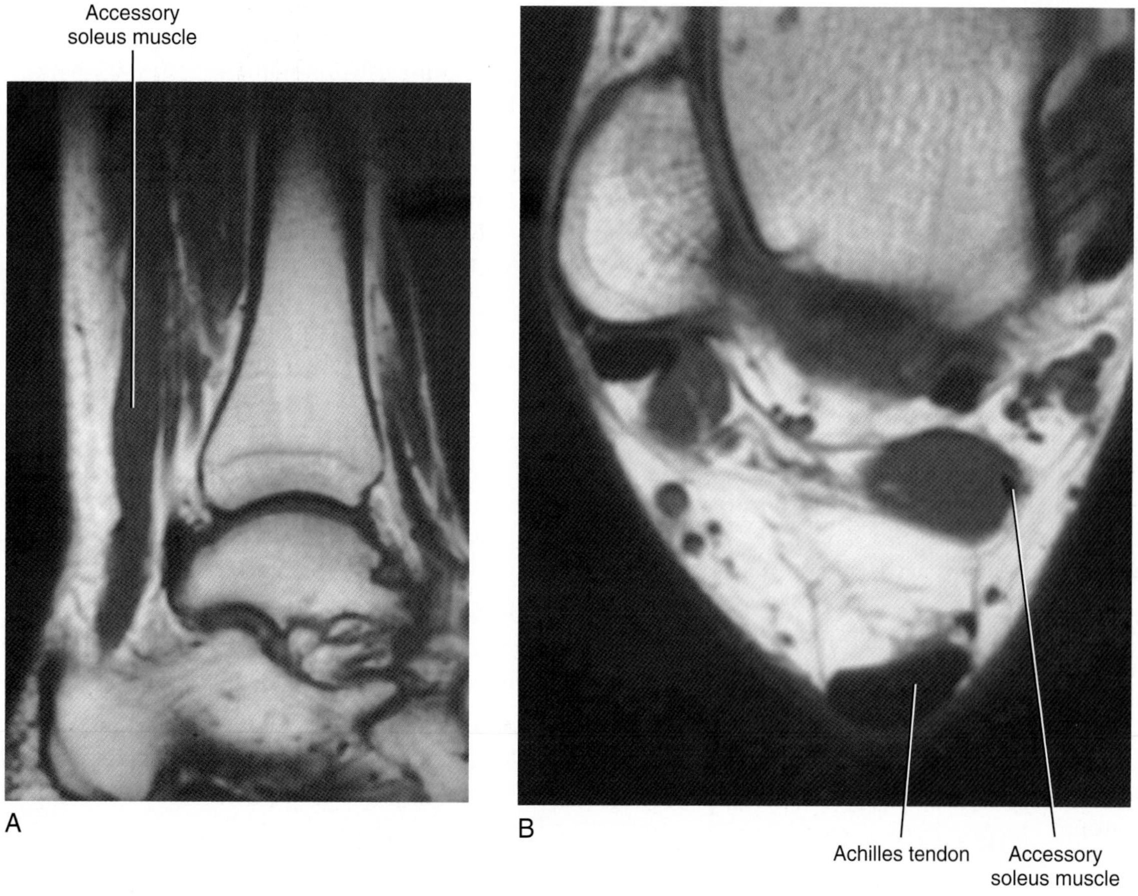
Accessory soleus muscle
A
B
Achilles tendon
Accessory soleus muscle

Figure 15-1 Accessory soleus muscle. Sagittal (**A**) and axial (**B**) T1-weighted images show an accessory soleus muscle located in the posteromedial compartment of the ankle. The location, appearance, and signal characteristics indicate that this represents an accessory muscle rather than a soft tissue mass.

BOX 15-1 ANATOMIC VARIATIONS OF MUSCLES

Upper Extremity Entrapment Syndromes

Thoracic outlet syndrome (anterior scalene syndrome)
- Anterior scalene muscle hypertrophy
- Subclavian artery, brachial plexus (C5-T1)
- Variable upper limb pain, paresthesias, motor dysfunction, and vascular insufficiency

Dorsal scapular nerve syndrome
- Scalene medius muscle hypertrophy
- Dorsal scapular nerve (C5)
- Rhomboid, levator scapulae atrophy

Quadrilateral space
- Muscle hypertrophy (uncommon cause)
- Axillary nerve
- Teres minor, deltoid atrophy

Radial nerve compression
- Anatomic abnormalities of coracobrachialis, long head triceps muscles
- Radial nerve at level of axilla
- All sensory and motor fields of the radial nerve

Cubital tunnel (sulcus ulnaris syndrome)
- Anconeus epitrochlearis (accessory muscle)
- Ulnar nerve
- Paresthesias, atrophy ulnar nerve distribution

Cubital tunnel syndrome
- Anconeus epitrochlearis (accessory) muscle
- Ulnar nerve
- Paresthesias in sensory dermatome ulnar nerve/atrophy late

Pronator teres muscle syndrome
- Two heads of pronator teres muscle, myositis, dynamic compression
- Median nerve
- Motor: Wrist, thenar muscles, finger flexors; paresthesias palm

Anterior interosseous syndrome
- Variations of flexor pollicis longus and flexor digitorum superficialis muscles (uncommon cause)
- Anterior interosseous nerve (motor branch of median nerve)
- Motor: Thumb and index finger; inability to pinch

Carpal tunnel syndrome
- Flexor muscle extending into carpal tunnel (uncommon cause)
- Median nerve
- Paresthesias in median nerve distribution; thenar atrophy

Ulnar tunnel syndrome (Guyon's canal)
- Tendon of fourth digit flexor extending into tunnel
- Ulnar nerve
- Paresthesias in ulnar nerve distribution; hypothenar atrophy

Lower Extremity Entrapment Syndromes

Cutaneous femoris posterior nerve syndrome
- Piriformis muscle hypertrophy or prolonged spasm
- Cutaneous femoris nerve
- Paresthesias in posterior thigh to level of knee

Piriformis muscle syndrome
- Piriformis muscle spasm, inflammation (greater sciatic foramen)
- Sciatic nerve
- L4-5 and L5-S1 distributions

Popliteal entrapment syndrome
- Aberrant origin or accessory head (third head) gastrocnemius muscle; medially placed plantaris joins medial gastrocnemius head
- Popliteal artery and vein (no entrapment of tibial nerve); entrapment, thrombosis, aneurysm
- Intermittent claudication of young active individuals

Peroneal tunnel syndrome
- Herniation of peroneal musculature (uncommon cause)
- Common peroneal nerve
- Pain in common peroneal nerve dermatome; weakness on dorsiflexion/inversion

Tarsal tunnel syndrome
- Accessory flexor longus muscle (uncommon cause)
- Posterior tibialis nerve
- Pain and paresthesias in medial plantar nerve dermatome

Muscles Presenting as a Pseudomass

Palmaris longus—wrist
Accessory soleus muscle—posterior ankle
First dorsal interosseous muscle (hypertrophy)—first dorsal web space

Muscles Mimicking Other Pathology

Peroneus tertius muscle—mimic split peroneus brevis muscle

Absent Muscles

Poland syndrome—absent pectoralis minor and sternal portion of pectoralis major
Palmaris longus

MUSCLE INJURY

Delayed Onset of Muscle Soreness

Delayed onset of muscle soreness (DOMS) describes a condition of muscle pain or soreness that occurs after acute muscle overuse (e.g., weight-lifting or aerobic exercise) and is usually self-limiting. The soreness typically begins within 2 to 3 hours of the activity and peaks at 2 to 3 days. The pain is centered at the myotendinous junction, and the muscle damage is at the ultra-structural level and is reversible. Although it is unusual to image a person because of DOMS, it is possible that a person may demonstrate MR findings associated with DOMS while being imaged for other reasons. The MR findings of DOMS are nonspecific and show areas of increased T2 signal within the involved musculature, occasionally mimicking a low-grade muscle strain (Fig. 15-2). Abnormal T2 signal has been shown to persist for up to 3 weeks after resolution of symptoms, and differentiation between DOMS and a grade I muscle strain requires close correlation with the clinical history and presentation.

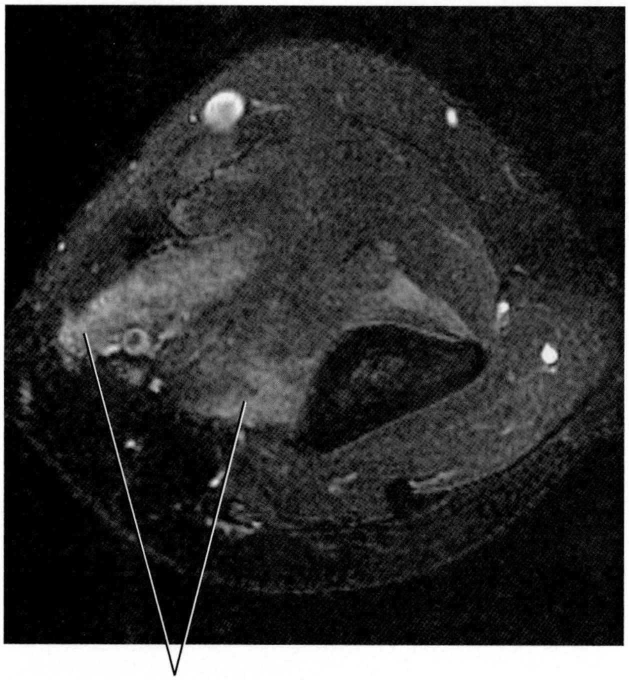
Areas of edema within the biceps and brachialis muscles representing changes associated with DOMS

Figure 15-2 Delayed onset of muscle soreness (DOMS). Axial T2-weighted image with fat saturation through the level of the mid forearm shows areas of edema involving the biceps and brachialis muscles associated with recent weight-lifting representing reversible changes of DOMS.

Acute Myotendinous Injury

Acute myotendinous injuries occur when the load placed on the myotendinous unit exceeds the tensile strength of the unit. Injury typically occurs during eccentric contraction (contraction that occurs while the muscle is lengthening) and often involves a muscle that crosses two joints, such as the rectus femoris, gastrocnemius, and sartorius. Onset of pain is acute at the time of activity (unlike DOMS, in which the pain begins 2 to 3 hours after the activity). The location of injury within the myotendinous unit is age-related, with the "weak link" of the unit changing as an individual ages (Box 15-2).

Apophyseal avulsion injuries typically occur in adolescent athletes (e.g., sprinters, long jumpers, cheerleaders, hurdlers, gymnasts) and result from violent muscular contractions. They are equivalent to a muscle pull in the mature athlete and most commonly occur in locations about the pelvis (Fig. 15-3). The elbow is another common location of apophyseal injury, often occurring in adolescent throwers (Fig. 15-4). Radiographs are usually sufficient to establish the diagnosis of an apophyseal avulsion injury when a cortical bone fragment is avulsed along with the tendon (Fig. 15-5). Occasionally, the tendon may avulse without an associated bone fragment, in which case MRI or ultrasound may be required to fully assess the extent of injury (Fig. 15-6; see also Fig. 15-4B). On MR imaging, a cortical avulsion fragment appears as a low-signal curvilinear structure on both T1- and T2-weighted images. Detection of the cortical avulsion fragment may be difficult because it is attached to the avulsed tendon, which also demonstrates low signal. A gradient-echo sequence or T1 sequence without fat saturation may be the most useful in detecting a small cortical avulsion fragment. After a complete avulsion, retraction of the torn

BOX 15-2 ACUTE MYOTENDINOUS UNIT INJURY AS IT RELATES TO AGE

Apophyseal injuries: Adolescents
Myotendinous injuries: Young adults <40 years of age
Tendinous injuries: Older adults >40 years of age

SECTION IV

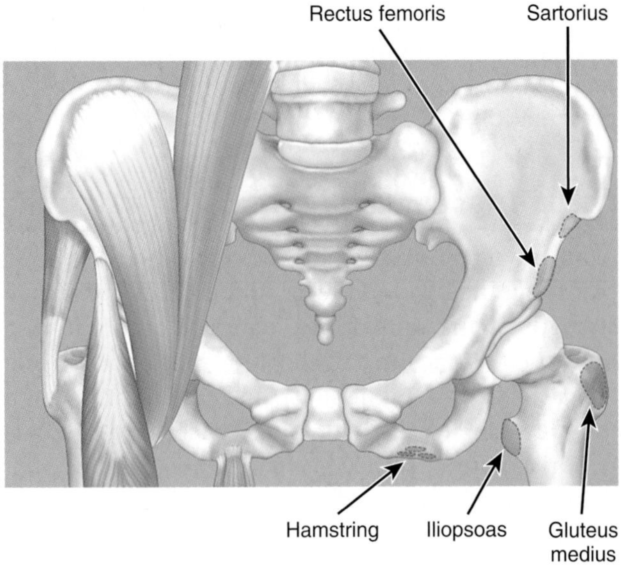
Rectus femoris
Sartorius
Hamstring
Iliopsoas
Gluteus medius

Figure 15-3 Muscle attachment sites in the region of the pelvis indicating the most common location of apophyseal avulsion injuries.

Table 15-1 Tendon Attachment Sites Around the Pelvis

Muscle	Attachment Site
Sartorius	Anterior superior iliac spine
Rectus femoris	Anterior inferior iliac spine
Hamstrings	Ischial tuberosity
Gluteus medius	Greater trochanter
Iliopsoas	Lesser trochanter
Gracilis	Inferior pubic ramus

tendon and adjacent osseous and soft tissue edema are often present. Although avulsion injuries can occur at nearly any location where a tendon attaches to bone, most apophyseal avulsion injuries in the adolescent patient occur in the pelvis, and knowledge of the specific attachment sites of various tendons can help establish the correct diagnosis (Table 15-1).

Two separate avulsion injuries deserve special caution. First, an avulsion fracture of the ischial tuberosity (hamstring origin) can result in a large displaced osseous fragment, which often results in extensive callous formation during the healing phase, thus mimicking an aggressive bone lesion (see Fig. 15-5C). The location of the abnormality should alert one to the possibility of a post-traumatic injury rather

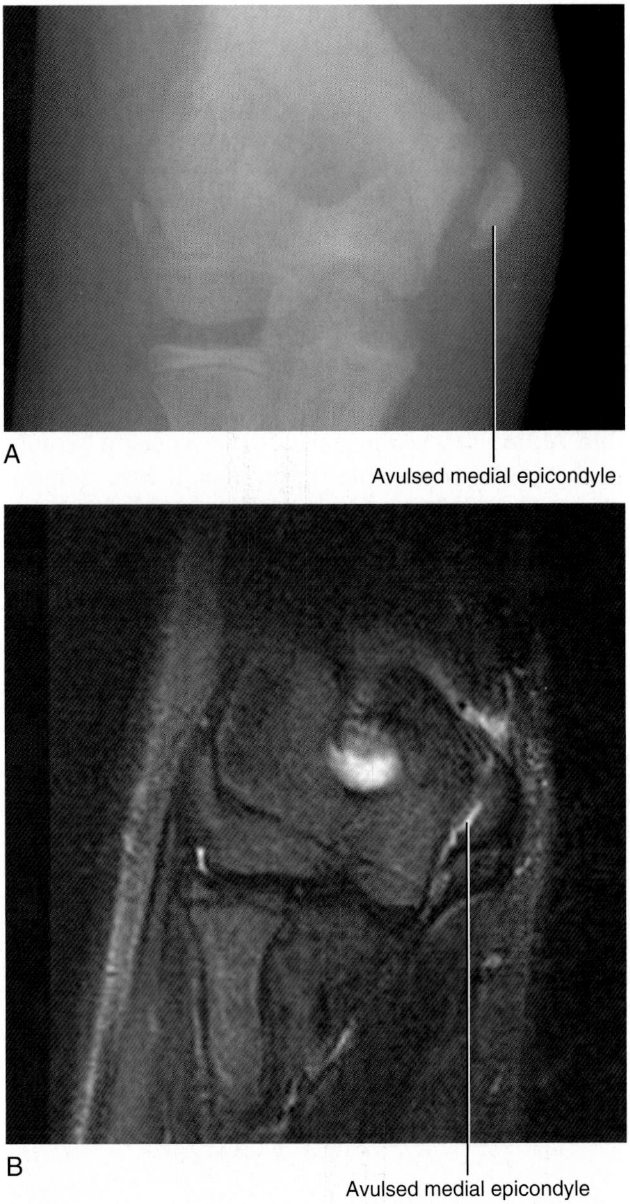
A
Avulsed medial epicondyle
B
Avulsed medial epicondyle

Figure 15-4 Avulsion injury of the medial epicondyle. A, Anteroposterior (AP) radiograph of the elbow demonstrates a displaced avulsion fracture of the medial epicondyle in an adolescent pitcher. The fragment is displaced, and there is overlying soft tissue swelling and associated medial elbow pain. **B,** Coronal T2-weighted image with fat saturation shows a nondisplaced avulsion injury of the medial epicondyle in a different adolescent pitcher. There is fluid within the apophyseal growth plate, indicating a Salter type I injury of the medial epicondyle.

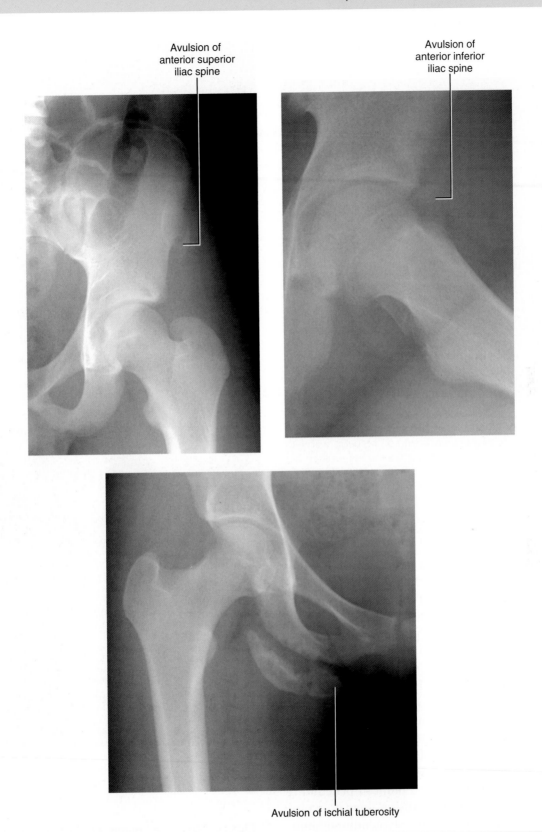

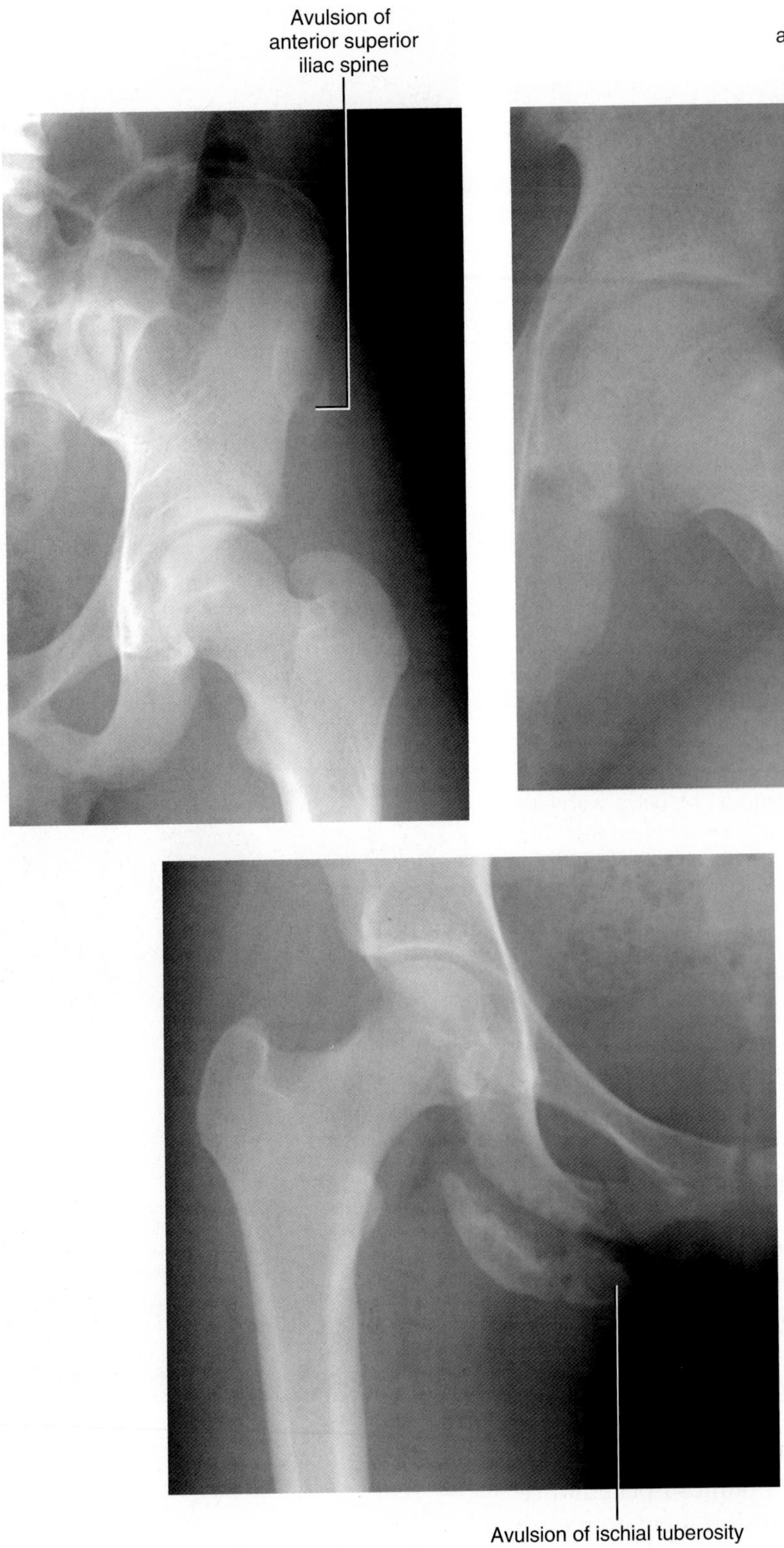
Avulsion of anterior superior iliac spine
Avulsion of anterior inferior iliac spine
Avulsion of ischial tuberosity

Figure 15-5 Osseous avulsion injuries at the typical location of tendon attachment sites.

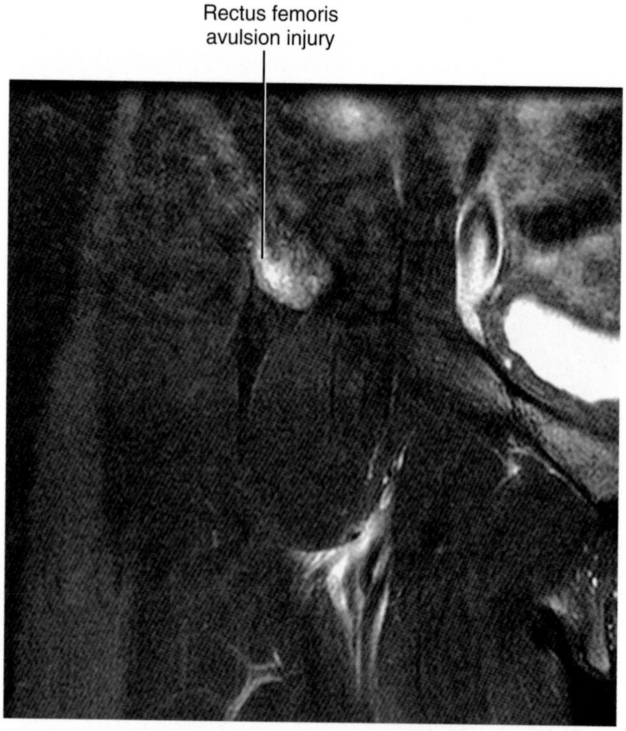
Rectus femoris
avulsion injury

Figure 15-6 Avulsion of the rectus femoris tendon. T2-weighted coronal image of the pelvis with fat saturation shows a high-grade partial-thickness avulsion of the rectus femoris tendon from the anterior inferior iliac spine. There is no cortical disruption, and the radiographs of the pelvis were normal.

than a neoplastic process. The second avulsion injury deserving special attention is that of an avulsion fracture of the lesser tuberosity of the proximal femur in an adult. An avulsion fracture in this lesion should be considered pathologic until proven otherwise because this is a very common location for metastatic disease (Fig. 15-7). An avulsion injury of the lesser tuberosity in the adolescent, however, is not usually associated with underlying bone pathology.

Acute muscle injuries are most common in young adults under 40 years of age and can be broadly subdivided into two basic types of injury: *muscle belly* and *myotendinous junction*. Muscle belly injuries most commonly are caused by direct blunt or penetrating trauma and may result in contusion, hematoma, or laceration of the muscle belly. Myotendinous injuries, on the other hand, result from the indirect forces exerted during sudden eccentric contraction of the muscle. Chronic repetitive stress-related overload of the muscle may also result in injury to the myotendinous junction. Muscle injuries are graded on a

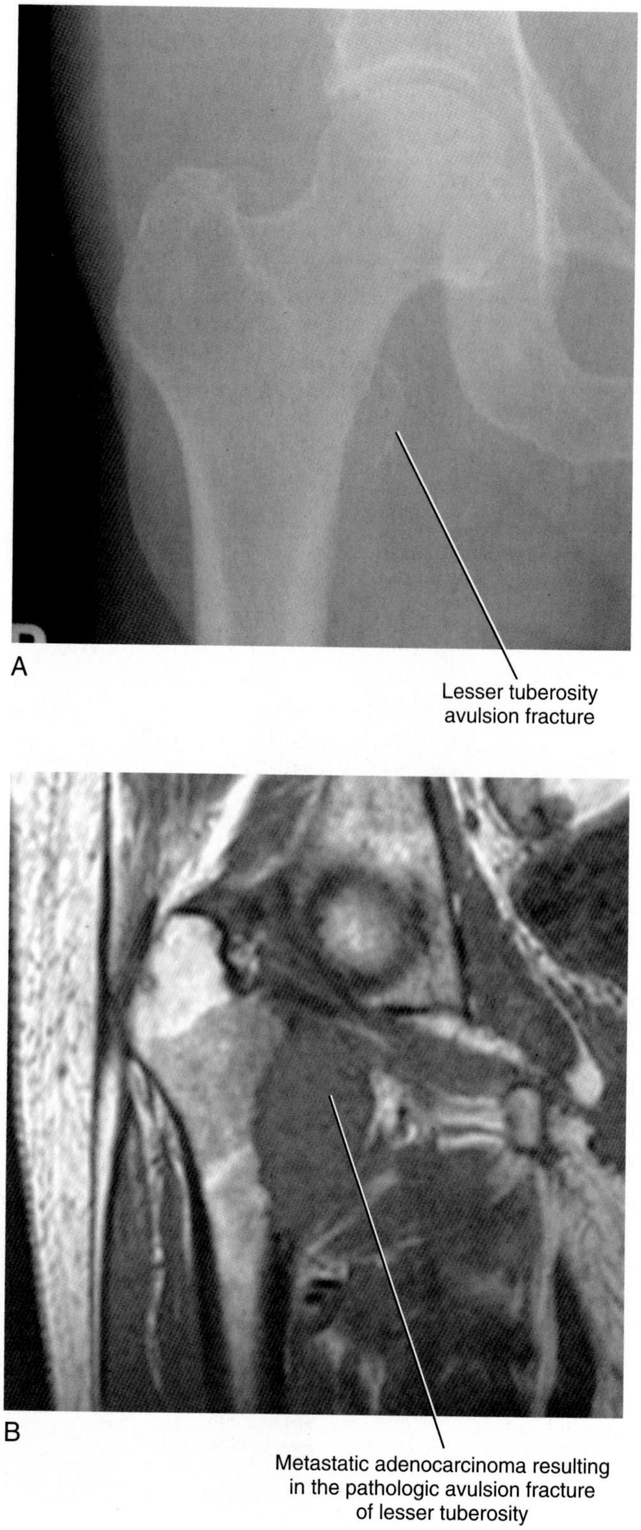
A
Lesser tuberosity
avulsion fracture
B
Metastatic adenocarcinoma resulting
in the pathologic avulsion fracture
of lesser tuberosity

Figure 15-7 Pathologic avulsion fracture of the lesser trochanter. A, Radiograph shows a minimally displaced avulsion fracture of the lesser tuberosity. **B,** Coronal T1-weighted image reveals a mass in the region of the lesser trochanter that was shown to be metastatic adenocarcinoma.

Table 15-2 Grading Scale of Acute Muscle Injury

Grade	Injury	MR Appearance	Clinical Significance
1	Strain	Feathery edema at musculotendinous junction	Pain, but no risk for propagation of injury
2	Partial tear	Feathery edema along musculotendinous junction with some disruption of fibers; intramuscular hematoma common	Pain, decreased strength, and risk for propagation of injury
3	Complete tear	Complete disruption and retraction of myotendinous unit; retracted muscle may present as palpable mass	Pain, decreased strength; often requires surgical repair

three-point scale (Table 15-2). MR imaging can be used to accurately grade acute muscle injury, which in turn can be helpful in guiding appropriate treatment and in predicting whether the individual is at risk for progression of the muscle injury (Fig. 15-8). A complete full-thickness muscle tear with musculotendinous retraction (grade III injury) requires surgical repair to prevent rapid-onset irreversible fatty atrophy of the involved muscle (Fig. 15-9).

Injuries isolated to the tendon most commonly occur in patients over 40 years of age and in most instances are related to weakening of the tendon that occurs with chronic overuse and aging. Injuries in this category include tears of the rotator cuff, Achilles tendon, or quadriceps tendon. These injuries are covered in detail under their respective joint chapters.

Muscle Hemorrhage

There are several potential causes of intramuscular hemorrhage. The most common is trauma associated with either a contusion or myotendinous junction injury. Other less common etiologies include bleeding diathesis and anticoagulation therapy. A spontaneous intramuscular hematoma in an individual without a history of trauma or risk factors for bleeding should prompt a thorough search for an underlying soft tissue neoplasm. Intramuscular hemorrhage can be described as either focal or diffuse. Focal bleeding results in an intramuscular hematoma, whereas diffuse bleeding results in an imaging appearance similar to that of intramuscular edema. Both MRI and ultrasound can accurately determine the size and location of a soft tissue hematoma and may help determine whether aspiration is necessary to prevent compartment syndrome.

The MRI appearance of an intramuscular hematoma is variable depending on the age of the bleed. In the acute setting (within the first 24 to 48 hours), a hematoma is usually isointense to muscle on T1-weighted images and bright on T2-weighted images. The subacute hematoma (longer than 48 hours) often appears mixed or heterogeneous with areas of bright T1 signal secondary to increased levels of methemoglobin. This MR appearance can persist for several weeks to months, and most intramuscular hematomas are imaged during this time period. The typical MR appearance of a heterogeneous mass with areas of mixed increased T1 signal combined with the history of recent trauma is usually diagnostic of an intramuscular hematoma (Fig. 15-10). Finally, in the chronic stages of an intramuscular hematoma, resorption of the blood products may lead to the formation of a seroma, which will demonstrate low T1 and bright T2 signal. At this stage, there may also be a low signal intensity rim, indicating the presence of hemosiderin. This low signal intensity ring may be accentuated (blooming artifact) by the use of gradient-echo imaging.

Myositis Ossificans

Myositis ossificans is a benign lesion of heterotopic bone formation that occurs in the soft tissues and is found most frequently in young athletes who participate in contact sports such as football and rugby. A significant number of patients may have no history of direct trauma. Myositis ossificans can also occur in patients with debilitating diseases such as poliomyelitis and paraplegia and in those with conditions that demonstrate a propensity for bone formation such as diffuse idiopathic skeletal hyperostosis. Numerous other terms have been used to describe myositis ossificans, such as heterotopic ossificans, myositis ossificans circumscripta, and ossifying hematoma.

The individual typically presents with a painful tender mass in the region of the upper arm or thigh with a history of direct trauma to the area. Although

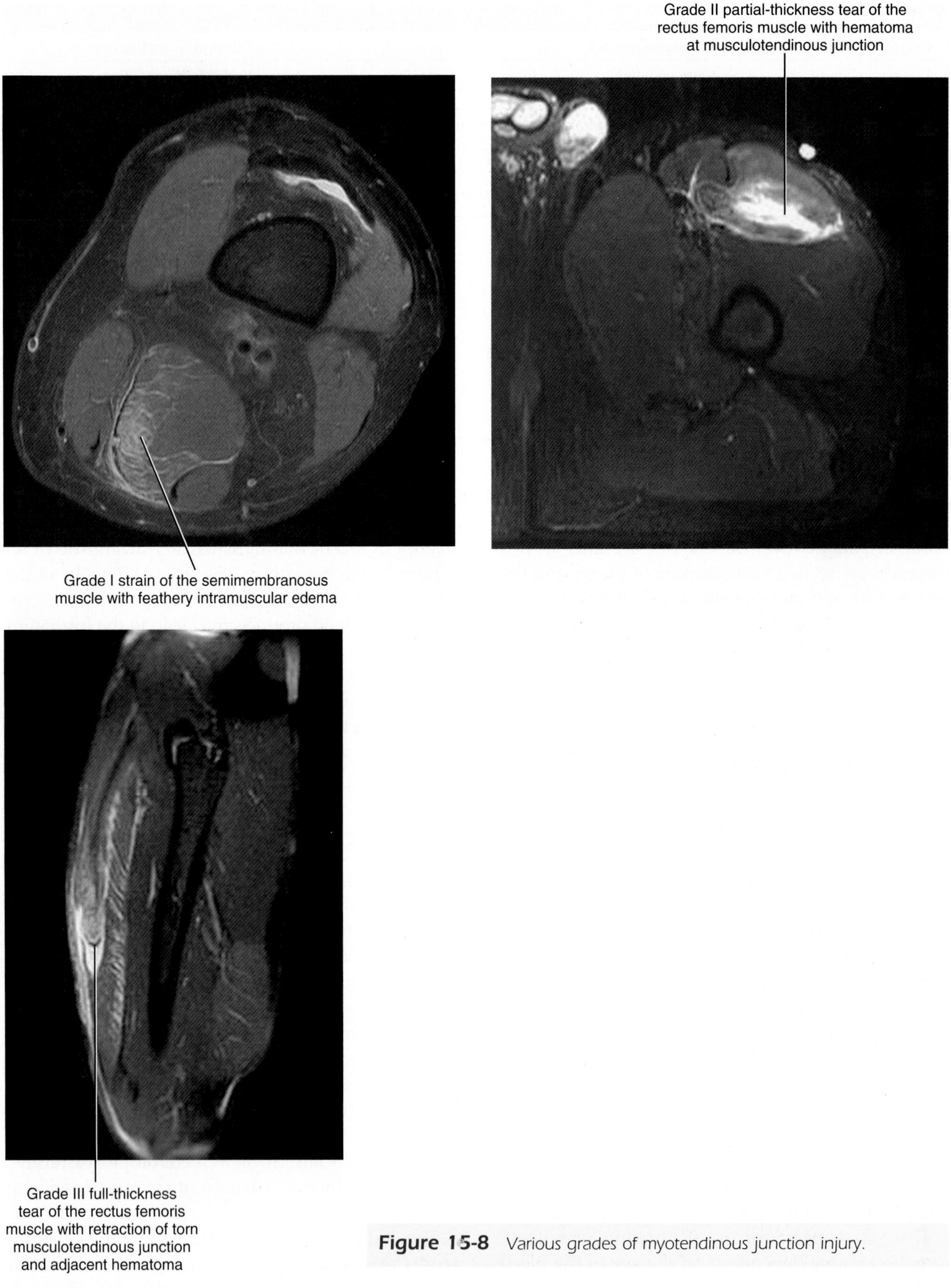
Grade II partial-thickness tear of the rectus femoris muscle with hematoma at musculotendinous junction
Grade I strain of the semimembranosus muscle with feathery intramuscular edema
Grade III full-thickness tear of the rectus femoris muscle with retraction of torn musculotendinous junction and adjacent hematoma

Figure 15-8 *Various grades of myotendinous junction injury.*

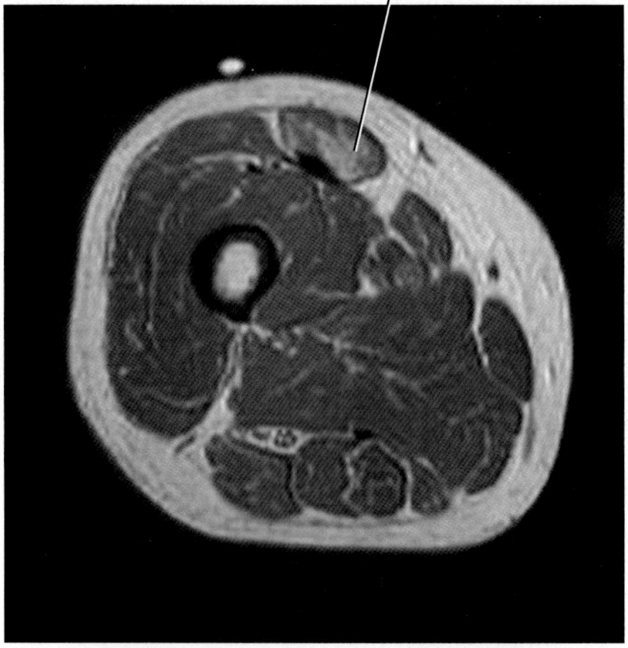
Fatty atrophy or rectus femoris muscle
as a sequela of old Grade III muscle injury

A

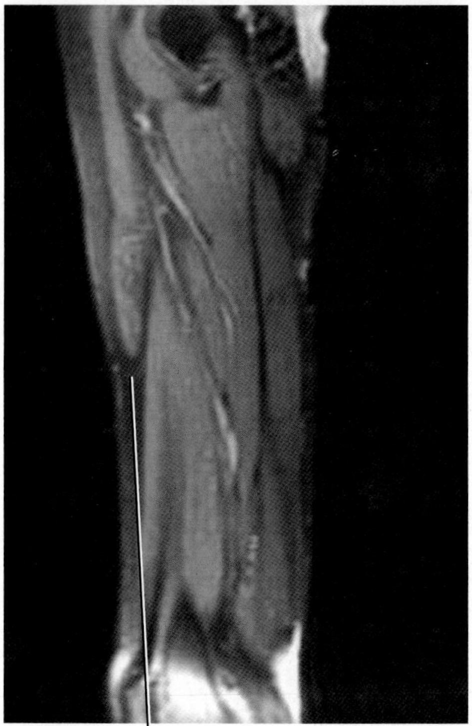
Old Grade III rectus femoris
muscle injury with
retraction and fatty atrophy

B

Figure 15-9 Chronic grade III tear of the rectus femoris muscle with axial T1-weighted images (**A**) shows fatty atrophy of the muscle, and sagittal T2-weighted image (**B**) shows chronic retraction of the muscle.

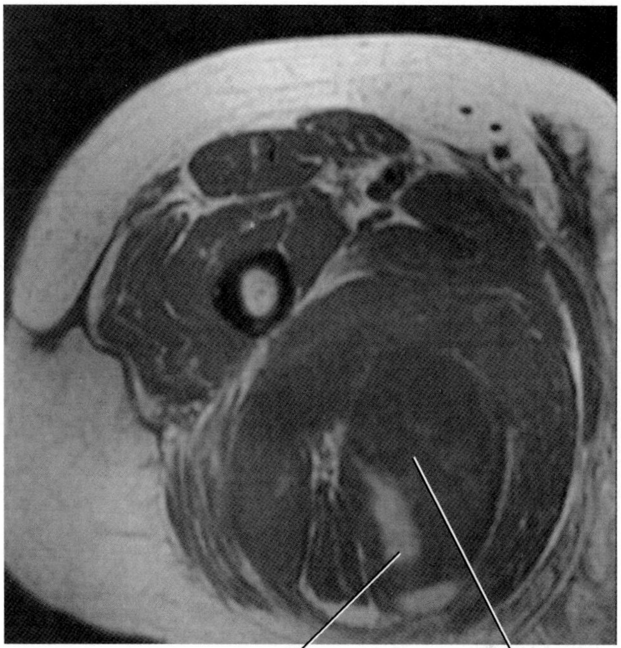
Bright T1 signal indicating
areas of methemoglobin
Intramuscular
hematoma

Figure 15-10 Intramuscular hematoma. Axial T1-weighted image shows a complex mass within the posterior musculature of the thigh in a patient on anticoagulation therapy. The mass shows focal areas of bright T1 signal representing methemoglobin.

the majority of lesions are located within skeletal muscle, they can also present in a periosteal or parosteal location. The most common diagnostic difficulty is distinguishing myositis ossificans from a soft tissue sarcoma; depending on the specific imaging characteristics, differential diagnosis may include synovial cell sarcoma, periosteal sarcoma, parosteal sarcoma, osteochondroma, and juxtacortical chondroma. During the acute phase of injury, infection (pyomyositis) may also be a diagnostic consideration.

The imaging appearance of myositis ossificans evolves over time, reflecting the changing histopathology of the injured soft tissues. During the acute phase following an insult to the muscle, inflammatory cells including fibroblasts and osteoblasts infiltrate the area and give rise to a painful soft tissue mass. Osteoblasts then begin to lay down osteoid, which over time gives rise to the zonal phenomenon of mature cortical bone.

Radiographs may demonstrate soft tissue swelling, but are otherwise negative during the first 2 to 3 weeks of symptomatology. During this acute phase, MRI demonstrates an ill-defined soft tissue mass with increased T2 signal with surrounding soft tissue edema. T1 signal is usually isointense to muscle, but may be variable because of the presence of blood products. At about 2 to 3 weeks after onset of symptoms, radiographs begin to demonstrate faint peripheral calcifications, which are better depicted on CT imaging (Fig. 15-11). During this subacute phase of myositis ossificans, MRI imaging shows variable internal signal on both T1 and T2 with early rim calcification and rim enhancement after administration of intravenous gadolinium. Dense peripheral calcification is usually visible by 6 to 8 weeks and progresses to mature bone formation by 4 to 6 months. CT imaging can nicely depict the zonal phenomenon of mature osteoid. The mature lesion demonstrates a well-demarcated mass with a low signal intensity rim on MRI (Fig. 15-12).

Early symptomatic lesions are treated with ice packs, rest, and nonsteroidal anti-inflammatories. Excision during the acute phase may result in aggressive recurrence, resulting in more extensive involvement of the soft tissues and ensuing long-term disability. If symptoms persist after complete maturation of the heterotopic bone, then surgical excision is recommended. The primary use of bone scintigraphy is to determine the maturity of myositis ossificans for purposes of surgical excision. Once the lesion completes maturation and has been stable for 6 months, the risk of recurrence after excision becomes minimal, and bone scan at this stage will demonstrate uptake similar to that of adjacent bone.

It is critical to differentiate myositis ossificans from a soft tissue sarcoma on the basis of clinical and imaging criteria, because biopsy of the cellular portion of myositis ossificans closely resembles osteogenic sarcoma histologically and can result in an erroneous diagnosis. Early resection also increases the risk of recurrence and long-term disability. Differentiation can usually be made between myositis ossificans and a soft tissue neoplasm on the following basis: Myositis ossificans most often presents in a young athletic individual with a history of trauma to the area. With myositis ossificans, the pain and mass usually decrease over time, whereas both increase over time in a soft tissue neoplasm. Myositis ossificans most frequently overlies the diaphyseal region of the bone, whereas osteogenic sarcoma usually overlies the metaphyseal region of the bone. With myositis ossificans, imaging shows early peripheral calcification that progresses to mature osteoid over time, whereas calcification within a soft tissue sarcoma demonstrates a pleomorphic appearance that is dense centrally rather than peripherally. If myositis ossificans is considered in the differential diagnosis, then close clinical and imaging follow-up (repeat imaging in 2 to 3 weeks) with the above criteria in mind, rather than biopsy, is recommended.

Compartment Syndrome

Compartment syndrome has been defined as a condition in which increased tissue pressure within a closed fascial space compromises the local circulation and leads to compromised neuromuscular function. Compartment syndrome can occur in any closed fascial space of the upper or lower extremity, but most often occurs in the leg as the result of trauma. It may be acute or chronic. The syndrome is usually first suspected on the basis of clinical presentation. For example, the individual typically presents with pain out of proportion to the physical examination, swelling and tension in the compartment, and pain with passive stretching. Pulselessness is a late sign of compartment syndrome that may not occur. Compartmental pressure of more than 30 mm Hg is diagnostic of compartment syndrome.

Acute compartment syndrome most often results from trauma and is most frequently seen in the lower leg after tibial fracture. Other potential causes are crush injury, hematoma, vascular injury, circumferential burns, and infection. Although compartment pressure measurements are the gold standard for diagnosing compartment syndrome, MRI may play a helpful role in the evaluation of atypical cases and in precisely defining the extent and location of abnormality. MR imaging demonstrates diffuse increased T2 signal within the muscles of the involved compartment along with mild swelling of the muscles within the involved compartment (Fig. 15-13). The underlying cause of compartment syndrome may also be obvious on MRI and includes fracture, hematoma, or evidence of concurrent infection and abscess formation.

Chronic compartment syndrome has also been described as *exercise-induced compartment syndrome.* The exact pathophysiology is unclear but appears to be related to muscle hypertrophy and overexertion. Chronic compartment syndrome occurs most often in runners, and the typical clinical presentation is one of an asymptomatic patient in the off season with

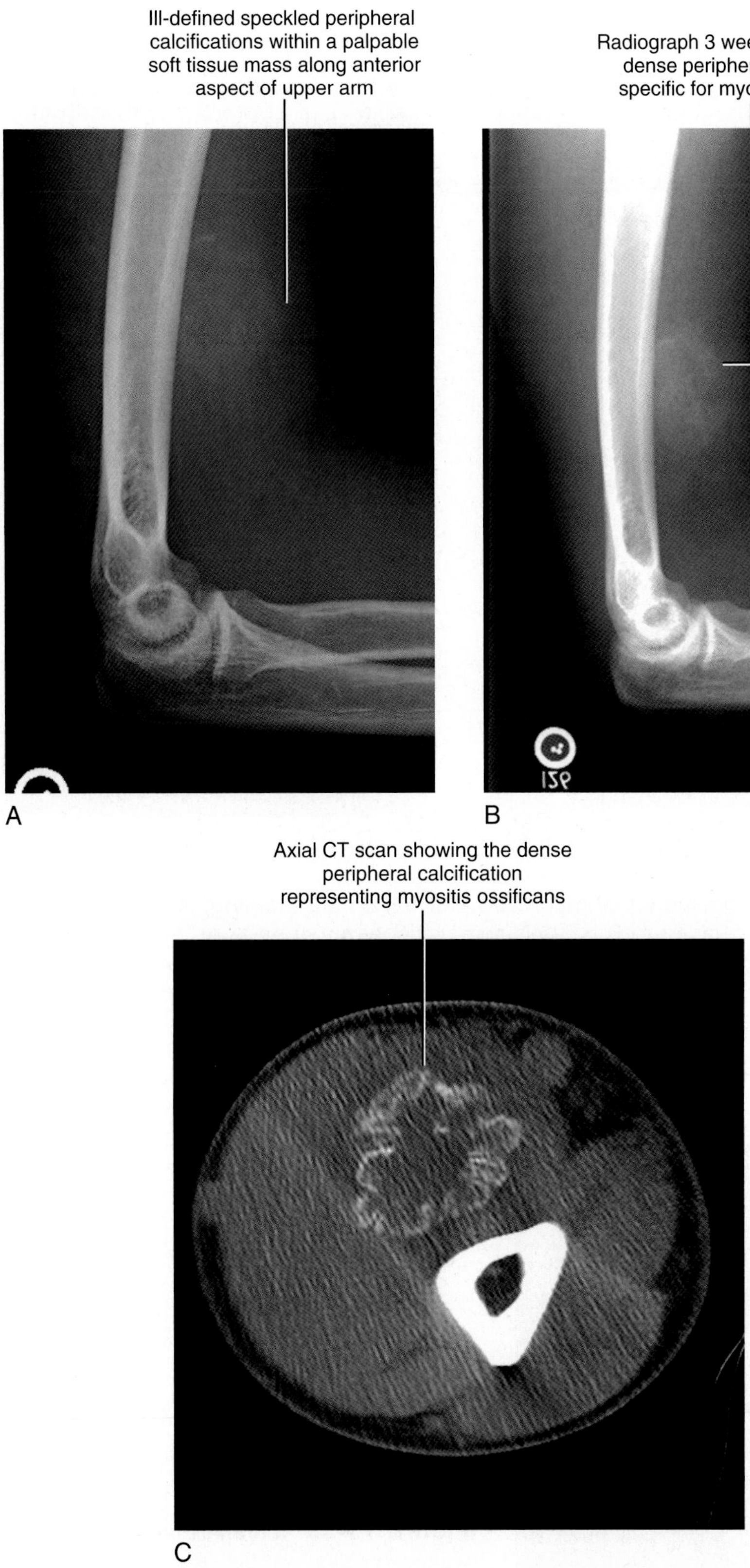
Ill-defined speckled peripheral calcifications within a palpable soft tissue mass along anterior aspect of upper arm
Radiograph 3 weeks later showing dense peripheral calcification specific for myositis ossificans
A
B
Axial CT scan showing the dense peripheral calcification representing myositis ossificans
C

Figure 15-11 Progressive appearance of myositis ossificans on radiographs and CT. Lateral radiograph (**A**) shows speckled peripheral calcifications, whereas a radiograph 3 weeks later (**B**) reveals dense peripheral calcification representing maturing myositis ossificans. **C,** Axial CT examination shows the dense peripheral rim of calcification, which is specific for myositis ossificans.

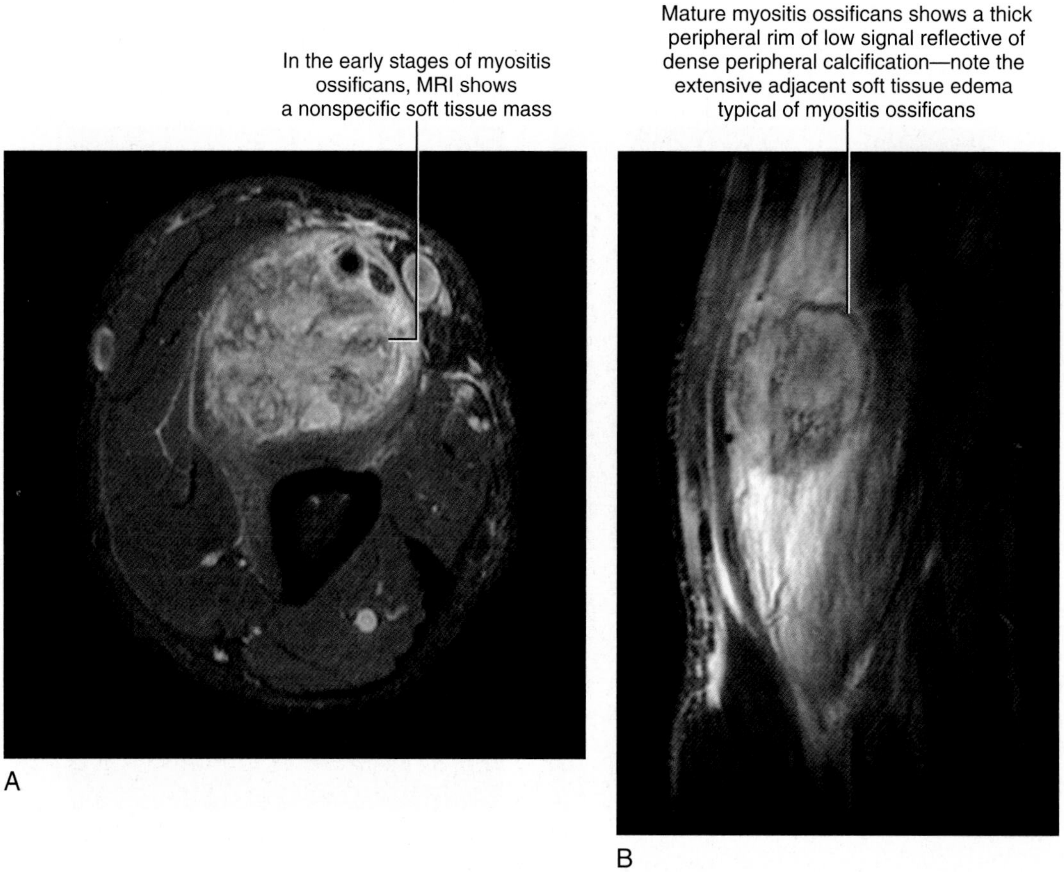
In the early stages of myositis ossificans, MRI shows a nonspecific soft tissue mass
Mature myositis ossificans shows a thick peripheral rim of low signal reflective of dense peripheral calcification—note the extensive adjacent soft tissue edema typical of myositis ossificans
A
B

Figure 15-12 Progressive appearance of myositis ossificans on MR imaging. A, Axial T2-weighted image with fat saturation shows a nonspecific soft tissue mass within the anterior aspect of the upper arm. **B,** Coronal T2-weighted image with fat saturation approximately 3 weeks after the initial MR study shows a thick rim of peripheral low signal representing dense peripheral calcification. This finding is specific for myositis ossificans.

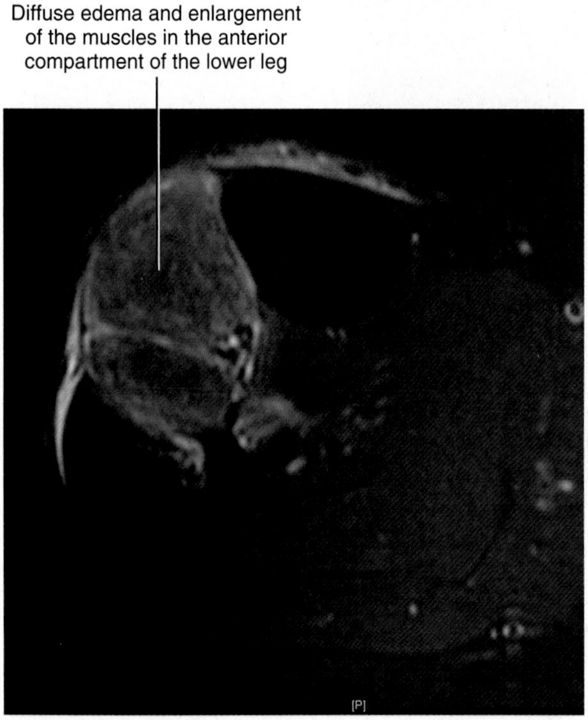
Diffuse edema and enlargement of the muscles in the anterior compartment of the lower leg
[P]

Figure 15-13 Compartment syndrome. Axial T2-weighted image with fat saturation shows diffuse swelling and edema involving all the muscles of the anterior compartment of the lower leg. The patient was a 22-year-old soccer player who presented with anterior leg pain 2 hours after a game. Surgery revealed gray, poorly perfused musculature of the anterior compartment.

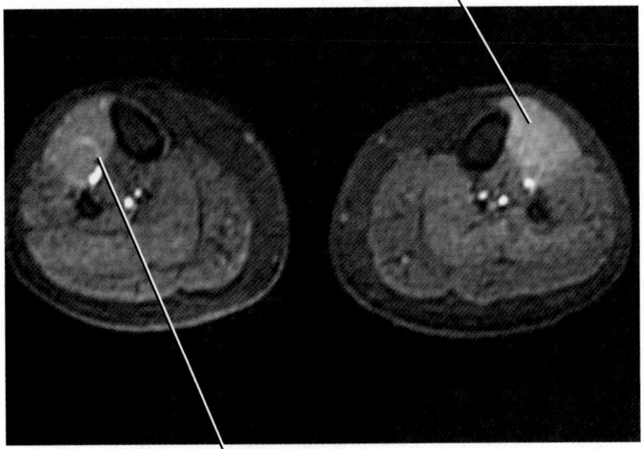
Minimal edema and swelling
of anterior compartment in
a patient with exercise-induced
compartment syndrome
Similar but milder changes
noted in the anterior compartment
of the contralateral leg

Figure 15-14 Exercise-induced compartment syndrome. T1-weighted post-gadolinium images with fat saturation demonstrate enhancement and mild swelling of the anterior compartment musculature. Enhancement is due to recovery phase. Pain and swelling were exacerbated in this patient by long-distance running.

pain gradually increasing during the running season. The pain is described as an aching sensation that begins while running and as the training progresses, the symptoms may persist for up to a day after activity. Clinical diagnosis is confirmed when pre-exercise pressure measurements are less than 15 mm Hg, 1-minute postexercise pressure is more than 30 mm Hg, and 5-minute postexercise pressure still exceeds 20 mm Hg. MRI findings parallel the clinical course in chronic compartment syndrome, demonstrating increased T2 signal and increased muscle girth in the involved compartment (Fig. 15-14). The findings are more significant in the immediate postexercise period. Chronic findings may include muscle atrophy and loss of muscle bulk, fibrosis, and even mature myositis ossificans in the affected compartment.

Muscle Herniation

Muscle herniation is a condition in which muscle herniates through a fascial defect. This is typically post-traumatic in origin and often occurs as the result of a rent in the fascial tissues allowing herniation of muscle through the defect. Fascial herniations of muscle usually occur in the region of the calf or thigh and often occur after blunt trauma to the affected area. The patient may present with a focal palpable mass that is intermittent and usually more noticeable during exercise. The herniation may result in focal pain, but it is often asymptomatic. When symptomatic, the pain is usually induced or exacerbated by exercise. The diagnosis is often made on the basis of history and clinical examination, but when imaging is required, MRI is the most sensitive imaging modality to correctly establish the diagnosis. MRI can reveal a focal area of muscle protruding through a defect in the overlying fascia. Because the herniation is often intermittent, MRI may be normal and demonstrate no evidence of herniation. When this occurs, repeat MR scanning with the patient contracting the suspected muscle may result in a positive MRI finding. However, this can be technically difficult and often leads to significant motion artifact. MRI usually fails to demonstrate the fascial defect unless muscle is seen protruding through the defect.

Myonecrosis

Myonecrosis or infarction of skeletal muscle occurs when the blood supply is inadequate to maintain muscle viability. Numerous potential causes exist, but uncontrolled insulin-dependent diabetes and sickle cell anemia are two of the most common. Inadequate blood supply to a muscle flap after reconstructive surgery or amputation may lead to myonecrosis and death of the entire flap. Trauma-induced myonecrosis can occur following direct injury and massive contusion of the musculature. Finally, pressure-induced devascularization of muscle can lead to myonecrosis. This form of myonecrosis is most often seen in the bedridden patient and usually occurs beneath a large decubitus ulcer with involvement of the muscles in the region of the buttocks or thigh.

Diabetic myonecrosis is most often seen in poorly controlled longstanding cases of insulin-dependent diabetes and results from occlusion or thrombosis of small- or medium-sized arterioles. Patients who develop myonecrosis often manifest other significant end-stage complications of diabetes including retinopathy, neuropathy, and nephropathy. In diabetic myonecrosis, involvement of the thigh and calf musculature is most common with up to one third of all patients demonstrating bilateral involvement at the time of initial presentation. The history of diabetes combined with the typical distribution can be important clues in establishing the correct diagnosis.

Regardless of the cause, patients with myonecrosis usually present clinically with severe pain and swelling of the affected muscles. MRI is often performed in these patients to investigate the source of pain. Typical MR findings include diffuse edema with high T2 signal within the involved musculature. Extensive reactive edema is usually present in the overlying subcutaneous fat and adjacent fascial planes, and it is not uncommon to see involvement of muscles in more than a single compartment. The infarcted muscle demonstrates edema and swelling during the acute phase with focal intramuscular fluid collections (liquefaction of muscle) developing later. Intravenous gadolinium will demonstrate intense enhancement of the involved muscles with rim enhancement of areas of necrotic liquefied muscle (Fig. 15-15).

It is not always possible to exclude infection in the presence of myonecrosis solely on the basis of MRI, and other diagnostic measures may be required such as aspiration and culture. It is important to note that the white blood cell count is usually normal in patients with uncomplicated myonecrosis. Proper clinical history is helpful in suggesting the diagnosis of diabetic or sickle cell-induced myonecrosis. Following trauma or pressure-induced myonecrosis, infection is nearly always included in the differential diagnosis and is often excluded on the basis of aspiration and culture. The location and pattern of muscle and soft tissue involvement, combined with a high index of clinical suspicion and proper clinical history, usually lead to the correct diagnosis.

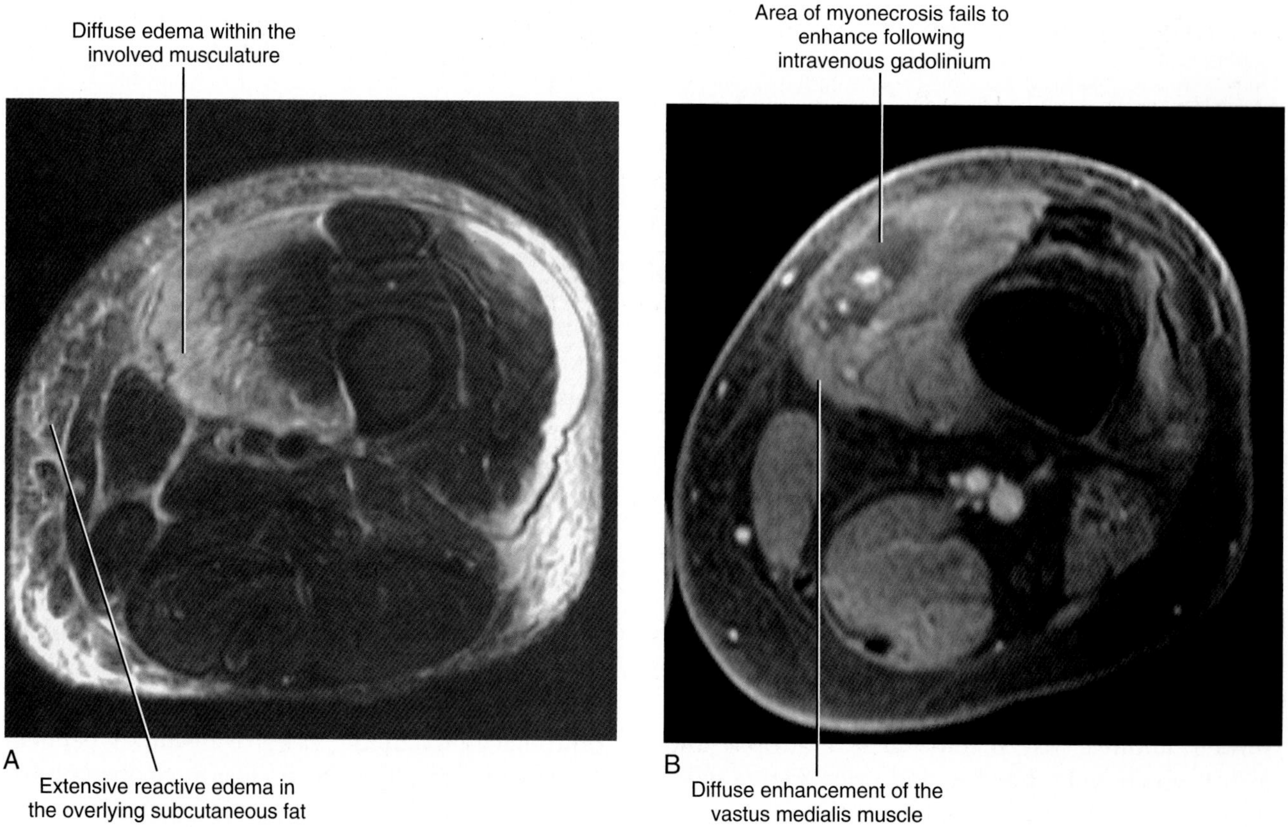
Diffuse edema within the involved musculature
Extensive reactive edema in the overlying subcutaneous fat
A
Area of myonecrosis fails to enhance following intravenous gadolinium
Diffuse enhancement of the vastus medialis muscle
B

Figure 15-15 Diabetic myonecrosis. Axial T2-weighted (**A**) and T1-weighted postgadolinium (**B**) images with fat saturation show extensive high T2 signal within the vastus medialis and enhancement following administration of intravenous gadolinium. A focal area of nonviable muscle within the central aspect of the vastus medialis demonstrates a lack of enhancement. Note the extensive overlying reactive subcutaneous soft tissue edema, which is a common MR finding in myonecrosis.

Rhabdomyolysis

Rhabdomyolysis is a condition characterized by widespread muscle cell death and lysis, resulting in the release of muscle components into the circulatory system. Numerous potential causes exist, which can be broadly categorized into hereditary and acquired. The hereditary causes are uncommon and are generally related to one of numerous enzyme deficiencies. Most cases are acquired rather than hereditary with exertional rhadomyolysis and heat stroke being the two most common causes. Clinical presentation is frequently that of an out-of-shape individual who undertakes strenuous physical training, such as a new military recruit or an individual who begins demanding training for athletic participation. Other potential causes are extensive muscle damage secondary to a crushing injury, extensive burns, alcoholism, and a broad range of drugs and toxins. The common pathway of this diverse set of causes is large-scale cellular damage resulting in increased cellular membrane permeability, leading to cell death, necrosis, and finally the release of cellular components into the circulatory system. Creatine phosphokinase (CK) and myoglobin are the two most notable cellular components and if intravascular quantities are sufficient, they can lead to cardiac arrest, disseminated intravascular coagulation, compartment syndrome, or acute renal failure.

Diagnosis of rhabdomyolysis is suspected on clinical presentation of muscle pain and weakness, fever, tachycardia as well as nausea and vomiting. Laboratory findings confirm the diagnosis showing a markedly elevated CK of at least five times the normal serum value and elevated levels of urinary myoglobin (myoglobinuria). Treatment is primarily supportive and consists of aggressive rehydration with intravenous fluids.

Imaging plays only a minor role in the diagnosis of rhabdomyolysis, which is usually established on the basis of clinical presentation and laboratory values. MRI is the most sensitive of our current imaging modalities with regard to identifying abnormalities of the muscle associated with rhabdomyolysis. Areas of rhabdomyolysis demonstrate diffuse increased T2 signal within the areas of myonecrosis, and MRI can show both the extent and the location of muscle damage (Fig. 15-16). The extent of muscle involvement as demonstrated on MRI has been shown to correlate with the severity of clinical symptoms and also parallels the clinical course of the disease with areas of increased T2 signal diminishing in intensity as the clinical symptoms resolve.

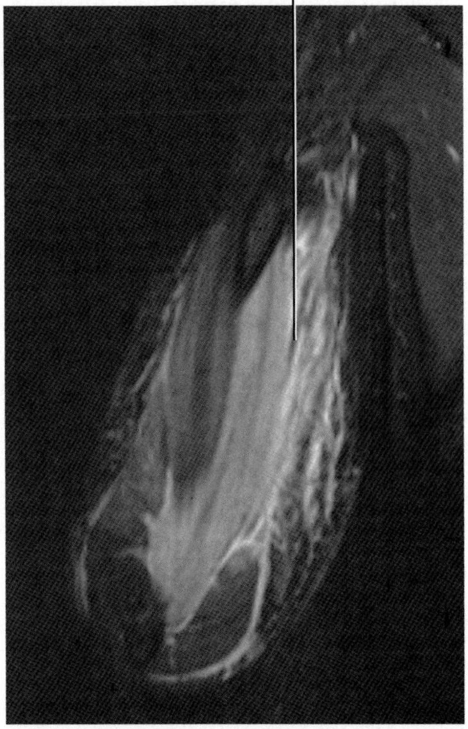
Diffuse increased T2 signal within the muscles of the upper arm

Figure 15-16 Rhabdomyolysis. Coronal T2-weighted image shows nonspecific diffuse increased T2 signal within the muscles of the upper arm in a patient with a clinical diagnosis of rhadomyolysis

MUSCLE INFLAMMATION

Several relatively uncommon conditions affecting muscle can result in myositis or inflammation of the muscle. These include infectious agents, such as bacterial, viral, and fungal, and noninfectious agents, such as sarcoid and autoimmune disorders. The idiopathic inflammatory myopathies include dermatomyositis, polymyositis, and sporadic inclusion body myositis.

Infectious Myositis

Pyomyositis

Pyomyositis is a focal area of bacterial infection of the muscle and can result from either hematogenous spread or from penetrating trauma. Although nearly any organism can result in pyomyositis, *Staphylococcus aureus* is the most commonly identified organism. Pyomyositis is rare in the healthy individual and usually occurs in a person with an underlying immunosupression such as HIV infection or in a person on immunosuppressive therapy for cancer or as part of a regimen following organ transplantation. Hematogenous seeding of muscle usually occurs in an area of injured muscle such as within a hematoma after blunt trauma or contusion. Patients typically present with focal symptoms of pain, swelling, redness, fever, and elevated white blood cell count. Most cases involve the large muscles of the buttocks, thigh, or calf and present with a single site of infection, although multifocal myositis can occur in a small percentage of cases.

Imaging of pyomyositis is best accomplished with MRI, which demonstrates a nonspecific area of increased T2 signal within the affected areas of the muscle. The muscle is often swollen and enlarged, and fluid is usually noted tracking along the adjacent fascial planes. In more advanced cases of pyomyositis, abscess formation can occur, which appears on MRI as a fluid collection within the muscle. Intravenous gadolinium results in enhancement of the involved areas of the muscle and in rim enhancement surrounding the fluid within an abscess. Fluid within an abscess typically does not enhance. Although unusual, gas can also be seen occasionally with soft tissue infection (Fig. 15-17). The primary role of MRI is to determine the extent of muscle involvement and to evaluate for complications such as abscess formation and underlying osteomyelitis. Other potential complications include compartment syndrome and the development of areas of necrosis. Treatment usually consists of administration of proper antibiotics targeted for the specific organism

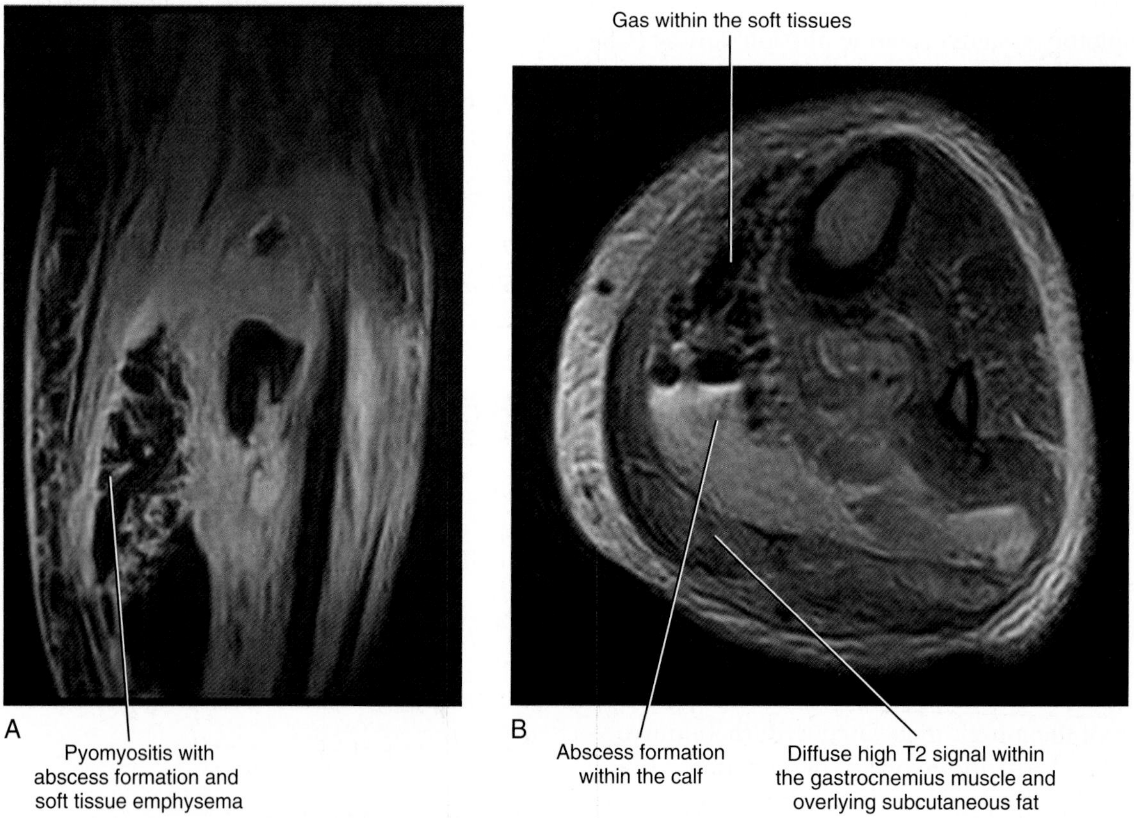
A
Pyomyositis with abscess formation and soft tissue emphysema
Gas within the soft tissues
B
Abscess formation within the calf
Diffuse high T2 signal within the gastrocnemius muscle and overlying subcutaneous fat

Figure 15-17 Pyomyositis with abscess formation. Coronal STIR (**A**) and axial T2-weighted image without fat saturation (**B**) show diffuse increased T2 signal throughout the musculature of the calf with abscess formation and extensive gas within the soft tissues. Pyomyositis developed after contusion and soft tissue injury to this region of the calf, and the patient presented with progressive pain, swelling, and erythema of the calf.

and abscess drainage. Necrotic muscle may need to be debrided.

The MR findings of pyomyositis are usually nonspecific without proper clinical history, and differential diagnosis includes contusion (with or without intramuscular hematoma), muscle strain, compartment syndrome, cellulitis, soft tissue neoplasm (with or without central necrosis), and diabetic muscle infarction. Patients with idiopathic inflammatory myopathies (discussed in the section, Idiopathic Inflammatory Myopathy) typically present with diffuse bilateral muscle involvement. Although the imaging characteristics may appear similar early in the disease process, the diffuse and bilateral distribution of muscle abnormalities noted in the idiopathic inflammatory myopathies should help to differentiate between infectious and noninfectious myositis.

Necrotizing Fasciitis

Necrotizing fasciitis refers to a rapidly progressive often fatal infection of the fascial planes between muscles. Although group A hemolytic streptococci and *Staphylococcus aureus* are often responsible for the initial infection, most necrotizing soft tissue infections also contain a mix of anaerobic and aerobic gram-negative organisms. Occasionally, other organisms such as viral infection can be a source of necrotizing fasciitis. Idiopathic cases of necrotizing fasciitis can occur, but most cases develop in an environment of local tissue hypoxia following trauma, surgery, or medical compromise. Early disease may be difficult to differentiate from cellulitis or less severe soft tissue infections, but necrotizing fasciitis progresses very rapidly and patients quickly develop signs of systemic toxicity.

Radiographs and CT demonstrate soft tissue swelling and indistinctness of the normal fascial planes and may also show gas within the soft tissues. MRI, however, is the modality of choice in suspected cases of necrotizing fasciitis because it clearly delineates the extent of disease. The classic MRI appearance is that of edema within the overlying subcutaneous fat in combination with fluid tracking along the fascial planes between the various muscles (Fig. 15-18). The underlying musculature may demonstrate edema, but it is unusual to have concurrent pyomyositis. Administration of intravenous gadolinium results in enhancement of the subcutaneous fat and fascial planes. Absence of enhancement indicates areas of necrosis and abscess formation. Because of the high mortality rate associated with necrotizing fasciitis, early diagnosis and aggressive treatment are required. Appropriate antibiotics and surgical debridement of necrotic tissue are essential, and MRI can play an important role in determining the extent of debridement that may be necessary.

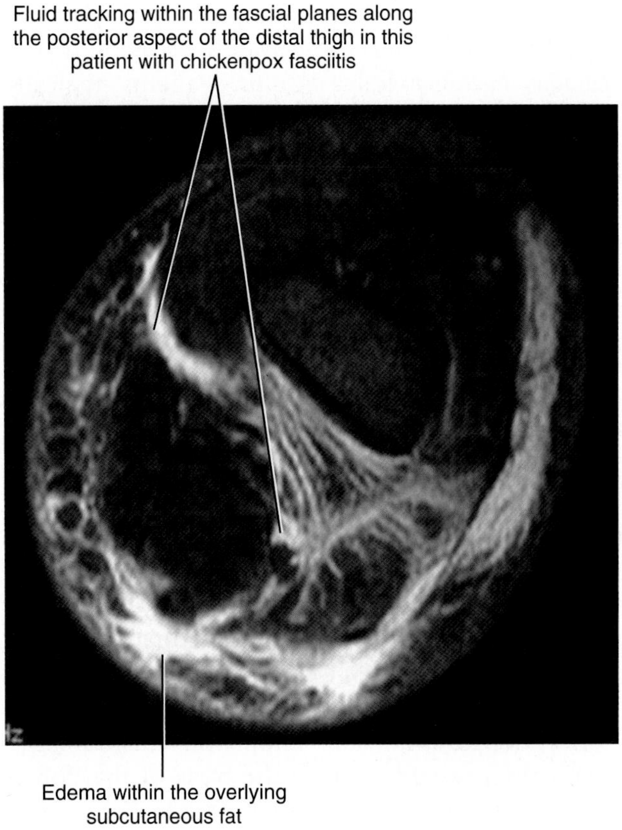
Fluid tracking within the fascial planes along the posterior aspect of the distal thigh in this patient with chickenpox fasciitis
Edema within the overlying subcutaneous fat

Figure 15-18 Chicken pox fasciitis. Axial T2-weighted image shows extensive fluid tracking along the facial planes of the posterior thigh in this patient with chickenpox fasciitis. There is minimal edema within some of the musculature; however. the predominant finding is that of fluid and edema within the fascial planes and in the overlying subcutaneous fat.

Findings on MRI alone are nonspecific, and differential diagnosis includes muscle strain or injury, contusion, and cellulitis. There is usually little doubt clinically regarding the diagnosis of necrotizing fasciitis, and MR imaging is performed to determine the extent of disease and to determine the extent of surgical debridement that may be necessary.

Idiopathic Inflammatory Myopathy

The idiopathic inflammatory myopathies are a rare group of autoimmune disorders that affect skeletal muscle. The most common idiopathic inflammatory myopathies include *dermatomyositis, polymyositis,* and *sporadic inclusion body myositis.* Patients typically present with progressive muscle weakness of the involved muscle groups. Dermatomyositis and polymyositis are symmetric in distribution and tend to involve the proximal muscle groups of the upper and lower extremities, whereas muscle atrophy associated with sporadic inclusion body myositis is more asymmetric in distribution and tends to involve the distal muscle groups rather than the proximal muscle groups of the extremities. Vague complaints of myalgias, tenderness, and fatigue often accompany the progressive muscle weakness, and other connective tissue diseases such as scleroderma, systemic erythematosus, or rheumatoid arthritis may coexist with dermatomyositis or polymyositis. Adults developing an idiopathic inflammatory myopathy are more likely to develop a malignancy during the first 2 years of the disease and should be closely screened for a coexisting malignancy.

The diagnosis of an idiopathic inflammatory myopathy is established on the basis of the Bohan and Peter diagnostic criteria. A probable diagnosis of polymyositis is made when a person has progressive bilateral muscle weakness of the extremities, elevated serum levels of muscle enzymes, and a myopathic pattern on electromyography. A definitive diagnosis is made when these three criteria are met and when muscle biopsy shows the typical pathologic changes. A diagnosis of dermatomyositis is made using the identical criteria when the typical skin changes are also present. Histologic changes of the muscle vary slightly with sporadic inclusion body myositis when compared with polymyositis or dermatomyositis, and the distribution of muscle weakness is more distal. In addition, progression of the disease and symptoms are usually more refractory to standard treatment, resulting in a more progressive muscle weakness and atrophy.

MRI is the imaging modality of choice in the evaluation of a suspected idiopathic inflammatory myopathy. During the acute phase of the disease, MRI shows increased T2 signal within the involved muscle groups. Use of a fat-saturation technique increases the conspicuity of the muscle edema. Abnormal T2 signal is usually bilateral and symmetric and is indicative of active inflammation (Fig. 15-19). MRI is useful in directing muscle biopsy during the acute phase of the disease, since areas of active inflammation are more likely to demonstrate the diagnostic histopathologic changes. A random, non–imaging-guided muscle biopsy has up to a 25% false-negative rate. Burned-out disease results in atrophy of the involved muscles, and MRI shows loss of normal muscle bulk and increased T1 signal representing fatty atrophy (Fig. 15-20). Subcutaneous inflammation in the patient with dermatomyositis manifests as areas of increased T2 signal within the subcutaneous fat. These areas of subcutaneous inflammation constitute the precursor to soft tissue calcinosis, which manifests on radiographs as sheetlike areas of calcifications within the subcutaneous soft tissues and is nearly diagnostic of dermatomyositis.

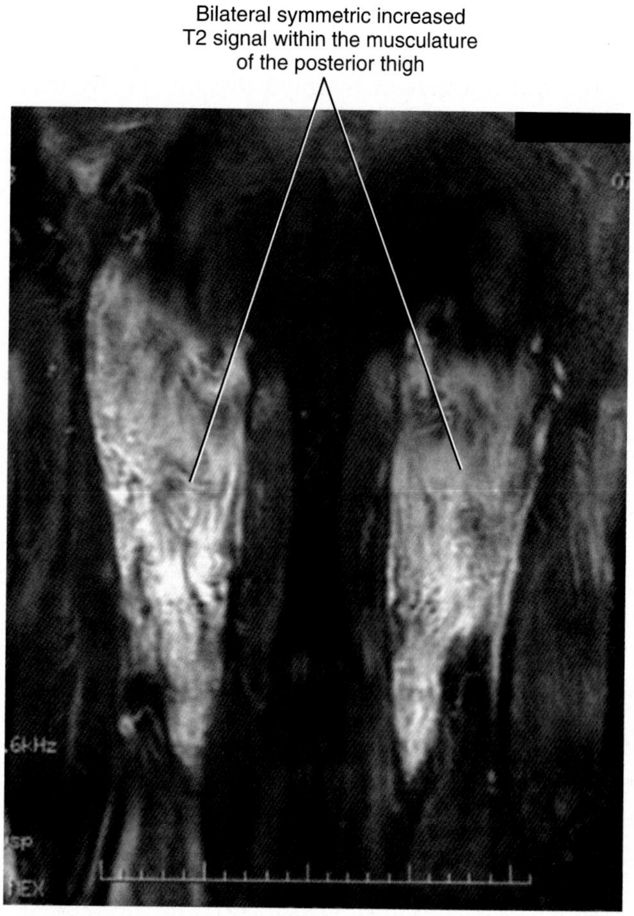
Bilateral symmetric increased T2 signal within the musculature of the posterior thigh

Figure 15-19 Active polymyositis. Coronal T2-weighted image with fat saturation of the thighs bilaterally demonstrates diffuse bilateral and symmetric increased T2 signal within the posterior musculature. MRI can be used to accurately show areas of active disease, thereby increasing the chance of obtaining tissue that will provide an accurate diagnosis.

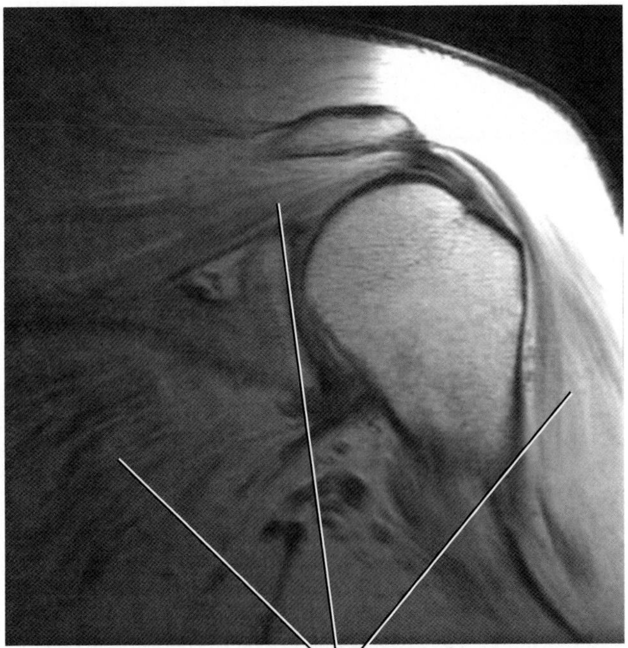
Diffuse fatty replacement of the muscles of the shoulder girdle

Figure 15-20 Chronic dermatomyositis. Coronal T1-weighted image of the shoulder shows diffuse fatty atrophy and replacement of the all of the muscles of the left shoulder girdle. This patient presented with progressive bilateral shoulder pain and weakness.

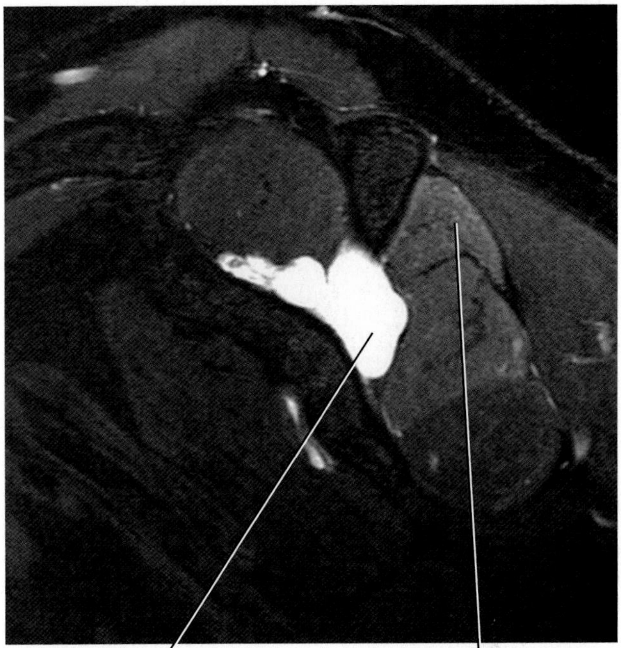
Paralabral cyst dissecting into the spinoglenoid notch causing compression of the suprascapular nerve
Diffuse increased T2 signal isolated to the infraspinatus muscle indicating neurogenic edema

Figure 15-21 Early neurogenic edema of the infraspinatus muscle. Sagittal T2-weighted image with fat saturation shows a large paralabral cyst dissecting into the spinoglenoid notch and resulting in compression of the suprascapular nerve and subsequent neurogenic edema of the infraspinatus muscle.

Muscle Atrophy

Muscle atrophy can involve a single muscle or can involve all of the musculature of a single extremity. Potential causes are numerous and varied (Box 15-3). Sources of muscle atrophy range from neurogenic abnormalities, such as stroke and nerve impingement, to trauma or diseases of the muscle. The distribution and extent of muscle atrophy often provide a clue to the specific cause.

BOX 15-3 COMMON CAUSES OF MUSCLE ATROPHY

Post-traumatic (crush injury, tendon tear)
Neurogenic (multiple sclerosis, paralysis, nerve damage, or nerve impingement)
Ischemia
Diabetes
Idiopathic inflammatory myopathy
Muscular dystrophy
Radiation therapy

Although radiographs, CT, and ultrasound all can demonstrate longstanding muscle atrophy, MRI is the most sensitive imaging modality and can reveal early muscle atrophy even before loss of muscle bulk.

In the acute stages of atrophy, increased T2 signal representing edema and increased extracellular water content are first noted within the muscle. These changes are best seen on T2-weighted images with fat saturation or short tau inversion recovery (STIR) imaging. The edema is often confined to a single muscle or a group of muscles. The distribution of atrophy is one of the key factors in establishing the correct differential diagnosis, especially if it corresponds to the enervation pattern of a specific nerve (Fig. 15-21). This MR appearance with increased water content can last for up to 1 year. Over time,

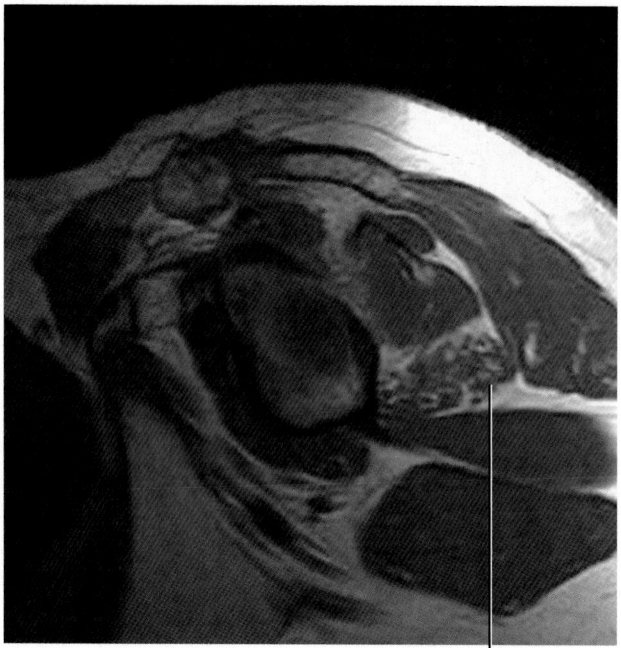
Decreased bulk and high
T1 signal indicates chronic
fatty atrophy isolated to the
teres minor muscle

Figure 15-22 Chronic denervation atrophy of the teres minor muscle. Sagittal T1-weighted image of the shoulder shows extensive loss of normal bulk and fatty replacement of the teres minor muscle. This indicates a remote injury to the axillary nerve.

however, the muscle begins to lose bulk and demonstrates a return to the normal intramuscular T2 signal. If the insult continues, the muscle eventually undergoes fatty replacement, during which time the muscle begins to show increased T1 signal and an overall decrease in the bulk of the muscle belly when compared with the contralateral muscle group or with adjacent muscles in the same extremity (Fig. 15-22). Once fatty atrophy has occurred, the muscle injury is considered irreversible.

Suggested Readings

Armfield DR, Kim DH, Towers JD, et al. Sports-related muscle injury in the lower extremity. Clin Sports Med 2006;25: 803–842.

Boutin RD, Fritz RC, Steinbach LS. Imaging of sports-related muscle injuries. Magn Reson Imaging North Am 2003;11: 341–371.

De Smet AA, Norris MA, Fisher DR. Magnetic resonance imaging of myositis ossificans: analysis of seven cases. Skeletal Radiol 1992;21:503–507.

Fleckenstein JL, Canby RC, Parkey RW, et al. Acute effects of exercise on MR imaging of skeletal muscle in normal volunteers. AJR Am J Roentgenol 11988;51:231–237.

Fugitt JB, Puckett ML, Quigley MM, Kerr SM. Necrotizing fasciitis. RadioGraphics 2004;24:1472–1476.

Kattapuram TM, Suri R, Rosol MS, et al. Idiopathic and diabetic skeletal muscle necrosis: evaluation by magnetic resonance imaging. Skeletal Radiol 2005;34:203–209.

Koulouris G, Connell D. Hamstring muscle complex: an imaging review. RadioGraphics 2005;25:571–586.

Marcantonio DR, Cho GJ. Focus on muscle in orthopedic MRI. Semin Musculoskelet Radiol 2000;4:421–434.

May DA, Disler DG, Jones EA, et al. Abnormal signal intensity in skeletal muscle at MR imaging: patterns, pearls, and pitfalls. RadioGraphics 2000;20:S295–315.

Palmer WE, Kuong SJ, Elmadbouh HM. MR imaging of myotendinous strain. AJR Am J Roentgenol 1999;173:703–709.

Park JH, Olsen NJ. Utility of magnetic resonance imaging in the evaluation of patients with inflammatory myopathies. Curr Rheumatol Rep 2001;3:334–345.

Verleisdonk EJ, van Gils A, van der Werken C. The diagnostic value of MRI scans for the diagnosis of chronic exertional compartment syndrome of the lower leg. Skeletal Radiol 2001;30: 321–325,.

Verrall GM, Slavotinek JP, Barnes PG, et al. Diagnosis and prognostic value of clinical findings in 83 athletes with posterior thigh injury: comparison of clinical findings with magnetic resonance imaging documentation of hamstring strain. Am J Sports Med 2003;31:969–973.

Index

Note: Page numbers followed by b indicate boxed material; those followed by f indicate figures; those followed by t indicate tables.

B